Wound Care

A Collaborative Practice Manual

THIRD EDITION

Edited by

Carrie Sussman, PT
Owner and Operator
Sussman Physical Therapy, Inc.
Wound Care Management Services
Torrance, California

Barbara M. Bates-Jensen, PhD, RN, CWOCN
Barbara M. Bates-Jensen PhD, RN, CWOCN
Assistant Professor
School of Nursing & Department of Medicine, Division of Geriatrics
University of California, Los Angeles
Los Angeles, California
and Veterans Administration Greater Los Angeles Healthcare System
Geriatric Research Education Clinical Center
Sepulveda, California

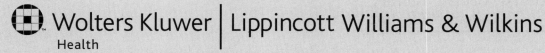

Wolters Kluwer | Lippincott Williams & Wilkins
Health

Philadelphia · Baltimore · New York · London
Buenos Aires · Hong Kong · Sydney · Tokyo

Acquisitions Editor: Peter Sabatini
Managing Editor: Andrea Klingler
Production Editor: Anne Seitz/Hearthside Publishing Services
Designer: Doug Smock
Compositor: Hearthside Publishing Services
Printer: Courier

Library of Congress Cataloging-in-Publication Data

CIP data may be located on the Library of Congress of website:
<http://cip.loc.gov/>http://cip.loc.gov/

The publishers have made every effort to trace the copyright holders for borrowed material. If they have inadvertently overlooked any, they will be pleased to make the necessary arrangements at the first opportunity.

To purchase additional copies of this book, call our customer service department at (800) 638-3030 or fax orders to (301) 223-2320. International customers should call (301) 223-2300.

Visit Lippincott Williams & Wilkins on the Internet: http://www.LWW.com. Lippincott Williams & Wilkins customer service representatives are available from 8:30 am to 6:00 pm, EST.

06 07 08 09 10
1 2 3 4 5 6 7 8 9 10

This book is dedicated to the memory of my dear husband and best friend Robert (Bob) J. Sussman with love and gratitude for the limitless collaboration, contributions, and unwavering support he provided for the development and production of all three editions of this book and whose constant encouragement has been the wind behind my achievements.

CARRIE SUSSMAN

Bob was a strong and forceful presence in the preparation of all three editions of our book. He was a lifesaver on the details and never hesitated to lend a hand with organization of materials and resources. He had a wonderful generous spirit and it is an honor to dedicate this third edition to him.

BARBARA BATES JENSEN

Preface

A New Name for the Third Edition

The third edition of *Wound Care: A Collaborative Practice Manual for Health Care Professionals* is a new title suggested by our readers to reflect the utility of the book to the multidisciplinary wound team. Our audience has given the first and second editions of this book overwhelmingly positive response. One way in which the text reflects the multidisciplinary readership is the use of two conceptual models of care throughout. The reader will see terminology that is reflective of the traditional medical model: "etiology," " pathogenesis," "diagnosis," and "prognosis" in its presentation of disease along with the disablement model used by rehabilitation professionals including "interventions," "functional outcomes," "impairments," and "disabilities."

Features of the Third Edition

The basic structure and organization of the book has not been changed. There is a logical and consistent format to each chapter. All chapters have updated and extensive referencing, clinical wisdoms, new and revised charts, new case studies, and procedures on how to apply treatment in a safe and effective manner to enhance patient outcomes.

In this revision there are two entirely new chapters, Management of Wound Pain and Wound Management with Negative Pressure Therapy; an expanded chapter on photo stimulation to include LASER; as well as updates to all chapters to reflect current information about basic medical science and wound management that have occurred since publication of the second edition. There are also new contributors from different disciplines including podiatry.

A very special key feature of this book is the section of 89 colored photographs that are carefully marked to illustrate characteristics for wound assessment, assessment of darkly pigmented skin, identification of wound pathology, anatomy, diagnosis, and the results of treatment. Black and white photo illustrations and drawings are liberally distributed throughout. The appendix at the back of the book lists wound dressing products by categories and their sources for quick reference.

Collaboration with the Multidisciplinary Team

Early in the development of this textbook we, the editors, recognized that just as in the real world, the skills and expertise of a multidisciplinary team were needed to provide the scope of information needed for preparing a text on successful wound management. The contributions of the text contributors reflect the expertise drawn from many disciplines including medicine, surgery, podiatry, nursing, physical therapy, research, orthotics, prosthetics, pharmacy, nutrition and dietetics, and occupational therapy. Collaboration was used in the writing of chapters that were coauthored by individuals from different disciplines. Two contributing authors are from outside the United States. Reference materials were used throughout that were published in many countries. Wound management is a global problem and a multidisciplinary challenge. We encourage collaboration across all borders. Yes, at times collaborating was challenging, but it has also been very rewarding. It seemed logical that this effort should set the stage for the collaborative practice encouraged by this book.

Organization of the Book

The book is organized into four parts. Part I, Introduction to Wound Diagnosis, reviews the diagnostic process used by health care professionals when evaluating a patient with a wound. The use of the diagnostic process provides clarity in communication and fosters collaborative practice. Clear communication assists with accountability and greater professional autonomy. After reviewing the diagnostic process in Chapter 1, the rest of Part I reviews implementation of the diagnostic process and includes the chapters: Wound Healing Physiology and Chronic Wound Healing, Nutritional Assessment and Treatment, Assessment of the Skin and Wound, Wound Measurements, Tools to Measure Wound Healing, and Vascular Evaluation. Together these chapters provided an assessment foundation for the patient with a wound. Chapters include procedures, forms, case studies, referral criteria, flow diagrams,

Part II, Management by Wound Characteristics, as indicated by the title, contains separate chapters that describe, in depth, wound management by specific wound characteristics: Management of Necrotic Tissue, Management of Wound Exudate and Infection, Management of Edema, Management of the Wound Environment with Dressings and Topical Agents, Management of the Wound Environment with Advanced Therapies (growth factors, living skin equivalents, etc), Management of Wound Pain, and Management of Scar. Each chapter begins with a definition of the characteristic, assessment parameters, the significance of the findings, interventions appropriate for treatment of the wound characteristic and ends with outcome measures, procedures and for specific interventions, self-care teaching guidelines for patients as appropriate, case studies and referral criteria for the specific wound characteristic, and resources.

Part III, Management by Wound Etiology chapters focus on the etiology of the wound and how that affects the wound management strategy and outcome. Etiologies presented include: Acute Surgical Wound Management, Pressure Ulcers: Pathophysiology and Prevention, Management of Pressure by Therapeutic Positioning, Diagnosis and Management of Vascular Ulcers, Management of the Neuropathic Foot, Management of Skin and Nails, Management of Malignant Wounds and Fistulas. As in all other sections and chapters, there is evidence-based supporting information, tables, clinical guidelines, forms, expected outcomes, self-care teaching guidelines, and resources.

Part IV, Management of Wound Healing with Biophysical Agents includes the following chapters: Electrical Stimulation for Wound Healing, Induced Electrical Stimulation: Pulsed Radio Frequency and Pulsed Electromagnetic Field Therapy, Photostimulation for Wound Healing, Therapeutic and Diagnostic Ultrasound, Whirlpool, Pulsed Lavage with Suction, and Negative Pressure Therapy. It must be pointed out that the use of biophysical agents are supplemental to other treatment regimens such as dressings and topical agents when the use of the agent is impacted by other treatments this is addressed, however those treatments are dealt with in other sections. Longer than other section introductions, the Introduction to Part IV presents guidelines for choice of the biophysical agent, candidacy of the patient for different agents, expected outcomes, and how to do a cost benefit analysis. Each chapter introduces the intervention, explains the science and theory of the intervention based on the evidence in the literature as it relates to wound healing along with animal and clinical studies. Most chapters feature tables summarizing clinical studies pertaining to the biophysical agent. Procedures and treatment protocols follow.

Users

Based on reader comments, this book serves as a reference for seasoned and beginning wound clinicians, researchers, and industry representatives, as well as a textbook for students in various health care fields dealing with wound management and care.

Carrie Sussman
Barbara M. Bates-Jensen

Contributors

Karen Wientjes Albaugh, PT, MPH, CWS
The Center for Advanced Wound Care
Reading, Pennsylvania

Neil Christopher R. Apeles, MSN, RN, PHN
Education Specialist, Critical Care and Pediatrics Department of Education Valley Presbyterian Hospital
Van Nuys, California

Barbara M. Bates-Jensen, PhD, RN, CWOCN
Assistant Professor
UCLA School of Nursing & Medicine, Division of Geriatrics
VA Greater Los Angeles Healthcare System,
Geriatric Research Education Clinical Center
Los Angeles, California

Autumn Bell , MPT, CLT
Center for Advanced Wound Care
Wyomissing, Pennsylvania

Michelle Cameron, PT, MD, OCS
Physical Therapy Consultant
Health Potentials
Portland, Oregon
and Resident Neurologist
Department of Neurology
Oregon Health and Sciences University
Portland, Oregon

Stanley Newell Carson M.D., F.A.C.S. (deceased)
Private Practice of Vascular and General Surgery and
Wound Management
Medical Director Fountain Valley Regional Hospital
Wound Care Program
Fountain Valley, California

Joan E. Conlan LVN, CPED
Glenmar, Mt. Shasta, California

Teresa Conner-Kerr, PhD
Chair and Professor
Winston-Salem State University
School of Health Sciences
Dept. of Physical Therapy
Winston-Salem, North Carolina

Carlos E. Donayre, MD
Associate Professor of Surgery
Division of Vascular and Endovascular Surgery
Harbor-UCLA Medical Center
David E. Geffen School of Medicine
University of California, Los Angeles
Los Angeles, California

Mary Dyson, PhD, LDH (Hon), FAIUM (Hon), FSCP (Hon), CBiol, MIBiol
Centre for Cardiovascular Biology and Medicine
Guy's Hospital Campus
Kings College
University of London
England, United Kingdom

William J. Ennis D.O.,MBA,FACOS
Clinical Professor of Surgery, Midwestern University
President-elect Association for the Advancement of Wound
Care (AAWC)
Medical Director Comprehensive Wound and Disease
Management Center
St. James Hospital and Healthcare Centers
Olympia Fields, Illinois

Nancy Elftman, CO, CPed
Certified Orthotist, Certified Pedorthotist
Cosmos Extremity/Hands on Foot
LaVerne, California

Evonne Fowler, MN, RN, CETN
Wound/Ostomy/Skin Care Specialist
Bellflower Kaiser Hospital
Bellflower, California

Allen Gabriel, MD
Senior Resident Plastic Surgeon
Loma Linda University Division of Plastic Surgery
Loma Linda, California

Mark Granick, MD, FACS
Philadelphia Plastic Surgeons, PC
Bala Cynwyd, Pennsylvania

Subhas C. Gupta, MD, PhD, FRCS
Loma Linda University Medical Center
Loma Linda, California

Elizabeth Hiltabidel, RN, MSN, CWOCN
Advance Practice Nurse, Wound and Ostomy Care
Loma Linda University Medical Center
Loma Linda, California

Teresa J. Kelechi, PhD, RN, CWCN
Assistant Professor College of Nursing
Medical University of South Carolina
Charleston, South California

Diane L. Krasner, PhD, RN, CWOCN, CWS, FAAN
Wound & Skin Care Consultant
York, Pennsylvania

Harriett B. Loehne, PT, DPT, CWS, FCCWS
Clinical Educator
Archbold Center for Wound Management
Archbold Medical Center
Thomasville, Georgia 31792

Liza G. Ovington, Ph.D
Regional Clinical Liaison Director
Johnson & Johnson Wound Care
Allentown, Pennsylvania

Roland A. Palmquist, DPM
Chief Podiatrist
Department of Health and Human Services, Indian Health
    Service,
Colorado River Service Unit, Parker Indian Health Center
Parker, Arizona

Gregory K. Patterson , MD
South Georgia Surgical Associates
Thomasville, Georgia

Mary Ellen Posthauer, RD, CD,LD
President
M.E.P. Healthcare Dietary Services, Inc.
Evansville, Indiana

Laurie M. Rappl, PT, CWS
Clinical Support Manager
Span-American Medical Systems, Inc.
Greenville, South Carolina

Susie Seaman, MSN, FNP, CETN
Nurse Practitioner,
Wound Healing Center
Grossmont Hospital, Sharp Healthcare
La Mesa, California

Lilly Shimahara, DPM, MPH, MSHS
Podiatrist
Department of Health and Human Services,
    Indian Health Service
Colorado River Service Unit, Parker Indian Health
    Center
Parker, Arizona

Carrie Sussman, PT, DPT
President
Sussman Physical Therapy Inc. and Wound Care Management Services
Torrance, California

Geoffrey Sussman, PhD, MPS, MSHPA, AFAIPM, MSMA, JP
Victoria College of Pharmacy
Monash University
Parkville campus
Parkville, Victoria, Australia

Nancy Tomaselli, RN, MSN, CS, CRPN, CWOCN
President/CEO
Premier Health Solutions. LLC
Cherry Hill, New Jersey

Matthew J. Trovato, MD
Plastic Surgery Resident
Division of Plastic Surgery, Department of Surgery
University of Medicine and Dentistry of New Jersey
New Jersey Medical School
Newark, New Jersey

Adela Valenzuela RN, MN, CWON
Loma Linda Veterans Administration Medical Center
Loma Linda, California

R. Scott Ward, PhD, PT
Associate Professor
Division of Physical Therapy
University of Utah
Salt Lake City, Utah

Lynda D. Woodruff, PT, PhD,
College of Health Sciences
Alabama State University
Montgomery, Alabama

Nina Woolfolk, RN, MSN
Manager of Clinical Education, Telemetry Services
Desert Regional Medical Center
Palm Springs, CA 92263

Acknowledgments

The third edition has grown up on the shoulders of the work done on the prior two editions and therefore we would like to express our appreciation to the many individuals who have made all *three* editions of this book possible.

- The outstanding and dedicated individuals who have contributed their considerable clinical and academic knowledge by authoring the chapters of this book.
* The staff of Aspen Publishers, Inc., our first publisher, who set us on course with preparation of the first and second editions.
* The staff of Lippincott Williams & Wilkins, Inc. including Susan Katz, Peter Sabatini, Karen Ruppert, Allison Noplock, Jennifer Clements, and Andrea Klingler, without whom the third edition would not have come to fruition.
* Anne G. Seitz of Hearthside Publishing Services managed the project from manuscript through to bound books. She has been our pillar of support during the preparation phase of the book.
* Support persons for the first and second editions : Kris Johnson, Erin McEntyre For all three editions: Debbie Denton. For the third edition Kristine Smith. These individuals took care the many not so small details associated with preparation of the manuscript.
* The reviewers and consultants whose suggestions were invaluable during development of the first, second and third editions: Michelle Cameron PT, OCS, MD; Linda Frankenberger MS, PT; Deborah Hagler, PT; Robert Kellogg, PhD, PT; Marko Markov, PhD; Gretchen Swanson, MPH, PT, DPT; Eleanor Price, PhD; Nancy A. Stotts, EdD, RN; Rebecca Lethwaite, PhD; Luther Kloth, MS, PT, FAPTA; and Arthur Pilla, PhD.
* Clinician supporters who have shared their expertise and their work for inclusion in the third edition including: Christine Newcomer, MSN, RN, WOCN,PhD Student, University of Virginia; Catherine Ratliff, PhD, GNP, CWOCN,CS; Berish Strauch, MD; and Mary Verhage, RN, BSN, CWOCN.
- The authors, publishers, companies, and colleagues who have allowed us to publish their artwork, photographs and tables to illustrate the information.

To our husbands and children: Robert Sussman, in whose memory we have dedicated the book, Ronald, Holly, and Thomas Jensen, who have sweated the big and small stuff with us during the preparation of all three editions and without whom completion of this project would not have been possible.

Carrie Sussman
Barbara M. Bates-Jensen

Contents

Color Plates

PLATES 1–6
Progression Through Three Phases of Wound Healing

The patient is a 97-year-old resident of a long-term care facility with stage IV pressure ulcers in the bilateral rib cage and sacral area.

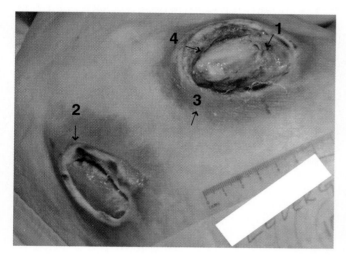

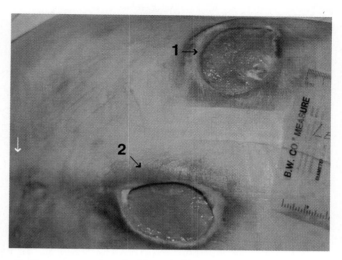

1. Chronic wound converted to acute inflammatory phase. Note:
(1) Yellow, stringy slough
(2) Edema
(3) Skin color changes (red), erythema
(4) Rib bone noted in superior ulcer
Wound healing phase diagnosis: acute inflammatory phase. Wound severity diagnosis: Impaired integumentary integrity secondary to skin involvement extending into fascia, muscle, and bone (stage IV pressure ulcer).
(Copyright © C. Sussman.)

2. Same wound as in Plate 1. Note:
(1) Rolled epidermal ridge around granulation base
(2) Brown hemosiderin staining (hemosiderosis)
Wound healing phase: proliferative phase.
(Copyright © C. Sussman.)

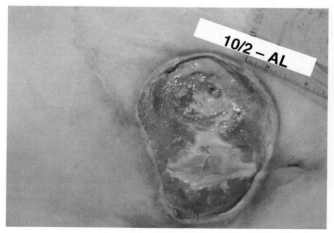

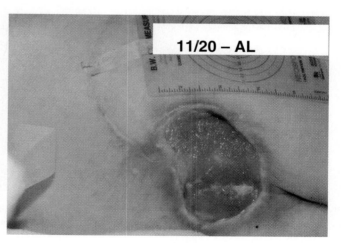

3. Same patient as in Plate 1. Chronic wound: converted to acute proliferative phase. This is a sacral wound with stringy, yellow slough evident. Note example of epidermal ridge formation. Predominant wound healing phase diagnosis: Proliferative phase. Wound severity diagnosis: same as in Plate 1.
(Copyright © C. Sussman.)

4. Same wound as in Plate 3, progressing through the proliferative phase. The wound is contracting and proliferating. Note changes in size, shape, and depth, as well as new healthy granulation tissue compared with Plate 3.
(Copyright © C. Sussman.)

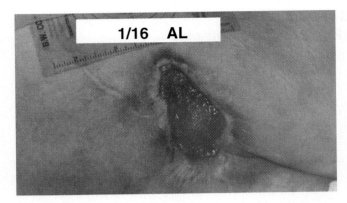

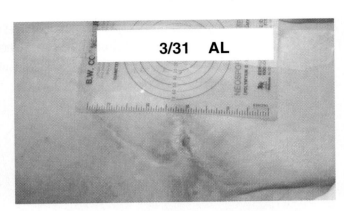

5. Note sustained wound contraction evident in Plates 4 and 5. Note epithelialization and proliferative phases. (Copyright © C. Sussman.)

6. The wound is completely resurfaced and is in the re-modeling phase. (Copyright © C. Sussman.)

PLATES 7–9
Progression Through Proliferative Phase

Plates 7–9 show a sacral pressure ulcer progressing from the chronic inflammatory phase through the proliferative phase of wound healing in a dark-skinned patient. In Plates 8 and 9, the wound edges demonstrate epithelial migration, with new epidermis clearly visible as bright pink.

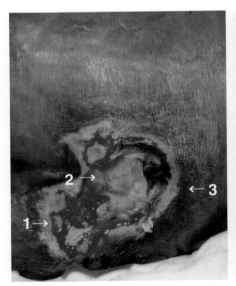

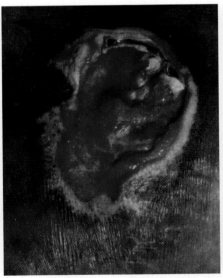

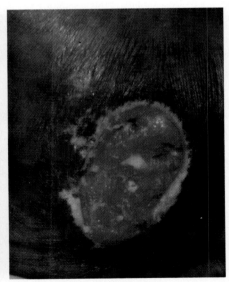

7. Chronic inflammatory phase. Note the following wound characteristics:
(1) Sanguineous drainage
(2) Muscle exposure
(3) Hemosiderin staining surrounding the wound
(Copyright © B.M. Bates-Jensen.)

8. Acute proliferative phase. Note the attached wound edges from the 12:00 to 6:00 positions and how well vascularized granulation tissue fills up one side of the ulcer. A new pink border of epithelium surrounds the granulation tissue. (Copyright © B.M. Bates-Jensen.)

9. All of the wound edges are now attached to the wound base. Note the presence of fibrin (yellow) within the granulation tissue. Ready for epithelialization phase. (Copyright © B.M. Bates-Jensen.)

PLATES 10 and 11
Abnormal Proliferative Phase

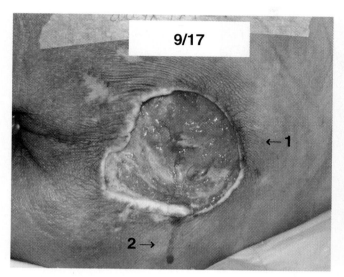

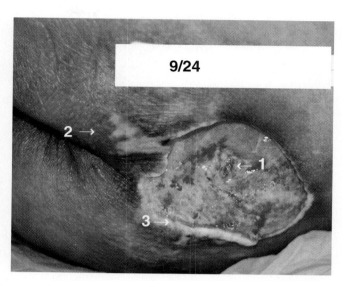

10. Acute proliferative phase. Note:
   (1) Hemosiderin staining
   (2) Sanguineous drainage
   (Copyright © B.M. Bates-Jensen.)

11. Chronic proliferative phase with attributes of infection. Note:
   (1) Hemorrhagic area of trauma
   (2) Hypopigmentation
   (3) Dull, pink granulation tissue
   (Copyright © B.M. Bates-Jensen.)

PLATE 12
Wound in Remodeling Phase

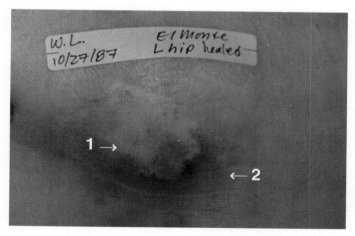

12. An example of a wound in the remodeling phase of wound healing. Note:
   (1) New epithelium (scar)
   (2) Hyperpigmentation (hemosiderin staining)
   (Copyright © B.M. Bates-Jensen.)

Plate 13
Anatomy of Soft Tissue

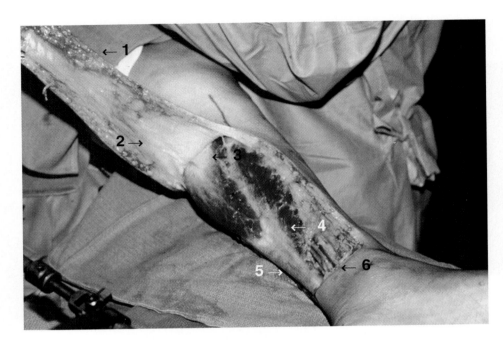

13. Full-thickness skin resected from calf. Note:
(1) Vascularized dermis
(2) Yellow, healthy fat tissue
(3) White fibrous fascia
(4) Dark red muscle tissue
(5) Tendon covered with peritenon
(6) Blood vessel
(Copyright © J. Wethe.)

PLATES 14–18
Wounding of the Skin

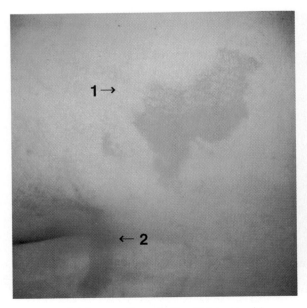

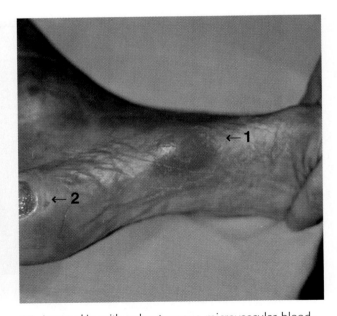

14. Superficial wounding of skin. This wound is perineal dermatitis and would be classified as a stage I pressure ulcer. Note its location over the rectum.
(Copyright © B.M. Bates-Jensen.)

15. Intact skin with subcutaneous microvascular bleeding (unblanchable erythema), suggesting deeper trauma located over a bony surface. This wound would be classified as a stage I pressure ulcer. Note maceration of the periwound skin.
(Copyright © B.M. Bates-Jensen.)

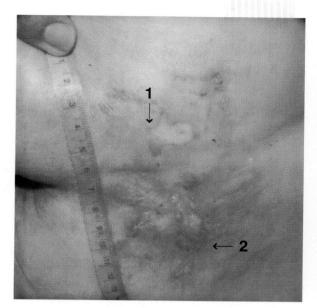

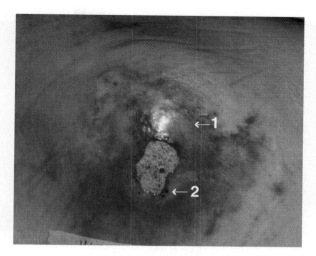

16. Perineal dermatitis with classic differentiating characteristics of diffuse erythema across the buttocks and perineal area, and partial-thickness skin loss. This wound is in the acute inflammatory phase and was not staged. Note:
(1) Multiple, partial-thickness lesions with irregular borders
(2) Lesions occur across the area singly and in groups, and may or may not be over a bony prominence
(Copyright © B.M. Bates-Jensen.)

17. Acute inflammatory phase, partial-thickness stage II pressure ulcer located over bony prominence. Note:
(1) Erythema and edema
(2) Reticular layer of dermis
(Copyright © B.M. Bates-Jensen.)

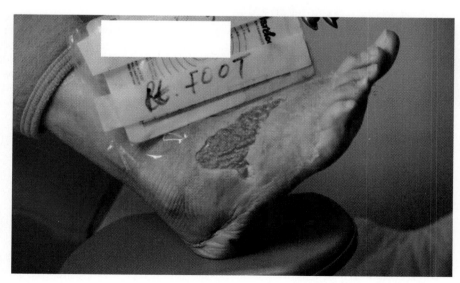

18. Full-thickness skin loss in the acute proliferative phase. The wound was not caused by pressure and was not staged. Wound edges are soft and flexible to touch.
(Copyright © C. Sussman.)

PLATES 19–22
Assessment of Darkly Pigmented Skin

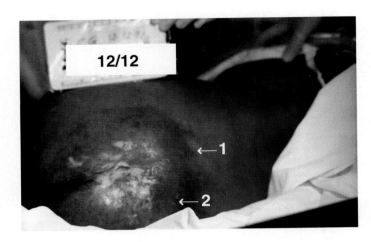

19. Pressure ulceration with multiple, small, stage II open areas. Wound is in acute inflammatory phase. Note onset date 12/12. Note:
(1) Clear line of demarcation between healthy tissues and inflamed tissues
(2) Evidence of discoloration, edema, and induration, suggesting underlying tissue death. Assess tissue temperature and pain.
(Copyright © C. Sussman.)

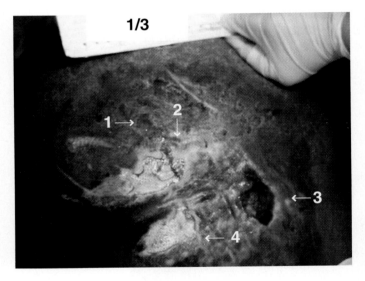

20. Same pressure ulceration as in Plate 19. Three weeks later, the skin shows evidence of the severe tissue destruction that occurred at the time of trauma. Note delayed manifestation of injury at the skin level. The date was 1/3. Note:
(1) Continued demarcation of inflamed tissue
(2) Irregular, diffuse wound edges
(3) Black and adherent eschar
(4) Partial-thickness skin loss; there is enlargement of stage II ulcers compared with those in Plate 19.
The correct staging for this sacrococcygeal pressure ulcer is at minimum a stage III. Once eschar is removed, the true depth of tissue loss can be determined. Documentation should reflect a combined area of wounding, including all three visible ulcers and the area of inflammation; this is the overall size estimate for the pressure ulcer. Inflammation is now chronic.
(Copyright © C. Sussman.)

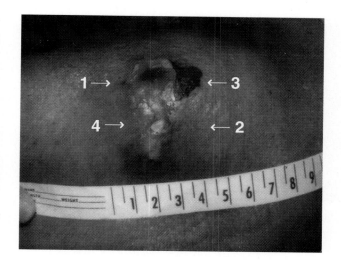

21. Assessment of inflammatory phase attributes in darkly pigmented skin. Note:
  (1) Erythema gives skin a reddish brown glow
  (2) Hemorrhage of microvasculature gives skin a purplish gray hue
  (3) Eschar-note tissue texture change to hard black
  (4) The color of adjacent skin is used as reference for normal skin tones
(Copyright © B.M. Bates-Jensen.)

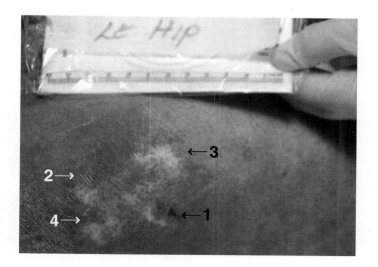

22. Assessment of epithelialization and remodeling attributes in darkly pigmented skin. Note:
  (1) New epithelial tissue is light red
  (2) New scar tissue lacks melanin and is bright pink
  (3) Old scar tissue lacks melanin and is silvery white
  (4) Residual hemosiderin staining
(Copyright © C. Sussman.)

PLATES 23–25
Abnormal Wound Attributes

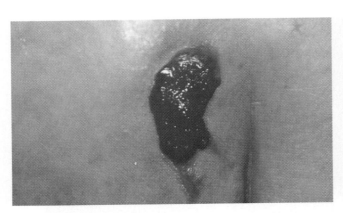

23. Wound is in chronic proliferative phase. Note hyper-granulation tissue and absence of epithelialization phase.
(Copyright © B.M. Bates-Jensen.)

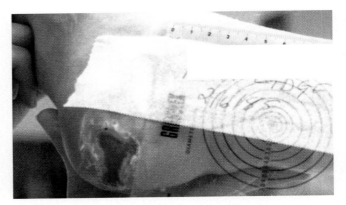

24. There is an absence of the epithelialization phase. Hyperkeratosis on heel ulcer of a 100-year-old woman. (Copyright © C. Sussman.)

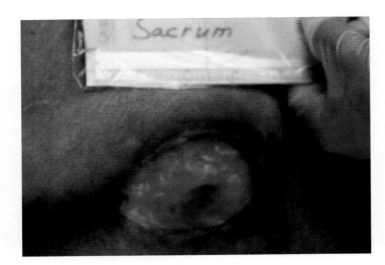

25. Wound is in chronic proliferative phase. Note:
   (1) Trauma to granulation tissue caused hemorrhagic spot that may go on to necrose
   (2) Hemosiderin staining from prior bleeding surrounds ulcer
(Copyright © C. Sussman.)

PLATES 26–32
Necrotic Tissue Types

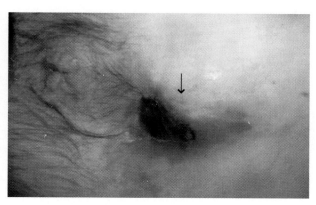

26. Hard, leathery eschar in the chronic inflammatory phase. Note how the eschar appears similar to a scab.
(Copyright © B.M. Bates-Jensen.)

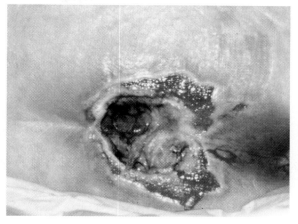

27. Soft, soggy, black eschar in the absence of an inflammatory phase.
(Copyright © B.M. Bates-Jensen.)

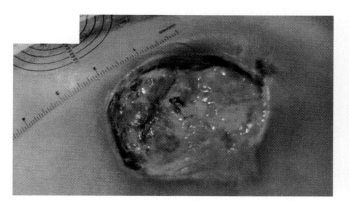

28. Chronic wound converted to acute inflammatory phase with yellow, mucinous slough.
(Copyright © C. Sussman.)

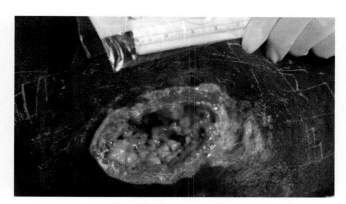

29. Necrotic fatty tissue.
(Copyright © C. Sussman.)

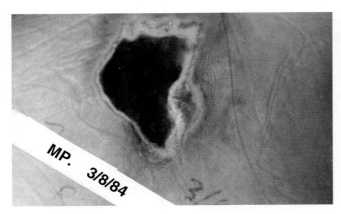

30. Eschar before debridement. Absence of inflammatory and proliferative phases.
(Copyright © C. Sussman.)

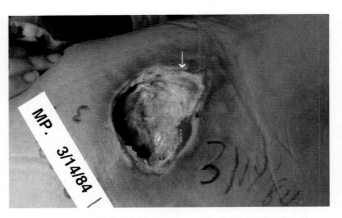

31. Eschar after debridement. Necrotic fat and fascia often called slough. Restart of inflammatory phase. Absence of proliferative phase.
(Copyright © C. Sussman.)

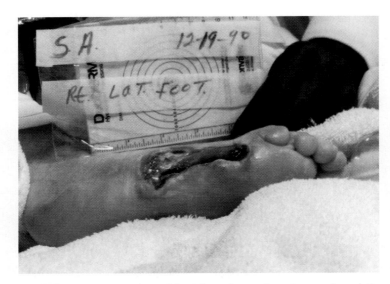

32. Soft, soggy necrosis and bruising often referred to as "purple" ulcer. Foot shows signs of cellulitis and edema. Acute inflammatory phase.
(Copyright © C. Sussman.)

PLATES 33–36
Wound Edges

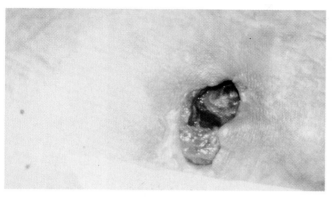

33. Absence of proliferative phase. Wound with no epithelialization present. The wound is clean, but nonproliferating. (Copyright © B.M. Bates-Jensen.)

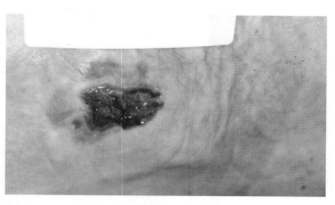

34. Same wound as in Plate 33. Wound is in acute proliferative phase with evidence of new epithelial migration. (Copyright © B.M. Bates-Jensen.)

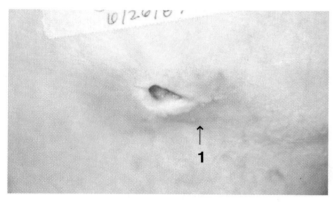

35. There is an absence of the epithelialization phase due to chronic fibrosis and scarring at the wound edge. Edges achieve a unique, grayish hue in both dark and lightly pigmented skin. Note rolled and thickened attributes. Chronic proliferative phase. (Copyright © B.M. Bates-Jensen.)

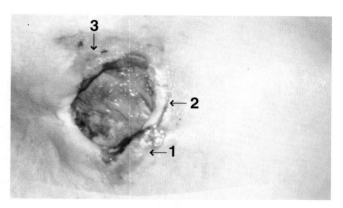

36. Example of knowledge gained from careful examination of the wound edge. This is a chronic, deep ulcer that does not bleed easily. Wound is in chronic proliferative phase. Note:
(1) New pressure-induced damage (hemorrhage)
(2) Maceration from wound fluid
(3) Friction injury with signs of inflammation
(Copyright © B.M. Bates-Jensen.)

PLATES 37 and 38
Surgical Dissection for Tunneling

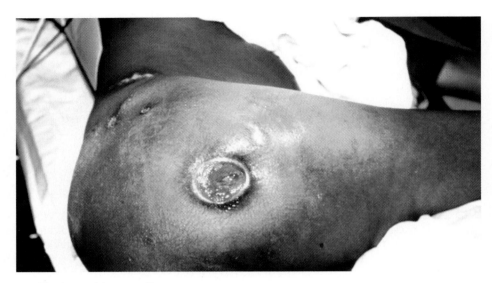

37. Unobservable tunneling.
(Copyright © J. Wethe.)

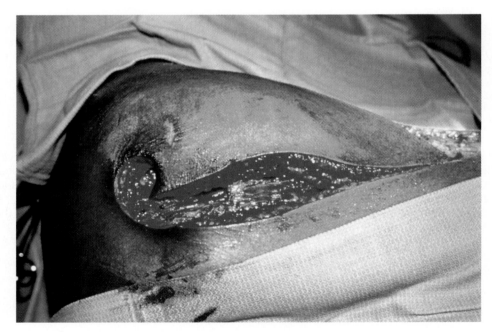

38. Same wound as in Plate 37 with surgical dissection demonstrating the extent of the tunneling process, forming a sinus tract.
(Copyright © J. Wethe.)

PLATES 39–41
Undermining and Tunneling

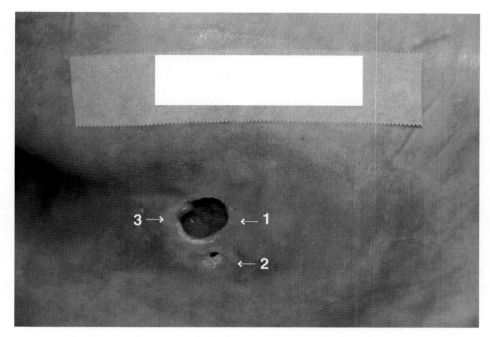

39. Wound with tunneling before insertion of a cotton-tipped applicator. Note:
(1) Ulcer reoccurrence at site of old scar tissue
(2) Skin bridge between two open ulcers
(3) Surrounding skin has unblanchable erythema; wound edges rolled under demonstrate chronic inflammatory phase
(4) Absence of proliferative phase
(Copyright © B.M. Bates-Jensen.)

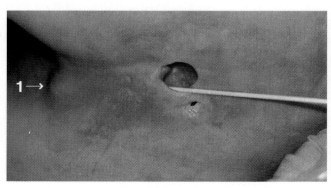

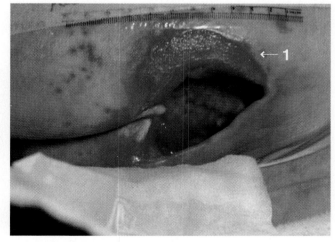

40. Same wound as in Plate 39. The wound's overall size is much larger than the surface open area. Tunneling is present. Note the bulge from the end of the cotton-tipped applicator.
(Copyright © B.M. Bates-Jensen.)

41. Undermined wound. Note the shelf.
(Copyright © C. Sussman.)

PLATES 42–47
Reading the Dressing: Wound Exudate Assessment

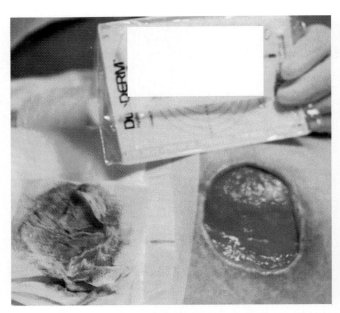

42. Wound appears "clean," but it is in the chronic proliferative phase. The quantity of exudate is determined by the amount of dressing saturated by the drainage. Note:
(1) Moderate to large amount of sanguineous exudate
(2) Moderate to large amount of purulent exudate
Evaluate for infection.
(Copyright © C. Sussman.)

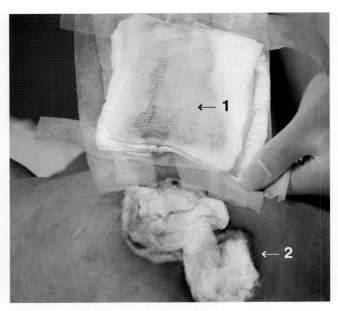

43. Wound with packing still present. Note:
(1) Moderate amount of serous exudate on dressing
(2) Green color of exudate suggests possible infection
(Copyright © C. Sussman.)

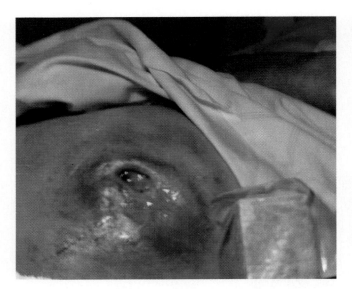

44. Wound with composite dressing. Dressing shows moderate amount of serosanguineous exudate. The wound bed shows a gelatinous mass that may be gelatinous edema. Bright pink skin is scar tissue. Evaluate for trauma.
(Copyright © C. Sussman.)

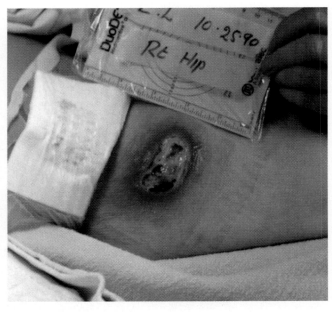

45. Wound with composite dressing shows scant amount of serous exudate. Wound is in chronic inflammatory phase. There is an absence of proliferative phase. Wound is stage III pressure ulcer.
(Copyright © C. Sussman.)

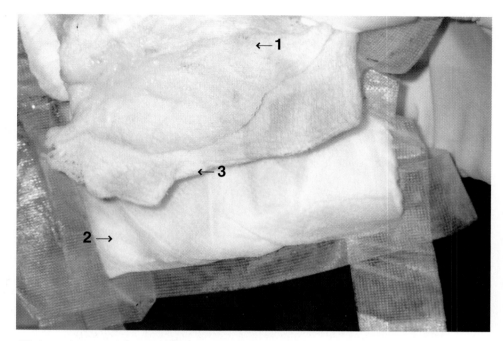

46. Large amount of serous drainage. Note:
(1) Drainage flows into secondary dressing
(2) Green tinge to edges of dressing, suggesting anaerobic infection (e.g., pseudomonas). Monitor for a degenerative change in exudate type from present serous to purulent (e.g., greener, thicker, and more opaque).
(Copyright © C. Sussman.)

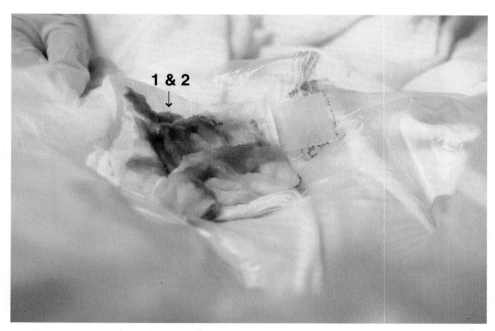

47. Large amount of purulent exudate. Note:
(1) Thick, opaque, cloudy appearance
(2) Green color
Assess for odor.
(Copyright © C. Sussman.)

PLATES 48–51
Scar Attributes

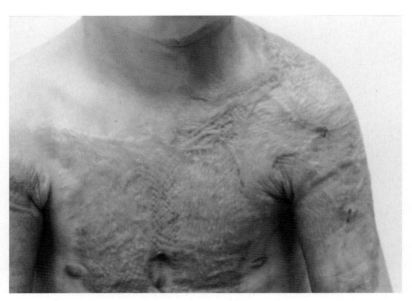

48. Hypertrophic scar.
(Copyright © 2001, R. Scott Ward.)

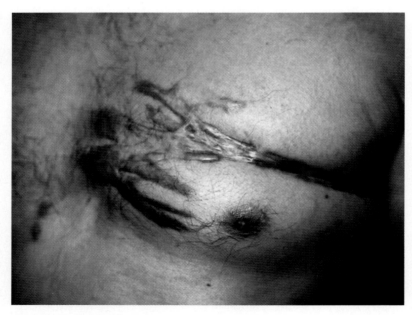

49. Immature keloid scar.
(Copyright © 2001, R. Scott Ward.)

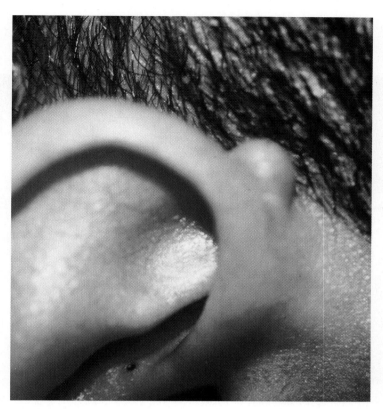

50. Keloid scar.
Copyright © 2001, R. Scott Ward.)

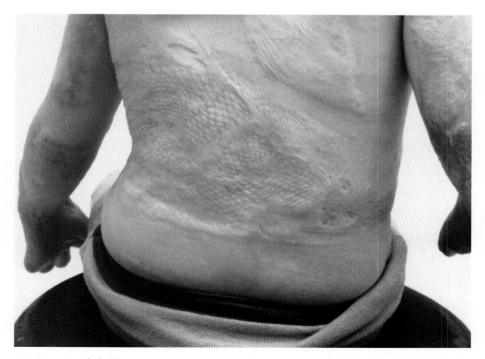

51. Maturing keloid scar.
(Copyright © 2001, R. Scott Ward.)

PLATES 52–54
Arterial Ischemic Wounds

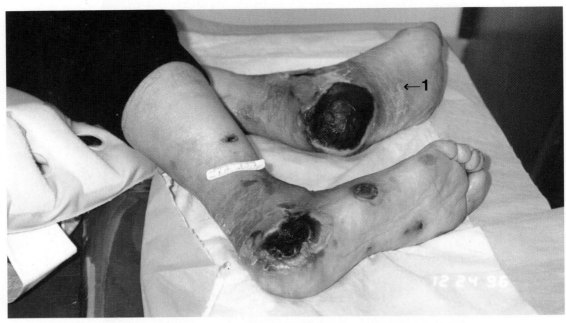

52. Severe arterial ischemic disease with multiple ischemic ulcers below the ankle bilaterally. There is an absence of the inflammatory phase with hard, dry, black eschar covering. Note trophic changes on foot, evidence of scaling. Do not debride.
(Copyright © E. Fowler.)

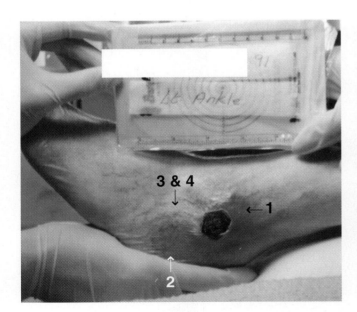

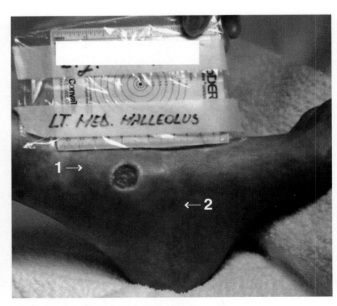

53. Classic ischemic ulcer. Note:
(1) Chronic inflammation with cellulitis
(2) Punched-out ulcer edges
(3) Covering of dry, black eschar
(4) Location over lateral malleolus
(Copyright © C. Sussman.)

54. Ischemic ulcer in chronic proliferative phase and absence of epithelialization phase. Note:
(1) Punched-out ulcer appearance with rolled wound edges
(2) Dependent rubor
(Copyright © C. Sussman.)

PLATES 55–60
Venous Disease

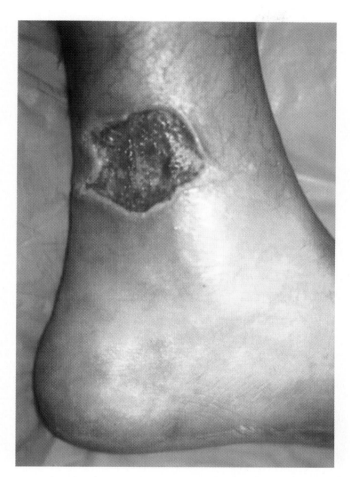

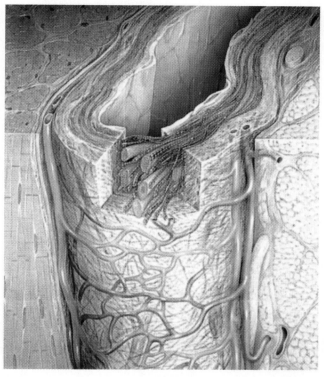

55. Ischemic ulcer in a 55-year-old male smoker with a 4-month history of having "blistered" his ankle with subsequent formation of a painful ulcer. He was diagnosed with venous stasis ulcer and treated with wet-to-dry dressing changes three times per day. Despite good compliance, his ulcer failed to improve. Physical exam revealed absent femoral, popliteal, and pedal pulses with an ABI of 0.35. The ulcer edge was irregular, but the base was clean with adequate granulation tissue. Although the ulcer was located proximal to the medial malleolus (the typical location of chronic venous stasis ulcers), this patient did not exhibit the physical signs of chronic venous insufficiency, such as brawny edema, hyperpigmentation, or stasis dermatitis. See Chapter 17 for the angiogram on this patient (Figure 17-4).
(Copyright © C. Donayre.)

56. Structure of the venous wall. Cross-section of a venous branch of the lower extremity reveals a relatively standard wall structure. The intima is covered by uninterrupted endothelium, which is connected to a thin connective tissue layer. The media is structured much more loosely than corresponding arteries, and is composed of distinct layers of collagenous and elastic fibers, between which narrow strips of smooth muscle are found.
(Copyright © C. Donayre.)

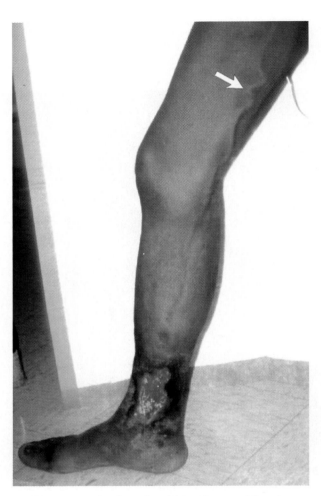

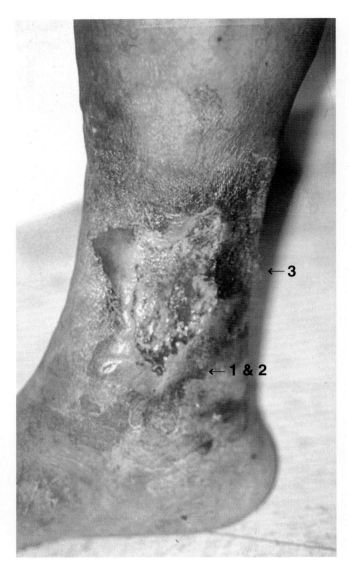

57. Venous stasis ulceration. This 49-year-old male with a 3-year history of recurrent venous ulceration was being treated with Unna boot changes once a week. Physical exam revealed patent femoral, popliteal, and pedal pulses. An enlarged, dilated, and tortuous greater saphenous vein was easily visualized with the patient in a standing position (white arrow). A duplex scan confirmed isolated greater saphenous vein incompetence, with a normal deep and perforator vein system. (Copyright © C. Donayre.)

58. Shallow and irregularly shaped lesion with a good granulating base. The associated physical signs of chronic venous insufficiency, such as hyperpigmentation, chronic scarring, and skin contraction in the ankle region, are readily identified. Note the classic characteristics of venous disease:
(1) Irregular edges
(2) Shallow ulcer
(3) Evidence of hyperpigmentation (hemosiderin staining) surrounding ulcer
(4) Location above the medial malleolus
(Copyright © C. Donayre.)

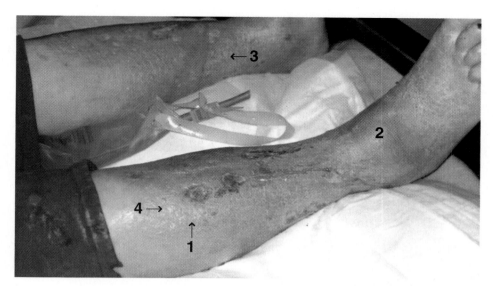

59. Stasis dermatitis. There is an absence of the epithelialization phase. Note evidence of:
(1) Brawny edema
(2) Trophic skin changes
(3) Hemosiderin staining (hyperpigmentation)
(4) Multiple shallow ulcers
(Copyright © B.M. Bates-Jensen.)

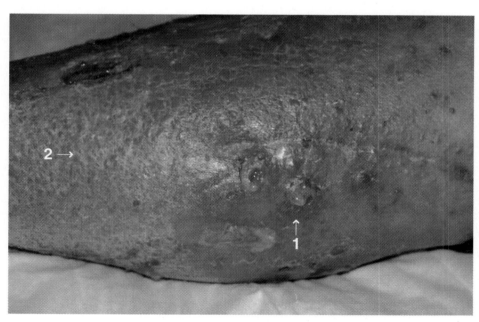

60. Close-up view of same leg as in Plate 59. Note evidence of:
(1) Edema leakage through wounds
(2) Scaling and crusting (trophic changes) due to lipodermatosclerosis
(Copyright © B.M. Bates-Jensen.)

PLATES 61–65
Malignant Cutaneous Wounds

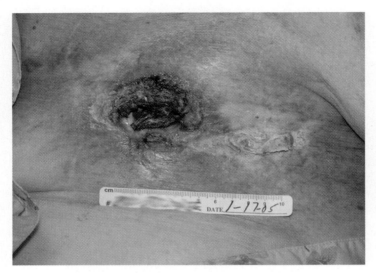

61. Cutaneous metastasis of breast cancer, four years post mastectomy and radiation therapy. Note thick, dry eschar with dried exudate covering the moist underlying wound. Significant odor.
(Copyright © S. Seaman.)

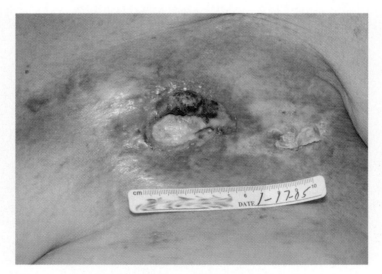

62. Immediately following sharp debridement of eschar and thorough cleansing with skin cleanser. Note fungating area at superior edge of wound with friable tissue, as well as slough and exposed rib in wound bed. Fragile surrounding skin is secondary to radiation therapy, and surrounding redness is due to high vascularity of area.
(Copyright © S. Seaman.)

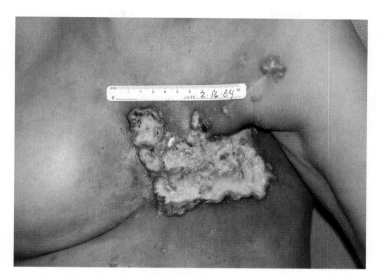

63. Eight years post mastectomy with ulcerative malignant lesion.
Note:
(1) Necrotic center and friable edges
(2) New metastatic nodule forming above ulcer
(Copyright © S. Seaman.)

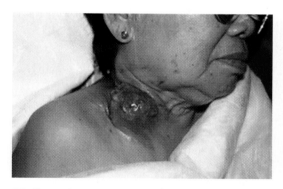

64. Fungating tumor secondary to metastasis of head and neck cancer. Note extreme friability of tissue. Requires extreme care to reduce bleeding with wound care.
(Copyright © G. Thomas.)

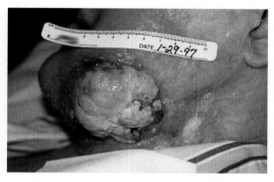

65. Fungating tumor from local invasion of oral cancer. Significant drainage and odor. Later developed an oral-cutaneous fistula.
(Copyright © G. Thomas.)

AU: Should this be electrical stimulation (ES)?

PLATES 66 and 67
Wound Healing with Electrical Stimulation-Chapter 21

Patient with vascular ulcer treated with ED and high-voltage pulsed current (HVPC) (see Chapter 21 for details).

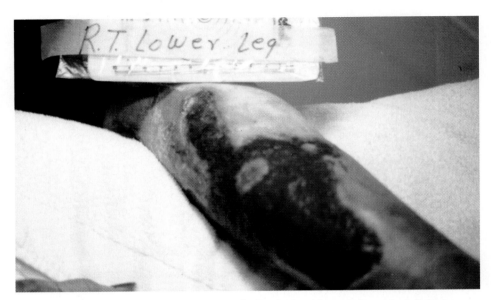

66. Note beefy, red granulation tissue and island of epidermal tissue in full-thickness wound. The wound was in the acute proliferative phase on 12/28.
(Copyright © C. Sussman.)

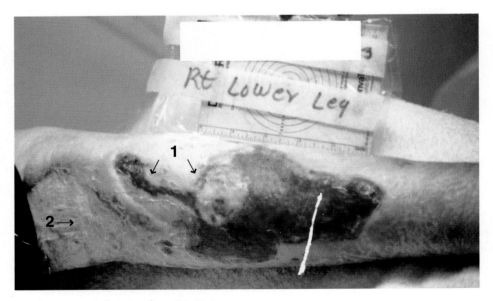

67. Same wound as in Plate 64. Note:
(1) Epidermal migration from wound edges, island, and wound shape changes
(2) Progression to the acute epithelialization phase by 2/17
(3) Hyperkeratotic skin changes due to old burn wounds and poor circulation
(Copyright © C. Sussman.)

PLATES 68–70
Wound Healing with Pulsed Short-Wave Diathermy: Case Study 1-Chapter 22

Patient with pressure ulcers treated with pulsed short-wave diathermy (PSWD) (see Chapter 22 for details).[x-ref]

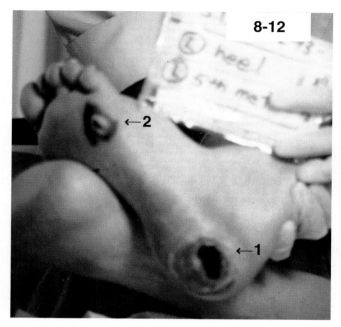

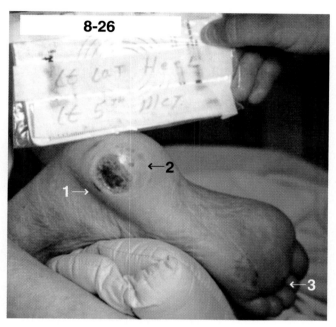

68. Patient with pressure ulcers. PSWD was begun on 8/16. Note:
(1) Black eschar on heel wound surrounded by partial-thickness skin loss; there is an absence of inflammatory phase
(2) Black eschar over the 5th metatarsal head; there is an absence of inflammatory phase
(Copyright © C. Sussman.)

69. Same ulcer as seen on heel in Plate 68, 10 days after start of PSWD. Note:
(1) Eschar removed to soft necrosis
(2) Reepithelialization of partial-thickness skin loss
(3) Eschar removed 5th metatarsal, and wound healed
(Copyright © C. Sussman.)

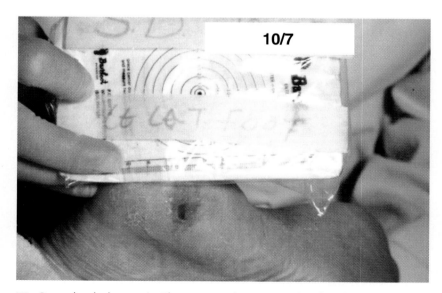

70. Same heel ulcer as in Plates 68 and 69, on 10/7. The ulcer healed and is shown in the remodeling phase.
(Copyright © C. Sussman.)

PLATES 71 and 72
Wound Healing with Pulsed Radiofrequency Stimulation: Case Study 2-Chapter 22[x-ref]

Patient with incisional wound treated with pulsed radiofrequency stimulation (PRFS) (see Chapter 22 for details).[x-ref]

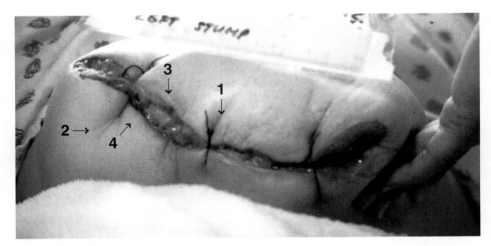

71. Patient with the incision from an above-the-knee amputation left open for delayed primary intention healing. Wound is in acute inflammatory phase. Start of treatment with PRFS began 8/3. Note:
(1) Sutures placed
(2) Edema
(3) Erythema and tissue tension
(4) Yellow, mucinous slough in incision line
(Copyright © C. Sussman.)

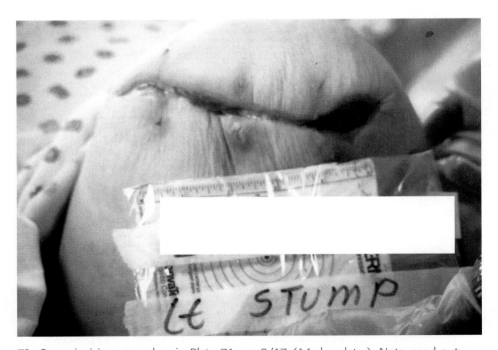

72. Same incision wound as in Plate 71, on 8/17 (14 days later). Note good outcomes: edema-free, necrosis-free, wound contraction, and granulation. The wound is in acute proliferative and epithelialization phases.
(Copyright © C. Sussman.)

PLATES 73–75
High-Resolution Ultrasound Scans

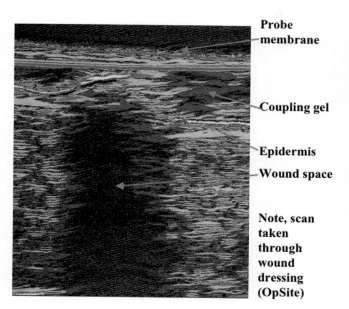

Probe
membrane

Coupling gel

Epidermis

Wound space

Note, scan
taken
through
wound
dressing
(OpSite)

73. Punch Biopsy Wound, day 3.
(Copyright P. Wilson.)

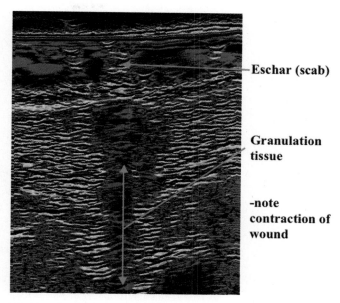

Eschar (scab)

Granulation
tissue

-note
contraction of
wound

74. Punch Biopsy Wound, day 14.
(Copyright P. Wilson.)

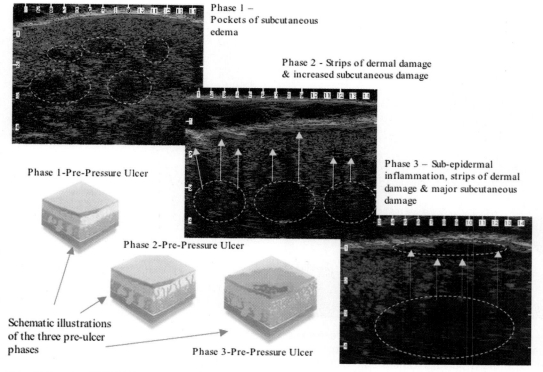

Phase 1 –
Pockets of subcutaneous
edema

Phase 2 - Strips of dermal damage
& increased subcutaneous damage

Phase 3 – Sub-epidermal
inflammation, strips of dermal
damage & major subcutaneous
damage

Phase 1-Pre-Pressure Ulcer

Phase 2-Pre-Pressure Ulcer

Schematic illustrations
of the three pre-ulcer
phases

Phase 3-Pre-Pressure Ulcer

75. Using the EPISCAN, pressure ulcers have been found to develop in the subcutaneous tissue over a hard prominence, typically a bone, and then spread out through the dermis to the epidermis, where at some point, an open wound often develops. Studies have shown that the early phases of pressure ulcer development shown below can be used to initiate earlier and more targeted intervention, and that this can significantly and cost-effectively reduce the occurrence of open pressure ulcers.
(Copyright P. Wilson.)

PLATES 76–78
Wound Healing with Ultrasound: Case Study 1-Chapter 24[x-ref]

Patient with a venous ulcer 24 hours after onset (see Chapter 24 for details).[x-ref]

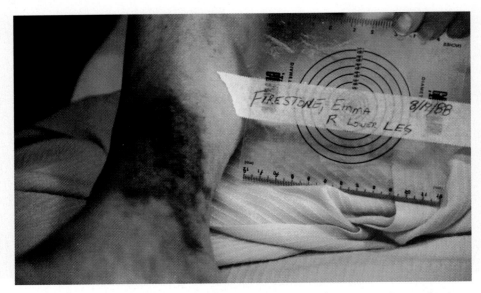

76. Wound is in acute inflammatory phase and shows subcutaneous hemorrhage (ecchymosis) associated with venous disease.
(Copyright © C. Sussman.)

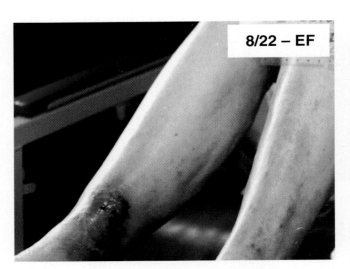

77. Same wound as in Plate 76, 4 days after 2 treatments with ultrasound. Shows absorption of the ecchymosis seen earlier. There is partial-thickness skin loss. The wound is in acute inflammatory phase.
(Copyright © C. Sussman.)

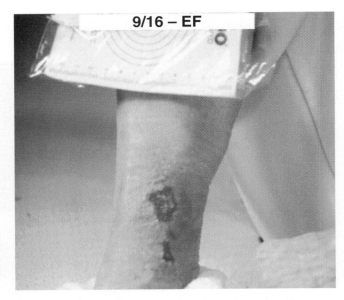

78. Same ulcer as in Plates 76 and 77, 4 weeks after start of ultrasound. Note wound contraction compared with that in Plate 77. There are soft, irregular wound edges and new epithelization. The wound is an epithelialization phase.
(Copyright © C. Sussman.)

PLATES 79–82
Wound Healing with Ultrasound: Case Study 2-Chapter 24 [x-ref]

Patient with blood blister on heel secondary to pressure, treated with ultrasound (US).

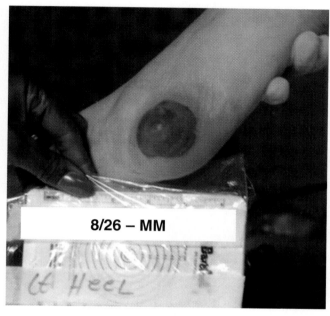

79. Acute inflammatory phase. Blister with bloody fluid at day of identification.
(Copyright © C. Sussman.)

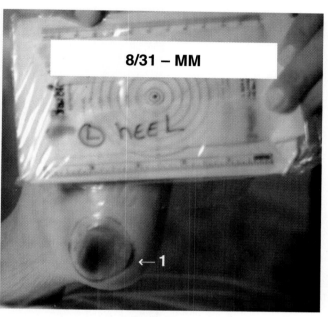

80. Same wound as in Plate 79 without blister roof. The periwound skin was treated with daily US for 4 days prior. Note area of apparent necrosis and hematoma. There is an absence of inflammatory phase.
(Copyright © C. Sussman.)

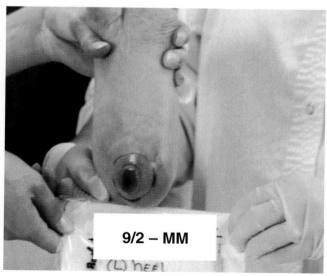

81. Same wound as in Plates 79 and 80 after 2 additional periwound US treatments. Note absorption of hematoma by reduced size of necrotic area and mild erythema surrounding the area of necrosis. The wound is acute inflammatory phase.
(Copyright © C. Sussman.)

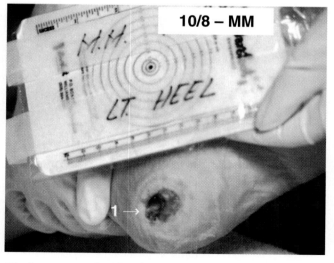

82. Same wound as in Plates 79-81. Note focal area of necrosis, and the time of change in treatment to electrical stimulation (ES) and sharp debridement. The wound shows the start of proliferative phase.
(Copyright © C. Sussman.)

PLATES 83 and 84
Venous Ulcer with Soring Sonica 180AU: Cannot find term, please confirm: Case Study

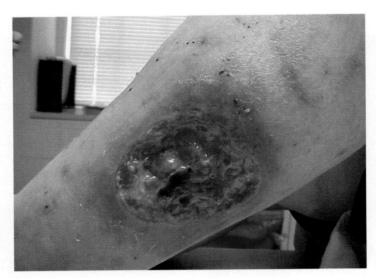

83. Before debridement.

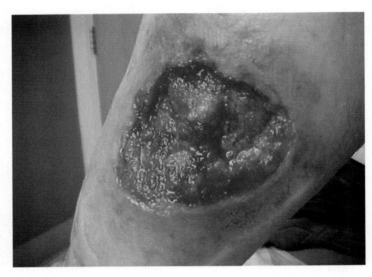

84. After debridement.

PLATES 85–87
Wound Healing with Pulsatile Lavage with Suction-Chapter 26

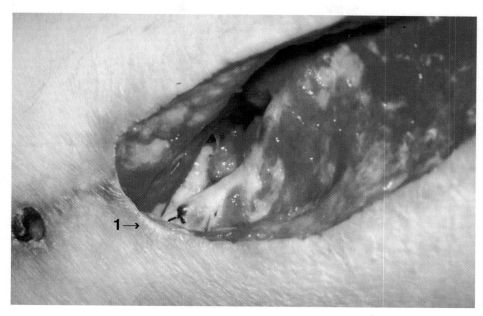

85. Exposed artery in infected bypass graft donor site in lower leg.
(Copyright © H. Loehne.)

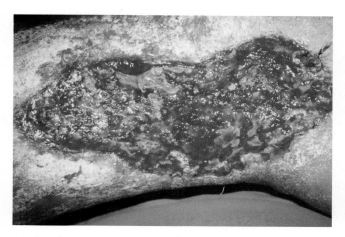

86. Pyoderma gangrenosum ulcer on medial lower leg of 8-year duration. Chronic epithelialization phase.
(Copyright © H. Loehne.)

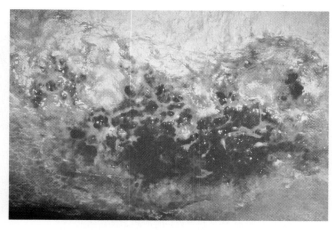

87. Pyoderma gangrenosum ulcer (same ulcer as in Plate 82 **AU: Should be Plate 86?**) on medial lower leg after 2 weeks of treatment with Pulsavac® System. Note epithelialization progressing to cover wound surface.
(Copyright © H. Loehne.)

PLATES 88 and 89
Pressure Mapping

Pressure mapping uses color and numbers to show areas of high pressure. Red and yellow (warm colors) are areas of high pressure, whereas green and blue (cool colors) are areas of low pressure. Mapping is evaluated by color distribution, not by numbers. Here, the same subject (5'10" and 175 lb) was placed on two different seat cushions. Note the different pressure loading patterns of the buttocks on the two cushions.

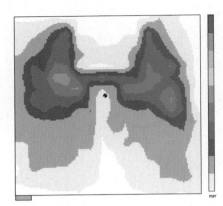 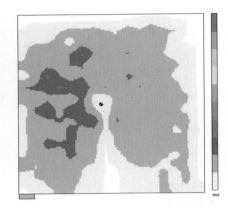

88. Foam cushion with sized ischial cut-out eliminates pressure over the ischial tuberosities and redistributes pressure over the femurs.

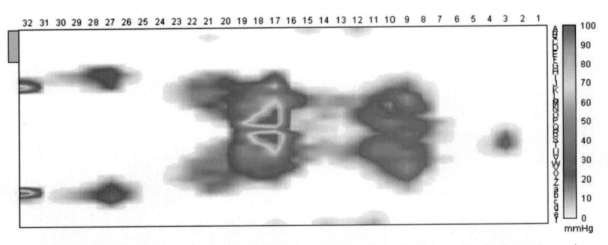

89. Four-inch high air-filled cushion takes some of the pressure off the ischials and redistributes it evenly over the surface of the cushion.

PART

I

Introduction to Wound Diagnosis

Carrie Sussman

Development of diagnoses to direct and guide treatment by nurses and physical therapists has grown over the past 15 to 20 years. Both disciplines recognize that use of a diagnostic process allows professional nurses and physical therapists to apply their skills and knowledge to the appropriate treatment of client situations that they can and should treat legally and independently. The role of diagnostician is unfamiliar to many, and practice experience in the area of diagnosis varies from nonexistent to full-practice integration for many years. Because the incorporation of diagnosis into the health-care professions is still in its infancy, there is much variance in understanding of the process. Therefore, there are a number of questions that need to be answered as the process begins:

- What does a diagnosis really mean?
- What kind of information needs to be collected to yield a diagnosis?
- How are diagnoses differentiated from one another?
- How is a diagnosis tailored to a patient's functional problem or human response to health or illness?
- How does diagnosis relate to prognosis and outcomes?
- How does the nursing or physical therapy diagnosis direct interventions?

Advanced clinicians who are familiar with classification systems and diagnostic methods will have additional questions:

- Can and should the medical diagnosis be part of the physical therapy diagnostic statement?
- What kind of functional diagnostic statement should be written for a person at risk for wounds?
- What is the difference between diagnosis and classification?

Part I begins with an introduction to the diagnostic process. It seeks to answer these questions and provide specific information about wound diagnosis. Guidelines for writing functional diagnoses that are meaningful and related to the prognosis and treatment interventions are included for both the physical therapy and nursing disciplines.

It is clear that the diagnostic processes and terminology are very similar for nurses and physical therapists. Both incorporate functional impairment and disability into the diagnostic process. For example, a nurse determines the client's response to health or illness as positive functioning, altered functioning, or at risk for altered functioning.[1] Nurses use a diagnosis that incorporates risk, which could work equally well for a physical therapist. Nursing diagnosis specifically identifies collaborative problems, then, the health care practitioner needed for joint management. The most appropriate joint manager for wounds may be the dietitian, the physician, or the physical therapist. Nurses already have taxonomy for *impaired tissue integrity* and *impaired skin integrity*. Physical therapists use disablement terminology, including the terms *impairment, disability*, and *handicap* in their management model.[2]

Functional diagnosis requires an understanding of functional impairment. Functional impairment differs from the pathogenesis or etiology of the problem and describes a functional change as physiologic, anatomic, structural, or functional at the tissue, organ, or body system level.[3] Functional impairments are the system or organ impairments that prevent normal function.[4] In impaired wound healing, a functional impairment occurs at the system, organ, or tissue level in the body.

Chapter 2 describes acute wound healing physiology and chronic wound healing factors, as well as intrinsic, extrinsic, and iatrogenic factors that can influence chronic wound healing. Assessment, examinations, tests, and measurements are an integral part of establishing a diagnosis. Chapters 3–7 describe methods and procedures for collecting information and interpreting the findings.

At the conclusion of Part I, clinicians will understand acute and chronic wound healing physiology. They will be able to perform the required tests and measures necessary to determine a functional wound diagnosis, develop a prognosis, select appropriate interventions, and document the diagnostic process and findings with a functional outcomes report. In Parts II, III, and IV, the clinician will learn the management skills and appropriate interventions required for different wound-related problems.

REFERENCES

1. Carpenito LJ. *Nursing Diagnosis: Application to Clinical Practice.* 6th ed. Philadelphia: J.B. Lippincott, 1994.
2. American Physical Therapy Association. A guide to physical therapy practice, I: a description of patient management. *Phys Ther.* 1995;75:707–764.
3. World Health Organization. *International Classification of Impairments, Disabilities, and Handicaps.* Geneva, Switzerland: WHO Publications Centre USA, 1980.
4. Jette AM. Physical disablement concepts for physical therapy research and practice. *Phys Ther.* 1994;74:380–386.

The Diagnostic Process

Carrie Sussman and Barbara M. Bates-Jensen

CHAPTER OBJECTIVES

At the completion of this chapter, the reader will be able to:
1. Describe each step in the diagnostic process.
2. Identify key data to collect during the assessment process.
3. Differentiate between behavioral and functional outcomes.
4. Explain the importance of determining prognosis during the diagnostic process.
5. Describe the process of evaluation using outcomes.

This chapter describes the diagnostic process used for management of patients with chronic wounds. Nurses and physical therapists employ essentially the same decision-making process in diagnosing patient problems, although the descriptive terminology may differ slightly. Nurses use the nursing process and nursing diagnosis as the framework for planning and evaluating patient care. The nursing process includes the following steps: assessment, diagnosis, goals, interventions, and evaluation. Physical therapists use a process that includes the steps of assessment, examination, diagnosis, prognosis, and outcomes.

To simplify terminology and guide the reader, the diagnostic process has been broken down in this textbook into four steps, each with two or three parts:

1. Assessment—includes review of the reason for referral, history, systems review/physical assessment, and wound assessment
2. Diagnosis—includes examination strategy, evaluation, and diagnosis
3. Goals—includes prognosis, goals, outcomes and evaluation of progress
4. Intervention—described in subsequent chapters

Examinations and specific measurements, as well as special test procedures, are found in Chapters 3, 4, 5, and 7, as well as in other chapters.

Step 1: Assessment Process

The assessment process assists in clinical decision making by preventing undirected care and inappropriate treatment. Assessment is performed for all patients before determining the need for special testing examinations and interventions. For nurses, this process begins when the patient is admitted to the agency. For physical therapists, this process begins with the reason for referral, which is part of the patient history.

The assessment process involves gathering data from the patient history and physical examination. The patient history determines which relevant systems reviews should be included in the physical examination. For physical therapists, the history and systems review determine whether the patient is a candidate for services; for nurses, the history and systems review determine the direction of the treatment plan.

Many physical therapists believe that a referral automatically constitutes candidacy for wound care. However, the reality is that not all patients are appropriately referred for physical therapy. For all providers, proper utilization management is mandatory in today's health-care environment.

Utilization management, which is part of the process of prospective management, is designed to ensure that only medically necessary, reasonable, and appropriate services are provided. Utilization management influences the treatment pathway to ensure optimal clinical outcomes.[1] For nurses, the assessment process provides the framework for planning comprehensive wound care, incorporating utilization management, and possibly making a referral for physical therapy.

Utilization management for a patient with a wound and comorbidities and coimpairment is a separate, but related, issue. Collaborative interdisciplinary management of comorbidities and coimpairments reduces the iatrogenic effects caused by inappropriate selection of interventions or handling of a wound, and lessens the extrinsic and intrinsic complications (see Chapter 2). The interdisciplinary nature inherent in caring for a patient with a wound requires clinicians to carefully determine candidacy for services before initiating referral or treatment. For example, a physical therapist may determine that a patient is not a candidate for whirlpool therapy as ordered by the physician, and may instead send the findings with an alternative recommendation to the referring physician.

The use of standardized forms is the best method of collecting assessment data quickly and efficiently, thus ensuring that important information is not lost. Use of forms that the clinician and patient complete ensures data maintenance from the interview. Partnering with or engaging the patient in his or her own care from the beginning is essential to achieving mutually satisfactory outcomes. A self-administered patient history form helps the clinician focus the interview and can save time. Samples of a self-administered patient history form and a focused assessment form for physical therapists and nurses are presented in Appendixes 1-A and 1-B. Some information can be found in the patient's medical record, but the patient, caregiver, or significant other can often provide additional insights and information not otherwise available.

Review of Admission/Referral

It is essential for a physical therapist to know the reason a patient was referred, because the referral is the first step in documenting patient history. The initial referral for wound care management is usually made to a nurse; if the nurse determines the need for physical therapy services, the physical therapist is brought into the team. It is critical for nurses to understand the expectations of and projected outcomes from a physical therapy referral in order to refer appropriately. In some health-care settings, a wound care team decides which services are necessary for wound management and makes the appropriate referrals. Patients referred to a physical therapist for wound healing have usually not shown signs of normal wound repair. Most often, other treatment interventions are in use or have been attempted with limited or no success. Physical therapy services usually involve an additional fee.

A referral to physical therapy is typically regarded as an attempt to maximize and enhance wound repair. However, referrals can be made for reasons beyond improved wound healing. For example, a patient may be referred for help in cleaning and debriding a necrotic wound, for enhancement of the inflammatory process, to reinitiate wound repair, or for recurrent infection. For the patient who presents with factors that impair wound healing, the reason for referral is to achieve a clean, stable wound that can be managed effectively by the nurse or caregiver at home. In other cases, pain management can be the reason for referral, with physical agents and electrotherapeutic modalities prescribed to help control pain.

For both nurses and physical therapists, wound closure may not be the highest priority. They must understand the reason for the referral and the expected outcomes, and the selected intervention must match the expected outcomes to meet the referral objectives. For example, a patient with a foot ulcer secondary to pressure and insensitivity is fearful of amputation and loss of ability to walk. The patient's main concern is limb salvage, and expectations are high. In contrast, the family of a debilitated long-term care patient may desire only comfort for their family member, with no expectations of wound closure. Family and caregiver perceptions of various interventions may differ from the clinician's view. What are perceived by one family member to be heroic and painful measures may, to the clinician, be considered normal procedures. The nurse must address these issues before making a referral to physical therapy.

Patient History

Patient history information is commonly collected during an interview process with the patient, family, significant others, and caregivers; by consultation with other health-care practitioners; and by reviewing the medical record. Ideally, in the continuum of care, the patient's historical information is transmitted with the patient, but this is not always the case. The clinician may need to piece together the history from the many sources named above. If only a limited amount of medical and social information is available, the clinician may need to choose diagnostic options based on available data. It is simpler and more effective to plan appropriate care with a complete history.

CLINICAL WISDOM

Patient History Data Needed To Determine Care Direction

- Reason for admission or referral
- Expectations and perceptions about wound healing
- Psychosocial-cultural-economic history
- Present medical comorbidities
- Current wound status

Remember that one of the primary goals of the patient interview is to begin to develop a therapeutic relationship with the patient and family. History taking allows the clinician to assess and diagnose patient problems and to place the problems within the context of the individual patient's life. Important skills used by clinicians during the patient history include listening, observing, and asking questions.

Chief Complaint and Health History

Begin the patient history by determining the patient's chief complaint or major reason for seeking care, as well as the duration of the problem. Why is the patient seeking help at this time? The reason may be as simple as convenience or as complicated as a wound problem that has worsened. Investigate motivations the patient may have beyond the obvious problem by asking a question such as, "How did you hope that I could help you today?"

Explore the meaning of the wound to the patient. Questions such as, "What do you think caused your wound?" "Why do you think it started when it did?" and, "How long do you think the wound will last?" can reveal the patient's level of understanding of the health problem. Based on their answers, care can be planned that is sensitive to the patient's needs and level of understanding.

The clinician also seeks a complete understanding of the patient's symptoms, i.e., the subjective feelings of the patient, during the interview. Seven criteria can be used to describe symptoms:

1. Location
2. Character
3. Severity
4. Timing
5. Setting in which the symptom occurs
6. Antecedents and consequences of the symptom
7. Other associated symptoms

CLINICAL WISDOM

Questions to Elicit Extent of Wound Symptoms

- *Location:* Where do you feel the wound? Do you feel it anywhere else? Show me where it hurts.
- *Character:* What does it feel like?
- *Severity:* On a scale of 0–10, with 10 being the worst pain you could imagine, how would you rate the discomfort you have now? How does the wound interfere with your usual activities? How bad is it?
- *Timing/Duration:* When did you first notice the wound? How often have you had wounds?
- *Setting:* Does the wound occur in a certain place or under certain circumstances? Is it associated with any specific activity?
- *Antecedents and Consequences:* What makes it better? What makes it worse?
- *Other Associated Symptoms:* Have you noticed any other changes?

Answers to these questions should provide a thorough understanding of the patient's wound symptoms.

Review the patient's present health and present illness status to learn additional information about his or her reasons for seeking care. Describe the patient's usual health and then focus on the present problem, investigating the chief complaint thoroughly, as described above. For interpretation and analysis of the patient's problem, it is helpful to document the chief complaint data in chronologic order.

Next, review the patient's past health history. Information about management of and response to past problems provides an indication of the patient's potential response to treatment of the current problem. Much of this information may be available in the patient's medical record. If not, the following information should be obtained:

- Past general health
- Childhood illnesses, accidents or injuries with any associated disabilities
- Hospitalizations
- Surgeries
- Major acute or chronic illnesses
- Immunizations
- Medications and transfusions
- Allergies

Current health information includes allergies, health habits, medications, and sleep and exercise patterns. Investigate environmental, food, drug, animal, and other allergies, as specific allergies may impact which interventions are chosen for the patient's wound care regimen. Allergic reactions usually affect the gastrointestinal tract, respiratory tract, and skin. Some products used for wound care can contribute to an allergic reaction, such as latex, which is found in dressings, gloves, and plastic tubing. Tape is also often associated with skin allergies. Sulfonamide is a common drug allergen that is contained in silver sulfadiazine (Silvadene), a common topical therapy for wound care; in some cases, the clinician may need to choose another topical agent to accomplish the treatment goals. The clinician should be aware of warning signs and take necessary measures to control any offending allergen.

Evaluate current and past habits relevant to the health of the patient, including alcohol, tobacco, illicit substance, and caffeine use. Alcohol, tobacco, and illicit substance use, in particular, present significant problems for tissue perfusion and nutrition for wound healing.

Complete a full medication profile, including prescription and over-the-counter medications, names, dosages, frequency, intended effect, and compliance with the regimen. Many medications interfere with wound healing or may interact with wound therapy.

Evaluate the patient's usual routine to determine patterns of physical and sedentary activities. Ask the patient to describe a typical day's activities. Exercise patterns influence healing of several wound types, such as venous disease ulcers. Finally, investigate the patient's sleep pattern and whether he or she perceives the sleep to be adequate and satisfactory. Ask the patient where he or she usually sleeps. Patients with severe arterial insufficiency may sleep sitting up in recliner chairs because of the pain associated with the disease. Likewise, patients with chronic obstructive pulmonary disease (COPD) may sleep sitting up because of difficulty breathing in the supine position.

The family health history provides information about the general health of the patient's relatives and family. Family health information is helpful in the identification of genetic, familial, and environmental illnesses. Specific areas to target are diabetes mellitus, heart disease, and stroke, as these diseases can impair wound healing and are risk factors for further wounding. If the patient has a family history of any of these diseases, he or she may have early signs of the disease as yet undiagnosed and is at higher risk of eventual disease development.

Sociologic History

Diagnosis and management of a patient's wound is best accomplished within the context of the whole person. It is important to gather information about the patient's sociologic, psychologic, and nutritional status. Sociologic data fall into seven areas:

1. Relationships with family and significant others
2. Environment
3. Occupational history
4. Economic status and resources
5. Educational level
6. Daily life
7. Patterns of health care.

The area of relationships with family and significant others includes gathering information on the patient's position and role in the family, the persons living with the patient, the persons to whom the patient relates, and any recent family changes or crises. The role of the patient within the family can dictate treatment decisions. For example, a grandmother with venous disease ulcers may be the primary caregiver of young grandchildren; thus, it would be unrealistic to expect compliance with a therapeutic regimen that includes frequent periods of elevating lower extremities. The family support system is often a critical factor when determining wound care management programs, and answers to questions such as, "Who will change the wound dressing and perform procedures?" "Who prepares meals?" and "Who will transport the patient to the clinic?" can influence treatment options.

Environment plays a significant role in the health and illness of individuals. Ask questions about the home, community, and work environments. Home-care patients can present challenging environments for wound repair. For example, an elderly woman living alone with four cats in a two-room trailer with minimal bathroom facilities will require different management strategies than the middle-aged man living with a spouse and family in a three-bedroom house in the suburbs. The community environment may provide additional resources for the patient, such as senior citizen centers, health fairs, or a neighborhood grocery store that delivers to the home. The work environment, along with the occupational history, can identify health-risk jobs and provide information on the ability of a patient to eliminate certain risk factors for impaired healing. For example, a grocery clerk with a venous disease ulcer will need help with work adjustment to a job that does not require standing for long periods of time.

Information on economic status and resources is important to determine adequacy for therapy compliance. It is not necessary to know a patient's exact income, but ask whether the patient feels the income is adequate and elicit the source of the income. It is important to identify patients with inadequate resources and to make appropriate referrals for financial assistance. Assess the patient's health insurance resources, including the source of insurance coverage and resources available to obtain necessary dressing supplies. If prolonged wound healing is expected, a discussion of financial reserves may be desirable. Some patients have insurance coverage that pays for all dressing supplies, whereas other patients have insurance coverage that pays for only certain types of supplies (e.g., gauze, but not tape). Still other patients have no coverage for supplies at all. The patient's economic history is also needed to determine whether he or she has adequate resources available to pay for a caregiver if one is needed to help with caregiving or changing dressings.

The educational level of the patient and assessment of age-appropriateness of intellect is helpful in planning future education on self-care. Ask the patient to describe a typical day and identify any differences on the weekend. This daily profile allows the clinician to perceive the whole patient. Answers to questions about the social and recreational activities of the patient, as well as typical daily routines, provide valuable insights into the patient's lifestyle and possible health risks. Evaluation of previous health-care access and use can assist with clinical judgment of past health promotion and prevention activities, including whether there has been continuity of care.

Psychologic History

The psychologic history includes an assessment of the patient's cognitive abilities (including learning style, memory, and comprehension), responses to illness (coping patterns and reaction to illness), response to care (compliance), and cultural implications for care. At this point in the history taking, the clinician usually has some idea of the patient's comprehension, memory, and overall cognitive status. If mental function is still unclear, the clinician can administer a mental status examination, such as the mini-mental status exam. Previous coping patterns and reactions to illness provide insight into possible reactions to the current situation. Has the patient had difficulties with wound healing in the past? Is there a history of chronic wounds? How has the patient responded to previous chronic wounds? Information about the patient's response to previous care and compliance with other therapy regimens can identify potential difficulties with adhering to the current treatment plan.

Cultural History

In today's culturally diverse world, patients often have belief systems and rituals that are significantly different from those of the clinician. It is very important for clinicians to assume nothing and to routinely assess the patient's and caregiver's values and beliefs about health and wellness. Be particularly sensitive in the assessment of a patient's culture and values. As more information becomes available on the influence of one's culture and values on health and illness, it is essential that each patient's views on health and illness be explored prior to determining goals of care and the overall treatment plan.

Nutritional History

Nutrition plays a major role in wound healing (see Chapter 3). During the patient history, determine the patient's usual daily food intake, risk for malnutrition, and specific nutritional deficiencies. Evaluate the patient's weight in comparison with his or her usual weight. Ask the patient to recall all foods eaten in the past 24 hours and determine whether this is a normal eating pattern for the patient.

Systems Review and Physical Assessment

The systems review portion of the patient history and the physical assessment of each system provide information on comorbidities that can impair wound healing. The individual's capacity to heal can be limited by specific disease effects on tissue integrity and perfusion, patient mobility, compliance, nutrition, and risk for wound infection. Throughout the patient history, systems review, and physical assessment, clinicians should consider host factors that affect wound healing.

Respiratory System

The respiratory system is critical for delivery of oxygen and nutrients to tissues to promote wound healing and control infection. Pulmonary disease can be progressive in conditions such as cystic fibrosis, COPD, and lung cancer. Nonprogressive respiratory diseases to consider are pneumonia, postcardiac or post-thoracic surgery, and traumatic injury.

Chronic Obstructive Pulmonary Disease. Patients with COPD have difficulty with pulmonary secretion retention, i.e., pulmonary secretion fills alveolar sacks and reduces the surface area for transference of oxygen through the alveolar membranes into the bloodstream. Physical assessment of patients with COPD includes evaluation of pulse oximetry, pulmonary function tests, and mode and amount of oxygen delivery. Transcutaneous oxygen transport measurements are also helpful (see Chapter 7). If noninvasive vascular test results are not available, they should be considered as part of the examination strategy for these patients.

Oxygen delivery is severely reduced when an individual lies in the horizontal position. In the supine position, the diaphragm's excursion space is reduced, which decreases thoracic expansion and tidal volume of air into the lungs. Elevating the head of the bed and placing the patient in semi-Fowler's position can improve airflow into the lungs. However, skin over the sacrococcygeal area will be at risk for pressure ulcer formation due to the shearing and friction forces present in this position. Decreased mobility is often an additional complication of COPD because of poor endurance, deconditioning, and breathing difficulty during activity.

Pneumonia. The patient at highest risk for pneumonia is the elderly, frail, institutionalized patient with multiple health deficits. The stress of this illness and its related signs and symptoms lead to impaired wound healing. Wounds will generally plateau, fail to continue healing, or deteriorate until the pneumonia is resolved. Wound repair may not be an option for a patient with pneumonia until the underlying disease is under control. Maintaining current wound status and preparing the wound for healing may be sufficient goals for this time frame.

Asthma. Asthma is a group of respiratory symptoms caused by infections, hypersensitivity to irritants (e.g., pollutants and allergens), psychologic stress, cold air, exercise, and drug use. The symptoms of asthma can be controlled with medications, including steroids such as prednisone. Inquire about the time of onset of the asthma and the start of medication. Some individuals have a long history of steroid use, which will affect their ability to heal. Steroids repress the inflammatory response, and without inflammation, wound healing will not progress. The effects of steroids can be mitigated by use of oral or topical vitamin A. The physician should be contacted with recommendations for vitamin A administration as soon as possible.

Cardiovascular System

The heart is responsible for pumping oxygenated blood through the circulatory system to all body tissues. Patients with cardiac disease have poor pump function, so all body tissues suffer. Cardiac disease can involve dysfunction of the coronary arteries, valves, or the electrical conduction system. In general, any dysfunction of the cardiac system creates significant difficulties related to wound healing. Specific cardiac diseases that affect patients with wounds include coronary artery disease and congestive heart failure (CHF).

CLINICAL WISDOM

Pacemaker Caution for Physical Therapists

Some patients have pacemaker implants to compensate for the dysfunction of their cardiac system. This is important information for physical therapists to consider when selecting a treatment intervention with electrotherapeutic agents.

Coronary Artery Disease. In coronary artery disease, blood vessels can become clogged, producing signs and symptoms of angina pectoris or myocardial infarction. In either case, blood flow is diverted away from the periphery of the body, impeding circulation to the tissues, which reduces the oxygen and nutrients available to them.

Congestive Heart Failure. CHF is the heart's inability to pump enough blood for body functioning. In this disease, the right or left side of the heart can fail, but ultimately both sides are generally involved, and symptoms of both right-sided and left-sided failure relate to fluid overload. Pharmacologic therapy is commonly prescribed for fluid balance and to decrease the burden on the heart, thus improving the heart's pumping action. In evaluation of the patient with

CHF and concomitant lower extremity ulcers and edema, it is essential to differentiate the edema associated with CHF from that associated with venous disease. Treatment for edema in patients with both CHF and venous disease can differ from treatment of patients with edema related only to venous disease.

Gastrointestinal System

The GI system (including the esophagus, stomach, small intestine, and large intestine) is responsible for digestion and absorption of nutrients and fluids. Specific disorders of concern for patients with wounds include GI bleeding and problems with digestion and absorption of nutrients. GI bleeding weakens the patient and decreases blood supply. Any disease causing GI malfunction leads to poor absorption of nutrients and fluids. Patients with gastrostomy tubes receive enteral nutrition directly into the stomach, bypassing the mouth. These tube feedings may be accompanied by loose stools, which can irritate skin and seep into wounds in the pelvic area, resulting in wound contamination. A dietary consultation is helpful in the optimal management of patients with GI tube feedings or malnutrition related to GI pathology.

CLINICAL WISDOM

Diarrhea with GI Tube Feedings

Diarrhea associated with tube feedings warrants investigation. Sometimes, slowing the rate of the feeding infusion, diluting the formula, or using a formula containing fiber can decrease or eliminate the diarrhea. Wound therapy for patients with diarrhea from tube feedings includes attention to dressings that protect the wound area from fecal contamination.

Nutrition and Hydration. Nutritional screening is an important component of patient assessment because of the relationships among malnutrition, pressure ulcer development, and impaired wound healing. Nutritional data can be found in the medical record as a single assessment or as pieces of information that the clinician must pull together. A sample nutritional assessment guide and diagram can be found in Chapter 3. If no standardized nutrition assessment form exists within an agency or setting, the clinician should evaluate the following factors: current weight, prior weight, weight change, and percentage of change in weight, height, and body mass index. Body weight is a commonly used indicator of nutrition. An involuntary increase or decrease in weight of 5% is predictive of a drop in serum albumin, a measure of protein available for healing (normal level is greater than 3.5 mg/dL).[2] Other laboratory tests to evaluate include prealbumin levels and total lymphocyte count.

Hydration status can be determined by interpreting intake and output sheets. This data is often kept in the patient's room and may be documented by nurses or nurse assistants, depending on the health-care setting. Signs of dehydration include thirst, tongue dryness in non-mouth breathers, and decreased skin turgor. Dehydration affects wound healing by reducing the blood volume available to transport oxygen and nutrients to healing tissues. The state of hydration affects weight and albumin levels.

■ CASE STUDY

Malnutrition and Wound Management in End-Stage Illness

A malnourished patient with a pressure ulcer on the coccyx is in the end stage of life. The patient and family refuse tube feedings and understand the consequences of the minimally nourished and dehydrated condition. In this case, palliative and preventive treatment is indicated. The wound can be kept clean, dressed to control drainage and odor, and managed for pain. The patient is also a candidate for a pressure-relief mattress replacement or specialty bed for prevention of additional skin breakdown. A turning schedule and caregiver training are also part of the prevention intervention strategy.

Genitourinary System

The genitourinary system is divided into the upper tract (kidneys and ureters) and lower tract (bladder, sphincters, and urethra). Patients with kidney failure may require treatment involving some form of dialysis and a special diet that can impair wound healing. Patients with kidney failure often have multiple system failure; evaluation for other diseases, such as diabetes and hypertension, is warranted because they often coincide with kidney dysfunction.

Urinary Incontinence. Bladder dysfunction, outlet problems, and sphincter dysfunction can cause urinary incontinence. The implications for skin damage include maceration from moisture on the skin, softening and separating of the epidermal layers, and irritation related to increased friction and shearing. Wound contamination is also a risk for patients with sacrococcygeal wounds and concomitant incontinence.

Peripheral Vascular System

The peripheral vascular system includes the venous, arterial, and lymphatic circulatory systems. Chapter 17 describes the pathogenesis and differential diagnosis of peripheral vascular disease (PVD). Clinicians should pay close attention to all medical record notations and comments from the patient and family about vascular disorders, including history of hypertension, deep vein thrombosis, claudication, cold feet, and chronic swelling of the lower extremities. Patients with PVD are at high risk for developing chronic wounds and resultant impaired wound healing. The diagnosis of PVD guides the clinician's examination strategy for observational and noninvasive vascular testing (see Chapter 7, Vascular Evaluation).

Neurologic and Musculoskeletal Systems

An imbalance or insufficient movement of body segments, limbs, or the whole body, due to impairment or disability of the neurologic or musculoskeletal systems, are known factors for predicting certain wound development, such as pressure

---

CASE STUDY

Cognitively Impaired Patient with Leg Ulcers

A patient who was cognitively impaired with a history of venous disease and recurrent leg ulceration demonstrates how a change in nutritional status affected her recurrent ulcers. Emma was an elderly patient with a diagnosis of Alzheimer's disease who was confined for her safety to a secure medical unit within a long-term care facility. She was nicknamed "Mrs. Houdini" because she could free herself from any restraint, including climbing the bedrails. Emma walked all day long with negative consequences to her venous disease. Compression stockings were not an option, because she would not tolerate them. Emma was hyperactive and a very poor eater.

The nursing director decided to investigate her nutritional status. She reviewed Emma's weight status and found progressive weight loss over the previous 3–4 months. Consultation with her physician led to further evaluation, revealing a low albumin level of 2.5 mg/dL. Evaluation by a speech pathologist demonstrated a delayed swallowing response and resulted in a recommendation for videofluoroscopic examination.

The nutritional assessment and resultant recommendation for gastrostomy tube placement was shared with the family. Emma tolerated the procedure well. A benefit of the gastrostomy tube placement for Emma was that it was covered by her clothing (out of sight and out of mind), so she left it alone.

In a few weeks, the nutrition added to her diet made Emma much less irritable and hyperactive. She could be placed in a gerichair with a restraint tray, and her legs were elevated part of the day. She walked with assistance a few times a day. She was transferred from the secure unit to the long-term care custodial area of the facility and had more social interaction. She gained weight and had no further episodes of venous dermatitis or ulceration during the next year.

---

ulcers and neuropathic ulcers. Neurologic disorders and dysfunctions of the musculoskeletal system include a broad range of medical diagnoses, such as spinal cord injury, cerebrovascular accident, Parkinson's disease, arthritis, and multiple sclerosis. Chapters 16, 17, and 19 include information about the impact of movement disability on pathogenesis of pressure ulcers, pressure ulcer prevention, therapeutic positioning, and problems of the neuropathic foot. The neurologic or musculoskeletal deficit guides examination strategies for the clinician. For example, a nurse caring for a patient with limited body movements and neurologic deficits will perform a pressure ulcer risk assessment to evaluate risk factors for pressure ulcer development, which may trigger referrals for therapeutic positioning evaluation by a physical therapist, as well as a nutritional consultation. In another example, patients who have had a cerebrovascular accident or stroke can have decreased activity and mobility, increasing their risk for pressure ulcer development and reducing the healing capacity of current wounds.

Cerebrovascular Accident. Cerebrovascular accidents, or strokes, are caused by disruption in blood flow to the brain. They usually affect one hemisphere of the brain, causing deficits on the contralateral side of the body. Stroke can result in impaired ability to walk, impaired ability to use an upper limb, and inability to communicate, think, or see adequately. A patient's limited ability to move body parts places him or her at risk for developing pressure ulcers, skin tears, and friction and shearing injury.

Arthritis. Arthritic disorders affect the joints of the body. The two main types of arthritis are rheumatoid arthritis and osteoarthritis. Rheumatoid arthritis affects the joints of the hands and fingers, making self-care of wounds difficult or impossible. Osteoarthritis affects older adults and is associated with painful joints, particularly knees, ankles, and hips (i.e., weightbearing joints). Evaluation of a wound patient with arthritis can be more difficult because of pain on positioning for adequate view of the wound. Treatment of arthritis commonly includes nonsteroidal antiinflammatory drugs and steroids, both of which can impair or slow wound healing.

Hematologic System

Disease processes such as anemia, fluid and electrolyte imbalance, and other blood dyscrasia associated with medication side effects or disease pathology affect wound healing capacity. Evaluation of laboratory values to rule out anemia, electrolyte imbalance, and infections is the key to hematologic system assessment.

Endocrine System

The endocrine system includes numerous glands that secrete body-regulating hormones. One such gland is the pancreas, which controls insulin levels in the body. Diabetes mellitus is the disease of most concern in the endocrine system, because it impairs wound healing and poses significant risk for wound development. Glucose levels alter wound healing and immune system functioning to control infection. Check for a diagnosis of diabetes mellitus. Is it type I insulin-dependent or type II non–insulin-dependent? The type of diabetes dictates whether the patient will use insulin or diet and exercise to control glucose. Patients with type I diabetes require insulin for glucose management, whereas those with type II diabetes control glucose initially with diet and exercise; if unsuccessful, oral hypoglycemic agents or insulin are used.

A normal glucose level is 80 mg/dL; levels of 180–250 mg/dL or greater indicate that glucose levels are out of control. Glucose levels greater than 200 mg/dL are known to have an impact on wound healing.[3] Review of laboratory values is prudent to determine the level of glucose control. Look specifically for a fasting blood glucose level <140 mg/dL and a glycosylated hemoglobin (HbA_{1c}) of less than 7%. The HbA_{1c} helps to determine the level of glucose control the patient has maintained over the past 2–3 months.

Complications from diabetes generally correlate with the length of time the patient has had the disease. Patients with the relatively recent onset of diabetes may not exhibit neuropathic or vascular complications. Patients who have had diabetes for longer periods of time and those with type I diabetes are at higher risk for complications associated with the disease, such as neuropathy, retinopathy, and vascular changes. The diabetic patient with a wound should trigger examination of sensation in the feet and vision testing. Patients with diabetic neuropathy can present with ulcers on the soles of their feet, and care should be taken to examine the plantar surfaces for callus formation, cracking, and bony deformities. Additional information on management of patients with vascular and neuropathic disabilities related to diabetes is discussed in Chapters 18 and 19.

Although this review of systems with physical assessment guidelines is not inclusive, it provides a framework for assessment of those areas of most concern to clinicians who manage patients with wounds. A complete history and physical examination provides the context for the wound itself; after completing this, the clinician can begin to plan interventions. If the information gleaned from the history and physical assessment is very limited, the clinician will need to make a clinical decision about the appropriateness of the referral based on the reason for referral, expected outcomes, and personal observations of the patient. Clinicians can complete the general history, systems review, and physical assessment in about 30–40 minutes for a single wound. An experienced clinician can perform a basic physical assessment in 10–15 minutes. Typically, not all information is gathered at one time; portions of the history and physical assessment can be gathered over a period of several days after multiple clinic or home visits.

Wound Assessment

Wound assessment involves evaluation of a composite of wound characteristics, including location, shape, size, depth, edges, undermining and tunneling, necrotic tissue characteristics, exudate characteristics, surrounding skin color, peripheral tissue edema and induration, and the presence of granulation tissue and epithelialization (also see Chapter 4 on wound assessment, Chapter 5 on wound measurement, and Chapter 6 on tools).

Wound History

Following are key questions to elicit information about the history of the wound: "How long has the wound been present?" "Is there a history of previous wounds?" "What interventions have been used, and have they been successful?" "What types of health-care providers have been involved in the management of the wound?" If the patient has been seen by providers from several disciplines and has undergone multiple interventions without successful progress toward healing, the patient's candidacy for more aggressive

intervention is questionable. The patient's previous therapy and response to therapy must be carefully examined to avoid repeating unsuccessful interventions. Granted, some patients do not heal. However, evaluation of past interventions with attention to appropriateness of topical wound care, prevention strategies, risk factor and comorbidity management, and use of adjunct therapy, such as a whirlpool or electrical stimulation, can reveal inconsistencies in treatment approach.

Patient Candidacy for Physical Therapy Services

During the assessment process, the clinician focuses on how the medical history and systems review affect the candidacy of the patient. Physical therapists may determine the candidacy of the patient for services. This is not an option in nursing; the nurse typically has no role in determining whether to provide nursing services to the patient. However, the nurse may assist in determination of appropriate therapy for patients when other disciplines are involved.

Sometimes the medical history and systems review findings suggest to the clinician that the patient's problem requires consultation, i.e., that it is outside the scope of the clinician's knowledge, experience, or expertise. In other cases, the intervention originally suggested is deemed inappropriate. In physical therapy, the patient is then identified as a noncandidate for the referred service. It then becomes the responsibility of the clinician to refer the patient to another practitioner who is skilled and knowledgeable in a different area, or better equipped to manage the identified problem or recommend an alternative treatment and management strategy. Following are examples of criteria that would trigger a referral:

- Vascular testing should be considered if hair loss, skin pallor or cyanosis, or cold temperature of the feet are found on assessment.
- Callus and hemorrhagic spots on the callus indicate deeper tissue damage and warrant further assessment for high pressure.
- Toenail abnormalities should be referred if this is not an area of expertise for the examiner.
- An abscess in a tunnel or sinus tract requires immediate referral for surgical management.
- Undermining or tunneling (i.e., a black hole without a bottom) should be immediately referred for surgical management.
- Signs of granulation tissue infection (e.g., superficial bridging, friable tissue, bleeding on contact, pain in the wound, and regression of healing) require medical intervention.

Step 2: Diagnosis

Examination Strategy

At this point in the examination, the risk factors for impaired healing are identified, based on data collected during the history and systems review. Because the specific information about a patient determines the examination strategy, not all patients will receive the same examination. There are two parts to the examination: Part 1 includes testing for factors related to the patient's comorbidities, and Part 2 looks at key features of the wound assessment.

Examination: Part 1

The first part of the examination involves testing for factors related to the physiologic or anatomic status of the comorbidities that impair healing, such as vascular or sensory impairment. These tests carry significant weight in the prediction of healing and development of the prognosis. For example, a low ankle-brachial index score indicates severe occlusive disease and is a predictor of failure to heal without reperfusion. Loss of protective sensation in the feet indicates a high risk for ulceration from pressure or trauma and leads to an intervention strategy.

A patient with a low ankle-brachial index would not be considered a candidate for physical therapy services or aggressive wound healing interventions because of the severity of vascular system impairment. In this case, a nurse would manage the patient's wound and refer the patient to a vascular surgeon. A patient with an insensitive foot due to neuropathy would be a candidate for physical therapy because this condition would constitute a medical necessity, requiring the skills of a physical therapist. The physical therapist would predict a functional outcome of risk reduction following interventions of pressure elimination and stimulation, leading to healing.

In both cases, the ulcerations are related to underlying medical pathology. In the former case, the ulcer would not be expected to respond unless the underlying pathology were addressed. In the latter case, ulcer management would be appropriate, along with risk reduction management. The interpretation of the data from the history and physical examination sets the stage for functional diagnosis and allows for triage of cases that should be referred or managed conservatively.

Examination: Part 2

This part of the examination strategy looks at four key features of the wound assessment: evaluation of the surrounding skin, assessment of the wound tissue, observation of wound drainage, and size measurements.

The sequence of the examination depends on visual observation and palpation of the impaired tissues. The examiner chooses tests and measures that are specific to the wound situation. For example, temperature testing may be the best way to distinguish the presence of inflammatory processes in pressure ulcers in patients with darkly pigmented skin. A wound tracing may be the best method to measure the irregular shape of a venous ulcer.

After completing the examination portion of the diagnostic process, the clinician interprets the physiologic and anatomic systems information and wound assessment data, bringing all of the information together like the pieces of a puzzle to develop a functional diagnosis.[4]

Evaluation and Diagnosis

The evaluation aspect of the diagnostic process includes evaluation and analysis of findings collected previously, which leads to clinical judgments. "Diagnosis" refers to the process itself, as well as the conclusion reached after the evaluation data have been organized.[5] Physical therapists are expected to use the diagnostic process to establish diagnoses for the specific conditions requiring attention. If the findings of the diagnostic process are such that management of the patient is beyond the physical therapist's knowledge, experience, or expertise, the therapist refers the patient to an appropriate practitioner.[5] Nurses may reach the diagnostic conclusion that a referral to another practitioner is needed, but they typically cannot relinquish responsibility while waiting for a referral and must provide a plan of care for the patient in the interim.

The purpose of data analysis is to draw conclusions about a patient's specific problems and needs so that effective interventions can be implemented. Problem identification is a process of diagnostic reasoning in which judgments, decisions, and conclusions are made about the data collected to determine whether intervention is needed.[6] Diagnosis involves forming a clinical judgment by identifying a disease/condition or human response through the scientific evaluation of signs and symptoms, history, and diagnostic studies. In many respects, a diagnosis is analogous to a research hypothesis: A research hypothesis directs the research study, and a diagnosis directs the patient's care plan. Both a research hypothesis and diagnosis are chosen based on available data and information, and both can be proven correct or incorrect as the study or care plan progresses.

Physical therapy diagnosis is defined as "a label encompassing a cluster of signs, symptoms, syndromes, or categories."[5] The purpose of a diagnosis is to guide the clinician in determining the most appropriate intervention strategy for the individual. When the diagnostic process does not provide adequate information, intervention may be based on alleviation of symptoms and remediation of deficits.

Nursing diagnoses identify specific human responses to existing or potential health problems. These problems may be physical, sociologic, or psychologic. Both nurses and physical therapists base diagnoses on the symptoms or the sequelae of the injurious process, such as impaired wound healing. Physical therapists evaluate the functional implications of impairments and disabilities, leading to a functional diagnosis. Impairment is defined as loss or abnormality of psychologic, physiologic, or anatomic structure or function.[7] Impairment describes the loss of function of a body system or organ due to illness or injury.[8] An example is the loss of function of skin and underlying soft tissue due to wounding or underlying pathology. Additional impairment characteristics include the effect of pathology/disease without attributing cause or the loss of a body part, such as by amputation. Underlying pathology creates the susceptibility to loss of function, for example, "undue susceptibility to pressure ulcers" and "undue insensitivity to pain."[8]

The definition of disability is any restriction or lack of ability (resulting from an impairment) to perform an activity in the manner or within the range considered normal for a human being. Disability can result from impairment or the person's response to the impairment. It can be permanent, reversible, or irreversible. Disability reflects a deviation in performance or behavior within a task or activity.[8] Examples are an individual who has musculoskeletal disablement that leads to difficulty walking or moving, and an individual with integumentary disablement related to the inability of the body to progress from the inflammatory phase of healing to the proliferative phase.

Functional Diagnosis

Functional diagnosis is an assessment of the related impairments and associated disabilities that affect wound status and its ability to heal. Examples of functional diagnosis include the following:

- Impaired sensation (inability to detect pressure or light touch)
- Impaired circulation (ankle-brachial index below 0.8) of lower extremities
- Impaired lower extremity strength and joint range of motion (including manual muscle testing and range of motion), resulting in persistent pressure to buttocks
- Impaired healing associated with chronic inflammation phase

Physical therapists use functional diagnosis to describe the consequences of disease and to justify the medical necessity of management by a physical therapist. With respect to wounds, the wound healing phase can be used as a functional diagnosis to describe the status of wound healing (see wound healing phases described in Chapter 2).

Each phase of healing can be impaired. Impaired wound healing can be described as prolonged, chronic, or failure to occur (i.e., absent). For example, a wound with prolonged or chronic inflammation indicates impaired functioning of the body system(s) needed to progress to the next phase of repair. The particular phase of wound healing that is dysfunctional helps to determine the interventions needed to restart the repair process.[9]

The impairments in wound healing can be labeled with a diagnosis (see Exhibit 1-1). The *wound healing phase diagnosis* is a diagnosis of impaired status regarding the biologic phase of wound healing.

The biologic phase of repair is observed by examination of the wound. Wounds become chronic and lack the function necessary to progress to the next phase of repair. This can occur in any of the healing phases. For example, when wound edges curl in and become fibrotic, this demonstrates absence of epithelialization due to impairment in the epithelialization process. Wounds can become "stuck" in the proliferative phase when infection is present and impairs the proliferative process, thus demonstrating chronic proliferation. Wounds can become chronically inflamed when tissue trauma is prolonged. The wound healing phase diagnosis describes the current status of the wound and can predict how the wound healing should progress. This is logical because wound healing is an orderly series of events; a wound in one phase should progress to and through each successive phase (see Chapter 2 for information about the biologic cascade of healing).

EXHIBIT 1-1   12 Possible Wound Healing Phase Diagnoses

1. Acute Inflammation
2. Chronic inflammation
3. Absence of inflammation
4. Proliferation
5. Chronic proliferation
6. Absence of proliferation
7. Epithelialization
8. Chronic epithelialization
9. Absence of epithelialization
10. Remodeling
11. Chronic remodeling
12. Absence of remodelling

Identifying the wound healing phase diagnosis of a wound in transition from one phase to another is challenging, because the transition is usually gradual, and phases overlap. In such cases, describe the change by using a ratio of the *dominant phase* to the *recessive phase*. *Dominant* refers to the most active phase observed, and *recessive* refers to the less active phase. A ratio is simply the relationship between two variables—in this case, the relationship between two phases of healing. An example of using a ratio to describe a wound with the dominant phase of active inflammation and the recessive phase of active proliferation is: "The wound healing phase diagnosis is INFLAMMATION/proliferation." The use of upper-case letters for the dominant phase emphasizes its dominance, whereas lower-case letters show the relationship of the recessive phase. If the two phases are equal, they can both be written in upper case (e.g., INFLAMMATION/PROLIFERATION). The prognosis in this example is that the wound healing phase will progress from inflammation to proliferation.

Step 3: Prognosis and Goals

Once the diagnosis is established, the clinician predicts, or prognoses, the expected outcome and selects an intervention. Prediction is a useful tool for goal setting. Prediction of the maximal improvement expected from an intervention and how long it will take is the *prognosis*. Prognosis may include prediction of *improvement* at different intervals during treatment.[5]

Some clinicians are intimidated by the idea of predicting outcomes, however, they are in the best position to do so if they are knowledgeable about the effects of the interventions prescribed and administered. Patients would not expose themselves to interventions with unpredictable results, and payers would not reimburse providers for services with unexpected benefits and indefinite costs. Successful clinicians are able to predict the patient outcomes. In the current health-care environment, a sound understanding of prognosis and outcomes is important for all health care professionals.

Wound Prognosis Options

The prognosis options are limited for wounds. One system for evaluating secondary intention wound healing defines healing as *minimally, acceptably,* or *ideally* healed. An ideally healed wound results in return of the fully restored dermis and epidermis with intact barrier function. An acceptably healed wound has a resurfaced epithelium capable of sustained functional integrity during activities of daily living. A minimally healed wound is characterized by reepithelialization but does not establish a sustained functional result and may recur. In all of these definitions, complete closure of the wound is expected.[10]

For some individuals and some wounds, closure is not an option. Rather, the best prognosis is a change in the wound healing phase from an impaired or early phase of repair to a more advanced phase of repair. For example, a wound that is chronically inflamed is impaired from progressing to more advanced phases of healing, and the predicted outcome is that the chronic inflammation will progress to acute inflammation. The prognosis for an acutely inflamed wound is progression to a proliferative phase. Some wounds progress to the proliferative phase, and it is not expected—nor is it preferred—for the wound to close by secondary intention; the prognosis is a clean and stable wound or a wound prepared for surgical closure. A change in phase is a functional outcome prediction. This method monitors a real change in the organ function of the skin and soft tissues, which is a measure of reduced functional impairment.

The prognosis that a wound is not expected to improve based on the results of the diagnostic process can determine referral for other management. Nurses may be expected to care for the wound, but the patient may not be a candidate for physical therapy intervention. Prognosis is not an option for physical therapists—it is a requirement and part of utilization management of medical services. Medicare mandates that a functional outcome prediction be established by the physical therapist at the start of care.

Goals

Nursing Goals

Nurses must set priorities, establish goals, and identify desired outcomes for patients. Goals are important because they assist in determining outcomes of care and measuring the effectiveness of interventions. Goals must be measurable, objective, and based on the prioritized needs of the patient.

Short-term goals are typically actions that must be taken before a patient is discharged or moved to another level of care. Long-term goals may require continued attention by a patient and/or caregiver long after discharge. Short-term goals should move a patient toward the long-term goal.

Physical Therapy Goals

Physical therapists are also required to establish short-term and long-term goals. These goals should be measurable, objective, functional, and very specific. Traditionally, a short-term goal was one that would be achieved in 30 days or less and usually corresponded to the end of the billing period or length of stay. Long-term goals were those predicted to be met by the time of discharge. With the shift to

short lengths of stay in health-care settings, the time frames have changed to correspond to the settings. Currently, there is a terminology shift away from using the term *goal* and replacing it with *expected outcome*. A goal is the desired or expected result of an intervention, and an outcome is the result or status after the intervention.

Completing the diagnostic process with recommendations is one outcome of physical therapy services. Physical therapists target specific, measurable outcomes for specific interventions. To make them functional outcomes, they must meet the criteria described below. Target outcomes are short-term, specific expectations of a change in impairment status. *Prognosis* is the expected outcome after a course of care and represents the long-term goal.

Examples of wound healing prognoses include the following:

1. Ideally healed closure
2. Acceptably healed closure
3. Minimally healed closure
4. Clean and stable open wound
5. Wound ready for surgical closure
6. Not expected to improve

Evaluation of Progress and Outcomes

An *outcome* is the result of what is done and is patient-focused or wound-focused. The intervention or activity done to achieve the result is the *process*. How are outcomes measured? Performance indicators are objective measurements used to monitor change resulting from an intervention. Providers, payers, regulators, and clinicians all work toward establishing reliable performance indicators to report clinical outcomes. Exhibit 1-2 lists examples of wound-related performance indicators, with outcomes and functional outcomes for each. Patient outcomes provide nurses and physical therapists with a means of assessing how interventions alter problems. Two types of outcomes are behavioral and functional. Payer groups have an interest in both the behavioral and functional outcomes.[11]

Reporting Outcomes

The reporting of outcomes is frequently confused with process. There has been much discussion about outcomes, when what is being reported is mainly process. This section discusses some commonly misused terms and the appropriate way to report an outcome.

Prevention, or the process to reduce or buffer risk, is often the target of an intervention. Risk factors usually exist prior to or at the onset of a problem (e.g., immobility, deformities, and smoking). Buffers are attempts to reduce or intervene to alter the progression of an impairment, disability, or handicap (e.g., take pressure off a diabetic ulcer).[7] Many reliable performance indicators that measure risk and intervention-related changes are used by both nurses and physical therapists. As part of the initial assessment, apply instruments with performance indicators to test the current status, and then retest status after applying the chosen

EXHIBIT 1-2 Examples of Performance Indicators with Wound Outcomes and Functional Wound Outcomes

Performance Indicators	Wound Outcomes	Functional Wound Outcomes
1. Change in wound and surrounding skin attributes 2. Reduced severity of wound in depth or size 3. Change in wound exudate characteristics or undermining 4. Closure	Progression through the phases of wound healing (inflammation, proliferation, and epithelialization)	1. Clean, stable wound ready for surgical closure 2. Dressing changes needed biweekly instead of daily 3. Exudate managed; patient returns to work 4. Return to work/leisure activities
1. Temperature comparison 2. Transcutaneous partial pressure of oxygen level 3. Laser Doppler	Oxygenation or perfusion of tissue	1. Progress to next wound healing phase 2. Pain level no longer interferes with ADL
1. Girth measurements 2. Volume meter measurements 3. Palpation grading system	Edema reduced or controlled	1. Patient able to don compression hose 2. Leg ulcers are smaller, require less frequent dressing changes
1. Wound exudate characteristics 2. Wound and surrounding skin attributes 3. Culture	Infection controlled	1. Wound exudate odor controlled, able to return to community 2. Pain alleviated, patient resumes walking
1. Free of necrosis 2. Proliferation phase tissue attributes 3. Change in depth or size	Clean, stable wound	1. Frequency of visits reduced 2. Physical therapy intervention no longer required 3. Patient can now manage wound dressing changes
1. Braden Scale score 2. Functional activities performance 3. Comprehension testing	Reduced risk of pressure ulceration	1. Repositions self in bed 2. Patient performs self-care activities while in wheelchair 3. Patient demonstrates use of hand mirror to monitor skin
1. Wound closure 2. Functional activities performed related to use of scar tissue	Acceptably healed scar	1. Patient identifies risk factors for reulceration 2. Patient uses protective equipment correctly under scar tissue to perform functional activities in wheelchair

intervention to measure achievement of the predicted outcome. For example, instead of stating the prognosis as "prevention of pressure ulcers" or "minimized risk of pressure ulcers," it is more appropriate to state, "Risk of pressure ulcers will be reduced from high to moderate, based on the Braden Scale." The Braden Scale (see Chapter 16) is used to measure risk for development of pressure ulcers. Mobility is one element of the Braden Scale. If a patient on admission has a low mobility score on the Braden Scale, indicating complete immobility, he or she is considered at high risk for development of a pressure ulcer. After the patient receives an intervention for mobility training, the mobility score improves, and he or she is slightly limited in mobility and makes frequent changes in body position. In this example, there has been a functional change in the mobility of the

patient. The functional outcome is improved mobility status, which leads to reduced risk of pressure ulceration.

Reduced risk of infection is a topic of confusion, and clinicians must understand that it is not an outcome. Freedom from infection or reduction in exudate, odor, or culture results are measurable outcomes. For any of these outcomes to be functional outcomes, they must change the way the body system functions. Freedom from infection can be an outcome of wound cleansing, but it becomes a functional outcome when wound healing progresses to the next phase of repair. The functional outcome would be correctly written as, "The wound is infection-free, and the wound healing has progressed from the inflammatory phase to the proliferative phase."

A troublesome word in health care is *maintained*, which implies no change. *Controlled* should not be mistaken for *maintained.* For example, if edema has fluctuated from treatment to treatment, and then stabilizes as a result of intervention, the outcome is that edema is controlled. A functional outcome for controlled edema would be stated as, "The edema in the tissues surrounding the wound is controlled, and the wound is epithelializing." The functional outcome of control of the edema is that the wound progresses to the next phase of healing.

Maximized and *minimized* are similarly confused with outcomes. For example, "maximized participation in activities of daily living" does not reflect the functional outcome of an intervention with an orthotic device. A functional outcome reports the result of the intervention, such as, "The patient performs activities of daily living wearing/using orthotic equipment, and has returned to work and/or resumed leisure activities." An example of misuse of *minimized* as an outcome is "minimized stresses precipitating or perpetuating injury." Correct use is, "Functional outcome—patient/caregiver identified stress-reduction methods to minimize risk of injury."

Improved is defined as "to make better or enhance in value." This is a subjective measure, not a measurable outcome. An outcome reports the objective result of improvement. For example, increased vital capacity measured in liters (performance indicator) is a measurable change in the pulmonary system, with a result of increased oxygenation of tissues for wound healing. The functional outcome is "wound progresses to next phase of healing."

Provided is sometimes confused with an outcome, although it is an action by the clinician, not an outcome of the intervention. An example of improper use is "provided electrical stimulation to enhance circulation." This describes the rationale for the intervention, not the outcome.

Promoted is another inappropriately used term. For example, "promoted angiogenesis" is a process. Angiogenesis is an expected outcome of treatment and represents an attribute of wound healing. The performance indicators of angiogenesis are change in wound attributes, phase, or size. The outcome is wound progression through the proliferative phase.

Behavioral Outcomes. Behavioral outcomes include behaviors that can be observed or monitored to determine whether an acceptable or positive outcome is achieved within the desired time frame. Outcomes must be specific, realistic, time-oriented, objective, patient-centered, and measurable. Once established, outcomes serve as an evaluation tool.

Use measurable action verbs to describe behavioral outcomes. For example, the verb *understand* is not measurable; we cannot measure a person's understanding. The same is true for the verbs *feel, learn, know,* and *accept,* But *identify* is measurable; the patient can be tested to determine whether he or she can identify. Other appropriate action verbs include *list, record, name, state, describe, explain, demonstrate, use, schedule, differentiate, compare, relate, design, prepare, formulate, select, choose, increase, decrease, stand, walk,* and *participate.*

Examples of behavioral outcomes for a patient with a wound include: "The patient will describe the signs of wound infection and identify correct action within 24 hours" and, "The patient will demonstrate wound dressing application within 2 days." Correct documentation that the target outcome was met would include: "Patient is able to describe the signs of infection and list the steps for corrective action. Patient is able to demonstrate correct wound dressing application."

Functional Outcomes. A functional outcome helps to communicate a change in function to the patient, caregiver, and payer. Physical therapists usually work with patients who have experienced loss of functional abilities, and they use functional tests that measure physical attributes to predict the function that the patient is expected to achieve after a course of treatment. *Function* in this context refers to activities and actions that are meaningful to the patient or caregiver. Meaningful function is determined while completing the reason for referral portion of the assessment.

To constitute a functional outcome, the results must meet three criteria:[12]

1. The result is meaningful
2. The result is practical
3. The result can be sustained over time outside the treatment setting

Meaningful is defined as being of value to the patient, caregiver, or both. *Practical* means that the outcome is applicable to the patient's life situation. *Sustainable over time* refers to functional abilities achieved through an intervention that are maintained by the patient or caregiver outside the clinical setting (e.g., a patient demonstrates the ability to apply a dressing and stocking during two follow-up visits).[13]

Standardized tests and measurement tools are useful to monitor and track change over time. The Bates-Jensen Wound Assessment Toll (BWAT) formerly Pressure Sore Status Tool (PSST), and Sussman Wound Healing Tool (SWHT), described in Chapter 6, can be used to document the outcomes of changes in wound attributes by changes in test scores, and can then be applied to function. For example, using the BWAT to monitor exudate amounts, a change in score on that test item from 4 (moderate exudate) to 2 (scant exudate) would indicate reduced drainage. This outcome is measurable and objective, and meets the criteria for a valid outcome. However, this information alone does not constitute a functional outcome. To interpret this score as a functional outcome, a statement must connect the findings with meaning to the patient, practical effect, and sustainable result. A correct statement of functional outcomes is, "Wound exudates BWAT (formerly PSST score) has reduced from 4 (moderate) to 2 (scant) exudate, patient demonstrates ability to monitor for signs of infection and action to take, and patient is now able to return to work and will be seen for intermittent follow-up."

Functional outcomes should be documented throughout the course of care, not just at discharge. Factors that can be used to demonstrate intermittent functional change include change in patient lifestyle, change in patient safety, and adaptation to impairment or disability. These statements

EXHIBIT 1-3   Example of Functional Outcomes Documented Throughout Course of Care

- *Initial statement:* Patient is unable to sit in wheelchair without trauma to integument.
- *Initial target outcome:* Patient is sitting for 2 hours in adaptive seating system in 2 weeks.
- *Interim outcome after 1 week:* Patient sits for 1 hour in adaptive seating system.
- *Discharge statement:* Patient sits in adaptive seating system for 2 hours without disruption of integumentary integrity.

EXHIBIT 1-4   How To Write Outcome Statements and Functional Outcomes

When reporting outcomes, use the following guidelines:
1. An outcome expresses the *result* of an intervention—not the intervention or the process—to reach an outcome (e.g., wound resurfacing/closure).
2. A behavioral outcome can be learned information (e.g., demonstrates application of wound dressing). This outcome would follow an intervention of instruction.
3. Other coordination of treatment, interdisiplinary, communication, and documentation if care resyktsare outcomes used to ensure proper utilization management include.

Functional outcomes are written to describe results of treatment on function and include three parts:
1. Description of a meaningful functional change to a body system (e.g., progression through the phases of healing)
2. Description of a practical result of a change in a body system (e.g., wound is minimally exudative)
3. Description of the sustainable result or change in the impairment status or disability resulting from the intervention (e.g., pressure elimination allows the patient to sit up in wheelchair 2 hours twice a day)

should be patient-centered and measurable (Exhibit 1-3).

Change in wound tissue attributes and size can also be used as functional outcome, such as "Free of necrosis, reduced risk of infection, and size reduced 50%, wound is clean and stable, decreased frequency of visits required" (Exhibit 1-4).

The Functional Outcome Report

This chapter has described three of the four steps of the diagnostic process. The functional outcome report (FOR) developed by Swanson (described below) describes the diagnostic process.[4] Swanson's FOR helps the therapist document clinical reasoning that is clear, logical, and understandable. As previously explained, payers need information about functional outcomes, not wound measurements and tissue color. The FOR process helps to communicate treatment strategies to justify the intervention and lead to a predictable functional outcome.[13] Appendix 1-C is a completed example of the report. Additional examples of the FOR can be found in Chapter 16 and the case studies in Part IV.

The FOR document contains six parts. Part I, Patient History and Medical History, begins with the *reason for referral*. Here, the clinician establishes patient needs. The report will read in one of the following manners:

- Patient/family seek services for …
- The patient/family reports …
- The following medical problems are associated with this request for service …

It is not unusual for there to be residual impairments and disabilities following a course of therapy in conjunction with a meaningful functional outcome that is important to the patient (e.g., a clean, edema-free wound). This may be the most important goal and the reason for the referral because it is meaningful to the patient.

Part II, Systems Review, is an analysis of *functional limitations*. Function refers to many different activities and actions. With respect to wounds, it includes identification and analysis of the functional limits of the local tissues to perform the activities necessary to initiate repair. Function also implies that the body systems are able to perform the

repair. For example, assessment of the current status of the tissue identifies tissue activity (e.g., inflammation phase) and the circulatory system response to injury (e.g., erythema, edema, pain, and heat). Impaired circulatory system function will impair the healing process.

Clinicians complete this portion of the report with the following leads:

- The specific functional items that are causing the patient's need for service are… (e.g., impaired healing response)
- Patient's functional loss of healing is due to… (e.g., impairment of the circulatory system)
- The loss of function causes the following… (e.g., inability to progress through the phases of repair without intervention)
- Patient has improvement potential… (e.g., patient has improvement potential, but remains at risk for ischemic ulceration)

In Part III, Evaluation, *clinical assessment or diagnosis* is the clinical impression, based on the results of clinician-selected tests and measures that have performance indicators for wounds. This is different from the medical diagnosis because it focuses on the functional consequence of the disease, rather than the etiology (see the section on functional diagnosis above).

Part IV, Functional Diagnosis, is the justification of *need for skilled service for the therapy problem*. Utilization management requires identification of the specific elements that will change as a result of the intervention and, once changed, will improve the patient's functional status. An example of a wound problem that can be expected to change as a result of an intervention is a change in the phase of wound healing as a result of an intervention (e.g., whirlpool). Change can also be expected in the wound symptoms (e.g., free of erythema or pain), which will demonstrate improved functional status of the tissues.

In Part V, Prognosis, *prediction of a functional outcome* is expected because clinicians are responsible for knowing the effects of the selected treatment interventions. The functional outcome section of the report has three components: the activity that would occur, the performance expected, and the due date. With respect to wounds, the "activity" may be erythema-free, the "performance" a change to the proliferative phase, and the "due date" 2–4 weeks. This segment of the report promotes continuity of care when multiple clinicians are involved.

Part VI, the final step in the FOR, is to present the *treatment plan with rationale*. Subsequent chapters will provide the rationale for many different interventions, based on established theory and science. Here, clinicians document the clinical judgment used to select a treatment plan. For example, the clinician writes that the wound is in the chronic inflammatory phase related to a large amount of necrotic tissue, has failed to respond to prior treatment interventions, and requires debridement to initiate the healing process. This becomes the rationale for selecting the treatment strategy (e.g., pulsatile lavage with suction) to remove the necrotic debris.

Evaluation of Progress

Once the target outcomes and goals have been determined, the reevaluation process is quite simple. Clinicians use performance indicators to measure a patient's progress toward the outcome within the desired time frame. For example, if the target outcome is "Patient's wound will demonstrate 25% reduction in size within 2 weeks," the clinician would monitor wound size throughout the 2-week period of time, and then determine whether the wound had reduced in surface area by 25% at the end of week 2. If the wound decreased in size more than 25%, the outcome was exceeded. If the wound decreased in size by 25%, the outcome was acceptably met. If the wound failed to decrease in size by 25%, the outcome was not met, and the goals must be adjusted and interventions reviewed.

Failure to achieve goals can be related to a change in the patient's overall condition, ineffective therapy, or inadequate adherence to the treatment regimen. Reevaluation is an ongoing, dynamic process that regularly recurs following reexamination of the effects of treatment. At that time, goals and outcomes can be adjusted, new goals developed, and interventions modified.

Because utilization management attempts to influence the clinical path from the beginning, in order to reduce deviation from an expected course and produce optimal outcomes, the adjustment of goals and expected outcomes should be minimal. Multiple approximations to reach the target outcome are not tolerated by patients or third-party payers. For example, the *APTA Guide to PT Practice*[14] lists wound management guidelines regarding range of visits and length of episodic care by physical therapists for patients with wounds. This range represents the lower and upper limits of services that an anticipated 80% of patients/clients with such wounds will need to receive to reach the predicted goals and outcomes (prognosis).

Multiple factors can modify the duration of the episode of care, frequency, and number of visits. For example, wounds extending into fascia, muscle, or bone (integumentary pattern E) require 4–16 weeks (12–112 visits) for an episode of care (all types of etiologies included). The prognosis for wounds of this severity is that, over the course of 4–16 weeks of care by the physical therapist, one of the following will occur:

- Wound will be clean and stable
- Wound will be prepared for closure
- Wound will be closed
- Immature scar will be evident[14]

Conclusion

The diagnostic process described in this chapter is intended as a framework for clinicians working with patients with wounds; it will be especially helpful to clinicians who are new to the diagnostic process or unfamiliar with its use. The information may or may not be new, but review of this key material will likely be helpful. Use of clinical judgment with diagnostic reasoning is one of the essential practice tools that nurses and physical therapists use with the patients they serve.

REVIEW QUESTIONS

1. What are the steps in the diagnostic process?
2. What is the difference between a behavioral and functional outcome?
3. What are five areas for data collection during the assessment phase?

REFERENCES

1. Clifton DW. Utilization management: Whose job is it? *Rehab Manage.* June/July 1996;38:44.
2. Bergstrom N, Bennett MA, Carlson C, et al. Treatment of pressure ulcers. *Clinical Practice Guideline.* No. 15. Rockville, MD: US Department of Health and Human Services (DHHS), AHCPR Publication No. 95–0652, December 1994.
3. Hisch IB, White PF. Medical management of surgical patients with diabetes. In: Levin ME, O'Neal LW, Bowker JH, eds. *The Diabetic Foot.* Chicago: CV Mosby, 1993.
4. Swanson G. *The Guide to Physical Therapist Practice.* Vol 1. Presented at California chapter, APTA, October 1995; San Diego, CA.
5. American Physical Therapy Association. A guide to physical therapy practice, I: a description of patient management. *Phys Ther.* 1995;75:707–764.
6. Doenges MD, Moorhouse MF, Burley JT. *Application of Nursing Process and Nursing Diagnosis.* 2nd ed. Philadelphia: FA Davis, 1995.

7. Jette AM. Physical disablement concepts for physical therapy research and practice. *Phys Ther.* 1994;74:380–386.

8. Swanson G. *The IDH Guidebook for Physical Therapy.* Long Beach, CA: Swanson and Company, 1995.

9. Sussman C. Case presentation: patient with a pressure ulcer on the coccyx. Paper presented at APTA Scientific Meeting and Exposition, June 1996; Minneapolis, MN.

10. Lazarus GS, Cooper DM, Knighton DR, et al. Definitions and guidelines for assessment of wounds and evaluation of healing. *Arch Dermatol.* 1994;130:489–493.

11. Swanson G. What is an outcome? And what does it mean to you? *Ultra/sounds.* (California Private Practice Special Interest Group—California APTA). 1995;94(51):7.

12. Swanson G. Functional outcome report: The next generation in physical therapy reporting in documenting physical therapy outcomes. In: Stuart D, Ablen S, eds. *Documenting Physical Therapy Outcomes.* Chicago: CV Mosby, 1993:101–134.

13. Staley M, Richard R, et al. Functional outcomes for the patient with burn injuries. *J Burn Care Rehab.* 1996;17(4):362–367.

14. Guide to physical therapist practice. *Phys Ther.* 1997;77:1593–1605.

1A

Patient History Form

Medical Record # _____   Name _____

Street Address _____

City, State, Zip _____

Telephone Number   (_____) _____

Sex: M/F _____   Height: _____   Weight: _____

Religious Preference: _____

What is your primary reason for seeking wound care today? _____

_____

How long has your wound existed? _____

_____

Who referred you here? _____

Who has been treating you before today? _____

Can you describe what you have been using on your wound? _____

_____

Who has been helping you with your wound care? _____

How have you been paying for your supplies? _____

Have you ever had surgery? _____   Type: _____

Do you have any allergies? Medications (Sulfa, Penicillin) _____   Other? _____

Do you smoke? _____   Packs per day: _____   # of years: _____

Do you use recreational or illicit drugs? If so, how often? _____

Do you drink alcohol? If so, how often? _____

Do you have any pain? _____

On a scale of 0–10 (0 = No Pain, 10 = Severe Pain), what is your pain level now?   0 – 1 – 2 – 3 – 4 – 5 – 6 – 7 – 8 – 9 – 10

What over-the-counter medications do you take (Tylenol, aspirin, antacids, vitamins, etc.)? _____

_____

What prescription medications do you take? Please include drug, dose, and frequency: _____

_____

Have you ever been told you had or do you currently have any of the following:

	Past	Present		Past	Present
Stroke:			Hypertension:		
Gangrene:			Cancer:		
Problems with circulation:			Chemotherapy:		
Arterial:			Radiation therapy:		
Venous:			Alternative treatments:		
Diabetes:			Swollen glands:		
Parkinson's:			Muscle spasms:		
Alzheimer's:			Polio or post-polio syndrome:		
Congestive heart failure:			Quadriplegia/paraplegia:		
Problems sleeping:			Myelomeningocele:		
Emphysema:			Decreased sensation:		
Bronchitis:			Arthritis:		
Chronic obstructive pulmonary disease:			Decreased activity:		
Problems controlling urine:			HIV or AIDS:		
Problems controlling bowels:			Hepatitis B:		
Atherosclerosis/arteriosclerosis:			Decreased appetite:		
Malnutrition:			Problems with mobility:		
Dehydration:			Changes in weight greater than 10 pounds:		
Thyroid disorder:			Pacemaker:		

Source: Copyright © Dean P. Kane, MD, FACS, PA.

Focused Assessment for Wounds

Medical Record # _____ Name _____

Attending Physician: _____

Referral Source: _____ MD _____ Nurse _____ Other _____

Site: __ Office __ Acute Hospital __ Subacute Center __ Nursing Home __ Assisted Living __ Home __ Other

    Facility Name / Address / Pt. bed #: _____

Physical Exam: _____ year-old M F acquired non-healing wound(s) on   /   /   .

Prior wound management includes: _____

_____

Past Medical History is positive for the following:

Allergies _____		Alcoholism _____	
CVA _____		NIDDM _____	
Gangrene _____		Complications of DM _____	
PVD _____		Weakness _____	
Arterial insufficiency _____		Paraplegia/quadriplegia _____	
CAD _____		Immobility/contractures _____	
IDDM _____		Parkinson's _____	

Vitals: T/P/R _____   BP: L/R _____ (sit/stand/lying)

Braden Scale:

Sensory/MS	1. totally limited	2. very limited	3. slightly limited	4. no impairment
Moisture	1. constantly moist	2. very moist	3. occasionally moist	4. dry
Activity	1. bedfast	2. chairfast	3. walks w/assist	4. walks frequently
Mobility	1. 100% immobile	2. very limited	3. slightly limited	4. full mobility
Nutrition	1. very poor	2. <1/2 daily portion	3. most of portion	4. eats everything
Friction/Shear	1. frequent sliding	2. feeble corrections	3. independent correction	

Braden Scale Total: _____

Mental Status: <u>Alert & Oriented X3:</u> Other: _____

Skin: (moist, dry, flaky, scaly, condition of nails): _____ Turgor: <u>good / med / poor</u>

  <u>Rubor, cyanosis, atrophy, dermatitis, hair loss, rash, erythema.</u>

EENT (Eyes sunken, swollen lymph nodes): _____ Mucous Membranes Moist: _____

Neuro (Cranial nerves, sensation): _____

Endocrine (Blood sugar/other): _____

Respiratory: <u>Lungs Clear:</u>   Other: _____

Cardiac: <u>Regular Rate & Rhythm:</u> Other: _____

Abdomen: <u>G-Tube: Soft/Supple/Without Masses or Tenderness:</u> Other: _____

Perineal: Skin intact _____ Other: _____

Lower Extremities: Ankle-Brachial Index: L: _____ R: _____

  Pulses Palpable: Dorsalis Pedis _____ Posterior Tibial _____ Popliteal _____

  Pulse Quality: Bounding _____ Strong _____ Weak _____ Barely Palpable _____

  Doppler: L+ _____ : R+ _____

  Edema _____ Circumference: (L) _____ : (R) _____

Functional Assessment: ADLs: Independent _____ Minimal Assist _____ Mod Assist _____ Total Assist _____

Labs/Nutrition: Hct: _____ % TP: _____ Alb: _____ Prealbumin: _____ Other: _____

  WBC: _____ % O2 Sat: _____ Lytes: _____

Suggested Tests/Examinations: _____

Adapted with permission from Dean P. Kane, MD, FACS, PA.

Sample Case Report Using HCFA-700

DEPARTMENT OF HEALTH AND HUMAN SERVICES
HEALTH CARE FINANCING ADMINISTRATION

FORM APPROVED
OMB NO. 0938-0227

PLAN OF TREATMENT FOR OUTPATIENT REHABILITATION *(COMPLETE FOR INITIAL CLAIMS ONLY)*

1. PATIENT'S LAST NAME Luck	FIRST NAME George	M.I.	2. PROVIDER NO.	3. HICN
4. PROVIDER NAME	5. MEDICAL RECORD NO. *(Optional)*		6. ONSET DATE 10/09/01	7. SOC. DATE 11/27/01

8. TYPE: ☐ PT ☐ OT ☐ SLP ☐ CR ☐ RT ☐ PS ☐ SN ☐ SW

9. PRIMARY DIAGNOSIS *(Pertinent Medical D.X.)*
CHF, COPD, multiple decubitus, weakness, debility

10. TREATMENT DIAGNOSIS
2 wounds with impaired wound healing secondary to eschar and chronic inflammatory phase. Impaired mobility, transfers, gait (707; 710.7)

11. VISITS FROM SOC.
15

12. PLAN OF TREATMENT FUNCTIONAL GOALS

GOALS *(Short Term)* Tissue Attribute changes expected:
Necrosis-free and wound healing progression to proliferative phase
Wounds #1 & 2 — 21 days
Reduce risk of pressure ulcers (Reduce Braden score to 19/22) — 15 days
Transfers and Gait with FWW to bathroom SBA — 15 days

OUTCOME *(Long Term)*
Target Performance Status:
Patient has improvement potential: Wounds will heal following intervention. Functional independent bed mobility, transfer and gait with assist device will be restored to enable patient to return to prior living situation in 6 weeks.

PLAN
1. Wound not improving with routine dressing changes, pressure relief & enzymatic debridement
2. Wounds #1 & 2 require a) sharp debride b) HVPC (electrical stimulation) to stimulate cells of repair and circulation for healing
3. Ther ex., balance, gait training to reduce risk of pressure ulcers and enhance circulation for healing current ulcers

13. SIGNATURE *(professional establishing POC including prof. designation)*

14. FREQ/DURATION *(e.g., 3/Wk × 4 Wk)*
6x/wk daily x 6 wks (36 days)

I CERTIFY THE NEED FOR THESE SERVICES FURNISHED UNDER THIS PLAN OF TREATMENT AND WHILE UNDER MY CARE ☒ N/A

15. PHYSICIAN SIGNATURE

16. DATE

17. CERTIFICATION
FROM   THROUGH   ☒ N/A

18. ON FILE *(Print/type physician's name)* ☒

20. INITIAL ASSESSMENT *(History, medical complications, level of function at start of care. Reason for referral)*

19. PRIOR HOSPITALIZATION
FROM 10/08/01   TO 11/26/06   ☐ N/A

<u>Reason for Referral:</u> Loss of mobility (e.g., unable to reposition in bed or ambulate); necrotic pressure ulcers R upper back and coccyx. Wants to regain prior level of indep. Gait with cane. Heal pressure ulcers for return to retirement home.

Hx: Mild dementia, indep. in gait w/cane; fell in shower and was unable to move; sustained pressure ulcers R upper back and coccyx, CHF, COPD.

<u>Systems Review:</u> 1) Cardiopulmonary system disabilities affect oxygen transport to tissues for repair. 2) Musculoskeletal impairments due to weakness (MMS BLE 3-/5 limit bed mobility, inability to transfer or ambulate without assist of 2 w/4ww ? few feet. Diminished balance. 3) Neuromuscular impairment due to reduced cerebral oxygen causes mild functional loss of mentation, impaired mobility, and awareness of need to reposition. Risk of pressure ulcers is moderate (Braden Risk score 17/23).

<u>Results of test and measures:</u> Wound Severity Dx (stage) delayed until both wounds are debrided.

<u>Wound healing tissue assessment:</u> 1) R upper Back: presence of tissue attributes "good for healing"; adherence of wound edges; and "not good for healing": necrosis and depth of 0.2cm; 2) coccyx: presence of attributes "not for healing": erythema, necrosis, absence of attributes "good for healing."

<u>Wound Size:</u> R Up Back: 17.7cm^2 Coccyx: 4.3cm^2. depth >0.2

21. FUNCTIONAL LEVEL *(End of billing period)*   **PROGRESS REPORT**   ☐ CONTINUE SERVICES *OR* ☐ DC SERVICES

1) Change in Wound Status: a) R upper back: progressed to proliferative phase of healing. Wound is erythema-free, necrosis-free and has factors "good for healing": Contraction sustained ? 2 weeks, edges are adhered. Wound is reduced in size from 17.5cm^2 to 12.3cm^2 (decreased 25%), b) Coccyx: increased size and extent from 34.4cm^2 to 37.41cm^2 after debriding. Severity Dx: Stage IV pressure ulcer. Tissue attributes present: "not good for healing" include: Undermining at 9:00 position, necrosis and erythema; good for healing attributes include: granulation-significant reduction in depth from 2.0 cm to 1.5 cm, appearance of contraction and sustained wound contraction for 2 weeks (reduced size). Wound is at end of acute inflammatory phase and progressing to proliferative phase. 2) Change in Mobility Status: a) Braden risk score 19/23; b) Performs transfers and gait with min-assist using FWW for 15 feet; c) Change in balance improved from fair to fair+ with functional change. Reduced risk of falling and pressure ulcers.

22. SERVICE DATES
FROM 11/27/01   THROUGH 11/30/01

FORM HCFA-700 (11-91)
STF CCR0224F

Source: Reprinted from Department of Health and Human Services, Health Care Financing Administration.

Wound Healing Physiology: Acute and Chronic

Carrie Sussman and Barbara M. Bates-Jensen

CHAPTER OBJECTIVES

At the completion of this chapter, the reader will be able to:
1. List three acute wound healing models.
2. List the benchmarks of the four wound healing phases.
3. List the benchmarks of wound phase changes for acute and chronic wound healing.
4. Describe the role of basic science research in developing wound treatments.
5. Apply knowledge of the wound microenvironment to identification of factors that can impact the healing process.

Scientific study of wound healing physiology has progressed from understanding and developing an acute wound healing model to identifying the cellular physiology and microenvironment of acute wounds, to comparing acute wound healing mechanisms and the microenvironment with factors affecting wound chronicity.[1,2] All of these areas of study are works in progress, with basic science research continuing to provide information for both acute and chronic wound classifications. Clinicians need to apply the basic science of wound healing physiology of both acute and chronic wounds to the selection and expected outcomes of treatment interventions. Innovative scientists, engineers, and manufacturers are also applying the scientific knowledge learned about wound healing physiology to the development of products that promote positive outcomes and mitigate the negative factors in healing wounds. Negative factors for wound healing are discussed later in this chapter. Ideally, all of the information and resources can be transferred to the clinical setting as best practices in wound management.

The basic science presented in this chapter is not comprehensive, but it provides a guide to present assumptions about the physiological processes of wound healing that occur in healing models and how they may affect outcomes of clinical care. The chapter covers basic acute wound healing models, chronic wound healing, fetal wound healing, the physiology of acute and chronic wound healing by phase, causative factors that interrupt acute wound healing processes in the wound microenvironment leading to chronicity, and factors from the patient and wound macroenvironment that can impact the healing process. Chapter 4 connects the concepts of basic wound healing science to the clinical assessment.

Wound Healing Models

Five basic wound healing models for wounds are discussed in this book.

1. Superficial wound healing
2. Primary intention wound healing
3. Delayed primary intention wound healing
4. Partial-thickness wound healing
5. Full-thickness/secondary intention healing

There are similarities among all five models. This chapter discusses the superficial, partial-thickness, and primary intention, and full-thickness/secondary intention wound healing models. Chronic wound healing is then presented, followed by fetal wound healing. Chapter 15 covers the primary intention and delayed primary intention healing models

Superficial Wound Healing

Alterations in the superficial skin, such as those caused by pressure (e.g., in stage I pressure ulcers), first-degree burns, and contusions, activate an inflammatory repair process that is comparable to that of open wounds.[3] Superficial skin involvement can indicate deeper soft tissue trauma, which warrants investigation for changes in skin color, temperature (e.g., warmth, followed by coolness, indicating tissue devitalization), tissue tension or swelling, and sensation (indicating tissue congestion).

If deep tissue death occurs a few days after first observation, the tissues can rupture and become a deep cavity. This often occurs in stage I pressure ulcers and is referred to as the *erupting volcano* effect. This effect is now attributed to deep tissue injury that is manifested under the skin as a purple discoloration, leading to the name "purple ulcers." *Color Plates 19* and *20* show superficial and partial-thickness (stages I and II) pressure ulcers with signs of deep tissue injury that manifest the true degree of involvement 3 weeks after they are first diagnosed. (Chapter 4 discusses assessment of deep tissue injury.)

In superficial wound healing, the soft tissues usually heal by themselves over time, but intervention at this stage can hasten return to functional activities, such as work and homemaking. For example, athletes are often assessed and treated immediately for superficial soft tissue injuries, with reduced loss of playing time, less pain, and less tissue swelling from congestion in the tissues. Tissue swelling can limit functional activities, resulting in diminished mobility and placing the individual at risk for further wounding. Part IV of this book, Management of Wound Healing with Biole physical Agents, explains the benefits of intervention for superficial wounds (e.g., thrombolysis or reabsorption of hematoma for faster healing, including stage I pressure ulcers, "purple ulcers," and grade I neuropathic ulcers). *Color Plates 76-78* illustrate how early intervention reduces hematoma (signs of deep tissue injury) and hastens repair. Case studies are described in Chapter 25.

Partial-Thickness Wound Healing

Wounds with partial-thickness loss of the dermis heal principally by epithelialization, which is the resurfacing of a wound by new epithelial cells, which are mostly keratinocytes. Epithelialization is the body's attempt to protect itself from invasion or debris by beginning to close the wound; this process begins immediately following injury.

Epithelial cells at the wound edges, as well as from the dermal appendages—sebaceous glands, sweat glands, and hair follicles—provide a supply of intact epithelial cells to assist in resurfacing the wound by lateral migration.[4,5] If dermal appendages are present, islands of epidermis can appear throughout the wound surface and speed the resurfacing process. The resulting epithelium is often indistinguishable from the surrounding skin, and the normal function of the skin is restored. Examples of partial-thickness wounds are abrasions, skin tears, stage II pressure ulcers, and second-degree burns.

Primary Intention Healing

Primary intention healing is associated with surgical wound healing. Table 2-1 compares primary and secondary intention healing activities. The major activity in primary inten-

TABLE 2-1 Principal Mechanisms of Primary and Secondary Intention Healing

	Primary intention	Secondary intention
Contraction	0	+++
Epithelialization	+	+
Connective tissue deposition	+++	++
Granulation tissue production	0	+++

0, no effect; +, slightly increased; ++, moderately increased; +++, substantially increased

Reprinted with permission from M.D. Kerstein, et al., *The Physiology of Wound Healing.* The Oxford Institute for Continuing Education and Allegheny University of Health Sciences, 1998: page 7.

tion healing is connective tissue deposition and epithelialization. There is no granulation tissue formation or wound contraction. See Chapter 15 for more details about primary intention healing.

Full-Thickness or Secondary Intention Healing

Full-thickness or secondary intention healing is the most effective method of healing when the wound extends through all layers of the skin and/or when it extends into underlying tissues. For example, when a large amount of tissue is removed or destroyed, a gap occurs, and the wound edges cannot be approximated or nonviable wound margins are present; in these cases, the wound is left to close by secondary intention (see *Color Plates 18, 38, and 85*). Wounds with a high microorganism count, debris, or skin necrosis are also left to close by secondary intention.

Full-thickness secondary intention healing principally occurs by contraction. Repair of tissue by secondary intention involves scar tissue formation. In this process, the anatomic structure of the scar tissue does not replicate the tissue replaced (e.g., muscles, tendons, or nerves). In addition, the surface tissue will not be equal in elasticity or tensile strength to the original.[4]

Sometimes, defects are too small to close by primary intention, and healing by secondary intention is preferred. Some wounds are incompletely covered by split-thickness skin grafts and are also best healed by secondary intention. If a wound is located in an area where contraction will produce disfiguring or nonfunctional deformities, the process of healing by secondary intention can be allowed to develop a strong, healthy wound bed. Then it is interrupted, and a split-thickness skin graft is placed on the granulating wound bed. Full-thickness wound healing involves a process that is divided into four overlapping phases of repair: inflammation, epithelialization, proliferation, and remodeling. Figure 2-1 is a schematic representation of secondary intention wound healing.

Chronic Wound Healing

Secondary intention is the healing model that is associated with chronic wounds.[6] Lazarus defines chronic wounds as

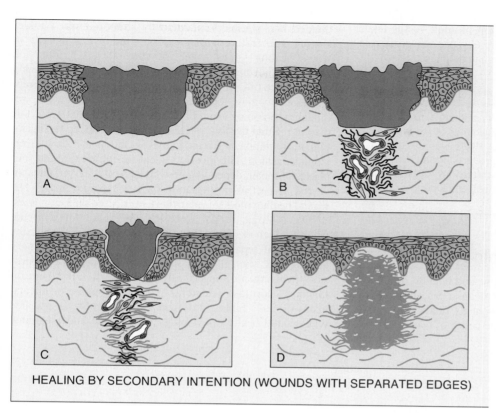

HEALING BY SECONDARY INTENTION (WOUNDS WITH SEPARATED EDGES)

FIGURE 2-1 Healing by secondary intention. **A.** A gouged wound, in which the edges are far apart and there is substantial tissue loss. **B.** This wound requires wound contraction, extensive cell proliferation, and neovascularization (granulation tissue) to heal. **C.** The wound is reepithelialized from the margins, and collagen fibers are deposited in the granulation tissue. **D.** Granulation tissue is eventually resorbed and replaced by a large scar that is functionally different than before wounding. (Adapted with permission from Rubin E and Farber JL. *Pathology.* 3rd Ed. Philadelphia: Lippincott Williams & Wilkins, 1999.

those that have "failed to proceed through an orderly and timely process to produce anatomic and functional integrity, or proceeded through the repair process without establishing a sustained anatomic and functional result."[6] *Orderly* refers to the progression of the wound through the biological sequences that comprise the phases of repair of acute wounds described below under Wound Healing Physiology. Orderliness can be interrupted during any of the phases of healing, but only recently have the causative factors for these interruptions been identified. Causative factors that affect the orderly progression of the healing process are presented in this chapter for each phase of wound healing.

Timeliness relates to the progression of the phases of repair in a manner that will heal the wound expeditiously. Timeliness is determined by the nature of the wound pathology, medical status of the patient, and environmental factors.[6] Those wounds that *do not* repair themselves in an orderly and timely manner are classified as chronic wounds; those that do are classified as acute wounds.

Fetal Wound Healing

Researchers are studying what can be learned from fetal wound healing. It has been known for some time that fetuses who undergo surgery in utero do not form scars.[7,8,9] Fetal wounds are continually bathed in amniotic fluid, which has a rich content of hyaluronic acid (HA) and fibronectin, as well as growth factors crucial to fetal development. HA is a key structural and functional component of the extra-cellular matrix (ECM), which fosters an environment that promotes cell proliferation and tissue regeneration and repair[5].[10] HA is laid down in the matrix of both fetal and adult wounds, but its sustained deposition is unique to fetal wounds.

An example of the effects of HA and amniotic fluid on healing of surgical wounds was reported by Byl et al in two studies.[11,12] Amniotic fluid, HA, and normal saline were applied to controlled incisional wounds. The surgeons were blinded to the fluids applied. Incisions treated with HA and amniotic fluid both healed faster than the saline-treated wounds; in fact, they appeared to close within minutes of application. The healing was quicker, and the quality of the scar was better in the HA and amniotic fluid incisions than in the saline-treated incisions. The tensile strengths of the wounds treated with amniotic fluid and HA were slightly weaker than those of the saline-treated group at the end of 1 week; however, after 2 weeks, all groups had equal tensile strength.

Many questions remain to be answered regarding fetal wound healing. There are many differences between fetal development and adult repair and regeneration. For example, the transplacental circulation provides a partial pressure of oxygen of 20 mm Hg, which is markedly lower than that in adults, signifying that the fetus lives in a hypoxic environment.[13] This is in marked contrast to the adult environment, where oxygen is a critical factor in prevention of infection and in the repair process. There are also differences in the fetal and adult immune systems, the histology of fetal skin during development, the function of adult versus fetal fibroblasts in collagen synthesis, the absence of myofibroblasts, and the absence of an inflammatory phase.[14,15]

Hyaluronic acid (HA) is a gel that is degraded in vivo and breaks down rapidly when applied to wounds. A wound dressing called Hyaff (ConvaTec, a Bristol Myers Squibb company, Princeton, NJ), has recently been produced from HA. When applied to the wound, this dressing creates an HA-rich tissue interface and moist wound environment conducive to granulation and healing (see Chapter 11).[16]

Wound Healing Physiology

The physiological process of acute wound healing in different phases was described by Hunt et al[17] as a cascade of overlapping events that occurs in a reasonably predictable fashion. Although the events overlap, the series of events can be divided into phases. A diagram by Hunt and Van Winkle[1] (Figure 2-2) features inflammation—the central activity of wound healing—in its center. On either side are proliferation and epithelialization, the concurrent events that occur as a consequence of injury. The lower portion of the diagram represents the coming together of the phases, leading to the remodeling phase of wound healing. The interpretation of this diagram is that the four phases—inflammation, epithelialization, proliferation, and remodeling—occur in an orderly, overlapping fashion. The literature identifies either three or four phases of repair, depending on whether epithelialization is included as part of proliferation or as a separate phase. The wound healing model used in this text is based on four phases.

The biologic repair process is the same for all acute wounds, open or closed, regardless of etiology. However, the sequence of repair is completed more quickly in primary healing and when there is superficial and partial-thickness skin involvement. Slower healing occurs when there is full-thickness skin loss extending into and through the subcutaneous tissue.[17] Table 2-2 defines key terminology associated with wound healing physiology to facilitate understanding.

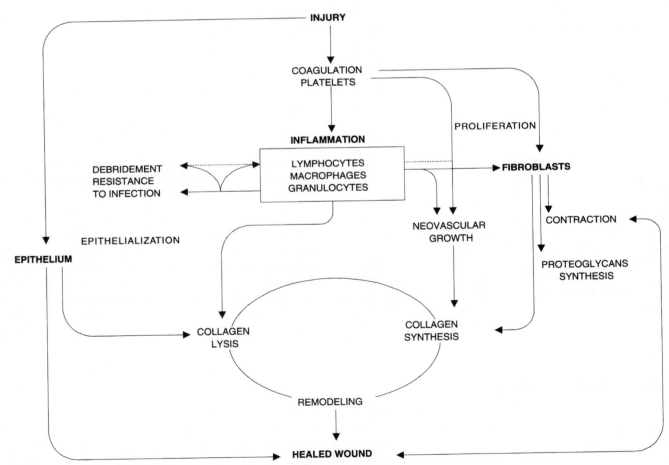

FIGURE 2-2 Diagram of wound repair. (Reprinted with permission from Hunt TK and Van Winkle W. *Fundamentals of Wound Management in Surgery, Wound Healing: Normal Repair.* South Plainfield, NJ: Chirurgecom, Inc, 1976.

TABLE 2-2 Terminology Associated with Wound Healing Physiology

Term	Definition (Reference)
Angiogenesis	Development of new blood vessels in injured tissues. Function of endothelial cells.
Apoptosis	A mechanism for cell deletion in the regulation of cell populations, as of B and T lymphocytes following cytokine depletion. Often used synonymously with *programmed cell death*.
Basement membrane	Thin layer of extracellular material found between the layers of the epithelia or between the epithelia and connective tissue. Also called *basal lamina*.[18]
Chemoattractants	Cause cell migration.
Chemotaxis	Attraction of a cell in response to a chemical signal.
Chronic wound	Wound that has "failed to proceed through an orderly and timely process to produce anatomic and functional integrity, or proceeded through the repair process without establishing a sustained anatomic and functional result."[6]
Collagenases	Enzymes that cleave (break) the bonds of the polypeptide chains in collagen at specific sites, aiding in its resorption during periods of connective tissue growth or repair.[18]
Complement system	11 proteins found in plasma with specific purpose of combating bacterial contamination. Also chemotactic for phagocytes; substances most responsible for acute inflammation.[4]
Extracellular matrix (ECM)	Intricate system of glycosaminoglycans (GAGs) and proteins secreted by cells; provides the framework for tissues.[18]
Free radicals	Highly reactive molecular species that have a least one unpaired electron in the outer shell. Attempt to react with other molecules to achieve an electrically more stable state in which the electron is paired with another. Important for normal cell functions, including metabolism and defense against infection.[42]
Galvanotaxis	Attraction of a cell in response to an electrical signal.
Glycosaminoglycans (GAGs)	Polysaccharides that contain amino acids, sugars, and glycoprotein. Termed *proteoglycans*.[73]
Growth factors (GFs)	Extracellular polypeptides—proteins able to affect cell reproduction, movement, and function. Term encompasses items c, d, and e, below. Regulators of the wound healing cascade. May be deficient in chronic wounds.[18]
a. Autocrine stimulation	GF produced by a cell acting on itself.
b. Paracrine stimulation	GF produced by one cell type acting on another in the local area.
c. Endocrine stimulation	GF produced by one cell type acting on distant cells.
d. Cytokines	Refers to diverse group of polypeptides and glycoproteins that are important mediators of inflammation. Anti inflammatory cytokines inhibit production of pro inflammatory cytokines, counter their action or both
e. Interleukins (ILs)	A group of pro inflammatory cytokines
f. Colony-stimulating factor	Term for GF used by hematologists.[21]
Hemostasis	Coagulation to stop bleeding and initiate the wound healing process.
Hydroxyproline (HoPro)	A polypeptide chain of insoluble collagen.
Integrins	Regulate a wide range of cellular functions during growth, development, differentiation, and the immune response Serve a critical function in cell adhesion and signaling during wound-healing, where they are fundamental to reepithelialization and granulation tissue formation.[71]
Ligand	A molecule that binds to another molecule, used especially to refer to a small molecule that binds specifically to a larger molecule.[153]
Matrix Metalloproteinases (MMPs)	Proteolytic enzymes that degrade proteins and ECM macromolecules. MMPs have the ability to degrade a variety of extracellular matrix components which is of benefit in the developmental and remodeling processes in healthy tissues.[71] Synthesized and secreted by multiple cell types involved in wound healing in response to biochemical signals.
Mitogens	Cause cell growth.
Mitogenic	Causing mitosis or cellular proliferation.
Neovascularization	Development of new blood vessels; another term for angiogenesis.
Phagocytosis	Ingestion, destruction, and digestion of cellular particulate matter.[18]
Proteases	Proteolytic enzymes that degrade proteins.[18]
Substrates	Substances acted upon by an enzyme, such as substances necessary for new tissue growth: protein, vitamin C, zinc.
Tensile strength	The most longitudinal stress that a substance can withstand without tearing apart.
Tissue inhibitors of metalloproteinases (TIMPs)	Secreted proteins that are widely distributed in tissues and fluids and serve as specific inhibitors for the MMPs. Synthesized and secreted by same multiple cell types as MMPs.[22]

Attributes that distinguish the healing of chronic wounds from that of acute wounds are continually being studied. After the process of normal wound healing by phase is explained below, the attributes and processes that may be responsible for chronic wound healing in each phase are presented. Table 2-3 summarizes factors and their effects on chronic wound healing during each phase of repair.

Inflammatory Phase

The classic observable signs and symptoms of inflammation are the benchmarks of the inflammatory phase and include changes in color in the surrounding skin (red, blue, purple), temperature (heat), turgor (swelling), sensation (pain), and loss of function (*Color Plates 1, 19*, and *21*). These attributes are only minimally manifested with normal healing; however, when present, these clinical manifestations should be regarded as clinical signs of excessive inflammation that are characteristic of impending infection.[18] The inflammation response is sometimes referred to as a "flare" because of the suddenness of the response, color, and associated temperature changes that are reminiscent of the flaring up of a fire.

Inflammation is the body's immune system reaction and is essential for orderly, timely healing. The physiology of inflammation is well-regulated in the normally healing acute wound and typically lasts 3-7 days. Acute inflammation begins soon after the injury, setting into motion a biologic cascade of events. The major goals of the inflammatory phase of healing are to provide for hemostasis and the breakdown and removal of cellular, extracellular, and pathogen debris; this produces a clean wound site for tissue restoration and initiation of the repair process. Signal sources, cytokines, and growth factors expressed at the time of injury within the wound communicate with and attract responder cells and regulate the repair process.

Figure 2-3 shows the progression of healing through a distinct but overlapping series of processes, leading to scar formation and normal wound healing. The following is a description of the key processes of the acute inflammatory phase, including:

- Coagulation cascade to achieve platelet activation and hemostasis
- Mitogenesis and chemotaxis of growth factors
- Controlled tissue degradation
- Role of perfusion
- Hypoxia and the regulatory function of the oxygen-tension gradient
- Complement system activation to control infection
- Neutrophil, macrophage, mast, and fibroblast cell functions
- Keratinocyte activation
- "Current of injury" stimulus for the repair process

After describing normal inflammation, the attributes and processes that may be responsible for chronic wound healing during the inflammatory phase are discussed.

Coagulation Cascade or Hemostasis

Clotting and vasoconstriction, or hemostasis, occur immediately after injury to reduce blood loss at the site of injury; this is called the *coagulation cascade*. Hemostasis is initiated immediately as the first major function of the platelets. Platelets, which are normally present in the intravascular space, are activated by collagen or microfibrils from the subendothelial layers that are exposed when injury occurs. The process, known as *platelet activation,* induces changes in platelet structure and function that are necessary for coagulation to occur, including thrombin, fibrin, and clot production, and, ultimately, hemostasis.[18] The fibrin clot becomes the primary foundation for collagen deposition and the pathway for the influx of monocytes and fibroblasts to the wound site.[19] Platelets within the fibrin clot release growth factors and cytokines, including *platelet-derived growth factor* (PDGF). The second, equally important function of the platelet is the secretion of cytokines and growth factors with multiple functions, including recruitment of leukocytes and fibroblasts to the injury site.[20]

Growth Factors and other Regulatory Proteins

The term *growth factor* (GF) includes all peptides that have growth-promoting activities; they are referred to as *cytokines* by cell biologists, *interleukins* by immunologists, and *colony-stimulating factors* by hematologists.[21] Research on the activities of GFs shows that they provide the key biochemistry for the wound healing process. Platelets and macrophages are the primary cells that produce and release GFs; as such, they are the critical components. Growth factors are naturally occurring proteins (polypeptides) that mediate and regulate tissue deposition. GFs can act on distant cells (endocrine stimulation), adjacent cells (paracrine stimulation), and themselves (autocrine stimulation).[18] Some GFs cause cell growth (mitogenesis), others cause cell migration (chemoattractants), and still others perform regulatory functions.

Each GF is involved in specific pathways; the name of the GF does not necessarily identify the only cells that produce it or the role it plays in healing. A key role of GFs and cytokines is to act as intercellular communicators. Transmission of the messages between cells of the same or different type requires a medium in which to disperse the message, and this can only occur in a moist environment. On the other end, there must be a receptor to receive the message.

Cell surface receptors on the target cell receive the message, bind to the cell, and produce a biological response in the receiving cell. The message may call for cell division, cell migration, or cell synthesis. Cells have the ability to increase (upregulate) or decrease (down regulate) their receptors in response to environmental signals. Cell receptors are not stationary on the cell surface, and their numbers can vary from time to time. They also can bind with one or more kinds of messages.[22]

GFs and cytokines differ in their functions. GFs deliver messages that are released to nonimmune cells and result in cell proliferation, such as the synthesis of granulation tissue.

TABLE 2-3 Summary of Factors and Effects during Each Phase of Wound Healing in Chronic Wounds

Chronic Inflammatory Phase	Chronic Epithelialization Phase	Chronic Proliferative Phase	Chronic Remodeling Phase
Different stimulus of repair a. From within b. Gradual c. Slowed	Diminished keratinocyte migration due to: a. Lack of moist environment b. Lack of oxygen c. Lack of nutritious tissue base d. Lack of stimulation by appropriate cytokine	Different composition of fibronectin: a. Partially degraded into fragments b. Fragments may perpetuate activity of matrix proteases c. Inhibit healing	Imbalance of collagen synthesis and degradation: a. Impaired scar tensile strength b. Overproduction of collagen: hypertrophic scarring c. Imbalance of fibrotic and antifibrotic cytokines: hypergranulation
Inadequate perfusion and oxygenation: a. Muted phase process b. Ischemic tissue barrier to angiogenesis	Keratinocyte migration obstructed by wound edges that are: a. Rolled b. Thickened c. Nonproductive	Excess activity of proteases causes: a. Accelerated rate of connective tissue breakdown b. Destruction of polypeptide-signaling molecules c. Production of metalloproteinases that do not lyse collagen	Hyperoxygenation: a. Hypertrophy of granulation tissue b. Impediment to epidermal cell migration
Free radicals and oxygen reperfusion injury: a. Large production of free radicals b. Disruption in normal defense against free radicals c. Capillary plugging by neutrophils	Keratinocyte migration slowed due to: a. Large gap b. Slow filling of "dead space"	Chronic wound fluid inhibition of: a. Cellular proliferation: endothelial cells, keratinocytes, fibroblasts b. Cell adhesion Repeated trauma and infection: a. Increases the presence of proinflammatory cytokines b. Increases the presence of tissue inhibitors (metalloproteinases) c. Lowers the level of growth factors Impediments to wound healing: a. Elevated levels of matrix metalloproteinases b. Imbalance between levels of matrix metalloproteinases and their inhibitors (TIMPs) Large tissue defect: a. Prolongs proliferation of tissue to fill the space Substrates relationship to stalling or plateauing: a. Inadequate substrates b. Bacterial competition for substrates necessary for tissue repair c. Continued lysis of new growth faster than synthesis of new material Long-term wound hypoxia effects: a. Negative effect on collagen production b. Decreased fibroblast proliferation c. Decreased tissue growth Impaired wound contraction: a. Wound remains large b. Delayed reepithelialization	Impairment of scar tensile strength: a. Wound breakdown b. Dehiscence

Adapted with permission from Bates-Jensen B. A Quantitative Analysis of Wound Characteristics As Early Predictors of Healing In Pressure Sores. Dissertation Abstracts International, Volume 59, Number 11, University of California, Los Angeles; 1999.

FIGURE 2-3 The phases of acute wound healing.

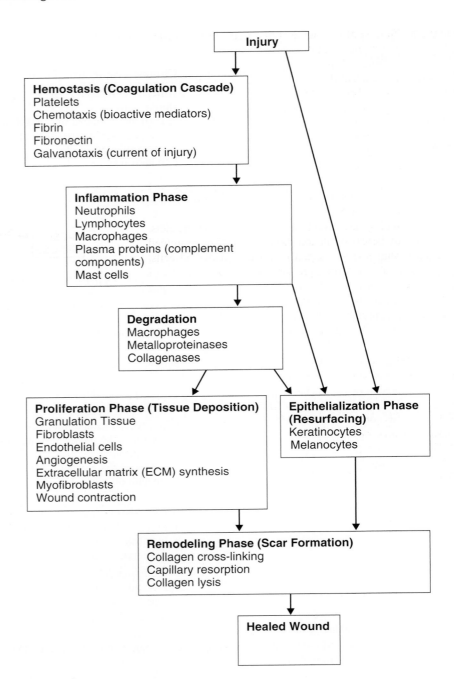

Cytokines communicate with immune system cells and attract those cells to the area of injury for the purpose of mounting an inflammatory response to destroy foreign organisms and debris. The same GF can have different biological roles, depending on the phase of healing or the degree to which it binds to a receptor.[22] Cytokines play a critical role in inflammation. They are divided into two groups: the proinflammatory and anti-inflammatory cytokines, which have powerful stimulatory and inhibitory actions on the inflammatory cells. In acute wounds, the level of proinflammatory cytokines peaks in a few days and remains low in the absence of infection.[23]

RESEARCH WISDOM

1. One reason that moisture-retentive dressings are a vital part of wound healing is because they provide the moist environment necessary for cellular communications.[22]
2. Although a moist wound environment is desirable for acute wound healing, chronic wound fluid has been shown to have an inhibitory effect on fibroblasts.[23] [24]

A third group of regulatory proteins is collectively named *chemokines*. Chemokines have two primary functions: regulate the trafficking of leukocyte populations during normal health and development, and direct the recruitment and activation of neutrophils, lymphocytes, macrophages, eosinophils, and basophils during inflammation.[23] Together GFs, cytokines, and chemokines are the key molecular regulators of wound healing. There is considerable overlap in target cell specificity and actions among the three groups.

Growth factors constitute a built-in check-and-balance system within the body to ensure that overproliferation does not occur. For example, extended exposure to some growth factors (at least 4 hours) is required before cell division can occur.[18] Other examples are endothelial growth factor (VEGF), which is a potent stimulus for angiogenesis, and endostatin, a potent inhibitor of angiogenesis; both are products of the platelets. The function of these two antagonists is to regulate programmed cell death (apoptosis) and speed removal of damaged cells, while endothelial cells work to restore the homeostatic state of the tissues as expeditiously as possible.[25] The critical balance between tissue deposition and tissue degradation is controlled by the activity of proteolytic enzymes, called proteases, during all phases of healing (their functions are discussed below). Figure 2-4 is a diagram showing current understanding of the GF pathways and interactions in the inflammatory phase of the wound healing cascade (see Table 2-4 for a key to acronyms).

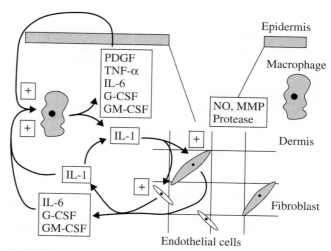

FIGURE 2-4 Inflammatory Phase. This simplified communication profile shows that the inflammatory phase is directed by inflammatory cells (first neutrophils and then macrophages) that release multiple cytokines. Adapted with permission from Goldman, R. Growth factors and chronic wound healing: past, present and future. *Advances in Skin and Wound Care.* 2004;17(1).

TABLE 2-4   Key to Acronyms Used in Figures 2-4 and 2-5

Cellular Sources	Cytokines	Function
Platelets	PDGF—Platelet derived growth factor	Chemotactic for neutrophils
	TGFβ—Transforming growth factor beta	Directs collagen matrix expression in late phase of wound repair
Macrophages	PDGF—Platelet derived growth factor	
	TNFα—Tumor necrosis factor alpha	Induces MMP transcription; Proinflammatory; Stimulates synthesis of Nitric oxide
	IL-1—Interlukin- 1	Proinflammatory; Stimulates synthesis of Nitric oxide (NO) Amplifies inflammatory response through increased synthesis of IL-1 and IL-6
	IL-6—Interlukin-6	Proinflammatory
	G-CSF—Granulocyte colony stimulating factor	Proinflammatory
	GM-CSF—Granulocyte-macrophage stimulating factor	Necrotic ECM degradation
Keratinocytes	IL-6—Interlukin-06	Stimulate Keratinocytes Induce Keratinocyte proliferation
	VEGF—Vascular endothelial growth factor	Potent stimulus for angiogenesis
Fibroblasts	KGF-2—Keratinocyte Growth Factor	Enable cellular migration the ECM; directs epithelialization
	IL-1—Interlukin 1	Proinflammatory; Amplifies inflammatory response through increased synthesis of IL-1 and IL-6
	TGF-β—Transforming growth factor beta	Directs collagen matrix exession Upregulates tissue inhibitors of MMPs
Endothelial cells	VEGF—Vascular endothelial growth factor	Potent stimulus for angiogenesis Upregulated in presence of NO

Wound healing involves a critical balance between controlled tissue deposition, mediated by the growth factors, and degradation, which is mediated by proteolytic enzymes. A family of 20 proteolytic enzymes, called matrix metalloproteinases (MMPs), has been identified as the critical group with the function of tissue degradation. Multiple cell types associated with wound healing (e.g., macrophages, epithelial, endothelial, neutrophils, and fibroblasts) receive specific chemical communication from proinflammatory cytokines (e.g., TNFα, IL-1, IL-6), which trigger synthesis of MMPs. To balance the activities of MMPs, there are endogenous enzyme inhibitors called *tissue inhibitors of metalloproteinase* (TIMPs). Four different TIMPs have been identified, and they are synthesized by the same cells that produce MMPs. MMPs require calcium ions for structural conformation and zinc ions in their active site for function. Collectively the MMPs are capable of degrading all components of the extracellular matrix (ECM). If the balance of MMPs and TIMPs is disrupted, a shift to high levels of MMPs can occur, resulting in excessive tissue degradation or destruction of other protein components in the ECM, including growth factors, cell surface receptors, and even the TIMPs.[22] This imbalance affects wound chronicity and chronic wound healing.

Platelet Activation

Activated platelets release biologically active substances, or signal sources, which are growth factors and cytokines. These include *platelet-derived growth factor* (PDGF), *epidermal growth factor* (EGF), *transforming growth factor-ß* (TGF-ß), *heparin-binding epidermal growth factor* (HB-EGF), and *insulin-like growth factor-1* (IGF-1), all of which facilitate cell migration of neutrophils and macrophages to the area of injury.[18,20] PDGF is a multifunctional, unique cytokine that plays multiple roles in wound healing, including release of endothelial growth factor (VEGF) and basic fibroblast growth factor (bFGF) early in the inflammatory phase. Angiogenesis occurs when endothelial cells respond to these GFs. The released growth factors regulate all phases of healing.

Hypothermia, often associated with surgery, inhibits platelet activation and increases bleeding time. Even a 0.2°C lowering of core body temperature will trigger peripheral vasoconstriction and tissue hypoxia.[26] Unless corrected, the coagulation cascade may not proceed normally, and there is increased risk of blood loss and infection. Rewarming of the blood will restore both platelet function and normal clotting time.[27,28] Hypothermia is often undetected.

CLINICAL WISDOM

Core body temperature should be monitored for hypothermia. This can be easily done with a tympanic membrane or liquid crystal strip thermometer.

Wound Space Hypoxia

Following vasoconstriction, the wound space becomes hypoxic. The process of hemostasis curtails blood flow directly to the site of injury to stop bleeding by creating fibrin clots in the local vessels. Lack of blood flow quickly depletes oxygen delivery to the wound space, producing an environmental change to the state of hypoxia. Hypoxia in the wound space immediately after wounding is a key factor in initiating the healing cascade. While hypoxia stimulates tissue repair, it also puts the tissues at risk for infection by impairing the function of neutrophils, lymphocytes, macrophages, and fibroblasts. Hypoxia is a signal that recruits endothelial responder cells and stimulates angiogenesis (the process of new blood vessel growth by the endothelial cells), which occurs during the proliferation phase. Local hypoxia also causes a shift to anaerobic glycolysis with increased lactate production, which is involved in activation of both angiogenesis and collagen synthesis. Lactate accumulation from white blood cells at the site contributes to the acidotic environment.[29] Thus, the hypoxic wound space becomes hyperlactic and acidotic.[17,30] Hypoxia, in conjunction with lactate produced through anaerobic metabolism and white blood cells, stimulates the release of angiogenic growth factors (AGFs) by macrophages to attract fibroblasts to the wound site.[31,32]

Infection and Oxygen

Soon after wounding, an oxygen-tension gradient develops across the wound that is used for regulatory purposes. If the normal gradient of oxygen is eliminated or a macrophage-free tissue space is created, the process of angiogenesis can be temporarily or permanently inhibited.[33] Oxygen is available in the blood in two forms: bound to hemoglobin and dissolved in plasma. The oxygen dissolved in plasma can be adequate for wound healing if tissue perfusion is satisfactory.[23] Oxygen is essential for preventing infection and meeting the metabolic demands of the tissues, as well as for the hydroxylation of proline necessary for useful collagen production in the remodeled wound. Although they are attracted to a hypoxic environment, once they arrive at the wound site neutrophils and macrophages require oxygen to kill bacteria. They do not function efficiently in a hypoxic environment, where microorganisms can proliferate at a faster rate than the neutrophils can phagocytose them, leading to infection.[34] Oxygen has been demonstrated to function equivalently to an "antibiotic" for prevention of wound infections.[35,36,37-39] Fibroblasts are aerobic cells that require oxygen for cell function, including division and collagen synthesis.[33] Signs of local hypoxia often go undetected. One example is the case of perioperative hypoxia-induced vasoconstriction and tissue hypoxia, which have been shown to triple the incidence of perioperative surgical wound infection.[26]

RESEARCH WISDOM

Facilitate delivery of oxygen to wound tissues by keeping the patient warm and well-hydrated.[33,40] Improve tissue oxygen levels by administering oxygen by nasal cannula at 5 L/minute.[35] Precaution: CO_2 retainers.

The Complement System

A noncellular (i.e., humoral) group of substances precedes the arrival of neutrophils to the wound space. This system, called the *complement system*, consists of approximately 11 proteins that normally reside in the plasma. Components of the complement system are responsible for acute inflammation through their ability to cause both humoral (i.e., protein) and cellular (i.e., phagocytic) defense mechanisms to move from the intravascular to the extravascular space, where bacteria accumulate. The primary function of the complement system is to facilitate bacterial destruction.

Complement activation occurs by way of several specific substances, most often bacteria. The complement system acts either through the classical pathway of lysing bacterial cell walls, thereby destroying the infecting organism, or the alternate pathway of opsonizing the invader (i.e., coating the antigen with antibody), which makes the invader more appealing and recognizable to the phagocytic cells. In addition, complement acts as a chemotactic agent for attracting phagocytic cells, neutrophils, and macrophages to the site of infection, and enhances their mechanism for oxidative killing.[4]

Two antibodies, IgG and IgM, directly activate the classical pathway of the complement system. These antibodies are produced by the lymphocytes located in the spleen, lymph nodes, and submucosa of the gastrointestinal, respiratory, and genital tracts. They produce specific antibodies in response to specific antigens. These antibodies can neutralize viruses and lyse gram-negative bacteria; as such, they are potent inhibitors of antigens.[4]

Neutrophils

Neutrophils (polymorphonuclear neutrophilic leukocytes) migrate into the wound space, usually within the first 24 hours after wounding, and remain from 6 hours to several days.[4] Neutrophils are granulocytic leukocytes that function as phagocytic cells to clean the site of debris and bacteria. Initially, neutrophils are the most prevalent type of white blood cell at the injury site. They use a special enzyme system to produce and employ free radicals to attack invading bacteria.[41] Neutrophils proliferate in hypoxic, acidotic environments and produce superoxide to fight bacteria and enhance the effectiveness of antibiotics. When the bacterial count is low or declines, the neutrophils stay at the site for only a minimal period of time. High bacterial counts prolong neutrophil activation and inflammation.[42]

The neutrophil is considered to be a primary cell responsible for cleansing wounds of microorganisms; therefore inadequate numbers of neutrophils will retard healing in infected wounds. When bacterial counts in the wound exceed 10^5 organisms per gram of tissue or ml of fluid, infection becomes apparent in the wound site. [5] The wound produces pus, which is the accumulation of dead neutrophils that have phagocytized debris in the wound. Neutrophils have a short life span because they cannot regenerate spent lysosomal and other enzymes used in the destruction of foreign substances. In addition to pus formation, neutrophils produce numerous toxic byproducts that, if there is excessive neutrophil activity due to high bacterial counts, negatively affect the wound tissue and even healthy tissue.[4]

When the wound is predominantly clean, neutrophil accumulation resolves. Whether it resolves or is prolonged (as may be the case in chronic wound healing), the monocyte becomes the primary white blood cell in the wounded tissues.[31] Once in the wounded area, monocytes are transformed into macrophages. The macrophages release cytokines, which amplify the inflammatory response by inducing fibroblasts and endothelial cells to synthesize and secrete more proinflammatory cytokines (interleukin-1 [IL-1] and interleukin-6 [IL-6]) and colony stimulating factors (G-CSF and GM-CSF).[2]

Macrophages

Macrophages are key players in both the inflammatory and proliferative phases of wound healing. They secrete a number of growth factors, including angiogenic growth factors (AGFs), transforming growth factor-ß (TGF-ß), tumor necrosis factor-((TNF-(), IL-1, and basic fibroblast growth factor (bFGF).[18] AGFs are signal sources that stimulate the budding of endothelial cells from the damaged blood vessels and subsequent angiogenesis. Reestablishment of the blood supply is essential for delivering nutrients to the newly forming tissue. The growth factors released by macrophages induce fibroblast proliferation, chemotaxis, and collagen deposition. Macrophage activity increases during the late phases of inflammation. The life span of the macrophage is estimated to be months to years; it is a component of wound fluid for a long period of time, transcending all phases of healing.[4]

Macrophages are the essential cells for transition from the inflammatory to the proliferative phase of healing because of these activities that initiate angiogenesis and granulation tissue formation.[32] Transforming growth factor-ß (TGF-ß) and platelet derived growth factor (PDGF) are specific chemoattractants for macrophages.[18] Both neutrophils and macrophages function in the low-oxygen, high-acidotic environment that is found in a hypoxic wound space.

In addition to initiating angiogenesis and granulation tissue formation, macrophages perform several important functions during the inflammatory phase, including:

1. Phagocytosis of debris and control of infection by ingestion of microorganisms and excretion of ascorbic acid, hydrogen peroxide, and lactic acid. The body interprets the buildup of these excreted byproducts as a signal to send more macrophages; the result of the increased macrophage population is a prolonged, more intense inflammatory response.
2. Autolytic debridement through synthesis and secretion of collagenases in preparation for the laying down of the new collagen matrix during the inflammatory phase and collagen degradation during the remodeling phase.[18]
3. Release of nitric oxide, which kills pathogens.

Nitric Oxide and Wound Healing

Nitric oxide plays many roles in human physiology, one of which is a regulator of wound healing. Nitric oxide (NO) is a small, gaseous free radical that is formed from the amino acid L-arginine by three distinct isoforms of nitric oxide synthase (NOS). L-arginine is a semiessential amino acid that is in short supply after injury, but it is the critical substrate for NO synthesis. Oxygen and L-arginine are combined by the enzyme NOS to form NO and citrulline.[43] The inducible isoform (iNOS) is synthesized in the early phase of wound healing by inflammatory cells, mainly macrophages.[44] NO synthesis occurs for 10–14 days following wounding, after which time it gradually decreases as the wound progresses towards healing.[44] NO can cross cell membranes without mediation of channels or receptors, which enhances its ability to act as a cellular signal for wound healing.[43] The NO reacts with peroxide ion O_2 radicals for pathogen killing. NO has been shown to kill *Staphylococcus aureus*, prevent replication of DNA viruses within cells, and serve as an immune regulator.[2]

Many cells participate in NO synthesis during the proliferative phase of healing, including fibroblasts.[45] NO released through iNOS regulates collagen formation and accumulation, cell proliferation, and wound contraction in distinct ways in animal models of wound healing.[46] The critical role of NO in fibroblast collagen synthesis is supported by the finding that in vivo NO inhibition results in reduced wound collagen accumulation Although iNOS gene deletion delays healing, and arginine and NO administration improves healing, the exact mechanisms of action of NO on wound healing parameters are still unknown [44,45,46]

NO role in wound repair has been of considerable interest because of findings that diabetic ulcer healing may be adversely effected by deficient NOS activity and the resulting NO deficiency.[43] There is also an increasing body of evidence that the overproduction of reactive nitrogen species (RNS)(NO^+) is implicated in the pathogenesis of inflammatory conditions and impaired healing.[24] Chapter 3 includes additional information about NO, its role in wound healing, and its relationship to L-arginine and protein nutrition.

Mast Cells

Mast cells are specialized secretory cells. In the resting state, mast cells contain granules which serve as histamine-binding sites. A number of biologically active substances exist in mast cell granules, including neutrophil chemotactic factor.[24] Mast cells promote fibroblast proliferation through the release of TNF-ß, which is a weak mitogen for fibroblasts. Mitogens cause cell mitosis and cellular proliferation.[18] Histamine, a vasoactive amine, is initially released from the mast cells after injury. It plays an important role in vascular dilation and permeability, inducing temporary mild edema. In low doses, histamine can stimulate collagen formation and healing.[24] Once the body has produced enough platelet and prothrombin reaction, the mast cell produces heparin. Heparin stimulates the migration of endothelial cells.

Other substances in the mast cells, eosinophil and neutrophil chemotactic factors, attract leukocytic cells. These cells act as chemical signals for the recruitment of macrophages, which leads to a modulation of the inflammatory phase. Macrophages promote later phases in the repair process through recruitment of fibroblasts.[47,48] The effect of heparin is to accelerate the activity of the leukocytes (neutrophils and eosinophils) in the thrombolysis of the hematoma that occurs in the wound following damage to the blood vessels at the time of wounding.[49]

Perfusion

Circulatory activities that follow wounding are manifested by temperature changes in the wound and surrounding tissues. Humoral and neurogenic factors, such as bradykinin, histamine, and prostaglandins, are responsible for causing vasodilation of the surrounding tissues. Increased perfusion increases local tissue temperature, a response known as *hyperemia*. Hyperemia is not an inflammatory reaction. Pain, as a consequence of the trauma to the tissues, irritates nerve endings and produces reflex hyperemia.[50] The vasodilation aids in movement of inflammatory cells from the vasculature into the site of injury. Vasodilation of adjacent vessels follows vasoconstriction at the wound site and is accompanied by perfusion, increased capillary pressure, and permeability of small blood and lymphatic vessels. This permits the plasma protein molecules to migrate into the surrounding tissues with consequent edema, erythema, and stimulation of the pain afferents. Fibrin plugs seal off the lymphatic flow to prevent spreading of infection. Increased perfusion or blood flow brings needed nutrients to meet the increased metabolic demands of the tissues.

Increased metabolic activities and blood flow raise the temperatures of the wound and surrounding tissues; higher vascularity results in higher tissue temperatures. A regular temperature pattern of healing can be determined by taking daily measurements of local skin temperatures following tissue injury. The measurements can be obtained using liquid crystal strips (see Chapter 4). If the zone of warmth does not decrease in width by the fourth postoperative day, the possibility of wound infection and disturbed healing exists.[50] This series of events is the physiologic basis for the classic signs and symptoms of inflammation: reddening of the surrounding tissues (or, in individuals with darkly pigmented skin, a purple or violaceous discoloration), pain, heat, and edema. The rise in tissue temperature provides an environment favorable for cell mitosis and enhanced cellular activities.[51,52]

Current of Injury

Endogenous biologic electrical currents are another component of healing. All body cells, including bone, skin, muscle, and nerve, possess injury currents. In the 1960s, Becker demonstrated the existence of a direct-current electrical system that controls tissue healing, which he named the *current of injury*.[53] The human body has an average charge on the skin surface of -23 mV.[54] Multiple experiments have demonstrated that a negative charge exists on the surface of the skin with respect to the deeper skin layers. This results in weak electrical potentials across the skin, creating a "skin battery" effect. The battery is driven by a sodium ion pump, initiated by the sodium ions passing through the cells of the epithelium via specific channels in the outer membrane. Once in the cell, they diffuse to other cells of the epithelium. Then, they are actively transported from these cells via electrogenic "pumps" located in all of the plasma membranes of the epithelium except the outer membrane. The result is the transport of NA$^+$ from the water bathing the epithelium to the internal body fluids, as well as generation of a potential of 50 mV across the epithelium.[55] If there is a break in the integrity of the skin, there is a net flow of ionic current through the low-resistance pathway of the injured cells and fluid exudate that line the wound; if the wound space becomes dry, the voltage gradient is eliminated.[38,39,37] Use of moist wound healing methods represents the clinical application of this theory.[56]

The ionic current flowing between the normal and injured tissue stimulates the repair process. During the repair process, there is a distinct pattern of current flow and polarity switching; when healing is complete, the current ceases. The bioelectric repair process is polarity-regulated, and cells of repair are attracted to the positive or negative poles, which is called *galvanotaxis*. Macrophages and neutrophils are attracted to the positive pole.[57,58]

Weiss et al[59] found reduced mast cell representation in wounds after positive polarity stimulation was seemingly inhibited by the positive pole, and suggested that as a mechanism for reduced fibrotic scarring. When the wound is inflamed or infected, neutrophils are attracted to the negative pole.[60] The negative pole also attracts fibroblasts,[61] which stimulate protein and DNA synthesis, and increase CA^{2+} uptake, fibroblast proliferation, and collagen synthesis.[62] Negative polarity facilitates migration of epidermal cells and is associated with suppression of bacterial growth.[63-67] It has been proposed that, in chronic wound healing, the current of injury fails to occur. One rationale for the use of exogenous electrical stimulation for wound healing is the theory that electrical stimulation mimics the current of injury and will restart or accelerate the repair process. Clearly, there are significant research data to support the concept that electrical current plays an important role in the cell physiology of wound healing (the use of electrical stimulation for wound healing is further explained in Chapter 22).

Fibroblasts

Fibroblasts respond to the chemotactic signals from growth factors released by platelets, macrophages, granulocytes, and keratinocytes. These growth factors stimulate fibroblast proliferation. Alignment of the fibroblast cells within the wound site during the inflammatory phase is an early indication of the strength that will eventually be imparted to the wound. Alignment of the fibroblasts along the wound axis and creation of cell-to-cell linkages aid in the contraction of the wound and the strength of the final scar tissue.[4] During the inflammatory phase, the fibroblasts differentiate into a specialized cell called the *myofibroblast*.

Inflammatory Phase in Chronic Wounds

Defining the critical attributes and benchmarks of chronic wound healing during the inflammatory phase is difficult because the differences between the normal acute wound healing process and that observed in chronic wound healing are only recently being recognized. Several factors have been identified as causing an interruption in the inflammatory phase of repair, including the stimulus for repair, inadequate perfusion and ischemia, free radicals and oxygen reperfusion injury, the balance of inflammatory cytokines and proteases, and the levels of growth factors present.[63]

Stimulus for Repair

One of the primary differences between acute and chronic wound healing is the stimulus for repair. In acute wounds, there is vascular disruption from the outside of the body to the inside of the body, initiating the hemostasis system and, thus, the wound healing cascade. In chronic wounds, the injury or stimulus for repair may come from within and can be gradual in onset. Suh and Hunt[34] used burn injuries as an example. After burn injury, the depth of the injury increases for 3–4 days as injured microvessels thrombose, slowing the sequence of repair and inflammation. These researchers suggest that the same mechanism may be responsible for the slower healing time in pressure wounds, in which the tissue dies back to where the blood flow is barely adequate to sustain life of the tissue. The vascular requirement for sustaining life may not be adequate for tissue healing.

Inadequate Perfusion and Ischemia

If the injury is caused by trauma, as with acute wounds, the condition and poor perfusion of the tissues in which the wounding occurs results in a slow and laborious course of healing.[29,64] Usually, chronic wounds are the result of underlying pathologic vascular insufficiency of some type and, because hemostasis is the stimulus for the wound healing cascade, the process is muted. Chronic wounds heal slowly; as the angiogenic stimuli become increasingly more removed from the initial wound edge, new blood vessels coalesce or drop out, resulting in a predominantly ischemic wound site.[64,29] In some cases, the ischemic tissue itself becomes an obstacle to healing because it is a barrier to angiogenesis.[29]

Inadequate perfusion often affects the healing of lower extremity wounds. Perfusion is affected by external as well as internal factors, including smoking, psychophysiological stress, and pain. All of these factors can increase the sympathetic tone of the vascular system and decrease tissue perfusion. Smoking also decreases microcirculation. Arterial ulcers are associated with macrovascular and microvascular disease that leads to tissue ischemia. Pressure ulcers are the consequence of compression of the base tissues and closure of the capillaries, also leading to ischemia. Diabetic foot ulcer healing is impaired because glucose inhibits proliferation of endothelial cells and there is a deficiency of angiogenic mediators. Infection also contributes to ischemia when neutrophils are deposited in the walls and lumen of the small vessels.[23]

Free Radicals and Oxygen Reperfusion Injury

Reactive oxygen species (ROS) is a collective term for oxygen-free radicals. Oxygen-free radicals take part in many metabolic processes, acting as part of the defense mechanism against infection. Free-radical species are generated during the process of oxidative phosphorylation and the electron transfer chain within the mitochondria. Normally, the free-radical species generated during these processes are used in a well-controlled manner; they serve useful functions in the cell metabolic processes, and do not escape to a significant degree from the mitochondria to other parts of the cell. Free radicals are chemically very reactive and can cause severe damage to many chemical compounds that are part of the cell, especially the lipids that make up the cell membrane. Enzymes within the cells usually catalyze the safe breakdown of oxygen-free radicals, thus protecting the cell from these compounds. In addition, tocopherol (a vitamin E component) in the lipid membrane and ascorbic acid (vitamin C) act as free-radical scavengers that can safely break down free radicals.[41]

Tissue ischemia triggers a series of events that includes the production of inflammatory mediators, mechanical capillary plugging by leukocytes, and oxygen metabolite formation, which leads to further tissue damage.[41,65] The wound healing process can begin with the entry of white blood cells into the damaged tissues from blood vessel disruption. However, even this process may be slowed. Once the injury is present, the leukocytes attempt to initiate the inflammatory stage of healing; however, many are unable to enter the wound tissue by passing through the capillary walls, due to increased rigidity of vessels and capillary plugging.[41] The leukocytes that do enter the wound tissue have difficulty performing bactericidal activities, due to decreased oxygen content in the wound bed from underlying tissue ischemia.[34,65] The mechanisms for capillary plugging by neutrophils and delayed entry into the wounded tissues are related to formation of oxygen-free radicals and reperfusion injury.

When blood flow is reestablished to the ischemic tissue, further damage to the tissues occurs from the disruption of the normal mechanisms of defense against injury from oxygen-free radicals. This is referred to as *reperfusion injury*. The mechanisms of reperfusion injury begin with ischemia and the conversion of the enzyme xanthine dehydrogenase to xanthine oxidase, which sets the scene for the generation of free radicals. When blood flow resumes to the ischemic site, the new availability of oxygen permits the production of large amounts of free radicals derived from xanthine oxidase.[41] These free radicals cause damage to the endothelium by lipid peroxidation. This overwhelms the normal free-radical defense mechanisms and leads to extensive injury of the endothelium, with ultimate destruction of the microcirculation. The consequence of these events is cell death.

In addition, an already difficult situation can be complicated by the escape of free radicals from the mitochondria.[41] Additional free radicals are released by neutrophils in response to activation of compounds released by endothelial cells during reperfusion. Both neutrophil activation and the availability of xanthine oxidase increase free radicals at the wound site, which results in increased endothelial damage.[24] When activated to produce free radicals, neutrophils lose their ability to deform to enter capillaries and adhere more easily to the endothelium, occluding capillaries.[41] Capillary occlusion and the neutrophils' inability to deform may explain the decreased levels of functioning neutrophils and macrophages present in chronic wounds.[41] Current research is focused on prevention of the most damaging features of ischemia and the resulting reperfusion injury. Clinicians need to be aware of the implications of new treatments that may be developed as a consequence of this research.

Epithelialization Phase

Benchmarks of the epithelialization phase are resurfacing of the wound and changes in the wound edges. Epithelialization, which protects the body from invasion by outside organisms, commences immediately after trauma and occurs concurrently with the other phases of wound healing (See Fig 2-5A and Table 2-4).[2] The process of resurfacing is the function of the keratinocytes (anatomy of the skin is explained in Chapter 4).

Keratinocytes

Keratinocytes make up the layers of the dermis and epidermis, as well as the linings of various body organs and dermal appendages (e.g., sebaceous glands, sweat glands, and hair follicles). Derived from epidermal stem cells that are located in the bulge area of the hair follicle, keratinocytes migrate from there into the basal layers of the epidermis and are capable of proliferating and differentiating to produce the epidermis. The epidermis is replenished by epidermal stem cells and progenitors arising from the keratinocytes. Keratinocytes synthesize insoluble proteins that cross-link to form a protective, cornified layer, the stratum corneum,

EPITHELIALIZATION PHASE

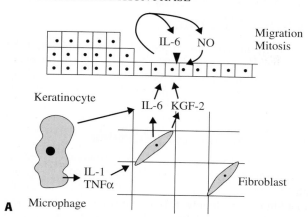

NEOANGIOGENESIS PHASE

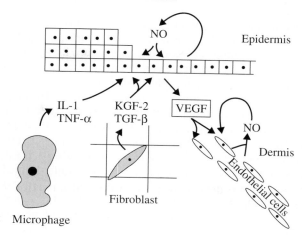

PROVISIONAL MATRIX PHASE

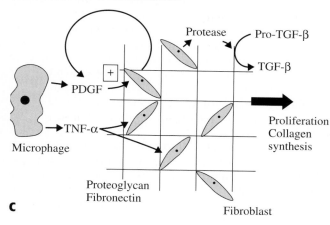

COLLAGEN MATRIX

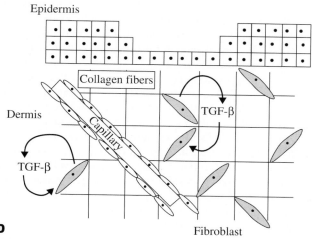

FIGURE 2-5 Overlapping Acute Wound Healing Phases. Early wound healing involves three overlapping phases: epithelialization, proliferation (neoangiogenesis and provisional matrix formation), and late proliferation.

A. 1) Epithelialization is directed by fibroblasts that express KGF-2 and IL-6, which direct keratinocytes to proliferate and migrate.
   2) Macrophages direct fibroblasts to express IL-1 and KGF-2.
   3) Later, keratinocytes self-express IL-6 and NO to perpetuate the process.

B. Keratinocytes direct neoangiogenesis at the wound edge by expression of VEGF. VEGF expression is upregulated in the presence of NO.

C. Macrophages initially direct provisional matrix formation (illustrated as a meshwork) by release of cytokines TNF-(and PDGF.

D. TGF-ß directs collagen matrix expression in later wound repair and collagen matrix formation. The illustrated meshwork is thicker, indicating deposition of collagen fibers over the provisional matrix network. Adapted with permission from Goldman, R. Growth factors and chronic wound healing: past, present and future. *Advances in Skin and Wound Care.* 2004;17(1).

which functions to keep pathogens out and water in.[66] Keratinocytes respond to signals from the macrophages, neutrophils, and the current of injury within hours after injury. As soon as the skin barrier is broken by a wound, the proin-

flammatory cytokine IL-1, which is stored in the cell, is released. The keratinocytes respond by entering an activation cycle.[66] Keratinocyte activation is transmitted to other neighboring cells (primarily fibroblasts), which in turn release multiple growth factors and initiate the wound healing cascade.[66]

Keratinocytes respond to signals from released growth factors by advancing in a sheet to resurface the open space. The leading edges of the advancing keratinocytes become phagocytic; they clean the debris, including clotted material, from their path. Cell sheets continue to migrate until the wound is covered and a new basement membrane is generated. Multilayered epithelial cells appear to migrate either as a moving sheet or in a complex "leapfrog" manner (also called *epiboly*)[18] A moist wound environment speeds the migration of keratinocytes toward one another from the edges of the wound and the dermal appendages.

Full-thickness skin loss injuries suffer loss of the dermal appendages, which are an important source of new keratinocytes. As a consequence, epithelial cells can migrate only from the wound edges. The advancing front of epidermal cells cannot cover a cavity, so they dive down and curl under at the edges. For example, full-thickness pressure wounds develop a buildup of epithelial cells at the wound edges, forming an epidermal ridge that curls under the edges and slows closure (as though the epithelial cells get tired of waiting for granulation tissue to fill in the wound defect, so they prematurely proliferate and migrate over the edge), as shown in *Color Plate 3*. The migration of epithelial cells is also oxygen-dependent; when there are low levels of oxygen, epithelial migration cannot debride the wound.

In surgical wounds that are sutured, epidermal migration begins within the first 24 hours. In healthy adults, it is usually complete within 48–72 hours postoperatively. In other wounds, skin trauma results in tissue degeneration, with broad, indistinct areas and edges that are difficult to see. This forms a shallow lesion, with more distinct, thin, separate edges. As tissue trauma progresses, the reaction intensifies, with a thickening and rolling inward of the epidermis. The edge is well-defined, sharply outlining the ulcer, with little or no evidence of new tissue growth. Repeated trauma and attempts to repair the wound edges result in fibrosis and scarring. The edges of the wound become indurated and firm,[67] which results in possible impairment of the migratory ability of the keratinocytes.[68]

Elasticity of the replaced epidermal layers affects the function of the skin as it overrides bony prominences and moving muscles or tendons. Once the wound has been resurfaced by epithelial cells, the cells begin the process of differentiating and maturing into type I collagen. The tensile strength of the remodeled skin will not exceed 70%–80% of the original. The quality of the scar tissue is an indication of the final outcome. The fact that closure has been achieved by epithelialization does not mean that the wound is fully healed. At this time, the new skin has a tensile strength of approximately 15% of normal. It must be treated carefully to avoid trauma, which can cause edema and infection, and can lead to reinflammation. Chronic inflammation causes a thickening of the skin and less elastic remodeled tissue.[69]

Epithelialization Phase in Chronic Wounds

As is true for interruption of the inflammatory phase, if the epithelialization process is interrupted or arrested, the result is a chronic wound. Causative factors that may arrest the epithelialization process by diminishing keratinocyte migration are discussed below.[63]

Diminished Keratinocyte Migration

Histological analysis of biopsies from chronic ulcers reveals a different appearance of the epidermis. It is mitotically active and hyperproliferative, however, these cells are unable to migrate. This is interpreted to mean that those keratinocytes at the chronic wound edge reveal only partially complete activation. The differentiation process is also incomplete and incapable of proceeding to full determination. One consequence is that cells grown from the nonhealing wound edge fail to respond to GFs and cytokines.[66]

Reepithelialization can be delayed in chronic wounds due to diminished keratinocyte migration from lack of a moist, oxygen-rich, nutritious tissue base, as is the case with debris-filled chronic wounds.[32] Decreased keratinocyte migration can also be due to a lack of stimulation, caused by failure of the appropriate cytokine to be released during the initial processes of the inflammatory phase of healing.[32,70]

Keratinocyte migration can be difficult in chronic wounds because of the rolled, thickened, nonproductive wound edge. Additionally, reepithelialization may be delayed until the wound has filled sufficiently with granulation tissue to provide a moist environment for keratinocyte migration. In wounds with significant tissue loss, epithelialization is slowed by virtue of the larger area requiring resurfacing. If wound contraction is impaired and the wound remains large, epithelialization is also affected because of the continued large area that must be resurfaced.

Research related to chronic wound healing in the epithelialization phase provides new insight into the process of epithelialization and identifies the weak links. Tissue engineers are taking advantage of the new science and developing products in the form of human skin equivalents that can be grown and combined with a patient's own keratinocytes to create skin that is reconstructed from an individual's own cells. The possibilities of growing customized skin replacements are huge.

Proliferative Phase

The proliferative phase of wound healing overlaps with and succeeds the inflammatory phase, beginning 3–5 days post injury and continuing for 3 weeks in wounds that heal by primary intention.[31] The goals of this healing phase are to fill in the wound defect with new tissue and restore the integrity of the skin. New tissue formation is the benchmark for the start of this phase. The processes involved in the proliferative phase are angiogenesis, collagen synthesis (extracellular matrix [ECM] formation), and wound contraction (see Fig. 2-5B and C.)[2]

In unwounded tissues, cells that are involved in repair are stationary; however, after wounding, they change into migrating cells. Migrating cells express specialized receptors called *integrins*.[22] Integrins serve a critical function in cell adhesion and signaling during wound healing, in which they are critical for reepithelialization and formation of granulation tissue because of their ability to recognize and respond to various components during formation of the ECM.[71]

As wound healing progresses from the inflammatory to proliferative phase, the synthesis of growth factors becomes the function of keratinocytes, fibroblasts, and endothelial cells. During this phase, GFs function to promote cell migration, proliferation, angiogenesis, and synthesis of the ECM components.[23] ECM is not a passive structure; rather, it is a complex environment in which interactions between the cells, GFs, and components of the ECM are critical to the successful progression of the healing process.

Angiogenesis

Restoration of vascular integrity is part of the proliferative phase; during this phase, angiogenesis, also known as *neovascularization*, takes place. Growth factors, primarily basic and acidic fibroblast growth factor (FGF) used as part of sentence defining role, TNF-α, EGF, and wound angiogenesis factor, play a major role in regulating angiogenesis.[18] Angiogenesis occurs as new capillary buds, arising from intact vessels adjacent to the wound, extend into the wound bed. As endothelial cells proliferate, grow into the wound space, and create capillaries, they connect to form a new network of vessels to fill the tissue defect. In the early stages of vessel growth, the vessels have loose junctions and gaps in the endothelial lining.[32] As a result, the initial capillaries are fragile and permeable, allowing passage of fluids from the intravascular to the extravascular space; thus, new tissue is often edematous in appearance.[32]

The thick capillary bed, which fills the matrix, supplies the nutrients and oxygen necessary for the wound to heal. To the naked eye, the capillary loops look like small granules, explaining the name *granulation tissue* (*see Color Plates 2, 4*, and *8*).[6] Granulation tissue first appears as pale pink buds; as it fills with new blood vessels, it becomes bright, "beefy," and red, as seen in *Color Plate 7*. The granulation begins at one side of the wound and "marches" across the wound bed, as shown in *Color Plates 8* and *9*. At this time, the granulation tissue is very fragile and unable to withstand any trauma. Trauma to the new tissue will cause bleeding that can reinitiate the inflammatory process and cause the laying down of excessive collagen; this results in poor elasticity and a less desirable scar. Protection of the new granulation tissue is very important. This tissue is structurally and functionally different from the tissues it replaces and will not differentiate into nerves, muscles, tendons, or other tissue.[4]

Fibroblasts

All connective tissue is composed of two major constituents: cells and extracellular material. The most important function of fibroblasts is the synthesis and deposition of the extracellular matrix (ECM) components—fibrous elements and ground substance. Fibrous connective tissue elements that give strength to the ECM include collagen, elastin, and reticulin. The nonfibrous portion includes ground substance that is primarily water, salts, and glycosaminoglycans (GAGs). GAGs are polysaccharides that contain amino acids, sugars, and glycoprotein (called *proteoglycans*). Types of GAGs found in skin include chondroitin sulfate, hyaluronic acid, and dermatan sulfate.[72] GAGs are hydrophilic substances, which causes them to attract large amounts of water and sodium. The turgor normally associated with connective tissue is a manifestation of the accumulation of fluid by the GAGs. Ground substance has semiliquid gel properties.[4]

Extracellular fibrous materials produced by fibroblasts include tropocollagen, a precursor to collagen. Tropocollagen is a soluble substance that is transformed into insoluble collagen by a process called *hydroxylation of proline*. This results in the polypeptide chain hydroxyproline (HoPro). In research, the measurement of HoPro is used to assess collagen deposition, with collagen estimated as seven times the value of HoPro.[73] In vitro and in vivo studies show that collagen hydroxylation, cross-linking, and deposition are proportional to the arterial partial pressure of oxygen.[33] Hydroxyproline deposition is proportional to wound tensile strength in rats.[33] Ferrous iron, a reducing agent (e.g., ascorbic acid), alpha ketoglutarate, and oxygen are required to achieve this transformation. Tropocollagen, thus transformed, is then combined with ground substance to form the scaffolding of repair.[4,72]

Elastin derives its name from its elastic properties. It is found in skin, lungs, blood vessels, and the bladder, and functions to maintain tissue shape.[3] A third fibrous connective tissue component is structural glycoprotein. Matrix proteins include fibronectin, integrins, collagen, and vitronectin; together, they form the basal lamina over which the keratinocytes migrate. Laminin is a component of the basement membrane that functions to inhibit keratinocyte migration.[23]

Matrix Formation

Granulation tissue fibroblasts, coated with a layer of fibronectin matrix, produce the matrix, or scaffolding, for collagen deposition that will support blood vessel growth by the endothelial cells.[33] The endothelial cells migrate and proliferate along the scaffolding, building new capillaries that are capable of providing oxygen and nourishment to the new collagen.[32,44] The optimal wound conditions for supporting fibroblast production of collagen and ground substances include the presence of cytokines (specifically, TGF-() produced by the macrophage and the fibroblast itself, and an acidic, low-oxygen wound bed. Fibroblasts secrete collagen until the wound is filled; then, collagen production ceases as the fibroblast is down-regulated. This process is called *fibroplasia*. Wound healing by fibroplasia requires that the wound be shaped like a boat or bowl to ensure that granulation tissue fills the base before the epithelial edges of the wound meet. Wounds that are not of this shape are at risk for premature surface healing, leaving a cavity under the skin that will subsequently break down (see Fig 2-5D).[2,74]

Cross-Linking of Collagen

Fibroblasts synthesize three polypeptide chains that coil to form a right-handed triple helix.[69] One of the polypeptide chains is HoPro. Now called *procollagen*, these spiraled chains are extruded from the fibroblast into the extracellular space. The next step is cleavage of the triple-helical molecule at specific terminal sites. Now the helix is referred to as a *tropocollagen molecule*. Tropocollagens then amass and convolve with other tropocollagen molecules to form a collagen fibril. Once the collagen fibrils are formed, they are very disorganized. This disorganization is why early scar tissue is weak with poor tensile strength. As the re-modelling phase of wound healing progresses the collagen is re-modeled into ordered, structured formations which increase the tensile strength of the scar tissue. The number of collagen filaments does not give the collagen matrix durability or tensile strength; rather, tensile strength depends on the microscopic welding, or bonding, of one filament to another. The sites at which these bonds occur are called *cross-links*. Intermolecular bonds are the major force holding the tropocollagen molecules together. The greater the number of these bonds, the greater the strength of the collagen filament. In an anoxic wound, cross-linking is inhibited.

Tropocollagen polymerizes (joins with many small particles to create a large molecule) to form various types of collagen.[3] Types I and III collagen are found in the dermis and are involved with wound healing. New tissue growth in the wound follows a pattern of fibronectin secretion, type III collagen production, and, lastly, type I collagen.[32, 44] The early immature type III collagen is gradually replaced with the normal adult type I collagen throughout the proliferation phase of healing and continuing through the remodeling phase of healing.

Type III collagen fibrils are small (40–60 nm), whereas type I collagen fibrils have a larger diameter (100–500 nm). The large-diameter fibers have less elasticity than do the small-diameter fibers. Approximately 80% of dermal collagen is type I, and these fibers provide the tensile strength to the tissue. The type III collagen fibers help the tissue withstand a load over time, which is referred to as *creep resistance*. The proportion of large to small fibrils changes over the life span, with type III gradually replaced by type I. The proportion of large-diameter to small-diameter fibrils determines the dermal tensile strength.[72]

Normally, collagen fibers are organized and arranged in parallel lines along mechanical stress points, giving tissue strength.[32] Type I collagen is the major component of normal adult dermis, but type III collagen is the predominant type of collagen synthesized in the wound.[44] Type III collagen is poorly cross-linked and not aligned in the same manner as type I collagen; as such, it provides minimal tensile strength to the new tissue.[32]

At this point, about 3 weeks after wounding, the greatest mass of collagen assembled by the tensile strength is roughly only 15% of normal. This new scar will not tolerate mobilization or rough handling, both of which will ultimately lead to creation of a new wound and further scarring.[69] Wound dehiscence and evisceration occur most frequently during this phase.[3]

Myofibroblasts and Contraction

Myofibroblasts contain an actin and myosin contractile system similar to that found in smooth muscle cells,[33] which allows them to contract and extend. The myofibroblast connects itself to the wound skin margins and pulls the epidermal layer inward. The myofibroblast ring forms what has been described as a "picture frame" beneath the skin of the contracting wound. The contracting forces start out equal in all wounds, but the shape of the "picture frame" predicts the resultant speed of contraction. Linear wounds contract rapidly, square and rectangular wounds contract at a moderate pace, and circular wounds contract slowly. One characteristic of pressure ulcers is that they take on a circular shape, which is an indicator that they will contract slowly.[69] Wound contraction is manifested by a change in wound shape and reduction in the open area of the wound. This occurs at the final stage of wound repair.

Myofibroblast function is mediated by growth factors. Wounds that heal by primary intention and partial-thickness wounds heal with very little wound contraction. However, in full-thickness wounds, contraction can account for up to a 40% decrease in wound size.[32,70] For successful healing, contraction needs to be balanced. A diminished level of contraction leads to delayed healing, with possible excess bleeding and infection. Conversely, excess contraction can lead to loss of function from tissue contractures.[32]

Wound contraction pulls the wound edges together for the purpose of closing the wound. In effect, this reduces the open area and, if successful, results in a smaller wound, with less need for repair by scar formation. Wound contraction can be extremely beneficial in the closure of wounds in areas such as the buttocks and trochanter, but it can be harmful in areas such as the hand and around the neck and face, where it can cause disfigurement and excessive scarring.

Rapid, uncontrolled wound contraction in these areas must be avoided. Tissue that draws together too tightly can cause deformity of the repaired scar and impairment of tissue function. Skin grafting is used to reduce contraction in undesirable locations. The thickness of the skin graft influences the degree of contraction suppression. Pressure garments are another method of controlling wound contraction (see Chapter 14).

Oxygen and nutrition demands remain very high to support the cells of repair (i.e., fibroblasts, myofibroblasts, endothelial cells, and epidermal cells), which reproduce at a rapid rate to create the collagen matrix. Nutrients, including zinc, iron, copper, vitamin C, and oxygen, are essential for fibroblast synthesis of the collagen matrix. The macrophages and neutrophils work to control infection as long as the wound remains open. The combination of these activities raises tissue temperatures. The wound needs warmth at this time to promote cellular division and manage infection.

RESEARCH WISDOM

Best Time to Apply Skin Grafts

Split-thickness skin grafts suppress contraction by 31%, and full-thickness skin grafts diminish contraction by 55%. The best time for application of skin grafts is during the inflammatory phase, before contraction begins.[69]

Proliferative Phase in Chronic Wounds

Several differences exist for the chronic wound in the proliferative phase.[63] Each of these processes and differences will be described, including:

- Fibroblast senescence
- Fibronectin composition
- Chronic wound fluid-inhibiting factors
- "Dead space" inhibition and prolongation of healing, stalling, or plateauing of healing
- Protracted inflammatory and proliferative responses
- Delayed reepithelialization, due to size of the "wound gap" or nonproductive wound edges

Fibroblast Senescence

Tissue samples biopsied from human pressure ulcers shows that there is variation in fibroblast response to GF, synthesis of GF, and deposition of ECM. Staining techniques were used that can identify senescent cells and differentiate them from necrotic or apoptotic cells. Vandeberge et al studied fibroblast senescence in pressure ulcers.[75] For this purpose, the study hypothesis defined cell populations as senescent when they failed to undergo 0.5 doubling after a one-week period.[75]

Findings from the research included: [75]

1. Fibroblast populations grown from normal, unulcerated skin undergo more doublings than those from the ulcer margin or wound bed before becoming senescent
2. Small fibroblasts have more doubling compared with large fibroblasts
3. Fibroblasts from patients of all ages become senescent after fewer population doublings than fibroblasts from adjacent normal skin
4. As fibroblast cell populations age, the number of senescent cells appear to increase, while cells in the proliferating pool decrease
5. Myofibroblasts appear to attempt wound contraction, but their efforts may be compromised by cellular senescence and/or necrosis

The literature review associated with this study pointed out that diabetic patients show premature fibroblast senescence and the decreased ability to divide; senescent fibroblasts lose their ability to produce collagen, instead producing high levels of procollagen and low levels of TIMPs; and fibronectin from senescent fibroblasts is structurally different from the fibronectin isolated from early passage cells and is not able to bind to collagen.[75] Cellular ineffectiveness is apparent from these studies, but the mechanisms responsible for this ineffectiveness are still unknown and under investigation.

Fibronectin Composition

Wysocki demonstrated differences in the composition of fibronectin (critical to the laying down of collagen) in chronic wounds, as compared with acute wounds.[76] The fibronectin in chronic wounds was partially degraded, whereas it remained intact in acute wounds. The small fibronectin fragments found in chronic wounds may perpetuate the activity of matrix proteases and inhibit healing.[77] Indeed, the excess activity of proteases, which breaks down connective tissue faster than it is formed and destroys important polypeptide-signaling molecules that coordinate healing, may play a role in persistent nonhealing wounds.[78]

Parks[79] has shown that chronic wounds exhibit production of two stromelysin (metalloproteinases that do not lyse collagen), which may represent the unregulated production of proteinase that contributes to the inability of some chronic wounds to heal.

Chronic Wound Fluid

The desire to learn more about the wound microenvironment has led researchers to look at wound fluid as a reflection of the microenvironment from which it was collected. Human studies of wound fluids are complicated by the inability to carefully control the variables related to the wound, the patient, and the way wound fluids are collected, leading to varied results. However, considerable efforts have been made by investigators to study fluid from both acute and chronic wounds.

It is fairly well-accepted that fluid from acute wounds is mitogenic for wound-associated cells, and fluid collected from chronic wounds is inhibitory to these cells of regeneration.[80,81] Analysis and study of wound fluid is providing important insight into the healing of chronic wounds. It has been suggested that chronic wound fluid analysis could be used to identify potential biomarkers of wound chronicity, leading to new treatment strategies and possibly customized treatment based on the identified biomarkers. This concept has already been applied to secreted biofluids of other chronic inflammatory conditions such as osteoarthritis and periodontal disease to determine disease and metabolic activity.[82]

Chronic wound fluid has been shown to inhibit proliferation of endothelial cells, keratinocytes, fibroblasts, and cell adhesion.[83,84] In nonhealing wounds, proinflammatory cytokines and proteases are present at high levels compared to the relatively low levels and narrower range of GFs present in healing wounds. When there is an increase in proinflammatory cytokines, there is an accompanying elevation of proteases production. This may be due to the presence of bacteria and their endotoxins, as well as the presence of platelet degranulation products.[22]

Recently the focus of chronic wound fluid research has been on the proinflammatory cytokines and proteases, but there is also interest in the potential of ECM components in wound fluid as biomarkers of wound healing pathology.[82]

Protracted Inflammatory and Proliferative Responses

Bennett and Schultz[85] suggested that, in chronic wounds, repeated trauma and infection increase the presence of proinflammatory cytokines and tissue inhibitors or metalloproteinases, and lower the level of growth factors. Other studies have shown lower levels of PDGF, bFGF, EGF, and TGF-β in chronic pressure sores, compared with acute wounds.[86,87] Yager et al reported elevated levels of matrix metalloproteinases and imbalance between the levels of matrix metalloproteinases and their inhibitors in the fluids of pressure ulcers, which may impede the healing of these wounds.[88] Initiation of healing following an intervention is accompanied by reduced levels of MMPs and an increase in TIMP activities.[82] The inhibitory effect of chronic wound fluid on fibroblasts was abolished by heating the wound fluid to 100°C, and heating it to 38°C had a significant effect.[81]

Dead Space or Large Tissue Gap

Full-thickness pressure ulcers often present with a "dead space" or "tissue gap," which prolongs proliferation because of the larger tissue defect that needs to be filled with new connective tissue and blood vessels.[34] Prolongation of the proliferative phase of healing can be observed in many chronic wounds. In these cases, the wound progresses to a certain point of new tissue growth and then "stalls" or "plateaus," with no further evidence of proliferation. The cessation of proliferation may be related to inadequate substrates necessary for new tissue growth, such as protein, vitamin C, and zinc.[29] Inadequate substrate availability may

be due to increased levels of bacteria in the wound environment or continued lysis of new growth faster than new material can be synthesized. The increased bacteria levels may compete with healthy cells for the substrates necessary for healing and thus prevent further tissue growth.[34]

Siddiqui and colleagues[89] suggested an alternate cause of decreased tissue proliferation. Using an in vitro system, their study demonstrated decreased collagen production and fibroblast proliferation in a chronically hypoxic wound environment, suggesting that long-term wound hypoxia exerts a negative influence on tissue proliferation.

Remodeling Phase

The final phase of wound healing is the remodeling phase, which begins as granulation tissue forms in the wound site during the proliferative phase and continues for 1–2 years postinjury until it reaches maturation.[32,90] During the remodeling phase, scar tissue is rebuilt to provide for increased tensile strength. The tensile strength increases from the 15%–20% strength associated with the initial scar tissue up to 80% of the original preinjury tissues by the end of the remodeling phase.[70,69] Remodeling involves a delicate equilibrium between collagen synthesis and lysis.

The remodeling phase shows most clearly the overlapping of all of the phases of wound healing. Typically, it is described as the end of the proliferative phase, which is about 3 weeks postinjury. Actually, collagen matrix formation and remodeling begin concurrently with the formation of granulation tissue. Unlike the other phases, no cell is predominant during remodeling.[3] Regulation of the remodeling process is the function of growth factors, primarily TGF-β, PDGF, and FGF, which are stimulated during tissue injury and repair by specific enzymes called *collagenases*. Collagenases are metalloproteinases (MMPs), which are proteolytic enzymes that degrade proteins and ECM macromolecules (i.e., GAGs).[18]

Matrix Remodeling

ECM and collagen deposition continuously and gradually changes from the time it is initially produced in the wound bed, and this process continues even after tissue integrity is restored.[32] Type III collagen, originally produced by the fibroblast, is gradually lysed by tissue collagenases, and type I collagen is produced to replace the lost tissues. The lysis of old collagen and production of new collagen lead to a change in the orientation of the scar tissue. The new type I collagen fibrils are laid down parallel to the lines of tension in the wound in an organized fashion, with strong crosslinking and bundle construction.[32] During this phase, the highly vascular and cellular granulation scar tissue is gradually replaced with less vascular and less cellular tissues.[34] Fibronectin and hyaluronic acid (part of the ECM ground substance), along with type III collagen, are reduced, and proteoglycans are deposited with the new type I collagen, increasing the wound's resilience to deformation.[32] Lysis of old collagen is accomplished by the action of bacterial collagenase, lysosomal proteases, and tissue collagenase synthesized by macrophages, epidermal cells, and fibroblasts.[32,70]

Matrix Metalloproteinases and Collagen Lysis or Degradation

Matrix metalloproteinases (MMPs) are a family of protein-degrading enzymes that play a key role in the remodelling of the ECM components through degradation of the ECM. Numerous proteases have been implicated in the proteolytic degradation of the ECM, most prominent among which are members of the MMP family. MMPs have been divided into collagenases, gelatinases, stromelysins, and matrilysins.[91]

Collagenase and other proteolytic enzymes are produced during the inflammatory phase and throughout the proliferative phase as regulators of fibroplasia. Proteolytic enzymes are proteases that degrade proteins (e.g., collagen). Collagenase can cleave, or break, the cross-linkage of the tropocollagen molecules, aiding in its reabsorption during periods of connective tissue growth or repair.[7] In a healthy wound, collagenase regulates the balance between synthesis and lysis of collagen. It is this ability to break down collagen that makes collagenase useful as a debriding agent. Breaking of the cross-linkage makes the tropocollagen molecule soluble so that it can be excreted from the body. The balance between collagen synthesis and collagen lysis is delicate, with a goal that one process should not exceed the other. However, as the wound matures during remodeling, collagen lysis increases. The organization of collagen fibers as they are laid down by the fibroblasts is part of this regulatory process; better organization produces a better functional outcome of more elastic, smoother, and stronger fibers for the repaired scar tissues.

Scar Formation

Clinical manifestations of the remodeling phase of healing include changes in the appearance of scar tissue. As collagen synthesis and degradation proceed, the vascularity and cellularity of the scar tissue diminish, with loss in scar tissue mass and obvious changes in the visual appearance of the wound site. The scar changes from bright red or pink to a silvery gray or white color, and the site becomes less bulky and flattens over time until a normotrophic scar is achieved.[34,90] Additionally, the scar tissue becomes more flexible as it matures.[34]

As long as the scar exhibits a rosier appearance than normal, remodeling or maturation of the immature scar is underway.[69] This process is an attempt by the scar to blend in, both cosmetically and functionally. An example is a surgical scar on the incision line. Initially it is bright red; then, over time, it blanches and conforms to the body contours. The entire process of wound remodeling until maturation takes from 3 weeks to 2 years postinjury.[69] Chapter 14 explains normal scar formation processes, complications, and

methods of managing scar formation for the most cosmetic and functional outcomes.

Remodeling Phase in Chronic Wounds

In chronic wounds, there appear to be similar mechanisms of dysregulation in collagen synthesis and degradation that produce hypertrophic scarring and hypergranulation. Hypergranulation creates a humping of the tissue, which inhibits the epidermal cell movements against gravity to cover and resurface the wound (see *Color Plate 23*). The reasons for this dysregulation are being investigated, and some research findings are described below. Hypertrophic scarring and keloid management are discussed in Chapter 14. *Color Plates 48-51* are photographs of hyptertrophic and keloid scars.

If collagen synthesis is impeded, the tensile strength of the wound is impaired, and the wound can break down or dehisce (reopen) after integrity has been restored. If collagen lysis is impaired, collagen is allowed to proliferate with no checks, and hypertrophy and keloid formation can result.[92,93] When both collagen synthesis and lysis are out of balance, they never seem to reach equilibrium; the result is proliferative scarring or excessive healing, and the repair process continues without an apparent "turn-off switch."[63] Imbalances are being traced back to the initial inflammatory phase of healing. Evidence indicates that MMP-8, a collagenase produced by neutrophils, experiences high activity during this phase, which may account for chronicity of the wound.[18] Evidence also implicates the imbalance of TFG-β isoforms.

Recent research has identified that there are several isoforms of TGF-β. Type 1 and 2 display similar fibrogenic behavior in vivo, but Type 3 plays an antagonistic, antifibrotic role that prevents scarring. In uncomplicated healing, TGFβ-1 is expressed early during the inflammatory phase. TGFβ-1 levels drop and TGFβ-3 levels rise during the late proliferative phase; the ratio of this activity is an important determinant of the progress of wound healing and formation of fibrotic scarring and hypergranulation tissue. In addition to GFs, their corresponding receptors are also expressed. These receptors, along with the corresponding TGF-β isoforms, decrease in density during granulation tissue remodeling when healing is well-regulated. However, excessive scarring is associated with dysregulation and the failure to eliminate TGF-β receptors, which are expressed by overactive fibroblasts during the remodeling phase. The result is persistent overproduction of matrix proteins and fibrosis.[14,15]

In the veterinary community, there has been significant interest in exuberant granulation because it is a frequent complication of wound healing on the legs of horses. The terms used to describe *hypergranulation* include *exuberant granulation or "proud flesh,"* and the three are used synonymously. Predisposing factors for hypergranulation in horses include tissue hypoperfusion, infection, trauma, and bandaging of wounds.[94,95,96,97]

In horses, the initial inflammatory reaction tends to be protracted, and this leads to the perseverance of TGFβ-1 well into the proliferative phase; this is suggested as the predisposing factor that leads to production of excessive granulation tissue. One study of horses reported findings that TGFβ-1 and TGFβ-3 expression in normal and exuberant wound healing are different. The latter tend to have higher concentrations of fibrogenic TGFβ-1 and lower concentrations of antifibrotic, antiscarring TGFβ-3. However, the differences were not statistically significant. Based on the study results, the authors suggest that production of exuberant granulation is related to bandaging of the wound, which is associated with higher concentration of fibrogenic TGFβ-1 and decreased expression of antifibrotic TGFβ-3. Healing appeared normal in wounds in which the TGFβ-3 concentrations were higher.[96]

Collagen synthesis is oxygen-dependent, but collagen lysis is not. Too much oxygen is believed to cause hypertrophy of the granulation tissues. Berry reported the sequence of events leading to exuberant granulation in horses under a moisture-retentive dressing as a moist wound bed that becomes purulent, followed by production of exuberant granulation tissue. The rationale for the exuberant granulation tissue was explained as: 1) bandaging decreases the ambient oxygen-tension gradient, which promotes angiogenesis and fibroplasia; and 2) the accumulation of exudate promotes persistent inflammation and increased granulation tissue formation.[95] This explanation is contrary to other research.

Different dressing types appear to be related to hypergranulation formation in horses.[98] Silicone gel dressings were found to prevent hypergranulation and improve tissue quality, possibly related to: 1) microvessel occlusion, which occurs significantly more often in wounds that were dressed with silicone; 2) gradual decrease in oxygen tension in the tissue until the point of anoxia, when fibroblasts no longer function adequately and undergo apoptosis, and the ratio of collagen synthesis to degradation is altered in favor of degradation minimizing fibrosis; 3) diminished expression of mutant p53, an indirect inhibitor of apoptosis also found in these wounds. In horses, exuberant granulation typically does not go on to wound closure.[29]

It is thought that the biochemistry is similar in humans, but human wounds close with hypertrophic scarring.[28] Dressing types are also reported to affect hypergranulation tissue development in humans. A report of clinical cases found an association between the use of occlusive dressings and hypergranulation.[99] A uncontrolled clinical trial found that use of a polyurethane foam dressing reduced hypergranulation tissue height by 2 mm of granulation tissue from initial measurements to measurements taken two weeks later, which was highly significant.[100]

Wound dressings, as described above, appear to play a significant role in exuberant granulation tissue formation and hypertrophic scarring related to prolonged contact of the wound tissue with wound fluid. Acute wounds benefit from contact with acute wound fluid which provides a moist environment for cell migration. Chronic wound fluid, on the other hand, contains destructive elements. Therefore, allowing wounds to bathe in chronic wound fluid such as occurs under an occlusive dressing, is no longer recommended as a method of moist wound healing, because of the potential for defective remodeling, as described.

New dressing materials are being developed with the purpose of controlling, removing negative elements from, and rebalancing the wound microenvironment to bias it toward a healing trajectory. For example, oxidized regenerated cellulose/collagen has demonstrated the ability to modify and rebalance the chronic wound environment by reducing the activity of proteases (see Chapter 11).

Acute wound healing has been studied extensively, and information learned over time has been extrapolated and applied to chronic wound healing based on the assumption that chronic wound healing is "abnormal." Research has identified chronic wound healing as a different process in many ways, as described in this chapter. The current thinking is that imbalances exist in the molecular environment of healing and nonhealing wounds. When the scales are tipped toward low levels of inflammatory cytokines and proteases, and mitotically competent cells are present, the balance will produce high mitogenic activity and healing. When high levels of inflammatory cytokines and proteases are present along with senescent cells, there is low mitogenic activity, and the result is a chronic wound.[23] Understanding the differences between acute and chronic wound healing is a work in progress; as scientists demonstrate new findings, this information is being used to customize treatment interventions. Other chapters in this book are devoted to those interventions.

Factors Affecting Wound Healing

A chronic wound is defined as one that deviates from the expected sequence of repair in terms of time, appearance, and response to aggressive and appropriate treatment.[101] When the response to wounding does not conform to the described cycle of wound recovery after a period of 2–4 weeks, the wound may have become "stuck" and unable to progress through the phases of healing without intervention.

The typical way to diagnose chronic wounds is to use the pathophysiology associated with ulcers. For example, there are ischemic arterial ulcers, diabetic ulcers (both vascular and neuropathic), pressure ulcers, vasculitic ulcers, venous ulcers, and rheumatoid ulcers, all of which are considered chronic wounds (Exhibit 2-1). Skin integrity and wound healing physiology are disrupted by the underlying pathology (intrinsic factors), environmental influences (extrinsic factors), and inappropriate management (iatrogenic factors), which influence whether the wound will go on to heal or become chronic or refractory. The following sections describe these factors that affect wound healing (Table 2-5). Chapter 5 describes how to use a wound healing trajectory to mon-

EXHIBIT 2-1   Examples of Chronic Wounds

- Ischemic arterial ulcers
- Diabetic vascular and neuropathic ulcers
- Venous ulcers
- Vasculitic ulcers
- Rheumatoid ulcers
- Pressure ulcers

itor timeliness of healing, and Chapter 12 discusses refractory wounds.

Health-care professionals who manage patients with wounds need to consider not only the wound but the whole patient, including his or her internal and external environment, for factors that contribute to poor healing response. Early identification of factors that contribute to impaired wound healing helps clinicians triage cases, reduces variability in cost and care, and improves the prognosis and outcomes for planned interventions.

Intrinsic Factors

Intrinsic factors are related to the patient's medical status and physiologic properties that can affect skin integrity and/or healing. Intrinsic factors include age, chronic disease, perfusion and oxygenation, immunosuppression, and neurologically impaired skin.

Age

Inflammation, cell migration, proliferation, and maturation responses slow with aging.[102,103] A major skin change that occurs with aging is thinning of the epidermis, which increases the risk of injury from shearing and friction, resulting in ulceration and skin tears. The skin also loses its impenetrability to substances in the environment, so irritants and certain drugs are more readily absorbed. The reproductive function of epidermal and fibroblast cells diminishes with age, and replacement is slowed. Elastin fibers are lost, and the skin becomes less elastic. The dermis atrophies, which slows wound contraction and increases the risk of wound dehiscence.[104] Wound dehiscence is two to three times higher in patients over age 60, yet, as Eaglstein[103] notes, the causative factors may be infection, inadequate protein intake, and other medical complications-not solely age. There is diminished vascularity of the dermis.[104]

Aging and chronic disease states often go together, and both delay repair processes; this is due to delayed cellular response to the injury stimulus, delayed collagen deposition, and decreased tensile strength in the remodeled tissue. The regeneration process can be diminished as a result of impaired circulatory function. Aging alone is not a major factor in chronic wound healing. Research now demonstrates that healing is only slightly retarded in elderly individuals without chronic disease states, compared with that of a young population.[105] Patient age did not significantly affect healing times for leg ulcers associated with venous

Table 2-5   Factors Affecting Wound Healing

Intrinsic Related to Medical Status	Extrinsic Related to Environment	Iatrogenic Related to Wound Management
Age	Medications	Local ischemia
Chronic Disease	Nutrition	Inappropriate wound care
Perfusion and oxygenation	Irradiation and chemotherapy	Trauma
Immunosuppression	Psychophysiologic stress	Wound extent and duration
Neurologically impaired skin	Wound bioburden and infection	

insufficiency[106] or for neuropathic foot ulcers using total contact casting.[107] However, age appears to affect the risk for skin breakdown in individuals who are older than 85 years; this group demonstrated a 30% risk of developing pressure ulcers.[108] Because chronic conditions are more common in older adults, age is at least a marker for conditions that predispose to chronic wounds, and it is typically identified as a cofactor in impaired healing.[109]

Chronic Disease

Chronic diseases of all kinds—renal, pulmonary, and other systemic diseases—affect the cardiopulmonary system and oxygen-transport pathway that delivers oxygen from the lungs to the tissues and removes carbon dioxide. The cardiopulmonary system is affected by hematologic, neuromuscular, musculoskeletal, endocrine, and immunologic conditions.[110] For example, depending on the location or level of a neuromuscular lesion, breathing functions can be compromised. This can contribute to reduced respiratory muscle function, which affects lung volumes, flow rates, inspiratory and expiratory lung functions, and the delivery of oxygen to and removal of carbon dioxide from the tissues that are required for healing. Impaired cardiopulmonary function affects mobility and is considered a risk factor for skin ulceration. In this case, the nurse and physical therapist must optimize the patient's positioning and mobility to compensate for the effects of chronic disease on the body.

Patients with diabetes are at risk for poor wound healing, due to the effects of high blood glucose levels on leukocyte function, with increased risk of infection.[111] The microvascular and neuropathic components of diabetes also place these patients at increased susceptibility to impaired healing.[112] In cases of immune suppression, such as is common in patients who have diabetes, cancer, human immunodeficiency virus (HIV) infection, and acquired immune deficiency syndrome, or those who are undergoing immunosuppressive therapy, the body lacks the ability to produce an inflammation phase, which is the body's immune response to injury. As described, the inflammatory response sets off the cascade of repair. Absence or impairment of inflammation at the onset of trauma will impair the healing cascade through all phases of healing.[113]

Perfusion and Oxygenation

All phases of wound healing require adequate perfusion, and the lack of perfusion is a barrier to healing. Oxygen is carried in the blood and dissolved in the plasma by red blood cells that are bound to hemoglobin. In anemia, there is reduced hemoglobin and reduced oxygen-carrying capacity of the blood. However, research data suggest that anemia does not impair wound healing when there is adequate *perfusion* and *blood volume*.[114]

Hypovolemia, the lack of adequate intravascular volume, has been shown to impair healing because there is insufficient volume to transport oxygen and nutrients to the tissues and remove waste products.[114] Prolonged hypovolemia impairs collagen production and diminishes leukocyte activities.[105] There are no external signs of mild hypovolemia; its diagnosis is made by measuring the transcutaneous partial pressure of oxygen in the blood. Hypovolemia should be considered in situations that are common to the chronic wound population, such as the use of diuretics, renal dialysis, and blood loss.

Fluid administration can correct hypovolemia, but care must be taken to maximize intravascular volume without causing fluid overload.[105] Hartmann and colleagues[115] reported that, according to measurements of subcutaneous oxygen tension, fluid replacement improved accumulation of collagen in healing wounds by day 7 in 29 patients after major abdominal surgery ($p < .05$).[115] Fluid replacement improves tissue perfusion,[116] although overhydration can lead to perfusion difficulties related to edema. Thus, wounded patients with fluid volume imbalance may be at risk for impaired healing.

Theories and research abound concerning why there is sometimes a failure to respond to the signals of injury. One theory of the etiology of venous ulcer chronicity attributes the problem to a dysfunctional fibrinolytic system.[117] According to this theory, lipodermatosclerosis is part of the pathogenesis of venous ulcers that impairs the progression of the inflammatory phase to the proliferative phase. Other theories that have been proposed to explain the effects of venous disease on wound healing include the trapping of cytokines in the tissues,[118] the anticirculatory effects of fibrin cuff formation at dermal vessels,[119] and free radicals.[41] Free radicals are also implicated in the development of leg ulcers, in which the protective mechanisms become deranged during ischemia and overwhelmed after reperfusion by the extent of free-radical production.[41]

Chronic venous hypertension leads to leukocyte accumulation in the skin and other tissues of the leg. There is strong evidence that neutrophils and monocytes initiate the damage that eventually leads to skin ulceration.[41] In addition to oxygen-free radicals, these cells replace proteolytic enzymes and inflammatory cytokines that lead to skin breakdown.[41] Oxygen-free-radical activity list of terms is elevated in individuals with diabetes mellitus and has been implicated in the

etiology of vascular complications.[41] Arterial ulcers result from severe ischemia and the mechanisms of ischemic reperfusion injury. Diabetes also leads to increased susceptibility to peripheral arterial atheroma, which leads to stenosis and occlusion that can cause ischemia and ulceration.[41]

Immunosuppression

Wound healing is also delayed in patients with HIV or cancer, in those undergoing immunosuppressive therapy, and in severely malnourished individuals.[120] Immunosuppression retards the inflammatory response, prevents any inflammatory response, and affects all phases of wound recovery.[113]

Neurologically Impaired Skin

Peripheral neuropathy is a common complication of chronic diabetes and alcoholism. There are three types of neuropathy: sensory, motor, and autonomic. Neuropathy affects the autonomic nervous system function of the sweat and sebaceous glands located in the skin, resulting in their impairment. When this function is impaired in the feet, the skin becomes dry and cracked, providing a portal of entry for infection. The skin acidity also changes, resulting in impairment of the ability to control surface bacteria. Patients with diabetes also have an impaired immune system that is simply unable to generate an inflammatory phase of repair and overcome infection. Combined, all of these functional impairments result in a chronically infected wound in patients with diabetes. Chapter 19 describes the examinations for testing for polyneuropathy, including photos of the consequences of the three types of impairment.

The central nervous system neuropathy associated with spinal cord injury (SCI) results in alteration of the functions of the autonomic nervous, motor, and sensory systems. If the lesion is above the 6th thoracic level, autonomic nervous system function is impaired in the early stages postinjury, and the individual is often unable to maintain a constant body temperature. This is due to loss of the ability to dissipate and retain heat from the interior of the body to the periphery via vasomotor responses to heating. Reflex sweating is also lost with injury at these levels, which places the individual with a SCI at risk for overheating.[121] Another complication of SCI is loss of vasomotor tone; this leads to dilation of the veins of the lower extremity, with resultant peripheral edema and frequent deep vein thrombosis.[122]

Neurologically impaired skin undergoes metabolic changes that can take 3–5 years to stabilize following injury.[121] These changes include:

1. An immediate, significant, and rapid increase in the rate of collagen catabolism
2. Decreased enzyme activity related to defective collagen biosynthesis in the skin below the level of injury; the increased rate of catabolism of collagen, coupled with defective collagen biosynthesis, produces fragile skin that is more subject to skin breakdown
3. Decrease in proportion of type I to type III collagen in the skin below the level of injury; properties of type III

collagen include thinner, weaker, more widely spaced fibrils that contribute to the fragility of the neurologically impaired skin

4. Decrease in density of adrenergic receptors in skin below the level of injury; this could be the cause of abnormal vascular reactions

5. Large increase in GAGs excreted in the urine, robbing the skin of the elasticity necessary to adapt to mechanical insults

Mechanical factors also affect skin integrity in individuals with SCIs. Muscle atrophy caused by paralysis reduces muscle bulk over bony prominences and exposes the skin covering them to mechanical forces; insensate skin cannot provide signals of impending damage. The combination of biochemical and mechanical changes increases the vulnerability of the skin to ulceration[121] and negatively affects ulcer healing.

Extrinsic Factors

Extrinsic factors come from sources in the environment that affect the body or wound, such as medications, nutrition, irradiation and chemotherapy, psychophysiologic stress, and wound bioburden and infection.

Medications

Many patients with chronic wounds have multiple comorbidities; they may be under treatment with anticoagulation (e.g., warfarin or heparin), antiplatelet aggregation (e.g., clopidogrel, aspirin, or other salicylates), or nonaspirin nonsteroidal anti-inflammatory (e.g., ibuprofen or cyclooxygenase [COX-2] inhibitors) medications. All of these drugs interfere with platelet activation.[123] Nonaspirin nonsteroidal anti-inflammatory drugs (NSAIDs), for example, inhibit angiogenesis through direct effect on endothelial cells, which in turn have deleterious effects on mitogenic activity of bFGF on fibroblasts. This results in decreased collagen production in the proliferative/angiogenic phase.[124] NSAIDs may be beneficial for their anti-inflammatory properties to control inflammation during the resolution of this phase. Early in the inflammatory phase, however, these drugs can have negative effects on progress of the proliferative phase when angiogenesis is occurring,[125] because they alter the balance of antiangiogenic and proangiogenic factors found in wound serum.

The ratio of proliferation to apoptosis is diminished with both classic NSAIDs and COX-2.[25] The effects of NSAIDs and aspirin on platelets is reversible, and the degree of intensity and duration of inhibition of platelet function by NSAIDs is dose-dependent. Platelet function returns to normal within 12 hours of administration of these drugs.[123] However, even a baby aspirin, 81 mg, can cause maximum inhibition of platelet function and primary hemostasis.[123] NSAIDs have other known side effects, including gastrointestinal bleeding and delayed healing of colonic anastomoses.[125]

The evidence of impaired healing associated with NSAIDS is based on laboratory and animal studies; no randomized, placebo-controlled studies have been published. Patients using these medications on a regular basis are observed to bruise easily, which may be related to less tissue tolerance for pressure, which results in deep tissue injury over bony prominences. Since platelet function is the key to initiation of the inflammatory response, that response may be blunted significantly and set the course for delayed wound healing. Clinical judgment is required to evaluate the risks and benefits of these medications for patients with wounds.

Steroids are immunosuppressive medications that can be applied topically or systemically. Steroids are prescribed for a diverse group of disorders, ranging from asthma to polymyalgia rheumatica. Steroids delay all phases of wound repair. They inhibit macrophage levels, reduce immunocompetent lymphocytes, decrease antibody production, and diminish antigen processing.[109,126] Applications of topical vitamin A and systemic vitamin A supplementation are effective in counteracting the effects of steroid medication.[127] Phenylbutazone and vitamin E also disrupt normal healing.[109] Data suggest that local anesthetics cause some cellular impairment of healing, but pain relief can be achieved with no clinically significant impairment in the rate of healing.[109]

Other common medications that can alter wound healing include immunosuppressive agents, antiprostaglandins, and antineoplastics.

Nutrition

Protein malnutrition and insufficient calories is a comorbidity related to chronic wound healing. Multiple studies cite malnutrition as a risk factor for wound healing.[128,129,130] A nutritional assessment should be considered for all patients with chronic wounds, and it is required for individuals who are unable to take food by mouth or who experience weight loss.

Chapter 3 discusses nutrition assessment, the effects of nutrition on wound healing, and nutrition interventions to prevent skin breakdown and promote healing.

Irradiation and Chemotherapy

The purpose of radiation therapy is to disrupt cell mitosis, and it has ongoing effects for the remainder of the individual's life.[109] The damage may not be visible on the surface and may have a suppressed or latent appearance. Thus, an individual who experienced radiation therapy may show signs of poor wound healing months or years after completion of the radiation therapy. Injuries to the cells of repair (fibroblasts and endothelial cells) and the vasculature of the area put tissues that have been irradiated at risk for breakdown and poor healing. The extent, dosage, frequency, and location of irradiation in relation to the wound site will determine its effect on wound healing. The effects of irradiation on tissue are not easily reversed.[104] Recovery depends on the dose of radiation and the half-life of the various cells.[109]

Chemotherapy is accomplished with anticancer drugs that damage DNA or prevent DNA repair. The primary effects of chemotherapy occur during the treatment period and immediately after it.[109] However, some drugs, such as methotrexate, are used for other medical reasons on a long-term basis and can interfere with tissue repair. Another consequence of chemotherapy is induced peripheral neuropathy with loss of protective sensation; this puts tissues, particularly those of the feet, at risk for breakdown similar to other peripheral neuropathies (see Chapter 19). As chemotherapeutic agents become more common, and individuals receive repeat episodes of care, the incidence of this type of neuropathy is likely to rise.

Psychoneuroimmunolgy and Psychophysiologic Stress

Psychoneuroimmunology (PNI), a multidisciplinary field of study that has the central premise that the nervous, endocrine and immune systems are components of an integrated system of body defenses was proposed by Ader about 30 years ago.[131] The PNI premise accounts for many of the current theories about the impact of stress on health outcomes. Mechanisms of action are under study and are only just beginning to be understood. The following is a brief description of how some of the identified mechanisms may affect healing outcomes as well as PNI interventions used to reduce the effects of stress.

Anatomically there is a close interaction between the nervous, endocrine and immune systems and studies demonstrate the existence of physical and chemical links between them at the cellular level.[132] Close communication between the body and mind occurs in both health and disease states.[133] The brain can start, influence and stop biologic skin events.[134] This is demonstrated by ways in which the skin acts as part of the "diffuse brain" in its ability to modify the quality of perceptions and feelings. For example, negative emotions such as those evoked by depression or anxiety have the ability to change the functions of the skin by producing signs such as pallor, sweat, horripilation, itch, and/or redness.[134]

Stress and depression induce the release of pituitary and adrenal hormones, adrenalin, noradrenalin and cortisol by the endocrine system that effects immune function. Cortisol is a key regulatory substance. Cortisol can up or down regulate proinflammatory cytokine production that appears to be a self maintaining phenomen associated with both chronic infection and delayed wound healing. Increased cortisol levels suppress migration of neutrophils and inhibit synthesis of proinflammatory mediators like Interlukin-1 (IL-1), Interlukin-6, and activation of metal metalloprotease enzymes like MMP-9, leading to decreased macrophage function and subsequent suppression of fibroblast proliferation and matrix degradation that affects the duration and strength of the wound.[135] Broadbent et al found that qualitative measures of high preoperative stress levels are predictive of post surgical reduction in levels of Interluken (IL) I and MMP 9, resulting in more painful, poorer, and slower healing.[135] Holden-Lund[136] examined the use of guided imagery for relaxation and wound healing of surgical patients, and demonstrated that stress, as measured by cortisol levels, and in-

flammation were reduced with use of guided imagery. This work parallels the subsequent findings by Braden that individuals with lower cortisol levels did not develop pressure sores.[137]

The interaction between stress and the growth hormone-somatomedin system is not entirely understood. Lee and Stotts reviewed the effect of the growth hormone-somatomedin system on healing, as well as the negative effects of sleep changes and stress on the system. They described the importance of the anabolic function of growth hormone on tissue repair and recommended interventions targeted at healthy functioning of the growth hormone-somatomedin system. Suggestions include promoting adequate time for uninterrupted sleep and encouraging exercise as a mild stressor to promote secretion.[138] North reviewed the effect of sleep on wound healing, concluding that sleep and relaxation may affect the physiological processes involved with wound healing.[139] The exploratory studies and reviews described here have focused on acute wound healing, but studies on the effect of stress as a causative factor in the development of chronic wound healing by interruption of the healing cascade would be useful.

It is estimated that 50%–80% of illnesses include some components of psychophysiological stress, which is recognized as a risk factor in addictions, obesity, high blood pressure, peptic ulcers, colitis, asthma, insomnia, migraine headaches, and lower back pain. Stress can be positive or negative. Positive stress allows us to perform all of our daily functions, whereas negative stress may weaken the immune system and requires management. An example of positive stress is exercise. Emery found that although cortisol levels in healthy elderly adults rose with exercise, this group demonstrated more rapid healing than a comparison group of sedentary healthy elderly possibly because the exercise activity increased blood flow to the area and improved tissue oxygen levels while enhancing neuroendocrine function.[140]

Further evidence that psychologic factors can play a negatve role in skin breakdown, is reported by Anderson and Andberg's[141] in early work with patients with SCI. These researchers looked at patient life satisfaction and incidence of pressure sores. In another study, paraplegics college students were found to have more skin breakdown during final examination periods than at other times of the school year.[142] Caregivers of Alzheimer's patients who experienced wounds were found to take longer to heal than individuals who did not live in such stressful situations.[143] Satisfaction with life activities has been inversely related to the incidence of pressure ulcer development.[144]

Several investigators have examined the role of stress in relation to wound healing.[137,136,144] Eller compared use of guided imagery with progressive muscle relaxation as interventions to reduce stress and found that both had positive effects on perceived quality of life but that there was more improved physiological change in the guided imagery group that persisted 6 months post treatment. Additionally, for an unexplained reason, the group of patients who were low frequency users of guided imagery practice had better outcomes than those who were more adherent to practice.[132] West also examined the role of stress, but looked at the effect of perioperative stress on the repair process, concluding that perioperative stress decreases tissue and wound oxygen tension via vasoconstriction related to high levels of circulating catecholamines.[144] Rice et al found that biofeedback relaxation training for patients with chronic leg ulcers increased tissue perfusion in the experimental group which had 87.5% healing compared to 44% healing for the control group.[145]

Noise as a stressor has also been explored in relation to wound healing. McCarthy and colleagues reviewed the potential impact of noise on wound healing.[146] Using an animal model, this group demonstrated impairment in leukocyte function in rats exposed to noise stress, compared with rats not exposed to noise stress. Wysocki demonstrated decreased healing in rats when they were exposed to intermittent noise.[147]

Byl suggested that there may be some learned element in nonhealing.[148] In Byl's neuroplasticity research there were findings that confirm the effects of negative learning on degradation of the representation of the hand on the somatosensory cortex.[149] Likewise, negative learning appears to have adverse effects on the cells of repair, maintenance of inflammation, adequate protein synthesis, and circulation. The patient may be able to reverse the adverse effects of stress through PNI interventions including hypnosis, progressive muscle relaxation, exercise, classical conditioning, self-disclosure, visual imagery, visualizing the process of healing (e.g., increasing blood flow to the affected area by imagining the phagocytic cells gobbling up bacteria and debris), and positive self-talk about healing.[134,140,145]

Bioburden and Infection

Excessive bioburden from necrotic tissue and infection has been identified as a barrier to preparing the wound bed for healing and the development of a chronic wound. For example, epidermal cells normally march forward as a sheet and lyse the necrotic debris from the wound edges; however, they are impaired in this process of phagocytosis if obstructed by a large quantity of devitalized material. Devitalized tissue and foreign matter debris contribute to the proliferation of bacteria in the wound, which, in turn, overwhelms the body with infection and can lead to sepsis. In such situations, the body cannot cleanse the wound without intervention. It is imperative to clean the wound down to healthy bleeding tissue to restart the inflammatory phase and the biologic cascade of healing. Bleeding creates a new acute inflammatory phase and serves as a signal source for the responder cells. However, if there is inadequate circulation, the response may fail to occur or be inadequate to initiate a new inflammation response.

Iatrogenic Factors in Chronic Wound Healing

Iatrogenic factors are related to the specific way that a wound is managed. These include local ischemia, inappro-

priate wound care, trauma, and wound extent and duration.[104, 105]

Local Ischemia

Local ischemia occurs in different ways, such as from pressure over a bony prominence or inappropriate application of compression to a limb with mixed venous and arterial disease. Individuals who smoke experience nicotine-induced vasoconstriction and tissue ischemia. Persons with a history of tobacco use are 76% more likely to develop a pressure ulcer than are nonsmokers.[150]

Inappropriate Wound Care

Inappropriate wound management includes the misuse of topical agents (e.g., antiseptics) or poor technique in the application of dressings and tape that results in tears and blisters on surrounding skin or the wound bed. Inappropriate wound care has been implicated as a factor in development of a chronic wound.[104,105] Wound desiccation from lack of a dressing or inappropriate dressing choice is not uncommon. Drying out of the wound interferes with the "current of injury" function,[151] as well as with the mitotic and migratory function of cells. Dressing changes and wound cleansing disrupt the wound environment, causing chilling of the wound and surrounding tissues. Lockfound that it takes up to 40 minutes for the tissues to regain their usual temperature, and chilling impairs cell mitosis for up to 3 hours.[152] Chilling also severely disrupts leukocytic activity and oxyhemoglobin dissociation.[153]

Containment of wound fluid on the wound with moisture-retentive dressings to maintain a moist wound environment for cell migration and communication has been part of wound management for many years. Although this may be useful for acute wounds, it has since been learned that bathing the wound in chronic wound fluid has a negative effect on the wound healing microenvironment, as described above.[23] For more information about wound care products, see Chapter 11.

Trauma

Trauma to wound tissue occurs frequently, impeding wound repair and influencing local wound infection.[154] Trauma retards the rate of healing, alters the tensions of respiratory gases in wounds remote from the injury site, and causes increased susceptibility to wound infection, probably due to decreased nutritive blood flow.[154] Trauma can be attributed to many different causes, including:

- High-pressure irrigation, such as in a whirlpool or with a Water Pik
- Sharp or mechanical debridement
- Improper pressure to new granulation tissue, traumatizing the fragile tissue and initiating a new inflammatory response, which retards healing and causes abnormal scarring
- Improper handling during removal of dressings, compression wraps, or stockings, causing trauma to venous ulcers whose surrounding skin is often extremely fragile

To address the problem of wound trauma, reducing dressings and adhesives have been developed.

CLINICAL WISDOM

Avoiding Adverse Treatment Effects

Careful evaluation of each treatment and technique, based on wound assessment, can avoid adverse treatment effects and change the course of the wound.

Wound Extent and Duration

There is evidence that supports the role of wound surface area and wound depth as factors in time to healing.[155-158] There is intuitive logic behind the belief injuries with large surface areas and multiple wounds, which also increase the surface area to be repaired, increase the need for oxygen, nutrients, and adaptive resources for healing because there is more damaged tissue to repair. Multiple sizable wounds present the host with a larger total surface area to repair.

Researchers looking at factors that can be used to predict wound healing have identified duration and size as two factors that are predictive of healing outcomes. Percentage of healing and ulcer area at week 3 were good predictors of 100% healing. Patients with venous ulcers that are initially large in size or who have moderate arterial insufficiency (ankle-brachial index of 0.5–0.8) have associated delayed healing times.[106] Shorter duration of ulceration and smaller size were predictive of time to heal.[159] Ulcers that are large, longstanding, and slow to heal after 3 weeks of optimal therapy are unlikely to change their course.[39] It is now possible to identify and diagnose correctly those ulcers that are unlikely to respond to standard care, and consideration should be given to introduce alternative therapies.[39]

The processes that occur throughout wound healing are complex and sensitive to internal and external environmental forces. The goals of wound care management are to provide interventions that mitigate the negative forces and progress wounds through the sequence of repair or regeneration in an orderly and timely manner. In order for healthcare clinicians to have successful wound healing outcomes, it is important to understand and recognize the key sequence of events. The ability to recognize the benchmarks of wound phase change is critical to monitoring the effects of treatment interventions and recognizing when an intervention is successful or not. Early identification that the wound has become "stuck" and unable to progress should trigger an appropriate response. Chronicity can occur during any phase of healing. A wound can also miss a phase of repair, such as when the body simply fails to initiate the phase (e.g., when there is inadequate circulation). These concepts are expanded upon in Chapter 4.

REVIEW QUESTIONS

1. Partial-thickness wounds involving only the epidermis heal by which of the following processes?
   a. contraction and granulation
   b. epithelialization or epidermal resurfacing
   c. epithelialization and granulation
   d. inflammation and remodeling

2. A clinician is assessing F.T.'s abdomen 3 days post abdominal-perineal resection surgery and notes erythema, slight edema, and slight increase in temperature at the incision site. These findings are most consistent with which of the following?
   a. These are normal signs of the inflammatory phase of wound healing.
   b. The wound is exhibiting early signs of impending infection.
   c. The wound is in the proliferative phase of wound healing.
   d. The wound is exhibiting signs of abscess formation.

3. Which of the following statements is *most* accurate about fibroblasts?
   a. They are responsible for phagocytosis of bacteria and wound cleanup.
   b. They are responsible for wound contraction and scar hypertrophy.
   c. They are responsible for collagen lysis in the remodeling phase of healing.
   d. They are responsible for angiogenesis and collagen synthesis.

4. Which following statements regarding the inflammatory phase of wound healing is correct?
   a. Inflammation is detrimental to wound healing.
   b. The overall effect of inflammation is a wound area free of debris because leukocytes break down necrotic tissue and phagocytose bacteria.
   c. Inflammation occurs only in dirty, infected wounds and indicates the need for antibiotics.
   d. Steroids enhance wound healing by blocking the inflammatory response.

5. Vitamin A may facilitate healing in some clients because:
   a. It is essential for cellular repair.
   b. It significantly affects blood and tissue oxygen levels.
   c. It can partially correct the effects of steroids on wound healing.
   d. It potentiates antibiotic therapy, thus reducing inflammation.

6. Which of the following appear to be principal mediators for full-thickness wound repair?
   a. Endothelial cells and fibroblasts
   b. Neutrophils and platelets
   c. Fibroblasts and neutrophils
   d. Platelets and macrophages

7. Contraction plays an important role in wound healing for:
   a. wounds healing by primary intention
   b. wounds healing by secondary intention
   c. superficial abrasions
   d. all wounds

REFERENCES

1. Hunt TK, Van Winkle W. *Fundamentals of Wound Management in Surgery, Wound Healing: Normal Repair.* South Plainfield, NJ: Chirurgecom; 1976.
2. Goldman Robert. Growth Factors and Chronic Wound Healing: Past,Present and Future. *Adv in Skin and Wound Care.* 2004;17(1):24-35.
3. Hunt TK, Hussain M. Can wound healing be a paradigm for tissue repair? *Med Sci Sports Exerc.* 1994;26:755-758.
4. Cooper DM. The Physiology of Wound Healing: An Overview. In: Krasner D, ed. *Chronic Wound Care: A clinical source book for healthcare professionals.* Vol 1. King of Prussia, PA: Health Management Publications; 1990:1-10.
5. Winter GD. Formation of the scab and the rate of epithelializatin of superficial wounds in the skin of the young domestic pig. *Nature.* 1962;193:293-294.
6. Lazarus GS, Cooper DM, Knighton DM, et al. Definitions and guidelines for assessment of wounds and evaluation of healing. *Arch Dermatol.* 1994;130:489-493.
7. Adzick NS, Harrison MR, Glick PI, et.al. Comparison of fetal, newborn and adult wound healing by histologic, enzyme-histochemical and hydroxyproline determination. . *J Pediatr Surg.* 1985;20:315.
8. Harrison MR, Langer JC, Adzick N, et. al. Correction of congenital diaphragmatic hernia in utero. V: Initial clinical experience. *J Pediatr Surg.* 1990:25:47.
9. Harrison MR, Adzick NS, Longaker MT, et. al. Successful repair in utero of a fetal diaphragmatic hernia after removal of herniated viscera from the left thorax. *N Engl J Med.* 1990;322:1582.
10. Mast B. The skin. In: Cohen I, Diegelmann, RF, Lindblad, WJ, ed. *Wound Healing Biochemical and Clinical Aspects.* Philadelphia: WB Saunders; 1992:344-355.
11. Byl N, McKenzie A, Stern R, et al. Amniotic fluid modulates wound healing. *Eur J Rehab Med.* 1993;2:184-190.
12. Byl N, McKenzie A, West J, et al. Pulsed micro amperage stimulation: A controlled study of healing of surgically induced wounds in Yucatan pigs. *Phys Ther.* 1994;74:201-218.
13. Hock RJ. The physiology of high altitude. *Aci Amer.* 1987;22:52.
14. Schmid P, Itin P, Cherry G, Bi C, Cox DA. Enhanced expression of transforming growth factor-beta type I and type II receptors in wound granulation tissue and hypertrophic scar. *Am J Pathol.* 1998;152(2):485-493.
15. Robson MC. Proliferative Scarring. *Surg Clin North Am.* 2003;83:557-569.
16. Edmonds M. Hyaluronic Acid in Reclcitrant Ulcers. Paper presented at: Evidence Based Outcomes in Wound Management; March 31, 2000; Dallas, TX.
17. Hunt TK, Heppenstall RB, Pines E, Rovee D, EDS. *Soft and Hard Tissue Repair: Biological and Clinical Aspects.* New York: Praegar Publishers; 1984.
18. Kerstein MD, Bensing KA, Brill LR, et al. *The Physiology of Wound Healing.* Philadelphia: The Oxford Institue for Continuing Education and Allegheny University of Health Sciences; March 1998.
19. Grinnell F, Billingham RE, Burgess L. Distribution of fibronectin during wound healing in vivo. *Journal of Investigative Dermatology.* 1981;76(3):181-189.
20. Doherty D, Haslett C, Tonnesen M, Henson P. Human monocyte adherence: A primary effect of chemotactic factors on the monocyte to stimulate adherence to human endothelium. *Journal of Immunology.* 1987;138(6):1762-1771.
21. Fylling CP. Growth Factors: A New Era in Wound Healing. In: Diane K, Kane D, eds. *Chronic Wound Care: A sourcebook for healthcare professionals.* second ed. Wayne, PA: Health Management Publications, Inc.; 1997:344-346.
22. Ovington Lisa G, Cullen Breda. Matrix Metalloprotease Modulation and Growth Factor Protection. *Wounds: a compendium of clinical research and practice.* 2002;14(June):1-13.
23. Schultz GS, Sibbald GR, Falanga V, et al. Wound bed preparation : A systematic approach to wound management. *Wound Repair and Regeneration.* March-April 2003;11(1):S1-S28.
24. Moseley R, Stewart JE, Stephens P, Waddington RJ, Thomas DW. Extracellular matrix metabolites as potential biomarkers of disease activity in wound fluid: lession learned from other inflammatory diseases? *British Journal of Dermatolgy.* 2004;150:401-413.
25. Sanchez-Fidalgo S, Martin-Lacave I, Illanes M, Motilva V. Angiogenesis, cell proliferation and apoptosis in gastric ulcer healing. Effect of a selective cox-2 inhibitor. *European Journal of Pharmacology.* 2004/11/28 2004;505(1-3):187-194.
26. Sessler DI. Mild Perioperative Hypothermia. *The New England Journal of Medicine.* June 12, 1997;336(24):1730-1736.
27. Michaelson AD, MacGregor H, Barnard MR, Kestin AS, Rohrer MJ, Valeri CR. Reversible inhibition of human platelet activatin by hypothermia in vivo and in vitro. *Thromb Haemost.* May 1994;71(5):633-640.
28. Valeri CR, Khabbaz K, Khuri SF, et al. Effect of skin temperature on platelet function in patients undergoing extracorporeal bypass. *J Thoracic Cardiovasc Surg.* Jul 1992;104(1):108-116.
29. Hunt T, Hopf H. Wound healing and wound infection: What surgeons and anesthesiologists can do. *Surgical Clinics of North America.* 1997;77(3):587-606.
30. Knighton DR, Silver IA, Hunt TK. Regulation of wound-angiogenesis: Effect of oxygen gradients and inspired oxygen concentration. *Surgery.* 1981;90:262.
31. Clark R. Wound repair: Overview and general considerations. In: Clark R, ed. *The Molecular and Cellular Biology of Wound Repair.* New York: Plenum Press; 1996:3-50.
32. Calvin M. Cutaneous wound repair. *Wounds: A compendium of clinical research and practice.* Jan 1998;10(1):12-32.
33. Byl N. Electrical Stimulation for Tissue Repair: Basic Information. In: Nelson R, Hayes KW, Currier DP, eds. *Clinical Electrotherapy.* third ed. Samford, CT: Appleton & Lange; 1999.
34. Suh D, Hunt T. Time line of wound healing. *Clinics in Podiatric Medicine and Surgery.* 1998;15(1):1-9.
35. Knighton DR, Halliday B, Hunt TK, et al. Oxygen as an antibiotic: The effect of inspired oxygen on infection. *Arch Surg.* 1984;119:199-204.
36. Hohn DC, et. al. Effect of O2 tension on microbicidal function of leukocytes in wounds and in vitro. *Surg Forum.* 1976;27:18-20.
37. Goodson WH, Andrews WS, Thakral KK, Hunt TK. Wound oxygen tension of large vs. small wounds in man. *Surg Forum.* 1979;30:92-95.
38. Goodson WH AW, Thakral KK, Hunt TK. Wound oxygen tension of large vs. small wounds in man. *Surg Forum.* 1979;30:92-95.
39. Phillips T, Machado F, Trout R, Porter J, Olin J, Falanga V. Prognostic indicators in venous ulcers. *J Am Acad Dermatol.* Oct 2000;43(4):627-630.
40. Jonsson K, Jensen J, Goodson Wd, et al. Tissue oxygenation, anemia, and perfusion in relation to wound healing in surgical patients. *Annals of Surgery.* 1991;214(5):605-613.
41. Coleridge-Smith PD. Oxygen, Oxygen Free Radicals and Reperfusion Injury. In: Krasner D, Kane D, eds. *Chronic Wound Care: A Clinical Source Book for Healthcare Professionals.* Vol 1. Wayne, PA: Health Management Publications, Inc.; 1997:348-353.
42. Knighton DR, 1988:188-193. HTIene. The defenses of the wound. In: Howard RJ SR, ed. *Surgical Infectious Diseases.* second ed. Stamford, CT: Appleton & Lange;; 1988:188-193.
43. Boykin Joseph V. The Nitric Oxide Connection: Hyperbaric Oxygen Therapy, Becaplermin, and Diabetic Ulcer Management. *Adv in Skin and Wound Care.* July August 2000;13(4):169-174.
44. Witte M, Barbul A. General principles of wound healing. *Surgical Clinics of North America.* 1997;77(3):509-528.
45. Schaffer MR, Tantry U, Efron PA, Ahrendt GM, Thornton FJ, Barbul A. Diabetes impaired healing and reduced nitric oxide synthesis: a possible pathophysiologic correlation. *Surgery.* May 1997;121(5):513-519.
46. Schaeffer MR, Tantry U, Gross SS, Wasserkrug HL. Nitric Oxide Regulates Wound Healing. *Journal of Surgical Research.* 1996;63:237-240.
47. Dyson M, Luke D. Induction of mast cell degranulation in skin by ultrasound. *IEEE Trans Ultrasonics, Ferroelectronics, Frequency Control.* 1986;33:194-201.
48. Dexter TM, Stoddart RW, Quazzaz STA, TA, Stoddart RW, Quazzaz STA. What are mast cells for? *Nature.* 1981;291:110-111.
49. Ross J. Utilization of Pulsed High Peak Power Electromagnetic Energy (Diapulse Therapy) To Accelerate Healing Processes. Paper presented at: Digest International Symposium, Antennas and Propagation Society; June 20-22, 1977; Stanford, CA.
50. Horzic Matija, Bunoza Davorka, Maric Kristina. Contact thermography in a study of primary healing of surgical wounds. *Ostomy/Wound Management.* Jan/Feb 1996;42`(1):36-42.
51. Lock PM. The effect of temperature on mitotic activity at the edge of experimental wounds. Paper presented at: Symposium on Wound Healing: Plastic, Surgical and Dermatologic Aspects, 1979; Molndal, Sweden.

52. Myers JA. Wound Healing and use of modern surgical dressing. *Pharm J.* 1982;229:103-104.

53. Becker RO. The significance of bioelectric potentials. *Med Times.* 1967;95:657-659.

54. Foulds IS, Barker AT. Human skin battery potentials and their possible role in wound healing. *Br J Dermatol.* 1983;109:515-522.

55. Vanable J Jr. Natural and applied voltages in vertebrate regeneration and healing. In: Liss AR, ed. *Integumentary Potentials and Wound Healing.* New York: 1989.

56. Jaffe LP, Vanable JW. Electric Field and Wound Healing. *Clinical Dermatology.* 1984(3):233-234.

57. Orinda N, Feldman JD. Directional protrusive pseudopodial activity and motility in macrophages induced by extracellular electric fields. *Cell Motil.* 1982;2:243-255.

58. Fukishima K, Senda N, Inui H, Miura H, Tamai Y, Murakami Y. Study of galvanotaxis of leukocytes. *Med J Osaka University.* 1953;4:195-208.

59. Weiss DS, et al. Pulsed electrical stimulation decreases scar thickness at split-thickness graft donor sites. *J Invest Dermatol.* 1989;92:539.

60. Kloth LC. Electrical stimulation in tissue repair. In: McColloch JM KL, Feeder JA, ed. *Wound Healing Alternatives in Management.* second ed. Philadelphia: F.A. Davis; 1995:292.

61. Erickson CA, Nuccitelli R. Embryonic fibroblast motility and orientation can be influenced by physiological electric fields. *Cell Biol.* 1981;98:296-307.

62. Bourguignon GJ, Bourguignon LYW. Electric stimulation of protein and DNA synthesis in human fibroblasts. *FASEB J.* 1987;1:398.

63. Bates-Jensen B. *A Quantitative Analysis Of Wound Characteristics As Early Predictors Of Healing In Pressure Sores. Dissertation Abstracts International, Volume 59, Number 11* University of California, Los Angeles; 1999.

64. Eaglstein W, Falanga V. Chronic wounds. *Surgical Clinics of North America.* 700 1997;77(3):689.

65. Wipke-Tevis D, Stotts N. Leukocytes, ischemia, and wound healing: A critical interaction. *Wounds.* 1991;3(6):227-238.

66. Tomic-Canic Marjana. Keratinocyte Cross-Talks in Wounds. *Supplement to Wounds.* September 2005:3-9.

67. Shea JD. Pressure sore: Classification and management. *Clin Orthop.* 1975;112:89-100.

68. Seiler WD, Stahelin HB. Implications for research. *Wounds.* 1994;6:101106.

69. Hardy MA. The Biology of Scar Formation. *Phys Ther.* December 1989;69(12):1014-1023.

70. Kirsner R, Eaglstein W. The wound healing process. *Dermatology Clinics.* 1993;11:629-640.

71. Steffensen B, Hakkinen L, Larjava H. Proteolytic events of wound-healing—coordinated interactions among matrix metalloproteinases (MMPs), integrins, and extracellular matrix molecules. *Crit. Rev. Oral. Biol. Med.* January 1, 2001;12(5):373-398.

72. Weiss EL. Connective tissue in wound healing. In: McCulloch J KL, Feedar J,, ed. *Wound Healing Alternatives in Management.* second ed. Philadelphia: FA Davis; 1995:26-28.

73. Byl N, McKenzie AL, West JM, Whitney JD, Hunt TK, Scheuenstuhl HA. Low-Dose Ultrasound Effects on Wound Healing: A Controlled Study With Yucatan Pigs. *Arch Phys Med Rehabil.* July 1992;73:656-663.

74. Harding KG, Bale S. Wound Care: putting theory into practice in the United Kingdom. In: Krasner D, Kane D, eds. *Chronic Wound Care: A Clinical Source Book for Healthcare Professionals.* Vol 1. second ed. Wayne, PA: Health Management Publications; 1997:115-123.

75. Vande Berg JS, Rudolph R, Hollan C, Haywood-Reid PL. Fibroblast senescence in pressure ulcers. *Wound Repair Regen.* Jan-Feb 1998;6(1):38-49.

76. Wysocki A. Fibronectin in acute and chronic wounds. *Journal of ET Nursing.* 1992;19(5):166-170.

77. Hynes R. Molecular biology of fibronectin. *Annual Review of Cell Biology.* 1985;1:67-90.

78. Grinnell F, Zhu M. Identification of neutrophil elastase as the proteinase in burn wound fluid responsible for degradation of fibronectin. *Journal of Investigative Dermatology.* 1994;103(2):155-161.

79. Parks W. The production, role, and regulation of matrix metalloproteinases in the healing epidermis. *Wounds.* 1995;7(5 Suppl A):23A-37A. XXX.

80. Staiano-Coico L, Higgins PJ, Schwartz SB, AJ Z, Goncalves J. Wound fluids: a reflection of the state of healing. *Ostomy Wound Management.* January 2000;46(1A):85S-93S.

81. Park H-Y, Shon K, Phillips T. The Effect of Heat on Inhibitory Effects of Chronic Wound Fluid on Fibroblasts in Vitro. *Wounds: A compendium of clinical research and practice.* November/December 1998;10(6):189-192.

82. Moseley R SJ, Stephens P, Waddington RJ, Thomas DW. Extracellular matrix metabolites as potential biomarkers of disease activity in wound fluid: lession learned from other inflammatory diseas? *British Journal of Dermatolgy.* 2004;150:401-413.

83. Bucalo B, Eaglstein W, Falanga V. Inhibition of cell proliferation by chronic wound fluid. *Wound Repair and Regeneration.* 1989;1(3):181-186.

84. Grinnell F, Ho C, Wysocki A. Degradation of fibronectin and vitronectin in chronic wound fluid: Analysis by cell blotting, immunoblotting, and cell adhesion assays. *Journal of Investigative Dermatology,* 1992; 98(4):410-416.

85. Bennett N, Schultz, GS. Growth factors and wound healing: Part II. Role in normal and chronic wound healing. *American Journal of Surgery.* 1993;166(1):74-81.

86. Cooper D, Yu EZ, Hennessey P, Ko F, Robson MC. Determination of endogenous cytokines in chronic wounds. *Annals of Surgery.* 1994;219(6):688-691.

87. Pierce G, Tarpley J, Tseng J, et al. Detection of platelet-derived growth factor (PDGF)-AA in actively healing human wounds treated with recombinant PDGF-BB and absence of PDGF in chronic non-healing wounds. *Journal of Clinical Investigation.* 1995;96(3):1336-1350.

88. Yager D, Zhang L, Liang H, Diegelmann R, Cohen IK. Wound fluids in human pressure ulcers contain elevated matrix metaloproteinase levels and activity compared to surgical wound fluids. *J Investigative Dermatology.* November 1996;107(5):743-748.

89. Siddiqui A, Galiano RD, Connors D, Gruskin E, Wu L, Mustoe TA. Differential effects of oxygen on human dermal fibroblasts: acute versus chronic hypoxia. *Wound Repair and Regeneration.* 1996;4(2):211-218.

90. Gogia P. Physiology of wound healing. In: Gogia P, ed. *Clinical Wound Management.* Thorofare, NJ: Slack; 1995:1-12.

91. Stamenkovic Ivan. Extracellular matrix remodelling: the role of matrix metalloproteinases. *The Journal of Pathology.* 2003;200(4):448-464.

92. Murray J. Scars and keloids. *Dermatologic Clinics.* 1993;11(4):697-708.

93. Stotts NA. Impaired wound healing. In: Carrieri-Kohlman V, Lindsay A, West C, eds. *Pathophysiological Phenomenon in Nursing.* second ed. Philadelphia, Pennsylvannia: WB Saunders Company; 1993:343-366.

94. Engelen M, Besche B, Lefay MP, Hare J, Vlaminck K. Effects of ketanserin on hypergranulation tissue formation, infection, and healing of equine lower limb wounds. *Can Vet J.* February 2004;45(2):44-49.

95. Berry DB 2nd, Sullins KE. Effects of topical application of antimicrobials and bandaging on healing and granulation tissue ormation in wounds of the distal aspect of the limbs in horses. *Am J Vet Res.* 2003;64.(1):88-92.

96. Theoret CL, Barber SM, Moyana TN, Gordon JR. Preliminary observations on expression of transforming growth factors beta 1 and beta 3 in equine rull-thickness skin wounds healing normally or with exuberant granulation tissue. *Vet Surg.* May-June 2002;31(3):266-273.

97. De martin I, Theoret CL. Spatial and Temporal Expression of Types I and II Receptors for Transforming Growth Factor TGF-β; in Normal Equine Skin and Dermal Wounds. *Veterinary Surgery.* 2004;33(1):70-76.

98. Ducharme-Desjarlais M, Celeste CJ, Lepault E, et al. Effect of a silicone-containing dressing on exuberant granulation tissue formation and wound repair in horses. *Am J Vet Res.* 2005;66(7):1133-1139.

99. Hawkins-Bradley B, Walden M. Treatment of a nonhealing wound with hypergranulation tissue and rolled edges. *J Wound Ostomy Continence Nurs.* 2002;29(6):320-324.

100. Harris A, Rolstad BS. Hypergranulation tissue: a nontraumatic method of management. *Ostomy Wound Manage.* 1994;40(5):20-22, 24, 26-30.

101. Mulder GD, Jeter KF, Fairchild PA, eds. *Clinician's Pocket Guide to Chronic Wound Repair.* Spartanburg, SC: Wound Healing Publications; 1991.

102. Jones PL, Millman A. Wound healing and the aged patient. *Nursing Clinics of North America.* 1990;25(1):263-277.

103. Eaglstein W. Wound healing and aging. *Clinics in Geriatric Medicine.* 1989;5(1):183-188.

104. Mulder G, Brazinsky BA, Seeley J. Factors complicating wound repair. In: McCulloch JM KL, Feeder JA, ed. *Wound Healing Alternatives in Management.* second ed. Philadelphia: FA. Davis; 1995:47-59.

105. Stotts NA, Wipke-Tevis D. Co-factors in impaired wound healing. *Ostomy/Wound Manage. Ostomy/ Wound Management.* March 1996;42(March):44-56.

106. Marston W, Carlin R, Passman M, Farber M, Keegy BA. Healing Rates and cost efficacy of outpatient compression treatment for leg ulcers associated with venous insufficiency. *J Vasc Surg.* 1999;30(3):491-498.

107. Sinacore DR, Muller MJ. Pedal Ulcers in Older Adults with Diabetes Mellitus. *Topics in Geriatric Rehabilitation.* December 2000;16(2):11-23.

108. Voss AC, Bender S, Cook AS, et al. Pressure Ulcer Prevention in LTC: Implementatin of the National Pressure Ulcer Long-term Care Study (NPULS) Prevention Program. Paper presented at: Symposium for Advanced Wound Care; April 2000; Dallas, TX.

109. Stotts N, Wipke-Tevis D. Co-factors in Impaired Wound Healing. In: Krasner D KD, ed. *Chronic Wound Care: A Clinical Sourcebook for Health Care Professionals*. Wayne, PA: 2nd ed.: Health Management Publications; 1997:64-71.

110. Dean E. Oxygen transport deficits in systemic disease and implications for physical therapy. *Phys Ther.* 1997;77:187-202.

111. Yue D, McLennan S, Marsh M, et al. Effects of experimental diabetes, uremia, and malnutrition on wound healing. *Diabetes.* 1987;36(3):295-299.

112. Rosenberg C. Wound healing in the patient with diabetes mellitus. *Nursing Clinics of North America.* 1990;25(1):247-261.

113. Norris S, Provo B, Stotts NA. Physiology of wound healing and risk factors that impede the healing process. *AACN.* 1990;1:545-552.

114. Hunt TK, Rabkin J, Von Smitten K. Effects of edema and anemia on wound healing and infection. *Curr Stud Hematol Blood Transf.* 1986;53:101-111.

115. Hartmann M, Jonsson K, Zederfeldt B. Effect of tissue perfusion and oxygenation on accumulation of collagen in healing wounds. Randomized study in patients after major abdominal operations. *European Journal of Surgery.* 1992;158(10):521-526.

116. Jonsson K, Jensen J, Goodson WD, West J, Hopf H, Hunt T. Assessment of perfusion in postoperative wounds using tissue oxygen measurements. *British Journal of Surgery.* 1987;74(4):263-267.

117. McCulloch JM. Treatment of wounds caused by vascular insufficiency. In: McCulloch JM KL, Feeder JA,, ed. *Wound Healing Alternatives in Management.* second ed. Philadelphia: F. Davis; 1995:216-217.

118. Falanga V, Eaglstein WH. The "trap" hypothesis of venous ulceration. *Lancet.* 1993;341(8851):1006-1008.

119. Burnand K, Whimster I, Naidoo A, Browse NL. Pericapillary fibrin in the ulcer-bearing skin of the leg: The cause of lipodermatosclerosis and venous ulceration. *British Medical Journal Clinical Research Education.* 1982;285(6348):1071-1072.

120. Mosiello G, Tufaro A, Kerstein M. Wound healing and complications in the immunosuppressed patient. *Wounds.* 1994;6(3):883-887.

121. Garber SL, Biddle AK, Click CN, et al. *Pressure ulcer prevention and treatment following spinal cord injury: A clinical practice guideline for health-care professionals.* Jackson Heights, NY: Paralyzed Veterans of America; August 2000.

122. Twist D. Acrocyanosis iln a spinal cord injured patient—effect of computer-controlled neuromuscular electrical stimulation: a case report. *Physical Therapy.* 1990;70:45:49.

123. Schafer Andrew I. Effects of Nonsteroidal Antiinflammatory Drugs on Platelet Function and Systemic Hemostasis. *J Clin Pharmacol.* 1995;35(3):209-219.

124. Jones KG, et. al. Inhibition of angiogenesis by nonsteroidal antiinflammatory durgs: insight into mechanisms and implications for cancer growth and ulcer healing. *Nat Med.* 1999;5(5):1418-1423.

125. Salcido R. Do Antiinflammatories Have a Role in Wound Healing. Paper presented at: Clinical Symposium on Advances in Skin and Wound Care; October 23-26, 2005; Las Vegas, NV.

126. Leiebowitch SJ, Ross R. The role of the macrophage in wound repair. *Am J Pathol.* 1975;78:71-91.

127. Hunt TK, Rabkin J, Von Smitten K. Vitamin A and wound healing. *J Am Acad Dermatol.* 1986;15:817.

128. Allman RM, Laprade CA, Noel LB, et. al. Pressure sores among hospitalized patients. *Ann Intern Med.* 1987;105:337-342.

129. Bergstrom N, Braden B. A prospective study of pressure sore risk among institutionalized elderly. *J Am Geriatr Soc.* 1992;40:747-758.

130. Breslow RA, Hallfrisch J, Goldberg AP. Malnutrition in tube fed nursing home patients with pressure sores. *J Parenter Enteral Nutr.* 1991;15:663-668.

131. Ader R. On the development of psychoneuroimmunology. *European Journal of Pharmacology.* 2000;405:167-176.

132. Eller LS. Effects of cognitive-behavioral interventions on quality of life in persons with HIV. *International Journal of Nursing Studies.* 1999;36:223-233.

133. Masek K, Petrovicky P, Ziˊdek Z, Frankovaˊ D. Past, present and future of psychoneuroimmunology. *Toxicology.* 2000;142:179-188.

134. Urpe M, Buggiani G, Lotti T. Stress and Psychoneuroimmunologic Factors in Dermatology. *Dermatologic Clinics.* 2005;23(4):609-617.

135. Broadbent E, Petrie KJ, Alley PG, Booth RJ. Psychological Stress Impairs Early Wound Repair Following Surgery. *Psychosomatic Medicine.* 2003;65:865-869.

136. Holden-Lund C. The effects of relaxation with guided imagery on surgical stress and wound healing. *Research in Nursing & Health.* 1988;11(4):235-244

137. Braden B. The relationship between stress and pressure sore formation. *Ostomy Wound Management.* 1998;44(3A 1Suppl):26S-36S.

138. Lee KA, Stotts Nancy. Support of the growth hormone-somatomedin system to facilitate healing. *Heart & Lung: Journal of Critical Care.* 1990;19(2):157-164.

139. North A. The effect of sleep on wound healing. *Ostomy Wound Management.* 1990;27:56-58

140. Emery CF, Kiecolt-Glaser JK, Glaser R, B. MW, Frid DJ. Exercise Accelerates Wound Healing Among Healthy Older Adults: A Preliminary Investigation. *Journal of Gerontology: Medical Sciences.* 2005;Vol. 60A,(11):1432-1436.

141. Anderson TP, Andberg M. Psychosocial factors associated with pressure sores. *Archives of Physical Medicine and Rehabilitation.* 1979;60(8):341-346.

142. Crenshaw R, Vistnes L. A decade of pressure sore research. *J Rehab Res Dev.* 1989;26:63-74.

143. Kiecolt-Glase JK, Marucha PT, Malarkey WB, Mercado AM, Glaser R. Slowing of wound healing by psychological stress. Lancet 1995;346, 1194-1196

144. West J. Wound healing in the surgical patient: Influence of the perioperative stress response on perfusion. *AACN Clinical Issues.* 1990;1(3):595-601.

145. Rice B, Kalker A, Schindler J, Dixon R. Effect of biofeedback-assisted relaxation training on foot ulcer healing. *J Am Podiatr Med Assoc.* March 2001;91(3):132-141.

146. McCarthy D, Ouimet M, Daun J. Shades of Florence Nightingale: Potential impact of noise stress on wound healing. *Holistic Nursing Practice.* 1991;5(4):39-48.

147. Wysocki A. The effect of intermittent noise exposure on wound healing. *Advances in Wound Care.* 1996a;9(1):35-39.

148. Byl N. The Doctor Within: The Inner Aspects of Healing. Paper presented at: American Physical Therapy Scientific Meeting; June 1997; San Diego, CA.

149. Byl NN, Merzenich MM, Cheung S, et al A Primate model for studying focal dystonia and repetitive strain injury: effects on the primary somatosensory cortex. Phys Ther 1977; 77 269-84.

150. Ross Products Division. *Executive Summary—Phase I prevention results: The national Pressure Ulcer Long-term care study.* Columbus, OH Sept 14, 1999.

151. Illingsworth C, Barker A. Measurement of electrical currents emerging during the regeneration of amputated finger tips in children. *Clin Phys Physiol Meas.* 1980:1:87.

152. Lock P. The effect of temperature on mitosis at the edge of experimental wounds. In: Lundgren A, Sover A, eds. *Symposia on Wound Healing: Plastic, Surgical and Dermatologic Aspects.* 1980; Molndal, Sweden.

153. Thomas ST. *Management and Dressings*: The Pharmaceutical Press; 1990.

154. Conolly WB, Hunt T, Sonne M, Dunphy JE. Influence of distant trauma on local wound infection. *Surg Gynecol Obstet.* April 1969;128(4):713-717.

155. Gorse G, Messner R. Improved pressure sore healing with hydrocolloid dressings. *Archives of Dermatology.* 1987;123:766-771.

156. Ferrell B, Osterweil D, Christenson P. A randomized trial of low-air-loss beds for treatment of pressure ulcers. *Journal of the American Medical Association.* 1993;269:494-497.

157. Gentzkow G, Pollack S, Kloth L, Stubbs H. Improved healing of pressure ulcers using dermapulse, a new electrical stimulation device. *Wounds.* 1991;3(5):158-169.

158. vanRijswijk L. Full-thickness pressure ulcers: patient and wound healing characteristics. *Decubitus.* Jan 1993;6(1):16-21.

159. Skene AL, Smith J, Dore CJ, Charlett A, Lewis JD. Venous Leg Ulcers: a prognostic index to predict time to healing. *British Medical Journal.* Nov 7, 1992;305(6862):1119-1121.

3

Nutritional Assessment and Treatment

Mary Ellen Posthauer, RD, CD, LD

CHAPTER OBJECTIVES

At the completion of this chapter, the reader will be able to:
1. Identify the guidelines for completing a nutritional screening and assessment.
2. Screen patients at risk for nutrition deficiency, using a nutritional screening tool.
3. Describe the role of nutrition in the process of wound healing.
4. Identify nutrients of particular importance to wound healing.

The role of nutrition is often the forgotten factor in wound healing. The identification of a client's nutritional status begins with a nutritional screening, followed by an assessment. A plan of care is then developed, based on the data derived from the assessment process.

As defined by the American Dietetic Association (ADA) Nutrition Care Process and Model, *medical nutrition therapy* involves a screening and referral system for identifying risk factors, which leads to the nutrition assessment. The assessment includes review and analysis of a patient's medical and diet histories, laboratory values, and anthropometric measurements. Based on the assessment, the nutrition modalities most appropriate to manage the condition or treat the illness or injury are chosen. The dietitian analyzes and interprets the data using evidence-based standards, and documents their use of these standards.

Nutritional Screening

Nutritional screening is the process of identifying characteristics known to be associated with nutritional problems. Its purpose is to pinpoint individuals who are malnourished or at nutritional risk. Intervention takes place after screening occurs. A screening involves interdisciplinary collaboration and can be completed by a member of the health-care team, such as the dietitian, dietetic technician, nurse, physician, or other qualified health-care professional. The Braden Scale for Predicting Pressure Sore Risk (see Chapter 15) includes nutritional screening information. A nutrition intervention to prevent wounds is included in Appendix 3-A at the end of this chapter.

Elderly clients often have multiple factors that place them at risk for pressure ulcer formation. Skin fragility, along with numerous other medical conditions that occur among the elderly, increases both risk and healing time.

Functional limitations, such as difficulty chewing or swallowing, affect the client's ability to ingest adequate calories and fluids. Immobility affects a client's ability to either prepare meals or travel to a dining room. Poor hearing and vision compromise a client's communication skills and can result in poor intake at meals. The saying, "We eat with our eyes," is illustrated when poor vision hampers eating. Altered mental status can limit a client's ability to feed himself or herself, or to comprehend the importance of consuming a balanced diet. Advanced dementia often results in weight loss, dysphagia, malnutrition, and pressure ulcers. The probability of developing pressure ulcers increases among clients who can no longer respond to their caregivers' attempts to assist in their nourishment.

The risk of pressure ulcers can also be increased by a patient's specific medical condition. For example, diabetes with chronic hyperglycemia can contribute both to the development of wounds and poor wound healing. High levels of glucose in the blood interfere with the transport of ascorbic acid into the cells, thereby inhibiting the deposition of collagen. Hip fractures and spinal cord injuries that restrict a client's mobility often result in increased pain and can interfere with eating.

Drug therapy can often cause side effects, such as nausea and gastric disturbances, which limit food and fluid intake. Corticosteroids increase the risk of wound complications such as infection, and inhibit protein synthesis.

This chapter is adapted with permission from Kathleen Neidert and Mary Ellen Posthauer. *The Role of Nutrition in Wound Healing,* (c) 1994, 1996, 1998, 2001, Mead Johnson and Company, Evansville, IN.

Corticosteroids cause depletion of vitamin A from the liver, plasma, adrenals, and enzymes, and interfere with collagen synthesis and resistance to infection.[1]

Clients with pressure ulcers or those identified as being at risk for developing pressure ulcers should be monitored at appropriate intervals. Many health-care organizations have wound-care teams that make weekly rounds to assess the condition of existing pressure ulcers and the implementation of care plans. Nutritional status should be assessed at minimum every 3 months for those clients at low risk, and monthly for those at high risk or who are already malnourished.

The treatment and prevention of pressure ulcers are key aspects of meeting the regulation concerning "quality of life" in the Omnibus Budget Reconciliation Act (OBRA) of 1987 (Public Law No. 101–239). This law focuses on providing care that enables nursing home clients to live a dignified existence and to maintain the highest degree of physical, mental, and psychosocial well-being possible.[2] See Exhibit 3-1 for definitions from the State Operations Manual (Pub. 100-07)/Provider Certification from the Centers for Medicare and Medicaid Services Manual System.

The Centers for Medicare and Medicaid Services (CMS), which regulates long-term care facilities in the United States, has targeted pressure ulcers, inadequate nutrition, and inadequate hydration as key survey issues. Surveyors at both the federal and state level utilize an Investigative Pressure Ulcer Protocol (Federal Tag F-314) to determine whether pressure ulcers are avoidable or unavoidable. The protocol investigates a facility's pressure ulcer treatment, prevention intervention, assessment (including nutrition), plan of care, and ongoing evaluations. The comprehensive assessment in long-term care

EXHIBIT 3-1 Federal Regulation Definitons: Medicare and Medicaid Requirements for Long Term Care Facilities

§483.25 Quality of Care
Each resident must receive and the facility must provide the necessary care and services to attain or maintain the highest practicable physical, mental, and psychosocial well-being, in accordance with the comprehensive assessment and plan of care.

Intent: §483.25
The facility must ensure that the resident obtains optimal improvement or does not deteriorate within the limits of a resident's right to refuse treatment, and within the limits of recognized pathology and the normal aging process.

Definitions: §483.25
• "Highest practicable" is defined as the highest level of functioning and well-being possible, limited only by the individual's presenting functional status and potential for improvement or reduced rate of functional decline. Highest practicable is determined through the comprehensive resident assessment by competently and thoroughly addressing the physical, mental or psychosocial needs of the individual.

Reprinted with permission from CMS Manual System, Pub 100-07 State Operations Provider Certification, 11/12/04.

includes the Resident Assessment Instrument (RAI), which evaluates the resident's skin condition, intrinsic risk, and other factors that can place the resident at risk for developing pressure ulcers or delay the healing of pressure ulcers.

CLINICAL WISDOM

Ensuring Optimal Nutrition

Maintaining or improving the nutritional status of elderly individuals who progress from one care setting to another presents a challenge for the health-care team. Identification of risk factors that contribute to undernutrition or malnutrition in long-term care facilities is essential. Federal regulations mandate that nursing facilities provide care that maximizes the resident's quality of life. Protein-energy undernutrition has been associated with the development of ulcers, cognitive problems, infections, and increased mortality. Optimizing nutrition screening and intervention helps to achieve positive outcomes for the resident. Often, reimbursement rates do not cover the cost of care. Liquid oral supplements or fortified foods are not reimbursable under state or federal regulations, but fall under the daily rate of care.

Examples of Risk Factors

• Impaired/decreased mobility and decreased functional ability
• Comorbid conditions, such as end-stage renal disease, thyroid disease or diabetes mellitus
• Drugs, such as steroids, that can affect wound healing
• Impaired diffuse or localized blood flow, e.g., generalized atherosclerosis or lower extremity arterial insufficiency
• A resident's refusal of some aspects of care and treatment
• Cognitive impairment
• Exposure of skin to urine and feces due to incontinence
• Undernutrition, malnutrition, and hydration deficits
• A healed ulcer[3,4,5]

The Agency for Health Care Research and Quality (AHRQ), formerly known as the Agency for Health Care Policy and Research (AHCPR), was established in 1989 under OBRA to enhance the quality, appropriateness, and effectiveness of health-care services and patient access to these services. AHCPR published a series of clinical practice guidelines related to pressure ulcers, including *Pressure Ulcer in Adults: Prediction and Prevention*[6] in 1992 and *Treatment of Pressure Ulcers*,[7] released in 1994. The guidelines assist the dietetic professional in assessment and development of action plans for the nutritional care of clients with pressure ulcers.

Nutritional Assessment

Nutritional assessment includes the interpretation of data from the screening process. The assessment process also includes a review of data from other disciplines (e.g., physical therapy and occupational therapy), which can affect the assessment process. Nutritional assessment precedes a care plan, intervention, and evaluation. *The Prevention of Pressure Ulcers: Nutrition Decision Tree* (Figure 3-1) and the recommendations made in Exhibit 3-2 can be used as guide-

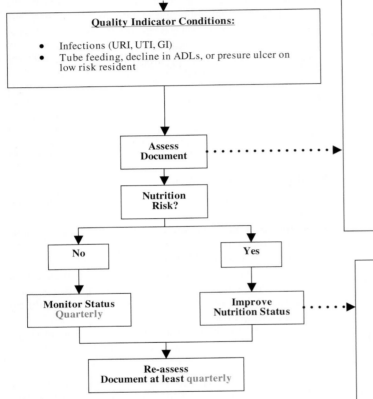

Trigger Conditions

- Undesired wt. loss: 5% in 30 days; 10% in 180 days
- BMI # 21 (705 x wt in lbs/ht in inches **or** wt in kilograms/ht in meters)
- Swallowing problems / dysphagia
- Resident leaves 25% or more of food uneaten at two-thirds of meals (in last 7 days)
- Immobility & selected conditions per master protocol

Quality Indicator Conditions:

- Infections (URI, UTI, GI)
- Tube feeding, decline in ADLs, or presure ulcer on low risk resident

Assess Document

Nutrition Risk?

No

Yes

Monitor Status Quarterly

Improve Nutrition Status

Re-assess Document at least quarterly

Dietitian Assess:
- Current weight/height
- Determine desirable body weight
- Body Mass Index (BMI)
- Interview for food preferences/intolerances
- Caloric needs
    1. Protein 1-1.2 g/kg
    2. Fluid 30 mL/kg or minimum of 1500 mL or per medical condition
- Laboratory values (within 30 days)
    1. Albumin
    2. Hb (Hemoglobin)
    3. Hct (Hematocrit)
    4. Prealbumin
- Risk factors for pressure ulcer development
    1. Medical history
    2. Validated risk assessment (i.e., Braden Scale)
    3. Medical treatments
    4. Medications (type of medications)
    5. Ability to meet nutritional needs orally (if inadequate, consider alternative method of feeding) consistent with patient's wishes
    6. Oral problems (i.e., chewing, swallowing)
- Pain

Considerations:
- Incorporate fortified foods at meals for weight gain
- Provide supplements between meals as needed
- Vary the type of supplements offered to prevent taste fatigue
- Provide preferred food/food substitutions
- At admission weigh weekly x 30 days and then monthly
- Monitor acceptance of food and/or supplements offered
- Evaluate lab values when available
- Provide assistance at meal time if needed
- Encourage family involvement
- Offer food/fluid at appropriate texture for condition
- Liberalize restrictive diets
- Consult with pharmacist and provide food and drugs at appropriate times and amounts
- Consider alternative method of feeding and if consistent with patient's wishes and goals of therapy:
    1. Provide tube feeding to meet needs per assessment
    2. Appropriate products provided and tolerance maintained
    3. Provide Total Parenteral Nutrition (TPN) when gut is non-functioning to meet needs per assessment

FIGURE 3-1 Nutrition Guideline: Policy for Prevention of Pressure Ulcers

EXHIBIT 3-2 Assessment Recommendations for Determining Proper Weight, Caloric Levels, and Degree of Nutritional Depletion

Recommended Weight for Height

Female: 100 lb per 5 ft + 5 lb per inch > 5 ft

Males: 106 lb per 5 ft + 6 lb per inch > 5 ft

Basal Energy Expenditure (BEE)

Female: 655 + (9.6 × wt. in kg) + (1.8 × ht. in cm) − (4.7 × age in years)

Male: 66 + 13.7 × wt. in kg) + (5.0 × ht. in cm) − (6.8 × age in years)

Estimated daily calorie levels are determined by multiplying the BEE and the appropriate injury and/or activity factor.

Injury Factors:

1.00–1.05	Postoperative (no complications)
1.05–1.25	Peritonitis
1.10–1.45	Cancer
1.15–1.30	Long bone fracture
1.20–1.60	Wound healing
1.25–1.50	Blunt trauma
1.30–1.55	Severe infection / multiple trauma
1.50–1.70	Multiple trauma with client on ventilator
1.60–1.70	Trauma with steroids
1.75–1.85	Sepsis

Burns (% total body surface):

1.00–1.50	0%–20%
1.50–1.85	20%–40%
1.85–2.05	40%–100%

Activity Factors:

1.2	For clients confined to bed
1.3	For ambulatory clients
1.5–1.75	For most normally active persons
2.0	For extremely active persons

Protein Needs for Adults

Condition:	Albumin Level: (g/dL)	Protein Requirement: (g/kg/d)
Normal nutrition	3.5 g/dL	0.8 g/kg/day
Mild depletion	2.8–3.5 g/dL	1.0–1.2 g/kg/day
Moderate depletion	2.1–2.7 g/dL	1.2–1.5 g/kg/day
Severe depletion	2.1 g/dL	1.5–2.0 g/kg/day
COPD		100–125 g protein/day total

Exceptions:

Renal failure	Protein requirement (g/kg/d)		
Non-dialyzed	0.5–0.6 g/kg/day	Hepatic failure	0.25–0.5 g/kg/day
Hemo-dialyzed	1.0–1.2 g/kg/day	Pulmonary compromised	1.2–1.9 g/kg/day (maintenance)
Peritoneal-dialyzed	1.2–1.5 g/kg/day		1.6–2.5 g/kg/day (repletion)

Another method to calculate protein needs: ratio of grams nitrogen to nonprotein calories (6.25 g protein–1 g N.)

Patient Conditions:	Ratio of Nonprotein kcal: 1 g N
Adult medical	125–150:1
Minor catabolic	125–180:1
Severe catabolic	150–250:1
Hepatic or renal failure	250–400:1

Reprinted with permission from Consultant Dietitians in Health Care Facilities, Practice Group of The American Dietetic Association, *Pocket Resource for Nutrition Assessment*, p. 50–53, (c) 2005.

Fluid Status
- Congestive heart failure/edema = 25 cc/kg of body weight
- Normal fluid status = 25–30 cc/kg of body weight
- 1 mL/kcal
- 100 mL/kg for first 10 kg body weight + 50 mL/kg for second 10 kg body weight + 15 mL/kg for remaining kg body weight
- OR shortcut to this method: (kg body weight − 20) × 15 + 1500 mL

Reprinted with permission from J.C. Chidester and A.A. Spangler, Fluid Intake in the Institutionalized Elderly. Copyright The American Dietetic Association. Reprinted by permission from *Journal of the American Dietetic Association*, Vol. 97, pp. 23–28, © 1997.

lines for performing a nutritional assessment. A Nutrition Risk Assessment form designed for long-term care facilities is included in Appendix 3-B. This risk assessment can also be utilized in other care settings, as the strategies and interventions apply to any health-care setting.

The dietitian reviews the screens and assessments from the various therapies to determine a nutritional care plan. The speech therapist determines the diet texture, including the need for any special feeding techniques, to be implemented by the dietary department. As an example, clients may require thickened liquids to prevent dehydration or aspiration. The occupational therapist often determines the need for self-help feeding devices, which promote eating independence. The dietitian is then responsible for ensuring that this special equipment is provided at meal time. Physical therapy sessions often result in the need for both increased calories and fluid, for which the dietitian will calculate and arrange provision at appropriate times.

Physical Conditions

Observe the client's skin condition, looking closely for signs of dehydration, edema, and/or ascites, which can be indicative of protein deficiency, renal disease, or hepatic disease. All of these signs have potential nutritional significance. Loose skin can be evidence of weight loss, and the interviewer should question the client about his or her usual weight. Make a visual scan for dry, flaky skin, skin that "tents" (which can reveal dehydration), and nonhealing wounds, purpura, or bruises.[9]

Older adults are particularly prone to pressure ulcers as a result of decreased mobility, multiple contributing diagnoses, poor nutrition, and loss of muscle mass. Often, the physiologic effects of aging also affect nutrition in older clients. The loss of skin elasticity and moisture, coupled with reduced sensation in susceptible areas, place older clients at risk for impaired skin integrity. Nutritional factors that contribute to skin breakdown include protein deficiency, creating a negative nitrogen balance; anemia, inhibiting the formation of red blood cells; and dehydration, causing dry, fragile skin. Dehydration can also increase the blood glucose level and slow the healing process.[10] With advancing age comes decreased skin response to temperature, pain, and pressure, which affects the skin's elasticity and the healing process.[11]

Dramatic changes in the skin occur with aging. Sweat glands decrease in number, and there is atrophy and thinning of the epithelial and fatty layers of tissue. In older individuals, there is little subcutaneous fat on the legs and forearms; this may be the case even if abundant abdominal or hip fat is present. One result of the general loss of fat from the subcutaneous tissue is the relative prominence of the bony protuberances of the thorax, scapula, trochanters, and knees. The loss of this valuable padding contributes to pressure ulcer risk in the aged.

Malnutrition is a condition of faulty or inadequate nutrition. Registered dietitians and other health-care professionals should examine clients for physical signs of malnutrition. Risk factors that can lead to undernutrition are noted in Exhibit 3-3. The term *malnutrition* is often used synonymously with the more descriptive and inclusive term *poor nutritional status*. Poor nutritional status has been defined by the Nutrition Screening Initiative as including "not only deficiency, dehydration, undernutrition, nutritional imbalances, and obesity, but other excesses such as alcohol abuse. Also included are inappropriate dietary intakes for conditions that have nutritional implications and the presence of an underlying physical or mental illness with treatable nutritional implications. Finally, poor nutritional status also encompasses evidence that a client's nutritional status may be deteriorating over time. Such evidence can be derived from objective clinical signs (Table 3-1), nonspecific clinical evidence, responses to direct, specific questions about diet and nutrition (even if complaints are not volunteered), and reliable reports from third parties (family, friends, caregivers, aides, social workers)."[12]

CLINICAL WISDOM

Pressure Ulcer

Warning Signs

The following are signs that an individual is at risk for or suffering from pressure ulcers:

- Subject to incontinence
- Needs help:
    moving arms, legs, or body
    turning in bed
    changing position when sitting
- Loses weight
- Eats less than half of meals/snacks served
- Is dehydrated
- Has discolored, torn, or swollen skin over bony areas

Report and Take Action

Below are some action steps to help individuals who are at risk for or suffering from pressure ulcers:

- Report observations and warning signs to nurse and dietitian.
- Check and change linens as appropriate.
- Handle/move the resident with care to avoid skin tears and scrapes.
- Reposition the resident frequently and properly.
- Use "unintended weight loss action steps" so resident gets more calories and protein.
- Use "dehydration action steps" so resident gets more to drink.
- Record meal/snack intake.

Adapted with permission from the Nutrition Screening Initiative, a project of the American Academy of Family Physicians, the American Dietetic Association, and the National Council on the Aging, Inc., and funded in part by a grant from Ross Products Division, Abbott Laboratories Inc.

EXHIBIT 3-3   Risk Factors that Can Lead to Undernutrition

Type of Risk	Examples
Social issues	Lack of socialization No help with meals Poverty
Mechanical barriers	Diminished/altered taste Eats slowly Ethnic preference not available Poor eyesight Poor health Poor hygiene Poor motor coordination Requires culturally accepted food

Medical conditions	Interference with eating due to:
	* Cholelithiasis
	* Congestive heart failure
	* Diabetic gastroparesis
	* Malabsorption syndromes
	* Increased energy needs due to:
	  * Burns
	  * Cancer
	  * Chronic obstructive pulmonary disease
	  * Fractures
	  * Infections
	  * Wounds

Psychological conditions	Anorexia Dementia Depression Late-life paranoia

Anthropometry

Anthropometry is the measurement of body size, weight, and proportions. These measurements are used to evaluate a client's nutritional status. Low body weight, when associated with illness or injury, increases the risk of morbidity. Obesity is common among nonambulatory clients whose caloric expenditure is low. Loss of height is an early indicator of osteoporosis.[13] The aging process causes changes in body composition, including a decrease in lean body mass, loss of height, and increased body fat.

Body Mass Index

Body mass index (BMI) is a weight-to-height ratio composed of body weight (in kilograms) divided by the square of the height in meters, or weight (lb)/ht (in^2) <tim> 705. BMI is used as an indicator of obesity and/or desirable body weight. It is highly correlated with body fat, but increased lean body mass or a large body frame can also increase the BMI. It is generally agreed that a normally hydrated person with a BMI of 30 would be obese, and a person with a BMI of more than 27 would be at major risk for obesity.[14] A BMI of = 21 with involuntary weight loss places a client at risk for developing pressure ulcers.

Height and Weight

Weight and body composition change with age. Weight tends to peak in the sixth decade, with a gradual decrease beyond the seventh decade. Body composition shifts, and the proportion of body weight that is fat increases, averaging 30% of the total body weight in the older adult, as compared with 20% of the total body weight in younger people.

Weight Variances

Variances in weight have a significant impact on nutritional health, and the degree of a person's weight change positively correlates with the impact on their health status. When evaluating the severity of weight variances (Exhibit 3-4), it is important to determine possible causes, such as recent surgery or any recently initiated treatments (e.g., radiation or diuretic therapy) that can affect weight status.

Malnutrition or poor nutritional status impacts the healing process. Malnutrition, dehydration, or unintentional weight loss whether secondary to poor appetite or other disease processes, places clients at risk for tissue breakdown and poor healing. Stress as a result of injury, surgery, burns, fractures, or wounds results in depletion of nutrient stores required for healing. The body's protective mechanism, the inflammatory response, alters blood flow to an injury or infection site during severe stress. Hypermetabolism mobilizes nutrients into glucose and amino acid pools. Glycogen stores and protein are used to produce glucose and stress factors. The total energy rate is high, as the metabolic rate increases and the body continues to deplete protein stores. Catecholamines and cortisol have the metabolic effect of increasing glycogen breakdown, mobilizing free fatty acids, and accelerating glucose production from amino acids. The storage of glucose, fatty acids, and protein declines with the continued glucose production from amino acids. Protein from the skeletal muscle, gut, and connective tissues supplies the glucose and amino acids necessary for the synthesis of stress factors and the immune cells (Figure 3-2).[15]

Therapeutic Diets

A highly restrictive diet order can contribute significantly to reduced food intake and a marked decline in nutritional status. The denial of favorite foods and/or enforcement of a therapeutic diet can also diminish a client's quality of life. Food is not nutritious unless eaten. Certain medical conditions require diet modifications, but these can often be met with simple adjustments and minimal restrictions.[17]

Treatments and Medications

Treatments and medications contributing to the risk for pressure ulcers include antidepressants, sleeping pills, drug-

TABLE 3-1 **Physical Signs of Malnutrition**

Signs	Possible Causes
Hair	
Dull, dry, lack of natural shine	Protein-energy deficiency
	Essential fatty acid (EFA) deficiency
Thin, sparse, loss of curl	Zinc deficiency
Color changes, depigmentation, easily plucked	Other nutrient deficiencies; manganese, copper
Eyes	
Small, yellowish lumps around eyes, white rings around both eyes	Hyperlipidemia
Angular inflammation of eyelids, "grittiness" under eyelids	Riboflavin deficiency
Pale eye membranes	Vitamin B12, folacin, and/or iron deficiency
Night blindness, dry membranes, dull or soft cornea	Vitamin A or zinc deficiency
Redness and fissures of eyelid corners	Niacin deficiency
Ring of fine blood vessels around cornea	Generally poor nutrition
Lips	
Redness and swelling of mouth	Niacin, riboflavin, iron and/or pyridoxine deficiency
Angular fissures, scars at corner of mouth	Niacin, riboflavin, iron and/or pyridoxine deficiency
Soreness, burning lips, pallor	Riboflavin deficiency
Gums	
Spongy, swollen, red; bleed easily, redness	Vitamin C deficiency
Gingivitis	Folic acid, vitamin B12 deficiency
Mouth	
Cheilosis, angular scars	Riboflavin or folic acid, pyridoxine deficiency
Soreness, burning	Riboflavin deficiency
Tongue	
Sores, swollen, scarlet, raw	Folacin or niacin deficiency
Soreness, burning tongue, purplish color	Riboflavin deficiency
Smooth with papillae (small projections)	Riboflavin, vitamin B12, or pyridoxine deficiency
Glossitis	Iron or zinc deficiency
Taste	
Sense of taste diminished	Zinc deficiency
Teeth	
Grey-brown spots	Increased fluoride intake
Missing or erupting abnormally	Generally poor nutrition
Face	
Skin color loss, dark cheeks and eyes, enlarged parotid glands, scaling of skin around nostrils	Protein-energy deficiency, specifically niacin, riboflavin, or pyridoxine deficiency
Pallor	Iron, folacin, vitamin B12 or vitamin C deficiency
Hyperpigmentation	Niacin deficiency
Neck	
Thyroid enlargement	Iodine deficiency
Symptoms of hypothyroidism	Iodine deficiency

(Continued)

TABLE 3-1   Physical Signs of Malnutrition   *(Continued)*

Signs	Possible Causes
Nails	
Fragility, banding	Protein deficiency
Spoon-shaped	Iron deficiency
Skin	
Slow wound healing	Zinc deficiency
Psoriasis	Biotin deficiency
Eczema	Riboflavin deficiency
Scaliness	Biotin deficiency, pyridoxine deficiency
Black and blue marks due to skin bleeding	Vitamin C and/or vitamin K deficiency
Dryness, mosaic, sandpaper feel, flakiness	Increased or decreased vitamin A
Swollen and dark	Niacin deficiency
Lack of fat under skin or bilateral edema	Protein-energy deficiency
Yellow-colored	Carotene deficiency or excess
Cutaneous flushing	Niacin
Pallor	Iron, folic acid deficiencies
Gastrointestinal	
Anorexia, flatulence, diarrhea	Vitamin B12 deficiency
Muscular System	
Weakness	Phosphorus or potassium deficiency
Wasted appearance	Protein-energy deficiency
Calf tenderness, absent knee jerks	Thiamin deficiency
Peripheral neuropathy	Folacin, pyridoxine, pantothenic acid, phosphate, thiamin deficiencies
Muscle twitching	Magnesium or pyridoxine excess or deficiency
Muscle cramps	Chloride decreased, sodium deficiency
Muscle pain	Biotin deficiency
Skeletal System	
Demineralization of bone	Calcium, phosphorus, vitamin D deficiencies
Epiphyseal enlargement of leg and knee Bowed legs	Vitamin D deficiency
Nervous System	
Listlessness	Protein-energy deficiency
Loss of position and vibratory sense, decrease and loss of ankle and knee reflexes, depression, inability to concentrate, defective memory, delirium	Thiamin, vitamin B12 deficiencies
Seizures, memory impairment, and behavior disturbances	Magnesium, zinc deficiencies
Peripheral neuropathy, dementia	Pyridoxine deficiency

Reprinted with permission from Consultant Dietitians in Health Care Facilities, CD-HCF Pocket Resource for Nutrition Assessment, 2005 Revision. Chicago, IL: Consultant Dietitians in Health Care Facilities; 2005:69-73

EXHIBIT 3-4   Severity of Weight Loss

Significant weight loss:[16]	Severe weight loss:
• 10% in 6 months	• > 10% in 6 months
• 7.5% in 3 months	• > 7.5% in 3 months
• 5% in 1 month	• > 5% in 1 month
• 2% in 1 week	• > 2% in 1 week

Reprinted with permission from American Dietetic Association. *Nutrition Care of the Older Adult.* Copyright 2004.

related immunosuppression, and steroid therapy. Many of the drugs designed to calm or reduce agitation can, in turn, reduce a client's mobility and activity levels, resulting in decreased food intake. The common side effects of some drugs, such as gastric disturbances, affect the intake of food and fluid. Radiation therapy, chemotherapy, and renal dialysis can result in increased nausea and vomiting, as well as decreased activity.

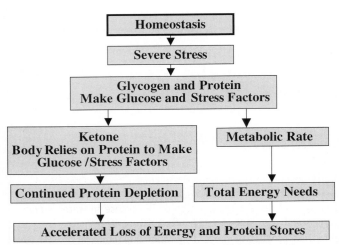

FIGURE 3-2 Metabolic Response to Severe Stress. (Reprinted with permission from Mary Ellen Posthauer, RD, CD, LD. Published in *Advances in Skin and Wound Care*, September 2005.)

CLINICAL WISDOM

Unintended Weight Loss

Warning Signs

- Needs help eating or drinking
- Eats less than half of meal/snack served
- Has mouth pain
- Has dentures that don't fit
- Has a hard time chewing or swallowing
- Coughs or chokes while eating
- Has sadness, crying spells, or withdrawal from others
- Is confused, wanders, or paces
- Has diabetes, chronic obstructive pulmonary disease (COPD), cancer, HIV, or other chronic disease

Report and Take Action

Below are some action steps to increase food intake, create a positive dining environment, and help individuals consume adequate calories:

- Report observations and warning signs to nurse and dietitian.
- Encourage the resident to eat.
- Honor food likes and dislikes.
- Offer many kinds of foods and beverages.
- Help individuals who have trouble feeding themselves.
- Allow enough time to finish eating.
- Notify nursing staff if the resident has trouble using utensils.
- Record meal and snack intake.
- Provide oral care before meals.
- Position individual correctly for feeding.
- If the resident has had a loss of appetite and/or seems sad, ask what's wrong.

Adapted with permission from the Nutrition Screening Initiative, a project of the American Academy of Family Physicians, the American Dietetic Association, and the National Council on the Aging, Inc., and funded in part by a grant from Ross Products Division, Abbott Laboratories Inc.

Medication should be checked for possible effects on nutritional intake, as well as any effect on the client's mental and physical status. Constipation and diarrhea are both risk factors that should be addressed in a nutritional assessment. Laxative abuse can induce a state of malabsorption. Chronic diarrhea can lead to dehydration and weight loss, which increase the risk for malnutrition and pressure ulcers.

Lab Values

Laboratory indexes for nutritional assessment primarily involve tests related to protein metabolism. Protein status can be evaluated through a nitrogen-balance study, visceral protein blood levels, and gross tests of immune functions such as total lymphocyte counts. Abnormal laboratory results can also reflect the effects of poor appetite and disease processes. Laboratory values indicating risk for poor wound healing are shown in Exhibit 3-5.

Laboratory values indicative of malnutrition include a serum albumin level below 3.5 g/dL, serum transferrin level less than 180 mg/dL, or prealbumin less than 17 mg/dL.[18] Serum albumin is a sensitive indicator of acute changes in clinical status from infection, hydration, starvation, or a combination of these factors. Sixty percent of total protein is albumin. Age and declining liver function affect the ability of the body to synthesize albumin. Serum albumin has a long half-life of roughly 20 days, so concentration falls slowly and is therefore not a good indicator of early malnutrition. Levels are shown with implications in Exhibit 3-6.

A serum cholesterol level of less than 160 mg/dL with poor intake and weight loss places a client at risk for pressure ulcers. A hemoglobin level less than 12 mg/dL and hematocrit level less than 33% are important indicators of anemia. Deficits in hemoglobin and hematocrit have been correlated with the risk of developing pressure ulcers. Prealbumin or thyroxine binding prealbumin levels are used to measure impaired nutrition status and the response to refeed-

EXHIBIT 3-5 Lab Values Indicative of Increased Risk for Delayed Wound Healing

Serum Transferrin < 170 mg/dL
Prealbumin < 16 mg/dL
Serum Albumin < 3.5 mg/dL with normal hydration status
Hemoglobin < 12 g/dL
Hematocrit < 33%
Serum Cholesterol < 160 mg/dL
Total Lymphocyte Count < 1800/mm
Serum Osmolality > 295 mOsm/L
BUN/Creatinine > 10:1

Reprinted with permission from *Treatment of Pressure Ulcers: Clinical Practice Guidelines, No. 15,* AHCPR Publication No. 95–0652, Agency for Health Care Policy and Research, U.S. Department of Health and Human Services, Rockville, MD, December 1994.

EXHIBIT 3-6 Laboratory Values and Implications

Test	Normal Values	Implications
Albumin (Alb)	3.5–5.0 g/dL 35–50 g/L (SI units)	**Function:** Maintain colloidal osmotic pressure, transport molecule for ions, hormones, some drugs, enzymes, fatty acids, amino acids, bilirubin, pigments **Site of Synthesis:** Liver **Half Life:** 12–18 days **Increased:** Dehydration **Decreased:** Overhydration, liver disease, severe burns, malnutrition, preeclampsia, malabsorption, CHF, nephritic syndrome, infection, stress, advanced malignancies, protein losing enteropathies, thyroid disease, renal disorders, pregnancy, vasculitis, ulcerative bowel disease, individuals : 70 years of age, trauma, sepsis, pernicious anemia, spinal cord injury, decubitus ulcer, cystic fibrosis, excessive administration of IV glucose in water, starvation, burns, surgery, MI, cytokine-induced inflammatory states
Blood Urea Nitrogen (BUN)	10–20 mg/dL 3.6–7.1 mmol/L	**Function:** Detoxified product of protein metabolism, indicates recent protein intake **Site of synthesis:** Liver **Increased:** Dehydration, increased protein intake, urinary obstruction, renal failure/insufficiency, increased catabolism of protein due to infection, tumors, starvation, stress, trauma, myocardial infarction, diabetes mellitus, increased age, steroid therapy, gastrointestinal bleeding, CHF, shock, GI hemorrhage, chronic gout, burns, sepsis **Decreased:** Overhydration, liver damage or advanced cirrhosis, low protein diet, malnutrition, pregnancy, impaired absorption
Cholesterol–Total	< 200 gm/dL < 5.20 mmol/L	**Function:** Used to form bile salts, hormones, and cell membranes **Site of synthesis:** Liver **Increased:** CVD, atherosclerosis, myocardial infarction, hypothyroidism, uncontrolled DM, biliary cirrhosis, pregnancy, hyperlipoproteinemia, nephritic syndrome, biliary obstruction, high cholesterol and/or saturated fat diet, hypertension **Decreased:** Hyperthyroidism, malnutrition, malabsorption, liver disease, anemia, stress, severe infection, cancer, pernicious anemia, cytokine-induced inflammatory states
Creatinine	Male 0.6–1/2 mg/dL 53–106 umol/L Female 0.5–1.1 mg/dL 44–97 umol/L	**Function:** Nitrogenous by-product in the breakdown of muscle creatine phosphate due to energy metabolism **Site of synthesis:** N/A **Increased:** Impaired renal function, shock, diabetic nephropathy, CHF, AMI, some cancers, dehydration, chronic nephritis, urinary tract obstruction, muscle disease, nephro-toxic drugs, gigantism, acromegaly, rhabdomyolysis **Decreased:** Overhydration, muscular dystrophy, pregnancy, eclampsia, scarcopenia or muscle wasting, severe wasting
Prealbumin (Prealb)	15–36 mg/dL 150–360 md/L	**Function:** Transport thyroxine, complexes with retinol-binding protein for vitamin A transport **Site of synthesis:** Liver **Increased:** Renal failure, dehydration, Hodgkin's, pregnancy **Decreased:** Liver disease, malnutrition, catabolic states, metabolic stress, inflammation, surgical trauma, hyperthyroidism, overhydration, protein losing enteropathy, infection, inflammations, cytokine-induced inflammatory states
Total lymphocyte count (TLC)	3000–3500 cells/mm3	**Increased:** Leukemia, infectious bacterial diseases, leukocytosis **Decreased:** Corticosteroid therapy, cancer, chemotherapy, radiotherapy, surgery, lymphopenia, malnutrition Degrees of depletion: mild = 1500–1800, moderate = 900–1500, severe < 900

Adapted with permission from *Pocket Resource for Nutrition Assessment*, 2005 rev., Consultant Dietitians in Health Care Facilities, a dietetic practice group of the American Dietetic Association, pp. 75-85.

ing. Pre-albumin levels decrease with infection, inflammation and cytokine induced inflammatory states.

Biochemical assessment data must be used with caution because it can be altered by hydration, medication, and changes in metabolism. Parameters for evaluating hydration status include assessing urine output (I/O), weight, blood urea nitrogen (BUN)/creatinine ratio (greater than 10 to 1), and skin turgor (Table 3-2).

Chewing and swallowing problems resulting in poor oral intake can lead to malnutrition and pressure ulcers. Edentulous clients or those who have loose dentures as a result of weight loss often avoid foods high in protein that are difficult to chew, such as meat or meat alternates. This restricts their overall intake, thus increasing the chance for weight loss. If untreated, clients with dysphagia become dehydrated, lose weight, and develop pressure ulcers. Loss of dexterity and/or the ability to self-feed is a risk factor for malnutrition because the result is often poor oral intake.

The Role of Nutrients in Wound Healing

With the spotlight on elaborate diagnostic tests, high-tech surgeries, and complex drug prescriptions, it is easy to lose sight of the basic concept of nutrition. More than just food, nutrition encompasses the many nutrients, calories, and fluids taken into the body, all of which are vital to the healing of wounds (Exhibit 3-7). References such as the *Nutrition Guideline: Policy for Treatment of Stage I-II and III-IV Pressure Ulcer* (Figures 3-3 and 3-4) can assist the health-care team in making appropriate nutrition intervention decisions to promote the healing of pressure ulcers. The guidelines for stages III and IV are more aggressive due to the complexity of the wounds.

Carbohydrates

Carbohydrates are supplied by starch in the form of grains, cereals, legumes (peas and beans), pasta, bread, and the natural sugars contained in fruits, vegetables, and milk. Added sugars also provide carbohydrates in the diet. Carbohydrates serve several functions, as shown in Exhibit 3-8.

Protein

All proteins consist of carbon, hydrogen, oxygen, and nitrogen atoms; proteins are the only nutrients containing nitrogen. Some proteins also contain phosphorus and sulfur. The body utilizes protein in numerous ways (Exhibit 3-9). Protein is responsible for the synthesis of enzymes involved in wound healing, cell multiplication, and the synthesis of collagen and connective tissue. Increased protein levels are linked to improved wound healing in patients with pressure ulcers.[19,20] The optimum protein range has not been established, but a range of 1.5–2.0 grams of protein a day per kilogram of body weight has been associated with proper wound healing.[21] Intakes beyond 2.0 g/kg can affect renal and hepatic functions.[22]

Protein is also a component of the antibodies necessary for proper immune system function. There are nine essential amino acids that must be supplied by the protein found in food consumed. Eleven nitrogen-containing amino acids (nonessential) can be made by the body. However, under conditions of stress, arginine and glutamine become conditionally essential amino acids. L-arginine, which is 32% nitrogen, stimulates the insulin-like growth factor that promotes healing. This stimulation of insulin secretion promotes the transport of amino acids into tissue cells and supports the formation of protein in the cells. Arginine is the substrate for nitric acid and a regulator of nucleic acid synthesis. Nitric acid production activates wound macrophages, which are rich sources of growth factors, cytokines, bioactive lipid products, and proteolytic enzymes necessary for the healing process.[23,24,25] The increased level of arginine promotes the conversion of arginine to ornithine, which is a precursor to proline. Proline is incorporated into collagen.[26,27,28]

Nutritional supplements formulated for wound care are often fortified with arginine and glutamine, as well as zinc and vitamins C and E. ß-hydroxy-ß-methylbutyrate (HMB),

TABLE 3-2 Useful Lab Values to Screen for Hydration Status

Lab Test	Normal Values	Dehydration	Over-hydration
Osmolality	280–303 mOsm/kg	> 303 mOsm/kg (critical)	> 320 mOsm/kg
Serum sodium	135–145 mEq/L	> 145 mEq/L	< 130 meEq/L
Albumin	3.4–5.4 g/dL	Higher than normal	Lower than normal
Blood urine nitrogen (BUN)	7–20 mg/dL	> 35 mg/dL	< 7mg/dL
BUN/creatinine ratio	10:1	> 25:1	< 10:1
Urine specific gravity	1.002–1.028 g/mL	> 1.028 g/mL	< 1.002 g/mL

Medline Plus Medical Encyclopedia
Reprinted with permission from *Healing Solutions, Hydration Care for Wound Prevention and Healing*, Novartis Medical Nutrition;2004:25.

EXHIBIT 3–7 Skin Integrity and Wound Healing: The Role of Nutrition

It has long been recognized but unappreciated that impaired nutritional status and inadequate dietary intake are risk factors for developing pressure ulcers. A well-balanced diet with adequate carbohydrate, protein, fat, water, vitamins, and minerals is necessary to maintain skin integrity.

Calories, protein, water, vitamin C, and zinc are often emphasized to promote wound healing. However, adequate intake of these nutrients or any nutrient alone does not facilitate healing. Sufficient calories plus all essential nutrients are required.

Calories

The body's first priority is for adequate energy. When the total amount of calories is too low, protein from both the diet and the patient's muscle stores will be used as an energy source; the patient will lose weight, and adipose tissue, as well as lean body mass, will be lost.

Every wound patient's calorie needs are unique. The caloric goal for patients with wounds is to prevent weight loss from occurring. In underweight patients, a slow, steady weight gain will increase the speed of wound healing. The three major nutrients—carbohydrate, protein, and fat—provide calories. Carbohydrates and fats are the preferred energy source for a healing wound.

Protein

Dietary protein is needed for tissue maintenance and repair. Protein depletion impairs wound healing by preventing a desirable wound bed from forming. Repletion of calorie and protein status in undernourished patients is associated with shorter time to heal and improved wound strength. In general, a wound patient's daily dietary protein needs (expressed as grams of protein) can be estimated by dividing the patient's weight in half. For example, a patient who weighs 100 pounds would need approximately 50 g of protein daily to heal wounds. Too high a protein intake will increase fluid needs, and wound healing will be reduced if fluid needs are not met.

Water

Water is an especially important nutrient for patients with wounds. Dehydration is a risk factor for development of wounds, and the water needs of patients with stages 3 and 4 pressure ulcers are very high. A good rule of thumb is to be sure that all patients receive a minimum of 1 mL of water for every kcal fed, or about 15 mL of water per pound of body weight per day. Wound patients need at least 2000–2500 mL of water a day (2 quarts or more).

Water and other household beverages are adequate sources of water in most cases and can be given orally or by feeding tube. These fluids, however, are not adequate to replace the fluid and electrolyte losses that accompany vomiting, diarrhea, or other sources of gastrointestinal fluid losses. In these cases, a rehydration solution, such as Equalyte(r) (Ross Products Division of Abbott Laboratories), which is specifically designed to match and replace these losses, is needed.

Vitamin C

Because nutritional deficiency has been associated with impaired wound healing, supplemental intake of vitamins and minerals is often thought to be important for wound healing. Although not appropriate for all patients, vitamin and mineral supplements are probably most beneficial for patients with a history of poor intake, who are, therefore, likely to have limited nutrient stores. A general one-a-day type vitamin and mineral supplement equal to 100% of the Dietary Reference Intake (DRI) for vitamins and minerals is prudent for patients with wounds.

Vitamin C is essential in collagen synthesis. Collagen and fibroblasts compose the basis for the structure of a new healing wound bed. A deficiency of vitamin C prolongs healing time, decreases wound strength, and contributes to decreased resistance to infection. There is no evidence, however, that human wound healing is improved by providing doses of vitamin C many times greater than the RDA. It is reasonable to increase vitamin C intake through consumption of fruits, vegetables, and juices for persons with extensive wounds who may rapidly exhaust their body reserves and for those with a history of poor intake.

Zinc

Zinc deficiency can occur through wound drainage or excessive gastrointestinal fluid losses, or can be due to long-term low dietary intake. Chronic, severe zinc deficiency results in abnormal function of white blood cells and lymphocytes, increased susceptibility to infection, and delayed wound healing. Large amounts of dietary zinc, however, interfere with copper metabolism and are not advisable. The amount of zinc in a multiple vitamin/mineral supplement is generally adequate. It is preferable and safer to provide the RDI in zinc through a one-a-day type of multiple vitamin and mineral supplement than to provide individual zinc supplementation at very high levels (such as zinc sulfate 200–300 mg daily or three times daily).

Courtesy of Ross Products Division, Abbott Laboratories, Columbus, Ohio.

arginine, and glutamine are the ingredients in one supplement. HMB is the metabolite of the amino acid leucine, which has a role in supporting the immune function. HMB serves as a precursor to cholesterol, which is a component of all cell membranes, and enhances the integrity of cells and reduces cell rupture under stress. Thus, lean body mass and muscle integrity are preserved.[29] Food sources of protein include meat, milk products, and legumes.

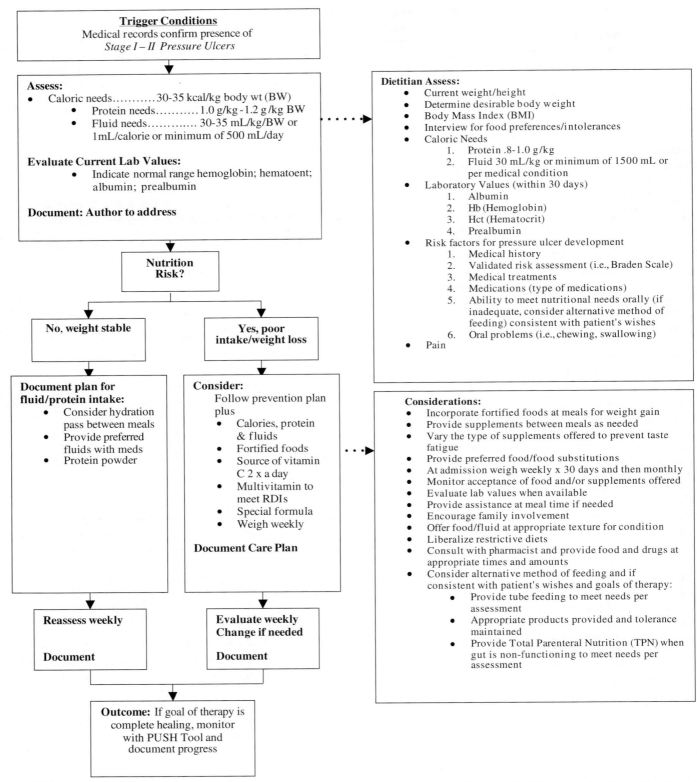

Trigger Conditions
Medical records confirm presence of
Stage I – II Pressure Ulcers

Assess:
- Caloric needs............30-35 kcal/kg body wt (BW)
  - Protein needs............1.0 g/kg - 1.2 g/kg BW
  - Fluid needs..............30-35 mL/kg/BW or
    1mL/calorie or minimum of 500 mL/day

Evaluate Current Lab Values:
- Indicate normal range hemoglobin; hematoent;
  albumin; prealbumin

Document: Author to address

**Nutrition
Risk?**

No, weight stable

**Yes, poor
intake/weight loss**

**Document plan for
fluid/protein intake:**
- Consider hydration
  pass between meals
- Provide preferred
  fluids with meds
- Protein powder

Consider:
  Follow prevention plan
  plus
- Calories, protein
  & fluids
- Fortified foods
- Source of vitamin
  C 2 x a day
- Multivitamin to
  meet RDIs
- Special formula
- Weigh weekly

Document Care Plan

Reassess weekly

Document

**Evaluate weekly
Change if needed**

Document

Outcome: If goal of therapy is
complete healing, monitor
with PUSH Tool and
document progress

Dietitian Assess:
- Current weight/height
- Determine desirable body weight
- Body Mass Index (BMI)
- Interview for food preferences/intolerances
- Caloric Needs
  1. Protein .8-1.0 g/kg
  2. Fluid 30 mL/kg or minimum of 1500 mL or
     per medical condition
- Laboratory Values (within 30 days)
  1. Albumin
  2. Hb (Hemoglobin)
  3. Hct (Hematocrit)
  4. Prealbumin
- Risk factors for pressure ulcer development
  1. Medical history
  2. Validated risk assessment (i.e., Braden Scale)
  3. Medical treatments
  4. Medications (type of medications)
  5. Ability to meet nutritional needs orally (if
     inadequate, consider alternative method of
     feeding) consistent with patient's wishes
  6. Oral problems (i.e., chewing, swallowing)
- Pain

Considerations:
- Incorporate fortified foods at meals for weight gain
- Provide supplements between meals as needed
- Vary the type of supplements offered to prevent taste
  fatigue
- Provide preferred food/food substitutions
- At admission weigh weekly x 30 days and then monthly
- Monitor acceptance of food and/or supplements offered
- Evaluate lab values when available
- Provide assistance at meal time if needed
- Encourage family involvement
- Offer food/fluid at appropriate texture for condition
- Liberalize restrictive diets
- Consult with pharmacist and provide food and drugs at
  appropriate times and amounts
- Consider alternative method of feeding and if
  consistent with patient's wishes and goals of therapy:
  - Provide tube feeding to meet needs per
    assessment
  - Appropriate products provided and tolerance
    maintained
  - Provide Total Parenteral Nutrition (TPN) when
    gut is non-functioning to meet needs per
    assessment

FIGURE 3-3 Nutrition Guideline: Policy for Treatment of Stage I–II Pressure Ulcer (Reprinted with permission from *Healing Solutions, A Team Approach for Pressure Ulcer Wound Care,* Novartis Nutrition, 2003.)

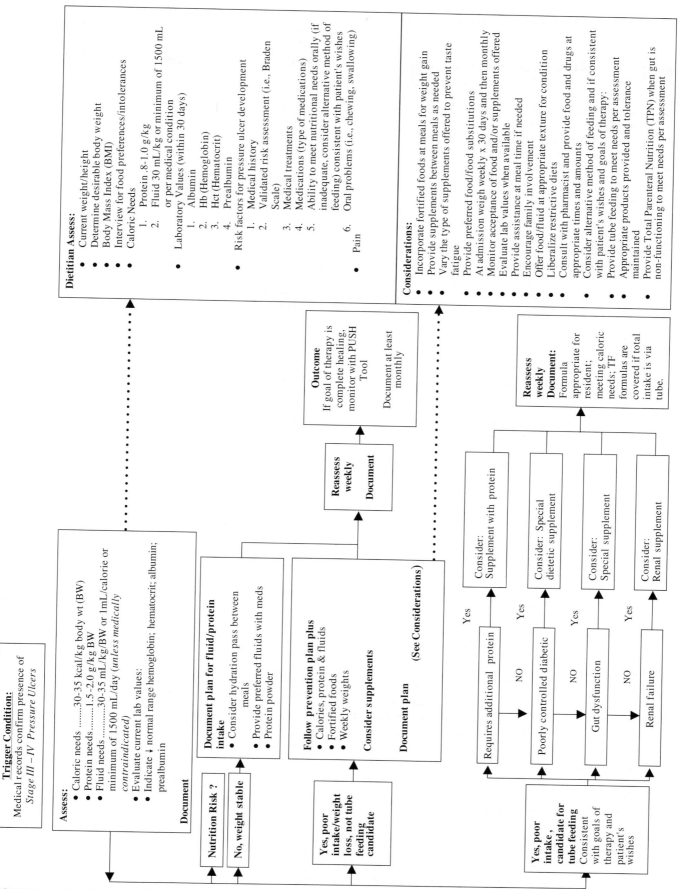

FIGURE 3-4 Nutrition Guideline: Policy for Treatment of Stage III – IV Pressure Ulcer: (Reprinted with permission from *Healing Solutions, A Team Approach for Pressure Ulcer Wound Care,* Novartis Nutrition, 2003.)

EXHIBIT 3-8   Functions of Carbohydrates

Carbohydrates serve the following functions:
- Serve as the most readily available source of energy for the body
- Spare protein for its primary use: building and maintaining tissue
- Provide cellular components for regulating metabolism
- Provide flavor, color, and variety to the diet
- Provide 4 kcal/g energy

CLINICAL WISDOM

Adding Protein and Calories

- Add dry milk to cream soups, mashed potatoes, casseroles, puddings, and milk-based desserts.
- Add 1/3 cup nonfat dry powdered milk to each cup of regular milk.
- Add cheese to vegetables, salads, potatoes, rice, noodles, and casseroles.
- Mix commercial supplements with ice cream or sherbet.
- Add yogurt to fruit and cereal.
- Add nuts, seeds, or wheat germ to casseroles, breads, muffins, pancakes, and cookies.
- Sprinkle nuts, seeds, or wheat germ on fruit, cereal, ice cream, and yogurt, or use in place of bread crumbs.
- Add peanut butter to sandwiches, toast, crackers, or muffins; use as a dip for vegetables and fruit; or add to milk and blend.
- Add dry beans to soups or casseroles.

Clients on dialysis or those with renal disease who require limited protein should be offered foods with high-quality protein, such as eggs, meat, fish, poultry, milk, and cheese. Proteins derived from animal sources are considered high-quality or complete proteins because they contain all of the amino acids essential to human nutrition in adequate amounts. The dietitian evaluates the appropriate quality and type of protein that will meet the diet order for clients with renal disease. Clients who are obese or those on low-cholesterol diets should select foods low in saturated fat, such as skim milk, lean fish, vegetable oils, and low-fat cheese.

Fats

Glycerides, which are composed of fatty acids and glycerol, are the most common fats in both the diet and the body. Fat is provided largely from meat, dairy products (e.g., milk, butter, cream, and eggs), fish and vegetable oils, nuts, and some fruits, such as olives and avocados. The functions of fats in the body and diet are shown in Exhibit 3-10.

Vitamins

A vitamin is an organic compound that the body requires in small amounts for proper functioning. The body cannot produce vitamins, so all vitamins must be obtained from food

EXHIBIT 3-9   Functions of Protein

Protein serves the following functions:
- Is involved in collagen synthesis, epidermal cell proliferation, skin integrity and resistance to infection, immune response, and gastrointestinal function
- Supplies structural and binding material of muscle, cartilage, ligaments, skin, hair, and fingernails
- Plays important roles as enzyme and hormone in chemical reactions and regulatory functions throughout the body and within cells
- Is a component of antibodies and immune system function
- Helps to maintain the fluid and mineral composition of various body fluids (fluid and electrolyte balance)
- Helps transport needed substances, such as lipids, minerals and oxygen, around the body
- Serves as building material for growth and repair of body tissues
- Provides 4 kcal/g

and beverages or from synthetic supplements. Vitamins facilitate various chemical reactions in the body, with different vitamins performing different functions. Vitamins play a key role in normal cell functioning and the cell's ability to use energy. Vitamins also participate in protein synthesis and cell replication. The functions of specific vitamins are best known by the results of their deficiencies.

Vitamin supplements are recommended if a client's diet is poor or limited in calories, or if a vitamin deficiency is suspected. A pharmacist or physician can determine the appropriate time to take a vitamin supplement in relationship to other medications. A daily high-potency multiple vitamin and mineral supplement is necessary if vitamin and mineral deficiencies are confirmed or suspected. Supplements should not be greater than 10 times the Recommended Dietary Allowance (RDA). Vitamins and their therapeutic properties are presented in Exhibit 3-11. Vitamins are divided into two groups, according to whether they are soluble in fat or water.

EXHIBIT 3-10   Functions of Fats

Fats serve several functions, including the following:
- Maintain normal cell membrane function
- Permit fat-soluble substances to move in and out of the cell
- Provide insulation under the skin from heat or cold
- Cushion the kidneys and other sensitive organs from shock and injury
- Provide flavor and aroma in food and carry the fat-soluble vitamins A, D, E, and K
- Serve as the most concentrated source of heat and energy, supplying 9 kcal/g
- Provide energy during long periods of food deprivation

EXHIBIT 3-11   Vitamins and their Therapeutic Properties

Vitamin A	Required for inflammatory response, although excessive amounts of this vitamin can exacerbate the inflammatory response
Vitamin B	Required for cross-linking of collagen fibers in rebuilding tissue
Vitamin C	Can increase the activation of leukocytes and macrophages to the wound site

Fat-soluble Vitamins

Vitamins A, D, E, and K are derived from the fatty and oily parts of certain foods. They remain in the liver and fat tissue of the body until they are used. Because the body does not excrete excess fat-soluble vitamins, there is some risk of toxicity from overdose resulting from over-accumulation.

Deficiencies of vitamin A have been associated with retarded epithelialization and decreased collagen synthesis. Because vitamin A is a fat-soluble vitamin and not excreted from the body, deficiencies are rare.

CLINICAL WISDOM

Nutritional Strategies

Nutritional supplements are frequently used to help achieve nutritional goals. For clients with pressure ulcers, weight gain and healing are often concurrent goals. Suggestions to achieve these goals include:

- Provide calorically dense supplements with a protein profile of 8 grams or higher and 200–250 kcal per 8 oz serving.
- Determine the client's flavor preferences and offer those preferred flavors. Clients often prefer a fruit-based product rather than the traditional milk-based products.
- Offer 2 fl oz of a nutrient-dense supplement 3 to 4 times daily, followed by 4 fl oz of water.
- Serve juice and/or fruit with meals to increase vitamin C intake.
- Offer supplements at least 1 hour before the next meal so client is hungry for the meal.
- Liberalize the diet when possible, as restrictive diets often reduce food intake. The American Dietetic Association has stated that liberalized diets for older adults in long-term care can enhance quality of life and nutritional status.[17]
- Consider nutritional support by tube feeding when the client cannot meet nutritional needs orally.
- Inform the client and/or caregivers of the risks and benefits of nutritional support. Ensure that nutritional support achieves the desired goals and is compatible with the wishes of the client and family.

Water-soluble Vitamins

Water-soluble vitamins include the vitamin B family and vitamin C, and are derived from the water components of foods. They are distributed throughout the water compartments of the body and, for the most part, are carried in the bloodstream. Unlike fat-soluble vitamins, they are not stored but are excreted in the urine when their concentration in the blood becomes too high. B vitamins are necessary for the production of energy from glucose, amino acids, and fat. Vitamin B6 (pyridoxine) helps maintain cellular integrity and form red blood cells. Thiamine and riboflavin are needed for cross-linking and collagenation.

Vitamin C (ascorbic acid) deficiency is associated with impaired fibroblastic function and decreased collagen synthesis, resulting in delayed healing, capillary fragility, and breakdown of old wounds. An age-associated decrease in ascorbic acid levels may increase the fragility of vessels and connective tissue, and lower the threshold for pressure-induced injury (Table 3-3).[30] Vitamin C deficiency is also associated with impaired immune function, decreasing the individual's ability to resist infection.[12] Because vitamin C is a water-soluble vitamin and cannot be stored in the body, deficiencies can develop quickly if adequate intake is not maintained. Vitamin C in doses exceeding therapeutic levels have not been demonstrated to accelerate wound healing.[31,32] If a client's diet is deficient in good sources of vitamins, an ascorbic acid supplement may be appropriate.

Water

Water, which constitutes about 60% of an adult's body weight, may be the most important nutrient of all. It is distributed in the body in three fluid compartments: intracellular, interstitial, and intravascular. Water serves many vital functions in the body (Exhibit 3-12).

Fluid requirements are met with 30 milliliters per kilogram of body weight or 1 mL/kcal, or a minimum of 1,500 mL/day (1.5 L) unless medically contraindicated. Additional fluids are needed for clients with draining wounds, emesis, diarrhea, elevated temperature, and increased perspiration. Clients on air-fluidized beds require 500 mL of additional fluids daily.

EXHIBIT 3-12   Functions of Water

Water serves many functions, including the following:

- Aids in hydration of wound site and oxygen perfusion
- Acts as a solvent for minerals, vitamins, amino acids, glucose, and other small molecules, and enables them to diffuse in and out of cells
- Transports vital materials to cells and carries waste away from cells
- Serves as a lubricant around joints
- Helps to maintain body temperature

Dehydration

Watch for Warning Signs

The following are signs that an individual may be at risk for or suffering from dehydration:

- Drinks less than 6 cups of liquid daily
- Has one or more of the following:
  dry mouth
  cracked lips
  sunken eyes
  dark urine
- Needs help drinking from a cup or glass
- Has trouble swallowing liquids
- Has frequent vomiting, diarrhea, or fever
- Is easily confused/tired

Report and Take Action

Most individuals need at least 6 cups of liquid to stay hydrated. Below are some action steps to help residents get enough to drink:

- Report observations and warning signs to nurse and dietitian.
- Encourage the residents to drink every time you see him or her.
- Offer 2–4 oz of water or liquids frequently.
- Record fluid intake and output.
- Offer ice chips frequently (unless the client has a swallowing problem).
- Check swallowing precautions; if appropriate, offer sips of liquid between bites of food at meals and snacks.
- Drink fluids with the residents, if allowed.
- Make sure pitcher and cup are near enough and light enough for the residents to lift.
- Offer the appropriate assistance, as needed, if the resident cannot drink without help.

Adapted with permission from the Nutrition Screening Initiative, a project of the American Academy of Family Physicians, the American Dietetic Association and the National Council on the Aging, Inc., funded in part by a grant from Ross Products Division, Abbott Laboratories Inc.

Clients with end-stage disease or severe congestive heart failure may require slightly less fluid intake, calculated at 20–25 mL/kg body weight.

Dehydrated patients have weight loss (2%, mild; 5%, moderate; 8%, severe), dry skin and mucous membranes, rapid pulse, decreased venous pressure, subnormal body temperature, low blood pressure, and altered sensation. Patients who are at risk of dehydration must be monitored carefully. Signs and symptoms of dehydration are listed in Exhibit 3-13. Daily body weight measurements can indicate large fluid losses or gains. For example, a weight loss of 2 kg in 48 hours indicates a corresponding loss of 2 L of fluid. Health-care providers should offer hydration more frequently to elderly clients whose sense of thirst is declining.

EXHIBIT 3-13 Signs and Symptoms of Dehydration

- If the client/resident is able to drink independently, keep water or other beverages at bedside so that they are easily accessible, and in a container that can be handled easily.
- If client/resident doesn't initiate drinking, offer water each time the client/resident is turned (every 2 hours).

Look for:
1. Dry skin
2. Cracked lips
3. Thirst (may be diminished in the elderly)
4. Poor skin turgor (The pinch test for skin turgor may be an unreliable indicator for dehydration in the elderly. If the test is used, use only the skin on the forehead or sternum. Pinch gently. If well hydrated, the skin goes back into place in 2 seconds.)
5. Fever
6. Loss of appetite
7. Nausea
8. Dizziness
9. Increased confusion
10. Laboratory values can indicate dehydration. Serum creatinine hematocrit, BUN, K^+, CL^-, osmolarity would be increased. Sodium can be increased, normal, or low, depending on the underlying cause of the dehydration.
11. Decrease in blood pressure
12. Increase in pulse
13. Constipation (recent diarrhea can offer an explanation for the dehydrated state, and constipation is a common occurrence when dehydration exists.)
14. Concentrated urine

Courtesy of Mary Ellen Posthauer, RD, CD, LD, President of Supreme-Care West, Inc., Evansville, Indiana.

Tips to Increase Fluids

- Hydration carts—offer fluids, such as juices, flavored water, or lemonade three times a day
- Popsicles
- Jell-O cubes
- Soups
- Sorbet/sherbet
- Ice cream
- Milk and milkshakes
- Ice chips
- Offer 4 oz of water between meals

Minerals

Minerals are inorganic elements that are needed by the cells to build body structures, maintain fluid balance, and activate enzyme systems. Once ingested, mineral salts usually dissolve in body fluids and form ions. The skeletal system depends on the minerals calcium, magnesium, and phosphorus for its structural rigidity.

Microelements

Microelements are trace minerals needed in very small amounts. These include iron, iodine, and zinc. Various minerals, such as iron, copper (Exhibit 3-14), manganese, and magnesium, play a role in wound healing, but the nature of their influence is unclear.[33] Zinc deficiencies have been associated with delayed healing, and appear to act by reducing the rate of epithelialization and fibroblast proliferation. Deficiencies require replacement, but there is no indication that supplemental zinc is useful if a deficiency does not exist.[33]

Some clients are able to maintain their nutritional status by oral intake of a balanced diet, supplemented with multiple vitamins and minerals. Having performed a nutritional assessment, the dietetic professional can devise an appropriate individualized nutrition plan for these clients, which involves collaboration between the dietetics professional and other health-care professionals.

Nutrition Based on Wound Etiology

Surgical Wounds

Acute surgical wounds result from operative procedures and typically progress in a timely fashion along the healing trajectory, with at least external manifestations of healing apparent early in the postoperative period. Key factors influencing healing include the systemic state of the client; nutritional status; presence of underlying medical conditions or malignancies; management of postoperative therapies such as wound care; and skin prep/type of suture material used.

Burns

Major burns result in severe trauma. In this state, energy requirements can increase as much as 100% above resting energy expenditure, depending on the extent and depth of the burn. This hypermetabolism is accompanied by exaggerated protein catabolism (i.e., breaking down of amino acids for energy) and increased urinary nitrogen excretion. Clients suffering from trauma such as burns are in negative nitrogen balance because they are forcing their bodies to use protein for energy (Exhibit 3-15).

Protein is also lost through the burn wound exudate. Wound management depends on the depth and extent of the burn, but the current trend is toward early excision and grafting. Metabolic needs are reduced slightly by the prac-

EXHIBIT 3-14   Functions of Zinc and Copper

Zinc is an essential cofactor for formation of collagen and protein synthesis.

Copper is required for cross-linking of collagen fibers in rebuilding tissue.

Exhibit 3-15   Nitrogen Balance

- Amount of nitrogen (*N*) consumed, compared with the amount excreted
- Nitrogen equilibrium: *N* in = *N* out
- Positive nitrogen balance: *N* in > *N* out
- Negative nitrogen balance: *N* in < *N* out

Reprinted with permission from Nitrogen Balance: Cataldo C, Debruyne, L., Whitney, E. *Nutrition and Diet Therapy*, p. 85, © 1999, Wadsworth Publishing.

tice of covering wounds as early as possible to reduce evaporative and nitrogen losses and prevent infection.

Skin Tears

Lacerations resulting from falls, bumps, or shearing forces due to poor lifting technique are often found in the frail elderly. Their skin is less elastic, has limited subcutaneous fat stores, is more susceptible to medication reactions, and is prone to tearing away. A skin tear that shows only limited improvement in 7–14 days requires the initiation of more aggressive nutrition therapy, such as the addition of protein, calories, and fluid.

Leg Ulcers

Many chronic, nonhealing ulcers occur on the lower legs and feet, particularly those of vascular origin. Management of lower-extremity ulcers is complex and resource intensive. It is essential that a multidisciplinary team manage clients with lower-extremity ulcers because they are typically associated with other pathologic conditions. It is extremely important to diagnose the cause of the wound, improve tissue perfusion by way of surgery if warranted, provide compression if needed, manage concurrent diseases, and provide support for possible alterations in life style (e.g., weight loss, proper diet, and smoking cessation).

Dermatitis

The yeastlike fungus *Candida albicans* lives with the normal flora of the mouth, vaginal tract, and gut. Pregnancy, oral contraceptives, antibiotic therapy, diabetes, skin maceration, typical steroid therapy, certain endocrinopathies, and factors related to depression of cell-mediated immunity can allow the yeast to grow, resulting in candidiasis.

In the adult, oral candidiasis occurs for several reasons. It may occur among diabetic clients with depressed cell-mediated immunity, the elderly, and those with cancer, particularly leukemia. Prolonged corticosteroid, immunosuppressive, and broad-spectrum antibiotic therapy, as well as inhalant steroids, can also cause infection.

Nutritional Support

The term "nutritional support" describes a variety of techniques available for use when clients are unable to meet the nutrient needs by normal ingestion of food. Nutritional support ranges from addition to the client's oral diet of a liquid nutritional supplement or various snack foods, to feeding by way of a tube placed into the gastrointestinal tract or, even more invasive, administering nutrients directly into the venous system (total parenteral nutrition) when the gastrointestinal tract is not functional.

Enteral and Parenteral Feeding

Nutritional support is used to place the client into positive nitrogen balance (i.e., the body maintains the same amount of protein in its tissues from day to day), in accordance with the goals of care and compatibility with the client's and family's wishes. Enteral feeding (tube feeding) can be initiated when the ability to chew, swallow, and absorb nutrients through the normal gastrointestinal route is compromised by conditions such as stroke, Parkinson's disease, cancer, and dysphagia, or when clients cannot meet their nutritional needs orally. Most enteral tube feeding formulas are nutritionally complete and designed for a specific purpose. Parenteral nutrition (delivery of nutrient solutions directly into a vein, bypassing the intestine) is necessary when enteral tube feeding is contraindicated, is insufficient to maintain nutritional status, or has led to serious complications. The *Prevention of Pressure Ulcers Nutrition Decision Tree* (Figure 3-2) can be used to determine when enteral and parenteral feeding should be considered.

Documentation in the Medical Record

Medical nutrition therapy documentation in the medical record should include:

- Amount of food consumed in both quantity and quality or type of food related to amount needed
- Average fluid consumed daily (mL), related to amount required
- Ability to eat: assisted, supervised, or independent
- Acceptance or refusal of diet, meals, and/or supplements
- Current weight and percent gained or lost
- New conditions affecting nutritional status, such as introduction of thickened liquids or new diagnosis
- New medications affecting nutritional status
- Current laboratory findings (past 3 months)
- Condition and/or stage of wounds
- Current calorie, protein, or fluid requirements
- Recommendation for plan of care

In order for supplies and services to be covered and reimbursed, they must be regarded as "medically necessary" and supported by physician's orders and documentation that illustrates medical need. A sample Minimum Data Set (MDS) progress note and tube feeding progress note for the dietetics professional to provide quality documentation are found in Appendices 3-C and 3-D at the end of this chapter. Most payers require that changes in a client's treatment plans are well documented and that such changes be based on nationally accepted practice guidelines, such as AHCPR clinical practice guidelines.

Adequate documentation by the health-care team should reflect the care required to prevent and treat pressure ulcers. Documented evidence of appropriate care includes:

- Regular assessment/reassessment of pressure ulcer risk factors
- Regular positioning schedule
- Pressure-reducing support surfaces—bed and chair
- Adequate nutritional intake—food/fluid intake
- Routine skin assessment and care
- Incontinence management
- Local wound care, including management of necrotic tissue, adequate cleansing and dressing that support moist wound healing, and monitoring of improvement or deterioration of each pressure ulcer
- Evaluation and reevaluation of the plan of care if pressure ulcer is not improving over time
- Change in clinical outcomes (e.g., lab values and weight status)

Documentation in the medical record must be consistent with the care that is actually provided.

Conclusion

Malnutrition impedes healing of both chronic and acute wounds.[34] Poor nutritional status has been shown to influence healing time negatively in clients with deep pressure ulcers.[18,35] Indeed, the development of a pressure ulcer or the failure of any type of wound to heal can be an indicator of malnutrition. In fact, malnutrition is one of the major risk factors for developing a pressure ulcer. The fact that aging is associated with both impaired healing[35] and reduced nutrient intake[36] sets the stage for the development and delayed healing of chronic wounds and slow to poor healing of acute wounds in the elderly.

Medical nutrition therapy can provide the means to meet these challenges. A diet that allows the client to enjoy favorite foods using oral nutrition supplements (if needed) or enteral and parenteral nutrition support can achieve optimal nutrition, thus having a positive impact on wound healing.

REVIEW QUESTIONS

1. Albumin levels are decreased with:
   a. Dehydration
   b. Increased protein intake
   c. Infection
   d. Edema
   e. All of the above
   f. Both C and D
2. The Center for Medicare and Medicaid Services (CMS) defines significant weight loss as:
   a. 7% in 60 days
   b. 5% in 30 days

c. 3% in 14 days

d. 10% in 180 days

e. All of the above

f. Both B and D

3. A client who weighs 140 lb with a stage IV pressure ulcer has a protein requirement of:

a. 83–95 grams of protein per day

b. 64–74 grams of protein per day

c. 51–74 grams of protein per day

d. 76–86 grams of protein per day

4. Identify the factor(s) associated with body's metabolic response to severe stress:

a. Metabolic rate slows

b. Conservation of energy/protein stores

c. Protein is the prime source for glucose

d. Accelerated loss of energy and protein stores

e. Both A and C

f. Both C and D

REFERENCES

1. Maklebust J, Sieggreen M. *Pressure Ulcers: Guidelines for Prevention and Management.* 3rd Ed. Springhouse, PA: Springhouse Corporation, 2001:356.

2. Omnibus Budget Reconciliation Act of 1987. Nursing Home Reform Legislation, 1987. Interpretive Guidelines: Transmittal #274, *State Operations Manual,* June 1995.

3. Ayello E, Braden B. (May-June 2002). How and why to do a pressure ulcer risk assessment. Adv Skin Wound Care 2002;15:125–132.

4. Bergstrom N, Braden B. A prospective study of pressure sore risk among institutionalized elderly. J Am Geriatr Soc 1992;40:747–758.

5. Gosnell S. An assessment tool to identify pressure sores. Nurs Res 1973;22:55–59.

6. Bergstrom N, Bennett MA, Carlson CE, et al. The Agency for Health Care Research and Quality (AHRQ), formerly known as the Agency for Health Care Policy and Research (AHCPR), Department of Health and Human Services (DHHS). *Pressure Ulcers in Adults: Prediction and Prevention: Clinical Practice Guideline.* AHRQ Publication No. 92–0047. Rockville, MD: AHRQ; May 1992.

7. Bergstrom N, Bennett MA, Carlson CE, et al. AHRQ, DHHS. *Treatment of Pressure Ulcers: Clinical Practice Guideline.* No. 15. AHRQ Publication No. 95–0652. Rockville, MD: AHRQ; December 1994.

8. Lacey K, Pritchett E. Nutrition care process and model: ADA adopts a road map to quality care and outcomes management. J Am Diet Assoc 2003;103:1061–1072.

9. Niedert K.,Dorner,B Nutrition Care of the Older Adult. Chicago: American Dietetics Association, 2004:125.

10. Maklebust J, Sieggreen M. Pressure Ulcers: Guidelines for Prevention and Nursing Management. 3rd Ed. Springhouse, PA: Springhouse Corporation, 2001:37.

11. Lewis T, Grant R. Observations upon reactive hyperemia in man. Heart (London). 1925;12:73–120.

12. Nutrition Screening Initiative, a project of the American Academy of Family Physicians, ADA, and the National Council on the Aging, and funded in part by a grant from Ross Products Division, Abbott Laboratories, Inc. Washington, DC: Nutrition Screening Initiative; 1993:2.

13. Dwyer JT. Screening Older Americans' Nutritional Health: Current Practices and Future Possibilities. Washington, DC: Nutrition Screening Initiative; 1991.

14. Report of the Dietary Guidelines Advisory Committee on Dietary Guidlines for Americans, 2000. Washighton DC: US Department of Agriculture, Agricultural Research Service;2000:3

15. Moldawer LL. Cytokines and the cachexia response to acute inflammation. Support Line April 1996:1–6.

16. Blackburn GL, Bristrain BF, Maini BS, et al. Nutritional and metabolic assessment of the hospitalized patient. J Parenter Enteral Nutr 1977;1:11–22.

17. Dorner B, Niedert C, Welch P. Liberalized diets for older adults in long-term care. J Am Diet Assoc 2002;102:1316–1323.

18. VanRikwsijk L, Polansky M. Predictors of time to healing deep pressure ulcers. Wounds. 1994;6:159–165.

19. Chernoff R, Milton K, Lipschitz E, et al. The effect of a high protein formula on decubitus ulcer healing in long term tube fed institutionalized patients. J Am Diet Assoc 1990(Suppl):A–130.

20. Breslow R, Hallfrisch J, Guy D, et al. The importance of dietary protein in healing pressure ulcers. J Am Geriatr Soc 1993;41:357–362.

21. Yarkony, GM. Pressure ulcers: a review. Arch Phys Med Rehabil 1994;75:908–917.

22. Kiy, AM. Nutrition in wound healing. A biopsychosocial perspecitve. Nurs Clin North Am 1997;32:849–861.

23. Steed D. The role of growth factors in wound healing. Surg Clin North Am 1997;77:575.

24. Martin P. Wound healing: aiming for perfect skin regeneraton. Science 1997;276:75.

25. Slavin J. Wound healing pathophysiology. Surgery 1999;17:i–v.

26. Albina JE, Mills CD, Barbul A. Arginine metabolism in wounds. Am J Physiol 1988;254:E459–E467.

27. Kirk JS, Barbul A. Role of arginine in trauma, sepsis, immunity. J Parenter Enteral Nutr 1990;14:226S–229S.

28. Schaffer MR, Tantry U, Ahrendt GM. Acute protein-calorie malnutrition impairs wound healing: a possible role of decreased wound nitric oxide synthesis. J Am Coll Surg 1997;184:37–43.

29. Nissen S, Aumbrad N. Nutritional role of leucine metabolite ß-hydroxy-ß-methylbutyrate (HMB) Journal of Nutritional Biochem1997;8:300–311.

30. Bergstrom N, Bennett MA, Carlson CE, et al. AHRQ, DHHS. *Treatment of Pressure Ulcers: Clinical Practice Guideline.* No. 15. AHRQ Publication No. 95–0652. Rockville, MD: AHRQ; December 1994:29.

31. Peter Riet G, Kessels AG, Knipschild PG. Randomized clinical trial of ascorbic acid in the treatment of pressure ulcers. J Clin Epidemiol 1995;48:1453–1460.

32. Vilter RW. Nutritional aspects of ascorbic acid: uses and abuses. West J Med 1980;133:485–92.

33. Bergstrom N, Bennett MA, Carlson CE, et al. AHRQ, DHHS. Treatment of Pressure Ulcers: Clinical Practice Guideline. No. 15. AHRQ Publication No. 95–0652, Rockville, MD: AHRQ; December 1994:30.

34. Maklebust J, Sieggreen M. Pressure Ulcers: Guidelines for Prevention and Nursing Management. 3rd Ed. Springhouse, PA: Springhouse Corporation, 2001:39.

35. Brylinksy C. Nutrition and wound healing: an overview. Ostomy/Wound Manage 1995;41:14–24.

36. Stotts N, Wipke-Tevis D. Co-factors in impaired wound healing. In: Krasner D, Kane D, eds. Chronic Wound Care: A Clinical Source Book for Healthcare Professionals. 2nd Ed. Wayne, PA: Health Management Publications, 1997:63–72.

SUGGESTED READING

Niedert K, Dorner B. Nutrition Care of the Older Adult. 2nd Ed. Chicago: American Dietetic Association, 2004.

Nutrition Intervention To Prevent Wounds

The first goal in preventing pressure ulcers is to identify at-risk individuals needing prevention and the specific factors placing them at risk. Analysis of data from the National Pressure Ulcer Long-Term Care Study (NPULS) has identified patients who are most likely to develop a pressure ulcer. The nutrition characteristics of residents of long-term care facilities and the nutrition processes of care that are highly associated with the development of new pressure ulcers include:

- Weight loss
- Dependence in eating
- Diabetes mellitus
- Poor meal intake
- Dehydration
- Oral problems associated with eating
- Missing diet order

Analysis of the NPULS data has also identified patients who are *less* likely to develop a pressure ulcer. These characteristics and processes of care are:

- Mechanical diet
- Fluid orders
- Oral commercial medical nutritional products (such as Ensure®, Ensure Plus®, Promote®)
- Enteral tube feeding (high-calorie and high-protein products, such as TwoCal® HN, and Ensure Plus® HN; and disease-specific products, such as Perative®)

In patients at risk for developing pressure ulcers or for worsening of ulcers, intensive therapy must be aimed at reducing risk factors. The following two levels of intervention and accompanying procedures will help health care providers to prevent and treat patients with wounds.

Level I Intervention—Oral Diet

Immediately:

- Remove restrictive diets.
- Limit use of non-supplemented liquid diets.

- Refer client to a registered dietitian.
- Order weekly weight measurements.
- Begin a 24-hour assessment of food and fluid intake.
- Evaluate the patient's ability to self-feed (consider use of finger foods, adaptive utensils, refeeding programs, increased time, or feeding assistance).
- Identify food preferences and intolerances.
- Optimize eating environment.
- Individualize meal times and patterns.
- Use medical nutritional products.
- Begin offering 2 ounces of high calorie supplement of 2 calories/ml with each medication pass. Begin a med pass program.

Within 7 days:

- Receive dietitian consultation or assessment that
  estimates nutritional needs
  evaluates weekly weight
  evaluates 24-hour intake for food and liquid
- Ensure good food quality and variety.
- Consider interdisciplinary assessment.
- Plan weekly reassessment of nutrition status and response to nutrition intervention.
- Document and reevaluate the plan of care.

Within 14 days, reassess goals of care:

- Advance to Level II intervention and begin tube feeding if nutrient needs are not met or weight loss continues.
- Begin palliative supportive care if aggressive nutritional therapy is not desired by patient, family, or health-care professionals.

Level II—Tube or Parenteral Feeding

For those patients who cannot maintain adequate dietary intake with Level I interventions and should not be allowed to decline:

- Begin tube feeding.
- Prevent tube feeding complications, such as pulmonary aspiration and glucose/electrolyte abnormalities.
- Reassess nutritional status.

Courtesy of Charlotte Gallagher-Allred, Ross Products Division, Abbott Laboratories, Columbus, Ohio.

- Reassess response to nutritional interventions.
- Document and reevaluate plan of care weekly.

Summary

Prevention, early intervention, and treatment programs are critical in caring for individuals with wounds. Aggressive nutritional management as part of a comprehensive plan of care contributes to reduced cost of care and decreased patient pain and suffering. The nutritional intervention strategies advocated in this exhibit will help the health-care provider provide care consistent with the following nutrition therapy goals and interventions identified by the Agency for Health Care Policy and Research:

1. Ensure adequate dietary intake.
2. Perform nutritional assessment.
3. Encourage dietary intake with oral supplements.
4. Tube feed if oral intake is inadequate.
5. Ensure adequate vitamin and mineral intake.

3B

Nutrition Risk Assessment

Strategies/Interventions: Weight Status

Rationale: Unintended weight changes are prevalent among extended-care residents and can lead to negative health outcomes. Along with accurately evaluating the resident's annual height and routine weight, the RD should review the medical record, interview the resident and/or the resident's family, and monitor the resident's dining performance. (MDS references J, K, E)

Strategies	Interventions to Consider
1. Communicate with nursing concerning residents with change in weight status.	1. Reweighing resident to verify weight change. 2. Consulting with nursing to identify possible causes.
2. Develop facility-wide weight policy.	1. Weighing on admission. 2. Weighing weekly for first month after admission. 3. Weighing residents with significant weight changes weekly for 4 weeks. 4. Instructing STNAs on how to accurately weigh residents. 5. Using consistent protocol when weighing. 6. Calibrating scales monthly.
3. Track weight trends.	1. Assisting in developing weight-tracking form. 2. Reviewing weights and communicating weight changes with nursing. 3. Alerting physician to unintended weight changes. 4. Identifying eating habits, food preferences, and consumption.
4. Determine possible causes of weight change. • Review for clinical signs, symptoms, and of malnutrition. • Review for increased nutrient needs. • Review lab tests indicating undernutrition. • Review clinical conditions that may cause unintended weight loss. • Review medications that cause anorexia, altered taste, and psychosocial needs.	1. Ordering high-calorie diet. 2. Determining a need for increased protein and calorie diet. 3. Offering nutrient-dense foods. 4. Observing for needed assistance in dining room. 5. Evaluating need for adaptive devices. 6. Encouraging exercise to increase appetite. 7. Offering appropriate substitutions at mealtimes.
5. Review multidisciplinary assessment.	1. Reviewing diet order to see if change in food consistency, liberalization, or fluid status might be warranted. 2. Assessing calorie and fluid needs. 3. Evaluating need for speech therapy screening. 4. Discussing advance directives with interdisciplinary team. 5. Communicating with STNAs assisting resident.
6. Review advance directives. Verify wishes and decisions regarding placement of tube feeding with resident/family.	1. If advance directives indicate comfort care only, RD may consider implementing aggressive comfort care measures to maximize quality of life. 2. If advance directives agree to placement of feeding tube, RD completes nutrition assessment and discusses recommendations with nursing who follows-up with MD.
7. Review and complete RAI.	1. Completing/reviewing MDS. 2. Completing RAPs. 3. Developing overall plan of care in cooperation with interdisciplinary team. 4. Determining if care plans are developed to provide consistent intervention by appropriate staff. 5. Determining if care plan has been implemented in accordance with professional standards of practice and changes. 6. Monitoring, reassessing, documenting, and modifying care plan. 7. Charting progress and changes as needed.

Strategies/Interventions: Oral/Nutrition Intake–Food

Rationale: If food intake is inadequate, unplanned weight loss can occur. Monitoring food intake is essential, and poor intake requires in-depth assessment, monitoring, and intervention. (MDS references AC, K)

Strategies	Interventions to Consider
1. Communicate with nursing concerning changes in food intake.	1. Reviewing meal intake records. 2. Reviewing changes in resident's food intake with staff.
2. Develop a procedure on meal intake.	1. Estimating caloric requirements of resident based on individual needs. 2. Interviewing resident/family to obtain diet history, food allergies/ intolerances, food preferences, cultural concerns. 3. Observing intake during meals.
3. Review risk factors for decreased intake based on the MDS.	1. Completing nutritional sections of MDS. 2. Weighing resident on admission/significant change, and as needed for monitoring. 3. Reviewing weight and relationship to UBW. 4. Using consistent weighing protocols. 5. Evaluating diet order for appropriateness. 6. Evaluating present intake based on individual needs. 7. Reviewing medical record for losses of nutrients. 8. Monitoring mental status. 9. Identifying residents who need assistance in preparing (opening cartons, cutting) and consuming foods. 10. Reviewing lab tests, if available. 11. Reviewing possible impact of medication on intake.
4. Determine possible causes of poor food intake, identify appropriate interventions, and monitor status of interventions.	1. Considering consistency modifications. 2. Exploring resident's cultural attitude toward food, identifying preferences, and providing favorite/comfort foods. 3. Scheduling routine snacks 3x/day or administer at least 6 small feedings if agreeable with resident. 4. Individualizing meal plan according to resident's wishes to encourage compliance. 5. Instructing STNA and family on importance of adequate nutrition intake. 6. Involving resident/caregiver/family in establishing intake goals. 7. Evaluating if resident/family may be restricting or exceeding calorie needs. 8. Arranging for foods to be provided at activities and in social setting. 9. Encouraging exercise to stimulate appetite and maintain muscle mass. 10. Discouraging medication passes in dining room during meal service. 11. Establishing mealtime routine in positive dining experience.
5. Review Advance Directives.	1. Verifying with resident/family wishes and placement for tube feeding. (Refer to Nutrition Therapy for Palliative Care if tube feeding not desired.)
6. Review and complete RAI.	1. Completing/reviewing MDS. 2. Completing RAPs. 3. Developing overall plan of care in cooperation with interdisciplinary team. 4. Determining if care plan interventions are developed to provide consistent intervention by appropriate staff. 5. Determining if the care plan has been implemented in accordance with professional standards of practice. 6. Monitoring, reassessing, documenting and modifying care plan. 7. Charting progress and changes as needed.

Strategies/Interventions: Oral/Nutrition Intake—Fluid

Rationale: Water accounts for 50-60% of total body weight. Humans can survive only a few days without water. Water regulates body temperature and is a medium for transport of nutrients and metabolic waste. Maintenance of fluid balance is essential to basic health and recovery from illness. (MDS references AC, J, K)

Strategies	Interventions to Consider
1. Communicate with nursing and physician changes in hydration status.	1. Suggesting I/O when fluid or electrolyte imbalance occurs.
	2. Consulting with nursing or physician to identify possible causes.
2. Develop a policy for hydration and fluid that addresses potential causes of dehydration.	1. Estimating fluid requirements per kg of body weight adjusted for clinical condition.
	2. Monitoring weight of residents on diuretics.
	3. Identifying and monitoring high-risk patients.
	4. Identifying interdisciplinary team responsibilities; monitoring and documenting care.
3. Review risk factors for dehydration based on the MDS.	1. Completing areas of MDS that relate to hydration.
	2. Monitoring status of rehydration therapy.
	3. Weighing resident as clinical condition requires. (See Weight Status Strategies/Interventions.)
	4. Observing clinical health and physical signs of hydration status.
	5. Monitoring I/O if applicable.
	6. Reviewing lab test if available to confirm hydration status.
4. Determine possible causes of dehydration and identify appropriate interventions: • Review other potential risk factors for dehydration. • Review for volume deficit. • Review for volume excess.	1. Individualizing hydration plan according to resident's wishes to encourage compliance.
	2. Instructing STNA/family on importance of adequate hydration and interventions to meet fluid requirements.
	3. Arranging for fluids to be provided at activities and in a social setting.
	4. Observing resident in dining environment.
	5. Exploring cultural attitude toward fluids.
	6. Reviewing resident's medications to assess possible impact on fluid electrolyte balance.
5. Review advance directives.	1. Verifying with resident/family wishes and placement for tube feeding. (Refer to Nutrition Therapy for Palliative Care if tube feeding not desired.)
6. Review and complete RAI.	1. Completing/reviewing MDS.
	2. Completing RAPs.
	3. Developing overall plan of care in cooperation with interdisciplinary team.
	4. Determining if care plans are developed to provide consistent intervention by appropriate staff.
	5. Determining if care plan has been implemented in accordance with Professional standards of practice and changes.
	6. Monitoring, reassessing, documenting, and modifying care plan.
	7. Charting progress and changes as needed.

Strategies/Interventions: Medications—Nutrition-Related

Rationale: Interactions between drugs and nutrients can alter drug or nutrient disposition, action, or toxicity. Drugs taken by older adults for disease and/or symptom management can impose a particularly high risk of causing drug and nutrient interactions. Since residents often take several medications and because other factors affect an individual's response to medications, nutrient and drug interactions need to be addressed by the interdisciplinary team. (MDS reference O)

Strategies	Interventions to Consider
1. Communicate with nursing and appropriate staff concerning medication regimen.	1. Reviewing medical record for routine drug use. 2. Interviewing resident and family. 3. Discouraging medication passes in dining room during meal service.
2. Evaluate nutrition implications of current medications and effect aging has on drugs prescribed. • Loss of appetite • Taste/smell dysfunction • Dry or sore mouth • Appetite stimulation or weight gain • Epigastric distress • Nausea • Diarrhea • Gastrointestinal gas • Constipation • Fluid loss • Mental status change	1. Identifying and documenting drugs that may impair senses or cause diuresis, anorexia, catabolism, nausea, vomiting, dry mouth, constipation, diarrhea, dysphagia, dyspepsia. 2. Identifying and documenting drugs that may stimulate appetite or cause edema or weight gain. 3. Identifying and documenting drugs that may have drug-nutrient interactions (DNIs) when compounded by alcohol use or pose significant risk when taken with alcohol. 4. Identifying and documenting potential DNIs caused by diet changes. 5. Identify and document drugs that may alter functional, cognitive, or emotional status. 6. Identifying and documenting side effects of drugs that may be reduced by altering timing and/or content of meals and snacks. 7. Reviewing possible side effects with interdisciplinary team and discussing recommendations with physician.
3. Review and complete RAI.	1. Completing/reviewing MDS. 2. Completing RAPs. 3. Developing overall plan of care in cooperation with interdisciplinary team. 4. Determining if care plan interventions (alternative fluid schedules, fluid options, etc) are developed to provide consistent intervention by appropriate staff. 5. Determining if care plan has been implemented in accordance with professional standards of practice. 6. Monitoring, reassessing, documenting, and modifying care plan. 7. Charting progress and changes as needed.

Strategies/Interventions: Relevant Conditions and Diagnoses

Rationale: Nutrition plays a role in many of the leading causes of death in the United States, including illnesses common in residents, such as heart disease, cancer, stroke, hypertension, and diabetes mellitus. Nutrition risk assessment is the first step in developing and providing disease-specific nutrition care options that are customized to meet the needs of the residents served. (MDS references E, H, I, J, M, P)

Strategies	Interventions to Consider
1. Communicate with nursing concerning changes in relevant conditions and diagnosis, causes of changes, and overall evaluation of the resident's condition.	1. Reviewing medical record. 2. Interviewing resident/family, investigating status prior to admission. 3. Reviewing with interdisciplinary team any significant change at moderate risk. (See Nutrition Risk Assessment form.) 4. Review with interdisciplinary team any significant change of condition/diagnosis placing resident at high risk. (See Nutrition Risk Assessment form.)
2. Evaluate nutrition implications for current relevant conditions and diagnoses.	1. Determining history of weight changes. 2. Determining previous treatment modalities. 3. Reviewing labs in light of diagnosis/condition. 4. Reviewing diet order, consistency, and overall intake including changes in fluid status. 5. Reviewing medications and potential drug-nutrient interactions. 6. Observing resident in current care setting. 7. Assessing edema, skin turgor, pressure ulcer/sore, and making appropriate nutrition interventions. 8. Recommending nutrition intervention as appropriate, e.g., liberalized diet based on resident's needs, alterations for food intolerances, enteral support, vitamin/mineral supplement.
3. Review and complete RAI.	1. Completing/reviewing MDS. 2. Completing RAPs. 3. Developing overall plan of care in cooperation with interdisciplinary team. 4. Determining if care plan is developed to provide consistent intervention by appropriate staff. 5. Determining if care plan has been implemented in accordance with professional standards of practice. 6. Monitoring, reassessing, documenting, and modifying care plan. 7. Charting progress and changes as needed.

Strategies/Interventions: Physical and Mental Functioning

Rationale: Physical and mental functioning play a significant role in the motivation and capacity of older persons to achieve and maintain nutritional health. Although numerous approaches, including feeding assistance and dietary supplementation, can be effective, proper assessment and intervention must be the first step to effective care. Assessment with appropriate intervention is key to identifying physical and mental conditions that can affect physical and emotional well-being and functional effectiveness. The involvement of the health care team is critical to improved nutritional health. (MDS references A, B, E, G, L, and P)

Strategies	Interventions to Consider
1. Communicate with nursing and all other disciplines involved in changes related to physical and mental functioning.	1. Reviewing medical record. 2. Interviewing resident and family. 3. Investigating status in previous living environment.
2. Develop restorative dining program.	1. Assessing resident's ability to eat independently. 2. Evaluating dining environment. 3. Using a team approach to determine restorative potential.
3. Evaluate for physical functioning abilities using the restorative dining program.	1. Observing resident in appropriate care setting. 2. Observing for depression, anxiety, sadness. 3. Identifying resident's general orientation: time, place, person. 4. Identifying what kind of assistance resident needs and why. 5. Identifying percentage of meal resident is eating without assistance. 6. Identifying total percentage of meal eaten. 7. Identifying need for use of adaptive devices. 8. Identifying time required for resident to finish meal. 9. Identifying need for special positioning devices. 10. Identifying physical and/or verbal cues resident needs to initiate and continue with meal. 11. Monitoring resident's response to program.
4. Evaluate oral status.	1. Reviewing guidelines for assessing oral cavity. 2. Completing oral cavity assessment. 3. Reviewing need for mechanically altered diet. 4. Reviewing multidisciplinary assessment.
5. Evaluate for signs and symptoms of dysphagia.	1. Educating caregivers on warning signs of dysphagia. 2. Consulting with speech language pathologist. 3. Altering food/fluid consistencies as appropriate.
6. Evaluate conditions and therapies associated with compromised nutrition and oral status.	1. Reviewing for polypharmacy, major surgery, poor dentition, cranial/facial abnormalities, disorder of taste/smell, salivary dysfunction, immunocompromising conditions.
7. Evaluate communicative barriers (vision, speech, hearing, cognitive status).	1. Educating staff on limitations of resident (plate placement, use of communication board, side of hearing deficit, etc.). 2. Providing appropriate cues as needed. 3. Developing standardized tray setup. 4. Consulting with appropriate rehabilitation therapist.
8. Review and complete RAI.	1. Completing/reviewing MDS. 2. Completing RAPs. 3. Developing overall plan of care in cooperation with interdisciplinary team. 4. Determining if care plan is developed to provide consistent intervention by appropriate staff. 5. Determining if care plan has been implemented in accordance with professional standards of practice. 6. Monitoring, reassessing, documenting, and modifying care plan. 7. Charting progress and changes as needed.

Strategies/Interventions: Lab Values

Rationale: Laboratory assessment can be prudently used to confirm suspected nutrition-related problems identified by clinical diagnosis, observation, history, and physical examination. Laboratory tests are recommended when plan of care warrants. (MDS reference P)

Strategies	Interventions to Consider
1. Communicate with nursing and appropriate staff concerning laboratory results.	1. Reviewing clinical diagnosis, history, and physical. 2. Determining whether requesting labs would affect outcome.
2. Evaluate nutrition implication of current lab results and effects of aging process.	1. Reviewing nutrition indications of lab data. 2. Identifying and documenting medications that could cause abnormal lab results. 3. Recommending and documenting changes in diet that could improve lab values. 4. Reviewing lab data with multidisciplinary team and recommending lab draws as appropriate. Before requesting labs, consider the following: • Will the outcome actually change the nutrition care plan? • Is the test cost-effective? • Is the nutrition goal for the resident consistent with treatment and advance directives?
3. Review and complete RAI.	1. Completing/reviewing MDS. 2. Completing RAPs. 3. Developing overall plan of care in cooperation with interdisciplinary team. 4. Determining if care plan (alternative fluid schedules, fluid options, etc) is developed to provide consistent intervention by appropriate staff. 5. Determining if care plan has been implemented in accordance with professional standards of practice. 6. Monitoring, reassessing, documenting, and modifying care plan. 7. Charting progress and changes as needed.

Strategies/Interventions: Risk Factor: Skin Conditions

Rationale: Pressure ulcers and other wounds are among the most challenging problems faced by caregivers in nursing facilities because of the frequency of occurrence and the cost to the resident and the facility physically, emotionally, and financially. Poor nutritional status is a risk factor for development of pressure ulcers; healing can be augmented with aggressive nutritional support. The cause of pressure ulcers is multifaceted, and intervention is best accomplished through an interdisciplinary team. (MDS reference M)

Strategies	Interventions to Consider
1. Communicate with nursing concerning all residents with skin impairments.	1. Reviewing skin assessment. 2. Reviewing medical record frequently for healing of pressure ulcers.
2. Review risk factors for pressure ulcers.	1. Completing and/or updating skin risk assessment with nursing. 2. Documenting factors that place resident at risk for impaired skin. 3. Reviewing medical treatments, laboratory values, and medications that may contribute to risk for pressure ulcers. 4. Reviewing lab values placing resident at possible risk for pressure ulcer development and poor healing.
3. Develop a skin care team.	1. Developing and implementing interdisciplinary pressure sore/ulcer protocol that includes: • Nursing measures such as skin checks, turning/positioning, applying barrier cream, offering fluids, and ordering specialty mattress. • Nutrition measures such as determination of calories, protein, fluid, vitamin and mineral needs. • Medical measures such as debridement or surgery, if medically appropriate. 2. Referring to AHCPR guidelines for suggestions on nutrition assessment and intervention. 3. Assisting skin care team in staff education related to pressure ulcer etiology, risk prevention, and treatment. 4. Setting up restorative dining program. 5. Providing family/resident education and counseling. 6. Involving therapists as needed.
4. Observe resident in dining environment.	1. Completing eating/dining performance evaluation. 2. Placing interventions into care plan. 3. Moving to appropriate dining environment. 4. Providing adequate devices as needed.
5. Review advance directives.	1. Verifying with family wishes for continued care and treatment. 2. If advance directives indicate comfort care only, skin and/or interdisciplinary team may consider implementing comfort care measures to maximize quality of life; follow-up with MD.
6. Review and complete RAI.	1. Completing/reviewing MDS. 2. Completing RAPs. 3. Developing overall plan in cooperation with interdisciplinary team. 4. Determining if care plans are developed to provide consistent intervention by appropriate staff. 5. Determining if care plan has been implemented in accordance with professional standards of practice and changes. 6. Monitoring, assessing, documenting, and modifying care plan. 7. Charting progress and changes as needed.

Nutrition Risk Assessment

Name_____ Adm Date_____ MR._____ Assess type_____

DOB_____ Age_____ Sex: M F   Advance Directive_____ Physician_____

Diagnosis_____

Ht (in)_____ Wt (lb)_____ Wt (kg)_____ Usual body wt range_____ BMI_____

BEE_____ Activity Factor _____ Injury Factor _____ Total cal _____ Total protein _____g (_____g/kg)

Total fluids _____cc (_____cc/kg) Fluid restriction_____

Diet order_____ Food allergies/sensitivities_____

Supplement/snacks_____ Cultural/religious preferences _____

Risk Factor	No/Low Risk (0 pts)	Moderate Risk (1 pt)	High Risk (3 pts)	MDS Ref	Pts	Comments
Weight status; loss or gain	BMI 19-27 No weight change	< 5% wt change in 30 days < 7.5% within 90 days; or < 10% within 6 mo	BMI <19 or > 27 ≦ 5% wt change in 30 days ≦ 7.5% in 90 days; or ≦ 10% within 6 mo	J,K,E		
Oral/nutrition intake; food	Intake meets 76-100% of estimated needs	Intake meets 26-75% of estimated needs	Intake meets = 25% of estimated needs	AC,J,K		
Oral/nutrition intake; fluids	Consumes 1500-2000 cc/day	Consumes < 1000-1499 cc/day	Consumes < 1000 cc/day	AC,J,K		
Medications; nutrition-related	0-1 drugs/day	2-4 drugs/day	5 or more drugs/day	O		
Relevant conditions and diagnoses	HTN, DM, heart disease, or other controlled diseases/ conditions	Anemia, infection, CVA (recent) fracture, UTI, alcohol abuse, drug abuse, COPD, edema, surgery (recent), osteoporosis, hx of GI bleed, food intolerance and allergies, poor circula-tion, constipation, diarrhea, GERD, anorexia, Parkinson's	Cancer (advanced), septicemia, liver failure, dialysis, ESRD, Alzheimer's, dementia, depression, dehydration, dysphagia, radiation/chemo, active GI bleed, chronic nausea, vomit-ing, ostomy, gastrectomy, fecal impaction, uncontrolled diseases or conditions	E,H,I, J,M,P		
Physical and mental functioning	Ambulatory, alert, able to feed self, no chewing or swallowing problems	Out of bed w/assistance, motor agitation (tremors, wandering), limited feeding assistance, supervision while eating, chewing or swallow-ing problems, teeth in poor repair, ill-fitting dentures or refusal to wear dentures, edentulous, taste and sensory changes, unable to communicate needs	Bedridden, inactive, total dependence, extensive or total assistance or dependence while eating, aspirates, tube feeding, TPN, mouth pain	A,B,E G,L,P		
Lab values	Albumin and other nutrition related lab values WNL	Albumin 3.0-3.4 g/dL, 1-2 other nutrition-related labs abnormal	Albumin < 3.0 g/dL, 3-5 other nutrition-related labs abnormal	P		
Skin conditions	Skin intact	Stage I/II pressure ulcers or skin tears not healing, hx of pressure ulcers, stasis ulcer, fecal incontinence	Stage III/IV pressure ulcers or multiple impaired areas	M		

Overall Risk Category: **0-2 points NO/LOW RISK 3-7 points: MODERATE RISK 8 points: HIGH RISK**

Total Points:_____   **Overall Risk Category:_____**

RD Signature:_____ Date:_____

CDM Signature:_____ Date:_____

Medical Nutrition Therapy Quarterly/MDS Progress Note

MEDICAL NUTRITION THERAPY QUARTERLY / MDS PROGRESS NOTE (MR#_____)

NAME:_____ GENDER: ❑ M ❑ F

TARGET WEIGHT _____ lb HEIGHT:_____ AGE:_____ years

1ST QUARTER	2ND QUARTER	3RD QUARTER
DIET ORDER:_____	Changed ❑ Y ❑ N	Changed ❑ Y ❑ N
SUPPLEMENT:_____	Changed ❑ Y ❑ N	Changed ❑ Y ❑ N
FORTIFIED FOODS:_____	Changed ❑ Y ❑ N	Changed ❑ Y ❑ N
TUBE FEEDING FLUSH_____	Changed ❑ Y ❑ N	Changed ❑ Y ❑ N
FOOD/FLUIDS % Intake _____ B _____ HS _____ L _____ Fluids _____ S _____ Supplement	_____ B _____ HS _____ L _____ Fluids _____ S _____ Supp	_____ B _____ HS _____ L _____ Fluids _____ S _____ Supp
FEEDING ABILITY ❑ Dependent ❑ Independent ❑ Limited Assist ❑ Set-up Only ❑ Self-Help Devices ❑ Type_____	Changed ❑ Y ❑ N	Changed ❑ Y ❑ N
ORAL STATUS ❑ Normal ❑ Mechanical Soft ❑ Requires modification to swallow solid foods and liquids, puree and thickened liquids ❑ Combined Oral and Tube Feeding ❑ No Oral Intake	Changed ❑ Y ❑ N	Changed ❑ Y ❑ N
MEAL LOCATION ❑ DR ❑ Room ❑ Restorative DR ❑ Other_____	Changed ❑ Y ❑ N	Changed ❑ Y ❑ N
COGNITIVE STATUS ❑ Alert/Oriented ❑ Depressed ❑ Cog. Impaired ❑ Disoriented / Confused ❑ Combative ❑ Wanders ❑ Comatose ❑ Other _____	Changed ❑ Y ❑ N	Changed ❑ Y ❑ N
CURRENT WEIGHT: _____ LBS _____% Change ❑ 30 days ❑ 90 days ❑ 180 days	_____ Wt _____% change ❑ 30 ❑ 90 ❑ 180	_____ Wt _____% change ❑ 30 ❑ 90 ❑ 180
PLANNED WEIGHT CHANGE: ❑ Yes ❑ No	❑ Yes ❑ No	❑ Yes ❑ No
CALORIC / HYDRATION REQUIREMENT: _____ Calories _____ Protein _____ Fluid	Changed ❑ Y ❑ N	Changed ❑ Y ❑ N
SKIN CONDITION ❑ Intact ❑ Burns 2nd/3rd degree ❑ Edema ❑ Reddened Areas ❑ Surgical Wounds ❑ Other: _____ ❑ Open Lesion/Infections _____	❑ Intact ❑ Burns 2nd/3rd degree ❑ Edema ❑ Reddened Areas ❑ Surgical Wounds ❑ Open Lesion/Infections ❑ Other:_____	❑ Intact ❑ Burns 2nd/3rd degree ❑ Edema ❑ Reddened Areas ❑ Surgical Wounds ❑ Open Lesion/Infections ❑ Other:_____
PRESSURE ULCER(S) ❑ YES ❑ NO STAGE: 1 2 3 4 LOCATION:_____ SIZE:_____	❑ YES ❑ NO STAGE: 1 2 3 4 LOCATION:_____ SIZE:_____	❑ YES ❑ NO STAGE: 1 2 3 4 LOCATION:_____ SIZE:_____
MEDICATIONS: Note new medications since last review		

Source: Mary Ellen Posthauer, RD,LD,CD

Appendix 3D

Monthly Medical Nutrition Therapy Tube Feeding Progress Note

Monthly Medical Nutrition Therapy Tube Feeding Progress Note F–74 (11/00)

NAME:_____ GENDER: ❑ M ❑ F

TARGET WEIGHT_____lb   HEIGHT:_____   AGE:_____years

	Date:_____	Date:_____
Date:_____		
TUBE FEEDING ORDER:	Changed Yes/No	Changed Yes/No
FLUSH:	Changed Yes/No	Changed Yes/No
FORMULA PROVIDES: Calories:_____ Protein:_____ Free H2O:_____ Flush:_____ Total Water:_____	Changed Yes/No Changed Yes/No	Changed Yes/No Changed Yes/No
DIET:_____ **PUMP:**_____ **NPO:**_____ **BOLUS:**_____	Changed Yes/No	Changed Yes/No
TOTAL CALORIES PER TUBE: ❑ 1%–25% ❑ 51%–75% ❑ 26%–50% ❑ 76%–100%		
NUTRIENT NEEDS: BEE_____ Injury Factor_____ Protein_____g/kg Fluid_____cc/kg Activity Factor_____ Total Calories_____ Total Protein_____g Total Fluids_____mL	Changed Yes/No	Changed Yes/No
SIGNIFICANT LAB VALUES: LABS	LABS	
WEIGHT:		
CURRENT WEIGHT:_____ % CHANGE:_____ ❑ Intact	Weight:_____ % Change:____ ❑ Intact	Weight:_____ % Change:____
SKIN CONDITION: ❑ Intact ❑ Edema ❑ Reddened Areas ❑ Edema ❑ Open Lesion/Infections _____ ❑ Pressure Ulcer Stage:_____	❑ Edema ❑ Red Areas ❑ Open Lesion/Infections ❑ PU Stage:____	❑ Red Areas ❑ Open Lesion/Infections ❑ PU Stage:_____

RECOMMENDATIONS:
RD SIGNATURE: _____   _____   _____

Mary EllenPosthauer, RD,CD,LD

Assessment of the Skin and Wound

Carrie Sussman

CHAPTER OBJECTIVES

At the completion of this chapter, the reader will be able to:
1. Identify structures that are part of the skin anatomy.
2. Apply classification systems to diagnose wound severity.
3. Perform tests and assess adjacent tissues and periwound status.
4. Perform tests and evaluate wound status.
5. Explain and apply the concept of wound phase diagnosis, based on the status of the phase of wound healing.

Chapter 4 continues the methodology of the diagnostic process described in Chapter 1 with Step 2: assessment of the skin and wound to develop a functional diagnosis of the wound.

For many years, it was assumed that the healing processes for acute and chronic wounds were equivalent, and that findings from one could be applied to the other. However, that opinion has shifted as more is understood about disruption in wound healing physiology and barriers to orderly healing. In this context, the search for the best method of wound assessment is ongoing. Groups of experts meet and publish reports on best practices for clinicians, such as the wound bed preparation approach to wound management, MEASURE, a proposed wound assessment framework.[1,2] There is consensus by these experts that global assessment is needed when wounds are not healing as expected in order to analyze the probable underlying causes. In these cases, a plan for management of the whole patient, not just the wound, needs to be prepared.

This chapter focuses on accurate and relevant assessment of adjacent skin, periwound skin, and wound bed. The assessment process presents many challenges, including lack of uniformity of terminology, lack of agreement about the key parameters to assess, and differences in the accuracy and reliability of available tests, measures, and techniques.[2] The data gleaned from this examination leads to two diagnoses introduced in this chapter—wound severity related to the depth of tissue impairment and the biologic phase of wound healing. These diagnoses then guide treatment decisions. Accepted terminology and the significance of tissue attributes are described and illustrated with color plates located in this book.

There is general agreement by wound healing clinicians that any consistently used assessment method is beneficial. Chronic wound management is a broad field with many factors to consider. Therefore, an assortment of examinations, tests, and measures are presented here that may not be applicable for all patients in all settings. Wound measurement and tracking healing with validated tools are found in Chapters 5 and 6.

Anatomy and Physiology of the Skin

Skin anatomy is reviewed here as a guide to the structures of the skin and the relationship between the depth of loss of skin integrity that occurs with wounding and the role of the structures of the skin in regeneration or repair. Wound severity is classified according to the level of skin structure loss. Several classification systems based on the level of loss of skin integrity are presented in the next section.

The skin is the largest organ in the body consisting of several layers. The epidermis which itself is composed of several layers beginning with the stratum corneum is the outermost layer. The innermost skin layer is the deep dermis. The skin has multiple functions, including thermal regulation, metabolic function (vitamin D metabolism), and immune functions. Also skin health is a mirror of general health, and skin failure often accompanies other system failures within the body. Figure 4-1 presents a diagram of skin anatomy.

Epidermis

Closing the wound quickly and efficiently is a function of the epidermis. When the epidermis is injured, the body is

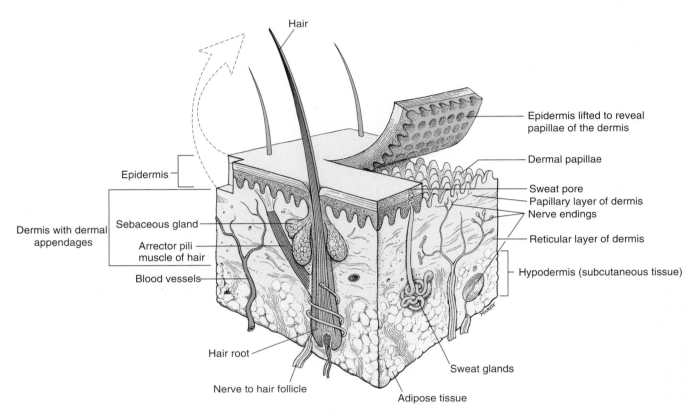

FIGURE 4-1 Anatomy of the skin. (Adapted with permission from Premkumar, K. The Massage Connection: Anatomy and Physiology. Baltimore: Lippincott Williams & Wilkins, 2004.)

subject to invasion by outside agents and loss of body fluids. Epidermal wounds heal primarily by cell migration. Clusters of epidermal cells migrate into the area of damage and cover the defect. These lead cells are phagocytic and clear the surface of debris and plasma clots. Winter[3] found that this cell migration progresses best in a moist environment. Repair cells originate from local sources that are primarily the dermal appendages (see below) and from adjacent intact skin areas. Healing occurs rapidly, and the skin is regenerated and is left unscarred. Blisters are examples of epidermal wounds. They may be small vesicles or larger bullae (greater than 1 cm in diameter).

Stratum Corneum and the Acid Mantle

Stratum corneum is an avascular, multilayer structure that functions as a barrier to the environment and prevents transepidermal water loss.[4] Recent studies have demonstrated that enzymatic activity is involved in the formation of an acid mantle in the stratum corneum. Together, the acid mantle and stratum corneum make the skin less permeable to water and other polar compounds, and indirectly protect the skin from invasion by microorganisms.

Normal surface skin pH is between 4 and 6.5 in healthy people; it varies according to area of skin on the body. This low pH forms an acid mantle that enhances the skin barrier function. Damage of the stratum corneum increases the skin pH and, thus, the susceptibility of the skin to bacterial skin infections.[5] For example, hand washing three times a day with cleansing agents alters the acid mantle for several hours, and multiple washings alters the barrier functions, including the skin pH, for up to 14 hours. Further damage is done by more washings. Diseases associated with increased skin surface pH include eczema, contact dermatitis, atopic dermatitis, perineal dermatitis and dry skin. Increased acidity is caused by perspiration or urine and stool from incontinence. Systemic diseases, such as diabetes, chronic renal failure and cerebrovascular disease, can also cause increased skin pH. Wound dressings and diapers have also been known to raise skin pH.[5]

If the pH of the skin shifts toward alkaline, it can become prone to secondary bacterial and fungal infections, which thrive in the perineal skin. Perineal skin lesions are associated with erosion of the skin and are seen frequently, but exactly how prevalent they are is not known.[6] This type of partial thickness skin erosion is often misdiagnosed as a stage II pressure ulcer. Some controversy exists about the difference between the two.

An association between wound surface pH and wound healing has been made. The pH of open wounds tends to be alkaline or neutral (range 6.5–8.5). As new epithelium is formed at the wound edges, the pH becomes similar to that of normal skin (approximately pH 5.9).[7]

Handwashing Effect on Skin Health of Health-care Professionals

Health-care professionals wash their hands between each patient, typically more than 3 times per day, and often develop eczema, contact dermatitis, atopic dermatitis and dry skin.

When removed, wound dressing adhesives strip the stratum corneum and cause noticeable transepidermal water loss.[4] The skin interprets this as trauma, and an inflammatory wound healing response, proportional to the amount of damage to the skin, is triggered.

Skin cleansers and moisturizers that have low or neutral pH are recommended for maintaining the acid mantle of the skin. Soaps, which are more alkaline than most synthetic detergents and nonionic surfactants (which are slightly acidic or neutral), may be the best choices to protect skin surface integrity,[5] but they should not be used to clean open wounds.

Skin Hydration and Lubrication

Stratum corneum hydration and lubrication are important in keeping the skin intact.. Extremes of either dryness or hydration are equally damaging. Halkier-Sorenson has done extensive research on the stratum corneum barrier function.[8] According to their findings, any disruption in the stratum corneum allows increased transepidermal water loss and an almost complete secretion of lamellar body contents from the uppermost granular layer into the intercellular spaces of the stratum corneum impairing the barrier function. Barrier disruption causes a localized inflammatory cascade, which is instrumental in the development of inflammatory skin diseases, such as eczema. Normal adult skin has the capacity to recover its barrier function within 6 hours. During recovery, there is an increase in lipid production within the stratum corneum. Recovery of the barrier is slower and more easily broken in aged skin. Application of effective moisturizer products containing the appropriate mix of lipids can reduce the epidermal water loss during the recovery period.

Oils and humectants can also be used to lubricate and hydrate the skin. Topical creams and ointments can benefit hydration and lubrication, but may also contain potential allergens. Understanding the mechanisms and sites of action helps in selecting skin care products that restore barrier function. Theoretically, moisturizers act on the epidermis on three different levels:

1. Stay on the surface of the stratum corneum
2. Penetrate into the intercellular spaces of the stratum corneum
3. Penetrate into the viable epidermis and eventually become incorporated into the cells and later secreted

Early application of skin barrier products will reduce transepidermal water loss and give the skin time to repair the stratum corneum. A good moisturizer can reduce the effect of the initial insult to the stratum corneum and block penetration of substances that can further injure the tissue. Petrolatum-based and lanolin-based skin care products have been shown to enhance barrier recovery by reducing water loss and inhibiting the inflammatory reaction of the cells. This leads to a significant decrease in skin breakdown and pressure ulcers in elderly residents of long-term care facilities.[8,9]

Other Layers of the Epidermis

Other layers of the epidermis below the stratum corneum include the stratum lucidum, stratum granulosum, and stratum germinativum and stratum basale. Each contains living cells with specialized functions (Fig. 4-2). For example, melanin, which is produced by melanocytes in the epidermis, is responsible for the color of the skin. Langerhans cells, are involved in immune processing.

Melanin and Skin Color

Although the structures of the skin are very similar, skin color varies greatly among humans,. Melanin produced from melanocytes accounts for the variation in pigmentation from very light to extremely dark. Although the number of melanocytes present in dark and light skin is similar, the size and activity of the melanocytes are greater in dark skin than in light skin. The melanin pigmentation is concentrated in a dark horny layer of the stratum corneum that can be wiped off when washing clean, dark skin. Of course, this does not mean that all the color is removed, just the superficial layer. The thickness of the stratum corneum in both dark and light skin is the same, but the cells in dark skin are more compact and have more cell layers. For this reason, dark skin is more resistant to external irritants. Healthy dark skin is usually smooth and dry, whereas dry dark skin can have an ashen appearance.[10]

Care of Darkly Pigmented Skin

Care of darkly pigmented skin requires keeping the skin lubricated. Petrolatum, lanolin-based lotions, and sparing use of soaps are recommended.[10]

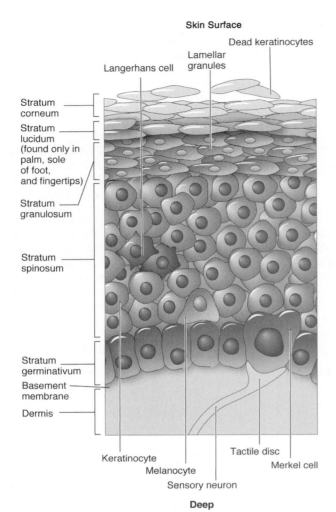

Skin Surface

Langerhans cell

Dead keratinocytes

Lamellar granules

Stratum corneum

Stratum lucidum (found only in palm, sole of foot, and fingertips)

Stratum granulosum

Stratum spinosum

Stratum germinativum

Basement membrane

Dermis

Keratinocyte

Melanocyte

Sensory neuron

Tactile disc

Merkel cell

Deep

FIGURE 4-2 Layers of the Epidermis. (Reprinted with permission from Premkumar K. The Massage Connection: Anatomy and Physiology. Baltimore: Lippincott Williams & Wilkins, 2004.

Dermal Appendages

Dermal appendages, which include hair follicles, sebaceous and sweat glands, fingernails, and toenails, originate in the epidermis and protrude into the dermis.[11] Hair follicles and sebaceous and sweat glands contribute epithelial cells for rapid reepithelialization of wounds that do not penetrate through the dermis (termed partial-thickness wounds). The sebaceous glands are responsible for secretions that lubricate the skin, keeping it soft and flexible. They are most numerous in the face and sparse in the palms of the hands and soles of the feet. Sweat gland secretions control skin pH to prevent dermal infections. The sweat glands, dermal blood vessels, and small muscles in the skin (responsible for goose pimples) control temperature on the surface of the body. Nerve endings in the skin include receptors for pain, touch, heat, and cold. Loss of these nerve endings increases the risk for skin breakdown by decreasing the tolerance of the tissues to external forces.

The *basement membrane* both separates and connects the epidermis and dermis. When epidermal cells in the basement membrane divide, one cell remains, and the other migrates

through the granular layer to the surface stratum corneum. At the surface, the cell dies and forms keratin.[11] Dry keratin on the surface is called scale. Hyperkeratosis (thickened layers of keratin) is often found on the heels and can indicate loss of sebaceous gland and sweat gland functions if the patient is diabetic.[12] Chapter 19 includes photos of hyperkeratosis on the heel of a patient with polyneuropathy. The basement membrane atrophies with aging; separation between the basement membrane and dermis is one cause for skin tears in the elderly.

Dermis

The dermis, or the true skin, is a vascular structure that supports and nourishes the epidermis.[11] In addition, there are sensory nerve endings in the dermis that transmit signals regarding pain, pressure, heat, and cold. The dermis is divided into two layers: the superficial dermis and deep dermis. The superficial dermis consists of an extracellular matrix (collagen, elastin, and ground substances) and contains blood vessels, lymphatics, epithelial cells, connective tissue, muscle, fat, and nerve tissue. The vascular supply of the dermis is responsible for nourishing the epidermis and regulating body temperature. Fibroblasts are responsible for producing the collagen and elastin components of the skin that give it turgor. Fibronectin and hyaluronic acid are secreted by the fibroblasts.

The deep dermis is located over the subcutaneous fat; it contains larger networks of blood vessels and collagen fibers to provide tensile strength.[11] It also consists of fibroelastic connective tissue, which is yellow and composed mainly of collagen. Fibroblasts are also present in this tissue layer. The deep dermis merges with the subcutaneous fat and fascia and can be confused with yellow slough. It should be evaluated for texture and vitality. A healthy reticular layer will be adhered and firm-not soft, mushy, or stringy, like slough. Often, granulation buds are seen protruding through the mesh of the reticular layer. *Color Plate 17* shows the reticular layer of the dermis, with red granulation buds poking through the mesh layer in a partial-thickness wound. The well-vascularized dermis will withstand pressure for longer periods of time than will subcutaneous tissue or muscle. The collagen in the dermis gives the skin its toughness. Dermal wounds, e.g., cracks or pustules, involve the epidermis, basal membrane, and dermis. Typically, dermal injuries heal rapidly. Cracks in the dermis can exude serum, blood, or pus, and lead to formation of clots or crusts. Pustules are pus-filled vesicles that often represent infected hair follicle.

Wound Classification Systems

Wound classification systems have been designed and researched with one specific wound type, they are often (sometimes inappropriately) used for any wound type. The five the wound classification systems presented in this chapter are:[13,14,15]

1. Classification by Depth of Tissue Injury.
2. National Pressure Ulcer Advisory Panel (NPUAP) pressure ulcer staging criteria
3. Wagner staging system for grading severity of dysvascular ulcers

4. University of Texas Treatment Based Diabetic Foot Classification System
5. Marion Laboratories red/yellow/black color system

The Classification by Depth of Tissue Injury, NPUAP pressure ulcer staging criteria, the Wagner staging system rank severity according to the level of tissue involvement. Classification by Depth of Tissue Injury is a generic classification and NPUAP and Wagner classifications are based on specific wound etiologies (pressure ulcers and dysvascular neuropathic ulcers). The University of Texas Treatment Based Diabetic Foot Classification System is used in situations in which neuropathy is present and where information is needed about infection, circulation (PVD), and the combination of infection and ischemia in order to assign risk and predict outcome.[14] Finally, Marion Laboratories in Europe has developed a system that classifies wounds based on the color of the wound surface-red, yellow, or black. Clinicians are cautioned that none of these wound classification systems should be used in reverse as a method of measuring wound healing.

Classification by Depth of Tissue Injury

Classification by depth of tissue injury—superficial, partial-thickness, or full-thickness skin loss-is a classification system commonly used for wounds that are not categorized as pressure ulcers or neuropathic ulcers, such as skin tears, donor sites, vascular ulcers (venous ulcers in particular), surgical wounds, and burns.

Wound thickness refers to a superficial wound with intact skin and partial-thickness or full-thickness loss of the skin including the epidermis and dermis that may or may not penetrate into subcutaneous tissues or deeper structures. Superficial wounds have intact skin that has been traumatized, such as a superficial burn wound or blister. These wounds are equivalent to the stage I pressure ulcer or, on the Wagner scale, a grade 0 dysvascular ulcer. Partial-thickness wounds extend through the first layer of the skin or epidermis and into, but not through, the second layer of the skin or dermis (1–4 mm). Full-thickness wounds extend through the epidermis, dermis, and beyond. Wounds deeper

than 4 mm are considered full-thickness wounds and can be further categorized according to depth of involvement by using the term *subcutaneous tissue wound*. These wounds extend into or through subcutaneous tissues and can extend into muscles, tendons, and possibly down to the bone. Classification according to the depth of injury identifies specific anatomic levels of the tissues involved, but does not report their condition or color.

Anatomic depth of tissue loss is predictive of healing.[16,17] Superficial wounds are often resolved by subcutaneous inflammatory processes, with the exception of wounds with intact skin that also have deep tissue injury and can manifest later as deep wounds. Partial-thickness wounds, which heal by epithelialization, heal faster than full-thickness and subcutaneous wounds. Full-thickness and subcutaneous wounds heal by secondary intention, a combination of fibroplasia or granulation tissue formation and contraction. Table 4-1 provides the definitions of partial-thickness and full-thickness skin loss.

National Pressure Ulcer Advisor Panel (NPUAP) Pressure Ulcer Staging System

Classification by stages is used by NPUAP to describe the anatomic depth of soft tissue damage observed after the pathology has declared itself.[13] The NPUAP pressure ulcer staging system is probably one of the most widely known wound classification systems. It is most often applied to pressure ulcers, but it is also used (sometimes inappropriately) to classify other types of wounds. It is best used for wounds with a pressure or tissue perfusion etiologic factor, such as with arterial/ischemic wounds and diabetic neuropathic ulcers.

The NPUAP and the Agency for Health Care Research and Quality (AHRQ, formerly known as the Agency for Health Care Policy and Research, AHCPR), used the initial pressure ulcer staging system proposed by Shea[18] as the basis for recommending a universal four-stage system for describing pressure ulcers using anatomic depth and the involvement of soft tissue layers. The pressure ulcer staging system is limited to a description of the anatomic tissue

TABLE 4-1   Classification by Depth of Tissue Loss

Thickness of Skin Loss	Definition	Clinical Examples/Healing Process
Superficial wounds	Effects only the epidermis	Sunburn, stage I pressure ulcer, stage 0 diabetic ulcer; heal by inflammation
Partial-thickness skin loss	Extends through the epidermis, into, but not through, the dermis	Skin tears, abrasions, tape damage, blisters, perineal dermatitis from incontinence; heal by epidermal resurfacing or epithelialization
Full-thickness skin loss	Extends through the epidermis and dermis into subcutaneous fat and deeper structures	Donor sites, venous ulcers, surgical wounds; heal by granulation tissue formation and contraction
Subcutaneous tissue wounds	Additional classification level for full-thickness wounds that extend into, or beyond, the subcutaneous tissue	Surgical wounds, arterial/ischemic wounds; heal by granulation tissue formation and contraction

loss; it is a diagnosis of severity of tissue insult before healing starts. The AHRQ adopted the NPUAP staging system for use in two sets of clinical practice guidelines.[19,20] It is widely accepted and commonly used to describe wound severity, organize treatment protocols, and select and reimburse treatment products for pressure ulcers. Table 4-2 presents the staging criteria for pressure ulcers, including the 1998 revised NPUAP definition of a stage I pressure ulcer.[21] The visual and nonvisual indicators that were included in the 1998 NPUAP stage I pressure ulcer definition have been validated.[22]

CLINICAL WISDOM

Reverse Staging or Back Staging of Pressure Ulcers

Reverse staging or back staging of pressure ulcers is an inappropriate way to define a healing wound. Once the ulcer is staged, the stage and wound severity diagnosis do not change; rather, correct terminology is *healing stage II, III, or IV.*

The pressure ulcer staging system is not ideal. It has many problems. For example, staging systems measure only one characteristic of the wound (the depth of tissue loss) and should not be viewed as a complete assessment independent of other indicators. Staging classification systems do not assess the healing process and, because of an inability to demonstrate change over time, hinder tracking of progress. The definition of a stage I pressure ulcer does not

TABLE 4-2 Pressure Ulcer Staging Criteria

Stage	Definition
I	An observable, pressure-related alteration of intact skin whose indicators, as compared with the adjacent or opposite area of the body, may include changes in one or more of the following: skin temperature, tissue consistency (firm or boggy feel), and sensation (pain, itching). The ulcer appears as a defined area of persistent redness in lightly pigmented skin; in darker tones, the ulcer can appear with persistent red, blue, or purple hues.
II	Partial-thickness skin loss involving epidermis and/or dermis. The ulcer is superficial and presents clinically as an abrasion, blister, or shallow crater.
III	Full-thickness skin loss involving damage or necrosis of subcutaneous tissue that can extend down to, but not through, underlying fascia. The ulcer presents clinically as a deep crater with or without undermining of adjacent tissue.
IV	Full-thickness skin loss with extensive destruction, tissue necrosis or damage to muscle, bone, or supporting structures (e.g., tendon, joint capsule).

Reprinted with permission from the NPUAP Statement on Reverse Staging of Pressure Ulcers, The Pressure Ulcer Staging System. NPUAP Report, Vol. 4, No. 2, September 1995. (c) National Pressure Ulcer Advisory Panel.

account for the severity of soft tissue trauma beneath the unbroken skin, such as that seen with purple ulcers. NPUAP proposes that this trauma should be referred to as "pressure-related deep tissue injury under intact skin" or "deep tissue injury."[23] The Panel is working on defining and naming stages for pressure ulcers that are not represented in the current stage structure.[24]

Furthermore, stage I lesions vary in presentation and pose validity concerns. For example, some stage I lesions indicate deep tissue damage that is just beginning to manifest on the skin, whereas others indicate only superficial insult in which damage may be reversible and may not be indicative of underlying tissue death. The European Pressure Ulcer Advisory Panel definition of a grade 4 pressure ulcer is: "Extensive destruction, tissue necrosis or damage to muscle, bone or supporting structures with or WITHOUT full thickness skin loss."[25] This definition appears to be addressing the issue of deep tissue injury and classifying it as a serious grade 4 lesion, which it may become.

There are also problems reliably assessing stage I ulcers in dark-skinned patients. In fact, in 1997, the NPUAP redefined stage I pressure ulcers to better reflect ethnic diversity in pressure ulcer patients (see Table 4-2). Not all of the indicators need to be present for a stage I diagnosis.[26] Identification and interpretation of skin color changes in darkly pigmented skin require special assessment strategies. These strategies are described in the section on assessment of the periwound and wound tissues. An ultrasound scanner image that can detect tissue damage and provide early identification of stage I pressure ulcers is demonstrated in (Color Plates 73–75).

Stage II pressure ulcers are lesions that are not necessarily caused by pressure, but are more likely due to shearing, friction, or incontinence. These ulcers should be distinguished from, and treated in a different manner than, pressure ulcers. Theoretically, pressure ulcer trauma starts at the bony tissue interface and works outward, eventually manifesting as damage on the skin. Conversely, stage II lesions start at the epidermis or skin and can progress to deeper layers. Stage II lesions are more often caused by friction or shearing of the tissues, which leads to superficial and partial-thickness damage to the epidermis and dermis.

EPUAP defines incontinence ulcers as: "Skin lesions not caused by pressure or shear."[25] Distinguishing features of lesions caused by incontinence include: location (not necessarily over bony prominences), edema, wet skin, incontinence of urine or feces, and color (more purple).[25] Be aware that a more purplish color can signify deep tissue injury and does not necessarily relate to incontinence.

Staging of pressure ulcers covered by eschar and necrotic tissue cannot be accomplished until removal of necrotic tissue allows for determination of the extent of depth of tissue involvement. Pressure ulcers with necrotic tissue filling the wound bed are full-thickness wounds, stage III or stage IV. The clinician cannot determine the level of tissue insult until the necrotic debris is removed. Likewise, with deep tissue injuries, the level of tissue insult cannot be staged until the full impact of the lesion manifests. It is also difficult to define stages in patients with supportive devices because of the difficulty in accurately assessing the wound without removal of the devices. Finally, accurate, meaningful communication is difficult, because clinicians may not have the experience necessary to recognize the various tissue layers that identify the stage or grade. In addition, clinicians may define stages differently. Staging requires practice and skill that develops with time spent examining wounds. Both the NPUAP and EPUAP have teaching aides for staging pressure ulcers available on their web sites.

Unfortunately, the staging system has been misinterpreted and misapplied in clinical practice as a way to monitor healing. It was not designed to do this. Biologically, wounds do not heal in the manner suggested by reversing the staging system. For example, a stage IV pressure ulcer cannot "heal" and become a stage II pressure ulcer. The purpose of staging pressure ulcers is to document the maximum anatomic depth of tissue involved (after all necrotic tissue is removed) and to determine the extent of tissue damage only. Staging can also aid examination of the *wound severity*, but not *wound healing*.

Elimination of reverse staging as a way to report and document wound healing quickly and efficiently has left a void in the system. The situation has been complicated further by the fact that the Center for Medicare and Medicaid Services (CMS, formerly known as the Health Care Financing Administration, HCFA), requires that providers continue to use reverse staging in order to comply with CMS regulations. Specifically, the Minimum Data Set (MDS) developed by CMS relies on the reverse staging of wounds, both pressure ulcers and venous ulcers, to demonstrate the progression of wound healing. This has created a dilemma for the conscientious practitioner. One pragmatic suggestion is to stage for the wound severity at baseline; then, upon subsequent reassessment, report decreasing stages as the wound shows attributes of healing (e.g., "Initial stage IV wound has attributes preventing healing of eschar, slough, and exposure of tendon, muscle, or bone indicators; progressing to a stage III wound with the presence of some healing attributes (absence of necrosis and presence of granulation tissue); progressing to a stage II reepithelialization beginning, and to stage I, healed").[27] Although this is a misuse of the staging system, it does have some merit. Until there is broad acceptance of a research-based tool to monitor healing and a change in the government reporting system, this may be the only route open to the thoughtful clinician. The Sussman Wound Healing Tool, Pressure Ulcer Scale for Healing (PUSH), and Bates- Jensen Wound Assessment Tool (BWAT) are tools for monitoring wound healing attributes described in Chapter 6.

Wagner Ulcer Grade Classification

The Wagner Ulcer Grade Classification system is used to establish the presence of depth and infection in a wound. This system was developed for the diagnosis and treatment of the dysvascular foot.[15] It is commonly used as an as-

sessment instrument in the evaluation of diabetic foot ulcers, and is also useful for neuropathic and arterial/ischemic ulcer classification. The system includes six grades, progressing from 0 to 5 in order of severity of breakdown in the diabetic, neuropathic foot (Table 4-3). The 0 classification evaluates for predisposing factors leading to breakdown; along with grades 1–3, it is used for risk management. Photos of the grades appear in Chapter 19.

The University of Texas Treatment Based Diabetic Foot Classification System

The University of Texas Treatment Based Diabetic Foot Classification System is used for situations in which neuropathy is present and information is needed about infection, circulation (PVD), and the combination of infection and ischemia in order to assign risk and predict outcome (Table 4-4).[14] Each ulcer is given both a numeric grade (o-III) and an alphabetic stage (A-D). Letter "A" denotes wound depth. Other letters denote ischemia and infection categories. However, it lacks consideration of biomechanics and neuropathy. Analysis of this system reveals that it is a better predictor of group outcome than of individual patient outcome.

Marion Laboratories Red, Yellow, Black Wound Classification System

Classification by color is a popular system because of its simplicity and ease of use. Three colors-red, yellow, and black-are used for assessing the wound's surface color.[28] The three-color system was originally conceived as a tool to direct treatment, with each color corresponding to specific therapy needs. The red wound is clean, healing, and granulating. Yellow signals possible infection, the need for cleaning or debridement, or the presence of necrotic tissue. The black wound is necrotic and needs cleaning and debridement. Red is considered the most desired characteristic, yellow is less desirable, and black is least desirable. If all three types are present, clinicians select the least desirable as the basis for treatment. Table 4-5 shows the red, yellow, and black classification system with clinical manifestations. Table 4-6 presents the four wound classification systems

TABLE 4-3 Wagner Ulcer Grade Classification

Grade	Characteristics
0	Preulcerative lesions; healed ulcers; presence of bony deformity
1	Superficial ulcer without subcutaneous tissue involvement
2	Penetration through the subcutaneous tissue; may expose bone, tendon, ligament, or joint capsule
3	Osteitis, abscess, or osteomyelitis
4	Gangrene of digit
5	Gangrene of the foot requiring disarticulation

Reprinted with permission from Wagner, FEW. The dysvascular foot: A system for diagnosis and treatment. *Foot and Ankle.* 1981;(2):64-122.

TABLE 4-4   University of Texas, San Antonio Classification

	Grade	0	I	II	III
S					
T	A	Preulcerative or postulcerative lesion; completely epithelialized	Superficial wound (not involving tendon, capsule or bone)	Wound penetrating to tendon or capsule	Wound penetrating to bone or joint
A	B	Infection	Infection	Infection	Infection
G	C	Ischemia	Ischemia	Ischemia	Ischemia
E	D	Infection and Ischemia	Infection and Ischemia	Infection and Ischemia	Infection and Ischemia

Reprinted with permission from Armstrong DG, Lavery L, Harkless LB. Validation of a diabetic wound classification system: the contribution of depth, infection, and ischemia to risk of amputation. *Diabetes Car PMID: 9589255 [PubMed - indexed for MEDLINE].* May 1998;21(5):855-859.

discussed in this section and the types of wounds most appropriate for use with each system.

Wound Severity Diagnosis

Wound diagnosis statements for physicians, nurses, and physical therapists are similar, in that all use diagnoses that reflect impairments of the involved tissues. In medicine, diagnoses are made based on identified pathological conditions. Nurses use nursing diagnoses to classify skin and tissue impairments, and to assist with developing care plans for wound care patients. Nursing diagnoses are expressed as specific diagnostic statements that include the diagnostic category and the "related to" stem statement. For example, *impaired tissue integrity* is a broad diagnosis that would be correctly applied to stage III and stage IV pressure ulcers. *Impaired skin integrity* is a subcategory that correctly applies to partial-thickness or full-thickness loss of skin. *Impaired skin integrity* should not be used as a diagnosis for surgical incisions or deep tissue wounds. The diagnosis of *risk for infection related to surgical incision* is more appropriate, because of the disruption of the skin during surgery, making it more vulnerable to infection.

The "related to" stem statements aid in communicating with other health-care professionals and planning care by targeting the defining characteristics for the diagnostic statement. For example, the diagnosis statement *impaired skin integrity* would be followed by a statement such as

impaired skin integrity related to friction and moisture from urinary incontinence. For nurses, the "related to" stem statement usually reflects etiologic factors in wound development and directs the plan of care and specific interventions.[29]

Physical therapists also use wound severity diagnoses that relate to depth of wound penetration. Wound diagnosis statements include a stem statement that indicates depth of skin involvement, such as *superficial skin involvement or partial-thickness skin involvement and scar formation, full-thickness skin involvement and scar formation,* or *involvement extending into fascia, muscle,* or *bone.* An example of a complete statement is: *impaired integumentary integrity secondary to partial-thickness skin involvement and scar formation.*[30] The statement refers to the functional impairment of the skin and different tissues, which has implications for disability.

The concept that the depth of tissue involvement or wound stage is a measure of wound severity is regularly accepted by all health care disciplines and this concept is used to select examinations, plan treatment, and predict functional outcomes.

The Assessment Process

Although the terms *assessment* and *evaluation* are often used synonymously, they are actually different. *Assessment* is the systematic process of assigning numbers or grades to events during the examination. Tests are the instruments or means by which events are assessed or measured, and examination is the process of determining the values of the tests. Evaluation is the process of making clinical judgments based on the data gathered from the examination. Skills of *evaluation* are necessary for interpreting what are appropriate tests and understanding the significance, reliability and validity of the tests and measurements,

Both assessment and evaluation require an understanding of the condition, the ability to recognize the importance and value of the information, and the skills to collect this information appropriately and methodically.[16] One thing

TABLE 4-5   Marion Laboratories Red, Yellow, and Black Wound Classification System

Color	Indication
Red	Clean; healing; granulation
Yellow	Possible infection; needs cleaning; necrotic
Black	Needs cleaning; necrotic

Data from Cuzzell JZ. The new RYB color code. *American Journal of Nursing.* 1988;88(10):1342-1346 And Stotts NA. Seeing red & yellow & black: the three color concept of wound care. *Nursing.* 1990;2:59-61.

TABLE 4-6   Wound Classification Systems and Wound Types

Wound Classification Systems	Pressure Ulcers	Venous Ulcers	Arterial and Ischemic Ulcers	Diabetic Ulcers (Neuropathic)	Other Wounds
Pressure ulcer staging	X		X (Those with a pressure component)	X (Those with a pressure component)	Stage II classification is appropriate for skin tears and tape damage
Wagner Ulcer dysvascular Classification System			X	X	
University of Texas Diabetic Classification				X	
Depth of tissue injury	X (full-thickness wounds require examination of deep tissue involvement)	X (full-thickness wounds require examination of deep tissue involvement)	X (full-thickness wounds require examination of deep tissue involvement)	X (full-thickness wounds require examination of deep tissue involvement)	Useful for skin tears, burns, and other skin wounds surgical secondary intention healing
Red, yellow, and black	X	X	X	X	

that differentiates assessment from evaluation is the scope of practice and skill set of the examiner. For example, performing tests and examinations and monitoring tissue attributes are within the scope of practice of physical therapist assistants and licensed practical/vocational nurses. Evaluation of the data is a skill that is in the purview of licensed physical therapists, registered nurses, nurse specialists, physician assistants, nurse practitioners, and podiatrists who have advanced skills and knowledge of wound management.

Purpose and Frequency

Wound assessment data are collected for five purposes:

1. Examine the severity (stage) of the lesion
2. Determine the status of wound healing
3. Establish a baseline for the wound
4. Prepare a plan of care
5. Report observed changes in the wound over time

Assessment data enable clinicians to communicate clearly about a patient's wound, provide for continuity in the plan of care, and allow for evaluation of treatment modalities.

Baseline assessment, monitoring, and reassessment are the keys to establishing a plan of care and evaluating the achievement of target outcomes and progress toward goals. Valid, significant tests and measurements should be selected for the assessment process. The same tests selected for initial assessment should be used throughout the course of care to evaluate progress and revise the treatment plan as required.

After the initial or baseline examination, wound attributes should be reassessed at regular intervals in order to measure any change in the status of the ulcer or in risk factors.[31] One study of stage III and stage IV pressure ulcers found that the percentage of reduction in the ulcer area after 2 weeks of treatment was predictive of healing time.[31] If, after 2–4 weeks of appropriate treatment, reassessment indicates that the wound has deteriorated or has failed to improve, the plan of care should be modified, and adjunctive treatment should be considered.[19]

Monitoring is a means of checking the wound frequently for signs and symptoms that should trigger a full reassessment, such as increased wound exudate or bruising of the adjacent or periwound skin. Monitoring includes gross evaluation for signs and symptoms of wound complications, such as erythema (change in color) of periwound skin and pus, which is indicative of infection. It should also include progress toward wound healing, such as granulation tissue growth (red color) and reepithelialization (new skin). Monitoring, unlike assessment, may be performed by unskilled caregivers, such as the patient's family or a nurse attendant. Monitoring takes place during dressing changes and other treatment applications.

Different care settings have different requirements that designate specific individuals to perform the assessment function. For example, in the home setting, a non-professional caregiver may monitor the wound attributes, but a nurse or physical therapist, assesses the findings. The caregiver may gather data at dressing changes and predetermined intervals, and reports changes to the nurse or physical therapist, who evaluates the results of the treatment plan. The professional wound case manager may see the patient's wound only intermittently for a complete reassessment. In a skilled nursing facility, requirements by federal licensing agencies typically prescribe intervals for reassessment. If the patient is in an acute or subacute setting where there are very short lengths of stay, there may be only a single assessment.

CLINICAL WISDOM

Monitoring Wound Progress

Teach family members and other caregivers to monitor the wound at each dressing change. Help them to identify signs of wound infection, such as large amounts of purulent exudate (pus), periwound erythema (reddish, purplish), warmth, increased tenderness or pain at the site, and elevated temperature. Caregivers should also be aware of healing characteristics, such as bright red color, new skin, and small amounts of clear drainage.

Procedures for Assessment of Skin and Wound

The following procedures are recommended for consistant and well organized assessment of the skin and the wound status. The section begins with the use of standardized data collection and documentation forms that list the significant skin and wound features at baseline assessment and that will be tracked over the course of care. Examples of tested forms are in Chapter 6. Next are procedures that use the senses of the clinician involved in the assessment process to assess the physical characteristics. Vision to observe the wound and surrounding tissues, smell to identify healthy from unhealthy tissues, touch using manual examination techniques to palpate contours and nervous system responses such as pain, protective sensation and thermal responses, and hearing to evaluate blood flow with a Doppler ultrasound and to listen to the patient's responses to tests and questions.

Data Collection and Documentation Forms

Information collection is easier, better organized, and more consistent when it is collected on a form, whether on paper or an electronic template. Although many forms exist, the most common is the skin care flow sheet used by nurses. Methods of recording assessment data should allow for the tracking of each assessment item over time, in objective and measurable terms that show changes in wound status. The Bates-Jensen Wound Assessment Tool (BWAT, formerly known as the Pressure Sore Status Tool, PSST) and the Sussman Wound Healing Tool (SWHT), can be used to record findings and measure each attribute objectively. Both forms, with instructions, are described in Chapter 6.

Useful forms for tissue assessment usually include the following items:

- periwound skin attributes
- wound tissue attributes
- wound exudate characteristics

Regardless of which instrument is used to collect findings, all attributes on the form should be considered. If the attribute is not applicable, the notation "N/A" should be made to fill the blank. If an attribute is absent, record a zero. If present, a grade or check is required. Leaving a blank space on the form implies that the attribute was not considered or assessed.

If the patient's medical diagnosis suggests possible related medical impairments associated with the wound and periwound skin (e.g., neuropathy or vascular disease), multiple forms may be required to report all the necessary elements relating to the patient's condition. Chapters 7 and 19 include forms specific to recording data related to those problems.

Policy, Procedures, and Documentation

Documentation requirements for wound assessment should be part of a facility's policies and procedures. Documentation should be accurate and clearly reflect the patient's condition, examinations performed, findings, care rendered, and proper notification of the physician of significant findings. Documentation of similar findings by practitioners in the same department or facility should be consistent and reflect facility policies.[32] Remember, medical records can be subpoenaed into court - sometimes several years after the assessment. "Documentation can be either your shield against a potential malpractice lawsuit or the sword that strikes you down."[32]

Assessment of Wound Attributes

Assessment encompasses examination of a composite of wound attributes. A single attribute cannot provide the data

■ CASE STUDY

Dangers of Differing Clinical Procedures and Facility Policies

A physical therapist (PT) debrided a toenail on a patient with a medical history of neuropathy associated with diabetes. The toe became infected, leading to below-the-knee amputation of the leg. The PT's action was called into question in a malpractice lawsuit. The debridement procedure followed by the PT was acceptable and documented, but it was the facility's policy to have a patient with diabetic neuropathy evaluated in the vascular laboratory for transcutaneous oxygen levels before debridement. The PT did not document an evaluation of the patient for circulatory status prior to performing the debridement procedure. As a consequence, the PT's action was called into question, and he became the defendant in a malpractice lawsuit.

EXHIBIT 4-1 Indexes for Wound Assessment

- Anatomic location
- Size: length, width
- Volume: depth (also stage if initial assessment; note if unable to stage)
- Undermining/tunneling
- Age of wound in weeks or months
- Attributes preventing healing: necrotic tissue (including eschar[87], hemorrhage (purple deep tissue injury), periwound erythema and edema, edges undermined (not connected)
- Attributes characteristic of healing: granulation tissue, new epithelium, attached wound edges
- Wound exudate: color, amount, odor, consistency
- Pain: to touch, pressure, tissue tension, all of the time or only during treatment
- Temperature: excess warmth, coolness, normal body temperature for the area

necessary to determine the treatment plan, nor will it allow for the monitoring of progress or degradation of the wound. The attributes for wound assessment include all of the following:

- Location
- Age of wound
- Size of the wound
- Stage or depth of tissue involvement
- Presence of undermining or tunneling
- Presence or absence of tissue attributes that prevent healing (e.g., necrotic tissue in the wound and erythema of the periwound tissue)
- Presence or absence of tissue attributes that aid healing (e.g., condition of the wound edges, granulation tissue, and epithelialization)
- Exudate characteristics

There are two schools of thought regarding tissue assessment: The first looks only at the wound tissue, whereas the second examines the wound tissue, periwound skin, and soft tissue structures. Because the periwound skin is intimately involved in the circulatory response to wounds, and the risk for infection, it is prudent to evaluate both areas. The examination of the wound and periwound skin provides data related to the wound healing phase diagnosis. Exhibit 4-1 lists the common indexes for wound assessment.

Wound severity assessment includes identifying the tissue layers involved in the wound. The more tissue layers that a wound penetrates, the more severe the wound is considered. This "wound severity diagnosis" impacts further wound assessment strategies, determines an appropriate treatment plan, and predicts healing time. For example, a partial-thickness wound would not be assessed for tunneling or undermining. This diagnosis also has impact on prediction of risk for nonhealing and on reim-

bursement. For example, a stage IV pressure ulcer requires more care and a longer length of stay than does a stage II pressure ulcer, and the risk of complications is greater.

Assessment of the wound is separate from assessment of the etiology of the wound, although the examinations chosen for the assessment can relate to or provide clues to the etiology. For example, wounds caused by venous insufficiency typically appear on the lower leg above the ankle; a brawny color is often seen in the adjacent tissues, edema is likely to be present, and the periwound skin may be fragile. A patient diagnosed with a diabetic ulcer and insensitivity will often have an ulcer on the plantar surface of the foot. There may be areas of callus over bony prominence, bony deformities, and hyperkeratosis of the heel, which are related to polyneuropathy. Therefore, soft tissues adjacent (i.e., tissues extending away from the periwound) to the area of wounding should be assessed for the attributes of location, sensation, circulation, texture, and color. These findings will be used to establish a treatment plan, and predict wound outcomes.

Observation and Palpation Techniques

Observation and palpation are classic components of physical diagnosis. They are used to determine alteration in soft tissue characteristics, including the skin, subcutaneous fascia, and muscles leading to a soft tissue or structural diagnosis.[33] Proper lighting and positioning of the patient and tissue to be assessed will improve observation.

Assessment Toolbox

A penlight, small mirror with a long handle, infrared and/or liquid crystal thermometer, and tuning fork are handy items to keep in the assessment toolbox.

Begin the tissue examination by evaluating for symmetry with the contralateral limb and adjacent structures, using both observation and palpation. Look for symmetry of tissue color, texture, contour, hardness/softness, and temperature. When compared with an area of normal skin and soft tissue, any differences in the skin, subcutaneous tissue, fascia, and muscle should be noted.

In palpation, the hands are important, sensitive diagnostic instruments. The clinician's hands should be clean, with the fingernails of appropriate length. It is important for the clinician to develop a palpatory sense in the hands. Different parts of the hands are valuable for different tests: the back of the hand is more sensitive to temperature; the palms of the hands are best used to detect changes in tissue contours (induration, edema); the thumbs are useful in applying pressure to check for hardness or softness at different tissue depths; and the finger pads are more sensitive to texture (fibrotic tissues) and fine discrimination. Techniques of palpation include the use of slow, light movements. Avoid pressing too hard and trying to examine the area too quickly, as this can provide confusing messages to the sensory receptors of the examiner's hands.

Palpation skills require practice to refine the practitioner's palpatory sense. The examiner should reduce other sensory inputs in the environment (noise, traffic, conversation), so as to concentrate and focus on the palpation examination. A common language with which to communicate the findings in easily understood terms is also important. Paired descriptors, such as *superficial-deep, moist-dry, warm-cold, painful-nonpainful, rough-smooth, hard-soft,* and *thick-thin* are useful to accurately describe findings. The state of tissue changes can be reported as acute, subacute, chronic (persistent), or absent. They can also be graded on a scale of 0–3+ as a way of diagnosing the severity of the problem. Familiar examples of this type of grading system are pitting edema and pulse strength. The use of a grading system is also helpful in reporting response to treatment intervention.

Requirements for a Successful Palpatory Examination

1. Concentration
2. Language to communicate findings
3. Light pressure
4. Slow movement

Assessment of Adjacent Tissues

The tissues surrounding and adjacent to a closed or open wound provide many clues that can identify the health of the skin, phase of wound healing, and the patient's overall health status. The term *adjacent* is used to describe tissues that may not show signs of wounding, but that are predictive of healing. *Periwound skin* refers to the tissues immediately surrounding the wounded tissue. Skin or trophic changes are important predictors of the body's ability to respond to wounding. The attributes of the adjacent tissues that should be assessed are described in the following sections, including:

- Skin texture (e.g., dryness, thickness, turgor)
- Scar tissue
- Callus
- Maceration
- Edema
- Color
- Sensation (pain, thermal, touch, protective, vibratory)
- Temperature
- Hair distribution
- Toenails
- Blisters

Skin Texture

Smooth, flexible skin has a feeling of fullness and resistance to tissue deformation that is called *turgor*. Turgor is a sign of skin health. Aging skin often shows signs of dryness due to atrophy and thinning of both the epithelial and fatty layers of tissue in the dermis. The feel of the skin reflects a loss of turgor. The areas most affected by loss of subcutaneous fat are the upper and lower extremities. This causes more prominent bony protuberances on the hips, knees, ankles, and bony areas of the feet, which results in a higher risk of pressure ulcer formation.

Elderly skin also loses elasticity due to shrinkage of both collagen and elastin. There is a weakening of the juncture between the epidermis and dermis, causing the skin layers to "slide" across each other and placing the person at risk for skin tears. Sebaceous glands and their secretions are diminished, which results in skin that is dry, often itchy, and easily torn.[34] Impaired circulation also contributes to changes in the skin; it is usually associated with aging, but can be due to a disease process, such as neuropathy associated with diabetes. This disease impairs the secretion of sweat and sebaceous glands, which in turn contributes to the slow resurfacing of partial-thickness dermal ulcers. Loss of sweat changes the pH of the skin, making it more susceptible to infection and bacterial penetration.

To assess skin texture, use observation and palpation. Look for evidence of dryness, such as flaking or scaling. To check skin turgor, gently pinch the tissues with thumb and forefinger, and observe how they respond. For example, in older patients, loss of elasticity can be exhibited by the tissues' slow return to normal after pinching. Tenting of the skin when pinched can be an early indicator of dehydration. In older patients, it is best to check for general skin turgor on the forehead or sternal area. Palpate by gently rubbing your fingers across the patient's skin and feeling for sliding of the epidermis away from the dermis.

Skin inspection is an opportunity to spot suspicious signs of early melanoma. If a suspicious skin lesion is noted, ask the patient how long the area of skin has been discolored, whether it has changed shape or size in the past 6 weeks to 6 months, and whether it has been examined by a physician. The ABCD rule with a 90% positive value is a valid screening tool for early melanoma.[35]

RESEARCH WISDOM

ABCD Rule

While checking the skin, observe for ABCD signs of early melanoma:

A: asymmetry—uneven edges, lopsided in shape
B: borders—irregular (scalloped, poorly defined)
C: color—black or shades of brown, red, white, occasionally blue
D: diameter—greater than 5 mm (larger than a pencil eraser)

Scar Tissue

Inspection of the adjacent skin should include checking for scar tissue. If present, scar tissue should be assessed for smoothness, flexibility, thickness, and toughness. Scar tissue that is mature has greater density and toughness, and is less resilient than surrounding skin. New scar tissue is thinner and more flexible than mature scar tissue, and is less resilient to stress. Wounding in an area of scarring will have less tensile strength when healed than will a new wound and will be more likely to break down (see *Color Plate 39*).

New scar tissue is bright pink in appearance. As the scar tissue matures, it becomes nearly the same color as the periwound skin, except in individuals with darkly pigmented skin. Hypopigmentation frequently follows injuries to dark skin. Loss of skin color can create more anxiety for individuals than the wound itself. If the wounding disruption is less than full-thickness loss of the epidermis, repigmentation will usually occur over time. However, new skin covering deeper lesions and new lesions will appear pink.[36] The scar area can even turn white. Hypopigmented areas are more susceptible to sunburn than are normally pigmented areas. For some individuals, burns and physical trauma can be followed by localized areas of hyperpigmentation. Like hypopigmentation, hyperpigmentation causes anxiety in many individuals.

Observe for abnormal scarring characteristics. Hypertrophic scarring results from excessive collagen deposition, causing a very thick scar mass that remains within the area of the original wound. These scars are unattractive and disfiguring, and can cause itching or pain that interferes with functional mobility (see *Color Plates 48*).

Hypertropic scars are differentiated from keloid scars, which are also thickened but extend beyond the boundaries of the original wound (see *Color Plate 50*).[37]Although keloids are found in people of all races, scarring is of special concern to African American individuals and some Asians, as opposed to other dark-skinned individuals, be-

cause of the frequency of keloid formation in these populations, which suggest a genetic factor. Frequency of occurrence is equal among men and women.

Keloids are similar to benign tumor growths in that they continue to grow long after the wound is closed and can reach a large size. Any attempt to cut or use dermabrasion to buff away a keloid will result in even more scarring.[36] In keloids, the mechanism of collagen deposition is totally out of control. Areas with keloids can be itchy, tender, or painful.[10] New therapies are being used to control this phenomenon, but if a patient reports a previous keloid or a familial tendency to form keloids, special attention should be made to address this problem at the time of initial assessment.

Hyperkeratotic scarring involves hypertrophy of the horny layer of the epidermis. It is commonly seen in diabetic patients and can be located in adjacent and periwound tissue (see *Color Plate 24* and Chapter 19).

Callus

The most commonly encountered calluses are located on the plantar surface of the foot, along the medial side of the great toe, over the metatarsal heads, and around the heel margin. Callus formation is a protective function of the skin to shearing forces of a prominent bone against an unyielding shoe surface. Neuropathy often leads to muscle imbalance and subsequent uneven weight distribution along the metatarsal heads, which results in callus formation in those areas. The location of the callus is a clue to the underlying bony pathologic condition.[38] Untreated, callus buildup will continue, creating additional shear forces between the bony prominence and soft tissues, and resulting in breakdown of the interposing soft tissues. Hemorrhage on a callus indicates probable trauma and perhaps ulceration beneath. The presence of a callus indicates the need for further assessment of the foot. Chapter 19 contains illustrations and more information about callus management.

CLINICAL WISDOM

Observation and Palpation of Calluses

Calluses often appear as thickened areas on the sole of the foot and are usually lighter in color (often yellow) than the adjacent areas. When palpated, the callus area will feel firm or hard to the touch. There may also be some scaling or flaking, roughness, or cracking of the callus. Cracked callus is a portal for infection. Build up of callus around a wound signals an area of high pressure, and further examination is required.

Maceration of Skin and Moisture Balance

There is no objective method of measuring skin moisture balance. The source of moisture that soaks and macerates the skin can be perspiration, soaking in a tub, wound exudate, or incontinence (urine or feces), as well as wound dressing products. *Maceration* is defined as "the softening of a tissue by soaking until the connective tissue fibers are so dissolved that the tissue components can be teased apart."[34]

When maceration occurs, the stratum corneum takes on a soft, white, spongy texture (see *Color Plate 15*). Softened tissue is easily traumatized by pressure and contributes to the development of pressure ulcers.[34] Moisture associated with incontinence is also a risk factor for pressure ulcers.

Determine the cause of the maceration. Macerated skin is thinner than adjacent skin. Palpate very gently to avoid trauma. Exposure to friction and shear should be avoided. Skin moisture barrier products can be used to reduce the impact of moisture on the skin, but they need to be evaluated based on the needs of the patient.

CLINICAL WISDOM

Good moisture balance of the skin can be achieved by choosing a dressing product that manages wound exudate and does not macerate the skin. The periwound skin can be protected by applying petrolatum or a zinc oxide paste combined with petrolatum to make it less stiff and easier to apply with a tongue depressor. The zinc oxide does not need to be removed during dressing changes. To ease removal of zinc oxide from the skin, apply petrolatum or oil.[39]

Excessive sweating can be related to medication, infection, or the environment, and may not be controllable.[40] "Excessive sweating is a problem in skin folds, such as under the breasts. Obese individuals have many skin folds that need to be examined because they are a common site of yeast infection. Absorbant products to control the moisture need to be evaluated to meet the requirements of the individual. Moisture control should include use of support surfaces and chair cushion coverings, because moisture and temperature affect tissue load tolerance. Moist skin has a higher coefficient of friction than dry skin; in that state, it has reduced tissue integrity. Cotton or air exchange covers for seat cushions are recommended because they can better dissipate moisture and heat on the surface, and promote better skin moisture balance.

As described, too much moisture can affect skin integrity. Likewise, a dry or desiccated wound is out of balance and slows keratinocyte migration. A dry state can be beneficial if the wound is located on the heel, has a dry eschar, and shows no signs of edema, erythema. flatulence, or drainage, yet needs daily monitoring.[41]

Edema

Edema is another example of moisture imbalance. Edema is "the presence of abnormally large amounts of fluid in the intercellular tissue spaces of the body, usually referring to demonstrable amounts in the subcutaneous tissues. It may be localized, due to venous or lymphatic obstruction or increased vascular permeability, or systemic, due to heart failure or renal disease."[42] The presence of edema can be associated with the inflammatory phase, the result of dependence of a limb, or an indication of circulatory impairment or congestive heart failure. One consequence of trauma is increased extracellular fluid in the tissues that both blocks the lymphatic system and causes increased capillary permeability. The function of edema following injury is to block the spread of infection. The result is a swelling that is hard; the application of pressure to the swollen area does not distort the tissues. The term *brawny edema* refers to this type of swelling and is associated with the inflammatory phase. Traumatic edema is usually accompanied by pain, whereas swelling resulting from lymphedema or systemic causes is usually painless.[43]

There are two types of edema: nonpitting and pitting. Nonpitting edema is identified by skin that is stretched and shiny, with hardness of the underlying tissues. Pitting edema is identified by firmly pressing a finger down into the tissues and waiting 5 seconds. If the tissues fail to resume the previous position after pressure is released, and an indentation remains, pitting edema is present. Pitting edema is often observed with dependence of a limb and with tissue congestion associated with congestive heart failure, venous insufficiency, and lymphedema. It is measured on a severity scale of 0–3+, where 0 = not present, 1+ = minimal, 2+ = moderate, and 3+ = severe.

When examining for edema, look for body symmetry and review the patient's medical history. Bilateral edema of the lower extremities can be a sign of a systemic problem, such as congestive heart failure, cirrhosis, malnutrition, or obesity. It may also be caused by dependence on or use of certain drugs. Drug-induced edema is often pitting edema and can be caused by hormonal drugs, including corticosteroids, estrogens, progesterones, and testosterone. Other drugs to consider include nonsteroidal antiinflammatory and antihypertensive drugs. Symptoms usually resolve if the drug is withdrawn.[43]

Systemic edema can extend from the lower extremities into the abdomen, which is termed ascites. Unilateral edema of the lower extremity of sudden onset can be due to acute deep vein thrombophlebitis and is a medical red flag that requires immediate referral to a physician. Other causes of unilateral edema include chronic venous insufficiency, lymphedema, cellulitis, abscess, osteomyelitis, Charcot's joint, popliteal aneurysm, dependence, and revascularization. Deep vein thrombophlebitis, chronic venous insufficiency, and lymphedema are the three most common causes.[43]

If the etiology of the edema is uncertain, consult with a physician before planning further testing or an intervention. If edema remains in the tissue, the large protein molecules can clog the lymphatic channels and cause fibrosis. Management of edema is another way to clinically manage moisture balance. Chapter 10 describes the management of edema with compression.

Measurement of Edema. Tissue volume increases when edema is present, stretching and expanding the tissue with a change in circumference or girth. Accurate assessment of edema is essential for early intervention and to evaluate the outcomes of treatment interventions. Edema is often evaluated and diagnosed by visual inspection, palpation for change in contour of the tissues, and by photographs. However, visual diagnosis is not as accurate as measurement.[44] Two methods used for measurement of the extent of edema formation are girth and volume.

After visual inspection, girth measurement of the limb is the most common method used in clinical practice because it is simple to perform. Research findings validate the sensitivity of girth measurements as a way to evaluate changes in edema over time.[44] Measurements should be taken at one or more reproducible reference points on the limb. Clinical variation in edema status is considered improved if the edema is diagnosed by girth measurement at the initial visit and then reduced at the follow-up visit, unchanged if girth is the same at both visits, and worsened if the measurement increases between the first and second assessments. A change of 1.5 cm between two measurements is reported as a valid, reliable estimate of improvement or worsening of edema. Smaller changes between assessments were evaluated but were less accurate.[44] A simple form, such as that shown in Exhibit 4-2, either handwritten or preprinted, that lists the measurements of both limbs side by side is a useful guide for consistency and completeness of the measurements. It is also useful for comparing baseline with retest measurements quickly and easily. Change in edema measurements is one way to assess treatment outcomes.

The procedure for girth measurements is as follows:

1. Mark and record the bony landmarks on the limb to guide the measurements, including the metatarsal heads, both malleoli, 3 cm above the lateral malleolus, 12 cm above the lateral malleolus, 18 cm above the lateral malleolus, and the lower edge of the patella.
2. Use a flexible tape measure to measure the circumference around these landmarks.
3. Measure both limbs.
4. Record measurements (for both limbs) side by side. Repeat at next assessment. Compare.

Volumetric measurement is made by using water displacement and is considered the gold standard. Volume meters are made of a heavy Lucite and come in different sizes for immersion of a foot and ankle, leg above the knee, or hand (Fig. 4-3). These meters are strong and durable. The water displacement method presents several problems, in-

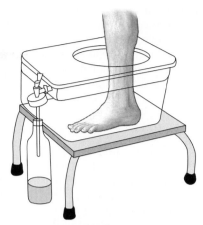

FIGURE 4-3 Volumetric edema measurement.

cluding the time to set up; transport of the apparatus. which may contain 1000 ml of water; inability to immerse the entire extremity in the tank; and unsuitable patient conditions, such as immersion of a limb that has an open wound.

The procedure for volume displacement measurement is as follows:

1. Fill volume meter with tepid water (approximately 95° F or 37°C).
2. Immerse the affected extremity in water.
3. Catch overflow in a graduated cylinder to measure volume displaced.
4. Repeat with both limbs.
5. Record volume displacements to both limbs side by side on a form.

Target Outcomes for Edema Interventions. The target outcomes are that the edema will be absent, reduced, or controlled. Baseline girth or volume measurements that were larger for the affected limb or area at baseline will be equal to or closer to the measurements of the unaffected limbs.

If both limbs are affected, it is not possible to do an opposite limb comparison, and measurements will be compared

EXHIBIT 4-2   Lower Extremity Girth Measurement Form

Date						
	Right	Left	Right	Left	Right	Left
Locations:						
Metatarsal heads						
Both malleoli						
3 cm ↑ lateral malleolus						
12 cm ↑ lateral malleolus						
18 cm ↑ lateral malleolus						
Lower edge of patella						

with the same limb or area. Palpation and observation, as well as decreased measurements, are used for evaluating changes in edema. Change in severity of pitting is another measurement with which to report changes in edema. Controlled edema means that, following an initial reduction, the edema has not returned to the prior level and remains in the tissues.

Color

Assessment of adjacent skin color provides a clues to skin and general health including circulation and is used clinically to indicate ischemia. Cyanosis would be suspected if the skin is bluish and would suggest need for further testing. Another way to use skin color for evaluation is to test for transient erythema a component of reactive hyperemia. Transient erythema can be detected in lightly pigmented skin by applying pressure to the skin. The pressure closes capillaries and induces a blanching of the skin color that returns to normal when pressure is released. Allow the area to be exposed to ambient room temperature and offloaded for 5-10 minutes before examining. If the color does not return or appear to be returning to that of the adjacent skin within 20-30 minutes after removal of pressure, it is considered *unblanchable erythema*, or *persistent erythema*.[22] Histology of unblanchable erythema shows erythrostasis in the capillaries and venules, followed by hemorrhage (see *Color Plates 14, 15, and 16*).[45] Unblanchable erythema is one of the hallmarks of stage one pressure ulcers. The same indexes cannot be used in *darkly pigmented skin*. Exhibit 4-3 has tips for assessing unblanchable erytherma.

Color Assessment for Darkly Pigmented Skin. Identification of stage I pressure ulcers has historically relied heavily on color changes in the skin. Erythema can sometimes be seen in darkly pigmented skin of lighter tones, but generally redness cannot be seen in these individuals.[36] Darkly pigmented skin is defined as skin tones that "remain unchanged (do not blanch) when pressure is applied over a bony prominence, irrespective of the patient's race or ethnicity."[46] Darkly pigmented skin is usually found in African Americans, Africans, Caribbean individuals, Hispanics, Asians, Pacific Islanders, Middle Easterners, Native Americans, and Eskimos

When assessing patients with darkly pigmented skin who are at high risk for pressure ulcers, careful attention should be paid to color changes at sites located over bony prominences. Look for color changes that differ from the patient's usual skin color (as described by the patient or those who are familiar with the patient's usual skin color, or as observed in an area of healthy tissue).[46] Consider conditions that can cause changes in skin color, such as vasoconstriction (pallor) caused by lying on a cold surface or hyperemia (redness or deepening of skin tones) from lying on a bony prominence. As with light-colored skin, remove pressure and allow the area to be exposed to ambient room temperature for 5–10 minutes before examining. When darkly pig-

mented skin is inflamed, the site of inflammation is darker and appears bluish or purplish (eggplant-like color; see *Color Plates 19* and *21*). This is comparable to the erythema or redness seen in persons with lighter skin tones.[46] Changes in color can indicate hemorrhage of the microvasculature in the skin or deep tissue trauma that will later rupture and form a crater. When there is an extremely high melanin content, the color of the skin can be so dark that it is difficult to assess any changes in color.[34]

Another complicating factor in identifying erythema in darkly pigmented skin is differentiating inflammation from the darkening of the skin caused by hemosiderin staining, which is a sign of wound chronicity or repeated injury. Hemosiderin staining usually occurs close to the wound edges, whereas injury-related color changes usually extend out a considerable distance and are accompanied by the other signs of inflammation. *Color Plate 10* shows hemosiderin staining at the margins of a wound in a dark-skinned person. The mechanism of hemosiderin staining is described later in this chapter.

Color changes are apparent around acute (inflamed—red or violet) and chronic open wounds (pigmentation—dark brown). If color is not a reliable indicator, use other clinical indicators, such as sensation (pain), temperature (heat or coolness), and tissue tension (edema or induration and hardness) to confirm the diagnosis of inflammation in darkly pigmented skin.

Assessment of tissue circulatory status by use of color is also difficult in darkly pigmented skin. Consider the effects of gravity on vasomotor changes in the tissues of the extremities in elevated and dependent positions. Color changes will appear more subtle than those in light skin. Assess the patient from a neutral position and then with

---

EXHIBIT 4-3   Tips for Evaluating Blanchable Erythema [25]

Blanchable Erythema "If the reddened area blanches when gentle pressure is applied, the microcirculation is intact." [25]	• Too little pressure: blanching may not occur • Too much pressure: further tissue damage is possible • Hard to determine blanching and nonblanching erythema if vascular refill time is short • Use of a transparent pressure disc makes it easier to observe whether the reddened area blanches when pressure is exerted. Use of the disc can standardize the amount of pressure.

the area elevated approximately 15° and dependent for about 5 minutes, and compare.[47] Assessment of capillary refill time for individuals with darkly pigmented skin should be attempted at the tips of the second or third fingers.[28] Also consider examining the nail beds. If they are not pigmented, apply pressure to the second or third fingers; if the skin under the nail blanches, it will provide a color comparison for assessing pallor or cyanosis. The speed of color return following the slow release of pressure is an indicator of the quality of vasomotor function. The slower the return of color, the more diminished is the vasomotor function. Compare the speed of return with that in your own nail bed or that of another person with normal vascularity.[47]

Proper lighting is important for accurate assessment. Avoid fluorescent light, which casts a blue color to the skin. Use natural or halogen lighting to assess skin tones. Flash photographs are recommended, because the flash makes the demarcation between normal skin tones and those that are traumatized easier to see, and the picture provides a visual record of the patient's skin status.[46] Notice the demarcation between normal skin tones and the traumatized area in *Color Plate 19*. The patient or a family member who is familiar with the patient's natural skin tones should be the primary person to provide information about skin color changes.

Deep Tissue Injury

Trauma to the skin and subcutaneous tissue causes rupture of the blood vessels and subcutaneous bleeding or hemorrhage, called *ecchymosis* (bruising); this is a sign of deep tissue injury. Ecchymosis appears as a purple discoloration in white skin and a deepening to a purple color in darkly pigmented skin. In the literature, these areas have been described as "purple ulcers."[48] Using the Sussman Wound Healing Tool (SWAT), 10 ulcer characteristics were evaluated as "good for healing" or "not good for healing," and after anlysis the presence of hemorrhage was ranked as the most significant predictor of "not good for healing".[49]

Purple ulcers cannot be classified according to the NPUAP staging system, and the significance of these ulcers is seldom recognized. NPUAP has attempted to raise awareness of this unstageable type of ulcer through a consensus conference of the pressure ulcer community[24] with an article by Ankrom et al [23] and a NPUAP white paper.[50] Ankrom reviewed the literature on the subject of pressure-related deep tissue injury under intact skin and identified limitations in the current staging systems' attempts to categorize these lesions.[23]

With purple ulcers, the skin over the hemorrhagic area can be taut, shiny, and edematous (see *Color Plate 32*). It can be intact or rubbed off.[48] The purple ulcer has been described as the end stage of nonblanchable erythema, and it always signifies full-thickness skin loss. Yet, the conundrum is that nonblanchable erythema under intact skin is also the

description used for stage I pressure ulcers, and these ulcers often manifest as stage III or IV.[23] Proper labeling for this class of pressure ulcers is important because they are dangerous lesions with the potential for rapid deterioration. Labeling provides the means for appropriate diagnosis and the development of efficacious interventions to address the problem. Staging is used to describe the depth of tissue injury. The term *unstageable* is often used to diagnose eschar-covered lesions, and it has come to be interpreted as wounds that will be staged once they are debrided. However, deep tissue injury lesions should *not* be debrided. As such, labeling a deep tissue "purple ulcer" as unstageable can have the unintended consequence of a care plan that does not include offloading.[50]

Biopsy specimens of purple ulcers show hemorrhage and early gangrenous changes.[51] Hemorrhage and clotting occur as a consequence of an acute injury, such as trauma from pressure, bumping, or shearing, as well as trauma to new granulation tissue and venous leakage from venous insufficiency (see *Color Plate 76*). Current management of a number of medical conditions with oral anticoagulant therapy increases the risk of hematoma.[52,53] In fact, some "purple" pressure ulcers may occur because of the increased use of these medications, which predispose tissues to subcutaneous hemorrhage with minimal amounts of pressure, friction, and shear.

Clotting cuts off oxygen to the tissues, with subsequent hypoxia and ischemia. Rapid deterioration of the tissues following injury can be a combination of "direct ischemic injury and reperfusion injury from oxygen free radicals, cytokines, and neutrophilic adhesion to microvascular endothelium.[50] When hypoxia is prolonged, the initial damage can be due to ischemia. However, a short period of ischemia followed by reperfusion can result in damage that is more severe than the injury itself. Typically, a stage I pressure ulcer is considered a minor lesion that is likely to heal with offloading. A deep tissue injury, if reperfusion injury is involved, may not respond to offloading to prevent further deterioration.[50] If the blood is not reabsorbed into the tissues in a timely fashion, tissue necrosis will occur. It is not known exactly how long clotted blood can remain in the tissues before necrosis occurs. In most cases, these ulcers are not reversible.

Witkowski described a topical regimen using locally applied nitrates to cause vasodilation and decreased adhesion and aggregation of cells, along with systemically administered hemorheologic agents, to clinically reverse the process.[51] However, there is no evidence that this is efficacious. Electrical stimulation, pulsed radiofrequency stimulation, and ultrasound facilitate thrombolysis, when started soon after injury (e.g., within 48–72 hours). However, in one reported case, therapeutic ultrasound was not started to treat a large rectus sheath hematoma until 9 days after the diagnosis, and hematoma was completely resolved following 20 sessions (5 times per week for four weeks).[52] Efficacy studies reported in the literature and photographs that show the effects of these interventions are described in Chapters 22, 23, and 25. Case studies with color photos are shown in *Color Plates 76–81*. Further research is needed to fully understand and reliably diagnose and predict the natural history of these lesions, the extent of tissue damage under the intact skin, and the viability of injured tissue, and to identify the most efficacious treatments for deep tissue injury.[50]

Rupture of the vessels around a wound and seepage from venous hypertension cause deposition of blood in the subcutaneous tissues. The blood stains the tissues by deposition of hemosiderin from lysed red blood cells, turning the skin a rust-brown color that is called *hemosiderosis*. Hemosiderosis is seen as a ring around pressure ulcers (see *Color Plate 2*) or a brown discoloration of the skin of the lower leg in patients with venous disease (see *Color Plates 55* and *56*). The discoloration can be permanent or gradually disappear.

CLINICAL WISDOM

Education of Health-care Workers about Deep Tissue Injury

Health-care providers need to be educated about the phenomenon of deep tissue injury and how to identify, describe, and document these lesions during the skin assessment.

Hair Distribution

Body hair is distributed over all four extremities, extending down to the digits. Over time, body hair diminishes and is eventually lost. The diminished presence of hair is seen in aging skin and in individuals with impaired circulation. As circulation in a leg decreases, hair is lost distally. Hair distribution can be used as an indicator of the level of vascular impairment and the need for vascular testing. Hair follicles are important to wound healing because as mentioned they contribute epidermal cells for resurfacing partial-thickness wounds. As such, the absence of hair is a factor in the prognosis of wound healing if there is a partial-thickness wound in an area where hair is usually found, such as the lower leg.

CLINICAL WISDOM

Assessment of Hair Distribution as an Indicator of Peripheral Circulation

1. An easy checkpoint for adequate tissue perfusion to the lower extremities is examination of the great toes for hair growth. Hair growth on the great toes implies adequate circulation to support the hair follicles. When working with female patients, remember to ask if they shave the hair on their great toes.

2. Move up the leg proximally from the ankle and assess the most distal point at which hair distribution stops. Next, palpate for skin temperature and pulses, and observe skin color in any areas denuded of hair for circulatory changes.

Toenails

Part of a comprehensive examination of the feet includes the toenails. Assess the color, thickness, and shape, and note any irregularities. Hypertrophic, thick nails are a commonly seen toenail pathology. Some toenails are shaped like a ram's horn. Ingrown toenails and fungal and pseudomonas infections, which give the toenail a green color, can also be observed. Findings of toenail abnormalities are considered referral criteria unless the clinician has knowledge and training in foot and nail care.[54] Chapters 19 and 20 include specific information that guides the assessment and care of feet.

Blisters

Trauma to the epidermis gives rise to blisters. Blisters can contain clear fluid or, if the trauma is deeper than the epidermis and ruptures blood vessels, the fluid can be bloody or brown (see *Color Plate 79*). The blister roof is nature's best dressing, but it can hide deep tissue damage. Removal of the blister roof is controversial. If the blister fluid is clear, tissue damage may not extend into the dermis or deeper; the wound will likely heal under the blister roof, and the epidermis will eventually fall off. The blister roof should not be disturbed and, in fact, may require protection. However, if the fluid is bloody, brown, or cloudy (see *Color Plate 79*), deep tissue damage may be present, and unroofing the blister can be the only way to determine the extent of trauma (see *Color Plate 80*). Ultrasound technology to identify depth of tissue edema and trauma, such as under a blister, is being tested with good outcomes. *Color Plates 73–75*.

Assessment of the tissue under the blister without breaking the blister is helpful in evaluating when the blister needs to be unroofed. The validity of using digital palpation to determine tissue resilience (i.e., less resilient or less stiff compared with adjacent tissue) has been demonstrated. Gently press down with a fingertip on the tissue beneath the blister roof and compress it. Release and feel for the resiliency of the subcutaneous tissues. If there is good resilience (i.e., it bounces back when the pressure is removed), the deep tissues may be mildly congested. However, if the tissue feels soft, spongy, or boggy, there is high probability of tissue congestion and probable necrosis.[22] The common term for this characteristic is "mushy" or "boggy." Practice and careful concentration are needed to perform this palpation examination. One tip is to try pressing the skin down on the contralateral location (e.g., on the heel) to compare the resiliency.

Sensation

Sensory testing procedures and expected outcomes are described in this section. They include pain, temperature, protective sensation, thermal sensation, and vibratory perception threshold (VPT).

Pain. Accreditation standards for health-care facilities in the United States require each patient's pain to be measured regularly and proper relief supplied.[55] Severe pain or tenderness, either within or around the wound, can indicate the presence of infection, deep tissue destruction, or ischemia. In recognition of the significant effect of pain on wound healing and wound management, Chapter 13 is devoted entirely to that topic, addressing the issues of wound pain and wound healing, including pain physiology, pain issues, pain assessment, and treatment strategies.

Temperature. Baseline skin temperature is one objective measurement of circulation that can be used to monitor circulatory response to treatment and evaluate inflammation. Local body temperature can be tested by palpation, with a liquid crystal skin thermometer, or with an infrared thermometer.

Thermography using a liquid crystal skin thermometer is a semiquantitative method that produces multicolor picture maps of the wound and adjacent tissues. These devices are reliable and have been clinically tested for evaluation of primary wound healing status of surgical wounds. The method is quick, simple, reliable, and inexpensive.[56]

Liquid crystal strips are available with different temperature ranges. Use of an inexpensive liquid crystal skin fever thermometer strip that changes color with temperature change is a simple, accurate. and useful way to assess the temperature of periwound skin. It is more sensitive to changes in temperature than the back of the hand. Strips are available with a range of 80°F—100°F (26°C—38°C). Skin thermometers usually have liquid crystal indicator lights in shades of brown, tan, green, and blue that respond to temperature shifts. The liquid crystal strip changes color in a few seconds after placing it on the tissue. To read the temperature, use the *highest* temperature window indicated by a color. Skin temperature is shown in 1°F intervals.

Normal skin temperature in areas of good circulation is usually approximately 95°F. An increase in temperature of the surrounding skin measured on the fever thermometer, compared with adjacent area temperature, is an indication of increased circulatory perfusion. This is the heat described as a classic sign of inflammation. The absence of an increase in periwound skin temperature compared with adjacent skin can be considered an indicator of wound chronicity.

Skin temperature is a useful measure for assessing many types of wounds, including surgical wounds. Changes in wound temperature are readily apparent during the first 8 postoperative days. During the first 3 postoperative days, the temperatures of the wound and adjacent tissues are typically the same. However, by postoperative day 4, there should be a discernible change, with the temperatures of the wound and surrounding tissues decreasing gradually. Zones of warmth around the wound become narrower, with significantly greater warmth over the incision than in the surrounding tissues. The heat measured in adjacent skin areas is not an inflammatory reaction; rather, it is reactive hyperemia. Hyperemia is the consequence of humoral substances released from cellular damage at the time of wounding—chiefly histamine—and pain that triggers neurogenic reactions, including vasodilation.[56] Only a narrow zone adjacent to the wound is due to inflammation. During the early postoperative period, the two areas are indistinguishable from one another. As the wound heals, the area of warmth narrows, decreases in temperature, and represents the area of true inflammation.

Wound temperature depends on the degree of vascularity of the tissues: a higher grade of vascularity will result in a higher tissue temperature.[56] If the expected outcomes (i.e., that the wound and adjacent skin temperatures decrease by the fourth postoperative day) are not met, this indicates that the wound is not healing by primary intention; secondary healing is imminent because of tissue necrosis or bacterial contamination.[56]

An increase in skin temperature of 4°F compared with the contralateral side[57] can indicate inflammation that has not manifested on the surface, such as a pressure ulcer over a bony prominence or the presence of infection (e.g., an abscess). It is a very useful tool for assessing inflammation and wounding in darkly pigmented individuals in whom the margins of erythema are difficult to see. Skin temperature can be measured at locations on the margins of discoloration and at the center over the bony prominence. The clock method (i.e., measuring the temperature at the 12:00, 3:00, 6:00 and 9:00 positions around the wounded tissue) is useful for recording this measurement in large wounds. Expect periwound temperature to decrease as the wound heals. [57]

The procedure for measuring skin temperature with a liquid crystal strip is as follows:

1. Ensure that the area of skin to be tested has been pressure-free and exposed to ambient air temperature for at least 5–10 minutes before testing. (A sheet can cover the patient for privacy and to avoid chilling.)
2. Dry the skin of sweat before each measurement, because moisture on the skin considerably modifies the image.[56]
3. Place a single layer of plastic against the skin as a hygienic barrier (this does not interfere with temperature accuracy). This step and the following can be eliminated if the strip is disposable. Strips can be reused for a single patient if the barrier is used.
4. Lay the temperature strip flat on the plastic barrier.
5. Hold the strip in place at both ends lightly, to avoid compressing capillaries. Wait for the color of the strip to change, allowing at least 1 full minute for the change to occur. In very inflamed tissues, color change can occur immediately, but it may change more as it is held for the full minute.
6. Read the temperature while the strip is still against the skin.
7. For large wounds, measure at the wound edge at the 12:00 and 6:00 positions and near the expected outer margin of the periwound erythema/discoloration. Repeat at the 3:00 and 9:00 positions.
8. For small wounds, measure by placing the liquid crystal strip across the wound diameter.
9. Record temperature at each point.

Temperature can also be measured using a thermistor, which is a probe placed against the skin that takes a reading, and a radiometer or infrared scanner, which determines temperature by measurement of surface reflection of infrared radiation. Any of the devices described here can reliably be used in the clinic with minimal training.

Infrared thermography is a reliable way to measure skin temperature gradients in patients who are at risk for or have neuropathic foot ulcers.[58,59] The impaired immune system response in this patient population blunts the typical signs of inflammation such as erythema; however, warmth can be detected with the infrared thermometer. In a randomized study group in which patients' nonulcerated limbs were the control, these individuals were found to have higher skin temperature initially in the ulcerated foot than the contralateral intact foot (91.1°F versus 84.2°F) After healing, the temperatures of both feet were equal. In the same group, toe cuff brachial index pressures >0.6 were associated with greater skin temperature gradients at the site of ulceration than those with higher pressure indices (9.4 +/−4.0 versus 5.8 +/−3.4 degrees F), reflecting the diminished circulation.[58]

Thermography has also been studied in a blinded, controlled study of 84 subjects with diabetic neuropathy who were at high risk for ulceration (Grade 2 or 3 on the Texas Classification System).[59] The object of the study was to evaluate the effective use of an infrared thermometer as a preventive tool in patients who met these criteria. Two groups of matched patients were given foot care protocols to follow at home. Neither group of patients had ulcerations at the time of enrollment. Both groups received standard care consisting of therapeutic footwear, diabetic foot education, and foot evaluation by a podiatrist every 10–12 weeks. The only difference in the protocols was twice daily infrared thermometry recordings by one group, called the enhanced therapy group. This group was instructed to call the clinic nurse if there was an increase of 4°F in temperature at the first metatarsal head.

At the end of the 6-month study period, 20% of the group that did not monitor temperature had developed complications. The enhanced therapy group had a 2% incidence of ulceration that occurred in one patient who did not follow the protocol as directed and did not report the temperature change.

Personal infrared thermometers may prove to be an effective means of reducing risk of ulceration in a high-risk group by providing an easy-to-use tool that encourages vigilant monitoring, provides immediate feedback about a pending problem, and empowers the patient to take action when change is measured.

Skin temperature is expected to increase when there is enhanced perfusion and vasodilation following superficial heating with whirlpool. Temperature changes in deeper tissues can occur following pulsed shortwave diathermy. However, the fever strip may not be sufficiently sensitive to measure these changes, in which case the infrared scanner thermometer is recommended.

To measure the effects of an intervention, take a baseline measurement before treatment and repeat the measurement after treatment. Skin temperature should rise after treatment with increased blood flow. If the target outcome of the intervention is to initiate the acute inflammatory phase, with resultant hyperemia and mild inflammation, measurement of tissue temperatures will help to verify the outcome.

The presence of coolness can also be used to assess circulation. Sometimes, there is an initial increase in skin temperature that is followed by coolness after trauma. Like warmth, coolness without trauma can be an indicator of circulatory status. Some areas of the body naturally have less warmth, such as the feet, toes, and fingers. The areas of the trunk or over well-perfused muscle tissues have greater warmth. If there is coolness in the digits or feet, other signs and symptoms, such as hair growth, skin color, pulses, and skin texture, should be evaluated for circulation. If those signs are also suggestive of circulatory impairment, further circulatory examination is warranted. Coolness can also be an indicator of impaired tissue viability or tissue death following ischemia.

A quantitative measure of tissue temperature as part of the assessment of wounds is not yet a standard of clinical practice. Journal articles describe temperature measurement as a useful method of assessment for inflammatory processes.[56,60,61,62,63] All of the procedures described in this chapter are simple, noninvasive, and quick. Most importantly, they have validity and clinical significance, and they are more reliable than clinical observation alone.[56]

RESEARCH WISDOM

A patient can have unapparent, mild core hypothermia that will affect wound healing and resistance to infection. The tympanic membrane temperature is an accurate measure of core body temperature.[56]

Protective Sensation. Testing for protective sensation is indicated if sensory loss is suspected. Neuropathy from many causes, including diabetes, Guillain-Barré syndrome, alcoholism, chemotherapy, and Charcot-Marie-Tooth disease, results in the loss of protective sensation.

A safe, accurate method for testing protective sensation has been developed using Semmes-Weinstein monofilaments.[64] The monofilaments come in different force levels. Levels 4.17, 5.07, and 6.10 are used to check for protective sensation. Force levels increase as the numbers increase. The object of the test is to determine if the patient can detect pressure when the monofilament is placed against the skin and the force applied is sufficient to buckle the monofilament. Testing is usually performed on the sole of the foot. The inability to sense the 5.07 monofilament is the threshold for loss of protective sensation. Many individuals with peripheral neuropathy do not feel the largest monofilament (6.10), which indicates a loss of protective sensation of 75g. This finding should trigger the prompt referral to a specialist for appropriate protective footwear and should be followed closely. The inability to detect the 5.07-level monofilament indicates a limited ability to use protective sensations. If the patient can distinguish this level of sensation at several points on the feet, the sensation is considered to be adequate to avoid trauma.[65]

Thermal Sensation. The test for thermal sensation is performed using test tubes or small narrow bottles filled with warm water. Be sure to test in a normal area before applying to possible insensate areas to avoid burns. Research reports that the lateral aspect of the foot is the area most sensitive to thermal sensation.[66] If a patient is unable to sense warmth, he or she is at high risk of burns if heat is applied to the skin. Testing for cold can be performed by applying a cold tuning fork. If a patient is unable to sense cold, he or she is at risk for injury from exposure to cold; the feet should be protected from frostbite if the patient is going to be exposed to very cold temperatures. Thermal allodynia can also be detected in hypersensitive areas.

Vibratory Perception Threshold (VPT). Vibratory perception threshold (VPT) is a measure of progressive peripheral neuropathy for aging adults and individuals with immune-mediated polyneuropathies and polyneuropathy including diabetes. In all groups, VPT is better perceived in the upper extremities compared with the lower. There is a significant age-related decline in VPT at all locations. VPT is recommended as a part of routine neurologic examination, including patients at risk for skin ulceration.[67,68] The International Working Group on the Diabetic Foot has developed guidelines to achieve global consistency and adequate diagnostic, preventive, and therapeutic strategies for patients with diabetes. VPT is one measure recommended by the Working Group.[69]

VPT testing is simple and easy to perform with a 128 Hz tuning fork.[67,68,70] The simplest method is the on/off method, which is reliable for testing VPT at the foot.[70] The test procedure is as follows:

1. Before testing the VPT at the foot, give the patient a preliminary test by placing the vibrating tuning fork on the sternum, so that the vibratory sensation can be readily recognized.
2. Ask the patient to shut the eyes and keep them closed.
3. Ask the patient to report the start of the vibration sensation and the cessation of vibration (on-off).
4. Strike the tuning fork and place it on the bony prominence on the dorsum of the great toe proximal to the nail bed.
5. Repeat the test eight times at the same location, recording the on/off report.
6. VPT is defined as "the total number of times the application of the vibrating tuning fork and the dampening of vibration was NOT felt. Scores can range from 0-8."[70]

In addition to VPT, protective sensation, ankle-brachial index, toe cuff pressures, and pedal pulses are widely accepted clinical testing measures that should be followed to prevent diabetic foot problems.

The clinical relevance of screening tests depends on validity, reliability, and practicality of use. The tests listed here meet those criteria as noted. Assessment is recommended annually for patients without neuropathy and every 6 months for individuals who do not have deformity or vascular disease. Patients who have neuropathy, deformity, or vascular disease diagnoses should be evaluated every 3 months. If ulceration is part of the patient history, evaluation should be performed every 1–3 months.[69] Any patient identified as having abnormal values at screening should be referred for further medical workup and special foot care education programs as described in other chapters. VPT results are a trigger to evaluate candidates for this intervention, as well as to validate the outcome of the intervention.

Evaluation of Wound Healing Status

Evaluation of wound healing status is described in the following sections. Chapter 2 presents acute and chronic wound healing physiology associated with the phases of wound healing and the reader is referred to this chapter for explanation of the mechanisms that may be apparent during the assessment. This information will be repeated minimally in this section. After the assessment the clinician will be able to evaluate the wound status with respect to the phase of wound healing and determine a wound healing phase diagnosis. A diagnosis is the summary of data collected during the assessment process. Wound "healing phase diagnosis" is a diagnosis of the functional status of healing based on the phase of the wound at the time of the assessment.[71]

Wound healing begins with the inflammatory phase, progresses to the proliferative phase and epithelialization phase and then the remodelling phase. Careful assessment of the wound and periwound tissue establishes the present, *predominant* wound healing phase benchmarks. This is done by examining and describing the signs and symptoms of one or more of three potential aspects of each healing phase: acute (progressing), chronic ("stuck" or plateaued), and absent (not apparent) for each phase of wound healing. Each aspect of each phase has benchmarks that are indicators of the phase status. These terms are explained further below. The *predominant* wound healing phase is the primary "phase diagnosis" for the wound at that time. The wound healing phase diagnosis is useful to demonstrate medical necessity for advanced interventions. These are described in the following section. There will also be benchmarks that signify transition to the next phase(s) or absence of the subsequent phases(s). During each phase, characteristics become apparent that identify the predominant phase. There is a close relationship between evaluation of the wound and periwound tissue signs and symptoms and diagnosis of the wound healing phase. Tables 4-7 through 4-10 list the "wound healing phase diagnosis" and related wound healing phase benchmarks.

Acute Phase

As normal acute wounds heal, there is an orderly, timely overlapping progression through the wound healing phases (inflammatory to proliferative/epithelialization, and remodeling).

Chronic Phase

Failure of the orderly, timely progression of healing through the successive phases results in a chronic wound. Chronic wounds can fail to initiate or stall in any phase of wound healing. When a wound stalls, plateaus, or simply gets stuck in one wound healing phase, the wound becomes chronic with respect to that phase. For example, wounds that experience repeated trauma from dressing changes or debridement often become stuck in the inflammatory phase of wound healing, thus the term *chronic inflammation*. Another example is the wound that fills with granulation tissue but does not stop proliferating, going on to form hypergranulation tissue *(Color Plate 23)*. At this point, the wound appears stuck building the collagen matrix and is unable to progress to the final stage of remodelling. This is termed *chronic proliferation*. A final example is the wound with chronic scar formation, such as with hypertrophy or keloid scars that do not stop laying down collagen and progress to remodelling, Here this is termed *chronic epithelialization.*

There is appropriate concern about wound chronicity during the phases of healing. Ennis and Meneses[72] used the term "stunned wound" to refer to wounds that begin the healing progression in an expected or "normal" trajectory, but then plateau or become recalcitrant and chronic. The term "stunned" is borrowed from the cardiology literature. Causes of "stunning" have been theoretically proposed to be related to repeated bouts of ischemia and reperfusion, or "senescent" cells. The authors of the paper encourage clinicians to think about the multiple factors on the cellular level and look for additional research to guide practice in this area. As more is learned, this phenomenon should be clarified. In the meantime, using a clinical perspective, the term

chronic phase, is used here to denote when the wound is stuck in a particular phase.

Absent Phase

The wound that fails to pass through a wound healing phase lacks attributes of that phase and is referred to as being in the *absence of inflammatory phase, absence of proliferative phase*, or *absence of epithelialization phase*. Wounds that fail to progress through a wound healing phase differ from those that get stuck or exhibit characteristics of chronicity in a phase. Wounds that are absent an inflammatory response, for example, do not demonstrate signs of inflammation, whereas wounds with chronic inflammation show signs of a continued inflammatory response. Absence of the wound healing phase indicates that the wound has not initiated the phase, for whatever reasons (e.g., lack of circulation). Absence of the wound healing phase signifies either the inability to heal or the need for help from an intervention to initiate the acute phase, leading to progression through phases (e.g., reperfusion through surgical intervention, debridement of senescent cells, or enhanced blood flow from a physical agent).

Identifying the Phase

Since phases overlap, benchmarks for multiple wound healing phases can be apparent at the same time. Because the phases of healing overlap, if the wound is transitioning from one phase to the next, the wound healing phase diagnosis is defined by the *primary* phase appearance. *Inflammatory* is the wound healing phase diagnosis if the identified attributes of acute or chronic inflammation are at least 50%–75% of what would be expected, (see Color Plate 1 and 7). A wound in the chronic inflammatory phase is also in absence of the proliferative phase and absence of the epithelialization phase. However, the chronic inflammatory phase would be the primary wound healing phase diagnosis. When the wound attributes of acute inflammatory are less than 50% of what are expected and there is significant proliferation of granulation tissue in the wound bed, the primary wound

TABLE 4-7   Wound Healing "Phase Diagnosis" and Prognosis

Wound Healing Phase	Acute Wound Healing "Phase Diagnosis"	Chronic Wound Healing "Phase Diagnosis"	Absence of Wound Healing "Phase Diagnosis"
Inflammatory Proliferative Epithelialization Prognosis	Acute inflammatory Acute proliferative Acute epithelialization Orderly, timely progression through phases of healing	Chronic inflammatory Chronic proliferative Chronic epithelialization Reinitiate acute phase, then progress through phases of healing. Progress to a clean, stable wound.	Absence of inflammatory Absence of proliferative Absence of epithelialization Initiate healing phase, if able, and progress through phases. Or progress to a clean, stable wound. If unable to initiate healing phase, refer.
Outcome	Healed wound	Healed wound clean stable wound	

phase diagnosis changes to proliferative phase (see *Color Plate 8*).

A wound healing phase diagnosis of *acute proliferative phase* means that most (50% or greater) of the wound surface appearance attributes (granulation tissue and contraction) are observed. If less than 50% of the proliferative phase attributes are identified, the wound is primarily in an inflammatory phase and has not yet reached the proliferative phase for diagnostic purposes. The diagnosis would be written *inflammatory phase/proliferative phase*. Some call this late inflammatory or early proliferative phase. A wound phase diagnosis of *epithelialization phase* is based on findings that the wound is resurfacing. Partial-thickness wounds that are resurfacing from the middle or edges are in the *epithelialization phase*. Wounds that are greater than 50% attached at the edges and do not have steep walls that are epithelializing also are diagnosed as being in the *epithelialization phase* (see Color Plate 5). Wounds in the acute epithelialization phase have an excellent prognosis for healing, whereas wounds in the chronic epithelialization phase need an intervention to restart the healing process. The prognosis then would be that the wound will heal with intervention. Wounds that have absence of the epithelialization phase of healing are at high risk for nonhealing unless contributing conditions can be altered, e.g., by reperfusion, application of moisture-retentive dressings, or stimulation with biophysical agents, as described in Part IV.

Inflammatory Phase

Assessment of the periwound and wound tissues during the inflammatory phase begins with assessment of four categories of wound attributes: periwound and adjacent tissue appearance, wound tissue appearance (color and texture), wound edges, and exudate characteristics (odor, type, and quantity). The major attributes of adjacent and periwound tissues that are observed and palpated in the inflammatory phase are color, temperature, firmness/texture, sensation, and ecchymosis (hemorrhage, bruising). In this section, the attributes of the wound and the periwound tissues that serve as benchmarks of the phase are described during acute inflammation, chronic inflammation, and absence of inflammation. The appearance of periwound and wound tissue changes as the wound progresses through the phases of healing. *Color Plates 1* and *2* show a wound that went from the chronic inflammatory phase to the acute inflammatory phase and subsequently progressed to the proliferative phase.

Acute Inflammation

Signs of acute inflammation (e.g., erythema, pain, edema, heat, loss of function) often extend well beyond the immediate wound and periwound tissues into adjacent tissues. Initially, they indicate a healthy response and are a prerequisite to normal healing. Use the characteristics observed during acute inflammation as a reference point for the evaluation of impaired responses.

Adjacent and Periwound Assessment

Skin Color. *Erythema* is one of the classic characteristics of the acute inflammatory phase. Initially, the adjacent skin can be erythematous due to reactive hyperemia. Erythema may not be evident in individuals with darkly pigmented skin (see previous discussion on skin color attributes found in light and darkly pigmented skin). Reddened skin with streaks leading away from the area can indicate cellulitis. If observed, check the patient's history for fever, chills, history of recurrent cellulitis, or medications being used to treat the condition. If no treatment has been initiated, these findings should be reported immediately to a physician.

Edema and Induration. The edema of the acute inflammatory phase is localized and brawny. It feels firm and distorts the swollen tissues, causing the skin to become taut, shiny, and raised from the contours of the surrounding tissues. This edema results from trauma (e.g., pressure ulcers, burns, and surgical debridement) and is related to the release of histamines. Histamines cause vasodilation and increase vascular permeability, resulting in the movement of fluid in the interstitial spaces. Edema is usually accompanied by pain.

Induration is abnormal hardening of the tissue at the wound margin from consolidation of edema in the tissues. A test for induration is to attempt to pinch the tissues gently; if induration is present, the tissues cannot be pinched. Induration follows reflex hyperemia or chronic venous congestion. [34]

Skin Temperature. Skin temperature should be palpated manually by using the back of the hand, a liquid crystal skin fever thermometer, or with an infrared scanner. During acute inflammation, expect the temperature of the wound and adjacent tissues to be the same. As healing progresses, the temperature of the adjacent wound tissue will gradually decline, and the area of increased temperature will narrow. [56]

Pain. Chapter 13 is devoted to wound pain with specific assessment guidelines. Therefore, this discussion is very limited. Spontaneous or induced pain in the adjacent tissues should be assessed by palpation or report, or both. Pain can indicate infection or subcutaneous tissue damage that is not visible, such as in pressure ulcers or vascular disease. Report of the sudden onset of pain accompanied by edema in a leg is a common indicator of deep vein thrombosis and wound infection. Unilateral edema accompanied by pain in the calf or palpation over a vein is an indicator of thrombophlebitis. Immediate referral should follow these findings. The absence of pain in an obviously infected or inflamed wound should be investigated as an indication of neuropathy and the need for further assessment of sensation. Refer to Chapter 13 for more information on pain assessment and treatment.

CLINICAL WISDOM

Excessive Inflammatory Signs and Infection

Excessive signs of acute inflammation should be considered a signal of impending wound infection. [73]

Wound Bed Tissue Assessment

Depth. A partial-thickness skin loss creates a shallow crater that looks red or pink, or shows the yellow reticular layer-a thin, yellow, mesh-like covering that constitutes the deep layer of the dermis (see *Color Plate 17*). If the crater is bright and shiny, it is healthy and viable and should be left intact. *Color Plate 13* shows the anatomy of the tissues beneath the skin. If the wound penetrates through the dermis into the subcutaneous tissue, it will appear as though it contains yellow fat (such as chicken fat) or white connective tissue, called *fascia*. Fascia is a connective tissue that covers and wraps around all muscles, tendons, blood vessels, and nerves. Wounds that extend through the subcutaneous tissue into the muscle can have a pink or dark red appearance with a shiny layer of fascia on top.

Undermining and Tunneling. Excavation of the subcutaneous tissues during debridement creates a "cave," or undermining, of the wound edges. Undermining can lead to separation of fascial planes (see *Color Plates 39–41*). Muscles lie together in bundles that are held together by fascia; when the fascia is cut, the muscle bundles separate. Separation of the fascial layers opens tunnels along the fascial planes between the muscles under the skin (see *Color Plates 39–41*). Tunnels can join together and form sinus tracts (see *Color Plate 38*). Infection can travel through these tunnels, leading to abscess.

Subcutaneous and Deeper Tissues. When debriding or treating deep or undermined wounds it is likely that muscle tissue or tendons will be exposed. Muscle tissue can be identified by appearance (striated) and by activity (it jumps or twitches when palpated). Muscles are connected to bones by tendons covered with white fascia and look like ropes. The sheath of fascia covering the tendon is called *peritenon*. Sparing the peritenon during wound care procedures will facilitate the growth of new granulation tissue over the intact peritenon to cover the tendon revised

Penetration of a wound into a joint can expose several anatomic structures, including ligaments, which are white and striated; joint capsule, which is white and shiny; and cartilage, which is white, hard, and smooth, and is located on the ends of bones. Bone is white and hard, and covered with a clear or white membrane called *periosteum*. The level of tissue exposed is used to stage or grade the wound severity, as described previously. Loss of peritenon or periosteum will compromise a skin graft. Wounds that can be probed to bone are considered to have osteomyelitis, and emergent referral is warranted.

Wound Edges. During acute inflammation, the wound edges are often indistinct or diffuse, and they change shape as wound contraction and epithelialization begins to cover the wound surface. Wound edges can be attached to the wound base or separated from it, forming walls with the base of the wound at a depth from the skin surface. This is considered a key factor in wound resurfacing. Wound edges should be palpated for firmness and texture. Observe the margins for curling. See *Color Plates 33–36* for an example of wound edges. When undermining occurs, the wound edge is not attached, and epithelialization cannot advance, because the keratinocytes are unable to advance across the gap. Repetitive injury to the wound edges can cause them to become firm, fibrotic, and indurated; this in turn can affect the ability of epithelialization to progress.[2]

Wound Drainage. Wound drainage during the acute inflammatory phase is an indication of the status of the clotting mechanisms and infection. Wound drainage that contains dead cells and debris is called *exudate* and is brown or grey and may be viscous and look like pus whereas clear fluid drainage is called *transudate*. During assessment, record the presence or absence, color, odor, quantity, and quality of the wound drainage.

Sanguineous Drainage. Initially, there is bleeding into the wound space that is controlled by clotting. Wounds that have bloody exudate are called *sanguineous*. Sanguineous wounds may have impaired clotting due to anticoagulant or antiplatelet pharmaceutical products (e.g., aspirin or Plavix) or disease processes, such as hemophilia. The amount of exudate will vary. Medical history, including a pharmacologic history, and systems review are indicated to determine the causes of the sanguineous drainage. Copious or persistent sanguineous drainage should be reported to a physician immediately as it may be a sign of internal bleeding.

Serous Transudate. Serous transudate is clear fluid that exudes from the wound. It is usually yellow and odorless, and is present in varying amounts during the inflammatory phase (see *Color Plates 43* and *46*).

Chronic Inflammation

Inflammation that persists for weeks or months is referred to as *chronic* or *persistent inflammation*. Chronic inflammation occurs when the macrophages and neutrophils fail to phagocytose necrotic matter, ingest foreign debris, and fight infection.[74] Therefore, necrotic matter and foreign debris is typically found in the wound bed. Chronic inflammation is also related to the release of histamine from the mast cells and reflex hyperemia associated with vasodilation of the surrounding vasculature. Repeated trauma to a wound can also develop into chronic inflammation.

Adjacent and Periwound Skin

Chronic inflammation in the periwound area appears as a halo of erythema in lightly pigmented skin and a dark halo in darkly pigmented skin. The latter may be easily mistaken because of its similar appearance to hemosiderin staining. There is minimal temperature change or cooling, compared with adjacent uninjured tissues. There may be some minimal firmness from edema in the periwound tissues. There is usually minimal pain response, or there can be intense pain associated with arterial vascular disease or infection. Arterial ulcers over the malleolus and pressure ulcers are frequently seen with a halo of erythema, but they lack the blood flow to progress the wound (see *Color Plate 53*).

Wound Bed Tissue

In wounds in the chronic inflammatory phase, necrotic tissue usually covers all or part of the wound surface. Necrotic tissue varies in color and may be black, yellow, tan, brown, or gray. Soft necrotic tissue, such as fibrin or slough, can be present in the wound bed. Fibrin forms on the wound surface of venous ulcers. Slough is necrotic fat and fascia adhering to the layer beneath it. See *Color Plates 26–32* for different appearances of necrotic tissue. Pale pink wounds can indicate chronic infection (see *Color Plate 11*).

In wounds that are chronically inflamed, a portion of the wound surface is often in the proliferative phase with granulation tissue present, but the proliferation fails to progress possibly due to infection. Not all pink tissue is granulation tissue and may be muscle tissue that lies beneath newly removed necrotic tissue is pink or dark red (see *Color Plate 13*). During assessment, record the presence and color of necrotic tissue. Wounds that are in the chronic inflammatory phase of healing often have a combination of several attributes. For example, a wound can have black and yellow necrotic tissue, as well as pink granulation tissue or healthy muscle tissue (see *Color Plate 7*).

Signs of acute inflammation may be absent. If, however, cellulitis or other infection is present, streaks of redness will often be seen in the periwound and adjacent skin extending away from the wound, and pain can become intense (see *Color Plate 53*). Signs and symptoms of systemic infection that can lead to sepsis, include fever of 101°F (39.4°C) or higher; chills; manifestation of shock, including restlessness, lethargy, confusion; and decreased systolic blood pressure.[28] These are red flags that require immediate medical follow up.

RESEARCH WISDOM

Wounds with early signs of infection are treated with a regimen of oral antibiotics for 2–4 weeks, and those that have late healing signs of infection are treated with topical antibiotics.[75] The prognosis is that the wound will resume progression through the phases of healing following intervention with antibiotics.

All chronic wounds are colonized with bacteria however, at times the bacteria overwhelm the host and become critically colonized and progress to infection. During assessment the clinician will identify certain attributes that may be indicators of infection. Cutting and Harding did an extensive literature review to determine criteria suggesting wound infection in granulating wounds. These criteria include what could be considered the traditional criteria for identification of infection with the addition of a list of phenomena not commonly recognized by health-care professionals.[76] These new criteria include:.

- Delayed or stalled healing compared with the norm for the site or condition
- Discoloration of the granulation tissue
- Friable granulation tissue that bleeds easily
- Unexpected pain or tenderness
- Pocketing at the base of the wound
- Bridging of the soft tissue
- Abnormal smell
- Wound breakdown.

CLINICAL WISDOM

Distinguishing Granulation Tissue from Muscle

To distinguish granulation tissue from healthy muscle, palpate the tissue with a gloved finger. Granulation tissue feels soft and spongy. It will not "jump" if pinched, but it may bleed. Muscle tissue is firm and resilient to pressure. It will jump or twitch if pinched or probed.

Chronic Wound Drainage

Wound drainage (exudate) characteristics including color and odor are often used as indicators of wound infection Wound exudate can be thick, yellow, tan, brown, or green with malodor. The amount of exudate can be moderate to large. Wound drainage that has a foul odor and/or comprises viscous yellow/gray or green exudate is often referred to as pus. Pus is a result of the demise of neutrophils after they have phagocytosed debris and excessive bacterial loads. When there is a high bacterial count (greater than 10^5), signs of active infection are seen. Prolonged, chronic inflammation is the result of a bacteria-filled wound.[74] A bacteria-filled wound infection that is of particular concern in chronic wounds is biofilm infection described in Exhibit 4-4.

Not all malodorous or yellow/gray exudate signifies infection. The odor and fluid can result from solubilization of necrotic tissue by enzymatic debriding agents or autolysis.

Cleanse exudate from the wound to determine whether the odor is transient or internal. If enzymatic or autolytic methods of debridement are used, the odor and debris should be removed by the cleansing. If odor remains, or the exudate that is expressed from the wound or adjacent tissues has color or odor, consider infection. Check for other symptoms of infection, such as heat, fever, and lethargy. Exudate color can suggest the type of infection. Normally, wound exudate is serous-a clear or light-yellow fluid. Green is usually associated with an anaerobic infection (see *Color Plates 42–47* and Chapter 9). Record the color, texture, and odor on the assessment form.

Exudate Volume. Exudate volume is considered an indicator of wound outcome.[31] The amount of wound exudate should be estimated as scant/minimal, small, moderate, or large/copious from examining the wound dressing or by expressing it from the wound. These methods are considered appropriate ways of estimating quantity. The absence of exudate or dryness of the wound bed can indicate desiccation and the need for adding moisture. During assessment, record the presence or absence, color, odor, and quantity of exudate. The BAWT includes a nominal Likert scale to rate each one of these aspects.

Gelatinous Edema. Following a secondary trauma to the wound bed, such as sharp or enzymatic debridement, wound edema forms as a result of leaking plasma proteins from damaged or irritated capillaries, which allows moisture to accumulate and form an opaque, gelatinous mass in the base of the wound. The edematous mass contains many substances, all of which contribute to sustaining the chronic inflammatory response. This mass is visible on examination and should

EXHIBIT 4-4 Biofilm Infections

One probable reason that chronic wound infection differs from acute wound infection is that biofilms play a significant role. It has recently been learned that the bacteria in chronic wounds are often protected from the host defenses by biofilms. Biofilms are survival strategies for infectious bacteria. Bacteria that are free floating are called planktonic, and these bacteria are readily killed by antibiotics. Bacteria that attach themselves to a surface are called sessile. In the sessile form, they collect together and form biofilms. Key characteristics of biofilm bacteria are protection from host defenses and tolerance to antimicrobials.[77] Bacterial biofilms are designed as an aggregation of one or more bacterial species into a slime-embedded community. The biofilm derives its defenses from an exopolysaccharide matrix formation that is resistant to host defenses and antibiotics. Biofilms are not only resistant to antibiotics, but they play a triple role in spreading antibiotic resistance in the following ways:

1. Treatment of biofilm-related infection requires long-term and frequently repeated episodes of antibiotic therapy.
2. Biofilm physiology enables embedded bacteria within the community to survive antibiotic exposure long enough to acquire specific resistance to the drug and to respond to the antibiotic with production of additional biofilm matrix and promotion of biofilm survival.
3. High cell density of the biofilm affects the genetic activity of the biofilm components by promoting efficient horizontal gene transfer. Horizontal gene transfer is very important within polymicrobial biofilms. In that environment, resistant genes can be transferred from apathogenic to highly virulent strains both within and beyond species borders. The effects of this behavior on the host have not been estimated, but potentially have significant consequences.[77]

Common examples of biofilm infections are dental caries, peritonitis, chronic tonsillitis, endocarditis, and osteomyelitis. Bacteria that form biofilms include *Pseudomonas aeruginosa,* staphylococci, and gram-positive and gram-negative cocci, Biofilm heterogeneity is well documented, as well as the fact that these biofilm bacteria can withstand many times the dosage of antibiotic sufficient to eradicate the planktonic form.[77,78]

What is the association of biofilms with wound infection? Investigators have studied the time needed for wound isolated *P. aeruginosa* to form a biofilm. They found that in just 5 hours after inoculation, a developing biofilm was visible with the characteristics of a mature biofilm obtained by 10 hours.[79] The findings that bacteria can quickly build this shield against antibiotics and immune cells early in the infection process are significant, suggesting the critical need to control infection as soon after wounding as possible. These findings may also explain why antibiotics are so ineffective against chronic wound infections.[79] See Chapter 9 for more on management of infection. Chapters 22–24 include information about the use of biophysical agents, electrical stimulation, pulsed electromagnetic fields, and ultrasound for enhanced biofilm destruction.

be recorded if present (see *Color Plate 44*).[80] It is considered a benchmark of the chronic inflammatory phase.

Absence of Inflammation

Absence of the inflammatory phase, or the inability of the body to present an immune response to wounding, can be due to many causes, including an immune-suppression state (e.g., human immunodeficiency virus infection/AIDS, cancer, diabetes, drug or radiation therapy, overuse of antiseptics, and severe ischemia). The absence of an inflammatory response prevents the wound from progressing through the biologic cascade of repair. It is different from chronic inflammation, with distinct signs and symptoms.

Lack of tissue perfusion is a common cause for an absent inflammatory phase. For example, a patient with an ulcer on an ischemic foot with an eschar over a wound on the heel has an absence of inflammation. Lack of perfusion is a barrier to healing. Unless reperfusion is an option, it may not be possible or appropriate in such a case to remove the eschar. In this case, the eschar is nature's best protection from the entry of infection. Protection of the eschar and the limb from trauma to prevent opening of the body to infection and new wounding is the preferred treatment strategy (see *Color Plate 52*).[19] In order for the wound to heal, in-

terventions are necessary to restart the inflammatory response. However, because of the comorbidity related to the problem, this may not be realistic.

Periwound Skin

The absence of an inflammatory phase is recognized by the absence of a vascular response to wounding, including the absence of color changes in the periwound skin and the absence of tension or hardness. However, there may be a boggy feeling and minimal temperature difference or coolness compared with adjacent tissue. Minimal pulses are palpable. Such findings should trigger further investigation of the vascular status of the patient. (see *Color Plate 52*).

Wound Bed Tissue

Wound bed tissue can be covered with hard, dry eschar to seal off debris and infection from the wound (see *Color Plate 52*).

Wound Drainage

Wound drainage can be scant, or the tissues can be dry. Dryness can be due to hemostasis sealing off the blood supply to the tissues without adequate profusion to progress the healing, ischemia reperfusion injury, or improper treatment.

TABLE 4-8 Wound Healing Phase Diagnosis: Tissue Characteristics and Benchmarks for Inflammatory Phase

Periwound Skin and Wound Tissue Characteristics	Acute Inflammatory Phase	Chronic Inflammatory Phase	Absence of Inflammatory Phase
Periwound skin color	• Unblanchable erythema in light-skinned patients • Discoloration or deepening of normal color in darkly pigmented patients • Ecchymosis (purplish bruising)	• Halo of erythema or darkening • Hemosiderin (rust-brown) staining • Hemosiderin staining • Ecchymosis	• Pale or ashen skin color • Absence of erythema or darkening • Hemosiderin staining • Ecchymosis
Edema and induration	• Firmness • Taut, shiny skin • Localized swelling • Consolidation (hardness) between adjacent tissues • Gelatinous edema may be seen on wound tissue	• Minimal firmness • Absent • May feel boggy	
Tissue temperature	• Elevated initially, decreases as inflammation progresses	• Minimal change or coolness	• Minimal change or coolness
Pain	• Present; wound is tender and painful unless neuropathy is present	• Minimal pain unless arterial etiology or infection, then can have intense pain	• Minimal or no pain unless arterial etiology, then can have intense pain
Wound tissue	• Blister with clear or bloody fluid • Shallow or deep crater with red to pink color • Red muscle • White, shiny fascia • Yellow reticular layer of dermis with granulation buds	• Necrotic; varies in color from yellow to brown to black • Necrotic tissue covering full or partial surface area • Soft or hard necrotic tissue • Yellow fibrin or slough • Portion of wound can have granulation tissue • Can also appear as clean, pale pink	• Covered with hard, dry eschar • Necrotic; varies in color from yellow to brown to black • Scab
Undermining/tunneling	• Can be present in deep wounds • Has potential for infection and abscess	• Can be present in deep wounds • Has potential for infection and abscess	• Can be present in deep wounds • Has potential for infection and abscess
Wound edges	• Diffuse, indistinct; can still be demarcating from healthy tissues	• Distinct; edges can be rolled or thickened • Is not continuous with wound bed if deep wound cavity	• Has distinct, well-defined wound edges • Can be attached to necrotic tissue

(Continued)

TABLE 4-8 **Wound Healing Phase Diagnosis: Tissue Characteristics and Benchmarks for Inflammatory Phase** *(Continued)*

Periwound Skin and Wound Tissue Characteristics	Acute Inflammatory Phase	Chronic Inflammatory Phase	Absence of Inflammatory Phase
Wound drainage	• Serous or serosanguineous	• Infection • Viscous • Malodor • Pus (yellow, tan, gray, or green) • Moderate to large amount	• Scant or dry
Color Plates	1, 14, 15, 17, 19	20, 25, 27, 36, 39, 42, 47	30, 52

Table 4-8 summarizes the findings during the inflammatory phase.

Proliferative Phase

The proliferative phase is divided into the acute proliferative (the active biologic process of proliferation, including, extracellular matrix [ECM] synthesis, granulation tissue formation and degradation, and wound contraction), chronic proliferative (the wound is stuck in the proliferative phase, hyperproliferating, or not progressing to the next phase of epithelialization and remodeling), and absence of proliferative phase (the wound bed lacks signs of ECM development or is not contracting). Characteristics of each of the three aspects of the proliferative phase are described.

Acute Proliferative Phase

Periwound Skin. During the proliferative phase, periwound skin regains color and contour symmetry with that of adjacent skin (edema resolved). If it is a recovering chronic wound, however, the clinician will likely see hemosiderin staining (pigmentation) around the wound margins (see *Color Plate 2*). Ecchymosis should be resolved. Skin turgor is normal and is not stretched or taut because the edema and induration are resolved (absent). Firmness is absent or minimal.

Periwound skin temperature, when palpated or measured with an LCD skin thermometer, is the same as the adjacent skin or slightly elevated, due to the enhanced perfusion of tissues and higher metabolic activities associated with healing. A temperature gradient of 4°F or greater indicates inflammation and possible infection, and further evaluation is needed.

Pain. Minimal pain is experienced during this phase and is absent in patients with neuropathy. Sudden onset of pain suggests possible infection.

Undermining and Tunneling. As previously described, wound undermining and tunneling occurs following de-

bridement of the skin and subcutaneous tissue (see *Color Plate 41*). The extent of undermining or tunnelling is a measure of the total soft tissue involved in the wound. Tunneling may be unobservable from the surface and yet have a great extent, as shown in *Color Plates 37* and *38* of the same wound. Undermining and tunneling close as the tissues reestablish continuity during the laying down of the collagen matrix and granulation tissue in the proliferative phase. Reduction of the extent of undermining/tunneling is a measure of the progression of proliferation and reduced overall wound size. Record findings of undermining and tunneling as part of the tissue assessment. If the tunneling extends beyond approximately 15 cm, notify the physician. Chapter 5 describes how to measure undermining/tunneling and calculate the extent of the overall wound.

Wound Bed Tissue. Tissue that develops during this phase is called granulation tissue because of the appearance of granules piled upon one another. Biologically, this tissue is the collagen matrix and new blood vessels. Granulation buds are clearly seen in *Color Plates 4* and *8*. Wounds that have a bowl-shaped cavity will fill with ECM and granulation tissue during the acute proliferative phase to create a surface across which epidermal cells can migrate. Note how the cavity is filling in those photos to create a level surface with the adjacent skin.

The acute proliferative phase starts when the wound bed tissue begins to show red or pink granulation buds and overlaps with the late inflammatory phase. The collagen matrix is laid down and is infiltrated by and supports the growing capillary bed, giving it a red color. Reduced depth in a full-thickness wound is a measure of proliferation activity. The collagen matrix does not replace the structures or functions of the tissues that occupied the cavity prior to injury; rather, this is scar tissue. The prevailing opinion is that this deep red color indicates a healthy, healing wound. A contrary opinion is explained later, in the section entitled Chronic Proliferative Phase.

Another feature that has been reported to appear during the acute proliferative phase of healing in a number of patients is the development of a yellow, fibrinous membrane on the surface of the granulation tissue. Removal of this membrane has been attempted, but it will recur in a few days. Wounds that develop this yellow membrane appear to be less susceptible to infection. These wounds continue to heal in a normal fashion. Recognizing this membrane during examination will prevent unnecessary disruption of the wound bed. [75]

Wound Edges. The wound edges are soft to firm and flexible to touch. Edges will roll in full-thickness wounds, but when the wound tissue fills the cavity to a point even with the edge of the wound, the edges will flatten, and epithelialization and contraction will continue together (see *Color Plates 3–5 and 8–9*). At this point, the wound acquires a distinctive wound shape or "picture frame." The cells that control the movement of the picture frame, the myofibroblasts, are located beneath the wound edge. The cells are contractile and will move forward, drawing the wound together, as in the drawing together of purse strings, shrinking the size of the open area measurably. The shape that the wound now assumes predicts the resulting speed of contraction. Linear wounds contract rapidly. Square or rectangular wounds contract at a moderate pace. Circular wounds contract slowly.

Wound contraction is a major activity of the acute proliferative phase of healing. Contraction reduces the areas that need to close by epithelialization. Contraction in areas such as the gluteals and abdomen is typically uncomplicated, but contracture is troublesome in areas such as the head, neck, and hand. Drawing together too tightly in those areas will cause a defect or contracture that can impair function and cosmesis. Wounds that would have a poor outcome if allowed to close by contraction warrant surgical intervention at the start of the proliferative phase. [81]

Wound Drainage. During the acute proliferative phase, the wound drainage is serosanguineous and of moderate to minimal quantity and odor.

Chronic Proliferative Phase

Periwound Skin

Color and Edema. Color of the skin at the wound edges can blanch or begin to draw together very tightly (see *Color Plate 36*). Gelatinous edema can be present, signifying an episode of trauma.

Skin Temperature and Pain. Compared with the temperature of the adjacent skin, periwound skin during the chronic proliferative phase can be cool or mildly elevated. There may be signs of intense pain, indicating that the wound has been traumatized and is undergoing another episode of acute inflammation, or infection may be present.

Undermining and Tunneling. Chronic proliferation develops when tissue integrity is not reestablished. Tunneling can extend a long distance and presents an opportunity for infection to travel up the fascial plane. Tissues in the tunnel can be necrotic. Tunneling can become a sinus tract, a cavity or channel underlying a wound that involves an area larger than the visible surface of the wound (see *Color Plates 37 and 38*). An abscess can form in the tunnel or sinus tract. [31] When undermining/tunneling persists in a proliferating wound and the assessment findings include a black hole that has no reachable bottom, the wound requires urgent medical management.

Wound Bed Tissue. Wound bed tissue in the chronic proliferative phase can exhibit attributes of infection, poor vascular supply, desiccation, or hypergranulation. Poor vascular supply appears as a pale pink, minimally granulating wound. A contrary opinion of some clinicians is that wounds that develop a livid red surface color may be infected and slow to heal (see *Color Plate 42*). Infection in granulating wounds is disruptive to healing. The features of infection that can be observed in granulating wounds include superficial bridging, friable tissue, bleeding on contact, pain in the wound, and a delay in healing. There are two stages in the proliferative phase when the granulation tissue can show these characteristics of infection: approximately 10 days postoperatively and at the end stage of healing, when the wound has progressed satisfactorily, but then becomes indolent. [75] *Color Plates 10 and 11* show the same wound. In *Color Plate 10*, the wound was progressing through the proliferative phase. Seven days later, it had attributes of infection, proliferation had ceased, and the wound was in the chronic proliferative phase.

Other factors that can contribute to chronic proliferation include the following: Poor vascular supply is indicated by pale pink, blanched to dull, and dusky red granulation tissue. Desiccated granulation tissue is dark, dull, and garnet red. Trauma to the fragile tissues such as hemorrhage from pressure. Hemorrhaging or bleeding of the granulation tissue vessels causes acute inflammation in the area and promotes scarring. The surface on the granulation tissue looks like a purple bruise. In *Color Plate 11*, note the small hemorrhagic area at the center of the wound, indicating rupture of blood vessels.

An imbalance of collagen synthesis and degradation can allow the collagen to proliferate unchecked, creating a hump of granulation tissue called "hypergranulation." Normally, the process of granulation and ECM formation decreases as the wound space decreases and wound integrity is recovered. The granulation tissue fills the wound space to the surface, and the epithelialization process ensues and covers the wound. However, when hypergranulation tissue overflows the wound bed, the epithelial cells cannot climb the hill of granulation tissue against gravity; the result is that the epithelialization process is halted. See *Color Plate 23* for hypergranulation. When hypergranulation develops, it is as if the proliferative "switch" is stuck and won't turn off, leaving the wound in a chronic proliferative phase. In this state, the tissue is predisposed to infection. There are some clinical case reports about the use of dressings to control hypergranulation that seem to offer a nontraumatic option of controlling the problem (see Chapter 2 for the case results).

Management of Hypergranulation

Because hypergranulation inhibits the reepithelialization of the wound surface, it must be prevented or controlled. Methods for preventing and controlling hypergranulation include:

1. Cauterization by applying silver nitrate sticks to the surface will necrose the superficial granulation tissue, which can then be wiped off.
2. Excess hypergranulation tissue can be trimmed by rubbing with a gauze sponge or snipping with scissors. This can trigger a new inflammatory cascade.
3. Hypertonic saline is a nontoxic method of reducing hypergranulation (see Chapter 11).
4. Wound dressings: silicone gel dressings have preventative potential,[82] and polyurethane foam-type dressings reduce hypergranulation.[83] Occlusive moisture-retentive dressings appear to enhance the development of hypergranulation.[84]

Wound Edges. One sign that a wound is in the chronic proliferative phase is when wound edges roll in and become hard and fibrotic, inhibiting further wound contraction. See *Color Plate 35* for an example of rolled fibrotic edges. Wounds of different pathogeneses develop this problem, including pressure ulcers and venous ulcers. This is apparently due to imbalances in the wound biochemistry that controls tissue deposition and degradation during the proliferative phase. This finding, another benchmark of the chronic proliferative phase, could suggest a referral to a physical therapist for a procedure such as ultraviolet light stimulation to restart the healing process.

Wound Drainage. Chronic proliferative exudate can be a yellow, gelatinous, viscous material on the wound granulation base, which indicates the wound has been traumatized. This appearance should not be confused with residue from wound dressings, such as amorphous hydrogels, or hyrocolloids or treatments, such as antimicrobial ointments. An infected wound in chronic proliferation can have a malodorous, viscous, reddish-brown, green, or gray exudate. *Color Plate 42* shows an apparently clean wound; however, the wound dressing shows signs of moderate to large amounts of sanguineous and purulent, reddish-brown exudate. This is a benchmark of the chronic proliferative phase and the wound needs treatment to recover.

Absence of Proliferative Phase

Periwound Skin: Color, Edema, Pain, and Temperature. The presence of hemosiderin staining or a halo of erythema surrounding the wound signifies a wound that is also in the chronic inflammatory phase. The skin can show signs of ecchymosis. Edema and pain are minimal or absent. Temperature is the same as adjacent skin, or coolness is present.

Wound Bed Tissue. A wound in an absence of proliferative phase is either not producing granulation tissue or not contracting (see *Color Plate 33*). The wound bed tissue can appear dry, dull red, and desiccated, like dried raw meat or it can contain pale pink granulation tissue. There is no change in wound depth in a two to four week time frame. Wounds that are in the chronic inflammatory phase or absence of inflammatory phase also have the absence of a proliferative phase, i.e., the wound is not progressing through the proliferative phase. These wounds often have a surface appearance of necrotic tissue and/or hemorrhage/ecchymosis. Any signs of ecchymosis signify a restart of the inflammatory process within the wound. The chronic inflammatory phase and absence of the proliferative phase can both be used as wound healing diagnoses for the same wound. The prognosis would be for the wound to progress to the acute proliferative phase. The medical history and systems review should guide the clinician to investigate the impairments to the proliferation process.

Wound Edges. Wound edges can be rolled or jagged, and the wound shape is irregular. The wound does not change shape, signifying lack of wound contraction. Deep wounds can lack continuity of wound bed and edges. The wound does not reduce in size.

Wound Drainage. Wounds lack exudate or have scant serous exudate. The wound in *Color Plate 45* is in the chronic inflammatory phase and has absence of a proliferative phase. Note the scant amount of serous exudate on the wound dressing. Treatment interventions should be reviewed to determine why the wound lacks moisture. Table 4-9 summarizes the findings during the proliferative phase.

Describing a Wound in the Proliferative Phase

The following is an example of a narrative note describing a wound in the acute proliferative phase:

Evaluation: The wound on the right hip has red granulation tissue. The wound edges are firm and soft. Wound is contracting into a rectangular shape.

Wound healing phase diagnosis: The wound healing phase diagnosis is proliferative phase.

Epithelialization Phase

Acute Epithelialization Phase

Periwound Skin. Because acute epithelialization begins at the time of wounding concurrently with the inflammatory phase and overlapping with the other phases, expect the signs of acute inflammation in the periwound skin. As the acute inflammatory process subsides, the periwound skin should return to the usual color for ethnicity and to the temperature of adjacent tissues. It should be firm, but not hard, edematous, or fibrotic. Maceration of the periwound skin and new epidermis can occur from leakage of wound exudate or the use of products that moisten the skin and saturate the cells. Maceration is especially damaging to new epithelium. Macerated skin appears pale and wrinkled, and feels soft and thin to touch, making it very susceptible to trauma, such as from pressure.

TABLE 4-9   Wound Healing Phase Diagnosis: Tissue Characteristics and Benchmarks for Proliferative Phase

Periwound Skin and Wound Tissue Characteristics	Acute Proliferative Phase	Chronic Proliferative Phase	Absence of Proliferative Phase
Periwound skin color	• Continuity with adjacent skin • Hemosiderin staining if recovering chronic wound	• Continuity with adjacent skin • Paler than adjacent skin	• Hemosiderin staining if chronic wound • Halo of erythema if in chronic inflammatory phase • Ecchymosis
Edema and induration	• Absent	• Hemosiderin staining • Gelatinous edema can be present, signifying trauma	• Minimal edema present
Tissue temperature	• Temperature can be minimally elevated if wound is well-perfused	• Minimal change	• Minimal change or coolness
Pain	• Pain-free or minimal pain • Inappropriate indicator in presence of neuropathy	• Painful, can indicate local inflammation; if intense, consider infection	• Minimal or absent • Intense if infection present
Wound tissue	• Shiny, bright red to pink granulation • Sustained reduction in wound depth • Sustained wound contraction • Reduced size • Covering of yellow fibrinous membrane on granulation tissue • Livid red	• Hypergranulation • Desiccation (dark red color) • Poor vascularization (pale pink) • Ecchymosis on granulation	• Necrotic tissue—stuck in chronic inflammatory phase • Ecchymosis on granulation inflammation restarting • Dull red—desiccated granulation • Pale pink granulation • Lacking change in wound depth • Unsustained contraction—no reduction in size of surface area
Undermining/tunneling	• Can be present in deep wounds • Closes as proliferation progresses	• Can be present in deep wounds • Fails to close or can extend • Has potential for infection and abscess	• Can be present in deep wounds • Fails to close or can extend • Has potential for infection and abscess • Unchanged size
Wound edges	• Soft to firm • Flexible to touch • Rolled if full-thickness • Change in wound shape from irregular to regular • Reduction in size of surface area • Drawing together • Adherence of wound edges by end of phase	• Tight drawing together to reduce size—contracture • Absence of continuity of wound bed and edges • Fibrotic • Fibrotic • Ecchymosis on wound edge	• Rolled or jagged, irregular edges • No change of shape—not drawing together • Absence of continuity of wound bed and edges
Wound drainage	• Serosanguineous or serous in moderate to minimal amount for wound size	• Yellow gelatinous following trauma	• Serous drainage, scant to minimal amounts

(Continued)

TABLE 4-9 **Wound Healing Phase Diagnosis: Tissue Characteristics and Benchmarks for Proliferative Phase** *(Continued)*

Periwound Skin and Wound Tissue Characteristics	Acute Proliferative Phase	Chronic Proliferative Phase	Absence of Proliferative Phase
		• Infection: viscous malodorous, red/brown, green, purulent	• Desiccated and dry
		• Large amount	
Color Plates	3 to 5, 8 to 10, 18	11, 23, 34, 35, 36, 42, 66	30, 31, 33, 39

CLINICAL WISDOM

Protection of Skin from Maceration

Skin barriers are products that can be used over the periwound skin and new scar tissue to protect them from maceration. ∎

Wound Edges and Wound Bed Tissue. Within hours of wounding, epithelial cells start migrating toward the center from the wound edges to cover the defect with new skin. Epithelialization occurs from several directions. The edges and hair follicles are sources of keratinocytes that cover the wound surface with epithelium. The wound edges must be adhered to the wound base for epithelial cell migration to cover the wound. The leading edge of the migrating cells is one cell thick. Gradually, the epithelium spreads across the wound bed, as shown in *Color Plates 5* and *6* of the same wound. The migrating tissue is connected to the adjacent skin and pulls it along to cover the opening.[81]

The new skin will be bright pink, regardless of normal pigmentation, and may never regain the melanin factors that color skin (see *Color Plates 8* and *22*). New skin is formed as a very thin sheet, and it takes several weeks for it to thicken. If the wound is less than full-thickness, islands of pink epithelium can appear in the wound bed from migrating cells donated by the dermal appendages, hair follicles, and sweat glands. Cells from these islands and edges spread out and cover the open area. *Color Plate 66* shows a wound with an island of epithelium. *Color Plate 67* of the same wound shows the migration of the epithelium across the wound from the edges and island. Notice how the edges of the new epithelium are jagged. Full-thickness wounds lose these island contributors, and they never regenerate.[85] Full-thickness wounds begin to epithelialize when the edges are attached and even with the wound so that there are no sides or walls, and the epithelial cells can migrate from the edge across the wound surface. Edges are soft to firm and flexible to touch, as shown in *Color Plate 18*. This wound went on to heal by epithelialization from the wound edges. The

wound environment is critical to a successful epithelialization phase. The wound must be kept warm, moist, and free of trauma at all times.

Wounds can bypass this phase of repair if it is necessary to place a skin graft or muscle flap to close the wound. Large wounds and wounds in areas where contraction will be harmful or will simply take too long to cover the wound can benefit from surgical repair. The wound shown in *Color Plate 67* was closed at that time by a split-thickness skin graft to speed the repair process.

CLINICAL WISDOM

Maintaining a Moist Wound Bed for Epithelialization

Amorphous hydrogel dressings are useful wound moisturizers. Along with moisture-permeable films and sheet hydrogels, they provide the warm, moist, homeostatic environment that is critical for epithelialization. Avoid Hydrocolloids or other srtong adhesives on new or fragile skin. ∎

Wound Drainage. A scant or small amount of serous or serosanguineous wound exudate is expected. The wound must be kept moist during this phase of healing, because desiccation will destroy the epithelial cells.

Chronic Epithelialization Phase

Periwound Skin. The characteristics of the skin can be the same as those seen in the chronic inflammatory and absence of inflammatory phases. The periwound skin can show signs of ischemia, such as a pale or ashen color in the elevated position that deepens to dark purple with dependence (rubor). Pain can be constant and throbbing, or intermittent claudication during walking, if it is associated with arterial occlusive disease. The appearance of the adjacent skin is usually dry, shiny, taut, and/or hairless. These characteristic indicate the loss of hair follicles and sweat and/or sebaceous glands, which benchmark the phase. The wound shown in *Color Plate 85* is in both the chronic epithelialization and chronic inflammatory phases. The appearance of adjacent and periwound skin changed as chronicity was altered and the acute epithelialization and proliferative phases were initiated (*Color Plate 87*).

Wound Edges. Epithelialization of deep wounds occurs only at the edges and can involve thickening and rolling under of the edges. When the cells cannot continue to migrate across the wound, they build up an epithelial ridge along the edge of the wound, as seen in *Color Plates 3 and 42*. Pressure ulcers typically develop a round shape when this occurs. In wounds in chronic epithelialization, the cells pile up on each other until the rolled, thickened edges become fibrotic. The wound edges need to be modified and the wound bed filled before wound epithelialization can be reinitiated. With full-thickness and deeper wounds, the process of healing by epithelialization at the wound edges will be arrested if 1) a large amount of wound debris interferes with epithelialization, or 2) the wound edges fall off into a deep wound bed with steep walls or do not adhere to the wound bed.

Hyperkeratosis (overgrowth of the horny layer of the skin) is another abnormality of the epithelialization phase. *Color Plate 24* shows a wound with hyperkeratosis and the irregular shape of a heel ulcer in a 100-year-old woman. Additional photos of hyperketatosis and the management of the problem are shown in Chapter 19.

Scar Tissue. The majority of wound closure in humans occurs by granulation tissue formation, followed by epithelialization.[85] New epithelium of scar tissue is bright pink, regardless of the pigmentation of normal skin. In darkly pigmented skin, the scar tissue may never regain pigmentation. The bright pink color may fade over time to a lighter shade of pink as the vascular system is fully reestablished.

Wound Bed Tissue. Wound bed tissue that is hypergranulating can develop a chronic epithelialization phase because the epithelial cells cannot migrate over the hump of granulation tissue against gravity (see *Color Plate 23*). In this case, the granulation tissue must be trimmed back to a level even with the periwound skin for epithelialization to resume.

Wound Drainage. The wound can be dry with no wound drainage. If no or only scant exudate is assessed, additional moisture may be needed to facilitate the migration of the epithelial cells; epidermal cells migrate best in a warm, moist environment. Wound dryness can be due to improper dressing selection, loss of dressing, dehydration of the wound or patient, or other iatrogenic conditions. On the other hand, there may be heavy exudate from a partial-thickness ulcer that should be epithelializing, but the exudate washes out the epidermal cells faster than they can migrate and attach to the wound surface. Excessive moisture associated with wound products can also cause this to occur and needs to be managed.

Absence of Epithelialization Phase

Absence of the epithelialization phase can be due to many factors such as failure of the wound to fill with the ECM, desiccation of the tissues, scar tissue from a prior wound that is not donating epithelial cells, repetitive trauma to the wound edges.

Periwound and Adjacent Skin. The color of the adjacent and periwound skin offers clues to the etiology of absence of the epithelialization phase. Absence of this phase can be related to a condition such as arterial obstructive disease (AOD). AOD limits blood supply and oxygen to the tissues and impairs the ability of the skin to repair itself. Examination of adjacent skin will reveal absence of hair, dependent rubor, and pallor on elevation. The wound will have a punched-out appearance and a very limited ring of epidermal tissue around it that does not migrate across the wound, as shown in *Color Plate 54*. If no prior vascular testing has been reported, further assessment of the vascular system is warranted.

Texture. Periwound skin that is dry, flaky, macerated, or has an irregular texture provides limited epidermal cells to resurface the wound. This wound will lack epithelialization activity.

Skin Temperature. Skin temperature is a reflection of blood supply. Skin temperature cooler than 92°F–96°F on the torso and lower in the extremities (75°F–80°F) indicates that blood supply to the skin may be limited; warmer skin can be due to infection.

Edema. Chronic edema caused by tissue congestion, such as lymphedema, congestive heart failure, or venous insufficiency, stretches the skin and fills the interstitial spaces with excess fluid, including large protein molecules. When the capacity of the tissue to hold fluid is exceeded, the fluid leaks through the skin. Because of the disease process, changes occur in the vascularity of the tissues, leading to the loss of dermal appendages and dry stasis eczema. These changes are known as *lipodermatosclerosis*.[86] Skin changes associated with this disease process are shown in *Color Plates 59* and *60*. Patients with lipodermatosclerosis can show absence of epithelialization phase. More information on lipodermatosclerosis is presented in Chapter 17.

Wound Edges. Another intrinsic factor that causes absence of epithelialization is decreased epidermal proliferation due to cellular senescence and delayed cellular migration, which are attributed to aging. In this case, there is slow or absent new skin growth from the edges or islands. Absence of epithelialization attributes include dry, flaky, hyperkeratotic skin at the wound edges. The dryness can be associated with a dry wound environment.

Wound Tissue. Hypogranulation results from the absence of the proliferative phase and failure to fill the wound bed and provide a surface for the epidermal cells to migrate across to cover the wound. Throughout the wound healing process, the epithelialization, inflammatory, and proliferative phases overlap, and attributes of each can be identified. Table 4-10 summarizes the findings during the epithelialization phase.

TABLE 4-10   Wound Healing Phase Diagnosis: Tissue Characteristics and Benchmarks for Epithelialization Phase

Periwound Skin and Wound Tissue Characteristics	Acute Epithelialization Phase	Chronic Epithelialization Phase	Absence of Epithelialization Phase
Periwound skin	• Early phase has same characteristics as acute inflammatory phase • Returns to normal color for ethnicity as inflammation subsides • Hemosiderin staining if chronic wound	• Can be same as chronic or absence of inflammatory phase • Can be ischemic (pale) or ashen • Can be purplish with dependency • Dry, flaky (hyperkeratotic—can be due to desiccation or aging skin) • Maceration: pale, wrinkled, soft, thin • Hemosiderin staining	• Scar tissue • Same as chronic or absence of inflammatory phase • Dry with hyperkeratosis or lipodermatosclerosis
Wound tissue	• Even with wound edges • Pink/red granulation • Reduction in wound surface area	• Not connected with wound edge • Hypergranulation	• Absence of resurfacing from edges or dermal appendages • Hypogranulation • Presence of scab or necrotic tissue
Undermining/tunneling Wound edges	• Steep walls limit migration • New skin moves out from wound edge and dermal appendages in irregular pattern • Bright pink color, regardless of usual skin pigmentation • Texture is soft to firm and flexible to touch, thin	• Steep walls limit migration • Epithelial ridge • Rolled under or thickened • Dry, flaky skin • Rounding off of wound shape	• Steep walls limit migration • Fibrotic wound edge • Rounding off of wound shape and edges • Macerated • Dry, flaky skin
Wound drainage	• Minimal to scant serous or serosanguineous	• Absent, dry; if hypergranulation, minimal/moderate	• Absent, dry
Scar tissue	• Thin layers of scar tissue • Thickens over time • Deep pink color initially; changes to bright pink color, regardless of normal skin pigmentation	• Hypertrophic scarring • Keloid scarring • Hyperkeratotic scarring	• Weak, friable epithelial tissue • Breaks or washes out
Color Plates	5, 22, 67	48–51	24, 33, 35, 48, 54, 58

EXHIBIT 4-5   Referral Sources

Physicians	Nurses		Allied Health Professionals
Dermatologist	Dermatology Nurse		Physical Therapist
Orthopedic Surgeon	Wound Ostomy Continence Nurse (WOCN)		Podiatrist
Plastic Surgeon	Geriatric Nurse Practitioner		Vascular Technician
Vascular Surgeon	Vascular Nurse		

CLINICAL WISDOM

Describing a Wound in the Epithelialization Phase

The following is an example of a narrative note describing a wound in the epithelialization phase:

Evaluation: A wound on the left medial ankle is adhered at 75% of the edges, and epithelialization is progressing over 50% of the open area.
Wound healing phase diagnosis: The wound is in the epithelialization phase.

Referral Criteria

A patient's problems must be identified and if indicated referred early to the medical provider who is most appropriate, according to the patient's wound severity or wound healing phase diagnosis. Referral should be made when there are findings that require the attention of another practitioner more skilled or more knowledgeable in management of the identified problem. Utilization management requires that this be done in an efficient and thoughtful manner. Referral depends on location, available resources, and other significant factors. For example, skin lesions such as scales, papules (e.g., warts and tumors), vesicles (e.g., chickenpox), shingles, and skin cancers are examples of skin conditions that can be seen on the adjacent skin and should be referred to a dermatologist. Wounds with a history of nonhealing for long periods of time can be cancerous, and they should be referred to a dermatologist for biopsy evaluation. Deep wounds that can be probed to the bone should be considered positive for osteomyelitis and require immediate referral to an orthopaedic surgeon. Wounds that are in the chronic inflammatory phase often need enhanced perfusion to heal. Vascular assessment would be a primary consideration, and a vascular surgeon may be the most qualified professional to evaluate and treat. A wound with deep tunneling should be referred to a plastic surgeon. Physical therapists are skilled in exercise, use of physical agents, and electrotherapeutic modalities, all of which enhance perfusion to tissues. Exhibit 4-5 lists possible referral sources, and Exhibit 4-6 lists red flags for referral.

Self-Care Teaching Guidelines for Skin and Wound Assessment

The skin and wound should be monitored by the patient or caregiver. A simple, 10-point observation sheet including the items below can be used.

Skin Monitoring Checklist

1. Changes in how the skin looks
2. Changes in the color of the skin over bony areas (learn to identify the color of skin that is normal for you)
3. Changes in the color of the wound tissue (more red, more yellow, more black)
4. Reddened areas where you have worn shoes or braces
5. Skin irritations, sores, or foreign bodies (check the soles of your feet with a mirror to see if there are any foreign items lodged there or areas of redness or tenderness)
6. Signs of excess moisture, redness, or cracking under skin folds (breast, stomach, around rectum, genitals)
7. Swelling of the feet and ankles
8. New blisters, scrapes, cuts, or bruises
9. Foul wound odor after wound is cleansed
10. Any pain in the wound or surrounding skin

Report any changes in the skin or wound to your healthcare provider. Research shows that contacting your healthcare provider at the first sign of a problem can prevent bad things from happening.

EXHIBIT 4-6   Red Flags for Referral

- Unilateral edema of the lower extremity of sudden onset; may be due to acute deep vein thrombophlebitis
- Findings of gross toenail abnormalities needing foot care
- Loss of protective sensation; requires prompt referral to a specialist for appropriate protective footwear and should be followed closely.
- Inability to initiate and progress through the phases of healing; prognosis for the wound is nonhealing
- Wounds that can be probed to bone; patient is considered to have osteomyelitis, and emergent referral is needed.
- Excessive signs of acute inflammation; should be considered as a signal of impending wound infection

Conclusion

Wound classification systems are used to identify wound severity by the depth of tissue impairment, leading to an impairment finding of *impaired skin integrity* (if the dermis is not penetrated) or *impaired tissue integrity* (if the wound extends through the dermis and deeper). Wound healing assessment by physiologic wound healing phase includes three aspects for each physiologic phase: acute, chronic, and absent. Each phase includes attributes and benchmarks for the acute, chronic, or absent state of the phase by symptoms found in the periwound skin and wound tissues. At the baseline assessment, clinicians need to know where in the trajectory of healing the wound is to plan treatment, make a diagnosis and prognosis of healing, select interventions, predict outcomes, and triage patients. Trajectories of healing are presented in Chapter 5.

The assessment is usually completed by the same clinician, but this is not always the case. The evaluator can be a person more highly skilled and trained in interpretive skills than the individual who collects data. For example, examination and recording of the different wound characteristics can be done by a properly trained physical therapist assistant or licensed practical nurse, with the evaluation of findings, wound healing diagnosis, and prognosis completed by a physical therapist, registered nurse, or wound ostomy continence nurse (WOCN). Collection tools to measure, grade, record, and monitor findings are described in Chapters 5 and 6.

Documentation requirements for wound assessment should be part of a facility's policies and procedures. Documentation should be accurate, clearly reflect the patient's condition, and consistent with documentation by other professionals in the same department or facility. If it is not documented, it did not happen.

REVIEW QUESTIONS

1. How do wound classification systems relate to the wound severity diagnosis?
2. What are the principle indexes for wound assessment?
3. What attributes of the adjacent tissues should be assessed?
4. What tests and measures are used to assess wound and adjacent tissue attributes?
5. How does assessment of darkly pigmented skin differ from that of lighter skin tones?
6. How would you apply the concept of wound healing phase diagnosis to the prognosis for a wound?

ACKNOWLEDGEMENT

Portions of this chapter also appear in Sussman, C Pattern 7B: Impaired integumentary Integrity Associated with Superficial Skin Involvement, Biggs-Harris Katherine Ed., Integumentary Essentials: Applying the Preferred Physical Therapist Practice Patterns [sm] Slack, Inc., Thorofare NJ, 2006 and are used with permission from Slack, Inc.

REFERENCES

1. Schultz GS, Sibbald GR, Falanga V, et al. Wound bed preparation : A systematic approach to wound management. *Wound Repair and Regeneration.* March-April 2003;11(1):S1-S28.
2. Keast David H, Bowering C, Keith EA, et al. MEASURE; A proposed assessment framework for developing best practice recommendations for wound asessment. *Wound Repair and Regeneration.* May-June 2004;12:1-17.
3. Winter GD. Formation of the scab and the rate of epithelializatin of superficial wounds in the skin of the young domestic pig. *Nature.* 1962;193:293-294.
4. Dykes P, Heggie R, Hill S. Effects of adhesive dressings on the stratum corneum of the skin. *Journal of Wound Care.* February 2001;10(2).
5. Yosipovitch G HJ. The importance of skin pH. *Skin & Aging.* Vol 11; 2003:88-93.
6. Gray Mikel. Influence of delivery vehicle on topical therapy for partial-thickness perineal wounds. *Wounds: a compendium of clinical research and practice.* May 2005(Supplement):2-6.
7. Schultz George S., Mozingo David, Romanelli Marco, Claxton Karl. Wound Healing and TIME; new concepts and scientific applications. *Wound Repair & Regeneration.* July/ August 2005;13(4):S1-11.
8. Halkier-Sorenson L. Understanding skin barrier dysfunction in dry skin patients. *Skin and Wound Care.* Vol 7; 1999:60-64.
9. Langemo D, Hunter S, Anderson J, Hanson D, Thompson P, Klug MG. Incorporating a body wash and skin protectant into skin care protocols reduces skin breakdown in two nursing homes. *Extended Care Products News;* 2003:36-37.
10. Makelbust J, Sieggreen M. Glossary. In: Makelbust J SM, ed. Pressure Ulcers: *Guidelines for Prevention and Nursing Management.* West Dundee, IL: S.N. Publications; 1996:8-9.
11. Sibbald RG CJ. Dermatological aspects of wound care. In: Krasner Diane RG, Sibblad RGary, ed. *Chronic Wound Care: A clinical Source Book for Healthcare Professionals.* third ed. Wayne, PA: HMP Communications; 2001:273-285.
12. Little J, Kobayashi G, Bailey T. Infection of the Diabetic Foot. In: Levin M E ONL, Bowker JH,, ed. *The Diabetic Foot.* Fifth ed. St Louis, MO: Mosby Year Book; 1993:181-198.
13. Panel NPUA. Pressure ulcst and risk assessment: consensus development conference statement. *Decubitus.* February 1989;2(2):24-28.
14. Armstrong DG LL, Harkless LB. Validation of a diabetic wound classification system. The contribution of depth,infection, and ischemia to risk of amputation. *Diabetes Care PMID: 9589255* May 1998;21(5):855-859.
15. Wagner FEW. The dysvascular foot: A system for diagnosis and treatment. *Foot and Ankle.* 1981(2):64-122.
16. Van Rijswijk L. Frequence of reassessmnet of pressure ulcers, NPUAP Proceedings. *Adv Wound Care.* July/August 1995;8(suppl 4)(July/August):19-24.
17. Ferrell BA, Osterweil D, Christenson P. A randomized trial of low-air-loss beds for treatment of pressure ulcers. *Journal of the American Medical Association.* 1993;269:494-497.
18. Shea JD. Pressure sore: Classification and management. *Clin Orthop.* 1975;112:89-100.
19. Bergstrom Nancy, Allman Richard M, Alvarez Oscar M, Bennet M Allison, Carlson Carolyn E, Frantz Rita. *Clinical Practice Guideline: Treatment of Pressure Ulcers.* Rockville MD: Us Department of health and Human Services Public Health Service Agency for health Care Policy and Research; 1994. 15.
20. Bergstrom Nancy, Allman Richard M, Carlson Carolyn E, et al. *Pressure Ulcers in Adults: Prediction and Preventions.* Rockville, MD: US Dept of Health and Human Services; May 1992. 3.
21. (NPUAP). NPUAP. *New Definition for Stage I Pressure Ulcers.* Buffalo, NY: 1998.
22. Sprigle Stephen, Linden Maureen, Riordan Brian. Analysis of Localized Erythema Using Clinical Indicators and Spectroscopy. *Ostomy/Wound Management.* Marech 2003;49(3):42-52.
23. Ankrom MA BR, Sprigle S, Langemo D, Black JM, Berlowitz DR, Lyder CJ, National Pressure Ulcer Advisory Panel. Pressure-Related Deep Tissue Injury Under Intact Skin and the Current Pressure Ulcer Staging Systems. *Advances in Skin and Wound Care.* January/February 2005;18(1):35-42.
24. Panel NPUA. Deep Tissue Injury. Paper presented at: Merging Missions Consensus Conference; February 25-26, 2005; Tampa, FL.

25. European Pressure Ulcer Advisory Panel (EPUAP). *Pressure ulcer classification* 2004.
26. Henderson C, Ayello C, Sussman Carrie. Draft definition of stage I pressure ulcers: inclusion of person with darkly pigmented skin. *Advances in Wound Care.* 1997;10:34-35.
27. Krasner D, Weir D. Recommendations for using reverse staging to complete the MDS-2. *Ostomy/Wound Manage.* 1997;43(3):14-17.
28. Cuzzell JZ. The new RYB color code. AJN. 1988;88(10):1342-1346.
29. Carpenito LJ. *Nursing Diagnosis, Application to Clinical Practice.* Vol 0. 6th ed. Philadelphia: JB Lippincott; 1995.
30. Metzger-Donovan Debra, Biggs Katherine, Sussman Carrie, Unger Pamela, Ward R Scott. Guide to Physical Therapist Practice, II. *Physical Therapy.* 1997;77:1163-1650.
31. vanRijswijk L, Polansky M. Predictors of time to healing deep pressure ulcers. *Ostomy Wound Management.* October 1994;40(8):40-42, 44, 46-48.
32. Abeln Susan. Reporting risk check-up. *PT Magazine.* Vol 5; 1997:38.
33. Greenman PE. Principles of structured diagnosis. *Principles of Manual Medicine.* second ed. Baltimore: Williams & Wilkins; 1996:13-20.
34. Makelbust J, Sieggreen M. Etiology and pathophysiology of pressure ulcers. In: Makelbust J SM, ed. *Makelbust J, Sieggreen M.* first ed. West Dundee, IL: S.N. Publications; 1991:19-27.
35. Nachbar F SW, Merkle T, Cognetta AB, Vogt T, Landthaler M, Bilek P, Braun-Falco O PG. The ABCD rule of dermatoscopy. High prospective value in the diagnosis of doubtful melanocytic skin lesions. *J Am Acad Dermatol.* Apr 1994;30(4):551-559.
36. Throne N. The problem of the black skin. *Nursing Times;* 1969:999-1001.
37. Weiss EL. Connective tissue in wound healing. In: McCulloch J KL, Feedar J,, ed. *Wound Healing Alternatives in Management.* second ed. Philadelphia: FA Davis; 1995:26-28.
38. Harkless LB, Dennis K. Role of the podiatrist. In: Levin ME ONL, Bowker JH,, ed. *The Diabetic Foot.* 5th ed. St. Louis, MO: Mosby-Year Book; 1993:516-517.
39. Sibbald RG, Cameron J. Dermatological aspects of wound care. In: Krasner Diane RG, Sibblad RGary, ed. *Chronic Wound Care: A clinical Source Book for Healthcare Professionals.* third ed. Wayne, PA: HMP Communications; 2001:273-285.
40. Sibbald RG, Williamson D, Orsted H. Preparing the wound bed—debridement, bacterial balance, and moisture balance. *Ostomy/Wound Management.* November 2000;46(11):14-35.
41. Bergstrom N, Allman RM, Alvarez OM, Bennet MA, Carlson CE, Frantz R. *Clinical Practice Guideline: Treatment of Pressure Ulcers.* Rockville MD: Us Department of health and Human Services Public Health Service Agency for health Care Policy and Research; 1994. 15.
42. Dorland. *Dorland's Illustrated Medical Dictionary. W.B. Saunders (Harcourt Health Services)* [electronic]. Available at: http://www .mercksource.com/pp/us/cns/cns_hl_dorlands. Accessed September 19, 2005, 2005.
43. Ruschhaupt WF III. Vascular disease of diverse origin. In: Young JR ea, ed. *Peripheral Vascular Diseases.* St. Louis, MO: Mosby-Year Book; 1991:639-650.
44. Berard Anick KX, Zuccarelli Francois,Abenhaim Lucien. Validity of the Leg-o-meter, an instrument to measure leg circumference. *Angiology.* 2002;53(1):21-28.
45. Parish CP, Witkowski JA. Decubitus ulcers: How to intervene effectively. *Drug Ther;* 1983:not numbered.
46. Bennett M. Report of the task force on the implications for darkly pigmented intact skin in the prediction and prevention of pressure ulcers. *Advances in Wound Care.* August 1995;8:34:35.
47. Roach LB. Assessment: Color changes in dark skin. *Nursing 77.* 1977:48-51.
48. Dailey C. Purple Ulcers. *J ET Nursing.* 1992;19:106.
49. Sussman C, Swanson G. The utility of Sussman Wound Healing Tool in predicting wound healing outcomes in physical therapy. *Adv Wound Care.* 1997;10(5):74-77.
50. Panel NPUA. *Deep tissue injury - White paper.* Washington, DC 2005.
51. Witkowski JA. Purple Ulcers. *J ET Nurs.* Vol 20; 1993:132.
52. Berna-Serna JD S-GJ, Madrigal M, Zuazu I, Berna-Mestre JD,. Ultrasound Therapy in Rectus Sheath Hematoma. *Physical Therapy.* April 2005;85(4):352-357.
53. Liefeldt L, Destanis P, Rupp K, Morgera S, Neumayer H-H. The hazards of whirlpooling. *The Lancet.* 2003/2/8 361(9356):534.
54. Fishman Tamara. Foot and Nail Care. Paper presented at: First Annual Wound Conference; October, 1995; Boca Raton, FL.
55. (JCAHO) JCoAoHO. Pain Management Standards (Standard RI 2.8 and PE 1.4). In: JCAHO, ed. *Comprehensive Accreditation Manual for Hospitals;* 2001.
56. Horzic Matija, Bunoza Davorka, Maric Kristina. Contact thermography in a study of primary healing of surgical wounds. *Ostomy/Wound Management.* Jan/Feb 1996;42`(1):36-42.
57. Armstrong DG LL, Liswood PJ, Todd WF, Tredwell JA,. Infrared Dermal Thermometry for the High -Risk Diabetic Foot. *Phys Ther.* February 1997;77(2):169-177.
58. Armstrong DG LL. Monitoring neruopathic ulcer healing with infrared-dermal thermometry. *J Foot Ankle Surgery.* Vol 35; 1996:335-338.
59. Lavery LA HK, Lanctot DR,Constantinides GP, Zamorano RG, ArmstrongDG, Athanasiou KA, C Agrawal CM,. Home Monitoring of Foot Skin Temperature to Prevent Ulceration. *Diabetes Care.* 2004;27:2642-2647.
60. Pernet A, Villano JB. Thermography as a preoperative and followup method for surgery of the hand. *Int Surg.* 1984;69(2):171-173.
61. Chan AW, MacFarlane IA, Bowsher DR. Contact thermography of painful diabetic neuropathic foot. *Diabetes Care.* 1991;10:918-922.
62. Benbow SJ, Chan AW, Bowsher DR, et al. The prediction of diabetic neuropathic plantar foot ulceration by liquid-crystal contact thermography. *Diabetes Care.* 1994;17(8):835-839.
63. Kohler A, Hoffmann R, Platz A, Bino M. Diagnostic value of duplex ultrasound and liquid crystal contact thermography in preclinical detection of deep vein thrombosis after proximal femur fractures. *Arch Orthop Trauma Surg.* 1998;117(1-2):39-42.
64. Birke James. Management of the Insensate Foot. In: Kloth LC MJ, ed. *Wound Healing: Alternatives in Management.* third ed. Philadelphia: FA Davis; 2001:385-408.
65. Cavanagh PR, Ulbricht JS. Biomechanics of the foot in diabetes mellitus. In: Levin ME ONL, Bowker JH,, ed. *The Diabetic Foot.* 5th ed. ed. St. Louis, MO: Mosby-Year Book; 1993:225.
66. Levin ME. Pathogenesis and management of diabetic foot lesions. In: Levin ME ONL, Bowker JH,, ed. *The Diabetic Foot.* 5th ed. St. Louis, MO: Mosby-Year Book; 1993:43.
67. Martina ISJ vKR, Schmitz PIM, van der Meché FGA,van Doorna PA for the European Inflammatory Neuropathy Cause and Treatment (INCAT) group. Measuring vibration threshold with a graduated tuning fork in normal aging and in patients with polyneuropathy. *J Neurol Neurosurg Psychiatry.* November 1998;65(November):743-747.
68. Merkiesa ISJ SP, van der Mechéa FGA, van Doorna PA, for the Inflammatory Neuropathy Cause and Treatment (INCAT) Group. Reliability and responsiveness of a graduated tuning fork in immune mediated polyneuropathies. *J Neurol Neurosurg Psychiatry.* May 2000;68(May):669-671.
69. Peters EJG LL. Effectiveness of the Diabetic Foot Risk Classification System of the International Working Group on the Diabetic Foot. *Diabetes Care.* 2001;24:1442-1447.
70. Perkins BA, Olaleye D, Zinman B, Bril V. Simple Screening Tests for Peripheral Neuropathy in the Diabetes Clinic. *Diabetes Care.* February 1, 2001;24(2):250-256.
71. Sussman Carrie. Case Presentation: Patient with a Pressure Ulcer. Paper presented at: American Physical Therapy Association Scientific Meeting,, 1996; Minneapolis, MN.
72. Ennis WJ, Meneses P. Wound Healing at the Local Level: The Stunned Wound. *Ostomy/Wound Management.* January 2000;46(suppl1A)(1A): 39S-48S.
73. Kerstein Morris D, Bensing Kathleen A, Brill Leon R, et al. *The Physiology of Wound Healing.* Philadelphia: The Oxford Institue for Continuing Education and Allegheny University of Health Sciences; March 1998.
74. Cooper Diane M. The Physiology of Wound Healing: An Overview. In: Krasner D, ed. *Chronic Wound Care: A clinical source book for healthcare professionals.* Vol 1. King of Prussia, PA: Health Management Publications; 1990:1-10.
75. Harding Keith G, Bale Sue. Wound Care: putting theory into practice in the United Kingdom. In: Krasner D, Kane D, eds. *Chronic Wound Care: A clinical Source Book for Healthcare Professionals.* Vol 1. first ed. Wayne, PA: Health Management Publications; 1990:115-123.
76. Cutting Keith F, Harding Keith G. Criteria to idenify wound infection. *Journal of Wound Care.* 1994;3(4):198-201.
77. Fux CA, Costerton JW, Stewart PS, Stoodley P. Survival strategies of infectios biofilms. *Trends in Microbiology.* January 2005;13(1):34-40.
78. Costerton J William, Ellis B, Lam K, Johnson Frank, Khoury Antoine E. Mechanisms of Electrical Enhancement of Efficacy of Antibiotics in

Killing Biofilm Bacteria. *Antimicrobial Agents and chemotherapy.* 1994;38(12):2803-2809.

79. Harrison-Balestra C, Cazzaniga AL, Davis SC, Mertz PM. A Wound-Isolated Pseudomonas aeruginosa Grows a Biofilm In Vitro Within 10 Hours and Is Visualized by Light Microscopy. *Dermatologic Surgery.* 2003;29(6):631-635.

80. Feedar Jeffrey A. Clinical management of chronic wounds. In: McCulloch J KL, Feedar J, ed. *Wound Healing Alternatives in Management.* 2nd ed. Philadelphia: FA Davis; 1995:140.

81. Hardy Maureen A. The Biology of Scar Formation. *Phys Ther.* December 1989;69(12):1014-1023.

82. Ducharme-Desjarlais M, Celeste CJ, Lepault E, et al. Effect of a silicone-containing dressing on exuberant granulation tissue formation and wound repair in horses. *Am J Vet Res.* 2005;66(7):1133-1139.

83. Harris A, Rolstad BS. Hypergranulation tissue: a nontraumatic method of management. *Ostomy Wound Manage.* 1994;40(5):20-22, 24, 26-30.

84. Berry DB 2nd, Sullins KE. Effects of topical application of antimicrobials and bandaging on healing and granulation tissue ormation in wounds of the distal aspect of the limbs in horses. *Am J Vet Res.* 2003;64:.(1):88-92.

85. Knighton D, Fiegel VD, Doucette MM. Wound repair: The growth factor revolution. In: D K, ed. *Chronic Wound Care: A Clinical Source Book for Health Care Professionals.* Wayne, PA: Health Management Publications; 1990:441-445.

86. Micheletti G. Ulcers of the lower extremities. In: Gogia PP, ed. *Clinical Wound Management.* Thorofare, NJ: Slack; 1995:100-101.

87. Porter JM, Moneta GL. International Consensus Committee on Chronic Venous Disease. Reporting standards in venous disease: An update. *J Vasc Surg.* 1995;21:635:645.

Wound Measurements and Prediction of Healing

Carrie Sussman

CHAPTER OBJECTIVES

At the completion of this chapter, the reader will be able to:
1. Explain the importance of wound measurement accuracy and consistency.
2. Apply the three most commonly used methods of wound measurement: linear, tracing, and photography, and describe the benefits and disadvantages of each.
3. Apply methods for clinical wound measurement of surface area, depth, and undermining/tunnelling, and describe the limitations of each.
4. Use wound measurements to calculate and track the rate of wound healing.
5. Use wound healing rates to predict the effectiveness of therapeutic interventions.
6. Describe the use of a validated tool that uses photography to measure wound healing.
7. Describe new technology used for measuring and reporting wound healing.

Wound measurement is an important component of wound assessment, as described in Chapter 4. Wound measurement looks quantitatively at three components: area, depth, and volume. These components are directly associated with the phases of wound healing and are therefore direct indicators of healing. As new granulation tissue develops, wound depth and volume decrease, the wound contracts, new epithelium covers the wound, and the area decreases in size.

The accuracy and consistency of measurements are critical to the objective evaluation of wounds in clinical practice and for research. Many studies and suggestions regarding the best way to measure wounds to achieve a reliable result have been published; however, no method reported is completely reliable.[1] At this point in time, there is no gold standard for wound measurement, which presents a dilemma for the wound management clinician. If the measurements are not reliable, how can the clinician ensure that the wound is healing and responding to the treatment interventions in a timely fashion?

Common methods of wound measurement using linear ruler measurements and wound tracings with planimetry are simple and easy to use. Each has its advantages, disadvantages, and level of reliability, which are discussed in this chapter, as well as complex methods applying photography. Step-by-step procedures for measuring wounds and the surrounding tissues, along with user-friendly hints and clinical "words of wisdom" are provided.

Wound volume measurements present special challenges. Although advanced technology of the future may improve their reliability, initially they will likely be too costly to implement in most wound care settings; they will probably be used first for quantifying research results more accurately with standardized measurements. However, the clinician should be aware of the direction that wound measurement is taking in order to evaluate research reports. Two currently available advanced technologies will be explained in this chapter.

Controlled clinical trials of many types of wound healing products use reduction in ulcer surface area as the dependent variable, and results are reported as a percentage of reduction in unit area per unit time (cm^2/mm^2 or %/day/week).[2] *Percentage of healing* refers to the decrease in wound area from the baseline to the day of measurement for each reevaluation period as a percentage of the wound size. The method of calculating this percentage is provided in this chapter. Percentage of healing reduction rates have been used to calculate the linear daily or weekly healing rates analyzed for different wound etiologies (pressure ulcers, venous ulcers, and diabetic ulcers). These rates are now becoming the standard predictor of whether the wound will heal, as

FIGURE 5-1 Trajectory of Healing for Healing and Non-Healing Diabetic Ulcers (Adapted from Robson MC, Hill D, Woodske M, Steed D. Wound healing trajectories as predictors of effectiveness of therapeutic agents. *Arch Surg.* July 2000;135(7):773-777.)

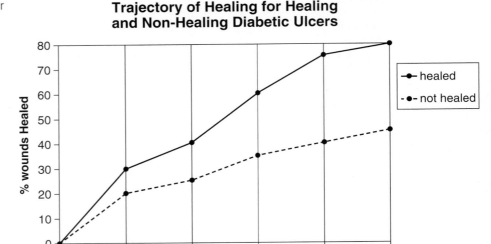

well as for comparing the results and costs of different interventions.[3–8]

Percentage of healing rates can be plotted on a graph (percentage of wound closure versus time of wound treatment) to show a trajectory of healing that identifies those patients whose wounds are on track to heal and those whose wounds are not healing. The points on the trajectory can be used as end points to compare results, rather than complete healing.[9] Figure 5-1 shows the trajectory of healing for healing and nonhealing diabetic ulcers. Preparation of a trajectory plot is included in this chapter.

Wound Location

Documenting the anatomic location of the wound is the first step in being able to reproduce measurements at that site. Record the anatomic name that clearly describes the wound location at the time of the wound measurement. For example, *trochanter* is a more precise descriptor than *hip* and signifies that the wound lies over the bony prominence. A circle over the anatomic site on the body diagram gives quick, easy identification of wound location on the completed wound measurement form.

The wound's anatomic location can be an indication of the wound etiology (Table 5-1). For example, wounds located over bony prominences are usually pressure wounds, wounds on the soles of the feet are often due to pressure and insensitivity (diabetic wounds), and wounds over the medial side of the ankle are often venous ulcers. Location also provides important information about the expected wound healing. Wounds in areas of diminished blood flow, such as over the tibia, heal slowly.

If several wounds are clustered close together in a location, they should be identified by either different letters or

TABLE 5-1   Common Locations of Chronic Wounds by Etiology

Arterial Ulcers	Pressure Ulcers	Neuropathic Ulcers	Venous Ulcers
Lower leg dorsum	Bony prominences:	Plantar surface of foot	Above the ankle
Foot	Occiput	Metatarsal heads	Medial lower leg
Malleolus	Ears	Heel	
Toe joints	Shoulder	Lateral border of foot	
Lateral border of foot	Scapulae	Midfoot deformities	
	Sacrum		
	Coccyx		
	Trochanter		
	Ischial tuberosity		
	Knees—condyles, patella		
	Tibia/fibula		
	Malleolus		
	Heel		
	Metatarsal heads		
	Toes		

EXHIBIT 5-1   Documenting Wound Location

Documenting Wound Location with Narrative Note
Example:
1. Single wound location: coccyx
2. Multiple wounds at a location:

   Initial note: *Three wounds are located upper, middle, and outer side on the right trochanter.*

The upper and middle wounds merge. Since they are upper to the outer wound, the same term upper is retained and the merger noted as in this example:

   Follow-up note: *The upper and middle wounds have merged and will in the future be referred to as the upper wound on the right trochanter.*

---

references such as *outer, inner, upper,* and *lower.* It is important to keep the same reference location ID for all of the wounds by name throughout the course of care. If one of the wounds in the cluster heals, this fact should be documented, and the same reference names for the remaining wounds should be retained for further documentation. If several wounds join together to become one, this information should be recorded, with a new ID name given to the revised wound site. Exhibit 5-1 shows an example of how to document wound location for multiple wounds.

Baseline and Subsequent Measurements

Measurement taken at the beginning of care establishes a baseline wound size; subsequent measurements are then performed at regular intervals depending on the health-care setting. For example, wound measurements are required weekly for the first four weeks in long-term care, usually every 48 hours in acute care, and at every visit in home care. The rationale for measurement is to quantify and measure the progression of wound healing and aid in predicting the treatment outcome.[10]

A policy and procedure (P&P) document concerning the frequency and method of wound measurement is necessary to set the standard for a particular facility and improve consistency across practitioners and disciplines. Comparison of wound measurements is only valuable if they are taken under the same conditions using the same methods. A standard for wound measurement also has legal and regulatory implications, since the baseline measurement and changes in wound size are the basis for judging change in wound status and compliance with regulation.

A section of the P&P can address the issue of who should perform wound measurements. For example, the policy could dictate that the baseline measurement be taken by the health professional and, after training, an unskilled individual in the home could take subsequent wound measurements and report to the skilled professional at a specified interval, such as weekly. Linear measurement of the size of the open surface area of a wound is an example of a type of measure that might be delegated to an unskilled individual. The significance of changes in wound size would be interpreted by the professional case manager.

A number of studies have found that baseline wound size, when accompanied by other risk factors for healing, is a significant predictor of response to treatment and 100% healing.[5–7,11] Larger ulcers were less likely than smaller ones to heal rapidly, even with optimal therapy; in the former case, the prognosis of the need for a longer time to heal should be documented, or a referral could be triggered.[7]

Measurements of wound size, extent, and changes are important to providers, payers, and regulators, as well as to the patient and the family. Well-documented wound measurements can be used as the best legal defense. The changes and progress toward recovery can also be considered positive feedback for the clinician, who can review the measurements and feel a sense of accomplishment. Measurements can also serve as the red flag that all is not well, triggering re-evaluation of the wound, patient, and treatment interventions. Because the information gathered is important to the interdisciplinary team, the language used requires uniform and consistent terminology to encourage good communication among the team members; such terminology is also beneficial for reimbursement.

Monitoring Wound Healing Measurements

Table 5-2 provides an overview of the three commonly used methods for monitoring wound healing.[12] The table highlights purpose, requirements, and information derived from each method. Many measurement methods and suggestions are included in this chapter, but not all will be useful in all settings. Different skills and interests will determine the methods and measurements used. Table 5-3 is a guide to the common usage patterns for wound measurements. Most clinical wound measurements are an approximation of size rather than precise measuring. Information about measuring with sophisticated computer-assisted or technologic equipment has been omitted from this chapter because these devices are usually research tools, rather than clinical practice approaches.

TABLE 5-2 Monitoring Recovery of Chronic Wounds: Photo, Tracing, Measurements

Purpose	Photo	Tracing/Planimetry	Measurements
Objective	Establishes baseline wound status and tracks changes throughout recovery	Records shape and size changes at baseline and throughout recovery	Linear: estimates size
	Wound size measurement	Wound size area	Perimeter: estimates boundary
	Records change in recovery phase or wound stage		Digitization: approximates surface area
Treatment planning	Validates overall treatment plan	Demonstrates short-term response to treatment plan	Demonstrates rate of recovery
Frequency	Baseline, weekly, or change in phase/condition, discharge	Baseline, weekly, or change in phase/condition, discharge	Baseline, weekly, or change in phase/condition, discharge
Time reference	Prospective	Prospective	Prospective
	Ongoing/interim	Ongoing/interim	Ongoing/interim

Requirements	Photo	Tracing	Measurements
Conditions	Correct light, body position, and device to indicate relative size; adjust for curvature and position	Use of standard anatomic landmarks and method to transfer tracing to medical record	Use of standard anatomic landmarks
Equipment	Camera and digial recording card or film	Tracing kit or digital tablet	Measurement tool and recording form
		Graph paper or grid	

Information	Photo and Flash	Tracing	Measurements
Type	Displays full-color picture	Gives black-and-white picture of size and shape	Provides numeric information
Comparison	Provides color comparison of phase, size, and tissue attributes	Represents topographic effects, size, and change	Summarizes quantitative changes for use in a graph
Use	Clinical medical review, program management, referral source, reports, survey team, legal, patient compliance	Clinical medical review, program management, referral source, reports, survey team, legal, self-care, patient compliance	Clinical medical review, program management, referral source, reports, survey team, legal, self-care, patient compliance

Table 5-3 Common Usage Patterns for Recording Wound Measurements

Always	Often	Sometimes	Rarely	New
L and W	Clock L X W area	Depth—greatest	Polaroid grid photo	Depth—four points of clock
L X W = area				
Tracing shape	Undermining—longest and "mapping"	Digital photography with computer technology	Stereophotography points of clock	Undermining/Tunnelling—four
Area size	Digital photo with flash	Planimetry	Video	Undermined estimate
				Area of erythema or discoloration in darkly pigmented skin
				Digital Tracing "wound map" with computed measurements

Measurement Forms

Examination and measurements must be consistent, complete, and accurate. One way to manage uniformity, consistency, and completeness is with the use of forms. Forms guide the examiner in a logical sequence and assist in organizing the information gathered. Forms can be paper-and-pencil instruments or electronic templates. They save time, because one simply completes the appropriate information on the preprinted form, which becomes a part of the documentation record.

There are numerous forms in use for documenting wound measurements. Exhibit 5-2 is a sample completed form for performing a wound measurement examination. A new form is used each week, and the forms are "tiled" onto pages of note paper with tape in the chart for easy reference to prior measurements. Keeping the measurements together in one place facilitates regular monitoring of the size changes. The

EXHIBIT 5-2   Completed Wound Measurement Form

Wound Measurements

Initial	___X___
Discharge	_____
OBWK#:	___O___
DC Status:	_____

Date: ____01/23/08_____   Patient Name: _____G. Lucky_____

Wound ID: _____R Trochanter_____   Med Rec#: _____0397_____

Wound Phase: _____Chronic inflammation_____

(all measurements in cm)

Linear Size: L(12:00–6:00) ____4.4____ X   W (3:00–9:00) _____3.3_____ = ___14.52 cm²___
Undermined: 12:00 (A1) _O_ 6:00 (A2) _0.5_   3:00 (B1) _1.5_   9:00 (B2) _O_

Overall Undermined
   Estimated Area   L + A1 + A2   X W + B1 + B2   = UEA
   (UEA):   (a) __4.9 (overall length)___ X (b) _4.8 (overall width)__   = __23.52 cm²__

Depth   12:00 _O___
              3:00 _0.3__
              6:00 _O___
              9:00 _O___

Erythema   12:00–6 :00 __6.5 cm__   X   3:00–9:00 __4.5 cm__   area = _29.25 cm²_
   (measured across wound surface)

Examiner: _____B Sweet, PT_____   (OBWK = the observation week # since start of care)

---

sample form uses the clock method (see below) for monitoring wound depth and undermining, and includes the following items:

- Wound anatomic location (called the *wound ID*)
- Size, including length by width open area, length by width area of erythema (color change), depth, undermining/tunneling, and overall wound size estimate (explained below)
- Period of the wound assessment: initial, interim observation week number (OB), and discharge (DC)
- Information about the wound healing phase (initials are inserted next to *wound phase* to identify the current wound phase—*I* for inflammatory, *P* for proliferative, and *E* for epithelialization, as described in Chapter 4)
- Discharge outcome status (healed or not healed)

The sample form works well when used in conjunction with the Sussman Wound Healing Tool (SWHT),[13] described in Chapter 6. Data can be entered into a computer database and program outcomes monitored.

Wound Size Measurement Accuracy and Reliability

Accurate, complete, uniform, and consistent wound measurements are required to establish a wound diagnosis, plan treatment, and document results. Careful measurement

records even small changes and shows improved wound status or deterioration.

Ways to maximize accuracy of wound size measurement include the following:

- Define specific procedures to determine the wound edge, total wound area, and description of areas of necrotic tissue (i.e., percentage of wound area).
- Be consistent. Take the measurement the same way each time from a noted reference point on the body; meaningful comparisons can only be made if a standardize measurement system is used.
- Use the same terminology and units of measure for each measurement.
- When possible, have the same person take repeat measurements.
- When possible, use an assistant to record measurements as they are taken and help position the patient.
- Use a prepared form, and fill in a measurement number at each space indicated on the form. This form can be preprinted or handwritten so nothing is forgotten. Record as soon as each parameter is measured; memory is not accurate.
- Record a zero if a characteristic is assessed and found absent to confirm that you observed the characteristic and assessed it. For example, partial-thickness wounds are superficial, so a zero should be written next to the depth measures spaces. A blank space does not show that this characteristic was assessed.

Wound Size Measurements

Measurements that track changes in wound size over time are described in this section, including surface area (SA) measurements (length multiplied by width), undermining or tunnels, and depth.

The most common wound measurements are length and width, which are measured from wound edge to wound edge. The wound edge is described by Schultz et al as nonadvancing or undermined.[14] Well-defined edges are clear and distinct, and can easily be outlined on a transparent piece of plastic. Edges that are not attached to the base of the wound imply a wound with some depth of tissue involvement (*Color Plate 33*). Chapter 6 more fully describes wound edges and their significance.

The *greatest length and greatest width method* of measurement refers to measurement across the diameter of the greatest length and greatest width of the wound. The length is multiplied by the width, which gives the estimated square area (SA) of the wound. The product is a single number that can be easily monitored for change in size. These two dimensions are always measured and can be the only measurement recorded. Less frequently measured are undermining/tunnels and depth.

The *clock method* is another way to measure wounds in which the face of a clock is used to guide the measurement. Select a 12:00 reference position on the wound; this position is usually toward the head of the body. Then, take the measurement from 12:00 to 6:00 and from 3:00 to 9:00. In situations such as severe contractures of the trunk and lower extremities, it may be more convenient and easier to reproduce the measurements if another convenient anatomic landmark is selected. For example, measurements in the foot may use the heel or toes as the 12:00 reference point. In a fetally contracted person, a trochanteric pressure ulcer may be more easily tracked if the 12:00 reference point is toward the knee.

The directions for measuring wound size on the NPUAP Pressure Ulcer Scale for Healing (Chapter 6) use a combination of the clock method and the greatest length and greatest width method. The directions specify using the longest length and the diameter perpendicular to it. Then, multiply length by width for surface area. Figure 5-2 is a graphic representation of measuring methods.

All of the described measurement methods are acceptable and widely used. It is important to remember two things when multiplying length by width to find wound surface area:

1. The geometric formula for the area of a rectangle (length times width), which is an approximation of the surface area, has been estimated to inflate the size of the wound by as much as 44% if the wound is irregularly shaped and large.[14]
2. All wound shapes are irregular so assume that this measurement will be inflated.

Choose a method that you are comfortable with and record which method is used. Then, use this method *consistently*. Exhibit 5-3 lists advantages and disadvantages of the clock method and the greatest length and greatest width method.

Supplies

Supplies needed for wound measurement should be assembled in advance to improve efficiency and reduce examiner and patient fatigue (see "Helpful Hints for Measuring"). These supplies include:

- Pen or pencil
- Disposable, plastic straight-edge ruler with linear measure ruled in centimeters
- Disposable gloves
- Normal saline
- Disposable syringe with 18-gauge needle or angiocatheter (for cleaning)
- Gauze paper, form, or pocket-sized notebook to record data (see Exhibit 5-2)

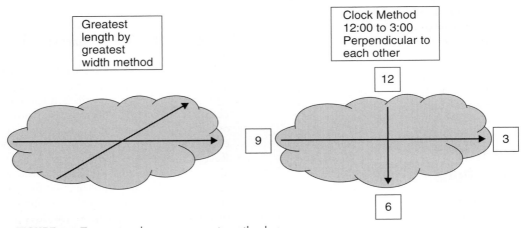

FIGURE 5-2 Two wound measurement methods.

EXHIBIT 5-3   Comparison of Two Wound Measurement Methods

Greatest Length by Greatest Width Method
Advantages
- Simple and easy to learn and use
- Most common method
- Reliable

Disadvantages
- Diameters change as size and shape change, so different diameters are measured each time
- Wound open area will be larger than in clock method

Clock Method
Advantages
- Simple and easy to learn and use
- Tracks same place on the wound over time
- More conservative measure of area

Disadvantages
- Requires more steps to perform
- More precision required to line up wound points along the clock "face"
- Less commonly used

How to Measure

Before measuring, the wound should be cleaned and examined closely. Look carefully at the edges to determine whether they are distinct so that you can measure from wound edge to wound edge. Take the following steps:

1. Position the patient.
2. Don gloves and remove wound dressing and packing.
3. Place dressing and packing in disposable infectious waste bag.
4. Clean wound with normal saline and syringe with 18-gauge needle or angiocatheter (see Chapter 9 for wound cleansing procedure).
5. Take measurements with disposable wound measurement ruler.
6. Measure the SA at greatest length and greatest width from wound edge to wound edge.
7. Record each measurement *as it is taken.*
8. Dispose of measurement instrument and gloves in infectious waste container.
9. Dispose of syringe with 18-gauge needle in sharps container.
10. Apply fresh dressing.
11. Calculate wound surface area.
12. Repeat weekly or more frequently, if indicated.

When using the clock method to measure surface area, replace step 6 above with the following (everything else remains the same):

6a. Establish the 12:00 position by choosing an anatomic landmark that is easy to identify and document it for all following measurements (example: ✓ 12:00 toward head).

6b. Mark 12:00 with arrow on the skin. Repeat with marks at 6:00, 3:00, and 9:00.
6c. Measure from wound edge at 12:00 to wound edge at 6:00 position.
6d. Measure from wound edge at 3:00 to wound edge at 9:00 position.

CLINICAL WISDOM

Using a Template to Improve Measurement Accuracy

To improve accuracy and better align the measurements, cut a circle from paper folded in half twice and mark the four clock points at the four paper folds. Place the circle over the wound to use as a template or guide, taping it to the peri-wound skin to keep it from shifting.[15] Take all measurements with the template in place to uniformly track the same wound locations for surface area, undermining, and depth (Figure 5-3).

Measurement of Undermining and Tunneling

Measurements of undermining (erosion under the wound edge) and tunnelling (a sinus) indicate the extent of wound damage into surrounding deep tissue. This condition occurs in an unknown number of wounds. It is often the consequence of wound debridement, i.e., when a body of necrotic tissue is removed, the fascial planes can separate during the probing action. Tunneling can progress to become a sinus tract and a pathway for infection. For this reason, any measurement of undermining and tunnelling requires careful, gentle probing to avoid further separation of the fascial planes. Some wound experts claim that the true extent of a wound is not known unless the undermining/tunnelling parameter is measured.[16] Figure 5-5 shows the difference in wound size when this parameter is measured and an undermined estimate of the total wound area is calculated, compared with measurement of the surface area alone. *Color Plates 37–38* demonstrate the extent of the tunnelling process in a trochanteric pressure ulcer. A measurement of extensive tunnelling is a red flag that indicates the urgent need to contact the physician and report the finding.

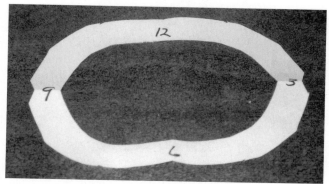

FIGURE 5-3 Using a template to improve measurement accuracy.

In a principal component analysis of the Pressure Ulcer Scale for Healing (PUSH) (See Chapter 6), the addition of a tunnelling measurement did not improve the validity and reliability of that tool; therefore, the measurement is not part of the tool components.[16] Facilities and health-care organizations need to determine if the measurement of undermining and tunnelling should be part of wound documentation and thus included in the wound care policies and procedures.

Three methods for measuring undermining and tunneling are described below. Choose one and use it consistently (see *Color Plates 39* and *40*).

Method 1

1. Map undermining around the *entire* wound perimeter by inserting a moist, cotton-tipped applicator into the length of the undermined/tunneled space and continuing around the perimeter. Dip the cotton tip into normal saline before insertion so it slides in easier and is less likely to cause tissue trauma (Figure 5-4).
2. At the end point, *do not force* further entry, but gently push upward until there is a bulge in the skin. Mark the points on the skin with a pen and connect them. Measure the length and width, and multiply these measurements to calculate the *overall undermined estimate* (explained below).

Method 2

1. The Sussman method for wound measurement applies the four cardinal points of the clock method to measurement of undermining and tunneling.[12] The 12:00 position is toward the head unless otherwise noted (see section on clock method of measurement, above).
2. Wet the cotton-tipped applicator with normal saline and insert gently into tunnel. Mark the place on the skin

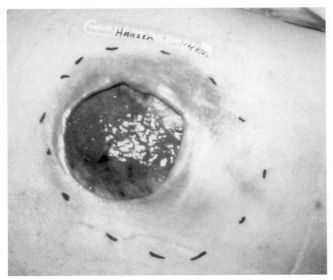

FIGURE 5-4 Mapping undermining around the entire wound perimeter. (Courtesy of Evonne Fowler, MN, RN, CETN.)

where the cotton tip causes a bulge, and withdraw the cotton-tipped applicator.
3. Grip the cotton-tipped applicator at the point at which the skin and wound edge meet, and withdraw it. This is the length of the tunnel.
4. Place the length of the cotton-tipped applicator up to the withdrawal point against a centimeter ruler or measure from wound edge to mark on skin as in method 1. Record the length measurement.

Method 3

1. Test the perimeter for undermining with a cotton-tipped applicator, and then select the longest tunnel to measure.
2. Use the clock method to identify the location(s) on the wound perimeter where tunneling is present, and then track the tunnel over time.

RESEARCH WISDOM

Accuracy and Reliability of Wound Undermining Measurements

Taylor[15] studied the variability of measurements of wound undermining among physical therapists trained in the Sussman wound undermining measurement method. Her findings show that the most significant variation occurred when the 12:00 position coincided with the greatest length of the wound's open surface area, which inflated the area measurements.

The results of studying measurements by 39 physical therapists over a 4-week period demonstrated several interesting findings. Three common errors occurred: misreading the measuring device, transferring the numbers, and calculating. As would be expected, there were more errors in measurement when the wounds were smaller. Overall, the coefficient of variation for open wound area measurements was 5% or less for intrarater replication for 69% of the physical therapists, and between 5% and 10% for the remaining therapists. The wound overall estimate had intertester variance of 10.5% or less for 100% of the study participants. Validation of the measuring technique was proven highly reliable, suggesting that this measurement can be used to document progress in the healing of undermined wounds.[15]

Overall Undermined Estimated Size

Undermining and tunnelling add to the extent of tissue involved in the wound. The linear measurement of the extent of wound undermining/tunnelling at the same four points on the clock is added to the SA length and width, becoming the overall length and overall width. Next, the overall length is multiplied by the overall width to derive an estimate of the *overall undermined estimated size* of the wound area (calculation below).[12] The product is a single number that can be monitored and graphed to show the trajectory of healing over time, as shown in Figure 5-5. This figure also shows graphically how the overall undermined estimated size compares with the SA estimate.[12] If only the open surface area is monitored for change in size, the wound appears significantly smaller than it actually is, and information about incremental changes in size is lost.

HELPFUL HINTS

Measuring

1. Wound Measurement Kit

   If wound measurements are taken frequently, assemble a kit made up of the supplies in the supplies list on page 128 for wound measurement. Keep it with you in a small plastic carrier.

2. Use an Assistant

   An assistant is helpful to:
   - Position patient
   - Comfort patient
   - Record measurements
   - Control wound "sagging" (see below)
   - Seek additional supplies or assistance

3. Patient Positioning

   It is easier for everyone if both the patient and measurer are comfortable during the procedure. Some patients and some wounds are difficult to position for accurate measurement. Once a convenient and comfortable position is found, record the position that works best. This will save time and effort and improve the uniformity of measurements over time.

   Example: Coccyx wound—position: right side-lying; heel wound—position: left side-lying.

4. Order of Measuring

   If measurements are always taken in the same order, the tracking of wound size will be more consistent. Take the length first, and the width second. If the clock method is used, take measurements in the 12:00, 6:00, 3:00, and 9:00 order for consistency.

5. Controlling Sagging Wounds

   Full-thickness wounds with undermining can sag from lack of subcutaneous support and the pull of gravity. Tension on the tissue is hard to maintain. Try to keep sagging to a minimum and maintain uniform tension for accurate length and width measurements.

6. Wound Measurement Recording Form (see Exhibit 5-2)

   A preprinted form is useful to guide consistency of wound measurements. The small sheets can be taped to a large sheet and placed in the medical record in a cascading fashion; in this way, numbers do not have to be rewritten, and errors are avoided. Measurements can also be entered into a computer, which is much more reliable than writing measurements on scraps of paper. A notebook is also useful to collect forms in one place.

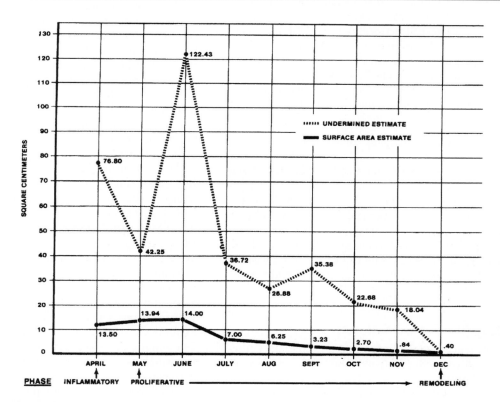

66-YEAR-OLD FEMALE
WOUND TYPE: PRESSURE WOUND
LOCATION: LEFT HIP

FIGURE 5-5 Wound healing trajectory: recovery of a pressure wound.

Extent of Wounding

Other information can be gleaned from the trajectory graph in Figure 5-5, for example, note the significant variations in the extent of the wound between May and July. However, notice the linear reduction in wound extent from September to December. As the wound healed, undermined/tunneled spaces closed, tissue integrity was restored, and the overall size was reduced. Graphing can also show how changes in the undermined estimate parallel the changes in wound phase. Note the abrupt jump in wound overall undermined estimate from 42.25 cm to 122.43 cm; this frequently coincides with the early proliferative phase. The expansion of the wound extent reflects the effects of wound debridement on loss of subcutaneous tissue integrity (the separation of fascial planes), producing tunneling. Loss of subcutaneous tissue integrity produces increased risk of infection, but subcutaneous tissue integrity is restored as the wound progresses through the proliferative phase to the remodeling phase.

Graphing the Trajectory of Healing

Graphs showing the wound healing trajectory, such as the one shown in Figure 5-5, are a very useful visual method for monitoring healing over time. The graph can be generated as part of a database program or manually drawn on graph paper. Graphing to visualize wound healing or deterioration is recommended for tracking the scores obtained using the Pressure Ulcer Scale for Healing (PUSH) tool (see Chapter 6). Recently, the wound healing trajectory has been suggested as a method for tracking significant points along the continuum of healing, rather than a single end point, when determining the efficacy of treatment interventions.[9]

Creating a trajectory of healing involves the following basic steps:

1. Perform the size measurements following a defined protocol.
2. Calculate the total wound area (cm²) or the percentage change in size.
3. Plot the wound healing curve on a graph. This requires two axes: horizontal and vertical. The horizontal axis represents time, and the vertical axis represents size in square centimeters or percentage of change. Time should be graphed at consistent intervals (e.g., weekly, with the baseline week 0). See Figures 5-5 and 5-6 for examples.

Calculating the Overall Estimate

1. Add the length of the SA from 12:00 to 6:00 to the undermined lengths at both 12:00 and 6:00. This is the overall length of the wound.
2. Add the width of the SA from 3:00 to 9:00 to the undermined lengths at both 3:00 and 9:00. This is the overall width of the wound.
3. Multiply the overall length by the overall width.
4. Document the overall size estimate of the wound.

Example: Overall Size Estimate

12:00–6:00 length + 12:00 undermining
+ 6:00 undermining = overall length

3:00–9:00 width + 3:00 undermining
+ 9:00 undermining = overall width

Overall length X overall width = overall estimated area

Wound Healing Rates as Predictors of Effectiveness of Therapeutic Interventions

Percentage reduction in wound size—rather than the actual size measurements—is a valid and useful method for predicting wound healing rates and tracking the healing of pressure ulcers, venous ulcers, and diabetic ulcers.[4,17,18] Two clinical studies found that full-thickness pressure ulcers that decreased 47% and 39% in size during the first 2 weeks of treatment were much more likely to heal and were distinguishable from those that did not heal.[3,4,19] Other clinical studies looked at leg ulcers for predictors of healing and found that a > 30% reduction in ulcer area after 2 weeks of treatment was a significant predictor of healing.[11,20] Phillips et al did a retrospective study of prognostic factors for venous ulcer healing. They found that ulcers with at least 40% healing by week 3 predicted more than 70% of the outcomes correctly. Kantor and Margolis report that the percentage of change in area over the first 4 weeks of treatment represents a practical and predictive measure of complete wound healing.[8] Sheehan and colleagues who studied diabetic foot ulcers found that ulcers with a 50% reduction in size at 4 weeks healed in 82% of patients, compared with those with a percent change of 25%, which failed to heal. Of equal importance, the sensitivity of the finding of 50% reduction was 91%, and the negative predictive value was also 91%. The high negative predictive value indicates that those who do not fall in the healer group have a high prediction for not healing.[18]

The conclusion supported by these studies is that pressure ulcers and leg ulcers (venous and diabetic) that do not reduce in size between 30% and 50% in a 2-week to 4-week period are not on a healing trend and are less likely to heal than ulcers that do reduce by these amounts. The clinician can calculate the percentage of change of the wound and use these numbers for comparison. Plotting the percentage of change on a graph will create a trajectory that shows whether the wound is following a course for healing or for nonhealing (see Figure 5-5). Review of the percentage of change becomes a pivotal clinical decision point that can be extremely valuable in the early identification of patients who require more aggressive and possibly more expensive interventions than those who are likely to heal with standard care.

Healing rates have additional implications for prediction of healing outcomes. Kantor and Margolis compared the healing rates of diabetic and venous ulcers and found that after 20 weeks of proper wound care, approximately 31% of diabetic neuropathic ulcers and 63% of venous ulcers will

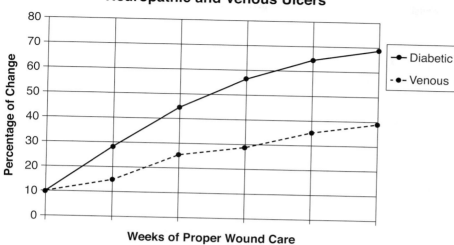

Trajectory of Healing for Diabetic Neuropathic and Venous Ulcers

FIGURE 5-6 Trajectory showing expected healing rates for venous and diabetic neuropathic ulcers. (Adapted with permission from Kantor J, Margolis DJ. Expected Healing Rates for Chronic Wounds. *Wounds: A compendium of clinical research and practice.* November/December 2000;12(6):155-158.

heal.[8] This study highlighted the differences in the rates of healing between venous and diabetic neuropathic ulcers. Venous ulcers showed an apparent healing rate that was twice that of diabetic ulcers for at least the first 12–16 weeks of treatment. Another finding was that wound duration, which has been identified as a risk factor for not healing, did not significantly slow the healing rates when compared with diabetic foot ulcers. Trajectory of healing from this study is shown in Figure 5-6.

It is clear that the precision of wound measurement and the method of calculating the rate of change can influence research outcomes and clinical decisions. Clinicians today are responsible for setting the goals of treatment and differentiating wounds that will go on to heal with standard care from those that should be triaged to adjunctive therapy.

CLINICAL WISDOM

Healing Rates

Healing rates should not be used to predict a specific anticipated healing date because factors that effect healing cannot be controlled. The rates should be used to help clinical decision making and identify effective and ineffective treatments. Accurate measurement of wound size is the basis for reliable predicting.

Application of Healing Rates

Clinicians must understand healing rate reporting, the method of calculation, and its application because of its newly identified importance. As described, the percentage of healing per unit of time (PHT), usually per week, is a valid way to identify healing and nonhealing wounds. PHT now appears as a frequent outcome measure in research reports, where it has been identified as a predictor of healing or nonhealing wounds.[2-4,7,11,20,21]

Methods of using PHT vary (see Exhibit 5-4 for an example.) The percentage of reduction in area from baseline calculation method presented here is the calculation method used to measure healing. However, this method can exaggerate the progress made by larger wounds relative to smaller ones, and the percentage of reduction in area can minimize the actual progress made by large wounds relative to the progress made in small wounds.[18] Wounds of different sizes and shapes present special problems. To compensate for these problems, Gilman[22] proposed a formula for measuring the wound perimeter change over time (Exhibit 5-5). The Gilman formula should be used if the population studied has a diversity of ulcer sizes.[21]

Margolis and colleagues[21] found the Gilman method of measurement useful for reporting the results of healing for venous ulcers, and they compared their results with those of other researchers looking at venous ulcers and diabetic leg ulcers. In all of the studies, the results were nearly identical: Venous ulcers that healed in 4 weeks or more had an initial healing rate of 0.049–0.065 cm/week, and diabetic ulcers had a rate of 0.063cm/week, suggesting that there may be a fairly uniform rate of healing for chronic ulcers, regardless of etiology.[21] Because repairing wounds appear to heal at the same rate, there should be no correlation between initial ulcer size and the rate of healing. Margolis et al[21] suggested using the 0.062 cm/week rate of healing for all chronic ulcers and recommended that a 4-week period be sufficient to establish a healing trend.

Before this recommendation can be used as a standard for all chronic wounds, consider the findings of Frantz and colleagues.[23] In an unpublished but reported study of pressure ulcers measured with stereophotogrammetry (SPG), they found that the trajectory for healing differed for partial-thickness and full-thickness ulcers. Linear advancement of the wound margin was 0.056 mm/day (0.0392 cm/week) for partial-thickness ulcers and 0.021 mm/day (0.0147 cm/week)

EXHIBIT 5-4   Calculating Percentage Rate of Change in Wound Size

One interesting way to determine how a wound is progressing is to look at the percentage rate of change. This is also an effective way to measure and predict successful outcomes. Percentage rate of change is a simple statistical calculation that uses the following formula:
1. Baseline (week 0) wound size (OA or overall OA size) measurement is used as the original size.
2. Subtract the next wound size OA or overall OA size measurement (interim) taken from the baseline.
3. Divide by baseline wound measurement and multiply by 100%.

Formula for computing rate of change in wound open area:

$$\frac{\text{Baseline open area (OA)} - \text{Interim open area (OA)}}{\text{Baseline open area}} \times 100\%$$

Example:

Wound open area (OA) baseline week 0	= 30 cm^2
Wound open area (OA) week 1 (interim)	= 28 cm^2
OA baseline – OA week 1 (interim)	= 30 – 28 = 2
Divide the remainder by the baseline OA	= 2/30 = 0.066
Multiply 0.066 X 100%	= 6.6% = Percentage rate of change

Note: A weekly percentage of change would use the prior week's size measurement instead of baseline. Wound size often changes significantly from week to week in the early phases of healing, and then the rate slows. Referring to the percentage rate of change on a weekly or biweekly basis is a reliable measure of how the wound is healing.

for full-thickness ulcers. Median time to healing for the partial thickness ulcers was 28 days, and it was 56 days for full-thickness ulcers. These findings suggest that norms for duration and rate of healing are specific to the level of tissue injury. More research on the rate of healing of a large population sample with chronic wounds is needed to substantiate the trend before using these numbers as benchmarks for the rate of healing for all chronic wounds (Exhibit 5-6).

Tallman et al[6] found that using initial wound size as the baseline for percentage of change in size calculation to determine the weekly healing rate gave healing rate instability from week to week, which decreased the ability to predict complete healing. They created another method to compare healing rates, which takes the mean of all previous healing rates between each visit (which becomes the mean adjusted healing rate) and uses that rate as the baseline size to calculate the percentage of change. This method improved healing rate stability from week to week and allowed pre-

diction of complete healing as early as 3 weeks from start of therapy ($p < .001$).[6] However, the sample in Tallman's study was small, including 15 elderly adults.

Polansky and vanRijswijk[2] suggest using the *median* time of healing for study groups, rather than the *mean* time to plot healing time curves. Median time is the time by which at least one-half of the patients have healed. The healing time curve provides a "moving picture" of healing and is developed using the Kaplan-Meir method called *survival analysis*. This methodology is particularly useful when there is a large study population and a significant number of patients who do not complete the entire study course; it may also be useful for prediction of healing of individual wounds.[9]

These healing time curves provide more information about healing than looking at the proportion of the population healed at the end of a study. Robson et al showed that healing trajectories are significantly different for healers

EXHIBIT 5-5   Gilman Method of Measuring Wound Healing Using the Wound Perimeter

$\bar{d} = \Delta A \bar{p}$

$\bar{d}$ = units of distance; $\bar{d}$ represents the average distance of advance of the wound margin over the study time T, in a direction toward the wound center

ΔA = the difference in area of the wound before and after the study time T

$\bar{p}$ = the average perimeter before and the wound perimeter after time T

Reprinted with permission from T.H. Gilman, Parameter for Measurement of Wound Closure, *Wounds: A Compendium of Research and Practice*, 1990;2(3):95–101. Health Management Publications.

EXHIBIT 5-6   Factors that Significantly Affect Healing Outcomes

- Initial surface area size: Larger ulcers take longer to heal.[4,7]
- Duration: Ulcers of short duration are most likely to heal.[7]
- Healing rate: A 30%–50% reduction in area size in the first 2–4 weeks predicts healing.[3,4,7,18]
- Circulation: Moderate arterial insufficiency (ankle-brachial index (0.5–0.8) increases risk of delayed healing.[5]
- Nutrition: Full-thickness pressure ulcers heal faster with proper nutrition.[4]

and nonhealers with diabetic ulcers (see Figure 5-1)[9]. Shifting of the wound healing trajectory from an impaired course to a more ideal course can be one way to evaluate the efficacy of the treatment plan. For more information about the measurement methods involved in doing survival analysis for wound healing in a clear and relatively easy-to-understand way, readers are encouraged to read the Polansky and vanRijswijk article.[2]

The healing rates for chronic wounds can be put into perspective when they are compared with the healing rates for acute wounds. Ramirez et al looked at the rate of healing of acute surgical wounds in normal adults in 1969.[24] The average surgical wound size was 10 cm^2, and there was a 50% reduction in wound size in 13 days, for an estimated healing rate of 0.37cm^2 per day. Wound closure was achieved in 21 days. Gilman calculated that this healing rate is about six times faster than chronic wounds make when making good progress.[25]

RESEARCH WISDOM

Healing rate during the first four weeks of observation has been validated as a predictor of healing outcome and is steady over the course of healing for venous, diabetic, and pressure ulcers.[3,4,6,7,17,21,26-28]

Measurement of Wound Depth

Wound depth is defined as the distance from the visible skin surface to the wound bed.[29] Initially wound depth is correlated with the depth/extent of tissue damage, and several staging systems use depth to categorize wound severity (see Chapter 4). As the wound heals, measurement of wound depth is a crude method of tracking the growth of granulation tissue in the wound base of deep wounds. It is also a way to measure early healing progress that may otherwise be missed, since depth reduction usually precedes the reduction in wound surface area.[30,31] Reduction in wound depth is accomplished through the formation of scar tissue that does *not* represent replacement of the tissue destroyed.

When measuring wound depth, it is common practice to try to find the deepest site in the wound bed. This method is difficult to reproduce from measurement to measurement because the wound bed fills in irregularly; what is the deepest spot one time may not be the same spot at the next measurement. Depth measurement accuracy is limited, regardless of how this measurement is made; however, the clock method allows for consistency in the measurement site that can be more closely reproduced at subsequent tests than the use of a single "deepest spot" method. There is controversy, especially among researchers, about the usefulness of depth measurements because of the inaccuracies recorded.[32]

Instead of a quantitative measurement of wound depth, some wound measurement tools observe the layers of tissue lost and rank the loss by an increasing numeric score that corresponds to greater depth of tissue lost. For example, a superficial ulcer may have a score of 1. A full-thickness wound with tissue loss to the bone may have a score of 4 or 5. Using the clock method for measuring wound depth is suggested as a method of tracking changes in depth at specific locations around the wound bed.[12] Reliability has not been validated. Recent rationale for considering a change in wound depth is the observation that "pocketing" at the bottom of a wound is a clinical indicator of critical wound colonization or infection. (See Chapter 6 Tools to Measure Wound Healing.)

The Clock Method

1. Cleanse the wound thoroughly before measuring.
2. Take depth measurements at the 12:00, 3:00, 6:00, and 9:00 positions.
3. Insert a cotton-tipped applicator perpendicular to the wound edge.
4. Hold the stick of the applicator with fingers at the wound skin surface edge.
5. Holding this position on the applicator stick, place applicator stick along a centimeter-ruled edge. Record for each of the four positions.
6. These depth measurements may or may *not* be at the deepest area of the wound.
7. A separate measurement may be taken and noted at the deepest area.

Partial-thickness wounds have a depth of less than 0.2 cm. Wounds with >0.2 cm depth are difficult to measure and should be recorded as > 0.2 cm. Measure the depth of full-thickness wounds of greater than 0.2 cm depth. When a wound is undergoing debridement of nonviable tissue, the wound depth usually increases; as the wound bed fills with granulation tissue, the depth decreases. Reduction in wound depth is a measurement of progression through the proliferative phase of healing.

Measuring Wound Volume

Measurement of wound volume is difficult and usually limited to research studies. Two methods of measuring wound volume have been reported. One method involves filling the wound with a measured amount of normal saline from a syringe. This works best for wounds that can be positioned horizontally so the liquid does not spill out. Still, accuracy is questionable because the amount of fluid absorbed by wound tissue or left in the wound cannot be measured.[33] Another method involves the use of Jeltrate, an alginate hydrocolloid used by dentists. By pouring the rapidly setting plastic into the wound, a mold of the wound is made. Jeltrate is reported to be well-tolerated by the wound tissue.[32] Regardless of which method of measuring wound volume is used, there are significant inaccuracies. Use of this parameter of measurement appears to be most appropriate in the research arena and of less value to the clinician.[32] Studies cited earlier in this chapter appear to support the idea that measurement of depth or volume may be superfluous, since percentage of change calculations based on surface have demonstrated validity for tracking healing.

Measurement of Surrounding Skin Erythema

Erythema of the skin surrounding a wound can be a measure of the inflammation phase of healing or a sign of infection. Chronic wounds often show a halo of erythema but lack the other signs of inflammation. The periwound erythema can be identified as unblanchable (See Chapter 4) redness or a darkening of the skin in darkly pigmented skin (see *Color Plates 19 and 20*). The "Clinical Wisdom" below addresses measurement of erythema in darkly pigmented skin. Streaking or significant signs of erythema projecting out a distance from the wound can indicate cellulitis, and medical measures are warranted. Measurement can be taken using the greatest length and greatest width method or the clock method.

The Clock Method

Supplies. Assemble all equipment needed:

- Two acetate measuring guides or one each plastic wrap over wound, topped by measuring guide
- Two pieces of plastic wrap, cut in approximately 6 in X 8 in pieces or larger, if wound plus periwound erythema is larger
- Fine-point transparent film-type marking pen so that ink won't bead up on the plastic (dark Pentel™ or Vis-a-Vis™)
- Paper towel, folded in half lengthwise
- Paper or graph form
- Transparent tape

How to Measure

1. Measure across the wound surface area from the 12:00 to the 6:00 position and to the outer margin of the periwound erythema.
2. Measure across the wound surface area from the 3:00 to the 9:00 position and to the outer margin of the periwound erythema.
3. Compute the periwound area of erythema.

Estimated Area of Erythema

12:00 to 6:00 length X 3:00 to 9:00 width = _____ cm^2

Example: 9:0 cm X 6.0 cm = 54 cm^2

Wound Tracings

Making a wound tracing, also known as the acetate method, is a popular and practical method for measuring wound area. A tracing is a drawing of the wound shape. Repeated tracings show changes in the size and shape of a wound over the course of recovery. When the tracing is made on metric graph paper, it is called *planimetry*. This method is most useful on wounds that are on flat surfaces, and it has limited usefulness for full-thickness wounds. Greater reliability using this method has been found for wounds with edges that begin to approximate over a bed of granulation tissue.[34] It is easy to learn, inexpensive, readily available, and requires minimal training.[35]

The method of measuring the wound area from transparency tracings and placing it on graph paper to determine

Measurement of Erythema in Darkly Pigmented Skin

Skin color changes reported by clinicians and in the literature[27] indicate that, when inflamed, the skin color of darkly pigmented individuals darkens to an eggplant/purplish color (see *Color Plates 19 and 20*). It can be difficult to differentiate darkening of inflammation from hemosiderin staining. When this is the case, proceed with temperature and edema examinations. For a full description of the assessment of darkly pigmented skin, see Chapter 3.

The following are guidelines for measuring the extent of inflammation/trauma in darkly pigmented skin:

- Use natural light or halogen light, not fluorescent light.
- Outline the margins of color change on the surrounding skin with a marking pen.
- Select a reference point for future measures.
- Measure using the greatest length and the greatest width or the clock method.
- Calculate the area of color change (as described for all length-by-width measurements).

size by counting the centimeters has shown high intratester and intertester reliability (0.99). Compared with linear measurements with a ruler, there is less overestimation of the real wound area, although some error can be expected. Using 1 cm graph paper to count squares has been reported to be quick and efficient.[34,36]

Tracings can be made on acetate measuring sheets supplied by manufacturers for this purpose or household plastic wrap with a plastic transparency marking pen (the ink does not bead up). Tracings taped to a sheet of paper can be stored in the patient record. However, because these tracings can come loose or become ragged, the tracing and form can be photocopied, with the photocopy stored in the chart.

Langemo and colleagues[34] compared the standard error of measurement for wounds of different shapes using four techniques: linear ruler length and width, planimetry, stereophotogrammetry (SPG) length and width, and SPG area. Both length and width measurements best measured circular wounds, tracing worked best for pear-shaped wounds, and SPG had the lowest standard error of measurement for L-shaped wounds. SPG incorporates the use of enhanced digital photography with a computer system using Wound Measurement System software (see Resources section at the end of this chapter).

Accuracy of measurement with the tracing method depends on how carefully the wound edges are followed as the tracing is drawn. Kloth and Feedar documented measurements using this method for patients in a research study.[37] Sussman suggested applying tracings to a graph form with a key for tissue assessment called *wound recovery form* for clinical practice reporting wound healing progression.[38]

Following are ways that tracings can be used:

- Tracings show change in the wound perimeter shape over time. Wound shape is a helpful indicator of the rate of healing. As described in Chapter 2, linear wounds contract rapidly, square or rectangular wounds contract at a moderate pace, and circular wounds contract slowly.[36]

- When placed on a metric graph form (planimetry), tracings show the wound size, as well as the shape of the healing wound (Exhibit 5-7).
- A tracing can become a "wound map," showing features of the wound bed, such as necrotic tissue, and adjacent

tissue characteristics, such as erythema (see Exhibit 5-7). Household plastic wrap is better than a grid sheet for this because it is clear.
- When placed on metric graph paper, features such as the *actual* amount of undermining/tunneling around the wound perimeter can be drawn on the wound map using the actual measurements and a ruler.
- The wound map tracing becomes the document on which assessment findings of tissue attributes are recorded. A

EXHIBIT 5-7   Wound Recovery Form with Tracing

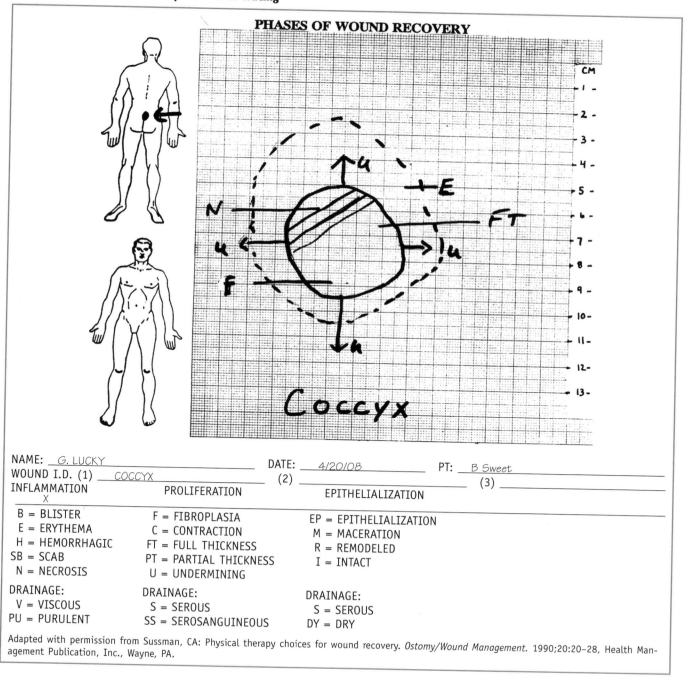

Adapted with permission from Sussman, CA: Physical therapy choices for wound recovery. *Ostomy/Wound Management.* 1990;20:20–28, Health Management Publication, Inc., Wayne, PA.

map key at the bottom of the graph form assigns letters to each tissue attribute, making this an easy way to describe the tissue in the drawing. The tracing is a paper-and-pencil instrument to track wound healing over time. *Note:* The tissue attributes on the wound recovery form are the same as those represented in the SWHT described in Chapter 6.

- The wound tracing can be scanned into a computer, making a digitized measurement of the wound. The area can be calculated, and the tracing can be stored on the computer.

How to Make a Wound Tracing

1. Place two acetate measuring guides or two pieces of plastic wrap over wound so that the bottom piece fits across the wound from 3:00 to 9:00, and the top piece fits from 12:00 to 6:00. This arrangement helps when separating the top layer from the bottom layer. Smooth each piece of plastic to remove wrinkles. Two layers are used to prevent contamination of the layer on which the tracing is made. The layer that was in contact with the wound is discarded with infectious waste after the tracing is completed.
2. Draw an arrow on the plastic wrap in the location and direction of the 12:00 position.
3. Trace the wound edges.

CLINICAL WISDOM

Tracings on Plastic Sandwich Bags

A plastic sandwich bag can be placed over the wound and a tracing can be made on the top layer, with the bottom layer of the bag acting as a wound barrier. Slit the bag in half and discard the contaminated layer with infectious waste. The top layer can be put on a graph form or placed in a zippered sandwich bag to keep for comparison measurements. This method is very useful for home care.

Optional Additions to Tracings

1. Draw any notable features within or around the wound surface area, such as an outline of the necrotic tissue or exposed bone. Label the features with a letter from the wound recovery form key.[26]
2. Mark areas of erythema or darkened darkly pigmented skin with broken lines around the wound surface area.
3. Mark areas of necrotic tissue or eschar with diagonal lines.
4. Mark other features with circles and dots, and label them with letters.
5. Place the tracing so that the 12:00 arrow is in the conventional 12:00 position on the graph form, and tape it onto the graph form. Make sure the plastic is taut and free of wrinkles. (See instructions for completing the wound recovery form below.)
6. Photocopy the wound tracing to create a permanent record. Discard the graph with the plastic tracing.
7. Mark wound features with lines drawn at right angles to the feature and label.

Wound Recovery Form

The wound recovery form[38] is a paper-and-pencil instrument that consists of a centimeter graph sheet, a linear measure aligned with the graph coordinates to show size, and anatomic figures (front and back) to mark location. The tissue characteristics are listed by phase: inflammation, proliferation, and epithelialization. The key assists the clinician in the evaluation and development of the wound phase healing diagnosis and to track the recovery of the wound by phase and wound characteristics. A completed form is shown in Exhibit 5-7.

Supplies

- Wound recovery form
- Wound tracing
- Transparent tape
- Fine-tip marking pen
- Photocopier (optional)

Using the Wound Recovery Graph

1. Prepare wound tracing (see above).
2. Place tracing on Recovery graph with the arrow aligned with lines at the 12:00 position.
3. Tape tracing in place unless it is adhesive-backed.
4. Draw lines that are exactly the same length as the length measurements taken from the undermining at clock points around the wound perimeter, starting at wound edges and moving outward.
5. Draw lines from the tissue characteristics out to the side of the graph and label with letter from key.
6. Print wound location at the bottom of the picture. Mark its location on anatomic figures.
7. This "wound map" is also a tissue assessment report.

Note: Tissue characteristics are described in Chapter 4.

CLINICAL WISDOM

Using the Wound Tracing for Positive Reinforcement

The wound tracing can also be a positive reinforcement in diabetic patients. Two wound tracings are made on acetate film or plastic wrap. A date is placed on the tracing next to the wound edge. One copy is placed in the patient records, and the other is given to the patient. The next assessment day, the patient brings in his or her copy, and the copy from the chart is presented. The wound is redrawn on both pieces of film and dated, so the size change can be visually compared. Patients receive positive reinforcement for their compliance by seeing their wounds get smaller (N. Elftman, *personal communication*, 1996).

HELPFUL HINTS

Tracings

A grid printed on acetate film that peels off a plastic backing sheet can be used to make wound tracings. The sheet acts as a barrier to infection and is discarded. The tracing is then ready to place in the medical record.

Digital Tracings

A portable handheld device is now available that improves the precision of wound measurement using wound tracings. This is the digital tracing tool by Smith and Nephew, called the Visitrak™ system (Figure 5-7A). Visitrak devices can calculate wound area and the percentage of change in size. The device is simple to handle, and nonskilled and semi-skilled individuals can learn to use it in less than 15 minutes.[39]

The device consists of a digital tablet and a tracing film, designed as a three-layer pack to minimize the risk of cross-contamination and secondary infection. The tracing film is transparent so the wound can be seen, and its edges are drawn with the stylus. The stylus transmits the information from the tracing to the digital processor of the digital tablet. The operator can select the way in which measurements are recorded, including width and length, grid squares, or planimetry. A probe is included for measuring depth, and this measurement can be added to length by width measurements for a wound volume measurement that is calculated by the device. Planimetry, as described above, provides the most accurate measurement of wound area for all sizes and shapes of wounds.

Visitrak is reported to have approximately 94% accuracy.[14] The clean layer with the tracing has an adhesive backing that can be separated from the contaminated layers and stored in the patient records. It has the same advantages as conventional tracings, including that of being able to show features of the wound, such as an area of necrotic tissue, with the additional advantage of being able to take an area measurement of the necrotic tissue area or areas and recording those. This device is a step between manual tracing methods and computer-assisted planimetry. The cost is reasonable and allows for improved accuracy, consistency, and reliability of wound measurements. Because the device is small and portable, it is practical for environments such as long-term care facilities and home care. The advantages of being able to document the rate of healing during the initial stages of care and identify nonhealing wounds have been described earlier in this chapter. The grid format is user-friendly with boxes and icons to cue the clinician to record all items needed for the evaluation of the wound progress (Figure 5-7B).

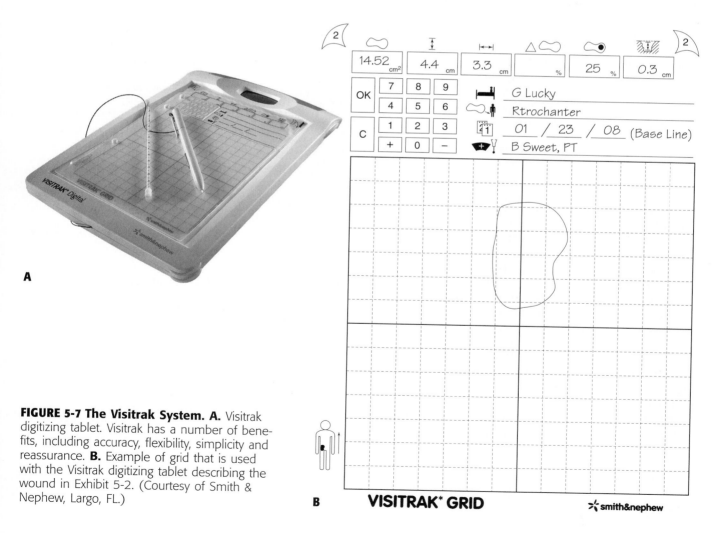

FIGURE 5-7 The Visitrak System. A. Visitrak digitizing tablet. Visitrak has a number of benefits, including accuracy, flexibility, simplicity and reassurance. **B.** Example of grid that is used with the Visitrak digitizing tablet describing the wound in Exhibit 5-2. (Courtesy of Smith & Nephew, Largo, FL.)

Wound Photography

"A picture is worth a thousand words" has often been used to describe the value of wound photography. Now that old adage can be modified to, "A picture of a wound is worth thousands of dollars."[1] Photo documentation is one way to prevent litigation in wound management. Wounds should be photographed if present on admission or when acquired and at discharge. The photograph serves as a permanent record of the wound at baseline and during its course of care. Unless consent for patient photography is part of the facility admission package, consent should be obtained before photography is used. In some facilities, the photographs of wounds are part of the patient's medical record; in others, they are stored separately. Wound photographs were reported to be part of the documentation procedures in 75% of the home-health care agencies in the United States.[40]

Serial color photographs document wound tissue characteristics. Lighting affects the color in several ways: Flash photography tends to give a blue tone to the photograph, and incandescent light gives a yellow tone. Photographs are used also to measure the wound size. The accuracy of wound measurement taken from a photograph is compromised by the problem caused by measuring wound area on curved surfaces.[35] Periodic photography is a method often used to validate the overall treatment outcome. Serial photos are effective teaching tools for in-services, referral sources, reimbursement, and patient encouragement. Photographs can be taken with simple instant cameras or with more complex camera equipment. However, with lower-end photo equipment, color and image quality may not accurately represent the wound.

The cost of digital camera equipment has decreased significantly in recent years as the quality of resolution of the images has improved. But using low-priced digital cameras still presents problems. Better resolution is now available using moderate-priced equipment, making this technology readily available to the average clinician. A real benefit is the ability to instantly view the photo to determine if it is a good representation of the wound. If not, it can be quickly and easily retaken. Dating features are included and are recommended.

Photographs can be downloaded into a computer where the records can be stored and photos printed. Identification information that protects patient privacy can be added to each photo for record keeping. Digital photos should not be retouched in order to maintain the validity of the original.

Digital photography with computerized planimetry is reliable and accurate when the computer software is designed to adjust for parallax. The Verge Videometer (VeV) system by Vista Medical is such a system. There are several advantages attributed to this system, including the fact that it is a noncontact method of photography and measurement that eliminates the risk of wound bed contamination and trauma, and avoids procedural pain.[31] The computer software is also designed as a database of wound information is available, but these systems are not yet a standard part of medical record keeping equipment in many facilities.

Scanning is yet another method for digitally storing photographs that has become more widely available. Again, the quality of photograph and scanner influence the quality of the computer image.

Complex camera equipment and computer systems are typically limited to use by researchers, but their availability to clinicians may increase as the standards for recording and documenting wounds are revised and use of telemedicine expands. Regardless of which method is used, the following are suggestions for taking high-quality photographs:

- Use a good light source.
- Position patient and wound carefully, ensuring that the patient's private areas are screened from the camera.
- Position a linear measure (ruler) in the photo to show relative size.
- Use a string of known length to measure distance from the camera to the wound for consistency of photos over time
- Use an identification sign with patient ID, wound location, and date in the photograph (unless dated by the camera).
- Select a camera with a zoom feature, if possible, to take close-up views of the wound.
- Use a ring flash attachment on a 35-mm close-up lens to eliminate shadows.
- Use an assistant to help maintain the patient's position and perhaps to position the marker.
- Record wound and patient position for repeated photographing sessions (example: "right side-lying").

HELPFUL HINT

Making an Identification Marker for Photographs

1. Tape plastic measuring sheet to a 3 in X 5 in index card.
2. Put card into a plastic sandwich bag.
3. Put two strips of white tape on the plastic sandwich bag.
   - Write patient ID and wound location on the first strip (example: W.J., coccyx).
   - Write date on second strip (example: 01/23/08).
4. Throw away the plastic bag.
5. Reuse the card.

Photographic Wound Assessment Tool

The Photographic Wound Assessment Tool (PWAT) is a modified version of the the Bates-Jensen Wound Assessment Tool (BWAT), formerly known as the Pressure Sore Status Tool (PSST) (see Chapter 6). It makes use of six domains of the BWAT that can be determined from photographs alone and do not require bedside assessment.[40] Each domain item of the PWAT is scored numerically, and a total score is calculated by adding the scores assigned to each of the six domains (Exhibit 5-8). The range of possible total PWAT scores is between 0 and 24, with zero representing a healed ulcer.[40]

The PWAT was applied and tested with pressure ulcers and leg ulcers and found to have high intertester and intratester reliability among experienced wound clinicians and

EXHIBIT 5-8   Six Domains of PWAT

1. Edges
2. Necrotic tissue type
3. Necrotic tissue amount
4. Skin color surrounding skin
5. Granulation tissue
6. Epithelialization

high concurrent validity, based on the degree of agreement between surface area calculation, obtained from the wound photograph (n = 46), and the surface area assessed, using wound tracings and linear measurements (the intraclass correlation coefficient [ICC] = 0.86 and 0.96, respectively). Serial photographs of 38 individuals were used to monitor changes in the wounds over time. Researchers were able to divide the ulcers into "healers" and "nonhealers," based on the changes in wound surface area, as measured by the PWAT. A comparison of PWAT scores revealed that there were almost statistically significant differences between the two groups (p = 0.07). The highest reliability was achieved when the PWAT was applied to pressure ulcers, compared with leg ulcers, probably reflecting its derivation from the BWAT, which was designed for assessment of pressure ulcers.

Limitations to its use are the added costs associated with wound photography, the need for consent before taking photographs, and the impact on the decision-making process by the clinician.[40] However, the PWAT may play an important role in the field of wound telemedicine. A tool that gives nurses and physicians a reliable and easy-to-use method of quantifying the status of wounds from photographs could potentially improve the quality of outpatient wound care. Trials of telemedicine using digital photography show that wound evaluation on the basis of viewing digital images is comparable to standard wound examination and results in similar diagnoses, most of the time.[41]

Video

Interactive video teleconferencing has also been pilot tested on patients with wounds that showed good potential for implementing telemedicine technology for patients with wounds who are unable to travel to health-care centers.[42] Video teleconferencing offers the benefit over still photography and digital imaging of allowing visualization of the wound from a variety of angles and positions with immediate feedback from the clinician, patient, other health-care practitioners, and family.[42] Although a number of barriers to implementation of this type of service exist, including proper lighting, a private space designated for the teleconference, funding for purchase of the equipment and telecommunication services, operator training, and others, this technology holds potential for enhancing patient access to and availability of health-care services.

Referral Criteria

As wound measurements are performed and repeated, it can become apparent that a wound is not progressing or is on a downward course, in which case a prompt referral for alternative or adjunctive treatment is necessary. The availability of advanced technologies for treatment, such as growth factors and tissue-engineered products, has made it very important to recognize and understand the criteria for referral. To do that, clinicians must have a valid and reliable way of measuring the efficacy of standard care. The standard care for chronic wounds has been well-developed and includes pressure relief off-loading or compression, debridement, moisture balance, bacterial balance, and proper nutrition. Referral should be considered when the following four criteria are met:[43]

1. Initial ulcer size and duration indicates that standard care is likely to fail (e.g., large, deep ulcer of longer than 1-year duration)
2. Rate of healing with standard care predicts failure (> 30% healing)
3. Wound fails to heal in predicted time, based on guideline of 30%–47% reduction in size in 2–4 weeks
4. Special circumstance exists, such as unusual diagnosis or patient demand

Emergent referral is warranted when:

- The extent of wound involves bone and/or deep subcutaneous spaces—may indicate osteomyelitis or other infection.
- There is an impending exposure of a named anatomic structure—wound extent should be evaluated medically
- There are black holes or tunnels that cannot be measured—high-risk situation
- Wound tunneling may perforate the peritoneal cavity in either the abdomen or rectum
- Wound size is enlarging more than expected.

Referral Sources

There are many health-care practitioners who have experience in complex wound management. One or more of these professionals should be contacted for follow-up management if any of the referral criteria listed above is met. Some choices include the following:

Physicians	Nurses	Health Professionals (Allied Health)
Dermatologist	Dermatology nurse	Physical therapist
Orthopedic surgeon	Wound ostomy continence nurse	Vascular technician
Plastic surgeon	Registered nurse	Podiatrist
Vascular surgeon	Geriatric nurse practitioner	
	Vascular nurse	

Self-Care Guidelines

In today's health-care environment, caregivers at many levels are used to measure and monitor the wound size parameters discussed in this chapter, as well as to report to the expert clinician their findings for interpretation. The most successful results occur when step-by-step instructions and repeated demonstrations are given to the designated data collector. Prepare an instruction sheet for measuring and/or tracing wounds, and create a chart such as that shown in Exhibit 5-9 for recording the data.

First, assess the individual's ability to follow directions. If the patient or lay caregiver is going to perform the measurements, limit the measurements to length and width. Teach the simple length by width method so that only one number needs to be reported. Many caregivers are capable of making wound tracings, which can also help them see that the wound is getting smaller as the report number decreases, or that the wound is changing in shape and size. This reinforces both the caregiver's and the patient's feeling of success. If the wound is not decreasing in size, this fact will be more obvious, triggering a change in treatment planning.

A form such as the one shown in Exhibit 5-9 can be faxed or sent electronically to the wound case manager to follow the progress of the wound if visits cannot be made on a frequent basis. If the person monitoring the wound is a paraprofessional, physical therapist assistant, or licensed practical nurse, additional wound measurements can be taught and performed with a high level of reliability and confidence.

Sample Instruction Sheet

Wound Measurements

Supplies
• Plastic measuring sheet
• Pen
• Plastic wrap
• Plastic sandwich bag (one or two)
• Handheld pocket calculator

Instructions
Wound measurements are taken once a week or biweekly.

1. Note the date.
2. Measure the longest diameter of the wound in each direction, head to toe (length) and side to side (width).
3. Record the length and width in the appropriate boxes on the form as the measurements are taken.
4. Multiply the two numbers together for a single total size measurement.

Instructions for Making a Wound Tracing at Home

1. Use either two pieces of plastic wrap or a plastic sandwich bag.
2. Place one layer of plastic against the clean wound. If the plastic becomes foggy, lift a corner of the plastic to allow the heat and moisture to escape, and the fog will go away.

EXHIBIT 5-9   Wound Measurement Record

Name: _____		Medical Record #: _____	
Date	**Length**	**Width**	**Total**
4/30/07	5 cm	3 cm	15 cm^2
5/15/07	4.5 cm	2.5 cm	11.25 cm^2
5/30/07	4.0 cm	1.75 cm	8.8 cm^2
6/15/07	2.5 cm	1.25 cm	3.13 cm^2

3. When you can see the edges of the wound, use a felt-tip marking pen to draw around the wound edges. Mark the date of the drawing next to the edge of the wound.
4. After the ink is dry (about 10 seconds), lift the top layer of plastic wrap or cut off the top layer of the plastic bag.
5. Save the wound tracing in another clean plastic lunch bag.
6. Discard the dirty plastic sheet.

Conclusion

This chapter described several measurement strategies for monitoring wound extent and healing by tracking change in six parameters of size: length, width, SA, undermining/tunneling, depth, and overall wound estimate. Obviously, performing all of the above measurements on all wounds is not realistic. All of the methods are common. One will appeal to one facility's practitioners, and another will be appropriate for another facility's, which provides an opportunity for collaboration. Hold a team meeting to decide on the method that meets the needs of the majority of practitioners and conveys the desired information. There is enough similarity among methods that the information communicated through the continuum of care can and will be readily interpreted. The keys to successful measurements are consistency and accuracy. Once a method is selected, incorporate it into the facility policies and procedures and then use it consistently by all clinicians.

REVIEW QUESTIONS

1. Describe two ways of taking linear wound surface area and depth measurements.
2. Describe the benefits of each of the three following types of wound measurements: linear, tracing with and without planimetry, and photography.
3. What is the benefit of performing the calculation of the percentage of change in SA at regular intervals?
4. How can an instrument to measure and score wound healing be useful in future health-care systems?
5. What are the criteria for referring a patient for adjunctive or alternative therapy?

RESOURCES

• The Wand and latex wound models: D. Taylor, Loma Linda University, School of Allied Health Professions, Loma Linda, CA

- Plastic/acetate measuring sheets are available from many wound care product manufacturers.
- Visitrak™ digital tablet: Smith & Nephew. For information and advice about products: web site: www.smith-nephew.com; e-mail: advice
- Verge Videometer System: Vista Medical, Winnipeg, Manitoba, Canada. Web site: www.vistamedical.org.

REFERENCES

1. Salcido R. The future of wound measurement. *Advances in Skin and Wound Care.* March/April 2000;13(2):54,56.
2. Polansky M, vanRijswijk L. Utilizing Survival Analysis Techniques in Chronic Wound Healing Studies. *Wounds: A compendium of clinical research and practice.* September/October 1994;6(5):15-58.
3. vanRijswijk L. Full-thickness pressure ulcers: patient and wound healing characteristics. *Decubitus.* 1993;6(1):16-21.
4. vanRijswijk L, Polansky M. Predictors of time to healing deep pressure ulcers. *Ostomy Wound Management.* October 1994;40(8):40-48.
5. Marston W, Carlin R, Passman M, Farber M, Keegy B. Healing rates and cost efficacy of outpatient compression treatment for leg ulcers associated with venous insufficiency. *J Vasc Surg.* 1999;30(3):491-498.
6. Tallman P, Muscare E, Carson P, Eaglestein W, Falanga V. Initial rate of healing predicts complete healing of venous ulcers. *Arch Dermatol.* October 1997;133(10):1231-1234.
7. Phillips T, Machado F, Trout R, Porter J, Olin J, Falanga V. Prognostic indicators in venous ulcers. *J Am Acad Dermatol.* October 2000;43(4):627-630.
8. Kantor J, Margolis DJ. Expected Healing Rates for Chronic Wounds. *Wounds: A compendium of clinical research and practice.* November/December 2000;12(6):155-158.
9. Robson MC, Hill D, Woodske M, Steed D. Wound healing trajectories as predictors of effectiveness of therapeutic agents. *Arch Surg.* July 2000; 135(7):773-777.
10. vanRijswijk L. Frequency of reassessment of pressure ulcers: National Pressure Ulcer Advisory Panel Proceedings. *Adv Wound Care.* July/August 1995: 19-24.
11. Arnold T, Stanley J, Fellows E, et al. Prospective multicenter study of managing lower extremity venous ulcers. *Ann Vasc Surg.* 1994;8(4):356-362.
12. Sussman C, Swanson, GH. A uniform method to trace and measure chronic wounds. Paper presented at Symposium for Advanced Wound Care, 1991; San Francisco, CA.
13. Sussman C, Swanson, GH, . The utility of Sussman wound healing tool in predicting wound healing outcomes in physical therapy. Paper presented at National Pressure Ulcer Advisory Panel Fifth Biennial Conference, 1997; Washington, DC.
14. Schultz GS, Romanelli M, Claxton K. Wound healing and TIME; new concepts and scientific applications. *Wound Repair & Regeneration.* July/August 2005;13(4):S1-11.
15. Taylor DR. Reliability of the Sussman method of measuring wounds that contain undermining. Paper presented at American Physical Therapy Association Scientific Meeting, April 1997; San Diego, CA.
16. Maklebust J. PUSH tool reality check: audience response. *Advances in Wound Care.* September 1997;10(5):102-106.
17. Pham HT, Falanga V, Sabolinski ML, Veves A. Healing rate measurement can predict complete wound healing rate in chronic diabetic foot ulceration. Paper presented at Symposium for Advanced Wound Care and Medical Research Forum on Wound Repair, May 2001; Las Vegas, NV.
18. Sheehan PJP, Caselli A, Gurini JM.,Veves A. Percent change in wound area of diabetic foot ulcers over a 4-week period is a robust predictor of complete healing in a 12-week prospective trial. *Diabetes Care.* 2003; 26:1879–1882.
19. vanRijswijk L. Full-thickness leg ulcers: patient demographics and predictors of healing. Multi-center leg ulcer study group. *J Fam Pract.* 1993;36(6):625-632.
20. VanRijswijk L. Group M-CLUS. Full-thickness leg ulcers: Patient demographics and predictors of time to healing. *J Fam Pract.* 1993;36(6):625-632.
21. Margolis DJ, Gross EA, Wood CR, Lazarus GS. Planimetric rate of healing in venous ulcers of the leg treated with pressure bandage and hydrocolloid dressing. *Journal of the American Academy of Dermatology.* March 1993;28(3):418-421.
22. Gilman TH. Parameter for measurement of wound closure. *Wounds: A compendium of clinical research and practice.* May/June 1990;2(3):95-101.
23. Frantz R, Bergquist S, Gardner S. Measurements of partial and full-thickness ulcers: critical parameters of healing. Paper presented at American Nurses Association Council of Nursing Research, June 1996; Washington, DC.
24. Ramirez AT, Soroff HS, Schwartz MS, Mooty J, Pearson E, Raben MS. Experimental wound healing in man. *Surgery, Gynecology & Obstetrics.* February 1969:283-293.
25. Gilman TH. Calculating healing rate of acute surgical wounds. In: Sussman C, ed. Torrance; 2001:email messages.
26. Pecoraro RE, H AJ, J BE, L SV. Chronology and determinants of tissue repair in diabetic lower- extremity ulcers. *Diabetes.* October 1991;40:1305-1313.
27. Cherry GW, Hill D, Poore S, Wilson J, Robson MC. Initial healing rate of venous ulcers: are they useful as predictors and comparators of healing? Paper presented at Symposium for Advanced Wound Care and Medical Research Forum on Wound Repair, May 2001; Las Vegas, NV.
28. Cukjati DRS, Karba R, Miclavici D. Modelling of chronic wound healing dynamics. *Medical and Biological Engineering & Computing.* 2000;38:339-347.
29. Hess CT. *Nurse's Clinical Guide, Wound Care.* Springhouse, Springhouse, PA; 1995.
30. Flanagan M. Wound measurement: can it help us to monitor progression to healing? *Journal of Wound Care.* May 2003:189-194.
31. Keast DH, Bowering CK, Evans AW, Mackeen GL, Burrows C, D'Souza L. CS MEASURE: A proposed assessment framework for developing best practice recommendations for wound assessment. *Wound Repair and Regeneration.* May-June 2004;12:1-17.
32. Gentzkow G. Methods for measuring size in pressure ulcers. National Pressure Ulcer Advisory Panel Proceedings. *Adv Wound Care.* July/August 1995:43-45.
33. Banks PBK, Washington MO, Stubblefield AM, Ho CH. Fluid volume measurements: the gold standard? Paper presented at 15th Annual Meeting and Exposition of the Wound Healing Society, 2005; Chicago, IL.
34. Langemo DK, Melland H, Hanson D, Olson B, Huneter S, Henly SJ. Two-dimensional wound measurement: comparison of 4 techniques. *Advances in Wound Care.* November/December 1998;11(7):337-343.
35. Harding K. Methods for assessing change in ulcer status. *Adv Wound Care.* July/August 1995:37-42.
36. Majeske C. Reliability of wound surface area measurement. *Phys Ther.* 1992;72:138-141.
37. Kloth Luther FJ. Acceleration of wound healing with high voltage, monophasic, pulsed current. *Phys Ther.* 1988;68:503-508.
38. Sussman C. Physical therapy choices for wound recovery. *Ostomy/Wound Management.* July/August 1990; 29:20-28.
39. Serana TE. A new electronic wound measurement device in clinical practice: is it practical? Paper presented at Clinical Symposium, 2004; Phoenix, AZ.
40. Houghton PE, Kincaid CB, Campbell K, Woodbury MG. Photographic assessment of the appearance of chronic pressure and leg ulcers. *Ostomy Wound Management.* April 2000;46(4):20-30.
41. Wirthlin D, Buradagunta S, Edwards R, et al. Telemedicine in vascular surgery: feasibility of digital imaging for remote management of wounds. *J Vasc Surg.* 1998;27(6):1089-1099.
42. Ratliff CR. Telehealth for wound management in long-term care. *Ostomy/Wound Management.* September 2005;51(9):40-45.
43. Eaglstein W. What is standard care and where should we leave it? Paper presented at Evidence Based Outcomes in Wound Management, March 2000; Dallas, TX.

SUGGESTED READINGS

Gilman TH. Parameter for measurement of wound closure. *Wounds.* 1990;2(3):95–101.

Polansky M, vanRijswijk L. Utilizing survival analysis techniques in chronic wound healing studies. *Wounds.* 1994;6(5):15–58.

Tools to Measure Wound Healing

Barbara M. Bates-Jensen and Carrie Sussman

CHAPTER OBJECTIVES

At the end of this chapter, the reader will be able to:

1. Explain the terms validity, reliability, sensitivity, and specificity as used for evaluating wound healing tools.
2. Review the wound characteristics commonly included in wound healing tools.
3. Describe the development and use of three wound healing tools:
   - Sussman Wound Healing Tool (SWHT)
   - Pressure Ulcer Scale for Healing (PUSH)
   - The Bates-Jensen Wound Assessment Tool (BWAT), formerly known as the Pressure Sore Status Tool (PSST)

Assessment of wound status to measuring healing should be performed at least weekly. Medicare requires a minimum of monthly reporting. How best to perform and document the wound assessment for the purpose of evaluating healing has not been agreed on, and several approaches have been proposed. Although there is general agreement that use of a systematic approach with evaluation of multiple wound attributes is helpful, there are no data available that demonstrate improved outcomes by using a standardized, research-based tool. However, it is prudent to use a systematic approach to increase communication among those involved in the wound care plan. Chapter 4 covered assessment of specific characteristics; Chapter 6 is devoted to tools that assess multiple characteristics in order for the clinician to evaluate healing. This chapter also includes information on instrument development and discusses tools used in evaluating wound healing.

While several instruments to evaluate pressure ulcers have been proposed,[1-8] only the Pressure Sore Status Tool, (now called the Bates-Jensen Wound Assessment Tool (BWAT)),[1] the Pressure Ulcer Scale for Healing (PUSH),[3,4] and the Sussman Wound Healing Tool (SWHT)[6] are currently in use for clinical practice or research. Table 6-1 shows the wound characteristics and scoring systems used by several of the proposed tools.

Measurements used to evaluate wound healing over time have included change in ulcer size or surface area, change in wound appearance, and stage of the wound. Use of a staging system has historically been very common as a method of evaluating healing. Although staging systems such as the NPUAP system[4] and the Wagner scale[9] (see Chapter 4) are appropriate for determining initial severity of tissue trauma, the systems have been misapplied as methods to measure healing by using the numerical classifications in reverse to downstage the ulcer to signify healing. Use of a single wound characteristic has not been helpful in monitoring healing, determining treatment response, and prescribing therapy or predicting outcomes. Thus, there is a clear need for tools that include multiple wound characteristics as measures of healing in a more biologically accurate manner.

Criteria for Evaluating Wound Healing Tools

Criteria to evaluate the appropriateness and utility of a tool include validity, sensitivity and specificity, reliability, responsiveness, and clinical practicality.

Validity

Validity is the accuracy with which an instrument or test measures what it purports to measure.[10] Validity is context-

TABLE 6-1   Comparison of Wound Healing Tools

Wound Characteristics and Format	Bates-Jensen Wound Assessment Tool (BWAT, previously PSST)	Pressure Ulcer Scale for Healing (PUSH)	Sessing Scale	Sussman Wound Healing Tool (SWHT)	Wound Healing Scale (WHS)	Photographic Wound Healing Tool (PWHT)	Pressure Ulcer Healing Process (PUHP—Japanese)
Size	X	X		X		X	X
Depth or Stage	X		X	X		X	X
Necrotic Tissue	X	X	X	X		X	X
Granulation Tissue	X	X	X	X	X	X	
Epithelial Tissue	X	X	X	X	X	X	X
Surrounding Tissue Characteristics	X			X		X	
Exudate	X	X	X		X	X	X
Undermining and Tunneling	X		X	X	X	X	X
Scoring Methods:							
Likert scale	X					X	X
Subscales with total score	X	X	X	X			X

specific, meaning that a tool that is valid in one study may not be valid for another study. For instance, a tool that is valid for measuring healing in pressure ulcers may not be valid for measuring healing in lower extremity vascular ulcers. Validity, as it relates to tool development, is a cyclical process. When indicated, information from validity testing may be used to change a tool to increase validity, then the newly revised tool is retested.[11] Validity is not a static quality and changes over time. Validity is not an "all-or-nothing" quality; it is usually a matter of degree. There are three main qualities in validity: content, criterion, and construct.

Content Validity

Content validity is the degree to which a test or instrument measures an intended content area. The match between the objective to be measured and the items (content) on a tool relates to content validity. Content validity is typically evaluated during an instrument or tool's development. Content validity may be determined using an expert panel whose members rate, in some manner, the items on the tool and the tool's ability to measure the objective. The panel's size depends on the specific type of procedures used. Guidelines are available for interpreting content validity but, in clinical practice, evaluation of how the tool was developed, who was involved, where knowledge of the tool's content was obtained, and the outcome of the expert panel is usually enough information. This is true because the ratings of the content specialists are only as good as their levels of expertise in the area measured.

Criterion Validity

Criterion validity evaluates the relationship between the instrument or tool and some other criterion. Criterion validity is concerned with the pragmatic issue: Is the tool a useful predictor? The functional usefulness of a tool is supported by criterion-related validity evidence.[10,11] There are two types of criterion available for evaluation—concurrent and predictive. Concurrent validity is testing the tool against present performance or status on a criterion. Predictive validity is testing the tool against future performance or status on a criterion. An example of concurrent validity for wound healing tools is the ability of a tool to separate partial- and full-thickness wounds, based on their scores on the tool. An example of predictive validity is the ability of a tool to predict healing or wound closure. Predictive validity is particularly important for wound healing instruments and bears further discussion. Predictive validity can be either positive or negative (for instance, a tool would be equally beneficial if it predicted those wounds that would not heal as it would if it predicted those wounds that would heal).

Predictive validity of tools involves the evaluation of the tool's sensitivity and specificity. Sensitivity is the true positive rate for the instrument and is calculated by dividing the number of those with a condition and a positive test by the total number of those with the condition. Specificity is the true negative rate for the instrument and is calculated by dividing the number of those without a condition and a negative test by the total number of those without the condition. Sensitivity and specificity are inversely related. Predictive validity is important. Screening tools that have predictive validity are based on the assumption that, after detecting specific variables, an intervention can be applied that would affect the predicted outcome.

Sensitivity and Specificity. Sensitivity is the number of true positives obtained when using the tool. Sensitivity involves using the tool and determining those with the condition that were obtained by using the tool versus all of those with the condition. For example, a sensitive wound healing tool should be able to determine all of the wounds that have improved. Sensitivity involves precision and accuracy of the instrument. Can the tool accurately identify those wounds that have improved? Ideally, a tool should be able to pick up 100% of those with the condition being measured. However, most tools sacrifice some degree of sensitivity for specificity.

Specificity is the number of true negatives obtained when using the tool. Specificity involves using the tool and determining those without the condition that were obtained by using the tool versus all of those without the condition. In an ideal world, a tool should be 100% specific to the condition being measured.

Construct Validity

Construct validity is the third quality of validity and refers to evaluation of the attribute that the tool is attempting to measure. This form of validity is more concerned with the underlying attribute than with any scores produced by the tool. Construct validity focuses on the tool's ability to function in accordance with the purpose for which it is being used. For instance, tools to measure wound healing should function by identifying wounds that are healing or nonhealing (the purpose for which the wound healing tool is being used).[11] Testing for this type of validity uses techniques such as known groups, where the researcher evaluates groups that are known to differ on the attribute being measured. If the tool being tested demonstrates different scores for the two groups, this supports construct validity. Likewise, the tool can be evaluated for construct validity by using a similar instrument that measures the same attribute; if both tools come up with similar scores, this would support the construct validity of the new tool. The final aspect of validity is reliability. A tool cannot be valid if it is not reliable. A tool can be very reliable and still not meet the criteria for validity, but it is not possible to have a tool that is valid and not reliable.

Reliability

Reliability of a tool is its ability to be used with minimal random error. Reliability reflects the consistency of the measure obtained and is concerned with accuracy, depending ability, consistency, and comparability of the tool. High reported reliability values on a tool do not guarantee that its reliability will be adequate in another sample or study.[10] As with validity, reliability estimates are specific to the population in the sample being tested. Reliability must be performed on each instrument used in a study. In clinical practice, this means that a wound healing tool that works for one organization may not work for another type of organization or another type of patient population. Each organization may have to test the tools to determine which work most reliably for them. There are several kinds of reliability tests for a tool.

Typically, three aspects of reliability are tested: stability, equivalence, and homogeneity. Stability reliability is also called *intrarater reliability* and evaluates the consistency of the tool with repeated measures. In this type of reliability, the same rater/observer uses the same tool on the same wound at different times. The goal is for the same rater to get the same score when observing the same phenomena repeatedly. This type of reliability may also be called *test-retest reliability*. Issues in wound healing tools with intrarater reliability relate to how much time should exist between measures. If the time period is long, the issue of concern is the possibility of different scores reflecting a true difference in the wound, and, if the time period is short, the concern exists regarding the possibility of the observer remembering a previous score.

Equivalence reliability may also be called *interrater reliability* and evaluates the multiple raters using the tool at the same time on the same wound. Interrater reliability is concerned with different raters getting the same score on the tool when evaluating the same wound. Adequate interrater reliability testing involves using at least 10 subjects or wounds and calculating the percentage of agreement between observers' scores on the tool or computing a Cohen's Kappa, which is a statistical analysis of agreements that mathematically corrects the data for chance agreements. Both percentage of agreement and Cohen's Kappa statistics are reported in literature on wound healing tools.

The final aspect of reliability is homogeneity. Homogeneity is the similarity or "sameness" of items within an instrument. The calculations behind homogeneity reliability are complex but the thinking is simple. Homogeneity testing examines the extent to which all the items on the tool consistently measure the same objective.[10] This form of reliability evaluates the correlation of different items within the same tool or a measure of the similarity of the tool items. This is reported as a measure of internal consistency, typically, Cronbach's alpha coefficient. Other approaches to testing internal consistency are to use Cohen's Kappa statistic, which determines the reliability of each item with the probability of chance taken out; correlations of each item with the total tool score for the instrument; and correlations of each item with each other item in the tool.[10] Factor analysis can also be used to evaluate an instrument's internal consistency. All forms of reliability may be reported for wound healing tools, so this basic discussion will help practitioners to understand better the use of an evidence-based instrument for wound assessment and healing.

Responsiveness

Responsiveness, or sensitivity to change, is another test criterion for a tool. An appropriate tool or method must be able to detect changes in the condition of the wound over time with repeated administrations. It is important for the instrument to be able to detect significant changes in the wound and to respond with a change in tool score. To some degree, sensitivity to change may be evaluated by assessing the tool's sensitivity and specificity. Responsiveness is the ability of the tool to respond quickly to changes in the wound status. One method of determining responsiveness of a tool is to evaluate change scores for reliability. Reliability of change scores is inversely dependent on the correlation between the initial score with the tool and the follow-up score.[11] If there is a strong correlation or relationship between the initial score and the follow-up score, the reliability of the change score will be lower. Likewise, if there is a weak relationship between the initial score and the follow-up score, the reliability of the change score will be much higher.

Clinical Practicality

Clinical practicality means that the tool must be simple, easy to learn, and easy to use, with clear instructions. It must be time-efficient and cost-effective. The tool must provide data that are meaningful enough to warrant the additional time and energy required to complete the assessment. Some aspects of clinical practicality can be evaluated during validity assessment, such as level of the language of the tool. The level of the language of the tool and the understandability of items should be reflective of the intended tool user. Similarly, scoring mechanisms and mathematical calculations must address the intended tool user.

Wound Characteristics

Most wound healing instruments include assessment of multiple wound attributes. This section provides a brief description of wound characteristics commonly included in instruments to measure healing. More comprehensive descriptions of wound characteristics are found in Chapter 4. The choice of which characteristics to include in a tool depends on the purpose of the instrument (prediction of healing, assessment of wound status, prescription of treatment, etc.) and, to some degree, the philosophy of the instrument developers.

Location

Assess the location of the wound by identifying where the lesion occurs on the patient's anatomy. Body diagrams are typically used to document wound location. Wound location has been shown to influence healing. However, which specific locations are beneficial or detrimental to healing are still to be determined.

Shape

As wounds heal, they often change shape and may begin to assume a more regular, circular/oval shape. The shape also helps to determine the overall size of the wound. Butterfly-shaped wounds occur in the sacrococcygeal area and are wounds with mirror images on each side of the coccyx. *Color Plates 3* and *4* show butterfly-shaped ulcers on the coccyx. The shape of the wound is determined by evaluating the perimeter of the wound. Shape of the wound is related to wound contraction. Wound contraction can be seen when the open surface area of the wound reduces and when the shape of the wound changes. Compare *Color Plate 3* with *Color Plates 4* and *5* to see the onset and progression of contraction and epithelialization. It is identified by a change in wound open area size and may be identified as a change in wound shape (e.g., from irregular to symmetric, such as the circular or oval formation and rounding off of the edges of the wound seen in pressure ulcers; see *Color Plate 2*).

Size

Most tools include some measure of size. The most commonly used method in determining size is to measure (in cm) the longest and perpendicularly widest aspect of the wound surface that is visible. The surface area can be determined by multiplying the length by the width. It can be difficult to determine where to measure size on some wounds, because the edge of the wound may be hard to visualize or the edge may be irregular. This is a skill that takes practice. Use of the same reference points for determining size improves the reliability and meaningfulness of the measures. (Chapter 5, Wound Measurements, has step-by-step procedures for measuring size, depth, and undermining.)

Depth

Measure the depth of the wound using a cotton-tipped applicator. Insert the applicator in the deepest portion of the wound, mark the applicator with a pen, and measure the distance from the tip to the mark, using a metric measuring guide. Multiple measures of depth within the wound can increase reliability of depth evaluation. Some tools evaluate wound depth using descriptive terms instead of numeric measurements.

Edges

The edges of the wound reflect some of the most important characteristics of the wound. When assessing edges, look for how clear and distinct the wound outline appears. If the edges are indistinct and diffuse, there are areas where the normal tissues blend into the wound bed. Edges that are even with the skin surface and the wound base are edges that are attached to the base of the wound. This means that the wound is flat, with no appreciable depth. Well-defined edges are clear and distinct and can be outlined easily on a transparent piece of plastic. Edges that are not attached to the base of the wound imply a wound with some depth of tissue involvement (*Color Plate 33*). The wound that is a crater or has a bowl/boat shape is a wound with edges that are not attached to the wound base (*Color Plate 41*). The wound has walls or sides. There is depth to the wound. As the wound ages, the edges become rolled under and thickened to palpation. The edge achieves a unique coloring. The pigment turns a grayish hue in both dark- and light-skinned persons (*Color Plate 35*). Wounds of long duration may continue to thicken, with scar tissue and fibrosis developing in the wound edge, causing the edge to feel hard, rigid, and indurated. Hyperkeratosis is the callus-like tissue that may form around the wound edges, especially with diabetic ulcers (see Chapter 19 and *Color Plate 24*). Evaluate the wound edges by visual inspection and palpation. *Color Plates 33–36* show wounds with different edges.

Undermining/Tunneling

Undermining and tunneling represent the loss of tissue underneath an intact skin surface. Undermining usually involves a greater percentage of the wound margins, with more shallow length than tunneling. Undermining usually involves subcutaneous tissues and follows the fascial planes next to the wound. Undermining is defined as erosion under the edge of the wound, and tunneling is defined as separation of the fascial planes leading to sinus tracts. An undermined area can be likened to a cave, whereas a tunnel is more like a subway. Tunneling usually involves a small percentage of the wound margins; it is narrow and quite long, and it seems to have a destination.

CLINICAL WISDOM

Tips for Assessing Wound Edges

Definitions for help in assessing wound edges:

- Indistinct, diffuse—unable to distinguish wound outline clearly
- Attached—even or flush with wound base, no sides or walls present, flat
- Not attached—sides or walls are present; floor or base of wound is deeper than edge
- Rolled under, thickened—soft-to-firm and flexible to touch
- Hyperkeratosis—callus-like tissue formation around wound and at edges

---

Assess for undermining by inserting a cotton-tipped applicator under the wound edge and advancing it as far as it will go without using undue force. Raise the tip of the applicator so that it may be seen or felt on the surface of the skin and mark the surface with a pen. Measure the distance from the mark on the skin to the edge of the wound. Continue this process all around the wound. Then use a trans-

parent metric measuring guide with concentric circles divided into four (25%) pie-shaped quadrants to help determine percentage of the wound involved (see *Color Plates 39–41*).

Necrotic Tissue Characteristics

Characteristics of necrotic tissue include *amount present, color, consistency,* and *adherence to the wound bed.* Choose the predominant characteristic present in the wound. Necrosis is defined as dead devitalized tissue. Color may be black, brown, gray, or yellow. Texture may be dry and leathery, soft, moist, or stringy. Odor may be present or absent. To determine whether the tissue being assessed is necrotic, see Chapter 8 and *Color Plates 3, 26–31, 52,* and *53.* One common error in assessing necrotic tissue is to assess all yellow and white tissue as necrotic. Yellow tissue may be either healthy yellow fat, the reticular membrane of the dermis, or a tendon. White tissue may be connective tissue, fascia, or a ligament. *Color Plate 13* shows healthy yellow and white tissue. Healthy tissue usually has a gleam not seen in devitalized tissue. Note, however, that the topical treatment or exudate is not the source of the "gleam." Healthy tissue is not friable and has resilience when compressed. Dead tissue tears and does not spring back when compressed. Waiting 24 hours helps to see whether the tissue changes color to gray or brown, indicating loss of vitality.

Necrotic tissue type changes as it ages in the wound, as debridement occurs, and as further tissue trauma causes increased cellular death. There are two main types of necrotic tissue: slough and eschar. Slough generally indicates less severity than does eschar. Slough usually appears as a yellow to tan mucinous or stringy material that is nonadherent to loosely adherent to the healthy tissues of the wound bed (*Color Plates 3, 28,* and *40*). Nonadherent material is defined as appearing scattered throughout the wound; it looks as though the tissue could be removed easily with a gauze sponge. Loosely adherent refers to tissue that is attached to the wound bed; it is thick and stringy and may appear as clumps of debris attached to wound tissue.

Eschar signifies deeper tissue damage. Eschar may be black, gray, or brown in color. Eschar is usually adherent or firmly adherent to the wound tissues and may be soggy and soft or hard and leathery in texture. A soft, soggy eschar is usually strongly attached to the base of the wound but may be lifting from and loose from the edges of the wound (*Color Plate 27*). Hard, crusty eschars are strongly attached to the base and the edges of the wound (*Color Plates 26, 30,* and *52*).

CLINICAL WISDOM

Eschar Appearance

Hard eschars are often mistaken for scabs. A scab is a collection of dried blood cells and serum on top of the skin surface, whereas an eschar is a collection of dead tissue and coagulated blood products within the wound.

Deep Tissue Injury

Sometimes, nonviable tissue appears prior to a wound's appearance. This can be seen on the skin as a white, gray, or purple area on the surface of the skin. The area usually demarcates within a few days, and the wound appears and interrupts the skin surface.

The amount of necrotic tissue present in the wound is evaluated by one of two methods. One method involves using clinical judgment to estimate the percentage of the wound covered with necrosis. Place a transparent measuring guide with concentric circles divided into four (25%) pie-shaped quadrants over the wound. Look at each quadrant and judge how much necrosis is present. Add up the total percentage from judgments of each quadrant; this determines the percentage of the wound involved. A second method involves actual linear measurements of the necrosis. Measure the length and width of the necrosis and multiply to determine surface area.

Exudate

Evaluating exudate type can be tricky because of the moist wound healing dressings used on most wounds. Some dressings interact with wound drainage to produce a gel or fluid, and others may trap liquid and drainage at the wound site. Before assessing exudate type, gently cleanse the wound with normal saline or water and evaluate fresh exudate. Pick the exudate type that is predominant in the wound, according to color and consistency. Remember that a wound with necrotic tissue present will almost always have an odor. Amount can also be difficult to assess accurately for the same reasons that it is difficult to determine the type of exudate in the wound. Moist wound healing dressings interact with wound drainage to trap drainage at the wound site. Others may absorb varying amounts of exudate. To judge the amount of exudate in the wound, observe two areas: the wound itself and the dressing used on the wound. Observe the wound for the moisture present. Are the tissues dry and desiccated? Are they swimming in exudate? Is the drainage spread throughout the wound? Use clinical judgment to determine how wet the wound is. Evaluate the dressing used on the wound for how much it interacts with exudate. *Color Plates 42–47* show different exudate characteristics.

Surrounding Skin Characteristics

The tissues surrounding the wound are often the first indication of impending further tissue damage. The color of the surrounding skin may indicate further injury from pressure, friction, or shearing. *Erythema* is defined as reddening or darkening of the skin, compared with surrounding skin. Erythema following trauma is due to rupture of small venules and capillaries or may be caused by inflow of blood to start the inflammatory process, or both events. Distinguishing between the two is often difficult. Erythema is usually accompanied by heat, but it may be accompanied by cooling, indicating devitalization of tissue.[10,11] Distinguishing and assessing erythema in darkly pigmented skin is described in detail in Chapter 4 (see *Color Plate 19*). The ability to see the margins of the change in skin color is enhanced by lighting and may be seen more easily in a photograph than in the living tissues, especially in very dark skin tones. *Color Plates 6, 14,* and *15,* and *19* show erythema in both lightly and darkly pigmented skin. Dark-skinned persons show the colors "bright red" and "dark red" as a deepening of normal ethnic skin color or a purple or blacker hue (*Color Plates 19–21*). As healing occurs in dark-skinned persons, the new skin is pink and may never darken. In both light- and dark-skinned patients, new epithelium must be differentiated from tissues that are erythematous. To assess for blanchability, press firmly on the skin with a finger; lift the finger and look for blanching (sudden whitening of the tissues), followed by prompt return of color to the area. Nonblanchable erythema signals more severe tissue damage.

Differentiation Between Erythema and Reactive Hyperemia

Erythema should be assessed after pressure has been relieved from the area, so as to eliminate effects of reactive hyperemia.

Edema

Edema in the surrounding tissues will delay wound healing in the pressure ulcer (*Color Plates 17–19*). It is difficult for neoangiogenesis, or the growth of new blood vessels into the wound, to occur in edematous tissues. Assess tissues within 4 cm of the wound edge. Nonpitting edema appears as skin that is shiny and taut, almost glistening. Identify pitting edema by firmly pressing a finger down into the tissues and waiting for 5 seconds; on release of pressure, tissues fail to resume normal position, and an indentation appears. Measure how far edema extends beyond the wound edges.

Induration

Induration is a sign of impending damage to the tissues. Along with skin color changes, induration is an omen of further pressure-induced tissue trauma. Assess tissues within 4 cm of the wound edge. Induration is an abnormal firmness of tissues with margins. Palpate where the induration starts and where it ends. Assess by gently pinching the tissues. Induration results in an inability to pinch the tissues. Palpate from healthy tissue, moving toward the wound margins. It is usual to feel slight firmness at the wound edge itself. Normal tissues feel soft and spongy; induration feels hard and firm to the touch.

Other Characteristics

Other characteristics that may be evaluated in the surrounding tissues include maceration and hemorrhage. *Maceration* is defined as a softening of connective tissue fibers by soaking until they are soft and friable. Macerated tissue loses its pigmentation, and even darkly pigmented skin looks blanched. This weakened tissue is highly susceptible to trauma, leading to breakdown of the macerated tissue and enlargement of the wound. *Hemorrhagic tissue* or *hematoma* is defined as a purple ecchymosis of wound tissue or surrounding skin (see *Color Plates 32, 75,* and *79*). The color plates show the deepening of tissue color or distinguishable purple ecchymosis that is an indicator of significant subcutaneous bleeding or hemorrhage. Wounds with hemorrhage have high probability of tissue death and, thus, enlargement of the wound. They are often referred to as "purple ulcers" or deep tissue injury.

CLINICAL WISDOM

Assessment of Hemorrhage or Hematoma Triggers Further Examination

The presence of hemorrhage or hematoma would be a trigger for further examination, including temperature testing, as described in Chapter 4, to determine tissue vitality. Hemorrhage would trigger a medical consultation. Hematoma is often reported in association with anticoagulation therapy, which is a fairly common treatment regime. The chapters in Part IV on electrical stimulation, pulsed electromagnetic fields, and ultrasound describe how these interventions effect thrombolysis and absorption of hemorrhagic material.

Granulation Tissue

Granulation tissue is a marker of wound health. It signals the proliferative phase of wound healing and usually heralds the eventual closure of the wound. Granulation tissue is the growth of small blood vessels and connective tissue into the wound cavity. It is more observable in full-thickness wounds because of the tissue defect that occurs with full-thickness wounds. In partial-thickness wounds, granulation tissue may occur so quickly and in concert with epithelialization that it is unobservable in most cases. Granulation tissue is healthy when it is bright, beefy red, shiny, and granular with a velvety appearance. The tissue looks bumpy and may bleed easily. Well-vascularized granulation tissue can be seen in *Color Plates 8, 9,* and *18*.

Epithelialization

Epithelialization is the process of epidermal resurfacing and appears as pink or red skin. Visualizing the new epithelium takes practice. *Color Plates 5, 6,* and *8* show the process of epidermal resurfacing. In partial-thickness wounds, the epithelial cells may migrate from islands on the wound surface or from the wound edges, or both. *Color Plates 68* and *69* show an example. In full-thickness wounds, epidermal resurfacing occurs from the edges only, usually after the wound has almost completely filled with granulation tissue. *Color Plates 5* and *6* show the same full-thickness wound as seen in *Color Plates 3* and *4*, with resurfacing evident from the

---

CLINICAL WISDOM

Appearance of Unhealthy Granulation Tissue

Unhealthy granulation tissue due to poor vascular supply appears as pale pink or blanched to dull, dusky red color (see *Color Plate 34*). Usually, the first layer of granulation tissue to be laid down in the wound is pale pink; as the granulation tissue deepens and thickens, the color becomes the bright, beefy red color, like *Color Plate 9*.

Try to judge what percentage of the wound has been filled with granulation tissue. This is much easier if there is history with the wound. If the same person follows the wound over multiple observations, it is simple to judge the amount of granulation tissue present in the wound. If the initial observation of the wound was done by a different observer or if the data are not available, simply use best judgment to determine the amount of tissue present.

---

wound edges. Epithelialization may first be noticed during the inflammation or proliferation phase of healing as a lightly pigmented pink tissue, even in individuals with darkly pigmented skin (*Color Plates 7–9*). Many people confuse new bright pink scar tissue or skin as erythema. *Color Plate 22* shows new pink scar tissue in a person with darkly pigmented skin. Use of a transparent measuring guide can be helpful to determine percentage of the wound involved in resurfacing and to measure the distance that the epithelial tissue extends into the wound from proliferative edges.

Wound healing tools include a combination of these wound attributes to measure healing, according to the theory on which the tool is based and the framework behind the instrument.

Tools to Monitor Wound Healing

This chapter describes three tools to monitor wound healing, the Sussman Wound Healing Tool (SWHT), the Pressure Ulcer Scale for Healing (PUSH), and the Bates-Jensen Wound Assessment Tool (BWAT) or Pressure Sore Status Tool (PSST) . There are similarities in some aspects of the tools: All evaluate tissue attributes of the wound, and two evaluate surrounding skin. Methods of assessment, format, and scoring are different. Copies of the three tools and instructions for use are found in this chapter's appendixes. The Photographic Wound Healing Tool (PWHT), which is derived from the PSST, is described in Chapter 5.

Introduction and Development of the Sussman Wound Healing Tool

The SWHT was developed by Sussman and Swanson[6] as a physical therapy diagnostic tool to monitor and track the effectiveness of physical therapy technologies used for pressure ulcer healing. The ability to predict pressure ulcer healing and treatment outcomes in physical therapy has yet to be done reliably. The monitoring and tracking of healing and treatment outcomes are essential for clinical decision making and triage, and provide payers and providers improved utilization management.

The basis for the SWHT is the acute wound healing model (see Chapter 2) that describes the changes in tissue status and size over time, as the wound progresses through the biologic phases of wound healing. Some attributes of the wound that are observed during each phase are considered to be related to failure to heal or "not good for healing," and others are considered to be indicators of improvement or "good for healing." For example, a tissue attribute such as necrosis is thought to be negative or not good for healing, whereas wound attributes such as granulation tissue (which represents fibroplasia) and adherence of the wound edges are considered good for healing. The concept of the SWHT is to benchmark the wound attributes as it recovers and progresses throughout the healing phases. For example, the "not good" attribute, necrosis, should change over time from present to absent, thus moving from "not good for healing" to "good for healing." The "good for healing" attribute, fibroplasia—significant reduction in depth—should be granulation observed as the wound heals and changes from absent to present, indicating improved tissue status.

The initial design of the SWHT is a qualitative instrument, meaning that a wound would be described as having certain tissue attributes. It is composed of 10 wound attributes, combined with 9 descriptive attributes of size, extent of tissue damage plus location, and acute wound healing phase, which are not measurable. The 10 wound tissue attributes described were each assigned a score as present or absent and ranked as not good or good for healing. Five attributes ranked as not good are hemorrhage, maceration, erythema, undermining, and necrosis. Five attributes ranked as good are adherence at the wound edge, fibroplasia, appearance of contraction, sustained contraction, and epithelialization.

Sussman Wound Healing Tool Attribute Definitions

Part I: Tissue Attributes

The first five attributes, hemorrhage, maceration, undermining/tunneling, erythema, and necrosis are all classified as not good for healing. The location of undermining is defined as undermining at any location around the wound perimeter. The extent of undermining/tunneling is not recorded or included as part of the assessment; only the presence or absence of this attribute is evaluated. The second five attributes—adherence at wound edge, granulation tissue, contraction, sustained contraction, and epithelialization—are all classified as good for healing. Several of the good-for-healing items require a brief explanation.

Adherence at the wound edge means that there is continuity of the wound edge and the base of the wound at any location along the wound perimeter (*Color Plates 8, 9, 69, and 87*). By definition, a partial-thickness wound will be adhered at the wound edge. A full-thickness or deeper wound will have closed by either granulation or contraction to the point where some area of the wound edge will be even with the skin surface. Granulation tissue, or fibroplasia, is evaluated by measuring wound depth, with a significant reduction in depth indicating proliferation of granulation tissue formation. A significant reduction in depth is defined as at least 0.2 cm change in linear depth measurements since the prior assessment. *Color Plates 7–9* show a significant reduction in depth. Contraction is assessed as being present when the open surface area size of the wound reduces. This item is scored at subsequent assessments as the contraction continues or if it has stopped. If the wound enlarges, however, this item would change from present to absent, and a new appearance of contraction would be required to have a score of "present" again. Sustained contraction means there is a continued drawing together of the wound edges that is measured by a reduction in wound surface open area size. It is usually accompanied by a change in wound shape. *Color Plates 3–5* show the same wound as it goes through wound contraction. Sustained contraction is scored zero at the appearance of the contraction benchmark, then scored 1 at subsequent reassessment, following the appearance of contraction. Occasionally, something interferes with the wound contraction, and the wound does not reduce in size or increases. This attribute would be marked zero—absent—if the wound size does not reduce or enlarges after the appearance of contraction.

The not-good-for-healing attributes are all related to the inflammatory phase of healing. The attributes that are good for healing are related to the proliferative and epithelialization phases of healing. As the wound attributes change from not good to good, the wound is progressing through the phases corresponding to those of acute wound healing.

Part II: Size Location and Wound Healing Phase Measures

Wound depth and undermining indicate extent of wound. If a wound has a depth less than 0.2 cm, it is scored as zero at all four points and at general depth. Depth and undermining are two indicators of "not good for healing."

11–15: Wound Depth. Five items on part II of the SWHT are related to presence of depth of at least 0.2 cm, both in general depth and at the four points of the clock—the 12, 3, 6, and 9 o'clock positions. Depth is measured as described in Chapter 4, and if it is at least 0.2 cm, it is recorded as present. Extent of depth is not significant for this assessment as long as it is at least 0.2 cm. (See *Color Plates 2, 7, 10,* and *31* for full-thickness depth.)

16–19: Tunneling/Undermining. Undermining and tunneling are measured at all four points of the clock, like depth. However, the objective measure used to report this attribute is also present or absent. With further testing and analysis, this attribute may prove to be redundant with part I. For the present time, it remains a part of the tool.

Additional Descriptive Attributes

Wound Location. Wound location is noted as the anatomic description most closely related to the wound site. Because lower torso and lower extremity wounds are most frequently seen, the locations have been broken down into the common sites for chronic wounds, and they have been clustered together for the upper body. Letters are also used to represent the wound location: *UB* for upper body, *C* for coccyx, *T* for trochanter, *I* for ischial, *H* for heel, and *F* for foot. Wounds in other locations can be added to the list if they are commonly seen in the practice setting by using letters on the form and adding a location descriptor to the key (e.g., *K* = knee, *A* = abdomen, *Th* = thigh). One needs to be sure to include the side of the body where the wound is located—right or left—by putting an *R* or an *L* next to the location letter.

Wound Healing Phase. The wound healing phase refers to the four biologic phases of wound healing: inflammatory, proliferative, epithelialization, and remodeling. Letters are used to represent the current wound healing phase: *I* for inflammatory, *P* for proliferative, *E* for epithelialization, and *R* for remodeling. As described in Chapter 4, the wound healing phase may be chronic, acute, or absent. Letters can be placed before the phase, such as the letter *C* before the phase for chronic, no letter before acute, or the letter *L* for lacking or absent, as modifiers of the current phase. A change in phase over time is an expected outcome. Chronicity of a phase should change to an active state of the phase, followed by progression to the next phase in the trajectory. Absence of a phase indicates need for investigation as to why the phase has not been achieved. This item is listed but unscored.

Testing the SWHT

One of the first questions applied to the SWHT was whether a tool design based on the four-phase acute wound healing model could be applied to chronic wounds, such as pressure ulcers. The SWHT is in the process of being tested on a data set of 112 pressure ulcer cases. All of the patients who were included in the data set were long-term care residents with pressure ulcers. Many experts consider pressure ulcers to be chronic wounds from the time of onset. The analyses are as yet incomplete.

SWHT for Monitoring and Tracking Wound Healing

The utility of the SWHT in the clinical setting for monitoring and tracking healing is easy and practical. Each of the attributes of the SWHT is scored as present or absent for wound tissue or surrounding skin. The total number of present not-good-for-healing attributes should diminish as the wound heals, and the total number of present good-for-healing attributes should increase. Change of score measures the change in healing and reduced severity of the wound. The scores are also useful for measuring the level of healing, indicating progress, lack of progress, or regression of healing. The SWHT has proven utility, both as a diagnostic tool that differentiates phases by assessment of healing attributes and as a tool for measurement of change in tissue status (e.g., tissue attribute) and size (e.g., change in depth and undermining) over time. Thus, the SWHT is designed to monitor and track healing, based on the acute wound healing model, and can be applied to acute or chronic wounds, such as pressure ulcers.

SWHT Reliability and Practicality

The SWHT has been clinically tested for reliability and clinical practicality by physical therapists (PTs) and PT assistants working in a long-term care facility during its 5 years of development and found to be very reliable for monitoring and tracking healing and nonhealing of pressure ulcers. It relies primarily on visual observation skills. No linear measurements, arithmetic calculations, or estimates of amount of tissue characteristic present are required. To health-care professionals who treat wounds, the SWHT information communicates clearly wound progress or risk. Documentation is very simple, and outcomes are visual. For example, it takes the clinician about 5 minutes to complete the assessment. In a trial educational session, a group of 10 PTs and PT assistants, who received 1 hour of classroom training followed by 1 hour of clinical practice on pressure ulcer patients, learned to use it well.

Assessment of Treatment Outcomes

Assessment of treatment outcome was the initial reason for development of the SWHT. Most patients are referred to the PT by the nurse for treatment after conventional treatments fails to heal the wound. To qualify for an intervention by the PT, the patient and the wound often need to meet a criterion of no progress, regression, or a halt of healing. Therefore, it is critical for the PT and the nurse to be able to set target outcomes, then to assess the response to the treatment intervention. A wound assessed with the SWHT as not progressing after a course of conventional care by the nurse would meet the criterion for referral. Once referred, the SWHT is useful for reporting wound outcomes associated with the intervention prescribed by the PT, such as physical therapy technologies. Response to treatment with these interventions should demonstrate consistent change in tissue status that corresponds to the biologic model for acute wound healing. A change in tissue status benchmarks the healing process and becomes a target functional outcome for reporting purposes, such as: the wound will be hemorrhage free, undermining free, necrosis free, and so forth. Reviewers can quickly determine a change in wound tissue status during the course of care because, as already described, the wound attributes should change from those that are not good for healing to those that are good for healing.

Using the SWHT
Two Parts of SWHT

Appendix 6-A shows the two parts of the long version of the SWHT and the procedure for using the SWHT. The SWHT is a paper-and-pencil instrument, comprising 19 attributes. Part I is the collection form of 10 tissue attributes. Part II is the list of 11 other attributes, including extent, location, and wound healing phase. All items on the SWHT are scored except location and the wound healing phase. Omission of a score indicates that the assessment was not completed. Scoring begins at baseline, week zero. The method of scoring for the tool is a number 1 for present and a zero for absent. This reporting format is readily compatible with computer technology and simplifies using the tool to build a database, such as the one described later. Completion of the form requires understanding of the definitions for each of the scored items. The assessment process is visual except for determining the presence of undermining/tunneling, which cannot be seen at the surface, and measurement of the open surface area of the wound.

SWHT Forms

Long Form

There are two forms of the SWHT, a long form (see Appendix 6-A) and a short form. Part I of the long form (Appendix 6-A) contains the 10 tissue attributes, listed in descending order of severity, next to definitions, followed by a column listing the rating option for the attribute as present or not present. The next column ranks the relationship to healing as not good or good. The last column is where the rating is listed as a score of present or absent. Part II lists measures and extent. The same scoring system of present or absent for 19 attributes of extent is applied. The attributes are the general depth of greater than 0.2 cm, the depth at the four clock points, and undermining at the four clock points. Date and week of care should be noted on the form. The benefit of the long form is having the definitions on the form. This would be helpful to a nurse or PT learning the system or for medical reviewers and surveyors looking for information about the rating system used for documentation.

Short Form

The short form of the SWHT is the same as the long form, except that the short form lacks the definitions printed on the form. The short form lists only the attributes and has columns to record data for multiple weeks. Part I can be printed on one side and part II on the other, and the paper can be cut to fit in a small, pocket-sized 4 × 6-inch loose-leaf notebook. Printing the forms as a pad punched with a hole pattern to match the notebook makes it easy and convenient to keep forms on hand. A set of the definitions and scoring can be printed on the same size paper, then kept in the notebook for reference. The notebook functions most smoothly if an alphabetic index the size of the notebook is used. The wound progress notebook can then be kept like a nursing treatment record book, with records alphabetically filed. The current patient wound healing records would then be readily available. The benefit of the notebook is that it will usually fit into a lab coat pocket and can be carried to the bedside or home. In a facility, it can be kept at the nurses' station, like the treatment record book, for easy reference. An additional benefit of the short form is that it is easy to see a complete history of the change in tissue status over multiple weeks of assessment. Reading the report over time provides a quick and clear evaluation to monitor wound healing progress.

Exhibits 6-1A and B show a completed case record. At the time of discharge or monthly, the completed record of wound attributes is taped in tiling fashion, like telephone order prescription sheets, onto a sheet of paper and filed in the medical record.

CLINICAL WISDOM

Use of Forms for Wound Measurement Along with the SWHT

Because wound measurement and tissue assessment or reassessment are usually done at the same time, it makes sense to record the information in the same record book. A wound measurement recording short form that fits in the same notebook as the SWHT meets this need. This form is used to record the size, depth, and undermining linear measurements. Each week, a new measurement form is added behind the SWHT form. By having the two forms together in the notebook, the examiner can check at a glance to see whether there is reduction in depth and open area. Chapter 5, Exhibit 5-2, shows a sample wound measurement form designed to fit this model.

Case Example Using the SWHT

Exhibits 6-1A and B show an example of a case where wound healing was monitored over a 5-week course of care, as reported on the short form of the SWHT, parts I and II. A summary (Exhibit 6-2) of the case example shows how the SWHT can be used to document a change in wound tissue status from a predominance of not-good-for-healing attributes to a predominance of good attributes. Exhibit 6-2 reflects the following:

- The patient had the presence at baseline, week zero, of hemorrhage, necrosis, and erythema, and absence of any attributes good for healing. The presence of these attributes at baseline is an indication that this wound will need aggressive intervention to improve.
- At week 2, there were multiple attributes that were indicators that this patient will be in the risk-for-not-healing group, including undermining and depth at all four clock points, further indicating the medical necessity for aggressive intervention to put the wound on a course of healing.
- Assuming that aggressive intervention was undertaken at week 2, the improvement in the wound tissue status from not good to good is significant by week 4.

Sussman Wound Healing Tool Database

Although the SWHT is a paper-and-pencil instrument, the SWHT wound database is maintained in a computer. The scoring system of using a 1 or a zero is computer-compatible for data management and data entry. The SWHT forms are printed on the computer as screens, and data are entered

EXHIBIT 6-1A   SWHT Part I: Wound Tissue Attributes

Week	0	1	2	3	4
Date: 2010	1/7	1/14	1/21	1/28	2/4
1. Hemorrhage	1	0	0	0	0
2. Maceration	0	0	0	0	0
3. Undermining	0	0	1	1	1
4. Erythema	1	1	1	0	0
5. Necrosis	1	1	1	0	0
6. Adherence	0	0	0	1	1
7. Granulation (decreased depth)	0	0	1	1	1
8. Appearance of contraction (reduced size)	0	0	1	1	1
9. Sustained contraction (more reduced size)	0	0	0	1	1
10. Epithelialization	0	0	0	1	1
Total "Not Good"	3	2	3	1	1
Total "Good"	0	0	2	5	5

Key: Present = 1. Absent = 0.
Copyright (c) 1997, Sussman Physical Therapy, Inc.

EXHIBIT 6-1B   SWHT Part II: Size, Location, Wound Healing Phase Measures, and Extent

Week	0	1	2	3	4
Date:	1/7	1/14	1/21	1/28	2/4
11. General depth > 0.2 cm	0	1	1	1	1
12. Depth @ 12:00 > 0.2 cm	0	1	1	1	1
13. Depth @ 3:00 > 0.2 cm	0	1	1	1	1
14. Depth @ 6:00 > 0.2 cm	0	1	1	1	1
15. Depth @ 9:00 > 0.2 cm	1	1	1	1	1
16. Underm @ 12:00 > 0.2 cm	0	0	1	1	0
17. Underm @ 3:00 > 0.2 cm	0	1	1	0	0
18. Underm @ 6:00 > 0.2 cm	0	1	1	1	0
19. Underm @ 9:00 > 0.2 cm	0	0	1	1	1
Location	RT	RT	RT	RT	RT
Wound healing phase	I	I	I	P	P

Key: Present = 1. Absent = 0. Location choices: upper body (UB), coccyx (C), trochanter (T), ischial (I), heel (H), and foot (F); add right or left (R or L). Wound healing phase: inflammation (I), proliferation (P), epithelialization (E), remodeling (R).

Copyright (c) 1997, Sussman Physical Therapy, Inc.

EXHIBIT 6-2 Summary of Wound Attribute Change over a 5-Week Course of Care

WEEK 0	WEEK 2	WEEK 4
"NOT GOOD" for healing	*"NOT GOOD" for healing*	*"NOT GOOD" for healing*
Hemorrhage Undermining Erythema Necrosis Depth 9:00	Necrosis Undermining Erythema Depth 12, 3, 6, 9:00 Undermining 12, 3, 6, 9:00	Undermining Depth 12, 3, 6, 9:00 Undermining 9:00
"GOOD" for healing	*"GOOD" for healing*	*"GOOD" for healing*
None	Fibroplasia Appearance of contraction	Fibroplasia Appearance of contraction Sustained contraction Adherence Epithelialization
Wound healing phase	*Wound healing phase*	*Wound healing phase*
Inflammatory phase	Inflammatory phase	Proliferative phase

Copyright (c) 1997, Sussman Physical Therapy, Inc.

either prospectively or retrospectively. Data reports can be printed, and the captured data can be analyzed on an individual patient basis or by group. Further testing of the SWHT is planned at different sites.

Summary

Clinicians can utilize the SWHT present/absent scoring system to assess healing, triage the case, guide treatment intervention, and report functional outcomes. The SWHT is a simple, easy-to-follow, and complete documentation system that provides payers and providers with improved utilization management.

Introduction and Development of the Pressure Ulcer Scale for Healing

In 1996, the National Pressure Ulcer Advisory Panel (NPUAP) in the United States convened a task force to address the practice of reverse staging of pressure ulcers that was encouraged by Medicare documentation requirements using the Minimum Data Set (MDS) system in long-term care facilities. The objective was to develop a biologically accurate and easy-to-use instrument to replace reverse staging. The task force developed and tested a tool to measure pressure ulcer healing, and the Pressure Ulcer Scale for Healing (PUSH) tool was presented in 1997 at the NPUAP biennial conference (see Appendix 6-B).

The PUSH tool incorporates three wound characteristics: surface area measurements, exudate amount, and surface appearance. These wound characteristics were chosen based on principal component analysis to define the best model of healing after following 37 pressure ulcers every 2 weeks for a total of 8 weeks[3,4] The three items identified in the model

for the proposed tool (surface area, exudate amount, and tissue type) were then tested on a new sample and performed similarly. The model explained 55%–65% of the variance at week zero through week 8 for the study sample.[12] The results demonstrated good discrimination among the time points, particularly the earlier times, compared with the later times.

Validity

Two retrospective studies have validated the original findings. A multisite retrospective study evaluated 273 pressure ulcers using the PUSH tool over 10 weeks. Ulcers in the study included both partial-thickness stage II and full-thickness stage III and IV (58%) ulcers. Results demonstrated 58%-74% of the variance over the 10 weeks was explained with the PUSH tool items. Inclusion of other variables did not contribute to the explanation of the variance. Pairwise comparisons showed evidence of sensitivity of the tool over time.[13]

The second retrospective study involved data from a sample of 2,490 nursing home residents, of whom 1,274 had a pressure ulcer at initial assessment.[14] However, only 269 ulcers met all criteria for study inclusion. All residents included in the study were participating in the National Pressure Ulcer Long-Term Care Study (NPULS).[15] The study demonstrated sensitivity of the tool over 12 weeks; however, only 40%-57% of the total variance was explained by the PUSH tool items. Additional multiple regression techniques indicated that the tool explained 49% of the variance over the first 7 weeks. Beyond 7 weeks, the tool explained 29% of the variance. Based on findings from the second study, the PUSH tool was revised to increase the sensitivity of the tool to changes over time. The current version of the PUSH tool includes dectiles (10 divisions of size) for the categorical size item instead of the original quintiles (5 divisions of size), and the largest surface area on the size item was increased to 24 cm². The revised definitions were tested on the 269 cases from the NPULS data set, and the findings remained consistent with the original findings, with respect to variance and sensitivity to change. The authors suggest that content validity, correlational validity, prospective validity, and sensitivity to change can be met by the proposed tool. PUSH allows a consistent, evidence-based methodology for reporting wound healing status among health care professionals. PUSH is not a comprehensive assessment instrument for pressure ulcers, nor is it a research tool for measuring healing and should not be used for those purposes. Although it was first developed as a way of measuring healing of pressure ulcers, the PUSH tool has since been evaluated as an instrument to assess progress of venous ulcer healing and was found to be sensitive to detect change over time.[16,17]

Use of the tool involves measuring size, evaluating exudate, and categorizing tissue type. The clinician measures the size of the wound, using length and width to calculate surface area (length × width) and chooses the appropriate size category on the tool (there are 10 size categories, from zero to 10). Exudate is evaluated as none (0), light (1), moderate (2), or heavy (3). Tissue type choices include closed (0), epithelial tissue (1), granulation tissue (2), slough (3), and necrotic tissue (4). The three subscores are then summed for a total score. Exhibit 6-3 shows total scores plotted on a graph. Note the different trajectories of healing and nonhealing pressure ulcers.[17] The PUSH tool offers assessment of three wound characteristics and is best used as a method of quantitatively reporting the direction of healing over time. The PUSH tool does not include items that may be relevant to treatment decisions. Assessment of additional wound characteristics with other tools, such as the SWHT or BWAT, could be used for baseline and more comprehensive assessment. The PUSH tool was designed for use as a trigger to identify when goals of treatment are being met and patients who need to be reevaluated. Inappropriate reporting of healing indirectly compromises the quality of life of patients with pressure ulcers. A simple sensitive instrument to monitor the efficacy of treatment methods of pressure ulcer care would presumably improve the quality of life.[17]

The PUSH tool may be used with an ulcer healing record form developed by the NPUAP that allows for recording of subscores and total score on a periodic basis. The advantage of this form is the ability to note quickly any progress or degeneration of the wound. Another method of monitoring PUSH scores over time is available as a graph. The value of using graphs to track ulcer scores is the ability to spot trends in wound recovery quickly, as well as failure to progress. Exhibit 6-3 contains an example of a PUSH healing chart.[15]

Utility of PUSH is beginning to be appreciated and to be reported. PUSH was selected as the outcome measure for a multidisciplinary set of 14 clinical decision trees to be used in long-term care facilities. The decision trees guide interaction between medicine, nursing, physical therapy and dietary. They work concurrently and are based on recognized best practice for pressure ulcer care. The decision trees use a consistent methodology of clinical problem solving, trig-

EXHIBIT 6-3 Example of PUSH Healing Chart

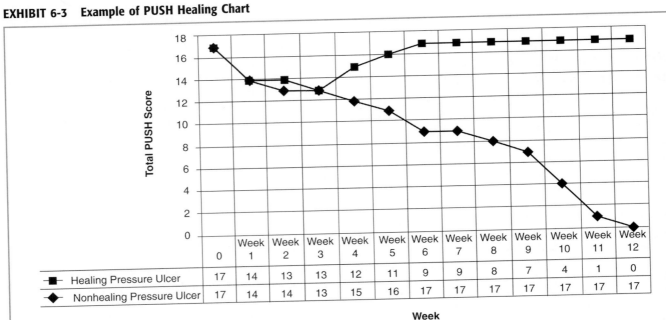

	0	Week 1	Week 2	Week 3	Week 4	Week 5	Week 6	Week 7	Week 8	Week 9	Week 10	Week 11	Week 12
■ Healing Pressure Ulcer	17	14	13	13	12	11	9	9	8	7	4	1	0
◆ Nonhealing Pressure Ulcer	17	14	14	13	15	16	17	17	17	17	17	17	17

Week

gers for care, and target outcomes. The same outcome measure, change in PUSH scores over time, is used for all.[18] Posthauer reported on the decision trees in action. A 3-month evaluation using the program was assessed after appropriate staff training at five long-term care facilities. The decision tree process was found to be useful in promoting collaboration between the disciplines.[19] Examples of the dietary decision trees are shown in Chapter 3.

PUSH was used as the primary outcome measure for a study of pressure ulcer healing in a randomized controlled product study involving 90 residents with stage II, III or IV pressure ulcers in multiple centers. Patients received either standard care plus placebo (N =33) or standard care plus the study product (N=56). Wound healing was assessed biweekly using PUSH version 3.0 over 8 weeks. Resulting PUSH scores were used as the quantitative outcome measure. The cumulative PUSH scores were found to be a sensitive measure of change in both groups and were used for comparison.[20]

Pompeo revised the way PUSH tool data collection instrument is used for the purpose of capturing system-wide wound outcomes data and validated its utility in a prospective study of long-term acute care hospitals.[21] Data were collected representing 13,737 patient days of care (374 patients with 989 wounds). The data recorded documented overall progress of healing for all wound patients, presumably with mixed wound etiologies, although this was not stated. Data were then used by the facility wound program to calculate healing as a function of time on a monthly basis as a tool to measure quality of care. The hospitals are now using the results of the study as a benchmark in the participating facilities to gauge the effectiveness of care.

As already mentioned, the PUSH tool is not used to provide information about specific interventions. Data must be carefully interpreted by thoughtful wound providers. Pompeo and colleagues suggest that the PUSH tool, as revised, was the best tool available for comparing healing outcomes. The same methodology and components of the original PUSH are kept intact. The revisions included: listing multiple wounds on one form using the original scoring grid, initial and end of stay or monthly summed PUSH score for all wounds, length of stay in days, change in total PUSH score, and the healing rate (PUSH score/total days of stay). Comparison was made only of initial and discharge or monthly PUSH Scores. Appendix 6-C is a copy of the Pompeo form. By combining the total wound scores, which has not been validated elsewhere, the score represented the wound severity and bioburden of all the wounds affecting the patient. Pompeo suggested that PUSH may have had limited adoption because weekly measurement and tracking as suggested by NPUAP for individual wound progress is time consuming. Alternative application of PUSH provides a broader picture of the progression of healing and of the severity of wound cases seen at the hospitals in the study where the data is used to benchmark wound outcomes as shown in Exhibit 6-4. Not all results are favorable compared to the benchmark. Many factors can account for the changes triggering evaluation of the components of the wound program to determine the factors responsible.

Pompeo postulated reasons why more clinics aren't using PUSH and decided that there are perceived time requirements about use of the tool itself, lack of familiarity with PUSH, an impression that it requires careful interpretation by skilled clinicians, and a perception that it has limited research support. More education is needed about the clinical utility and value of PUSH. Now that the sensitivity of PUSH for measuring healing is demonstrated, is it reasonable and appropriate to use the Pompeo method and combine all wounds into a total PUSH score to determine the wound bioburden and the rate of wound healing? By combining the data for different wound etiologies, would the healing rates be meaningful since wounds of different etiologies have different healing times? For example, venous ulcers heal twice as fast as diabetic ulcers, partial-thickness wounds heal faster than deep wounds, and forefoot ulcers heal faster than mid or heel ulcers in diabetics.[22-27] More research is needed to answer these questions. It would, however, meet the current documentation requirements of the Centers for Medicare and Medicaid Services (CMS) for reporting healing. The idea of PUSH was to develop a simple-to-use tool sensitive to change in pressure ulcer healing..

To summarize, PUSH is a valid tool for replacing "reverse staging"; monitoring pressure or leg ulcer healing or deterioration over time; providing a consistent, method for monitoring pressure ulcers; enhancing communication among health-care providers regarding changing wound status; and reporting efficacy of wound interventions and wound programs. Pompeo found that PUSH was best used in settings where care is provided over several weeks and used the PUSH score for a heterogenous mixture of wounds to track bioburden as well as healing rate.[16,17]

Introduction and Development of the Bates-Jensen Wound Assessment Tool (BWAT) or Pressure Sore Status Tool

The Bates-Jensen Wound Assessment Tool (BWAT) or Pressure Sore Status Tool (PSST) developed in 1990 by Bates-

EXHIBIT 6-4 How Can You Use PUSH in Your Clinical in Practice?

- For baseline measurements
- For weekly or 30 day documentation
- For 30 day comparison of results—CMS requirements (as suggested by Pompeo)
- To track rate of healing to determine trend of healing or nonhealing
- To track wounds of different etiologies
- To evaluate efficacy of a wound program
- To evaluate outcomes of patient care over time
- To market results of a clinical wound program

Jensen[1] and revised in 2001, evaluates 13 wound characteristics with a numerical rating scale and rates them from best to worst possible (see Appendix 6-D). The BWAT is recommended for use as a method of assessment and monitoring of pressure ulcers and other chronic wounds. It is a pencil-and-paper instrument comprised of 15 items: location, shape, size, depth, edges, undermining or pockets, necrotic tissue type, necrotic tissue amount, exudate type, exudate amount, surrounding skin color, peripheral tissue edema, peripheral tissue induration, granulation tissue, and epithelialization. Two items are nonscored: location and shape. The remaining 13 are scored items, and each appears with characteristic descriptors rated on a scale (1 best for that characteristic and 5 worst attribute of the characteristic). It is recommended that wounds be scored initially for a baseline assessment and at regular intervals to evaluate therapy. Once a lesion has been assessed for each item on the BWAT, the 13 item scores can be added to obtain a total score for the wound. The total score can then be monitored to "see at a glance" healing or degeneration of the wound. Total scores range from 13 (skin intact but always at risk for further damage) to 65 (profound tissue degeneration). The tool has a one-page sheet of instructions for use, in addition to the item descriptions (Appendix 6-D). The original PSST was developed as an assessment tool for both clinical use and research. Over the years, BWAT use has evolved to include measuring and predicting wound healing and is used in wounds beyond pressure ulcers. The BWAT has provided a basis for many other wound assessment tools and is the most widely used of the instruments presented. Only minor changes were made to the PSST to create the second generation tool, the BWAT. In addition to the name of the instrument, "none" category choices (for items previously without a "none" category) were added. The scoring and guidelines for use are the same.

Validity

The items on the original PSST were developed through the use of experts participating in a modified Delphi panel and the same items remain on the BWAT. The content validity of the tool was established with the use of a nine-member expert judge panel (mean overall content validity index = 0.91, $p = .05$). Content validity was established for each individual item on the tool and for the total tool with the panel. Concurrent validity was evaluated in a long-term care setting and involved comparing medical record documentation of pressure sore stage with the original PSST depth item for a Pearson Product Moment correlation coefficient of $r = .91$ ($p = .001$).[1]

In a later study, the total score was compared with recorded stage of the wound, and findings revealed a relatively strong positive relationship between the two scores (Pearson Product Moment correlation $r = .55$, $p = .001$). The study demonstrated little difference between the mean total scores of stage I versus stage II sores and for stage III versus stage IV sores, but significant difference between stage I and II versus stage III and IV scores (stage I and II

mean total score 23.35 versus stage III and IV mean total score 31.83; $p < .001$).[17,28]

Reliability

Reliability was demonstrated on adult patients in an acute care hospital with enterostomal therapy (ET) nurses or nurses with special training in wound management. The mean interrater reliability coefficient was 0.91.[29] Intrarater reliability estimates yielded a mean of 0.975. Although high reliability estimates had been established with expert nurses, a question remained as to the efficacy with practitioners who did not have extraordinary education or experience in wound assessment and management. Reliability of the original PSST, when used by "regular" health-care practitioners, was addressed in a long-term care facility. Fifteen practitioners with varied educational and experience backgrounds participated in the study. Two PTs, three licensed practical nurses, and 10 registered nurses participated in the study. Pairs independently assessed 16 wounds across a broad spectrum of severity on two occasions (2 hours apart). An expert nurse also independently assessed the same wounds as the practitioner pairs. Interrater reliability estimates were calculated between practitioners themselves and between practitioners and the expert rater. Intrarater reliability estimates were calculated in a similar manner, except that each rater's recordings were compared with a second assessment (taken within 2 hours of the first) for the same wound. Interrater reliability for the practitioners yielded a mean of 0.78. Reliability estimates for the practitioners versus the expert yielded a mean of 0.82. Intrarater reliability for the practitioners averaged 0.89.[16,29]

Because the BWAT involves a Likert-type ordinal scale and the probability of chance agreements between two raters is 0.20 for any item, the data were also subjected to analyses using a polychotomous data stratagem. Resulting kappa statistics for each item on the scale yielded coefficients above 0.60. Collectively, the results from the long-term care setting suggested that use of the original PSST by general health care practitioners resulted in lower reliability than did its use by ET nurses but certainly within an acceptable range.

Sensitivity and Specificity

Predictive validity of the original PSST was evaluated in a retrospective study of 143 pressure sores (51 partial-thickness wounds, 92 full-thickness wounds) over 6 weeks, with a minimum of three assessments per ulcer during the study period. The main outcome measure of the study was time to 50% healing, as measured by surface area. Data were analyzed with survival analysis techniques, with the main finding that surface area changes plus net PSST change at 1 week were most predictive of time to 50% healing. The positive predictive value of a net improvement in total PSST score at 1 week was 65%, whereas the positive predictive value of a net deterioration in PSST score at 1 week was only 31%. Sensitivity in this sample was 61%, and specificity was 52%.[30]

The BWAT is meant to be used once a pressure sore has developed; it is not a risk assessment tool. It is recommended that the pressure sore be scored initially for a baseline assessment and at regular intervals to evaluate therapy. Once a lesion has been assessed for each item on the BWAT, the 13 item scores can be added to obtain a total score for the wound. The total score can then be plotted on the pressure sore continuum at the bottom of the tool to see regeneration or degeneration of the wound at a glance. Total scores range from 13 (skin intact but always at risk) to 65 (profound tissue degeneration).

BWAT Scoring

The assessment and, ultimately, the quantification of clinical judgment forms the foundation for determining treatments and for evaluating effectiveness of therapy. After completing a full wound assessment using the BWAT, the individual 13 items' scores can be summed to create the total BWAT score. This total score can be monitored over time as an index of wound status and effectiveness of treatment. The total BWAT score can be plotted on the continuum at the end of the tool, along with the date of assessment and, thus, can provide a visual aid to determining healing or nonhealing of the wound. A retrospective study[30] suggests that changes in the BWAT score at 1 week plus changes in surface area measurements may have predictive value. A 1-week net decrease (improvement) in total BWAT score plus a decrease in surface area was the best predictor of time to 50% wound closure in 143 partial- and full-thickness pressure sores within a 6-week study period. Thus, the total BWAT score may provide a method of predicting outcomes. More research is needed in this area.

A PUSH score can be calculated from the BWAT tool. The following guidelines will convert BWAT subscale scores into PUSH subscale scores. Table 6-2 provides an example of conversion.

1. Wound size: It is best to use actual surface area measurements, length × width, to determine which PUSH size category is appropriate. If actual measurements are not available, the following guide may be helpful:
   - If BWAT size category = 1, then PUSH size category score = 0, 1, 2, 3, 4, 5, or 6
   - If BWAT size category = 2, then PUSH size category score = either 7 or 8
   - If BWAT size category = 3, then PUSH size category score = either 9 or 10
   - If BWAT size category = 4 or 5, then PUSH size category score = 10
2. Exudate amount:
   - If BWAT exudate amount score = 1, then PUSH exudate amount score = 0
   - If BWAT exudate amount score = 2 or 3, then PUSH exudate amount score = 1
   - If BWAT exudate amount score = 4, then PUSH exudate amount score = 2
   - If BWAT exudate amount score = 5, then PUSH exudate amount score = 3
3. Tissue type:
   - If BWAT Total Score = 13, then PUSH Type Score = 0 *OR* if Granulation = 1 *AND* Epithelialization = 1, then PUSH Type Score = 0
   - If Necrotic Tissue Type = 4 or 5, then PUSH Type Score = 4
   - If Necrotic Tissue Type = 2 or 3, then PUSH Type Score = 3
   - If Epithelialization < 5, then PUSH Type Score = 1
   - If Granulation < 5 *AND* Epithelialization = 5, then PUSH Type Score = 2

Assessment of Treatment Response

The BWAT tool allows for temporal tracking of individual characteristics, as well as the total score. Each characteristic is assessed as described above and given a value from

TABLE 6-2 Example of PUSH Score Derivation from BWAT Scores

BWAT Items	BWAT Scores	PUSH Items	PUSH Scores
1. Size	*4* (6.5 × 6.0 cm = 39 cm²)	*1. Size* A (724 cm²)	10
2. Depth	3		
3. Edges	2		
4. Undermining	1		
5. Necrotic Tissue Type	3		
6. Necrotic Tissue Amt.	4		
7. Exudate Type	4		
8. Exudate Amt.	5	*2. Exudate Amt.* (Heavy)	*3*
9. Skin Color	4		
10. Edema	1		
11. Induration	2		
12. Granulation	3	*3. Tissue Type** (Slough)	*3*
13. Epithelialization	4		
Total Score	**40**	Total Score	**16**

* Note that necrotic tissue is item 5 on BWAT and 3 on PUSH, where slough is not classified as necrotic tissue if all necrotic tissue is absent.

the Likert scale; thus, the scores can be monitored for improvement or deterioration in each characteristic. This quantification of observations allows for monitoring not only individual items and total score but also groups of characteristics. For example, the characteristics of necrotic tissue type and amount may be tracked with exudate type and amount to evaluate debridement or infection management.

Another benefit associated with the assignment of numeric values to items on the tool is the ability to set realistic goals. Clinical experience shows that not all pressure ulcers heal and certainly not always in the same setting. The BWAT allows for more realistic goal setting as appropriate to the health-care setting and the individual patient and pressure ulcer. For example, the patient with a large, necrotic, full-thickness ulcer in acute care will probably not be in the facility long enough for the wound to heal completely. However, the tool enables clinicians to set smaller goals, such as "The wound will decrease in type and amount of necrotic tissue."

CLINICAL WISDOM
Realistic Goal Setting

In some instances, a pressure ulcer may never heal because of host factors or other contextual circumstances. In this case, an example of a goal might be to maintain the total BWAT score between 20 and 22.

Pressure sore severity, as well as overall health status of the patient, can also determine the appropriate management approach for ulcer healing. Severity states are a method of differentiating or stratification of various degrees of symptom intensity. In the case of the pressure ulcer, it refers to some measure of the degree of the tissue insult. The total BWAT score can be used as a method of stratification to guide care planning. BWAT scores can be divided into four suggested severity states, with total scores of 13–20 indicating minimal severity, 21–30 mild severity, 31–40 moderate severity, and 41–65 extreme severity. The goals of pressure sore management are to decrease the overall severity status of the wound and to make this decrease in a timely fashion. Figure 6-1 displays the BWAT severity state groups.

The severity status groups can be useful in designing general treatment algorithms. An example of a treatment algorithm for one wound in each severity state is presented below. These treatment algorithms are derived from clinical practice guidelines.[31]

BWAT Minimal Severity Scores 13–20. Pressure sores with a BWAT total score of 13–20 are generally reversible stage I lesions, with intact skin at high risk for altered integrity, or shallow stage II, partial-thickness pressure sores. Figure 6-2 presents a generic algorithm for treatment for wounds in this severity state. The main goals for wounds in this severity state are to prevent further damage and to provide a moist wound environment for healing.

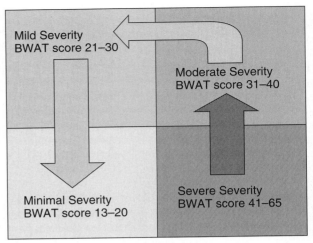

FIGURE 6-1 Severity states based on BWAT scores. The goals of therapy are: (1) to decrease the overall severity state of the wound and, thus, the BWAT score and (2) to make the decrease in a timely fashion. There is equal concern regarding severity of the wound and the duration of time that the wound spends in any severity state. (Copyright Barbara Bates-Jensen)

BWAT Mild Severity Scores 21–30. Pressure sores with mild severity include both partial-thickness and full-thickness wounds. Figure 6-3 presents a general treatment algorithm for partial-thickness wounds with mild severity scores. The goals of care for partial-thickness wounds with mild severity scores are to absorb excess wound exudate, maintain a clean wound bed, and maintain a moist environment. Full-thickness wounds with mild severity scores offer more options for treatment because the wound can present as a clean, full-thickness wound or as a wound filled with necrotic debris.[32]

BWAT Moderate Severity Scores 31–40. Figure 6-4 is a care plan for a full-thickness wound with necrotic tissue present. The goals of care for full-thickness wounds with moderate severity scores are to obtain/maintain a clean wound bed, provide a moist environment, absorb excess exudate, prevent premature closure, and reduce wound dead space. Wounds with moderate (and mild) severity scores have the most diverse presentations clinically, so choices regarding treatment are numerous.[32]

Figures 6-5, 6-6, and 6-7 demonstrate general treatment algorithms. These algorithms can be used to determine appropriate care for a variety of chronic wounds with moderate to extreme BWAT severity scores. Wounds in the moderate severity state are predominantly full-thickness wounds or stage III or IV pressure sores. Figure 6-5 presented the case of the full thickness wound with necrotic debris and large amounts of exudate. Treatment is focused on debridement and absorbing exudate. Figure 6-6 presents the case of the full-thickness clean wound with undermining or dead space, and the treatment focus is on eliminating the dead

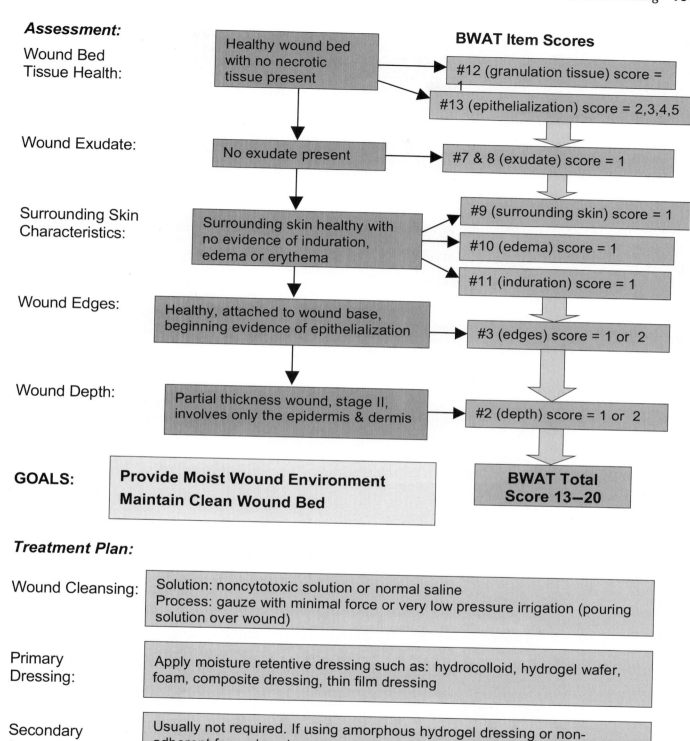

Assessment:

Wound Bed Tissue Health:

Wound Exudate:

Surrounding Skin Characteristics:

Wound Edges:

Wound Depth:

Healthy wound bed with no necrotic tissue present

No exudate present

Surrounding skin healthy with no evidence of induration, edema or erythema

Healthy, attached to wound base, beginning evidence of epithelialization

Partial thickness wound, stage II, involves only the epidermis & dermis

BWAT Item Scores

#12 (granulation tissue) score = 1

#13 (epithelialization) score = 2,3,4,5

#7 & 8 (exudate) score = 1

#9 (surrounding skin) score = 1

#10 (edema) score = 1

#11 (induration) score = 1

#3 (edges) score = 1 or 2

#2 (depth) score = 1 or 2

GOALS: Provide Moist Wound Environment Maintain Clean Wound Bed

BWAT Total Score 13–20

Treatment Plan:

Wound Cleansing: Solution: noncytotoxic solution or normal saline
Process: gauze with minimal force or very low pressure irrigation (pouring solution over wound)

Primary Dressing: Apply moisture retentive dressing such as: hydrocolloid, hydrogel wafer, foam, composite dressing, thin film dressing

Secondary Dressing: Usually not required. If using amorphous hydrogel dressing or non-adherent foam dressing may need dressing or tape to keep gel or foam in place.

OUTCOME: Wound 100% resurfaced with new epithelium

FIGURE 6-2 Minimal BWAT severity score treatment algorithm for mild, dry, partial-thickness wound. (Adapted with permission from ConvaTec, a division of Bristol-Myers Squibb, USA.)

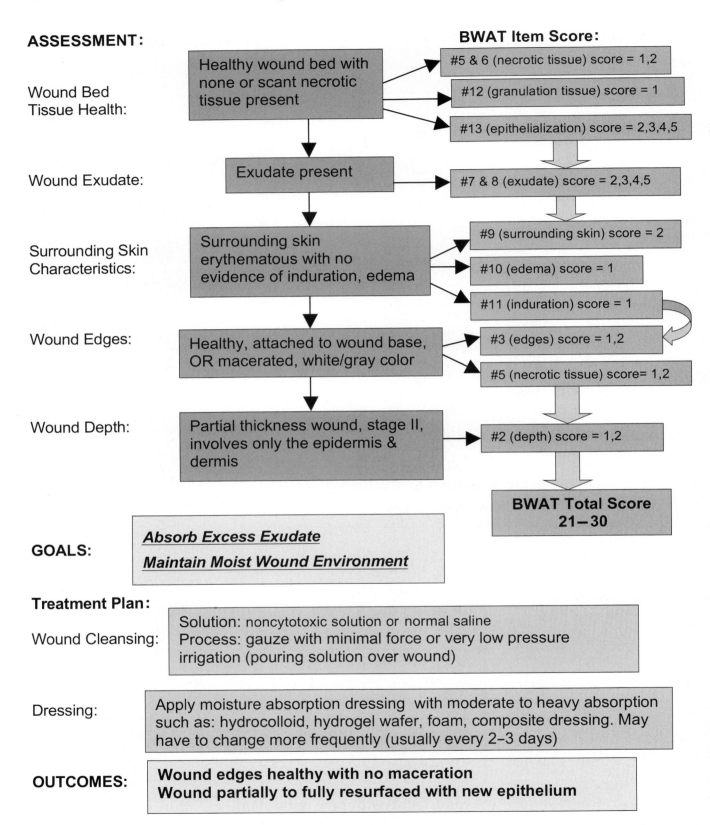

FIGURE 6-3 Partial-thickness wound with mild BWAT severity score treatment algorithm. (Adapted with permission from ConvaTec, a division of Bristol-Myers Squibb, USA.)

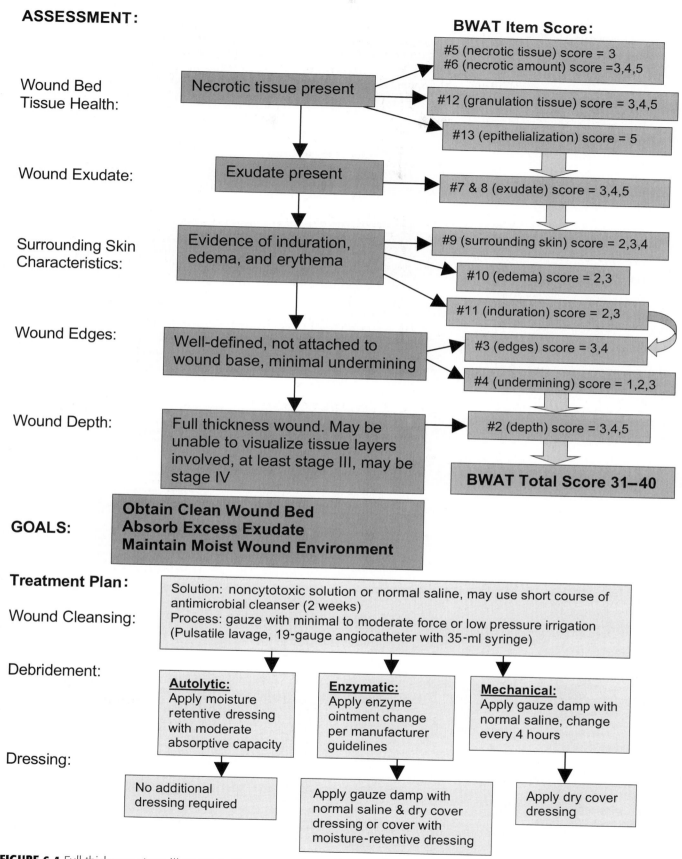

FIGURE 6-4 Full-thickness stage III or stage IV pressure ulcer with a moderate BWAT severity score treatment algorithm. (Adapted with permission from ConvaTec, a division of Bristol-Myers Squibb, USA.)

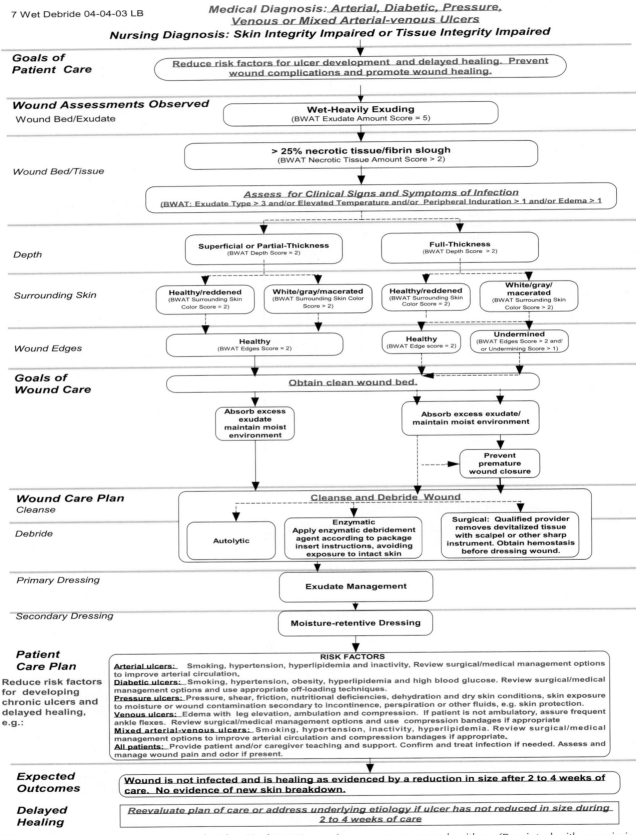

FIGURE 6-5 General full-thickness wound with critical BWAT severity score treatment algorithm. (Reprinted with permission from ConvaTec, a division of Bristol-Myers Squibb, USA.)

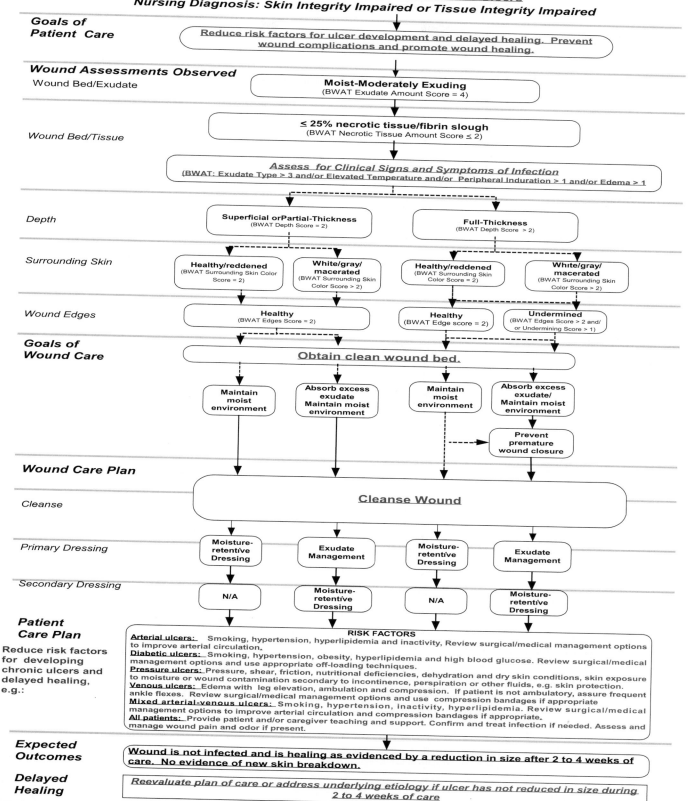

6 Moderate 04-04-03 LB

Medical Diagnosis: _Arterial, Diabetic, Pressure, Venous or Mixed Arterial-venous Ulcers_
Nursing Diagnosis: _Skin Integrity Impaired or Tissue Integrity Impaired_

Goals of Patient Care

Reduce risk factors for ulcer development and delayed healing. Prevent wound complications and promote wound healing.

Wound Assessments Observed

Wound Bed/Exudate

Moist-Moderately Exuding
(BWAT Exudate Amount Score = 4)

Wound Bed/Tissue

≤ 25% necrotic tissue/fibrin slough
(BWAT Necrotic Tissue Amount Score ≤ 2)

Assess for Clinical Signs and Symptoms of Infection
(BWAT: Exudate Type > 3 and/or Elevated Temperature and/or Peripheral Induration > 1 and/or Edema > 1

Depth

Superficial orPartial-Thickness
(BWAT Depth Score = 2)

Full-Thickness
(BWAT Depth Score > 2)

Surrounding Skin

Healthy/reddened
(BWAT Surrounding Skin Color Score = 2)

White/gray/ macerated
(BWAT Surrounding Skin Color Score > 2)

Healthy/reddened
(BWAT Surrounding Skin Color Score = 2)

White/gray/ macerated
(BWAT Surrounding Skin Color Score > 2)

Wound Edges

Healthy
(BWAT Edges Score = 2)

Healthy
(BWAT Edge score = 2)

Undermined
(BWAT Edges Score > 2 and/ or Undermining Score > 1)

Goals of Wound Care

Obtain clean wound bed.

Maintain moist environment

Absorb excess exudate Maintain moist environment

Maintain moist environment

Absorb excess exudate/ Maintain moist environment

Prevent premature wound closure

Wound Care Plan

Cleanse

Cleanse Wound

Primary Dressing

Moisture-retentive Dressing

Exudate Management

Moisture-retentive Dressing

Exudate Management

Secondary Dressing

N/A

Moisture-retentive Dressing

N/A

Moisture-retentive Dressing

Patient Care Plan

Reduce risk factors for developing chronic ulcers and delayed healing, e.g.:

RISK FACTORS
Arterial ulcers: Smoking, hypertension, hyperlipidemia and inactivity, Review surgical/medical management options to improve arterial circulation.
Diabetic ulcers: Smoking, hypertension, obesity, hyperlipidemia and high blood glucose. Review surgical/medical management options and use appropriate off-loading techniques.
Pressure ulcers: Pressure, shear, friction, nutritional deficiencies, dehydration and dry skin conditions, skin exposure to moisture or wound contamination secondary to incontinence, perspiration or other fluids, e.g. skin protection.
Venous ulcers: Edema with leg elevation, ambulation and compression. If patient is not ambulatory, assure frequent ankle flexes. Review surgical/medical management options and use compression bandages if appropriate
Mixed arterial-venous ulcers: Smoking, hypertension, inactivity, hyperlipidemia. Review surgical/medical management options to improve arterial circulation and compression bandages if appropriate.
All patients: Provide patient and/or caregiver teaching and support. Confirm and treat infection if needed. Assess and manage wound pain and odor if present.

Expected Outcomes

Wound is not infected and is healing as evidenced by a reduction in size after 2 to 4 weeks of care. No evidence of new skin breakdown.

Delayed Healing

Reevaluate plan of care or address underlying etiology if ulcer has not reduced in size during 2 to 4 weeks of care

FIGURE 6-6 General full-thickness wound with undermining or pocketing with moderate BWAT severity score treatment algorithm. (Reprinted with permission from ConvaTec, a division of Bristol-Myers Squibb, USA.)

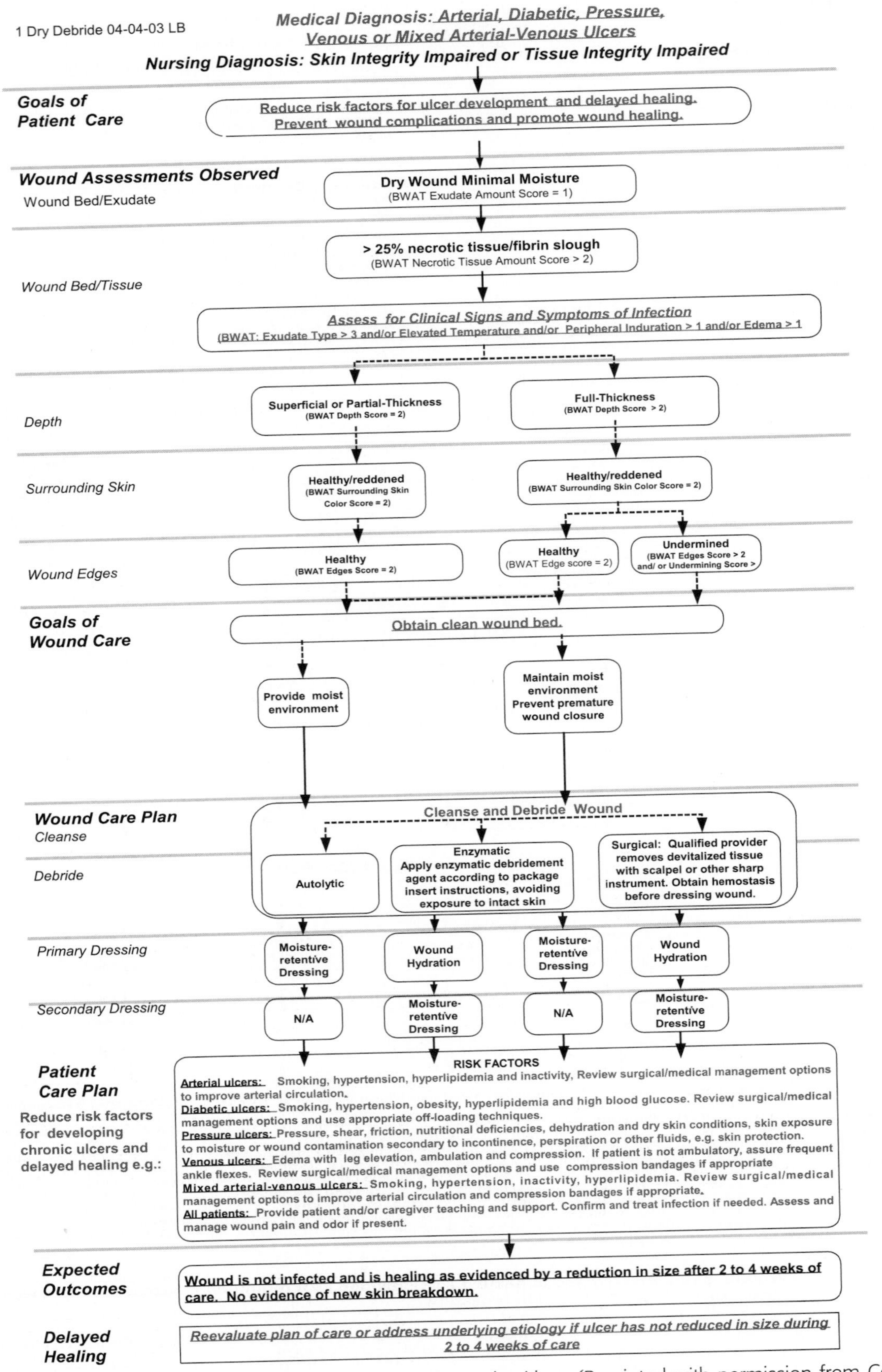

1 Dry Debride 04-04-03 LB

Medical Diagnosis: _Arterial, Diabetic, Pressure,_
Venous or Mixed Arterial-Venous Ulcers
Nursing Diagnosis: _Skin Integrity Impaired or Tissue Integrity Impaired_

Goals of Patient Care

> Reduce risk factors for ulcer development and delayed healing.
> Prevent wound complications and promote wound healing.

Wound Assessments Observed
Wound Bed/Exudate

Dry Wound Minimal Moisture
(BWAT Exudate Amount Score = 1)

Wound Bed/Tissue

> 25% necrotic tissue/fibrin slough
(BWAT Necrotic Tissue Amount Score > 2)

Assess for Clinical Signs and Symptoms of Infection
(BWAT: Exudate Type > 3 and/or Elevated Temperature and/or Peripheral Induration > 1 and/or Edema > 1

Depth

Superficial or Partial-Thickness
(BWAT Depth Score = 2)

Full-Thickness
(BWAT Depth Score > 2)

Surrounding Skin

Healthy/reddened
(BWAT Surrounding Skin Color Score = 2)

Healthy/reddened
(BWAT Surrounding Skin Color Score = 2)

Wound Edges

Healthy
(BWAT Edges Score = 2)

Healthy
(BWAT Edge score = 2)

Undermined
(BWAT Edges Score > 2 and/ or Undermining Score >

Goals of Wound Care

Obtain clean wound bed.

Provide moist environment

Maintain moist environment
Prevent premature wound closure

Wound Care Plan
Cleanse

Cleanse and Debride Wound

Debride

Autolytic

Enzymatic
Apply enzymatic debridement agent according to package insert instructions, avoiding exposure to intact skin

Surgical: Qualified provider removes devitalized tissue with scalpel or other sharp instrument. Obtain hemostasis before dressing wound.

Primary Dressing

Moisture-retentive Dressing

Wound Hydration

Moisture-retentive Dressing

Wound Hydration

Secondary Dressing

N/A

Moisture-retentive Dressing

N/A

Moisture-retentive Dressing

Patient Care Plan

Reduce risk factors for developing chronic ulcers and delayed healing e.g.:

RISK FACTORS

Arterial ulcers: Smoking, hypertension, hyperlipidemia and inactivity, Review surgical/medical management options to improve arterial circulation.
Diabetic ulcers: Smoking, hypertension, obesity, hyperlipidemia and high blood glucose. Review surgical/medical management options and use appropriate off-loading techniques.
Pressure ulcers: Pressure, shear, friction, nutritional deficiencies, dehydration and dry skin conditions, skin exposure to moisture or wound contamination secondary to incontinence, perspiration or other fluids, e.g. skin protection.
Venous ulcers: Edema with leg elevation, ambulation and compression. If patient is not ambulatory, assure frequent ankle flexes. Review surgical/medical management options and use compression bandages if appropriate
Mixed arterial-venous ulcers: Smoking, hypertension, inactivity, hyperlipidemia. Review surgical/medical management options to improve arterial circulation and compression bandages if appropriate.
All patients: Provide patient and/or caregiver teaching and support. Confirm and treat infection if needed. Assess and manage wound pain and odor if present.

Expected Outcomes

> Wound is not infected and is healing as evidenced by a reduction in size after 2 to 4 weeks of care. No evidence of new skin breakdown.

Delayed Healing

> _Reevaluate plan of care or address underlying etiology if ulcer has not reduced in size during 2 to 4 weeks of care_

FIGURE 6-7 Critical BWAT severity score with dry eschar treatment algorithm. (Reprinted with permission from ConvaTec, a division of Bristol-Myers Squibb, USA.)

space and prevention of premature wound closure. The goals of care for wounds in this severity state are to obtain/maintain a clean wound bed, absorb excess exudate, eliminate dead space to prevent premature wound closure, and provide a moist wound environment.

BWAT Critical Severity Scores 41–65. Wounds with BWAT total scores between 41 and 65 are generally deep full thickness wounds or stage III or IV pressure sores with more critical clinical manifestations, including undermining and necrosis. Figure 6-7 presents an algorithm for treatment for a wound necrotic eschar present. The goals of care for wounds in this severity state are to identify and treat infection, obtain a clean wound bed, absorb excess exudate, eliminate dead space to prevent premature wound closure, and provide a moist wound environment.[32]

The use of the BWAT score for determining severity state and guiding treatment offers a new approach to managing pressure ulcers. This approach may be useful in designing broad generic treatment guidelines, but individualization of the care plan must still occur, based on the clinician's judgment. The treatment plans presented based on the BWAT severity scores focus only on topical wound care, and the clinician must remember that attention to nutrition, adequate support surface use, and attention to the status of the whole patient is also part of the care plan.

Outcomes with Standardized Wound Assessment Using the BWAT

The BWAT was evaluated as part of a standardized assessment and treatment program in a prospective multicenter study of wound healing outcomes.[33] Wound healing outcomes from March 26 to October 31, 2001, were recorded on patients in three long-term care facilities, one long-term acute care hospital, and 12 home care agencies for wounds selected by staff to receive care based on computer-generated validated wound care algorithms. Figures 6-5 through 6-7 provide examples of the algorithms used to provide wound care. After diagnosis, wound dimensions and status were assessed using the BWAT. Pressure ulcer treatment was based on the BWAT item assessment scores with standardized protocols consisting of avoidance of gauze dressings, debridement, wound cleansing, and moist wound healing strategies. Most of the 767 wounds selected to receive the standardized-protocols of care were stage III-IV pressure ulcers (n = 373; mean healing time 62 days) or full-thickness venous ulcers (n = 124; mean healing time 57 days). A greater proportion of partial-thickness stage II pressure ulcers healed (61% of 134 ulcers) compared to stage III/IV pressure ulcers (36% of 373 full-thickness ulcers) (P<.001). Partial-thickness pressure ulcers healed faster than same-etiology full-thickness pressure ulcers (mean 31 days, SD 54 versus 62 days, SD 41; P<.001)[33]. While the findings cannot be related to the standardized assessment alone, the study does provide beginning data on use of a standardized assessment and healing.

Availability and Clinical Use of the BWAT

The BWAT is available for use as part of a web-based software program designed to organize data and generate reports on pressure ulcer prevention programs in long-term care facilities (see the program at www.pressure.med.ucla.edu). The Pressure Ulcer Quality Assessment (PUQA) system is based on the pressure ulcer quality indicators derived from the Assessing Care of Vulnerable Elders (ACOVE) project.[34] The ACOVE quality indicators have also been used to inform the Minimum Data Set (MDS) quality indicators, which are used to judge the quality of care provided in nursing homes. The PUQA system is based on current clinical practice guidelines and is directed at care processes rather than outcomes. The system has been reviewed and validated by a panel of experts. The PUQA system is based on use of a pressure ulcer risk assessment on admission to the nursing home. All other assessments are initiated off of the initial pressure ulcer risk assessment. The PUQA system is designed to monitor and document consistent implementation of a pressure ulcer prevention programs for multiple facilities. Assessments are categorized into three types:

- Baseline: initial assessment
- Follow Along: quarterly (or more frequent if desired) assessments with the schedule determined by the initial risk assessment
- Quality Control: frequent, intermittent, shorter assessments designed to monitor and document consistent implementation of the prevention interventions

The system monitors pressure ulcer prevention in five general areas:

1. Risk Assessment
2. Skin & Pressure Ulcer Assessment
3. Support Surface Use and Scheduled Repositioning
4. Nutrition
5. Incontinence

All assessment screens include the ability to print paper forms for use in data collection and conducting the assessments. The BWAT forms the basis for the pressure ulcer assessment portion of the system. The BWAT portion of the program allows for tracking healing outcomes and generates reports for facility use in improvement programs as well as narrative reports on individual pressure ulcers. The BWAT narrative reports generated from the system include factors currently required by federal guidelines such as pressure ulcer pain, whether or not the wound dressing is intact, and notification of the physician and dietician. During initial feasibility trials of the program, time estimates for completing the assessments and entering data into the system were calculated based on research staff conducting all parts of the PUQA system.[35] These estimates will be refined as the system moves into more formal evaluation with nursing home staff completing the protocols in the system. Time required for licensed nurses to perform risk assessment and pressure ulcer assessments was calculated at 0.26 hour per week for one resident (based on mean time for risk assessment and pressure ulcer assessment).

Conclusion: Clinical Utility of Wound Healing Tools

Use of a wound healing tool should enhance communication between health-care professionals involved in wound healing. By providing a framework for assessment and documentation with an attempt at quantification, the communication process becomes more meaningful. An objective method of assessing wound healing and monitoring changes over time allows for evaluation of the therapeutic plan of care and may be used to guide and direct therapy. This is particularly true in a managed care environment. For example, if a specific treatment modality is in use and the patient's wound status, as determined with the wound healing tool, has not changed in 2 weeks, reevaluation of the plan of care is warranted. Some studies have demonstrated that wounds with a 50% reduction in surface area within 2 weeks healed more expediently than did those without a 50% surface area reduction.[21,22] These data become an expectation for chronic wound healing. Use of wound healing tools may uncover other outcome criteria that will help to identify critical attributes during the course of healing.

Use of a research-based wound healing tool, such as those described in this chapter, can improve health-care practitioner communication and the generalizability of research studies, can allow discrimination in studies dealing with treatment modalities, and may help to improve understanding of wound healing. It can provide increased sensitivity, allowing greater precision and clarity in studies related to the treatment and development of pressure ulcers. An instrument that is sensitive to change in wound status will be helpful in the development of critical pathways for pressure ulcers and is useful as an outcome measure.

REVIEW QUESTIONS

1. Describe content validity, criterion validity, and predictive validity.
2. Stability reliability can be evaluated using which of the following methods?
   a. Test-retest techniques
   b. Interrater and intrarater measurements
   c. Internal consistency measurements
   d. Split-half techniques
3. List and describe five common wound characteristics used in healing instruments to evaluate wounds.
4. Explain the criteria you would use to select a wound healing tool for clinical reporting.
5. Describe how plotting the wound healing progression can be used.
6. Describe the validity and reliability of the SWHT, the PUSH, and the BWAT.

REFERENCES

1. Bates-Jensen BM, Vredevoe, D, Brecht ML. Validity and reliability of the Pressure Sore Status Tool. Decubitus. 1992;5(6):20-28.
2. Ferrell BA, Artinian BM, Sessing D. The Sessing Scale for assessment of pressure ulcer healing. J Am Geriatr Soc. 1995;43:37-40.
3. vanRijswijk L. Full-thickness pressure ulcers: patient and wound healing characteristics. Decubitus. Jan 1993;6(1):16-21.
4. Thomas DR, Rodeheaver GT, Bartolucci AA, et al. Pressure Ulcer Scale for Healing: Derivation and validation of the PUSH tool. Adv Wound Care. 1997;10(5):96-101.
5. Krasner D. Wound Healing Scale, version 1.0: A proposal. Adv Wound Care. 1997;10(5):82-85.
6. Sussman C, Swanson G . The utility of Sussman Wound Healing Tool in predicting wound healing outcomes in physical therapy. Adv Wound Care. 1997;10(5):74-77.
7. Houghton PE, Kincaid CB, Campbell K, Woodbury MG. Photographic assessment of the appearance of chronic pressure and leg ulcers. Ostomy/Wound Management. 2000;46(4):20-30.
8. Ohura T. Assessment of Pressure Ulcer Healing Process. Oral presentation. Paper presented at International Pressure Ulcer meeting, New York, June 2000.
9. Wagner FEW. The dysvascular foot: A system for diagnosis and treatment. Foot and Ankle. 1981(2):64-122.
10. Burns N, Grove SK. The concepts of measurement. In: Burns N, ed. The Practice of Nursing Research: Conduct, Critique & Utilization, 4th ed. Philadelphia: WB Saunders, 2000: 389-410.
11. Waltz CF, Strickland OL, Lenz ER. Reliability and validity of criterion-referenced measures. In: Waltz CF, Lenz ER, ed. Measurement in Nursing Research, 2nd ed. Philadelphia: FA Davis, 1991:229-257.
12. Bartolucci AA, Thomas DR Using principal component analysis to describe wound status. Adv Wound Care. 1997;10(5):93-95.
13. Stotts NA, Bartolucci A. Testing the Pressure Ulcer Scale for Healing (PUSH) and Variations of PUSH. Paper presented at: Symposium for Advanced Wound Care and Medical Research Forum on Wound Repair, Miami Beach, FL, 1998.
14. Stotts NA, Thomas DR, Frantz R, Bartolucci A, Sussman C, Ferrell BA, Cuddigan J, Maklebust J. An instrument to measure healing in pressure ulcers: Development and validation of the Pressure Ulcer Scale for Healing (PUSH). J Gerontol Series A. 2001;56(12):M795-799.
15. Voss AC, Bender S, Cook AS, et al. Pressure Ulcer Prevention in LTC: Implementation of the National Pressure Ulcer Long-term Care Study (NPULS) Prevention Program. Paper presented at: Symposium for Advanced Wound Care, Dallas, TX, April 2000.
16. Ratiliff CR. Use of the PUSH Tool to measure venous ulcer healing. Ostomy/Wound Management. 2005;51(5):58-63.
17. Sussman C, Cuddigan J, Ayello E, Lyder C, Langemo DK. Measuring Pressure Ulcer Healing is Critical to Quality of Life. Paper presented at: Partnership for Health in the New Millenium: Launching Healthy People 2010, Washington, DC, 2000.
18. Sussman C, Myer A. Clinical Decision Trees for Pressure Ulcer Prevention and Treatment. Paper presented at: Symposium for Advanced Wound Care; Las Vegas, NV, April 29, 2003.
19. Posthaur ME. Nutrition: A key link in clinical decision trees. Adv in Skin and Wound Care. 2004;17(9):474,476.
20. Lee S, Kwon PME, Dorner B, Redovian V, Maloney MJ. Pressure Ulcer Healing with a Concentrated, Fortified Collagen Protein Hydrolysate Supplement: A Randomized Controlled Trial. Paper presented at: Clinical Symposium on Advances in Skin and Wound Care, Las Vegas, NV, October 23-26, 2005.
21. Pompeo M. Implementing the PUSH tool in clinical practice: Revisions and results. Ostomy/Wound Management. August 2003 2003;49(8):32-46.
22. Kantor J, Margolis DJ. Expected healing rates for chronic wounds. Wounds: Compendium Clinical Research Practice. 2000;12(6):155-158.
23. Cherry GW, Hill D, Poore S, Wilson J, Robson MC. Initial Healing Rate of Venous Ulcers: Are They Useful as Predictors and Comparators of Healing? Paper presented at: Symposium for Advanced Wound Care and Medical Research Forum on Wound Repair, Las Vegas, NV, May 2001.
24. Pham HT, Falanga V, Sabolinski ML, Veves A. Healing Rate Measurement can predict complete wound healing rate in chronic diabetic foot ulceration. Paper presented at: Symposium for Advanced Wound Care and Medical Research Forum on Wound Repair; Las Vegas, NV, May 2001.

25. VanRijswijk L, Polansky M. Predictors of time to healing deep pressure ulcers. Ostomy Wound Management. 1994;40(8):40-42, 44, 46-48.

26. Sinacore DR. Healing times of diabetic ulcers in the presence of fixed deformities of the foot using total contact casting. Foot Ankle International. 1998;19(9):613-618.

27. Tallman P, Muscare E, Carson P, Eaglestein W, Falanga V. Initial rate of healing predicts complete healing of venous ulcers. Arch Dermatol. 1997;133(10):1231-1234.

28. Bates-Jensen BM& McNees, P. The wound intelligence system: Early issues and findings from multi-site tests. Ostomy/Wound Manage. 1996;42(Suppl 7A):1-7.

29. Bates-Jensen B& McNees, P. Toward an intelligent wound assessment system. Ostomy/Wound Manage. 1995;41(Suppl 7A):80-88.

30. Bates-Jensen B. A quantitative analysis of wound characteristics as early predictors of healing. In: Pressure Sores. Dissertation Abstracts International, Vol. 59, No. 11, Los Angeles: University of California, 1999.

31. Bergstrom N, Allman RM, Alvarez OM, Bennet MA, Carlson CE, Frantz R. Clinical Practice Guideline: Treatment of Pressure Ulcers (AHRQ Publication No. 95-06-0652). Rockville MD: US Department of Health and Human Services, Public Health Service Agency for Health Care Policy and Research (AHCPR) now Agency for Health Care Research and Quality (AHRQ), 1994.

32. Sanada H, Bates-Jensen BM. Updating Pressure Ulcer Care [Japanese]. Tokyo, Japan: Shorinsha Publishers, 1999.

33. Bolton L, McNees P, Van Rijswijk L, de Leon J, Lyder C, et al. Wound-healing outcomes using standardized assessment and care in clinical practice. J Wound, Ostomy, Continence Nursing, 2004; 31(2):65-71.

34. Bates-Jensen BM. Quality indicators for prevention and management of pressure ulcers in vulnerable elders. Annals Internal Medicine, 2001;135(8)Part2:744-751.

35. Bates-Jensen BM, Cadogan M, Jorge J, Schnelle JF. Standardized quality assessment system to evaluate pressure ulcer care in the nursing home. J American Geriatrics Society 2003;51:1195-1202.

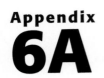
Long Form SWHT and Procedures for Using the SWHT

Sussman Wound Healing Tool (SWHT)
WOUND ASSESSMENT FORM

NAME: _____ MEDICAL RECORD NO.: _____

DATE: _____ EXAMINER: _____

CIRCLE WEEK OF CARE: B 1 2 3 4 5 6 7 8 9 10 11 12

SWHT Variable	Tissue Attribute	Attribute Definition	Rating	Relationship to Healing	Score
1	Hemorrhage	Purple ecchymosis of wound tissue or surrounding skin	Present or absent	Not good	
2	Maceration	Softening of a tissue by soaking until the connective tissue fibers are soft and friable	Present or absent	Not good	
3	Undermining	Includes both undermining and tunneling	Present or absent	Not good	
4	Erythema	Reddening or darkening of the skin compared to surrounding skin; usually accompanied by heat	Present or absent	Not good	
5	Necrosis	All types of necrotic tissue, including eschar and slough	Present or absent	Not good	
6	Adherence at wound edge	Continuity of wound edge and the base of the wound	Present or absent	Good	
7	Granulation (Fibroplasia—significant reduction reduction in depth)	Pink/red granulation tissue filling in the wound bed, reducing wound depth	Present or absent	Good	
8	Appearance of contraction (reduced size)	First measurement of the wound drawing together, resulting in reduction in wound open surface area	Present or absent	Good	
9	Sustained contraction (more reduced size)	Continued drawing together of wound edges, measured by reduced wound open surface area	Present or absent	Good	
10	Epithelialization	Appearance and continuation of resurfacing with new skin or scar at the wound edges or surface	Present or absent	Good	

MEASURES AND EXTENT (Depth and Undermining: Not Good)

	Depth/Location	SCORE	Undermining/Location	SCORE	Other	Letter
11	General depth >0.2 cm		16	Underm @ 12:00	Location	
12	General depth @ 12:00 >0.2 cm		17	Underm @ 3:00	Wound healing phase	
13	General depth @ 3:00 >0.2 cm		18	Underm @ 6:00	Total "Not Good"	
14	General depth @ 6:00 >0.2 cm		19	Underm @ 9:00	Total "Good"	
15	General depth @ 9:00 >0.2 cm					

Key: Present = 1. Absent = 0. Location choices: upper body (UB), coccyx (C), trochanter (T), ischial (I), heel (H), foot (F); add right or left (R or L). Wound healing phase: inflammation (I), proliferation (P), epithelialization (E), remodeling (R).

Copyright © 1997, Sussman Physical Therapy Inc.

Location _____

Wound healing phase _____

Total "Not Good" _____

Total "Good" _____

Procedure for Using the SWHT

Completion of the SWHT is by observation and physical assessment, as follows:

1. Each wound of each patient needs its own SWHT attributes form.
2. Write the patient's name, medical record number, and date of assessment at the top of the form.
3. The examiner signs the document.
4. As the wound is assessed, the rater marks a 1 or a 0 to signify present or absent on the form next to each of the 19 attributes. The squares in the column must be marked with one of the two scores.
5. The wound location and the current wound healing phase are marked with the appropriate letter. Choose the appropriate letter to represent the anatomic location of the wound and place it in the square at the time of the initial assessment and subsequent reassessments. The location will not change.
6. Letters are also used to represent the current wound healing phase: mark an *I* for inflammatory, *P* for proliferative, *E* for epithelialization, and *R* for remodeling. In the appropriate box, the phase is noted initially and at each reassessment. The wound healing phase should change as the wound heals.
7. Undermining and depth require some physical assessment to determine presence or absence.
8. Make open area measurements and list them on a separate form (see Chapter 5), then compare them with subsequent measurements to determine contraction and sustained contraction, measured as reduction in linear size.
9. Score part I. Add the number of "not good for healing" attributes and the number of "good for healing" attributes listed. The score of "not good for healing" attributes should diminish as the wound heals, and the score of "good for healing" attributes should increase.
10. A summary of the change is shown in Exhibit 6-4.

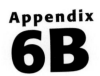
Pressure Ulcer Scale for Healing and Instructions for Use

PUSH Tool 3.0

Patient Name:_____ Patient ID#:_____

Ulcer Location: _____ Date:_____

DIRECTIONS:

Observe and measure the pressure ulcer. Categorize the ulcer with respect to surface area, exudate, and type of wound tissue. Record a subscore for each of these ulcer characteristics. Add the subscores to obtain the total score. A comparison of total scores measured over time provides an indication of the improvement or deterioration in pressure ulcer healing.

Length	0	1	2	3	4	5	
	0 cm²	< 0.3 cm²	0.3−0.6 cm²	0.7−1.0 cm²	1.1−2.0 cm²	2.1−3.0 cm²	
x Width		6	7	8	9	10	**Subscore**
		3.1−4.0 cm²	4.1−8.0 cm²	8.1−12.0 cm²	12.1−24.0 cm²	> 24 cm²	
Exudate Amount	0	1	2	3			**Subscore**
	None	Light	Moderate	Heavy			
Tissue Type	0	1	2	3	4		**Subscore**
	Closed	Epithelial Tissue	Granulation Tissue	Slough	Necrotic Tissue		
							Total Score

Length × Width: Measure the greatest length (head to toe) and the greatest width (side to side) using a centimeter ruler. Multiply these two measurements (length × width) to obtain an estimate of surface area in square centimeters (cm²). Caveat: Do not guess! Always use a centimeter ruler and always use the same method each time the ulcer is measured.

Exudate Amount: Estimate the amount of exudate (drainage) present after removal of the dressing and before applying any topical agent to the ulcer. Estimate the exudate (drainage) as none, light, moderate, or heavy.

Tissue Type: This refers to the types of tissue that are present in the wound (ulcer) bed. Score as a "4" if there is any necrotic tissue present. Score as a "3" if there is any amount of slough present and necrotic tissue is absent. Score as a "2" if the wound is clean and contains granulation tissue. A superficial wound that is reepithelializing is scored as a "1." When the wound is closed, score as a "0."

    4-Necrotic Tissue (Eschar): black, brown, or tan tissue that adheres firmly to the wound bed or ulcer edges and may be either firmer or softer than surrounding skin.
    3-Slough: yellow or white tissue that adheres to the ulcer bed in strings or thick clumps, or is mucinous.
    2-Granulation Tissue: pink or beefy red tissue with a shiny, moist, granular appearance.
    1-Epithelial Tissue: for superficial ulcers, new pink or shiny tissue (skin) that grows in from the edges or as islands on the ulcer surface.
    0-Closed/Resurfaced: the wound is completely covered with epithelium (new skin).

Version 3.0: 9/15/98
©National Pressure Ulcer Advisory Panel

PRESSURE ULCER HEALING CHART
(To Monitor Trends in PUSH Scores over Time)
(Use a separate page for each pressure ulcer)

Patient Name:_____   Patient ID#: _____

Ulcer Location: _____   Date: _____

Directions: Observe and measure pressure ulcers at regular intervals using the PUSH tool. Date and record PUSH Subscale and Total Scores on the Pressure Ulcer Healing Record below.

PRESSURE ULCER HEALING RECORD

DATE														
Length × Width														
Exudate Amount														
Tissue Type														
Total Score														

Graph the PUSH Total Score on the Pressure Ulcer Healing Graph below (see Exhibit 6-4)

PUSH Total Score	PRESSURE ULCER HEALING GRAPH												
17													
16													
15													
14													
13													
12													
11													
10													
9													
8													
7													
6													
5													
4													
3													
2													
1													
Healed 0													
DATE													

PUSH Tool Version 3.0: 9/15/98

Instructions for Using the PUSH Tool

To use the PUSH tool, the pressure ulcer is assessed and scored on the three elements in the tool:

- Length × Width = scored from 0 to 10
- Exudate Amount = scored from 0 (none) to 3 (heavy)
- Tissue Type = scored from 0 (closed) to 4 (necrotic tissue)

Ensure consistency in applying the tool to monitor wound healing. Definitions for each element are supplied at the bottom of the tool.

Step 1: Using the definition for length × width, a centimeter ruler measurement is made of the greatest head-to-toe diameter. A second measurement is made of the greatest width (left to right). Multiply these two measurements to get square centimeters, then select the corresponding category for size on the scale and record the score.

Step 2: Estimate the amount of exudate after removal of the dressing and before applying any topical agents. Select the corresponding category for amount and record the score.

Step 3: Identify the type of tissue. Note: If there is ANY necrotic tissue, it is scored a 4. If there is ANY slough, it is scored a 3, even though most of the wound is covered with granulation tissue.

Step 4: Sum the scores on the three elements of the tool to derive a total PUSH score.

Step 5: Transfer the total score to the Pressure Ulcer Healing Graph. Changes in the score over time provide an indication of the changing status of the ulcer. If the score goes down, the wound is healing. If it gets larger, the wound is deteriorating.

Pompeo Individual Patient Pressure Ulcer Scale for Healing Form[21]

Patient:	Admit Date:	# of Days:
Hosp. #.	DC Date:	

Patient Discharges for Month of:	Scoring Completed by:

Identifiers: (circle if wound acquired)		Admit PUSH Scores				Discharge PUSH Scores			
		Initial Subscores			Total	Final Subscores			Total
	Wound Location	Size	Exudate	Tissue	■	Size	Exudate	Tissue	■
A									
B									
C									
D									
E									
F									
G									
H									
I									
J									
■		Sum of initial Total PUSH Scores ↓				Sum of final Total PUSH Scores ↓			

Length	0 0 cm[1]	1 <0.3 cm^2	2 0.3-0.6 cm^2	3 0.7-1.0 cm^2	4 1.1-2.0 cm^2	5 2.1-3.0 cm^2	
x Width		6 3.1-4.0 cm^2	7 4.1-8.0 cm^2	8 8.1-12.0 cm^2	9 12.1-24.0 cm^2	10 >24.0 cm^2	**Subscore**
Exudate Amount	0 None	1 Light	2 Moderate	3 Heavy			**Subscore**
Tissue Type	0 Closed	1 Epithelial Tissue	2 Granulation Tissue	3 Slough	4 Necrotic Tissue		**Subscore**
							Total score

Number of acquired wounds: _____

Change in PUSH = ☐PUSH = PUSH initial − PUSH final = _____
(HEALING Score)

Healing Rate = ☐PUSH/Total Days = _____ / _____ = _____

Form 1: Individual Patient Pressure Ulcer Scale for Healing
(may be reproduced without permission)

Pompes M. Implementing the PUSH Tool in Clinical Practice: Revisions and Results. Ostomy/Qound Management. 2003;49(8):32–46.

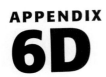
Bates-Jensen Wound Assessment Tool

Instructions for Use

General Guidelines

Fill out the attached rating sheet to assess a wound's status after reading the definitions and methods of assessment described below. Evaluate once a week and whenever a change occurs in the wound. Rate according to each item by picking the response that best describes the wound and entering that score in the item score column for the appropriate date. When you have rated the wound on all items, determine the total score by adding together the 13 item scores. The higher the total score, the more severe the wound status. Plot total score on the Wound Status Continuum to determine progress.

Specific Instructions

1. **Size:** Use ruler to measure the longest and widest aspect of the wound surface in centimeters; multiply length × width.

2. **Depth:** Pick the depth, thickness, most appropriate to the wound using these additional descriptions:

   1 = tissues damaged but no break in skin surface
   2 = superficial, abrasion, blister or shallow crater; even with and/or elevated above skin surface (e.g., hyperplasia)
   3 = deep crater with or without undermining of adjacent tissue
   4 = visualization of tissue layers not possible due to necrosis
   5 = supporting structures include tendon, joint capsule

3. **Edges:** Use this guide:

Indistinct, diffuse	=	unable to clearly distinguish wound outline
Attached	=	even or flush with wound base, *no* sides or walls present; flat
Not attached	=	sides or walls *are* present; floor or base of wound is deeper than edge
Rolled under, thickened	=	soft to firm and flexible to touch
Hyperkeratosis	=	callous-like tissue formation around wound & at edges
Fibrotic, scarred	=	hard, rigid to touch

4. **Undermining:** Assess by inserting a cotton tipped applicator under the wound edge; advance it as far as it will go without using undue force; raise the tip of the applicator so it may be seen or felt on the surface of the skin; mark the surface with a pen; measure the distance from the mark on the skin to the edge of the wound. Continue process around the wound. Then use a transparent metric measuring guide with concentric circles divided into four (25%) pie-shaped quadrants to help determine percentage of wound involved.

5. **Necrotic Tissue Type:** Pick the type of necrotic tissue that is *predominant* in the wound according to color, consistency and adherence using this guide:

White/gray nonviable tissue	=	may appear prior to wound opening; skin surface is white or gray
Nonadherent, yellow slough	=	thin, mucinous substance; scattered throughout wound bed; easily separated from wound tissue
Loosely adherent, yellow slough	=	thick, stringy, clumps of debris; attached to wound tissue
Adherent, soft, black eschar	=	soggy tissue; strongly attached to tissue in center or base of wound
Firmly adherent, hard/black eschar	=	firm, crusty tissue; strongly attached to wound base *and* edges (like a hard scab)

6. **Necrotic Tissue Amount:** Use a transparent metric measuring guide with concentric circles divided into four (25%) pie-shaped quadrants to help determine percentage of wound involved.

7. **Exudate Type:** Some dressings interact with wound drainage to produce a gel or trap liquid. Before assessing exudate type, gently cleanse wound with normal saline or water. Pick the exudate type that is *predominant* in the wound according to color and consistency, using this guide:

Bloody = thin, bright red
Serosanguineous = thin, watery pale red to pink
Serous = thin, watery, clear
Purulent = thin or thick, opaque tan to yellow
Foul purulent = thick, opaque yellow to green with offensive odor

8. **Exudate Amount:** Use a transparent metric measuring guide with concentric circles divided into four (25%) pie-shaped quadrants to determine percentage of dressing involved with exudate. Use this guide:

None = wound tissues dry
Scant = wound tissues moist; no measurable exudate
Small = wound tissues wet; moisture evenly distributed in wound; drainage involves ≤ 25% dressing
Moderate = wound tissues saturated; drainage may or may not be evenly distributed in wound; drainage involves > 25% to ≤ 75% dressing
Large = wound tissues bathed in fluid; drainage freely expressed; may or may not be evenly distributed in wound; drainage involves < 75% of dressing

9. **Skin Color Surrounding Wound:** Assess tissues within 4 cm of wound edge. Dark-skinned persons show the colors "bright red" and "dark red" as a deepening of normal ethnic skin color or a purple hue. As healing occurs in dark-skinned persons, the new skin is pink and may never darken.

10. **Peripheral Tissue Edema & Induration:** Assess tissues within 4 cm of wound edge. Nonpitting edema appears as skin that is shiny and taut. Identify pitting edema by firmly pressing a finger down into the tissues and waiting for 5 seconds. On release of pressure, tissues fail to resume previous position and an indentation appears. Induration is abnormal firmness of tissues with margins. Assess by gently pinching the tissues. Induration results in an inability to pinch the tissues. Use a transparent metric measuring guide to determine how far edema or induration extends beyond wound.

11. **Granulation Tissue:** Granulation tissue is the growth of small blood vessels and connective tissue to fill in full-thickness wounds. Tissue is healthy when bright, beefy red, shiny, and granular with a velvety appearance. Poor vascular supply appears as pale pink or blanched to dull, dusky red color.

12. **Epithelialization:** Epithelialization is the process of epidermal resurfacing and appears as pink or red skin. In partial thickness wounds it can occur throughout the wound bed as well as from the wound edges. In full thickness wounds it occurs from the edges only. Use a transparent metric measuring guide with concentric circles divided into four (25%) pie-shaped quadrants to help determine percentage of wound involved and to measure the distance the epithelial tissue extends into the wound.

BATES-JENSEN WOUND ASSESSMENT TOOL   NAME: _____

Complete the rating sheet to assess wound status. Evaluate each item by picking the response that best describes the wound and entering the score in the item score column for the appropriate date.

Location: Anatomic site. Circle, identify right (**R**) or left (**L**) and use "**X**" to mark site on body diagrams:

_____ Sacrum & coccyx   _____ Lateral ankle
_____ Trochanter   _____ Medial ankle
_____ Ischial tuberosity   _____ Heel   _____ Other Site

Shape: Overall wound pattern; assess by observing perimeter and depth. Circle and date appropriate description:

_____ Irregular   _____ Linear or elongated
_____ Round/oval   _____ Bowl/boat
_____ Square/rectangle   _____ Butterfly   _____ Other shape:

Item	Assessment	Date Score	Date Score	Date Score
1. Size	1 = Length × width < 4 sq cm 2 = Length × width 4—16 sq cm 3 = Length × width 16.1—36 sq cm 4 = Length × width 36.1—80 sq cm 5 = Length × width > 80 sq cm			
2. Depth	1 = Nonblanchable erythema on intact skin 2 = Partial thickness skin loss involving epidermis &/or dermis 3 = Full thickness skin loss involving damage or necrosis of subcutaneous tissue; may extend down to but not through underlying fascia; &/or mixed partial & full thickness &/or tissue layers obscured by granulation tissue 4 = Obscured by necrosis 5 = Full thickness skin loss with extensive destruction, tissue necrosis or damage to muscle, bone or supporting structures			
3. Edges	1 = Indistinct, diffuse, none clearly visible 2 = Distinct, outline clearly visible, attached, even with wound base 3 = Well-defined, not attached to wound base 4 = Well-defined, not attached to base, rolled under, thickened 5 = Well-defined, fibrotic, scarred or hyperkeratotic			
4. Under-mining	1 = None present 2 =Undermining < 2 cm in any area 3 = Undermining 2–4 cm involving < 50% wound margins 4 = Undermining 2–4 cm involving > 50% wound margins 5 = Undermining > 4 cm or Tunneling in any area			
5. Necrotic Tissue Type	1 = None visible 2 = White/gray nonviable tissue &/or nonadherent yellow slough 3 = Loosely adherent yellow slough 4 = Adherent, soft, black eschar 5 = Firmly adherent, hard, black eschar			
6. Necrotic Tissue Amount	1 = None visible 2 = < 25% of wound bed covered 3 = 25% to 50% of wound covered 4 = > 50% and < 75% of wound covered 5 = 75% to 100% of wound covered			

Item	Assessment	Date Score	Date Score	Date Score
7. Exudate Type	1 = None 2 = Bloody 3 = Serosanguineous: thin, watery, pale red/pink 4 = Serous: thin, watery, clear 5 = Purulent: thin or thick, opaque, tan/yellow, with or without odor			
8. Exudate Amount	1 = None, dry wound 2 = Scant, wound moist but no observable exudate 3 = Small 4 = Moderate 5 = Large			
9. Skin Color Surrounding Wound	1 = Pink or normal for ethnic group 2 = Bright red &/or blanches to touch 3 = White or gray pallor or hypopigmented 4 = Dark red or purple &/or nonblanchable 5 = Black or hyperpigmented			
10. Peripheral Tissue Edema	1 = No swelling or edema 2 = Nonpitting edema extends < 4 cm around wound 3 = Nonpitting edema extends ≥ 4 cm around wound 4 = Pitting edema extends < 4 cm around wound 5 = Crepitus and/or pitting edema extends ≥ 4 cm around wound			
11. Peripheral Tissue Induration	1 = None present 2 = Induration, < 2 cm around wound 3 = Induration 2–4 cm extending < 50% around wound 4 = Induration 2–4 cm extending ≥ 50% around wound 5 = Induration > 4 cm in any area around wound			
12. Granulation Tissue	1 = Skin intact or partial thickness wound 2 = Bright, beefy red; 75% to 100% of wound filled &/or tissue overgrowth 3 = Bright, beefy red; < 75% & > 25% of wound filled 4 = Pink, &/or dull, dusky red &/or fills ≤ 25% of wound 5 = No granulation tissue present			
13. Epithelialization	1 = 100% wound covered, surface intact 2 = 75% to < 100% wound covered &/or epithelial tissue extends > 0.5cm into wound bed 3 = 50% to < 75% wound covered &/or epithelial tissue extends to < 0.5cm into wound bed 4 = 25% to < 50% wound covered 5 = < 25% wound covered			
TOTAL SCORE				
SIGNATURE				

WOUND STATUS CONTINUUM

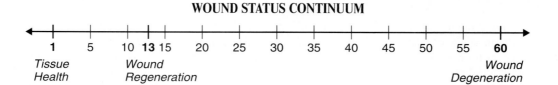

Plot the total score on the Wound Status Continuum by putting an "X" on the line and the date beneath the line. Plot multiple scores with their dates to see regeneration or degeneration of the wound at a glance.
© 2001 Barbara Bates-Jensen

CHAPTER 7

Vascular Evaluation

Gregory K. Patterson

CHAPTER OBJECTIVES

At the completion of this chapter, the reader will be able to:

1. Describe two techniques for noninvasive vascular testing.
2. Compare and contrast vascular evaluation methods.
3. Describe the technique for obtaining an ankle brachial index.
4. Describe the technique for performing a venous refill time.

Introduction

The initial evaluation of the wound care patient should always contain a thorough vascular assessment. Many of the patients referred to wound care specialists have wounds that are of vascular etiologies. These include arterial, venous, and diabetic wounds. Despite all of the modern wound care therapies, almost all of these wounds will not heal unless the underlying cause is assessed and treated or confirmed to be not significant. If wounds do heal without treatment of their etiology, they most assuredly have a high rate of recidivism, especially in the case of venous ulcers and underlying chronic venous insufficiency.

History and Physical Examination

The evaluation of any patient, including the patient with wounds, begins with an adequate history. Exhibit 7–1 lists areas of medical history used to identify risk factors for vascular disease, both arterial and venous. It goes beyond the general medical history discussed in Chapter 1 and focuses on specific vascular-related events. The history and physical examination should include past medical and surgical histories, including the known presence of peripheral vascular disease (PVD), atherosclerotic cardiovascular disease, diabetes mellitus, renal disease, prior deep vein thrombosis,

varicose veins, chronic venous insufficiency and history of elevated cholesterol and triglycerides. Thorough surgical history includes all previous operations, especially vascular procedures, including peripheral arterial and venous procedures. Cardiac procedures should also be included, secondary to the fact that the greater saphenous vein is often utilized for bypass procedures. This can cause significant wounds, especially in the diabetic population, and can aggravate the patient with long-standing venous insufficiency. Medications are of importance, especially the use of steroids, rheologic agents, antihypertensive medications, anticoagulants, antiplatelet agents, and aspirin.

Critical evaluation of the patient's symptomatology can often distinguish the cause of the wound. In the discussion of symptoms with the patient with suspected arterial problems, attention should be given to the presence of pain. Typical *claudication* (Greek for "to limp") is pain in the calf only, with walking some distance. This pain should rapidly diminish after the activity is stopped. If this does not occur for long periods of time or if the pain is helped by positional changes, a neurologic cause, such as spinal stenosis or disk problems, should be entertained. This is the so-called pseudoclaudication or neuroclaudication. Rest pain is pain across the forefoot, mainly associated with positional elevation. Typical patients will state that, to relieve the pain at night, they will "hang" their feet over the side of the bed.

EXHIBIT 7–1   Past Medical History

Risk Factors for Peripheral Vascular Disease[1]
Cardiac history

- Heart disease (cardiac catheterization? results?)
- Heart attack (date of last event)
- Chest pain (note location of the pain, how is pain relieved? onset?)
- Stroke (date of event, note location of weakness or speech deficit)

Hypertension (severity, medications, age at onset, highest blood pressure reading)

Hyperlipidemia (last cholesterol level, medication, number of years)

Smoking history (number of packs per day × years smoked = number of pack-years) (For example: a patient smoking two packs per day for 20 years has a 40-pack-year smoking history.) (quit? year quit)

Diabetes (number of years, medications)

Concomitant illnesses (renal disease, collagen vascular disease, arthritis, pulmonary disease, malignancy [type of malignancy], back [spine] problems, etc)

Family history of arterial disease

Risk Factors for Venous Disease
Trauma (type, date)
Deep vein thrombosis (date, anticoagulants)
Prolonged inactivity or standing activity
Multiple pregnancies
Family history of venous disease or varicose veins
Obesity
Clotting disorders

Past Surgical History
Vascular surgery (date of procedure, indication)
Angiogram/venogram (dates, indication, intervention?)
General surgery (date of procedure, indication)

This will increase gravity's assistance of blood flow, thus relieving pain. With the venous patient, history of pain or "tiredness" should be discussed. Also swelling that tends to increase during the day or during long periods of standing. With female vein patients, an obstetrical history should be elicited. This is to assess for presence of varicosities during pregnancy, secondary to the effect of high levels of estrogen on the vein walls or pelvic congestion from the gravid uterus "pressing" on the iliac veins.

The physical exam is extremely important and is aided by a thorough knowledge of the arterial and venous anatomy, including the lymphatic system. The examination should include inspection, palpation, and special diagnostic physical exam maneuvers. Inspection should include the size and symmetry of the limb in question. It should be compared with the contralateral limb. Edema or swelling should be assessed. The color and texture of the skin, including the nail beds and capillary refill, should be checked. Texture should also be assessed for the presence or absence of hair, which

is highly suggestive of arterial disease, as is muscle wasting. The overall venous pattern should be checked, and the presence of and location of all varicose veins should be documented. Scars, rashes, and pigmentation changes, such as hemosiderin deposits seen in chronic venous insufficiency, should be noted. See Table 7–1 for details concerning the differential between arterial disease and venous insufficiency.

CLINICAL WISDOM
Trophic Changes
Trophic changes are skin changes that occur over time in patients with chronic arterial insufficiency. Trophic changes include absence of leg hair; shiny, dry, pale skin; and thickened toenails. These symptoms are due to the chronic lack of nutrition from a good blood supply to the extremity. Some of these changes occur naturally in elderly patients.

The next step of the physical exam should be palpation of all major pulse points and the assessment for any audible harsh sounds, called bruits. This can be done with a regular stethoscope. The major pulses checked should include the radial and brachial in the arm, the carotid artery in the neck, and the femoral pulse in the groin (Figure 7–1). The popliteal pulse is often difficult to assess from the anterior approach (Figure 7–2) but should be checked routinely, secondary to the rare but well-known problem of popliteal artery aneurysm. The popliteal can be assessed with the patient in the prone position, using the posterior approach (Figure 7–3). The dorsalis pedis and posterior tibial arteries are assessed (Figures 7–4 and 7–5). Wound assessment of all ulcers and wounds should be completed as with all wound patients.

CLINICAL WISDOM
The pulse exam includes locating and grading bilateral femoral, popliteal, dorsalis pedis, and posterior tibial artery pulses. The following system should be used to grade pulses:
- 0 = No pulse
- 1+ = Barely felt
- 2+ = Diminished
- 3+ = Normal pulse (easily felt)
- 4+ = Bounding, aneurysmal ("pulse hits you in the face")

Vascular Testing–Introduction

Beyond the standard history and physical, if further investigation of a patient's vascular status is needed, more objective data in the form of vascular testing should be obtained. This testing can be in the form of noninvasive or invasive testing. Noninvasive testing, as the name implies, uses some form of external non-skin piercing imaging or method of measurement of the structure and physiologic function to determine information on some aspect of the vascular system. The most commonly used technique is that of ultrasound and its many derivatives. In the area of invasive test-

TABLE 7-1 **Comparison of Arterial and Venous Disease**

	Arterial Insufficiency	Venous Insufficiency
Pain	Intermittent claudication, may progress to rest pain Chronic, dull aching pain, progressive throughout the day	
Color	Pale to dependent rubor, a dull to bright, reddish color, more common with advanced disease	Normal to cyanotic, more common with advanced disease
Skin Temperature	Piokilothermic, taking on the environmental temperature. Much cooler than normal body temperature	Usually no effect on temperature
Pulses	Diminished to absent without Doppler stethoscope	Usually normal, may be difficult to palpate, secondary to significant edema
Edema	Usually not present unless combined disease or can be related to cardiac disease and congestive heart failure	Present from mild to severe pitting edema. Can have weeping edema fluid from open wounds
Tissue Changes	Thin and shiny. Hair loss. Trophic changes of the nails. Muscle wasting.	Stasis dermatitis with flaky, dry, and scaling skin. Hemosiderin deposits—brownish discoloration. Fibrosis with narrowing of the lower legs, "bottle legs"
Wounds	Distal ulceration, especially on toes and in between in the web spaces. May develop gangrene and severe tissue loss.	Shallow ulcers in the gaiter distribution of the foot and ankle, usually the medial surface.

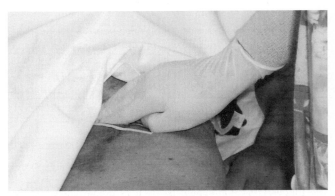

FIGURE 7-1 Palpation of femoral artery. Courtesy of Archbold Wound Care Center, Thomasville, Georgia.

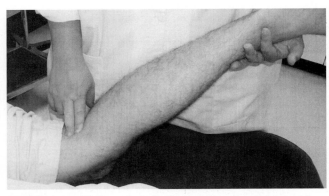

FIGURE 7-3 Palpation of popliteal artery (posterior approach). Courtesy of Archbold Wound Care Center, Thomasville, Georgia.

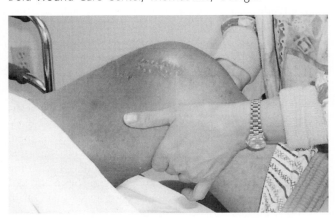

FIGURE 7-2 Palpation of popliteal artery (anterior approach). Courtesy of Archbold Wound Care Center, Thomasville, Georgia.

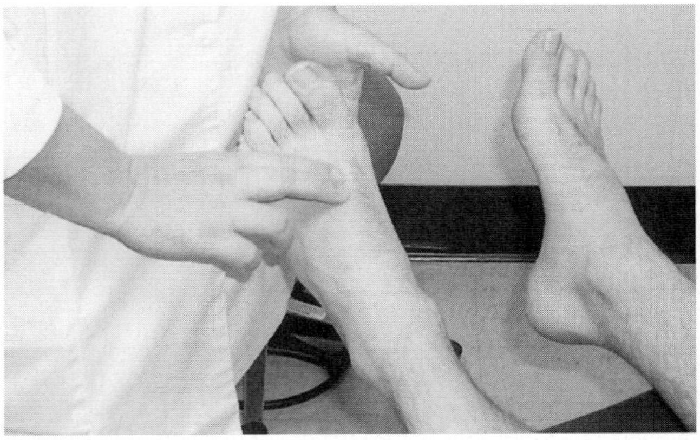

FIGURE 7-4 Palpation of dorsalis pedis artery. Courtesy of Archbold Wound Care Center, Thomasville, Georgia.

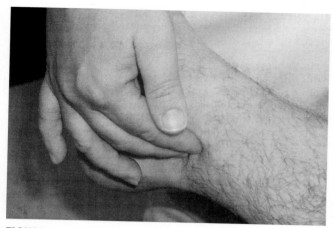

FIGURE 7–5 Palpation of posterior tibial artery. Courtesy of Archbold Wound Care Center, Thomasville, Georgia.

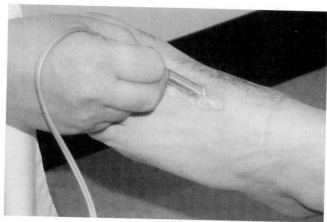

FIGURE 7–6 Continuous wave Doppler probe assessing dorsalis pedis artery. Courtesy of Archbold Wound Care Center, Thomasville, Georgia.

ing, contrast injection and data acquisition, usually in the form of radiographs, are the most commonly employed. Familiarity with the various tests available and their limitations is essential to wound care professionals. This is important, especially if the wound care specialist is the person ordering and interpreting the tests.

Continous Wave Doppler and the Ankle Brachial Index

In 1842, Christian Johann Doppler, a physicist, discovered the Doppler effect. This principle states that, when a sound source and a reflector are moving toward one another, the sound waves are spaced closer to one another. When the two are moving apart, the sound waves are farther apart. A modern example of this principle is that, as a train approaches, the whistle's pitch is higher, and as it passes, the pitch becomes lower. By using this principle today, we can determine the velocity and direction of blood flow. This is the basis of many of the modern noninvasive tests.

The most widely used noninvasive instrument is the continuous wave Doppler. This utilizes a piezoelectric crystal in a hand-held "pencil" probe. This crystal emits a sound wave that is reflected by the traveling red blood cells in the vessel of interest. This sound wave is reflected back to the probe and is transformed into an audible signal, which we can listen to subjectively or record on a graphic analyzer (Figure 7–6).

The continuous wave Doppler gives us a phasic flow pattern. The normal flow is triphasic. The first sound represents forward flow during systole; the second sound is a negative deflection. This represents a reversal of flow during diastole. The third and smallest sound represents a return of forward flow, caused by elastic recoil of the artery. As disease progresses, this triphasic flow diminishes to a biphasic flow. This is due initially to the loss of elastic recoil caused by "hardening" of the arteries. If the disease progresses further, the flow will decrease to a monophasic signal as the flow loses its pulsatile nature (Figure 7–7).

The phasic flow patterns are mainly a subjective test. When we apply a blood pressure cuff and occlude the flow in the artery, then use the Doppler to access the return of flow as the pressure is decreased in the blood pressure cuff, we have obtained a Doppler blood pressure. The most common form of this is the ankle-brachial index (ABI). This compares or indexes the ankle pressure to the arm pressure. This value is obtained by first assessing the highest arm pressure, then placing the blood pressure cuff just above the ankle and obtaining the systolic number with the Doppler probe. Both the posterior tibial artery and the dorsalis pedis artery values are observed. The ankle pressure is then divided by the arm pressure, giving a percentage value. In a

FIGURE 7–7 Phasic flow patterns.

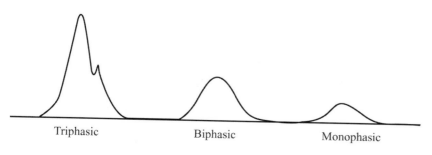

Triphasic   Biphasic   Monophasic

normal patient, this value is greater than 1.0. There is some disease present when the number falls below 0.90–0.95. However, the patient usually becomes symptomatic with claudication pain at around 0.70. Rest pain usually occurs at 0.4–0.5. Tissue loss occurs at 0.3 and below. Table 7–2 presents ABI data on prediction of wound healing, and the ABI values and their significance are presented in Exhibit 7-2.

One must remember that a patient describes claudication when walking. If a patient's symptoms are consistent with claudication and the ABIs are not, this may be because they were obtained at rest. Therefore, one can make a patient exercise by walking, thus increasing vascular demand, decreasing vascular resistance, and decreasing overall relative blood flow. Utilizing this exercise testing will uncover some marginal patients. This is well described by Dr. S.T. Yao, in his classic 1970 article in the *British Journal of Surgery* 1970.[1] Some of the flaws in obtaining ABIs are operator error, placing the cuff too high on the lower leg, and dividing the arm pressure by the foot pressure, instead of vice versa.

CLINICAL WISDOM

Diabetic Patients

The ankle-brachial index can be falsely elevated in patients with diabetes. This is due to the calcification of the inner layer of the artery, i.e., the cuff is unable to compress calcified distal vessel(s). This phenomenon is referred to as *noncompressible vessels*. Instead of ABI, one should use the next unaffected vessels, the digital arteries. This *toe-brachial index* or TBI is normal at 0.75 or greater.

EXHIBIT 7-2   Significance of Ankle-Brachial Index Values

ABI	≤ 0.5	Referral to vascular specialist (compression therapy contraindicated)
ABI	$= 0.5-0.8$	Referral to vascular specialist. Intermittent claudicant indicating peripheral arterial occlusive disease (compression therapy contraindicated)
ABI	$= 0.8-1.00$	Mild peripheral arterial occlusive disease (compression therapy with caution)
ABI	$= > 1.00$	Referral to vascular specialist. Indicates calcified vessels if diabetic

Segmental and Digital Plethysmography

An expansion of the standard ABI is the segmental plethysmography or lower extremity arterial study (LEA). This utilizes blood pressures along the entire leg in either a three- or four-cuff system. This obtains pressures from the high thigh, low thigh, below the knee, and above the ankle. All pressures are indexed again to the brachial artery or arm blood pressure. A significant decrease between two cuffs indicates an arterial lesion between these two locations, thus allowing for localization of arterial disease. This may be somewhat difficult to interpret if there is multifocal disease. Segmental plethysmography, or segmental pressures, as they

TABLE 7–2   Table of ABI Values

Dopplex® Ankle Pressure Index (API) Guide

Ankle Pressure (mmHg)

Brachial Pressure (mmHg)

Brachial\Ankle	30	35	40	45	50	55	60	65	70	75	80	85	90	95	100	105	110	115	120	125	130	135	140	145	150	155	160	165	170	175	180	185	190	195	200	
180	.16	.19	.22	.25	.27	.30	.33	.36	.38	.41	.44	.47	.50	.52	.55	.58	.61	.63	.66	.69	.72	.75	.77	.80	.83	.86	.89	.92	.94	.97	1.00					180
175	.17	.20	.22	.25	.28	.31	.34	.37	.40	.42	.45	.48	.51	.54	.57	.60	.62	.65	.68	.71	.74	.77	.80	.82	.85	.88	.92	.94	.97	1.00						175
170	.17	.20	.23	.26	.29	.32	.35	.38	.41	.44	.47	.50	.52	.55	.58	.61	.64	.67	.70	.73	.76	.79	.82	.85	.89	.91	.94	.97	1.00							170
165	.18	.21	.24	.27	.30	.33	.36	.39	.42	.45	.48	.51	.54	.57	.60	.63	.66	.69	.72	.75	.78	.81	.84	.87	.90	.93	.96	1.00								165
160	.18	.21	.25	.28	.31	.34	.37	.40	.43	.46	.50	.53	.56	.59	.62	.65	.68	.71	.75	.78	.81	.84	.87	.90	.93	.96	1.00									160
155	.19	.22	.25	.29	.32	.35	.38	.41	.45	.48	.51	.54	.58	.61	.64	.67	.70	.74	.76	.80	.83	.87	.90	.93	.96	1.00										155
150	.20	.23	.26	.30	.33	.36	.40	.43	.46	.50	.53	.56	.60	.63	.66	.70	.73	.76	.80	.83	.86	.90	.93	.96	1.00											150
145	.20	.24	.27	.31	.34	.37	.41	.44	.48	.51	.55	.58	.62	.65	.69	.72	.75	.79	.82	.86	.90	.93	.96	1.00												145
140	.21	.25	.28	.32	.35	.39	.42	.46	.50	.53	.57	.60	.64	.67	.71	.75	.78	.82	.85	.89	.92	.96	1.00													140
135	.22	.26	.29	.33	.37	.40	.44	.48	.51	.55	.59	.62	.66	.70	.74	.77	.81	.85	.88	.92	.96	1.00														135
130	.23	.27	.30	.34	.38	.42	.46	.50	.53	.57	.61	.65	.69	.73	.77	.80	.84	.88	.92	.96	1.00															130
125	.24	.28	.32	.36	.40	.44	.48	.52	.56	.60	.64	.68	.72	.76	.80	.84	.88	.92	.96	1.00																125
120	.25	.29	.33	.37	.40	.45	.50	.54	.58	.62	.66	.70	.75	.79	.83	.87	.91	.95	1.00																	120
115	.26	.30	.34	.39	.43	.48	.52	.56	.60	.65	.69	.74	.78	.82	.86	.91	.95	1.00																		115
110	.27	.31	.36	.40	.45	.50	.54	.59	.63	.68	.72	.77	.81	.86	.90	.95	1.00																			110
105	.28	.33	.38	.42	.47	.52	.57	.61	.66	.71	.76	.80	.85	.90	.95	1.00																				105
100	.30	.35	.40	.45	.50	.55	.60	.65	.70	.75	.80	.85	.90	.95	1.00																					100

GREATER THAN 1.00

Huntleigh Healthcare, a world leading manufacturer of pocket Dopplers, offers an extensive range of bi-directional pocket Dopplers with visual flow and rate display, together with a wide range of interchangeable probes for both vascular and obstetric applications.

WARNING: False high readings may be obtained in patients with calcified arteries because the sphygmomanometer cuff cannot fully compress the hardened arteries. Calcified arteries may be present in patients with history of Diabetes, Arteriosclerosis and Atherosclerosis.

Courtesy of Huntleigh Diagnostics Ltd., Cardiff, United Kingdom.

are also known, are typically accompanied by pulse volume recordings (PVR). PVRs show the volume of change in the limb with each pulse beat. These are obtained with the same equipment, including the blood pressure cuffs, as with the segmental pressures. The cuffs are inflated to occlude arterial flow, then deflated to just below systolic pressure, so that only arterial flow is maintained in the limb. The readings are then obtained. These readings usually have a sharp upstroke, indicating systolic flow. They also have a corresponding dicrotic notch, indicating elastic recoil of the artery wall. With mild disease, there is loss of the dicrotic

notch. With moderate to severe disease, there is decrease in the upstroke of the waveform. With severe disease, there is loss of the volume beneath the curve (Figure 7–8).

Digital plethysmography, or "toe pressures," is the same as segmental pressures, except that a special, small-sized cuff is used and placed on the toe, usually the great hallux. Because of the small-sized digital arteries and the increase in vascular resistance through these arteries, these pressures are reduced. When compared with or indexed to the brachial pressure as a toe brachial index, the normal value is greater than or equal to 0.75. TBIs are extremely useful with dia-

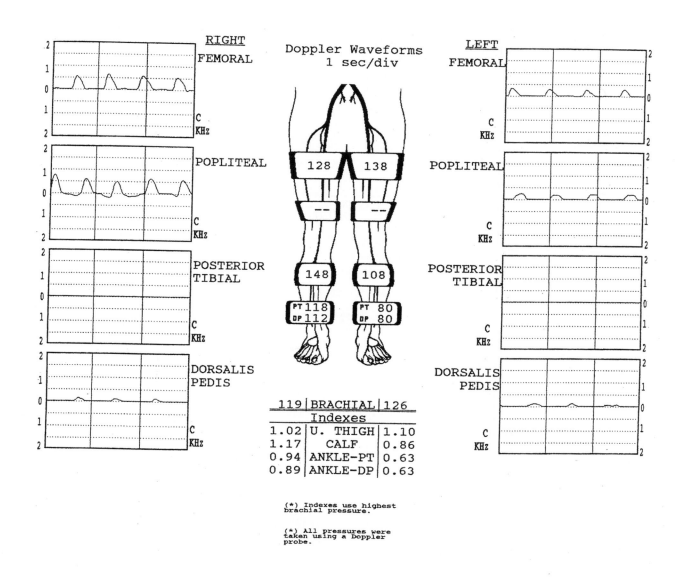

119	BRACHIAL	126
	Indexes	
1.02	U. THIGH	1.10
1.17	CALF	0.86
0.94	ANKLE–PT	0.63
0.89	ANKLE–DP	0.63

(*) Indexes use highest brachial pressure.

(*) All pressures were taken using a Doppler probe.

EVIDENCE FOR MILD OCCLUSIVE DISEASE ON RIGHT AT REST. SEVERE ON LEFT, PROBABLY SUPERFICIAL FEMORAL ARTERY IN NATURE. ABNORMAL TBI BILATERALLY.

FIGURE 7–8 Segmental pressure study with pulse volume recordings.

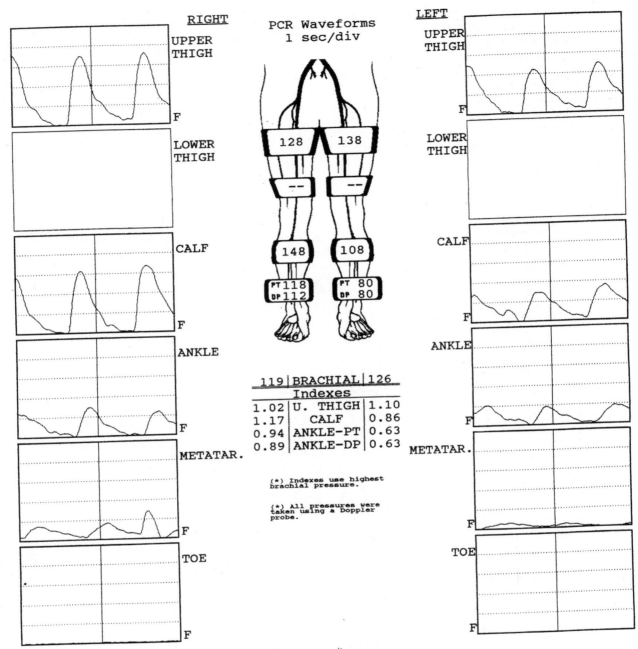

FIGURE 7–8 Segmental pressure study with pulse volume recordings.

betic patients because of the process of medial calcific stenosis (MCS), which is a process where the media of the vessel wall is calcified. This causes a standard segmental pressure study to have values that are falsely elevated (greater than 1.2) or they become non-compressible because the vessel in question cannot be occluded to obtain a true systolic blood pressure. MCS does not affect digital arteries; therefore, they will be more indicative of arterial disease in diabetic patients.

Arterial and Venous Duplex

Duplex scanning is a combination of B-mode ultrasound scanning (gray scale ultrasound) and pulsed Doppler flow detector and spectral analyzer. B-mode ultrasound can show anatomic details with the assistance of color flow Doppler, which shows blood direction. When there is a blockage, there is reversal of flow with a mosaic color pattern. With the pulsed gated Doppler, the Doppler signal can be set to analyze inside the vessel only, so that the readings are not confused with other surrounding structures. In the case of arterial stenosis, the velocity or speed of the blood increases through the stenosis and is recorded in centimeters per second (cm/sec).[2–4] A good example of this is when you place your finger over the end of a water hose. The more of the opening you cover, the faster the water will come out.

In venous duplex scanning, B-mode scanning is used to detect any echogenic material, such as thrombus. The probe is pushed down on the vein to see whether it will collapse. Normally, a vein will compress easily, and an artery, because of its thick wall, will not. In the case of thrombosis, the vein will not compress easily. Color flow Doppler is used to assess for flow in the vein or around a thrombus. It is also used to assess for reflux, or backward flow due to chronic venous insufficiency.[5,6]

Transcutaneous Oxygen Measurements

The end result of all vascular studies concerns the delivery of blood to the individual cells, but, in reality, the end result is the delivery of oxygen to the tissues. With this in mind, the actual measurement of oxygen at the skin level mirrors the delivery on the cellular level. Measurement of transcutaneous oxygen ($tcPO_2$) levels utilizes an airtight fixation ring affixed to the site in question. An electrode inside the ring is then heated above body temperature to 41° C. This allows diffusion of oxygen from the capillary level to the skin level and a measurement in millimetres of mercury is made. If the $tcPO_2$ is less than 20 mm Hg, the wound or ulcer will not heal. If the $tcPO_2$ is greater than 30 mm Hg, the wound or ulcer should heal without problems. This is also true of an ulcer that needs to be debrided. Safe debridement may be carried out if the $tcPO_2$ is greater than 30 mm Hg. In the case of amputation, less than 5 mm Hg indicates insufficient levels of oxygen for healing.[7]

CLINICAL WISDOM

Accuracy of tcPO2 Measurements

Transcutaneous oxygen measurements are not reliable in patients with swelling or infection! Do not test these patients. The patient can be tested when the infection is clear and the swelling is gone.

Transcutaneous oxygen measurements have been shown to be predictive for healing of ulcers and amputation wounds,[8] and for determining the extent of chronic ischemia in limbs with and without wounds.[9,10] As mentioned earlier, the diabetic patient with PVD presents some difficulty in evaluating because of MCS. Toe pressure of digital plethysmography is the test of choice but, as is often the case, if the toes are involved, extensively calloused, or have been removed with minor amputation, $tcPO_2$ measurements are very useful. Transcutaneous oxygen measurements do have disadvantages. The reproducibility of the test and the fact

that it takes approximately 30 minutes to perform at one level unless one has access to the newer four to six channel machines.

Skin Perfusion Pressures and the Laser Doppler

Often, the skin in many vascular patients seems to become the "first victim" of critical limb ischemia. With this in mind, the actual skin perfusion pressure (SPP) has been looked at for a prediction of critical ischemia. This is well published, mainly in the Scandinavian literature. There is a problem with the widespread use of this technique. Traditionally, SPP is performed using a Xenon radioisotope single-pass washout technique. This requires special equipment; the patient must keep the limb in question immobile for at least 20 minutes, and the procedure can be painful, necessitating analgesics.

New techniques of measuring SPP with a laser Doppler (Figure 7–9) have been developed in the past several years. The laser Doppler uses a low-energy laser probe, secured in the bladder of a blood pressure cuff. These cuffs come in a variety of sizes, from large cuffs for thigh measures to tiny cuffs for toe digital SPP measurements (Figure 7–10). The

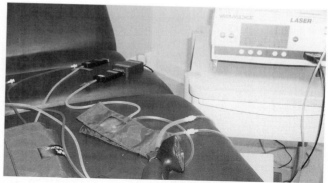

FIGURE 7–9 Laser Doppler unit with transducer cuffs. Courtesy of Archbold Wound Care Center, Thomasville, Georgia.

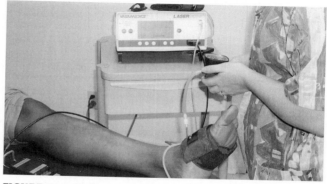

FIGURE 7–10 Patient undergoing laser Doppler exam. Courtesy of Archbold Wound Care Center, Thomasville, Georgia.

cuff is inflated to stop skin perfusion; after an adequate baseline is obtained, the cuff is slowly deflated. The skin perfusion is measured in volume percent units (LD1); the SPP is the reading that increases at least 40% over baseline (Figure 7–11). The laser Doppler can also obtain pulse volume recordings of skin perfusion, thus allowing for further assessment of a patient's vascular status. In the case of newer machines, they often have both a laser Doppler and a tcPO$_2$.

The laser Doppler has been shown to be 80% accurate at predicting critical limb ischemia.[11,12] It has also been shown to be a good predictor of healing of amputation wounds.[13] Castronuovo and colleagues' study of SPP in the diagnosis of critical limb ischemia used logistic regression analysis to predict the probability of healing versus the SPP (mm Hg). This revealed a sigmoid-shaped curve. Patients with an SPP greater than 45 mm Hg had a 100% healing rate. The 50% healing rate was for approximately 25 mm Hg.[11]

MAGNETIC RESONANCE ANGIOGRAPHY

The use of magnetic resonance imaging (MRI) has been applied to vascular studies in the form of magnetic resonance angiography (MRA). MRA has become a functional addition to invasive angiography.[14] MRA has advanced over the last 15 years and now can visualize all of the same vessels

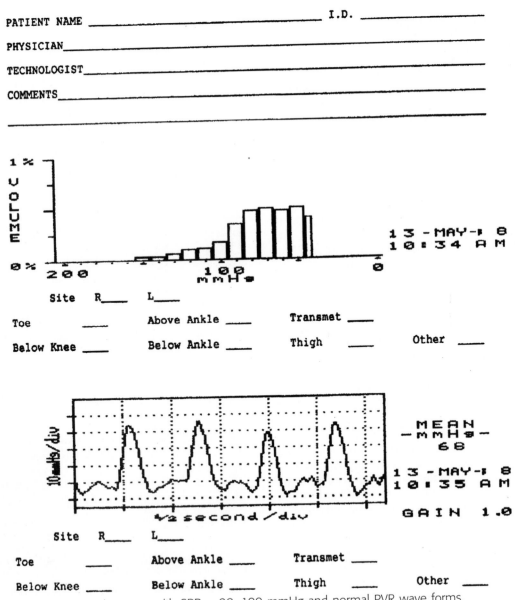

FIGURE 7-11 Normal laser Doppler exam with SPP = 90–100 mmHg and normal PVR wave forms.

and hemodynamically significant stenoses seen on contrast angiography. It has been very useful in imaging both the extracranial and intracranial cerebral circulation, as well as the heart and thoracic and abdominal aorta.[15]

MRA has several advantages over traditional contrast angiography. It is noninvasive for the most part. If contrast is used, it is a nonionic contrast, which does not cause any nephrotoxicity. It also has nonvisualization of cortical bone, which has been reduced in digital subtraction angiography but not completely eliminated. Probably the single greatest advantage is it can readily identify target recipient vessels not always identified on conventional contrast angiography.[16] This problem of visualizing occult distal vessels because of contrast washout may increase amputation rates before vascular reconstruction is attempted. MRA is also comparable in overall cost to contrast angiography.

MRA does have some disadvantages. It is experience dependent by both radiologist and surgeons. This leads to "overreading" or overcalling the severity of the stenoses. It also needs the availability of a MRI unit, including specialized software and coils. Despite this, it is replacing angiography in some centers.

Computed Tomography Angiography

One of the newer applications of an existing radiologic test is that of computed tomography (CT) angiography. This test employs ultrafast helical CT scanners to obtain multiple serial images enhanced with contrast. These images are then reconstructed into a three-dimensional projected image. Many of the newer-generation CT scanners and the available software allow for some of the most "contrast-enhanced angiogram"-like pictures, when compared with true angiography. The acquisition of these images is relatively fast for the patient, but the problem lies in the reconstruction of these images. This process takes some highly sophisticated computer software and hardware and is recently more widely available. Future computer and reconstructive developments will undoubtedly move CT angiography to the forefront of all non-interventional vascular imaging.

Invasive Studies and Contrast Angiography

Invasive vascular studies, as the name implies, require some invasive component beyond the standard intravenous aspect of the study. In the case of contrast enhanced angiography, this usually requires a femoral artery puncture or brachial artery cutdown. Catheters are then manipulated, which can cause plaques to break off and embolize or even to sustain inadvertent vessel wall damage. Serious complications can occur from the procedures, including heart failure, contrast-induced renal heart failure, and even death (0.05%).[17–19] Despite these complications, angiography remains the "gold standard" for vascular evaluation. If angiography is entertained, all patients should be in the care of a general or vascular surgeon. Angiography has definite advantages over other studies, which include anatomic landmarks for better localization of vessels in question, thus smaller incisions and directed approaches during revascularization. Endo-luminal intervention, such as angioplasty, is also a significant advantage beyond pure diagnostic tests, thus changing the role of angiography to a therapeutic modality.

One technically significant disadvantage of angiography is nonvisualization of distal runoff vessels. Several studies have shown that up to 70% of patients have failure to opacify the small distal runoff vessels during angiography.[14–21] This is due to a dilution effect of the contrast traversing multiple segments of stenoses. In some cases, there is not enough contrast to visualize the smaller vessels. Therefore, the vessels should be explored before amputation is considered or before patients undergo "on-table" intraoperative angiography and, in some cases, MRA.[20–23]

Venous Imaging

Diagnostic evaluation for chronic venous insufficiency can include both non-invasive tests, which can include duplex ultrasound and plethysmography tests. The two primary assessments of these tools is to look for both venous obstruction from previous thrombosis or congenital obstruction, as well as external compression from either a mass effect from something such as a tumor, or from scarring from other problems. The other assessment includes that of reflux which is categorized by abnormal flow past the existing valves in veins which were designed to decrease the overall pressure in the vein itself.

If one is evaluating the overall vascular system, it seems to be somewhat designed backwards as in the heart is pumping blood downhill to the legs in a high pressure system. As the return system is a low pressure system, this would cause significant increased pressures at the ankle level. But by having valves placed in the veins, this allows for decreasing individual pressure to just the pressure in the isolated column of the vein between two subsequent valves. If a valve goes bad, it causes that column of blood to send its pressure to the next column of blood and so on throughout the leg which causes ambulatory venous hypertension, or the main pathophysiologic problem associated with chronic venous insufficiency. The above mentioned tests, again, evaluate both for obstruction which can cause increased pressure by not allowing blood to flow out of the venous system, but also incompetent valves causing reflux which will cause increased pressure as well.

The tests can be divided into two main divisions. One is that of physiologic tests, which gives some type of quantitative measure of the overall venous hemodynamics that are seen. The other is an anatomic evaluation which gives a qualitative assessment of the overall function or dysfunction of the venous system. Physiologic tests include ambulatory venous pressure monitoring, photo plethysmography (PPG), air plethysmography (APG), light reflective rheography (LRR), and volumetric studies of the lower leg. These tests can be useful in the serial evaluation both prior to treatment and after treatment to assess the overall improvement on a quantitative level of the overall venous hemodynamics.

Venous Pressure Measurements

Venous pressure monitoring in the form of ambulatory venous pressure monitoring is a true hallmark, especially in overall experimental and physiologic studies of chronic venous insufficiency as it actually records the true pressure that is seen in the veins while the patient ambulates. This typically is performed utilizing a small butterfly needle, such as a 20 or 21 gauge needle. This is placed in a superficial vein on the foot in a sterile fashion, and it is then connected to a pressure transducer and recording device. The patient can do provocative maneuvers which can include dorsaflexion of the foot up on the "tip toes". Both static pressure measurements are obtained while the patient is still and then, with the provocative maneuvers, dynamic pressure is recorded. Also, the evaluation in overall time for the pressure to return to a resting level can also be calculated in this fashion. In a normal leg, the active dorsaflexion of the foot will cause blood to be pumped out of the lower leg and you should see a normal venous pressure drop. When the activity is stopped, the pressure will slowly rise as the arterioles fill through the capillary system back into the venous system. This usually takes approximately up to 2-5 minutes, but typically can be seen in one minute. If the pressure returns to baseline much quicker, usually less than 30 seconds, there is some evidence of reflux through the veins which will increase the pressure, not through the arterial system, and this is considered abnormal. Also, a resting ambulatory venous pressure of greater than 30mmHg is considered abnormal in a static situation. The extent of chronic venous insufficiency does correlate with the higher the venous ambulatory pressure found. Studies have shown a correlation between the amount of increased ambulatory venous pressure and the overall incident of ulceration.

Photo Plethysmography (PPG)

PPG essentially measures the venous refill time. The time that it takes for the vein to refill through the normal arterial capillary system, and abnormalities are seen in reflux where it fills directly back in a backwards fashion through the overall veins. This is done through light absorption through the skin to estimate the overall venous pressures. This is done through light absorption on the wavelength of hemoglobin through a light emitting diode in a photoelectric cell that measures the light reflected from the skin as it changes color with filling of micro vasculature. A diode is placed approximately 10-15cm from the medial malleolus to a self-adhesive tape ring. The machine is calibrated and zeroed, and then the patient is asked to perform passive dorsaflexion of the foot to again cause venous pumping through the calf sinusoids emptying the lower leg veins. After approximately eight passive dorsaflexions of the foot which are

done on a rhythmic basis, the foot is relaxed. Utilizing both paper tracing and an audible change in tone emitted by the machine, the examiner can measure the rapidity in which the veins refill, again obtaining a quantitative venous refill time. Refill times greater than 24 seconds are considered normal. Rapid refill times can be quantified on the overall severity of chronic venous insufficiency (Table 7-3)[24]. False negatives can occur if there is any significant arterial inflow disease which may hamper normal filling of the vessels through the arterial circuit, as well as significant decrease in ankle mobility as to show decrease calf muscle pumping of venous blood out of the venous circuit.[25]

Light Reflective Rheography (LRR)

LRR is a variation of PPG which uses infrared light but, as opposed to PPG, has three light diodes which reduces the overall effect of external light and surface reflection, in theory giving a much more accurate study. Both PPG and LRR have both been discussed at national wound care meetings as screening tools for large scale wound care populations. Both of these have been shown to be effective in this avenue.

String Gauge Plethysmography

String gauge plethysmography is a similar variation of plethysmography to study venous refill times, as well as overall venous emptying. This uses a string gauge to encircle the leg and sense tension changes caused by the calf with exertion. This can also add additional information as a small specialized blood cuff can be utilized to occlude superficial venous structures and may actually normalize the venous return, indicating isolation of superficial disease. Overall, it is not widely used anymore as newer techniques have come into more use, such as air photoplethysmography which is discussed in the next paragraph.

Air Photo Plethysmography (APG)

APG utilizes air cuffs to show volumetric changes in the leg which can be quantified to again reveal venous reflux times. Again, a patient undergoes active motion of the calf to pump blood out of the venous circuit with refill times being obtained through the cuff and air chambers that are connected to a pressure transducer and a computerized recorder. Tourniquets may be used at above the ankle, below the ankle, below the knee, and above the knee to stop abnormal refill times and show corrected refill times which can isolate disease, both to the superficial system differentiating

TABLE 7-3 Venous Refill Times & Levels of Venous Disease

	Normal	> 25 sec
Level 1	Mild	20–24 sec
Level 2	Moderate	10–19 sec
Level 3	Severe	< 10 sec

These correlate with the overall severity of Chronic Venous Insufficency between the greater saphenous and lesser saphenous vein, as well as the perforator system, and finally on to the deep system .

Outflow tract obstruction can also be evaluated with positional changes to show any evidence of a more proximal occlusion from a previous clot or anatomic abnormality.

Foot volumetry has been utilized in the past as an evaluation of venous insufficiency. It is not used widely at this time except in experimental purposes, and utilizes displaced water in an open box with a photoelectric sensor showing change in water levels.

Duplex Ultrasound

Continuous wave Doppler ultrasound along with color flow and power Doppler settings is the gold standard in detecting reflux in the outpatient setting. Assessment of the vein is performed not only from an anatomic standpoint, as well as to assess for clot from deep vein thrombosis, but also whether there is sluggish flow indicating engorgement of the vessels to abnormal flow indicating reflux. The duplex ultrasound machine can be programmed for both arterial and venous settings. Venous settings typically show blood flow away from the transducer in blue, indicating venous return from the foot to the heart in direction with abnormal "reflux" flow being shown as red flow, or flow back toward the transducer. The vessels are noted for their compressibility with manual compression of the vessel through the subcuticular and muscle tissues with the transducer. A vein is easily compressible; arterial structures are not. And if a vein has a previous thrombosis present, it is also non-compressible. A complete venous duplex ultrasound should show not only the patency of the vessels, but any anatomic abnormalities, accessory vessels, and vessels with reflux, and should isolate these to what system of veins are involved. A full assessment should include all the deep system vessels, including the common femoral vein, superficial femoral vein, profunda femoral vein, popliteal vein, posterior tibial and peroneal veins, and occasional insonation of the anterior tibial veins. Superficial veins should include not only the greater saphenous vein and lesser saphenous vein, but accessory pathways such as the vein of Giacomini. Perforator vessels should be elicited as well with the standard criteria being if reflux is not visualized, then reflux may be present in a dilated perforator greater than 3 mm in size. Perforators should be typically identified in relationship to a known anatomic spot, such as the medial malleolus, and distance from the top of the medial malleolus should be given in centimeters so that isolation of these areas are obtained.

Duplex can also be utilized to evaluate an ulcer bed, but caution should be taken to protect the transducer head so that cross-contamination of patients does not occur. Methods to perform this are to cover the transducer head with either a commercially available sterile bag, whereby ultrasound gel is placed in the bag, the transducer is then placed in the bag, and additional sterile gel is placed in the wound itself and the wound is then scanned with the covered ultrasound probe. A sterile glove may also be substituted for covering of the transducer head in these cases. Vessels running underneath the ulcer or within 2 cm of the periphery are considered the veins responsible for the ulcerated area and correspond to known anatomic vessels. Typically, depending on the location of the wound such as medial lower leg wounds above the medial malleolus, these are branches from the greater saphenous vein, the posterior arch system, the posterior tibial veins, and potentially the peroneal veins. Other ulcer locations correspond to other vessels, including laterally placed ulcers and anterior placed ulcers corresponding to the short saphenous vein, peroneal veins for lateral ulcers, and the anterior arch to greater saphenous vein and anterior tibial system for the anterior located veins.

Invasive tests for chronic venous disease can include both invasive venography, similar to contrast angiography. But, in the case of leg veins, the valves must be considered. Therefore, both descending venography to assess for valvular function and ascending venography to evaluate for obstruction must be done. Typically, these need to be done on separate days secondary to contrast loads can be nephrotoxic and damage kidneys, as well as access points usually being in the deep femoral vessels in descending venography, and multiple superficial access points in ascending venography.

Other Studies

Just as in an arterial system, other studies may include magnetic resonance venography (MRV) or CT venography. But, these tend to be difficult sometimes to obtain secondary to exact timing of the venous phase of contrast injections so that there are not arterial vessels still present causing "arterial contamination".

New Venous Studies

Intravascular ultrasound (IVUS) is a new method initially employed in arterial evaluation, but is gaining more favor in venous evaluation including invasive venous procedures such as bedside placement of inferior vena cava filters being placed with the assistance of an IVUS catheter without typical x-ray studies. Typically, the catheter has either a tiny rotating vascular ultrasound head at the end of the catheter, or multiple arrays in a circumferential pattern that give a full picture of the vessel wall. Stenoses may be correlated with a change in diameter as well as the course of obstruction and anatomy, including branches for visualization of tributaries as well branches for anatomic landmarks for use in performing interventions as with the above mentioned IVC filters. It may also be utilized for interventions of venous vessels, such as stent placements for stenosis and obstruction. This may show length and size of available stents to utilize, and follow up immediate evaluation following stent placement without having to use contrast material.

Lymphoscintigraphy

Lymphoscintigraphy using Technetium 99M-Sulfur colloid is utilized to diagnose lymphedema. A portion of Technetium 99M-Sulfur colloid is administered through an intradermal and subcutaneous injection at the first web space of the leg. A picture is obtained with a gamma camera or taken of both the legs and pelvis at certain times; 10, 20, 30, and 60 minutes. The patient walks before, during, and in between the examinations to provide normal venous return. Normally, radioactive material should flow toward the cephalad direction from the foot with early nodes being visualized in the groin at 10 minutes and well visualized at 20 minutes. Abnormal studies show faint or delayed uptake at 30 minutes, and no uptake at 60 minutes showing absence of lymphatic activity. Further causes of lymphedema should be assessed once lymphedema is diagnosed, including lymphatic obstruction or overwhelming venous obstruction leading to so-called phlebolymphedema or venous-caused lymphedema. If the nodes are visualized well at 10 and 20 minutes, further study can be concluded as essentially normal.

Conclusion

Due to the high incidence of vascular etiologies for wounds, each wound care patient should undergo a thorough history and physical examination. Once a major etiology is considered, further investigation by noninvasive vascular testing should be entertained. Secondary to the myriad noninvasive vascular testing available, each wound care specialist should familiarize himself or herself with the testing that is available at the institution, including the institution's accuracy for this testing. Each wound care specialist should be familiar with and readily apply the ABI, and should include this as part of physical examination and assessment. If definitive diagnosis is reached with noninvasive testing or if invasive testing such as angiography is entertained, a directed consultation with a general or vascular surgeon is needed.

Referral Criteria

The following indicators guide referral to a vascular surgeon or the vascular lab:

1. ABI greater than 1.0, tcPO$_2$ measurement greater than 30 mm Hg: semiurgent vascular appointment
2. Gangrene present: urgent vascular appointment
3. ABI
   a. Greater than 0.8: routine vascular appointment
   b. Between 0.5 and 0.8: semiurgent vascular appointment
   c. Below 0.5: urgent vascular appointment
4. Exposed bone or tendon at base of ulcer: urgent vascular appointment
5. Gross infection or cellulitis: urgent vascular appointment
6. ABI less than 1.0 with diminished or absent pulses: semiurgent vascular appointment
7. Nonhealing wounds despite 3+ pulses and good wound care: semiurgent vascular appointment

When in doubt, refer to vascular lab for further evaluation

Self-Care Teaching Guidelines

The key to prevention of vascular diseases is patient education. Education is the key to preventing debilitating circulatory problems. Patients must learn the correct way to avoid added stress on their circulatory systems and when to notify their physician if there is a problem.

Self-Care Teaching Guidelines Specific to Arterial Insufficiency

1. Do not smoke! Even one cigarette a day can decrease circulation.
2. Follow physician's directions for controlling blood pressure, diabetes, and high cholesterol.
3. Inspect legs and feet daily, and report any signs of redness, pain, or ulceration immediately. Be sure to inspect between toes.
4. Wash and dry feet every day.
5. Lubricate skin to avoid cracks.
6. The first thing to go into the shoe in the morning should be a hand. Check to make sure there are no foreign objects that could injure the foot.
7. Cut toenails straight across. If possible, have a podiatrist cut the toenails.
8. Do not wear tight shoes.
9. Test bath water with a hand or thermometer (<98° F) to avoid burns.
10. Do not walk barefoot at any time, either inside or outside the home.
11. Wear comfortable, wide-toed shoes that cause no pressure (orthotics, if necessary).
12. Do not wear constricting clothes.
13. Wear clean cotton socks with smooth seams or without seams

Self-Care Teaching Guidelines Specific to Venous Insufficiency

1. Do not smoke!
2. Wear support stockings as prescribed.
3. Avoid crossing legs.
4. Elevate legs when sitting.
5. Inspect legs and feet daily, and report any increased swelling, new or larger ulcers, increased pain, redness, or infection.
6. Avoid trauma to legs, such as bumping or scratching.
7. Keep legs and feet clean.
8. Eat a well-balanced nutritional diet that is low in sodium.

REVIEW QUESTIONS

1. Taking segmental pressures is a noninvasive diagnostic test for arterial competence. In a comparison of lower extremity pressures with upper extremity pressures, which

of the following is associated with a poor prognosis in terms of lower leg wound healing?

  a. Ankle/brachial index of 1.1

  b. Ankle/brachial index of 0.9

  c. Ankle/brachial index of 0.8

  d. Ankle/brachial index of 0.5

2. Which of the following descriptions is MOST characteristic of venous disease ulcers?

  a. Commonly occur on the tips of toes or over the malleolar head, with minimal exudate.

  b. Usually pale ulcer base, with necrotic tissue present.

  c. Wound edges are punched out and regular in appearance, and wound is usually painful.

  d. Commonly occur on the gaiter area, with irregular wound edges and moderate exudate.

3. Which of the following best reflects adequate tissue perfusion and oxygenation to support wound healing?

  a. Capillary refill time greater than 35 seconds

  b. Transcutaneous oxygen tension greater than 40mm Hg

  c. Albumin levels greater than 2.5

  d. Palpable dorsalis pedis and posterior tibial pulses

REFERENCES

1. Yao ST. Haemodynamic studies in peripheral arterial disease. *Br J Surg.* 1970;57(10):761–766.
2. Kohler TR., Nance DR, Cramer NM, Vandenburghe N, Strandness DE Jr. Duplex scanning for diagnosis of aortoilliac and femoropopliteal disease: A prospective study. *Circulation.* 1987;76(5):1074–1080.
3. Edwards JM, Coldwell DM, Goldman ML, Strandness DE Jr. The role of duplex scanning in the selection of patients for transluminal angioplasty. *J Vasc Surg.* 1991;13(1):69–74.
4. Malone JM, Anderson GG, Lalka SG, et al. Prospective comparison of noninvasive techniques for amputation level selection. *Am J Surg.* 1987;154(2):179–184.
5. Heijborer H, Buller HR, Lensing AW, Turpie AG, Colly LP, Tencate JW. A comparison of real-time compression ultrasonography with impedance plethysmography for the diagnosis of deep-vein thrombosis in symptomatic outpatients. *N Engl J Med.* 1993;329(19):1365–1369.
6. Belcaro G, Labropoulos N, Christopoulos D, et al. Noninvasive tests in venous insufficiency. *J Cardiovasc Surg.* 1993;34(1):3–11.
7. Wagner WH, Keagy BA, Kotb MM, Burnham SJ, Johnson G Jr. Noninvasive determination of healing of major lower extremity amputation: The continued role of clinical judgment. *J Vasc Surg.* 1988;8:703–710.
8. Wyss CR, Matsen FA III, Simmons CW, Burgess EM. Transcutaneous oxygen tension measurements on limbs of diabetic and nondiabetic patients with peripheral vascular disease. *Surgery.* 1984;95(3):339–345.
9. Ballard JL, Eke CC, Bunt TJ, Killeen JD. A prospective evaluation of transcutaneous oxygen measurement of diabetic foot problems. *J Vasc Surg.* 1995;22:485–492.
10. Franzeck UK, Talke P, Bernstein EF, Goldbranson FL, Fronek A. Transcutaneous PO_2 measurements in health and peripheralarterial occlusive disease. *Surgery.* 1982;91(2):156–163.
11. Castronuovo JJ Jr, Adera HM, Smiell JM, Price RM. Measurement is valuable in the diagnosis of critical limb ischemia. *J Vasc Surg.* 1997;26(4):629–637.
12. Castronuovo JJ. Diagnosis of critical limb ischemia with skin perfusion pressure measurements. *J Vasc Technol.* 1997;21(3):175–179.
13. Adera HM, James K, Castronuovo JJ Jr, Byrne M, Deshmukh R, Lohr J. Prediction of amputation wound healing with skin perfusion pressure. *J Vasc Surg.* 1995;21(5):823–828.
14. Carpenter JP, Owen RS, Baum RA, et al. Magnetic resonance angiography of peripheral runoff vessels. *J Vasc Surg.* 1992;16(6):807–815.
15. Edelman RR, Mattle HP, Atkinson DJ, Hoogewoud HM. MR angiography. *AJR Am J Roentgenol.* 1990;154:937–946.
16. Owen RS, Carpenter JP, Baum RA, Perloff LJ, Cope C. Magnetic resonance angiography of angiographically occult runoff vessels in peripheral arterial occlusive disease. *N Engl J Med.* 1992;326:1577–1578.
17. Shehadi WH, Toniolo G. Adverse reactions to contrast media: A report from the Committee on Safety of Contrast Media of the International Society of Radiology. *Radiology.* 1980;137:299–302.
18. Hessel SJ, Adams DF, Abrams HL. Complications of angiography. *Radiology.* 1981;138:273–281.
19. Waugh JR, Sacharias N. Arteriographic complications in the DSA era. *Radiology.* 1992;182:243–246.
20. Patel KR, Semel L, Clauss RH. Extended reconstruction rate for limb salvage with intraoperative prereconstruction angiography. *J Vasc Surg.* 1988;7:531–537.
21. Ricco JB, Pearce WH, Yao JS, Flinn WR, Bergan JJ. The use of operative prebypass arteriography and Doppler ultrasound recordings to select patients for extended femoro-distal bypass. *Ann Surg.* 1983;198:646–653.
22. Scarpato R, Gembarowicz R, Farber S, et al. Intraoperative prereconstruction arteriography. *Arch Surg.* 1981;116:1053–1055.
23. Flanigan DP, Williams LR, Keifer T, Schuler JJ, Behrend AJ. Prebypass operative angiography. *Surgery.* 1982;92:627–633.
24. Sarin S, Shields DA, Scurr JH, et al: Photo Plethysmography: A Valuable Non-Invasive Tool In the Assessment of Venous Dysfunction? J Vasc Surg 16:154-162, 1992.
25. Schroeder PJ, Dunn E: Mechanical Plethysmography and Doppler Ultrasound Diagnosis of Deep Vein Thrombosis. Arch Surg 117:300-303, 1982.

SUGGESTED READING

Bates, Barbara. *A Guide to Physical Examination and History Taking.* 6th ed. Philadelphia: Lippincott Company; 1995.

Moore WS. *Vascular Surgery: A Comprehensive Review.* 4th ed. Phildelphia: Saunders; 1993.

Sussman C. Circulatory system disease and ulcers. *Wound Care Patient Education and Resource Manual.* Gaithersburg, MD: Aspen Publishers; 1999.

Management by Wound Characteristics

Barbara M. Bates-Jensen

The Bates-Jensen rules for wound therapy are as follows: *If the wound is dirty, clean it. If there's leakage, manage it. If there's a hole, fill it. If it's flat, protect it. If it's healed, prevent it.*

Understanding the impact of wound characteristics on treatment options provides a template for intervention. Often, the physical appearance of the wound is the driving force behind treatment options. Part II presents management of wound healing by examination of physical characteristics commonly observed in wounds. Specific interventions by the clinician are required by the presence of necrotic tissue; exudate and infection; and edema. Clean, proliferating wounds; refractory wounds; and scar tissue present additional opportunities and obstacles for optimal therapy.

Part II begins with a chapter on management of necrotic tissue. A description of the significance and pathophysiology of necrotic debris in the wound bed opens the discussion. Specific necrotic tissue characteristics of consistency, color, adherence, and amount, as well as how necrotic tissue presents in wounds of different etiology are described. The characteristics of necrotic tissue in various wound types and the clinical presentation of slough and eschar are described.

There are five methods of wound debridement to manage necrotic tissue: mechanical, enzymatic, sharp, autolytic, or biosurgical. Chapter 8 presents each debridement method with indications for use, contraindications, advantages, disadvantages, and procedures for implementation. Outcome measures based on the color and amount of necrotic tissue in the wound are presented to measure the effectiveness of debridement. The chapter concludes with self-care teaching guidelines for other health-care workers, family caregivers, and patients.

Chapter 9 reviews management of exudate and infection. The significance and pathophysiology of wound exudate are presented and discussed for various wound types. The definition and significance of wound infection are presented. Misdiagnosis of wound infection occurs frequently in clinical practice. Differentiation of infection and colonization of the wound is not a simple task for most clinicians. Comparing characteristics of the infected wound with the inflamed wound reveals significant similarities, as well as some key differences. Wound culture is one of the primary methods of differentiating between infection and inflamma-

tion. Ovington and Bates-Jensen provide background and discussion on wound cultures with tissue biopsy, needle aspiration, and quantitative swab techniques and includes a procedure for each technique. The rising incidence of resistant organisms is presented with reference to methicillin-resistant *Staphylococcus aureus*.

One method of management of exudate and infection is wound cleansing. Wound cleansing and irrigation are discussed in relationship to use of antimicrobial cleansers, and specific cleansing procedures for various wounds are presented. The use of topical antimicrobials (antibacterials, antifungals, and antiseptics) is presented, with discussion on management of exudate with moist wound dressings completing the management interventions. Outcome measures for evaluating exudate management in terms of amount and type of exudate are presented. The chapter ends with self-care teaching guidelines for use with other health-care workers, family caregivers, and patients.

Chapter 10 focuses on the management of edema. Fowler and Carson discuss the etiologies associated with edema and strategies directed toward edema management. Management of edema includes a description of the procedures for managing edema and the parameters to measure to determine intervention outcomes. Edema assessment and edema measurement and control are presented as two primary categories of quantitative and qualitative findings. Quantitatively, leg circumference and leg volume can be measured to give a reference range of leg size, and, with care, pitting edema can also be measured and quantified. Procedures and guidelines for determining quantitative measurements are included. Qualitative assessment includes general appearance of the skin and leg, and patient statements about the edema.

Elimination and control of edema may be accomplished through leg elevation, exercise, and the use of compression therapy. Leg elevation facilitates the removal of fluid by utilizing gravity in assisting venous return. Compression therapy works with exercise to facilitate the movement of excess fluid from the lower extremity. Included as appropriate for edema management are the following procedures: leg elevation, elastic wraps, tubular bandages, paste bandages, graduated compression stockings, intermittent sequential compression devices, and exercise. The chapter details expected outcomes for each user-friendly method and helpful hints. The chapter concludes with a case study emphasizing the principles of edema management and self-care teaching guidelines, including a sample patient contract.

The next two chapters in Part II examine wound management of the clean wound and advanced wound therapy for the refractory wound. Geoffrey Sussman provides discussion on wound management of the clean wound with topical wound care products for moist wound healing. Discussion includes inert and passive products such as gauze, lint, and fiber products and modern moist wound dressings. The features of an "ideal" wound dressing are presented. Generic wound product categories of film dressings, foams, hydrocolloids, hydrogels, alginates, hydroactive dressings, and combination/miscellaneous dressings are then presented. Each wound category includes a definition of the products, the composition and properties of the dressing, indications and contraindications for use, procedures for application and removal of the dressings, and expected outcomes. Discussion of wound cleansing and use of topical antimicrobials is presented in relation to the clean wound. This chapter is supplemented with an appendix by Krasner on dressing categories for easy reference by the clinician.

Chapter 12 presents advanced wound therapies for the refractory wound. The chapter begins with a definition of the refractory wound. Then background, indications, and contraindications for use of growth factors and biological skin substitutes are presented. The section on growth factors is extensive and covers a wide variety of growth factors. This chapter provides the clinician with a quick reference for determining appropriate use of advanced therapy for wound care.

New to this section is Chapter 13: Management of Wound Pain. This comprehensive discussion of wound pain includes an extensive section on wound pain physiology, as well as practical tools for assessing and treating wound pain. Sussman and Bates-Jensen present general guidelines for evaluating pain from different chronic wounds and specific strategies for assessing pain in a variety of populations. Management of wound pain is covered for a variety of different wounds in conjunction with generic management principles. An extensive section on self-care teaching guidelines completes this chapter.

The final chapter in this section, Chapter 14, focuses on management of scar tissue. Scott Ward provides a thought-provoking evaluation of methods to manage scars. The chapter begins with a review of scar tissue formation and dysfunctional scarring, such as keloid formation and hypertrophic scars. The interactions between scarring, contraction, and functional ability are discussed. Measurement and methods of scar assessment are presented. The chapter covers scar interventions including surgery (realignment and use of tissue expanders), pharmaceutical agents, and use of physical agents to reduce pressure and skin tension on the scar site. Pressure therapy using molded splints and pressure garments is discussed. Noncustom pressure therapy, as with elasticized cotton tubular bandages, elastic wraps, or self-adherent stretch wraps, is discussed in relation to management of the scar. Exercise, silicone, massage, and other methods are also presented. The chapter includes self-care teaching guidelines and provides the clinician with an easy reference for management of scar tissue.

The chapters on wound management by wound characteristics in Part II all include tools, such as procedures for specific interventions, self-care teaching guidelines, and guidelines for measuring outcomes. The procedures and guidelines included in these chapters provide the clinician with a "toolbox" for daily practice in wound management. Each chapter focuses on simplifying the often-complex task of determining which interventions are appropriate for patients with wounds. Each follows the simple rules for therapy stated at the beginning of Part II. If the wound is dirty or if necrotic debris and infection are present, clean the wound. Debride the devitalized tissue and identify and treat infection. If the wound is leaking excess exudate or if edema is present, manage the drainage. Control the edema and contain excess exudate. Provide for a moist wound environment, not a wet wound environment. If there is a hole or if significant tissue has been lost at the wound site, provide for tissue replacement with a wound dressing, or fill the hole. If the wound is flat, in the process of reepithelialization, or scarring, protect it from external trauma and complications related to scarring. Finally, if the wound is healed, prevention of future wounds is critical.

Management of Necrotic Tissue

Barbara M. Bates-Jensen and Neil Christopher R. Apeles

CHAPTER OBJECTIVES

At the completion of this chapter, the reader will be able to:

1. Define the terms *eschar* and *slough*.
2. Describe two outcome measures for management of necrotic tissue.
3. Identify indications for sharp debridement.
4. Describe two advantages and disadvantages for sharp, autolytic, enzymatic, mechanical, and biosurgical debridement.

Significance of Necrotic Tissue

As tissues die, they change in color, consistency, and adherence to the wound bed. As necrotic tissue increases in severity, the color progresses from white/gray to tan or yellow, and finally, to brown or black. Consistency of the necrotic tissue changes as the tissues desiccate or dry. Initially consistency may be mucoid with a high water or moisture content. Later the material becomes more clumpy and stringy in nature. Eventually, the tissues appear dry, leathery, and hard. Consistency of the necrotic debris is related to retaining moisture in the wound bed. As the wound is exposed to air, the necrotic debris dehydrates, becoming leathery, dry, and hard. The level of tissue death and the wound etiology also influence the clinical appearance of the necrotic tissue. As subcutaneous fat tissues die, a collection of stringy, yellow slough is formed. As muscle tissues degenerate, the dead tissue may be more thick or tenacious. Histologic studies of human skin during pressure sore development demonstrate that, as the insult to the tissue progresses, the level of necrosis deepens.[1,2] Hard, black eschar represents full-thickness destruction, possibly occurring from prolonged ischemia and anoxemia or from a sudden large vessel disruption from shearing forces.[2] Fat and dermal necrosis and the formation of a slough may be compounded by infection from previous contamination by normal skin flora.[1,3,4] The debris may appear as yellow slough or a mucoid substance.[4,5] Prolonged ischemia may cause necrosis of underlying tissues and manifest as a gray area,

blueness of the skin, or white devitalized tissue.[1,5,6] Tissue color varies as necrosis worsens, from white/gray nonviable tissue to yellow slough, and finally, black eschar.

Consistency refers to the cohesiveness of debris (i.e., is it thin or thick? stringy or clumpy?). Consistency also varies on a continuum as necrosis deepens. The terms *slough* and *eschar* refer to different levels of necrosis and are described according to color and consistency.[1–3] Slough is described as yellow (or tan) and thin, mucinous, or stringy; eschar is described as brown or black and soft or hard, and represents full-thickness tissue destruction.[1,2] The more water content present in the necrotic debris, the less the debris adheres to the wound bed. *Adherence* refers to the adhesiveness of the debris to the wound bed and the ease with which the two are separated. Necrotic tissue tends to become more adherent to the wound bed as the level of damage increases and as moisture in the wound decreases. Clinically, eschar is more firmly adherent than yellow slough. The boxed table on the next page refers to color plates for necrotic tissue assessment. Plate captions give more information.

Necrotic tissue retards wound healing because it is a medium for bacterial growth and a physical barrier to epidermal resurfacing, contraction, or granulation.[7–9] The more necrotic tissue present in the wound bed, the more severe the insult to the tissue and the longer the time required to heal the wound.[1] In the process of treating the necrotic wound, the amount of necrotic tissue present leads to modification of treatment and debridement techniques. In addition, determining the severity of the tissue insult may be postponed if the amount of necrotic debris is sufficient to obscure visualization of the total wound. Necrotic tissue may be observed in chronic wounds with various etiologic factors.

Arterial/Ischemic Wounds

Necrotic debris in the ischemic wound may appear as dry gangrene. It may have a thick, dry, or desiccated black/gray appearance. It is usually firmly adherent to the wound bed. It may be surrounded with an erythematous halo (see *Color Plates 47* and *53*).

Neurotrophic Wounds

Neurotrophic wounds usually do not present with necrosis but often have hyperkeratosis surrounding the wound. This hyperkeratosis looks like callus formation at the wound edges. The wound edges need to be decallused or saucerized frequently (see Chapter 19, Figures 19-15B, 19-15C, and 19-21).

Venous Disease Wounds

Venous disease wounds may have either eschar or slough present. Often, venous wounds will appear with yellow fibrinous material covering the wound. Eschar may be attributed to desiccation of the wound and the necrotic debris (see *Color Plate 56*).

Pressure Sores

The necrotic debris that occurs in pressure sores relates to the amount of tissue destruction. In the early stage of pressure sore formation, the tissues may appear hard (indurated), with purple or black discoloration on intact skin. This is indicative of tissue death, and the necrosis appears as the wound demarcates. Exhibit 8-1 presents a critical thinking model, or guideline, for assessment of necrotic tissue and may be helpful in determining the best intervention.

Interventions

The therapeutic intervention for necrotic tissue presenting in the wound is debridement. Once the wound is predominantly clean and free of necrosis, debridement is no longer indicated. A variety of debridement choices are available to clinicians. Debridement choices often hinge on the appearance of the wound, the type of wound, and the type and amount of necrotic debris present in the wound. Some gen-

eral guidelines may be helpful. Appendix 8-A presents debridement choices for a variety of wounds and necrotic tissue types. There are five main types of wound debridement: mechanical, enzymatic or chemical, sharp, biosurgical, and autolytic. Debridement strategies typically involve use of more than one form of debridement. Reimbursement for debridement is available for clinicians under several CPT (current procedural technology) codes and ICD-9 *diagnostic* codes. Coding varies according to health-care professional status, and clinicians are advised to clarify codes specifically prior to billing for debridement services. In general, CPT codes 11040–11044 relate to full-thickness debridement as performed by physicians and physician extenders (nurse practitioners, clinical nurse specialists, or physician assistants). The CPT codes must be used in conjunction with ICD-9 *diagnostic* codes for Medicare billing. Code 86.22 is used when physicians perform the debridement procedure and code 86.28 should be used when the procedure is performed by nonphysicians. CPT codes 97601 and 97602 provide a mechanism for reporting interventions associated with active wound care as performed by occupational and physical therapists. Code 97601 refers to selective debridement techniques without anesthesia, such as high-pressure waterjet; sharp selective debridement with scissors or scalpel; and topical applications including the enzymatic and autolytic agents. Code 97602 refers to nonselective debridement techniques without anesthesia, such as wet-to-moist gauze dressings or enzymatic agents. Reimbursement is constantly changing, and clinicians are advised to review current guidelines. Discussion of advantages and disadvantages of each debridement intervention follows.

Mechanical Debridement

Mechanical debridement involves the use of some outside force to remove the dead tissue. The most common types of mechanical debridement are wet-to-dry gauze dressings, wound irrigation (using syringe and needle or pulsatile lavage), and whirlpool (see Chapter 26). The advantages of mechanical debridement include the following:

- Mechanical debridement uses treatment options that are familiar to most health-care professionals.
- Wound irrigation can effectively decrease the bacterial burden on the wound, when done correctly, and it can be used in conjunction with other treatment options.
- Whirlpool may soften necrotic debris for ease of removal by other methods.

Assessment of Necrotic Tissue Types—Color Plates				
Color	Black/brown eschar	Tan/yellow slough	Yellow fibrinous	White/gray
Moisture content	Hard	Soft/soggy	Soft/stringy	Mucinous
Adherence	Firmly attached base and edges	Attached base only	Loosely attached	Clumps
Color Plate(s)	7, 20, 21, 26, 30, 52	1, 27, 31	3	28, 29, 31

EXHIBIT 8-1   Necrotic Tissue Assessment Guideline

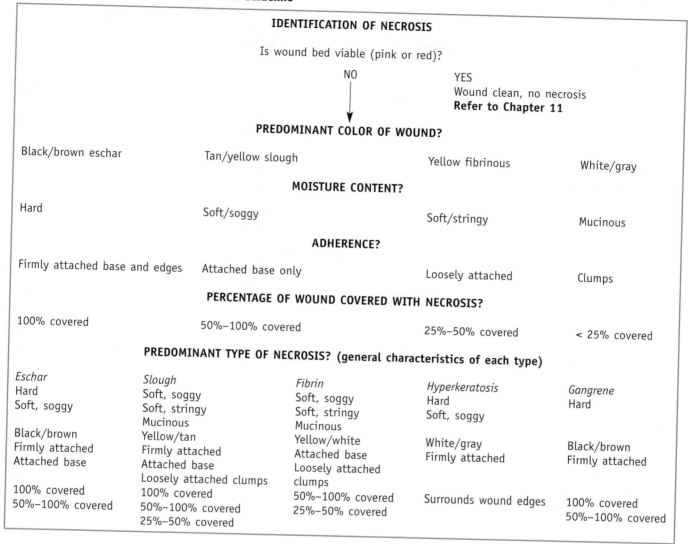

The disadvantages of mechanical debridement relate primarily to use of wet-to-dry gauze dressings and outweigh potential benefits; they include the following:

- Wet-to-dry gauze dressings as a form of mechanical debridement are nonselective, removing healthy tissue in addition to dead tissue.
- Wet-to-dry gauze dressings are rarely applied correctly.
- Wet-to-dry gauze dressings may cause pain on removal.
- Wet-to-dry gauze dressings may be more costly in terms of labor and supplies.
- Wet-to-dry gauze dressings may cause maceration of the skin surrounding the wound.
- Wet-to-dry gauze dressings may release airborne organisms and cause cross-contamination.[10]

Wet-to-dry gauze dressings continue to be the most commonly used debridement technique, despite the significant disadvantage of removing viable tissue, as well as nonviable tissue. The Agency for Healthcare Research and Quality (AHRQ), (formerly the Agency for Health Care Policy and Research [AHCPR]), panel's expert opinion recommendation is to use this method cautiously, because it can traumatize new granulation tissue and epithelial tissue, and to administer adequate analgesia when this method is employed.[10] When using wet-to-dry dressings for debridement, larger pore nonwoven cotton sponges are more effective. Mulder and colleagues found that of three different types, the sponge with the largest pores was more effective at removing necrotic tissue than sponges with smaller pores.[11]

Wound irrigation removes necrotic debris from the wound bed by using pressurized fluids. Pulsatile lavage (see Chapter 27) and high-pressure irrigation are two techniques for debridement. High-pressure irrigation involves the use of devices that deliver the irrigant solution to the wound at pressures between 8 and 12 pounds per square inch (psi). Use of a 35-mL syringe with a 19-gauge angiocatheter attached delivers fluids to the wound with high-pressure irrigation. This provides enough force to separate and remove necrotic tissue from viable tissue, yet not so much as to drive bacteria deeper into the wound tissues. The clinician performing high-pressure irrigation must use protective equipment to protect from potential bacterial contamination. Procedures for wet-to-dry gauze dressings and high-pressure irrigation are presented for reference and use.

Mechanical Debridement Procedures

Procedure: Wet-to-Dry Gauze Dressings

Equipment Needed:

- Sterile normal saline
- Gauze (rolled or 4 × 4-inch squares)
- Cover/topper sponges
- Sterile gloves (one pair)
- Clean gloves (two pairs)
- 35-mL syringe and 19-gauge needle
- Paper tape, trash bag

Frequency: Apply every 8 hours for wet-to-dry (see Chapter 11 for wet-to-moist gauze dressings).

Indications: Moist necrotic wounds (not effective on dry eschar).

Contraindications: Do not use on clean wounds because the healthy tissue will be debrided.

Precaution: Patient may need premedication for pain at the time of dressing change.

Procedure:

1. Explain dressing and procedure to patient and caregiver.
2. Wash hands.
3. Prepare dressing supplies.
   a. Open gauze and moisten with normal saline.
   b. Open cover sponges.
   c. Tear tape.
4. Apply clean gloves (to protect from cross-contamination).
5. Remove dirty dressing and dispose in trash bag.
6. Remove gloves and dispose in trash bag (gloves have been contaminated with the dirty dressing).
7. Apply clean gloves (to protect from cross-contamination).
8. Evaluate wound (see Chapter 4 for more on wound evaluation).
9. Clean wound.
   a. Use 35-mL syringe and 19-gauge needle to apply wound cleanser directly into wound.
   b. Use normal saline or a nonionic surfactant wound cleanser.
   c. Antimicrobial solutions, such as povidone iodine, destroy healthy wound tissues and should be used cautiously—*for short-term treatment, for appropriate bacterial flora only* (see Chapter 9 for more on wound cleansers and infection).
10. Remove gloves and apply sterile gloves (to prevent introduction of new bacteria into the wound). When wound care is being carried out in the home or long-term care setting, the procedure may be performed using only clean gloves.
11. Open the moistened gauze, fluff, and place in the wound loosely. Be sure to place some of the dressing in undermined or tunneled areas.
12. Cover the wound with the cover or topper sponges. Use one cover sponge for each gauze 4 × 4-inch square used in the wound or each 6–8 inches of rolled gauze used in the wound.
13. Secure the dressing with paper tape, write the date and time, and initial the tape.
14. Remove gloves and dispose in trash bag, dispose of the trash bag, and wash hands.
15. Review procedure with patient and caregiver.

Procedure: Wound Irrigation

Equipment Needed:

- Sterile normal saline
- Goggles, if splashing is anticipated
- Clean gloves (one pair)
- 35-mL syringe and 19-gauge needle or angiographic catheter
- Irrigation tray
- Trash bag
- Gauze sponges (4 × 4-inch squares or Kerlix super sponges) *or* cover/topper sponges

Frequency: Apply with each dressing change.

Indications: All wounds.

Contraindications: Use "gentle" irrigation on clean wounds and more vigorous irrigation on necrotic wounds (see Chapter 9).

Procedure:

1. Explain procedure to patient and caregiver.
2. Wash hands.
3. Prepare supplies.
   a. Open gauze or cover sponges.
   b. Fill syringe with irrigant.
      1) Use normal saline or a nonionic surfactant wound cleanser.
      2) Antimicrobial solutions, such as povidone iodine, destroy healthy wound tissues and should be used cautiously—*for short-term treatment, for appropriate bacterial flora only!* (See Chapter 9 for more on wound cleansers and infection.)
4. Apply goggles and clean gloves (to protect from splashing and cross-contamination).
5. Remove dirty dressing and dispose in trash bag.
6. Remove gloves, dispose in trash bag, and apply clean gloves (to protect from cross-contamination).
7. Evaluate wound (see Chapter 4 for more on wound evaluation).
8. Flush wound with irrigant. Hold needle/catheter 1–2 inches from wound bed.
   a. Irrigate forcefully to debride loose, necrotic tissue mechanically.

b. May attach a 14-French straight catheter to irrigate tunnels and large undermined areas.

c. Irrigate gently if wound is clean or free of necrotic debris.

9. Dry surrounding skin with gauze or cover sponges.
10. Apply prescribed dressing, according to procedure for dressing.
11. Remove gloves and dispose in trash bag, dispose of the trash bag, and wash hands.
12. Review procedure with patient and caregiver.

Enzymatic or Chemical Debridement

Chemical or enzymatic debridement involves applying a concentrated, commercially prepared enzyme to the surface of the necrotic tissue, in the expectation that it will aggressively degrade necrosis by digesting devitalized tissue. A physician's order is required, and manufacturer's guidelines should be followed. Enzymatic ointments are not active in dry environments, and most are not intended for use on dry eschar without proper preparation of the eschar. Eschar must be cross-hatched with a scalpel and the wound surface kept moist for the preparations to be successful. Enzymes require a specific pH range for best results, and many are inactivated by heavy metals (such as those often found in wound cleansers, topical dressings, and antimicrobial solutions). Frequency of dressing changes depends on the type of enzyme used and range from once to three times daily. Use of a secondary dressing is typically required, and most manufacturer guidelines recommend moist gauze dressings. Use of other moisture-retentive dressings may facilitate enzymatic debridement, but the choice of the dressing should match the expected dressing change frequency for the enzyme preparation. The surrounding skin must be monitored for potential maceration and the wound observed for potential infection. Enzymatic debridement is selective, only affecting the necrotic tissue and not damaging healthy wound tissues. However, once the wound is clean and free of necrotic debris, more appropriate dressings should be implemented because the enzyme preparations, although not harmful, are typically more costly.

There are three enzyme ointments available in the United States: collagenase, papain-urea, and papain-urea in combination with chlorophyllin. The AHRQ guidelines used collagenase as an example of a topically applied enzyme and cited studies indicating that enzymatic debridement could result in a clean granulating wound bed in 3–30 days.[12] A review of the literature related to debridement suggested that, if the enzyme was ineffective, the observed debridement may be due to autolysis instead.[13] As mentioned above, use of moist wound healing topical dressings can facilitate debridement with enzyme preparations. Martin and colleagues[14] found that a hydrogel alone can obtain results to similar to that of an enzymatic agent, with less expense. In this study, 17 patients were evaluated in a randomized, controlled trial of enzymatic debridement for necrotic wounds.[14] Investigators found a mean time of 8 days to debride stage IV pressure ulcers for those treated with an amorphous hydrogel dressing, compared with a mean time of 12 days for those treated with an enzymatic preparation containing streptokinase/streptodornase. Although the times were not significantly different, they did indicate that an agent without enzyme activity could produce an effect similar to one with enzyme activity.

There is no clear choice of recommended enzyme preparation; scientific research results vary in their conclusions. Research with animal models on the effectiveness of papain-urea, fibrinolysin and deoxyribonuclease (DNAse), and collagenase have been inconclusive, with some demonstrating more effectiveness with collagenase[15] and others finding papain-urea more effective.[16]

Two randomized clinical trials have evaluated enzymatic ointments in head to head comparisons. Alvarez and colleagues compared collagenase and papain-urea for pressure ulcer debridement in 26 nursing home residents with stable necrotic pressure ulcers followed weekly for 4 weeks[17,18]. The papain-urea ointment was significantly more effective than the collagenase ointment in reducing amount of necrosis present at each of the 3 week intervals (P=.016). Granulation tissue formation was enhanced in the papain-urea treated group also; however, these significant differences did not translate into differences in healing rates. The second trial by Pullen et al evaluated collagenase and fibrinolysin/deoxyribonuclease (DNASE) in 121 patients with pressure ulcers over 4 weeks.[19] There was no statistically significant difference in the two groups with 46.7% (28 of 60) of those in the collagenase group and 36.1% (22 of 61) of those in the DNAse group showing greater than or equal to 50% reduction in necrosis over the 4 week period. Enzymatic ointments have yielded consistently positive results for their efficacy in wound debridement. Debridement with enzymatic ointments is faster than with autolysis and more conservative than sharp debridement.

The advantages of chemical or enzymatic debridement include the following:

- It is selective, working only on necrotic tissue
- It is effective in combination with other debridement techniques, such as sequential sharp debridement and autolytic debridement.

The disadvantages include the following:

- Often, enzymatic use is prolonged more than necessary, increasing costs.
- Enzymatic debridement can be slow to achieve success: It may take from 3 to 30 days to achieve a clean wound bed.

Procedures for enzymatic debridement are included for reference and use.

Enzymatic Debridement Procedures
Procedure: Enzymatic Preparations
Equipment Needed:

- Sterile normal saline
- Enzymatic preparation
- Gauze (rolled or 4 × 4-inch squares) or cover/topper sponges

- Cleansing solution
- 35-mL syringe and 19-gauge needle
- Sterile gloves (one pair)
- Clean gloves (two pairs)
- Paper tape, trash bag

Frequency: Follow manufacturer's guidelines.

Indications: All necrotic wounds; moist necrotic wounds are best. If the wound has dry eschar, *cross-hatch* the eschar to improve healing. It is useful to match type of necrotic tissue to actions of enzyme activity, but not essential. For example, a venous disease ulcer will have more fibrin associated with the necrosis, and an enzyme that works on fibrin might be more effective.

Contraindications: Do not use on clean wounds, dry gangrene, or dry ischemic wounds, unless vascular consultation or ankle-brachial index (see Chapter 7) has been obtained and circulatory status determined.

Procedure:

1. Explain dressing and procedure to patient and caregiver.
2. Wash hands.
3. Prepare dressing supplies.
   a. Open gauze or cover/topper sponges and moisten with normal saline (most of the enzymatic ointments require a moist dressing for maximum effectiveness).
   b. Tear tape.
4. Apply clean gloves (to protect from cross-contamination).
5. Remove dirty dressing and dispose in trash bag.
6. Remove gloves and dispose in trash bag (gloves have been contaminated with the dirty dressing).
7. Apply clean gloves (to protect from cross-contamination).
8. Evaluate wound (see Chapter 4 for more on wound evaluation).
9. Clean wound (follow manufacturer's guidelines on use of cleaning solutions).
   a. Use normal saline or a nonionic surfactant wound cleanser.
   b. Use 35-mL syringe and 19-gauge needle to apply wound cleanser directly into wound.
   c. *Avoid* antimicrobial solutions, such as povidone-iodine, which destroy enzymatic activity in the enzyme preparations.
10. Remove gloves and apply sterile gloves (to prevent introduction of new bacteria into the wound). (When wound care is being carried out in the home or long-term care setting, the procedure may be performed using only clean gloves.)
11. Apply the enzymatic ointment with a tongue blade or cotton-tipped applicator to wound bed. As an alternative, the enzymatic ointment may be applied directly to the gauze dressing to be applied to the wound surface.
12. Open the moistened gauze, fluff, and place in the wound loosely. Be sure to place some of the dressing in undermined or tunneled areas.
13. Cover the wound with the cover or topper sponges. Use one cover sponge for each gauze 4 × 4-inch square used in the wound or each 6–8 inches of rolled gauze used in the wound. (May use a dressing other than gauze or cover/topper sponges for appropriate topical therapy as the secondary dressing for the wound.)
14. Secure the dressing with paper tape, write the date and time, and initial the tape.
15. Remove gloves and dispose in trash bag, dispose of the trash bag, and wash hands.
16. Review procedure with patient and caregiver.

Sharp Debridement

Sharp or instrumental debridement may be performed as a one-time debridement or as sequential conservative instrumental debridement. One-time surgical debridement is rapid and effective, and may convert the chronic wound to an acute wound. Laser debridement may be considered as a form of surgical debridement and may be effective on those patients who are not candidates for the operating room. Sequential conservative debridement involves removal of loose avascular tissue with sterile instruments. Because sharp debridement involves use of a scalpel, scissors, or other sharp instrument to remove nonviable tissue, it is the most rapid form of debridement. Sharp debridement is indicated over other methods for removing thick, adherent, and/or large amounts of nonviable tissue and when advancing cellulitis or signs of sepsis are present. Both registered nurses and physical therapists (PTs) may perform sharp debridement for wounds in most states. Health-care professionals who use sharp debridement must demonstrate their competence in sharp wound debridement skills and meet licensing requirements.[20] Check individual state practice acts before proceeding.

One multicenter, randomized, controlled trial noted the following effects of sharp debridement on the healing rates of diabetic ulcers.[21] (The trial was designed to compare the effects of a topical growth factor versus placebo on wound healing in 118 patients.) All patients received sharp debridement as needed throughout the study period. Analysis subsequently demonstrated that, independent of treatment, centers that used sharp debridement relatively frequently experienced better healing rates than did those that used sharp debridement less frequently. The highest degree of healing (83%) occurred in the center that used sharp debridement most frequently. This finding suggests that a relationship exists between sharp debridement and wound healing.

Of course, the main advantage of sharp debridement is the speed of converting a necrotic wound to an acute clean wound. When sharp debridement is performed as a one-time operative procedure, the chronic wound may convert to an acute wound, with resultant wound closure. Sharp de-

Licensing Issues

Registered nurses and PTs may perform sharp debridement. Nurses must (and PTs should) complete an education course on wound debridement and competence validation of wound debridement skills. Competence validation involves performing debridement skills on a wound model, such as a pig's foot, and demonstration of debridement skills on patients, with a qualified mentor to document competence. Some states do not allow nurses or PTs to perform sharp debridement, so it is wise to check with the state board of registered nursing, the state nursing practice act, and the PT licensing agency for validation of practice requirements for performing wound debridement.

bridement is a selective form of debridement when performed properly. Sequential conservative instrumental debridement is effective in combination with enzymatic, mechanical, and autolytic debridement and can speed the removal of necrotic debris when used in combination with other techniques. Conservative instrumental debridement can be performed in any health-care setting by nonphysician clinicians and does not require transfer to an acute facility. The disadvantages of sharp debridement include the following:

- Sharp debridement requires a level of experience or skill and specific education.
- There is often questionable reimbursement when sharp debridement is performed by nonphysicians (nurses). Reimbursement depends on individual state practice acts for nurses.
- Sharp debridement may be painful for the patient, and therefore, analgesia (topical or systemic) may be needed.
- There is a potential for blood loss and infection from the procedure.

There are special indications for sharp debridement in relationship to pressure ulcers. Sharp debridement should be performed when gross necrotic tissue, sepsis, or advancing cellulitis is present and should be done with physician collaboration and probable systemic antibiotic coverage. Ischemic wounds should not be debrided (by any means, but most certainly not with sharp debridement) unless the clinician is certain of collateral circulation by vascular studies or an adequate ankle-brachial index is present. Pressure ulcers on heels that present with black, hard eschar may be left intact, provided that they are inspected daily and are stable, nonerythematous, and nontender; if signs and symptoms of pathology develop (redness, sogginess, or mushy feel to the area or frank purulent drainage), they should be debrided immediately. Procedures for sharp debridement are presented for reference and use.

Safe Sharp Debridement

A key to successful, safe sharp debridement is knowledge of anatomy and assessment. The three-part Sharp Debridement of Wounds video series—Introduction and Technique, Anatomy and Assessment of the Torso, and Anatomy and Assessment of the Lower Extremity—is a training tool available to teach anatomy of common wound locations on the torso and lower extremities, assessment of necrotic tissue, instrument techniques, and procedures of sharp debridement.[22] Nearly all educational wound conferences offer preconference workshops in wound debridement. These conferences combine on-site didactic knowledge with expert instruction and skill attainment using animal models.

Sharp Debridement Procedure
Procedure: Sharp, Sequential Instrument Debridement
Equipment Needed:

- Silver nitrate sticks, Gelfoam, or hemostatic dressing (optional)
- Sterile normal saline
- 35-mL syringe and 19-gauge needle
- Gauze or cover/topper sponges
- Instrument set
- No. 10 and No. 15 scalpels and blades
- Wound dressing of choice
- Clamp (Kelly or mosquito)
- Suture removal set
- Sterile gloves (one pair)
- Clean gloves (one pair)
- Paper tape, trash bag
- Cotton-tipped applicators
- Scissors (small, fine, serrated; and large, with or without serrations)
- Forceps (Adson—with or without teeth—or Adson-Brown)

Frequency: Perform according to clinical judgment and physician's orders.
Indications: All necrotic wounds; moist necrotic wounds are best. If the wound has dry eschar, autolytic or enzymatic debridement may be used first to soften necrosis and facilitate sharp removal of debris.
Contraindications: Do not perform if you don't feel comfortable or don't know what you are cutting! Do not perform on clean wounds, dry gangrene, or dry ischemic wounds unless vascular consultation has been obtained and circulatory status determined.

Procedure:

1. Verify physician orders.
2. Explain procedure to patient and caregiver.
3. Premedicate patient for pain and relaxation.
   a. Topical: lidocaine (Xylocaine) spray or solution or benzocaine (Hurricaine) spray. Lidocaine spray can be used as a gauze compress directly to the wound

site for 10 minutes for effective topical anesthesia or may be locally injected.

  b. Systemic: oral, intramuscular, or intravenous as a preoperative/predebridement regimen. Administer approximately 30 minutes prior to therapy to increase patient tolerance and compliance with procedure.

4. Assemble equipment.
5. Arrange for an assistant.
6. Provide adequate lighting.
7. Position patient.
8. Wash hands.
9. Prepare clean field and equipment.
10. Apply clean gloves (to protect from cross-contamination).
11. Remove dirty dressing and dispose in trash bag.
12. Clean wound (follow manufacturer's guidelines on use of cleaning solutions). Warm solution to 96° to 100° F for patient comfort, if possible.
  a. Use 35-mL syringe and 19-gauge needle to apply wound cleanser directly into wound.
  b. Use normal saline or a nonionic surfactant wound cleanser.
13. Evaluate wound (see Chapter 4 for more on wound evaluation).
14. Remove gloves and dispose in trash bag (gloves have been contaminated with the dirty dressing). Open the suture removal kit and/or scalpel.
15. Apply sterile gloves (to prevent introduction of new bacteria into the wound). (When wound care is being carried out in the home or long-term care setting, the procedure may be performed using only clean gloves.)
16. Using the pickup forceps from the suture removal kit, lift the dead tissue or eschar that you are trying to debride and cut it with scalpel or scissors. Grasp dead tissue and hold it taut so that the line of demarcation is clearly visualized. Cut it with care and try to take it down in layers to prevent removal of healthy tissue. If indicated, use the clamp to hold back necrotic debris to help visualize the line of demarcation between healthy and dead tissue. Pain and bleeding are signs of healthy tissue.
17. Remove as much nonviable tissue as possible, but limit procedure to 15–30 minutes.
  a. Request reevaluation when any of the following are present:
    1) Elevated temperature or patient is on downhill course
    2) No wound improvement over several weeks
    3) Cellulitis *or* gross purulence/infection
    4) Impending exposed bone or tendon
    5) Abscessed area
    6) Extensively undermined area
  b. Aggressiveness of debridement should be guided by the following:
    1) The amount of necrotic tissue present
    2) Patient pain tolerance limits

    3) Time schedule and limits to avoid patient and provider fatigue (15–30 minutes)
18. Stop debriding when the following occur:
  a. There is impending bone or tendon.
  b. You are close to a fascial plane or other named structure.
  c. You get nervous.
19. Provide postdebridement care.
  a. Cleanse wound with normal saline.
  b. Apply wound therapy of choice.
  c. Document procedure.
20. Secure the wound therapy with paper tape if necessary, write the date and time, and initial the tape.
21. Remove gloves and dispose in trash bag, dispose of the trash bag, and wash hands.
22. Review procedure with patient and caregiver. (See Exhibit 8-2 for more information on self-care teaching guidelines for wound care with necrotic tissue.)

Autolytic Debridement

Autolytic debridement is the process of using the body's own mechanisms to remove nonviable tissue. Autolysis may be accomplished by use of any moisture-retentive dressing. Maintaining a moist wound environment allows collection of fluid at the wound site, which promotes rehydration of the dead tissue and allows enzymes within the wound to digest necrotic tissue. Autolytic debridement typically involves adequate wound cleansing to wash out the partially degraded nonviable tissue. It is more effective than wet-to-dry gauze dressings because it selectively removes only the necrotic tissue, and therefore, protects healthy tissues. Mulder and colleagues[23] evaluated 16 patients in a randomized, controlled trial of a hypertonic hydrogel versus wet-to-dry gauze for wound debridement.[23] Their results suggested that the hydrogel could safely facilitate removal of dry adherent eschar from wounds. All of the wounds were chronic, with at least 75% necrotic tissue present. Other investigators have also found amorphous hydrogels to be effective in digesting and removing necrotic debris from wounds.[24-26] Autolysis, when used in place of gauze or standard care, results in faster healing of diabetic foot ulcers.[27] Autolysis is facilitated by cross-hatching if the wound is covered with dry eschar. The AHRQ panel recommends autolytic and enzymatic debridement approaches as being better for patients in long-term care or home care settings and for those who cannot tolerate other methods.[12]

    Autolysis can be performed alone or in conjunction with other techniques, such as sequential conservative sharp debridement or enzymatic debridement. It is typically slower to achieve a clean wound bed, compared to sharp debridement, although progress should be seen within 6 days. It is essential to choose the appropriate dressing for autolysis. Dressing choice can be determined by the wound appearance. For instance, a wound that is covered with a dry eschar might be autolytically debrided using a thin film dressing, whereas a wound with obvious depth and moderate

EXHIBIT 8-2   Self-Care Teaching Guidelines

Self-Care Guidelines Specific to Necrotic Tissue	Instructions Given (Date/Initials)	Demonstration or Review of Material (Date/Initials)	Return Demonstration or Verbalizes Understanding (Date/Initials)
1. Type of wound and reason for necrotic tissue			
2. Significance of necrosis			
3. Topical therapy care routine:			
a. Clean wound			
b. Apply enzymatic preparation (if appropriate)			
c. Apply autolytic dressing—transparent film, hydrocolloid, or hydrogel			
d. Apply secondary dressing if using enzymatic preparation			
4. Frequency of dressing changes			
5. Expected change in wound appearance during debridement			
6. When to notify the health-care provider:			
a. Signs and symptoms of infection			
b. Failure to improve			
c. Evidence of undermining			
d. Impending bone or joint involvement			
7. Importance of follow-up with health-care provider			

exudate would not be treated with a thin film dressing (an alginate dressing or one with more absorptive capacity would be the better choice).

Autolysis is usually performed using one of the following dressing choices (but any moisture-retentive dressing can achieve autolysis):

- Transparent film dressings (best for dry eschar; because they are nonabsorptive, they rapidly create a fluid environment)
- Hydrocolloids (best for moist wounds with necrosis because they provide some absorptive capacity while maintaining a moist wound environment)
- Hydrogels (promote autolysis by maintaining a moist wound environment)

The advantages of autolysis are that progress can be determined quickly (there should be observed progress within 6 days). Autolysis is selective, of relatively low cost, and effective in combination with other debridement techniques. Autolysis has also been shown to be safe and effective on diabetic foot ulcers. Diabetic foot ulcer healing rates are faster when a hydrogel is used instead of a conventional gauze dressing.[21] Disadvantages include the caregiver education required for treatment compliance. The patient and caregiver must be informed and aware of the wound appearance, odor, and exudate under the dressing during autolysis since this can be disturbing. Procedures for autolysis using several dressings are presented for reference and use.

Autolytic Debridement Procedures
Procedure: Autolytic Debridement— Transparent Film Dressing
Equipment Needed:

- Sterile normal saline
- Skin sealant
- Transparent film dressing
- Clean gloves (two pairs)
- Sterile gloves (one pair)
- Paper tape, trash bag
- 35-mL syringe and 19-gauge needle

Frequency: Apply every 3–5 days. Always change dressing when drainage leaks out.

Indications: All necrotic wounds, but most beneficial for dry eschar; may cross-hatch eschar to facilitate autolysis.

Contraindications: Do not use for dry gangrene or dry ischemic wounds unless vascular consultation has been obtained and circulatory status determined.

Procedure:

1. Explain dressing and procedure to patient and caregiver.
2. Wash hands.
3. Prepare dressing supplies.
   a. Open transparent film dressing.
   b. Be sure that dressing size is at least 2 inches larger than wound area to be covered.
4. Position patient off of affected area.
5. Apply clean gloves (to protect from cross-contamination).
6. Remove dirty dressing and dispose in trash bag. (There is likely to be an odor, and the wound drainage may appear quite disturbing.)
7. Remove gloves and dispose in trash bag (gloves have been contaminated with the dirty dressing).
8. Apply clean gloves (to protect from cross-contamination).
9. Evaluate wound (see Chapter 4 for more on wound evaluation).
10. Clean wound (follow manufacturer's guidelines on use of cleaning solutions).
    a. Use 35-mL syringe and 19-gauge needle to apply wound cleanser directly into wound.
    b. Use normal saline or a nonionic surfactant wound cleanser.
    c. *Avoid* antimicrobial solutions, such as povidone-iodine, which destroy healthy wound tissues and should be used cautiously—*for short-term treatment, for appropriate bacterial flora only* (see Chapter 9 for more on wound cleansers and infection).
11. Remove gloves and apply sterile gloves (to prevent introduction of new bacteria into the wound). (When wound care is being carried out in the home or long-term care setting, the procedure may be performed using only clean gloves.)
12. Apply skin sealant to skin surrounding the wound and allow to dry until skin looks shiny (skin sealant protects the skin surrounding the wound from maceration and stripping during dressing removal).
13. Apply the transparent film dressing according to manufacturer's guidelines.
    a. When treating lesions in the sacral/coccygeal area, it is best to apply the dressing in a crisscross, overlapping fashion, using strips of the dressing.
    b. Avoid tension and wrinkling of the dressing.
14. Secure the dressing, write the date and time, and initial the dressing.
15. Remove gloves and dispose in trash bag, dispose of the trash bag, and wash hands.
16. Review procedure with patient and caregiver.

Procedure: Autolytic Debridement— Hydrocolloid or Hydrogel Wafer Dressings
Equipment Needed:

- Sterile normal saline
- Hydrocolloid dressing or hydrogel wafer dressing
- Skin sealant (optional)
- Clean gloves (two pairs)
- Sterile gloves (one pair)
- Paper tape, trash bag
- 35-mL syringe and 19-gauge needle
- Paper tape

Frequency: Apply every 3–5 days. Always change dressing when drainage leaks out.

Indications: All necrotic wounds. Dry eschar may benefit from cross-hatching to facilitate autolysis. This procedure is particularly effective in moist necrotic wounds with moderate amounts of exudate.

Contraindications: Do not use for cellulitis, documented wound infection, dry gangrene, or dry ischemic wounds unless vascular consultation has been obtained and circulatory status determined.

Procedure:

1. Explain dressing and procedure to patient and caregiver.
2. Wash hands.
3. Prepare dressing supplies.
   a. Open hydrocolloid/hydrogel dressing.
   b. Be sure that dressing size is at least 2 inches larger than wound area to be covered.
4. Position patient off of affected area.
5. Apply clean gloves (to protect from cross-contamination).
6. Remove dirty dressing and dispose in trash bag. (There is likely to be an odor, and the wound drainage may appear quite disturbing.)
7. Remove gloves and dispose in trash bag (gloves have been contaminated with the dirty dressing).
8. Apply clean gloves (to protect from cross-contamination).
9. Evaluate wound (see Chapter 4 for more on wound evaluation).
10. Clean wound (follow manufacturer's guidelines on use of cleaning solutions).
    a. Use 35-mL syringe and 19-gauge needle to apply wound cleanser directly into wound.
    b. Use normal saline or a nonionic surfactant wound cleanser.
    c. *Avoid* antimicrobial solutions, such as povidone-iodine, which destroy healthy wound tissues and should be used cautiously—*for short-term treatment, for appropriate bacterial flora only!* (See Chapter 9 for more on wound cleansers and infection.)
11. Remove gloves and apply sterile gloves (to prevent introduction of new bacteria into the wound). (When wound care is being carried out in the home or long-term care setting, the procedure may be performed using only clean gloves.)
12. Peel backing off the hydrocolloid or hydrogel wafer dressing and apply according to manufacturer's guidelines.

a. Apply strips of tape to the wafer edges in a picture-frame manner; use of a skin sealant under the tape is advised to protect from stripping.

b. Avoid use of skin sealants under hydrocolloid and hydrogel dressings.

13. Secure the dressing, write the date and time, and initial the dressing.

14. Remove gloves and dispose in trash bag, dispose of the trash bag, and wash hands.

15. Review procedure with patient and caregiver.

Biosurgical Debridement

Biosurgery, or larval debridement therapy (LDT), is the application of disinfected maggots to the wound to remove the nonviable tissue.[28] Fly larvae, either *Lucilia sericata* or *Phaenicia sericata*, are applied to the wound. The maggots secrete proteolytic enzymes that break down necrotic tissue and then ingest the liquefied tissue.[28,29] The secretions also have antimicrobial properties that are helpful in preventing bacterial growth and proliferation, including methicillin-resistant *Staphylococcus aureas*. In vitro studies have shown that the secretions also promote the growth of human fibroblasts.[29] This growth effect of maggot secretions contributes to improved granulation in wounds debrided by maggots.[30] Generally, the maggots are left in the wound from 1–4 days.[28–30]

Biosurgery has not been widely used in the past 50 years; it was reserved as a last resort for serious wounds that failed all other therapies.[31] However, maggot therapy is once again gaining popularity. Since only nonviable matter is liquefied and digested, biosurgery is considered a selective debridement method. Advantages are reduced bacterial burden and possible growth-stimulating effects. However, some disadvantages of biosurgery are:

- Availability
- Slower rate of debridement when compared to sharp debridement
- Removal and disposal of larvae
- Client and family preference and/or approval for larval treatment

The use of biosurgery as a method for debridement is not suitable for all wounds. There have been a limited number of studies on debridement and healing rates in specific wound types. Sherman[32] studied the effects of maggot therapy on lower extremity ulcers in 18 diabetic patients that failed to respond to conventional wound therapy. After five weeks the conventionally treated wounds still had 33% of their surface covered with necrotic tissue, whereas, the wounds treated with maggot therapy were completely debrided in 4 weeks. In this study, biosurgical debridement was effective at debriding lower extremity, nonhealing ulcers in diabetic patients. One randomized controlled trial of 12 subjects evaluated the cost effectiveness of biosurgical debridement on venous ulcers, and concluded that this method of debridement, when compared with hydrogel therapy, was cost-effective and efficacious.[33]

Maggots are effective in environments where fluid and oxygen are readily available and where wound pH is relatively stable. The ideal dressing for wounds treated with maggots allows oxygen exchange for the maggots, prevents maggots from escaping, and is appropriate for wound characteristics.[34] Since many patients and caregivers are uncomfortable with the notion of larval therapy, teaching must be done so that they completely understand the benefits and disadvantages of biosurgery. More studies are needed to evaluate the effects of biosurgery on wound healing in specific wound types and conditions.

Outcome Measures

Three appropriate characteristics for evaluating the effectiveness of debridement are the type of necrotic tissue, the amount of necrotic tissue, and adherence of necrotic tissue to the wound. Outcome measures for necrotic tissue are specific to the type of debridement used during treatment. For example, outcome measures for sharp debridement are typically achieved faster than the same outcomes when other, less aggressive debridement techniques are used. Changes in necrotic tissue are intermediate outcomes; the final outcome measure is healing.

Amount of Necrotic Tissue

The amount of necrotic tissue should diminish progressively in the wound if therapy is appropriate. The amount of necrotic tissue can be measured by linear measurements (measuring the length and width of the necrotic debris), by determining the percentage of the wound bed covered, and by photography. To determine the percentage of the wound bed covered, use a transparent measuring device with concentric circles. Draw a horizontal and a vertical axis through the circles, creating four quadrants (each equal to 25% of the wound) and use the device to help judge the percentage of the wound involved. The actual percentage of wound coverage may be documented, or a rating scale similar to the following may be used :

1 = None visible
2 = < 25% of wound bed covered
3 = 25–50% of wound covered
4 = > 50% and < 75% of wound covered
5 = 75–100% of wound covered

Type of Necrotic Tissue

The type of necrotic tissue should change as the wound improves and heals when conservative methods of debridement are used, including mechanical, autolytic, and enzymatic techniques. As the necrotic tissue is rehydrated, the appearance will change from a dry, desiccated eschar to a more soggy, soft slough and, finally, to a mucinous, easily dislodged tissue. The color usually changes as the necrosis

TABLE 8-1 Debridement Time Frames

Necrotic Tissue Type	Debridement Choice	Expected Outcomes	Time Frame Guide	Notes
Eschar	Autolysis	1. Eschar nonadherent to wound edges 2. Necrotic tissue lifting from wound edges 3. Necrotic tissue soft and soggy 4. Color change from black/brown to yellow/tan	14 days	Depending on type of dressing used for autolysis, may proceed at more rapid rate.
Eschar	Enzymatic preparations	1. Eschar nonadherent to wound edges 2. Necrotic tissue lifting from wound edges 3. Necrotic tissue soft and soggy 4. Color change from black/brown to yellow/tan 5. Change from eschar to slough	14 days	Requires compliance on dressing changes in order to be effective.
Eschar	Sharp	1. Removal/elimination of eschar, if done one time or significant change in amount and adherence, if sequential	Immediate if one time, 7 days if sequential	If sequential sharp debridement used in conjunction with enzymatic preparation or autolysis, may expect clean wound base in 7 days.
Slough or fibrin	Autolysis or enzymatic preparations	1. Necrotic tissue lifting from wound base 2. Necrotic tissue stringy or mucinous 3. Tissue color yellow or white 4. Change in amount of wound covered—gradual decrease to wound predominantly clean	14 days	Will require moderate amount of exudate absorption and protection of surrounding tissues from maceration.
Slough or fibrin	Sharp	1. Removal/elimination of necrotic slough if done one time or significant change in amount and adherence, if sequential	Immediate if one time, 7 days if sequential	If sequential sharp debridement used in conjunction with enzymatic preparation or autolysis, may expect clean wound base in 7 days.

is debrided. The black/brown eschar gives way to yellow or tan slough. Usually, eschar improves to slough material. Rating the type of necrotic tissue is best accomplished by the use of a scale similar to the following:

1 = None visible
2 = White/gray nonviable tissue and/or nonadherent yellow slough
3 = Loosely adherent yellow slough
4 = Adherent, soft black eschar
5 = Firmly adherent, hard black eschar

Adherence of Necrotic Tissue

Adherence of the necrosis should decrease as debridement proceeds. Initially, the necrotic tissue may be firmly attached to the wound base and all wound edges. As debridement proceeds, the necrosis begins lifting, loosens from the edges of the wound, and eventually disengages from the base of the wound, as well. Adherence is best evaluated using a rating scale similar to that for types of necrotic tissue.

General guidelines for debridement times are presented in Table 8-1.

Referral Criteria

Debridement in arterial/ischemic ulcers is contraindicated unless, and until, adequate circulatory status has been determined. If you don't feel comfortable or have limited or no experience in debridement, you may want to refer to a health-care provider with more experience. The following patients may warrant referral to the physician or an advanced practice nurse:

- Patients with dry gangrene or dry ischemic wounds (for vascular consultation for circulatory status determination)
- Patients with elevated temperature or those on a downhill course
- Patients with no wound improvement over several weeks (possible consultation with other health-care practitioners: PTs, dietitians, wound care nurses, enterostomal therapy [ET] nurses, and physicians)
- Patients with evidence of cellulitis *or* gross purulence/infection
- Patients with impending exposed bone or tendon present in the wound
- Patients showing evidence of an abscessed area or patients with extensively undermined areas present in the wound

Self-Care Teaching Guidelines

Patient and caregiver instruction in self-care must be individualized to the topical therapy care routine, the individual patient's wound, the individual patient's learning style and coping mechanisms, and the ability of the patient/caregiver to perform procedures. Exhibit 8-2 presents self-care teaching guidelines related to necrotic tissue management.

Conclusion

Debridement is a critical component of good wound care. Prompt, aggressive removal of non-viable tissue removes both a physical impediment to healing and a bacterial haven. A variety of debridement methods exist; sharp, mechanical, enzymatic, autolytic, and biotherapy. Sharp debridement is the method of choice in terms of time to achieve a clean wound bed and for those wounds with extensive and adherent necrosis. If signs of cellulitis are present then sharp debridement is the method of choice. Other debridement methods may be used in conjunction with sharp debridement between provider visits for continuous therapy. The key point to remember is the quicker a clean wound bed is obtained, the faster wound closure can be expected.

REVIEW QUESTIONS

1. Which of the following methods of debridement may be most useful with patients in long-term care facilities or in the home environment?
   a. sharp, enzymatic, and autolytic
   b. mechanical and autolytic
   c. sharp and mechanical
   d. autolytic and enzymatic
2. A client presents with a sacral wound that is 100% covered with thick, adherent black eschar. Which of the following debridement techniques is indicated?
   a. mechanical
   b. enzymatic
   c. autolytic
   d. sharp
3. Which of the following therapies could be classified as autolytic debridement?
   a. hydrogel dressings
   b. hydrocolloid dressings
   c. wet-to-dry gauze dressings
   d. thin film dressings
   e. a, b, c
   f. c and d
   g. a, b, d

REFERENCES

1. Shea D. Pressure sores: Classification and management. *Clin Orthop.* 1975;112:89–100.
2. Witkowski JA, Parish LC. Histopathology of the decubitus ulcer. *J Am Acad Dermatol.* 1982;6:1014–1021.
3. Enis JG, Sarmiento A. The pathophysiology and management of pressure sores. *Orthop Rev.* 1973;2:25–34.
4. Sather MR, Weber CE, George J. Pressure sores and the spinal cord injury patient. *Drug Intell Clin Pharm.* 1977;2:154–169.
5. Agris J, Spira M. Pressure ulcers: Prevention and treatment. *Clin Symp.* 1979;31:2–14.
6. Edberg EL, Cerny K, Stauffer ES. Prevention and treatment of pressure sores. *Phys Ther.* 1973;53:246–252.
7. Alterescu V, Alterescu K. Etiology and treatment of pressure ulcers. *Decubitus.* 1988;1:28–35.
8. Winter G. Epidermal regeneration studied in the domestic pig. In: Hung TK, Dunphy JE, eds. *Fundamentals of Wound Management.* New York: Appleton-Century-Crofts; 1979:71–111.

9. Sapico FL, Ginunas VJ, Thornhill-Hoynes M, et al. Quantitative microbiology of pressure sores in different stages of healing. *Diagn Biol Infect Dis.* 1986;5:31–38.

10. Lawrence JC, Lilly HA, Kidson A. Wound dressings and airborne dispersal of bacteria. *Lancet.* 1992;339(8796):807.

11. Mulder GD. Evaluation of three nonwoven sponges in the debridement of chronic wounds. *Ostomy/Wound Manage.* 1995;41(3):62–67.

12. Bergstrom N, Bennett MA, Carlson CE, et al. *Treatment of Pressure Ulcers.* Clinical Practice Guidelines No. 15. Rockville, MD: U.S. Department of Health and Human Services (DHHS). Public Health Service, Agency for Healthcare Research and Quality (AHRQ), formerly known as the Agency for Health Care Policy and Research (AHCPR) Publication No. 95–0652, December 1994.

13. Rodeheaver GT. Pressure ulcer debridement and cleansing: A review of current literature. *Ostomy/Wound Manage.* 1999;45(1A Suppl):80–86.

14. Martin SJ, Corrado OJ, Kay EA. Enzymatic debridement for necrotic wounds. *J Wound Care.* 1996;5(7):310–311.

15. Mekkes J, Zeegelaar J, Westerhof W. Quantitative and objective evaluation of wound debriding properties of collagenase and fibrinolysin/ deoxyribonuclease in a necrotic ulcer animal model. *Arch Dermatol Res.* 1998;290:152.

16. Hobson D, et al. Development and use of a quantitative method to evaluate the action of enzymatic wound debriding agents in vitro. *Wounds.* 1998;10(4):105.

17. Alvarez OM, Fernandez-Obregon A, Rogers RS, Bergamo L, Masso J, Black J. Chemical debridement of pressure ulcers: A prospective, randomised, comparative trial of collagenase and papain/urea formulations. *Wounds.* 2000;12(12):15–25.

18. Alvarez OM, Fernandez-Obregon A, Rogers RS, Bergamo L, Masso J, Black J. A prospective, randomised, comparative study of collagenase and papain-urea for pressure ulcer debridement. *Wounds.* 2002;14:293–301.

19. Pullen, R, Popp, R, Volkers, P, et al. Prospective randomized double-blind study of the wound-debriding effects of collagenase and fibrinolysin/deoxyribonuclease in pressure ulcers. *Age Ageing.* 2002;31:126–130.

20. Wound, Ostomy, and Continence Nurses Society. *Guideline for Prevention and Management of Pressure Ulcers: WOCN Clinical Practice Guideline Series.* Glenview: IL: Wound, Ostomy, and Continence Nurses Society; 2003.

21. Steed DL, Donohoe D, Webster MW, Lindsley L. Diabetic Ulcer Study Group. Effect of extensive debridement and treatment on the healing of diabetic foot ulcers. *J Am Coll Surg.* 1996;183:61–64.

22. Sussman C, Fowler E, Wethe J. *Sharp Debridement of Wounds* (video series). Torrance, CA: Sussman Physical Therapy, Inc. 1995.

23. Mulder GD, Romanko KP, Sealey J, Andrews K. Controlled randomized study of a hypertonic gel for the debridement of dry eschar in chronic wounds. *Wounds.* 1993;5(3):112–115.

24. Flanagan M. The efficacy of a hydrogel in the treatment of wounds with non-viable tissue. *J Wound Care.* 1995;4(6):264–267.

25. Bale S, Banks V, Haglestein S, Harding KG. A comparison of two amorphous hydrogels in the debridement of pressure sores. *J Wound Care.* 1998;7(2):65–68.

26. Colin D, Kurring PA, Quinlan D, Yvon C. Managing sloughy pressure ulcers. *J Wound Care.* 1996;5(10):444–446.

27. Smith J, Thow J. Update of systematic review on debridement – Wound care. *Diabetic Foot.* 2003;6(1):12–16.

28. Zacur H, Kirsner RS. Debridement: Rationale and therapeutic options. *Wounds: Compend Clin Res Pract.* 2002;14(7Suppl E):2E–7E.

29. Prete PE. Growth effects of Phaenicia sericata larval extracts on fibroblasts: Mechanism for wound healing by maggot therapy. *Life Sci.* 1997;60(8):505–10.

30. Mumcuoglu KY. Clinical applications for maggots in wound care. *Am J Clin Dermatol.* 2001;2(4):219–227.

31. Wollina U, Liebold K, Schmidt WD, Hartman M, Fassler D. Biosurgery supports granulation and debridement in chronic wounds—clinical data and remittance spectroscopy measurement. *Int J Dermatol.* 2002;41(10):635–639.

32. Sherman RA. Maggot therapy for treating diabetic foot ulcers unresponsive to conventional therapy. *Diabetes Care.* 2003;26(2):446–451.

33. Wayman J, Nirojogi V, Walker A, Sowinski A, Walker MA. The cost effectiveness of larval therapy in venous ulcers. *J Tissue Viability.* 2000;10(3):91–4.

34. Sherman RA, Hall MJR, Thomas S. Medicinal maggots: An ancient remedy for some contemporary afflictions. *Annu Rev Entomol.* 2000;45(1):55–81.

SUGGESTED READING

Black J, Black S. Surgical management of pressure ulcers. *Nurs Clin North Am.* 1987;22:429–438.

Davis JT. Enhancing wound-debridement skills through simulated practice. *Phys Ther.* 1986;66:1723–1724.

Fowler E. Instrument/sharp debridement of non-viable tissue in wounds. *Ostomy/Wound Manage.* 1992;38:26–33.

Gordon, B. Conservative sharp wound debridement. *J Wound Ostomy Continence Nurs.* 1996;23(3):137.

Haury B, Rodeheaver G. Debridement: An essential component of traumatic wound care. *Am J Surg.* 1978;135:238–242.

Thomaselli N. WOCN Position statement: Conservative sharp wound debridement for registered nurses. *J Wound Ostomy Continence Nurs.* 1995;22(1):32A.

Wound, Ostomy, Continence Nurses Society. *Guideline for Prevention and Management of Pressure Ulcers.* Glenview: IL: Wound, Ostomy, and Continence Nurses Society; 2003.

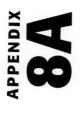

Debridement Choices for Chronic Wounds

Wound Type	Tissue Type	Consistency	Adherence	Amount of Debris	Debridement Choices	Rationale and Notes
Pressure sores	Black/brown eschar	Hard	Firmly adherent, attached to all edges and base of wound	75%–100% wound covered	1. *Autolytic*—best choice is transparent film dressing. May use hydrocolloid or hydrogel; score eschar with scalpel for more rapidresults. 2. *Enzymatic ointment with secondary dressing*—must score eschar with scalpel.	1. Transparent film dressings trap fluid at the wound surface with no absorptive capabilities, providing for more rapid hydra-hydration of the eschar and facil-itating autolysis. Hydrocolloid/hydrogel dressings have an absorptive capacity and may require more time for autolysis. 2. Enzymatic ointments effective against collagen and protein may be most effective.
	Black/brown eschar or Yellow/tan slough	Soft, soggy Soft, stringy	Adherent, attached to wound base, may or may not be attached to wound edges	50%–100% wound covered	1. *Autolytic*—best choices are hydrocolloids and hydrogels; composite dressings may also be beneficial. 2. *Enzymatic ointment with secondary dressing.* 3. *Sharp, sequential, or one time*—may be used alone or in conjunction with any of the above methods	1. Hydrocolloids and hydrogels provide for absorption of mild to moderate amounts of exudate while maintaining a moist wound environment to facilitate autolysis. 2. Enzymatic ointments effective against collagen and protein may be most effective. May need to protect intact skin from enzyme and excess exudate.
	Yellow/tan slough	Soft, stringy	Adherent, attached to wound base; may or may not be attached to wound edges or loosely adherent to wound base	Less than 50% wound covered	1. *Autolytic*—best choices are hydrocolloids and hydrogels. 2. *Enzymatic ointment with secondary dressing.* 3. *Sharp, sequential, or one time*—may be used alone or in conjunction with any of the above methods.	1. Hydrocolloids and hydrogels provide for absorption of mild to moderate amounts of exudate while maintaining a moist wound environment to facilitate autolysis. 2. Enzymatic ointments effective against collagen and protein may be most effective. May need to protect intact skin from enzyme and excess exudate.

Wound Type	Tissue Type	Consistency	Adherence	Amount of Debris	Debridement Choices	Rationale and Notes
	Yellow slough	Mucinous	Loosely adherent to wound base, clumps scattered throughout wound	50%–100% wound covered	1. *Autolytic*—best choices are hydrocolloids and hydrogels. 2. *Enzymatic ointment with secondary dressing.*	1. Hydrocolloids and hydrogels provide for absorption of mild to moderate amounts of exudate while maintaining a moist wound environment to facilitate autolysis. 2. Enzymatic ointments effective against collagen and protein may be most effective. May need to protect intact skin from enzyme and excess exudate. Should be discontinued when wound is predominantly clean.
Venous disease ulcers	Black/brown eschar	Hard	Firmly adherent, attached to all edges and base of wound	50%–100% wound covered	1. *Autolytic*—best choices are hydrocolloids and hydrogels. 2. *Enzymatic ointment with secondary dressing.*	1. Hydrocolloids and hydrogel dressings have absorptive capacity, which helps to prevent maceration of surrounding tissues and promotes autolysis. 2. Enzymatic ointments effective against fibrin may be most effective.
	Yellow slough	Soft, soggy, or fibrinous	Firmly adherent, attached to all edges and base of wound	50%–100% wound covered	1. *Autolytic*—best choices are hydrocolloids and hydrogels. 2. *Enzymatic ointment with secondary dressing.* 3. *Sharp, sequential, or one time*—may be used alone or in conjunction with any of the above methods.	1. Hydrocolloids and hydrogel dressings have absorptive capacity, which helps to prevent maceration of surrounding tissues and promotes autolysis. 2. Enzymatic ointments effective against fibrin may be most effective. May need to protect intact skin from enzyme and excess exudate. Should be discontinued when wound is predominantly clean.

Wound Type	Tissue Type	Consistency	Adherence	Amount of Debris	Debridement Choices	Rationale and Notes
Venous disease ulcers (cont.)	Yellow slough	Fibrinous or Mucinous	Loosely adherent Clumps scattered throughout wound	Any amount of wound covered	1. *Autolytic*—best choices are hydrocolloids and hydrogels. 2. *Enzymatic ointment with secondary dressing.*	1. Hydrocolloids and hydrogel dressings have absorptive capacity, which helps to prevent maceration of surrounding tissues and promotes autolysis. 2. Enzymatic ointments effective against fibrin may be most effective. May need to protect intact skin from enzyme and excess exudate. Should be discontinued when wound is predominantly clean.
Arterial ischemic ulcers	Black/brown eschar	Hard	Firmly adherent, attached to all edges and base of wound	50%–100% wound covered	1. *Autolytic*—best choices are hydrogels. 2. *Enzymatic ointment with secondary dressing.*	Must be certain of circulatory status prior to initiating debridement. 1. Hydrogel dressings have absorptive capacity, which helps to prevent maceration of surrounding tissues and promotes autolysis. The amorphous hydrogels are nonadherent and require a secondary dressing. 2. Enzymatic ointments: may need to protect intact skin from enzyme and excess exudate. Should be discontinued when wound is predominantly clean.
		Soft, soggy	Adherent, attached to wound base; may or may not be attached to wound edges	50%–100% wound covered	1. *Autolytic*—best choices are hydrogels. 2. *Enzymatic ointment with secondary dressing.* 3. *Sharp, sequential, or one time.*	1. Hydrogel dressings have absorptive capacity, which helps to prevent maceration of surrounding tissues and promotes autolysis. The amorphous hydrogels are nonadherent and require a secondary dressing. 2. Enzymatic ointments effective against protein and collagen may be most effective. May need to protect intact skin from enzyme and excess exudate. Should be discontinued when wound is predominantly clean.

Wound Type	Tissue Type	Consistency	Adherence	Amount of Debris	Debridement Choices	Rationale and Notes
Neurotrophic/ diabetic ulcers	White/gray	Hard	Hyperkeratosis, callus formation at wound edges	Involves all/partial wound edges	1. *Sharp, sequential, or one time*—saucerization or callus removal. 2. *Autolytic*—best choices are hydrocolloids and hydrogels.	1. Saucerization may be required at each dressing change. 2. Hydrocolloids and hydrogels soften the callus formation, and this may facilitate removal as the dressing is removed.

Management of Exudate and Infection

Barbara M. Bates-Jensen and Liza G. Ovington

CHAPTER OBJECTIVES

At the completion of this chapter, the reader will be able to:

1. Describe the differences between wound colonization and wound infection.
2. Explain the effects of antimicrobial cleansing solutions on the wound environment.
3. Describe wound cleansing procedures.
4. Discuss issues related to obtaining wound cultures.
5. Describe methods of managing exudate.

Wound exudate (also known as *wound fluid* and *wound drainage*) is an important wound assessment feature because the characteristics of the exudate help the clinician to diagnose wound infection, evaluate effectiveness of topical therapy, and monitor wound healing. Wound infection retards wound healing and must be treated. Proper assessment of wound exudate is also important because it confirms the body's brief, normal, inflammatory response to tissue injury. Thus, accurate assessment of wound exudate and diagnosis of infection are critical components of effective wound management.

Significance of Exudate

The healthy wound normally has some evidence of moisture on its surface. Healthy wound fluid contains optimal ratios of endogenous chemicals, including enzymes, cytokines and growth factors, which play a role in promoting the efficient deposition of granulation tissue, regrowth of blood vessels, and reepithelialization of the wound.[1] The moist environment produced by wound exudate allows efficient migration of epidermal cells and prevents wound desiccation and further injury.[2,3]

In acute wounds that are healing by primary intention, exudate on the incision line is normal during the first 48–72 hours. After that time, the continued presence of exudate is a sign of impaired healing. Infection and seroma are the two most likely causes. In chronic wounds, increased exudate is a response to the inflammatory process or infection. In-

creased capillary permeability causes leakage of fluids and substrates into the injured tissue. When a wound is present, the tissue fluid leaks out of the open tissue. This fluid is normally serous or serosanguineous.

Evaluation of the wound type, number and type of organisms present, and condition of the patient are important in determining risk for infection. Evaluation of wound type includes assessment of whether the etiology of the wound is acute or chronic, whether the wound tissues are necrotic versus clean, and whether the wound is currently healing or nonhealing. The number and type of organisms present in the wound tissues are evaluated for burden on the wound, possible bacteria-produced toxins, and pathogenicity of the organisms. Patient condition relates to status of the immune function and local host defenses.

In an infected wound, the exudate may thicken, become purulent, and remain in moderate to copious amounts. An example of exudate character changes in infected wounds is the presence of *Pseudomonas* organisms, which produce a thick, malodorous, sweet-smelling, green drainage,[4] or *Proteus* infection, which may produce an ammonia odor. Wounds with foul-smelling drainage are generally infected or filled with necrotic debris, and healing time is prolonged as tissue destruction progresses.[5] Wounds with significant amounts of necrotic debris will often have a thick, tenacious, opaque, purulent, malodorous drainage in moderate to copious amounts. True wound exudate should be differentiated from necrotic tissue that sloughs off of the wound secondary to debridement; this exudate is commonly attached to or associated with the necrotic debris. However, frequently, the only method of differentiation is adequate debridement of necrotic tissue from the wound. Necrotic tissue becomes more soluble, most often as a result of enzymatic or autolytic debridement. Often, the removal of the necrotic tissue dramatically reduces the amount of exudate and changes its character.

Wounds can become edematous when excessive amounts of plasma proteins leak from damaged capillaries and pervade the local tissue environment. The fluid of wound edema contains proteolytic enzymes, bacteria and bacterial toxins, prostaglandins, and necrotic debris, all of which contribute to chronic inflammation. Exudate also drains valuable and needed substrates, such as growth factors, from the wound bed and impairs the healing process. Excess exudate losses drain substrates and energy that could be used for wound healing processes.[4]

The character and amount of exudate change as pressure ulcers heal, which has been found by some researchers to be predictive of healing.[6,7] Xakellis and Chrischilles[6] examined 39 patients with pressure ulcers in a clinical trial and found that, when exudate was present at baseline, wounds healed more slowly, regardless of treatment. The healing rate of wounds was reduced by two-thirds when exudate was present at baseline. In contrast, other researchers have not found exudate amount at baseline to be a significant predictor of healing.[8,9] However, most acknowledge the negative effects of large amounts of exudate on healing outcomes.

Assessment of Wound Exudate

Characteristics of exudate that can be evaluated in the clinical setting are color, consistency, adherence, distribution in the wound, presence of odor, and the amount present.[10] The color and consistency of wound exudate can vary, depending on the type of wound, degree of moisture in the wound, wound healing phase, and presence of organisms in the wound. Table 9-1 presents various types of wound exudate and associated characteristics. *Color Plates 42–47* (reading the dressing and wound exudate characteristics) will help

the clinician to identify exudate types and make an appropriate assessment of their significance.

Estimating the amount of exudate in a wound can be difficult because of wound size variability. What might be considered a significant amount of drainage for a smaller wound may be considered a minor amount of drainage for a larger wound, making clinically meaningful assessment of exudate more difficult. This difficulty can be compounded by the type of topical dressing in use. Certain dressing types interact with or trap wound fluid, which can then mimic certain characteristics of exudate, such as the color and consistency of purulent drainage. For example, both hydrocolloid and alginate dressings can mimic a purulent drainage upon removal of the dressing.

Preparation of the wound site for appropriate exudate assessment involves removal of the wound dressing and cleansing to remove dressing debris in the wound bed. Then evaluate the wound for true exudate. Cooper[10] suggests estimating the percentage of exudate in the wound by clinical observation. This approach works if the wound exudate is thick and can be observed in the wound bed. When wound exudate character is more serous in nature, clinical observation of the wound alone is insufficient to quantify the amount of drainage. For thinner wound exudate, the amount of drainage is estimated by noting the number of dressings saturated during a period of time. Clinical judgment of the amount of wound drainage requires some experience with expected wound exudate output in relation to the type of wound and current phase of wound healing, as well as knowledge of the absorptive capacity and normal wear time of different topical dressings.

Although not part of exudate assessment, evaluation of the wound dressing provides the clinician with valuable data about the effectiveness of treatment. Evaluation of the percentage of the wound dressing saturated or involved with wound drainage during a specific time frame is helpful for clinical management, including dressings beyond traditional gauze. In estimating the percentage of the dressing involved with the wound exudate, clinical judgment is quantified, and the clinician must put a number to visual assessment of the dressing. For example, the clinician might determine

TABLE 9-1   Wound Exudate Characteristics

Exudate Type	Color	Consistency	Significance
Sanguineous/bloody	Red	Thin, watery	Indicates new blood vessel growth or disruption of blood vessels
Serosanguineous	Light red to pink	Thin, watery	Normal during inflammatory and proliferative phases of healing
Serous	Clear, light color	Thin, watery	Normal during inflammatory and proliferative phases of healing
Seropurulent	Cloudy, yellow to tan	Thin, watery	May be first signal of impending wound infection
Purulent/pus	Yellow, tan, or green	Thick, opaque	Signals wound infection; may be associated with odor

that 50% of a hydrocolloid dressing was involved with wound drainage over a 4-day wearing period. Based on the above data, the clinician might quantify his or her judgment for this type of dressing, length of dressing wear time, and wound etiology, concluding a "minimal" amount of exudate was present.

Appropriate wound exudate assessment requires consideration of wound etiology. Independent of exudate differences related to etiology of the wound, certain characteristics of exudate indicate wound degeneration and infection. If signs of cellulitis (erythema or skin discoloration, edema, pain, induration, and purulent drainage) are present at the wound site, the exudate amount may be copious and seropurulent or purulent in character. With further wound degeneration, the amount of exudate remains high or increases, and its character may change to frank purulence. Wound infection must be considered in these cases, regardless of etiology.

Arterial/Ischemic Wounds

Exudate in the ischemic wound may vary in amount and character. Arterial/ischemic wounds are often dry or have only a scant to small amount of serous exudate.

Neuropathic Wounds

Neuropathic wounds generally present with minimal exudate, possibly due to a limited inflammation response because of concomitant vascular disease and immune status changes from diabetes. The exudate is usually serous or serosanguineous in character.

Venous Disease Wounds

Venous disease wounds usually are highly exudative, both on initial presentation and throughout the course of healing. The pathophysiology of venous disease usually involves the development of lower extremity edema, caused by leakage of blood components into surrounding tissues secondary to chronic ambulatory venous hypertension. As such, a key component in the management of venous disease wounds is application of sustained, external, gradient compression to manage the edema. This compression is essential for the healing of the venous wound. As the venous ulcer heals, edema is lessened, and the wound exudate increases as the excess fluid takes the path of least resistance—in this case, the wound bed. Often, venous wounds appear with yellow fibrinous material covering the wound, which must be differentiated from true exudate.

Pressure Sores

Pressure sores present with a variety of wound exudate characteristics and amounts. In partial-thickness pressure sores, the wound exudate is most likely to be serous or serosanguineous in nature, and presents in minimal to moderate amounts. Similarly, in clean full-thickness pressure sores there are generally minimal to moderate amounts of serous to serosanguineous exudate. As healing progresses in the clean, full-thickness pressure sore, the character of the exudate changes and may become bloody if the fragile capillary bed is disrupted and lessens in amount. For full-thickness pressure ulcers with necrotic debris, wound exudate is dependent on the presence or absence of infection and the type of therapy instituted. The quantity of exudate may appear moderate to large; in fact, it is related to the amount of necrotic tissue present and the liquefaction of the debris in the wound. Typically, a necrotic full-thickness pressure ulcer presents with serous to seropurulent wound exudate in moderate to large amounts (Figure 9-1). With appropriate treatment, the wound exudate amount can temporarily increase, although the character gradually assumes a serous nature.

Significance of Infection

Bacteria are present in all chronic wounds and do not in themselves constitute an infection. The presence of bacteria in wounds is often described as meeting one of three conditions: contamination, colonization, or infection. These three conditions vary with respect to the behavior and loca-

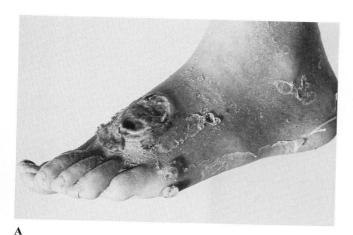

A

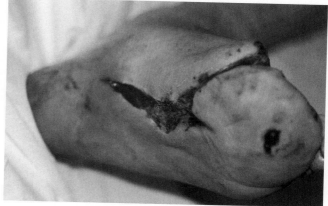

B

FIGURE 9-1 Obvious signs of infection.

tion of the bacteria in the wound, as well as the effect on and response from the host.

Bacterial *contamination* refers to the presence of nonproliferating bacteria on the wound surface with no injury to or visible signs of immune response from the host (e.g., erythema, edema, pain, heat, and purulent exudate). Bacterial *colonization* refers to the presence of proliferating bacteria on the surface of the wound, again with no injury to or immune response from the host. Bacterial *infection* refers specifically to the presence of proliferating bacteria within viable tissues—i.e., they are no longer only on the superficial tissue but have invaded living tissues—to such an extent that injury to tissues occurs and a host immune response is evoked and visible. When host and wound conditions are favorable, infection can occur.

Basically, infection represents an imbalance between bacterial numbers and/or virulence and the host's ability to defend itself. If bacterial numbers are high, the combination of bacterial species is right, or the host immune response is depressed, even in the absence of clinically observable signs of infection, wound healing can be delayed. Microbiologic research has shown that the presence of four or more bacterial groups in a wound is associated with delayed healing.[11] Wound infection extends the inflammatory response, delays collagen synthesis, retards epithelialization, and causes more injury to the tissues. Bacteria not only compete with fibroblasts and other cells for limited amounts of oxygen and other nutrients, but they produce and release a variety of deleterious chemicals into the wound environment, such as toxins and proteases.[12]

Large acute wounds generally react to bacterial burden differently than in small, chronic, ulcerative wounds. Acute wounds, in particular those with prolonged inflammatory responses, are more susceptible to bacterial invasion by skin flora.[8] Wounds involving the loss of large amounts of body surface area (15% of surface area or greater) are also at a greater risk for bacterial invasion. Sufficient numbers of skin flora organisms will cause acute wounds such as grafts and flaps to fail and, if untreated, lead to sepsis. In contrast, a chronic leg ulcer may remain unchanged for months or years, showing no signs of infection or sepsis, with the same or larger numbers of organisms present.[13] The same organisms that pose serious threat of infection and sepsis in some acute wounds present a different pictures in the small chronic wound, which may go on to heal despite the presence of these organisms. Chronic wounds are often contaminated with skin flora, such as *Enterococcus, Staphylococcus, Bacillus*, or, occasionally, gram-negative organisms.[13]

High levels of bacteria are found in chronic wounds presenting with necrotic debris. The number and density of aerobes and anaerobes are greater in necrotic wounds and in those with undermining.[5] The presence of a foul odor is usually associated with anaerobic organisms. Sharp debridement of necrotic tissue virtually eliminates the anaerobic organisms (such as *Bacteroides, Streptococcus, Enterobacter*, and *Escherichia coli*) and decreases the aerobic organisms (such as *Staphylococcus aureus*) present in the wound.[5]

Methicillin-resistant *Staphylococcus aureus*

Methicillin-resistant *Staphylococcus aureus* (MRSA) is of special concern for patients with wounds. *S. aureus*, which is part of normal skin flora, is on the skin of approximately 20%–50% of healthy adults and can persist in wounds.[14] Patients at the highest risk for developing MRSA colonization and infection are those with a history of injection drug abuse, the presence of chronic disease, previous antimicrobial therapy, previous hospitalization, admission to an intensive care unit, or a prolonged stay in a health-care institution.[15] All forms of *S. aureus*, including MRSA, can quickly invade and infect breaks in skin integrity, making wounds one of the most common sites of *S. aureus* and MRSA colonization and infection.

In the early 1940s, penicillin was found to be effective against *S. aureus*. Soon after its initial use, however, some strains of *S. aureus* began to produce the enzyme penicillinase, which inactivates antimicrobials, such as ampicillin, other penicillins, and cephalosporins. Methicillin was the first penicillinase-resistant semisynthetic penicillin; it continues to be used to treat *S. aureus* infections. The late 1960s and early 1970s saw the emergence of MRSA, with the first reports of outbreaks in both acute and long-term care facilities.[14] MRSA infections are of concern because resistance to methicillin is associated with resistance to other antimicrobials. A gene on the bacterial chromosome that codes for abnormal penicillin-binding protein (PBP) carries resistance to methicillin.[14] This abnormal PBP has a lower affinity for all penicillin, so very little methicillin binds to it. Therefore, all penicillins, which must bind to the PBP site in order to kill the bacteria, are ineffective in treating MRSA.

Some strains of MRSA mutate and become resistant to other antimicrobials as well. Of particular concern is the recent discovery of the potential for MRSA to acquire the gene-conferring vancomycin hydrochloride (Vancocin HCl) resistance from vancomycin-resistant enterococci (VRE), leading to vancomycin-resistant *S. aureus*.[14] Because vancomycin is the drug of choice for treating MRSA, resistance to vancomycin would present critical problems.

Treatment of an MRSA wound infection involves antimicrobial therapy and prevention of cross-contamination. Topical antimicrobial therapy specifically designed for MRSA-infected or MRSA-colonized wounds must be used cautiously for routine wound infections so that the antimicrobial will be available if the patient develops MRSA. Mupirocin (Bactroban) is specific for MRSA and can be used topically for wounds infected with the organism.

Prevention of cross-contamination between patients requires significant patient and caregiver education at all levels in the use of universal standard precautions and good hand-washing procedures. Care must be taken to prevent not only contamination of multiple patients with the organisms, but also multiple body systems within the same patient. An alternative method of controlling MRSA is the use of ultraviolet light (see Chapter 23).

Wound Colonization Versus Infection

Distinguishing between colonization and infection in chronic wounds is often difficult. Although colonization has traditionally been described as causing no injury to or response from the host, it has recently been suggested that an elevated or "critical" level of surface colonization can delay wound healing without eliciting a host immune response.[16] The process of differentiating between a critically colonized wound and an infected wound is an important part of better understanding of treatment choices. The treatment of infection usually involves the use of systemic antibiotics and sometimes the concomitant use of topical antimicrobials.

A topical antimicrobial agent alone will not address a true invasive tissue infection. However, it has recently been determined that systemic antibiotics rarely reach adequate levels in the granulation tissue of chronic wounds to effectively control superficial proliferating bacteria.[17] Topical antimicrobial agents may therefore play an important role in the treatment of wounds with high surface levels of proliferating bacteria or critical colonization, and may even prevent the eventual invasion of viable tissue, which causes infection. Improved topical antiseptics have recently become available to wound clinicians in the form of dressings that provide a sustained release of the antiseptic agent at the wound surface while maintaining wound moisture levels and managing wound exudate.

Most clinicians agree that greater than 10^5 organisms per gram of tissue indicate wound infection, but there is no specific number to indicate critical colonization. Laboratories use different references, so what may be considered colonization in one facility may be considered infection in another facility. The overall condition of the patient also enters into the diagnostic process. Infection is usually signalled by a systemic reaction to the microorganisms that have invaded the tissues, whereas colonization merely indicates the presence of microorganisms on the wound surface, which can occur without a systemic reaction. Systemic signs of infection include elevated temperature and white blood cell count, as well as confusion in the older adult.

The classic local signs of infection—erythema, edema, pain, heat, and purulence—are usually reliable in acute wounds, but may be of less value in assessing chronic wounds such as pressure sores, diabetic foot ulcers, and venous ulcers. In these cases, the patient's overall condition may include the presence of a disease or medication that impairs the immune response. These chronic wounds may, however, still exhibit more subtle indicators of an imbalance of bacteria relative to the host's ability to defend against them. Gardner[18] recently validated signs and symptoms of infection in chronic wounds. Increasing pain, friable granulation tissue, foul odor, and wound breakdown were found to be more valid indicators of local infection in chronic wounds than were the classic signs. Additionally, increasing

pain and wound breakdown were found to be sufficient indicators, with a specificity of 100%.

Wounds with continuing moderate to large amounts of seropurulent or purulent exudate and signs and symptoms of infection should be evaluated for infection. Local signs of wound infection include erythema or skin discoloration, edema, warmth, induration, increased pain, and purulent drainage, with or without a foul odor. Table 9-2 gives local and systemic characteristics of wound infection.

Assessment of Wound Infection

Assessment of wound infection involves assessment of the patient's overall condition, observation of the wound and surrounding tissues to differentiate wound inflammation versus the infected wound, and wound cultures to determine colony count. Clinical signs of inflammation are often mistaken for infection. Table 9-3 presents clinical manifestations of both inflammation and infection for comparison. Immunocompromised patients can fail to demonstrate any signs of infection, or the signs may be significantly diminished. For example, in older adults, confusion or agitation may be the first indicator of infection, with elevated temperature occurring much later in the course of the illness. In some cases, a wound simply fails to progress, without obvious signs of infection.

In immunocompromised patients, identification of the organism may be critical to treatment inasmuch as the responsible organism may be opportunistic in nature and not the typical culprit in wound infections.[19] Immunocompromised

TABLE 9-2 Characteristics of Wound Infection

Local Signs of Infection (acute and chronic wounds)	Systemic Signs of Infection (acute and chronic wounds)
Erythema or skin discoloration	Elevated temperature
Edema	Elevated white blood cell count
Warmth	Confusion or agitation in older adults
Induration	Red streaks from wound
Increased pain	
Purulent wound exudate	

Local signs specific to chronic wounds

Friable granulation tissue
Wound breakdown
Foul odor

TABLE 9-3 **Comparison of Wound Characteristics in Inflamed and Infected Wounds**

Wound Characteristic	Inflammation	Infection
Erythema	Usually presents with well-defined borders. Not as intense in color. May be seen as skin discoloration in dark-skinned persons, such as a purple or gray hue to the skin, or a deepening of normal color.	Edges of erythema or skin discoloration may be diffuse and indistinct. May present as very intense erythema or discoloration with well-demarcated and distinct borders. Red stripes or streaking up or down from the area indicates infection.
Elevated temperature	Usually noted as palpable increase in temperature at wound site and surrounding tissues.	Systemic fever (may not be present in older adult populations). Look for acute confusion in older adults, as usually occurs prior to fever.
Exudate: odor	Any odor present may be due to necrotic tissue in the wound, solubization of necrotic tissue, and the type of wound therapy in use, not necessarily infection.	Specific odors are related to some bacterial organisms, such as the sweet smell of *Pseudomonas* or the ammonia odor associated with *Proteus*.
Exudate: amount	Usually minimal; if injury is recent, should see gradual decrease in exudate amount over 3–5 days.	Usually moderate to large amounts; if injury is recent, exudate amount will not decrease; amount remains high or increases.
Exudate: character	Bleeding and serosanguineous to serous.	Serous and seropurulent to purulent.
Pain	Variable. In acute stages may be very tender and painful.	Pain is persistent and continues for an unusual amount of time. Must take wound etiology and subjective nature of pain into account when assessment is performed.
Edema and induration	Slight swelling, firmness at wound edge may be detected.	May indicate infection if edema and induration are localized and accompanied by warmth.

patients may also exhibit signs of infection when the bacterial burden is less than that required for producing infection in immunocompetent patients.

CLINICAL WISDOM

Cellulitis and Wound Infection

Advancing cellulitis indicates that the offending organism has invaded tissue surrounding the ulcer and is no longer localized. Advancing cellulitis begins as a small red or discolored area that is indurated, edematous, and warm to touch, and progresses to involve other tissues. Left uncontrolled and untreated, cellulitis can result in sepsis.

The common method of confirming clinical infection is by colony count. Clinicians diagnose infection based on clinical signs and symptoms, and obtain cultures to aid in determining the appropriate antibiotic therapy. For example, in outpatient clinics, the usual sequence involves the clinician diagnosing the wound infection based on signs and symptoms, and obtaining a culture to confirm the correct selection of antibiotics for treatment. For inpatients diagnosed with infection, antibiotic therapy is generally initiated immediately, and the culture reports are used to adjust or modify the antibiotic regimen.

Colony counts higher than 100,000 (10^5) organisms/mL are considered confirmation of clinical infection. A heavy bioburden (bacterial colonization in the wound) or compromised host resistance (e.g., immunocompromised or diabetic patients) can both result in bacterial colony counts higher than 100,000 organisms/mL. Chronic wounds do not have to be sterile in order to heal. However, when the bacterial burden in a wound is over 10^5 organisms per gram of tissue, wound healing is impaired or delayed.[5,12] Wounds colonized with (β-hemolytic streptococcus can exhibit impaired healing with colony counts less than 100,000/mL.[12] There are also wounds that heal uneventfully in the presence of bacterial colony counts greater than 100,000/mL.

It is clear that the determination of infection involves critical evaluation of the wound, patient, and pathogen. Evaluation of the pathogen occurs by colony count and provides the documentation of infection. Documentation of infection is based on the amount of the bacteria present in the wound tissue.

Quantitative Wound Culture

As traditionally performed, swab cultures detect only surface contaminants and may not reveal the organism causing the tissue infection.[20] Quantitative wound culture is recommended for determination of infection. According to Stotts,[21] if a standardized technique is used, a quantitative swab technique can accurately document the bacterial burden in wounds. The technique for obtaining the culture specimen should capture bacteria in the wound tissue, not simply bacteria on the wound surface.

Tissue biopsy, needle aspiration, and the quantitative swab technique are the most frequently used methods of quantitative wound culture. Each has an important place in clinical practice.

Tissue Biopsy

Tissue biopsy is the removal of a piece of tissue with a scalpel or by punch biopsy. Before performing a tissue biopsy for wound culture, the area is cleansed with sterile solution that does not contain antiseptic. The area may be treated with topical anesthetic or injected with local anesthetic. The biopsy is performed and pressure applied to the area to control bleeding. The biopsy tissue is promptly transported to the laboratory, where it is weighed, flamed to kill surface contaminants, ground and homogenized, and plated in various media in varying dilutions. Findings are expressed in number of organisms per gram of tissue.[22,23]

Needle Aspiration

Needle aspiration involves insertion of a needle into the tissue to aspirate fluid that contains organisms.[24] Intact skin next to the wound is disinfected with a substance such as povidone-iodine and allowed to dry. A 10-mL disposable syringe with 0.5 mL of air in it and a 22-gauge needle are used. The needle is inserted through intact skin; suction is achieved by briskly withdrawing the plunger to the 10-mL mark. The needle is moved backward and forward at different angles for two to four explorations. The plunger is gently returned to the 0.5-mL mark, the needle is withdrawn and capped, and the specimen is transported to the laboratory. In the laboratory, the aspirated fluid is diluted in broth and plated. Data are expressed in colony-forming units (CFU) per volume of fluid. If tissue is extracted by this technique, the weighing and grinding described for tissue biopsy processing also need to be done and, in this case, the data generated are in number of organisms per gram of tissue.

CLINICAL WISDOM

Performing Tissue Biopsy and Needle Aspiration

By physical therapy practice acts, physical therapists are not allowed to perform tissue biopsy or needle aspiration procedures. Physical therapists must work collaboratively with nursing to obtain these samples as required.

Quantitative Swab Technique

The swab technique has been criticized as a method that produces information about colonization of the ulcer surface, rather than in the tissue. One of the problems with the routine swab technique for culturing a wound is that it has been performed in a variety of ways and, therefore, cannot be relied on to address the issue of bioburden in the tissues. There is controversy on how to obtain a swab culture. Some recommend culturing the exudate in the wound prior to wound cleansing.[25,26] Others recommend that, after cleansing of the wound is complete, the culture be obtained using a Z technique (side to side across the wound from one edge to the other).[27,28] Others suggest irrigation of the wound with sterile water or saline and pressing of the swab against the wound margin or ulcer base to elicit fresh exudate.[29]

The recommended method of quantitative swab culture involves cleansing the wound with a solution that contains no antiseptic solution. The end of a sterile, cotton-tipped applicator stick is rotated in a 1-cm^2 area of the open wound for 5 seconds.[29] Pressure is applied to the swab to cause tissue fluid to be absorbed in its cotton tip. The swab tip is inserted into a sterile tube containing transport medium and sent to the laboratory. The end of the applicator that is not sterile is not inserted into the tube for culture. Serial dilutions of the organisms are made on agar plates. A swab moistened with normal saline without preservative provides more precise data than does the use of a dry swab.[30] Results are expressed as organisms per swab, CFU per swab, or in a semiquantitative manner, such as scant, small, moderate, or large (1+ to 4+) bacterial growths.

Tissue biopsy, needle inspiration, and the quantitative swab technique are used to evaluate the bacteria present in wound tissue, rather than on the surface of the wound, in the exudate, or in necrotic tissue. They are used to examine tissue for aerobic and anaerobic organisms. They also can be used to obtain a specimen for Gram stain, a method recognized as a rapid diagnostic technique of infection.[30,31] For a Gram stain, the tissue fluid is placed on a slide, treated with various stains, and viewed under the microscope. In wounds in which swabs yielded less than 10^5 organisms, the Gram stain is considered to show no bacteria.

Data show that the tissue biopsy, needle aspiration, and quantitative swab techniques are comparable in terms of sensitivity, specificity, and accuracy.[21] The following section describes how the procedures are performed.

Procedures for Quantitative Wound Culture

Equipment Needed

- Gloves (clean and sterile)
- Sterile saline (nonbacteriostatic)
- Container to transport specimen
- Lab requisition
- Appropriate dressing materials

Culture Technique-Specific Equipment Needed

- Punch biopsy/scalpel
- Wound culture swab
- Anaerobic medium, if required
- 10-mL syringe with 22-gauge needle
- Cork

Procedure Preparation—For All Methods

1. Wash hands. (Reduces transmission of microorganisms.)
2. Don clean gloves (and gown, if necessary). (Maintains universal precautions.)
3. Remove soiled dressings and discard in plastic bag. Then remove and discard gloves. (Prevents contamination and spread of microorganisms.)

4. Clean wound and surrounding skin with normal saline. (Removes contaminated debris.)

Procedure: Swab Method

1. Don sterile gloves and remove swab from culturette tube, taking care not to touch swab or inside of tube. (Maintains universal precautions and aseptic technique.)
2. Swab wound area 1 cm^2 with sufficient pressure to obtain wound fluid. (Ensures collection of a good specimen.)
3. Use separate swabs if taking more than one specimen. Swab only a 1-cm^2 area of wound with each swab. (This ensures good culture specimen and prevents cross-contamination. Care must be taken to swab the wound instead of the wound edges to prevent contamination by skin flora and contaminated debris.)
4. Carefully place swab into culturette tube without touching swab or the inside, outside, or top of container. (Prevents contamination and keeps those areas free of pathogens that could be spread to others who handle the tube.)
5. Crush ampule of medium in culturette and close securely, making sure swab is surrounded by medium. (Keeps specimen from drying out and provides supporting medium.)

Procedure: Anaerobic Swab Culture Method

1. If collecting a specimen for anaerobic culture, take care to keep the anaerobic transport culture tube in an upright position to prevent carbon monoxide from escaping. Close container securely after swab is placed in tube. (Maintains anaerobic environment.)

Procedure: Syringe Method

1. Disinfect intact skin with antiseptic and allow skin to dry for 1 minute. (Anaerobic specimens are obtained from deep inside wounds.)
2. Place 0.5 mL of air in 10-mL disposable syringe with 22-gauge needle. Insert needle into intact skin adjacent to wound. Withdraw plunger to achieve suction and move the needle back and forth at different angles. (Prevents contamination at needle withdrawal site.)
3. Return the plunger gently to the 0.5-mL mark; do not insert drainage into the tissues. (This ensures a good specimen and prevents contamination from skin flora. Syringe method is used when large amounts of pus or drainage are present or for collecting tissue.)
4. Cork needle to send syringe/needle to laboratory as one unit . Do not recap or attempt to disconnect needle from syringe. (This maintains universal precautions and prevents injury from needle stick and spread of microorganisms.)

Procedure: Tissue Biopsy

1. Don sterile gloves. Obtain a biopsy specimen using a 3–4 mm dermal punch or a scalpel. (This allows for determination of the tissue level of microorganism contamination. Biopsy is usually performed by a physician or advanced practitioner.)
2. Place specimen in sterile container. (Prevents spread of microorganisms.)

Procedure: Final Steps—All Methods

1. Remove and discard gloves in plastic bag. (Reduces transmission of microorganisms.)
2. Wash hands.
3. Don sterile gloves and apply sterile dressing to the wound. (Dressing absorbs drainage and immobilizes and protects the wound.)
4. Label specimen container(s) with patient name, room number, date, time, and exact source of specimen. (This ensures proper identification of specimen. Proper source of specimen is important for laboratory to rule out normal flora from location.)
5. Place container in clean plastic bag, and have specimen transported to laboratory as soon as possible. (Plastic bag prevents spread of microorganisms. Immediate transport prevents overgrowth of microorganisms that can occur if specimen is left at room temperature for an extended length of time.)
6. Dispose of soiled equipment into appropriate receptacle. (Maintains universal precautions.)
7. Wash hands. (Reduces transmission of microorganisms.)

Management of Exudate and Infection

Management of exudate and infection includes wound cleansing, the use of topical antimicrobials, antiseptics, and antifungals, the use of antimicrobial dressings, and management of exudate with topical dressings.

Wound Cleansing

Effective wound cleansing removes debris that supports bacterial growth and delays wound healing. Wound cleansing delivers cleansing solution to the wound by mechanical force, aids with separation of necrotic tissue from healthy wound tissues, and removes bacteria and dressing residue from the wound surface. The process of wound cleansing involves selecting a cleansing solution and a method of delivering the solution to the wound. Exhibit 9-1 presents the guidelines for pressure ulcer cleansing recommended by the Agency for Health Care Research and Quality (AHRQ, formerly known as the Agency for Health Care Policy and Research [AHCPR].[20] These principles extend to the cleansing of all wounds.

Cleansing solutions should be chosen based on their efficacy and safety for use in a particular type of wound. Isotonic normal saline is generally preferred because it is physiologic, nontoxic, and inexpensive. Saline does not contain preservatives and must be discarded 24–48 hours after opening.[32] Commercial solutions are available to assist in wound cleansing for wounds requiring more cleansing capacity to

EXHIBIT 9-1   Recommended Guidelines for Pressure Ulcer Cleansing

1. Cleanse wounds initially and at each dressing change.
2. Use minimal mechanical force when cleansing ulcer with gauze, cloth, or sponges.
3. Do not clean wounds with skin cleansers or antiseptic agents (povidone-iodine, sodium hypochlorite solution, hydrogen peroxide, and acetic acid).
4. Use normal saline for cleansing most ulcers.
5. Use enough irrigation pressure to enhance wound cleansing without causing trauma to the wound bed. Safe and effective ulcer irrigation pressures range from 4 to 15 psi.
6. Consider whirlpool treatment for cleansing ulcers that contain thick exudate, slough, or necrotic tissue. Discontinue whirlpool when ulcer is clean.

Reprinted with permission from N. Bergstrom, M.A. Bennett, C.E. Carlson, et al. Treatment of Pressure Ulcers, Clinical Practice Guideline No. 15, December 1994, U.S. Department of Health and Human Services, Public Health Service, Agency for Health Care Policy and Research, AHCPR Publication No. 95-0652.

remove adherent debris from the wound surface. These wound cleansers contain surfactants that act to lower surface tension and to loosen matter from the wound surface.[32] Nonionic surfactant wound cleansers are recommended as generally safe for use on healing wounds.

CLINICAL WISDOM

Normal Saline for Wound Cleansing

Two useful strategies for obtaining normal saline for wound care in the home setting:

1. Saline can be made at home by adding two teaspoons of table salt to 1 L of boiling water. Be sure to discard after 24 hours.
2. Pressurized saline sold for contact lens care may also be used. This preserved saline may be used for a longer duration, and the pressure from the canister is not sufficient to cause wound trauma.

For healthy, clean wounds, cleanse with normal saline and do not use antimicrobial solutions or skin cleansers. Clean wounds do not need to be cleansed with antimicrobial solutions, because the goal of care is to clear low levels of contaminants from the wound. In fact, antimicrobial solutions may be harmful in a clean wound. Solutions such as povidone-iodine, acetic acid, hydrogen peroxide, and sodium hypochlorite (Dakin fluid) are toxic to fibroblasts *in vitro*. Use of antimicrobial agents have traditionally been contraindicated in the healthy proliferative wound because of the potential damage to the healthy tissues.[20,33,34] Contraindication of the use of antiseptic and antimicrobial solutions for cleansing clean pressure ulcers is based on *in vitro* laboratory studies of the toxicity of topical wound cleansers.[35,36]

More recent *in vivo* research has, however, shown that traditional antiseptic solutions such as povidone iodine, 0.25% acetic acid, 0.25% sodium hypochlorite, and 5% mafenide acetate (Sulfamylon solution) can be used safely in wounds for short periods (4–7 days) to control bacterial levels, without compromising the healing process.[37] The study in question examined the effects of 5 different antiseptic solutions, compared with saline controls in a study on the healing of partial-thickness wounds in swine. The wounds were treated topically with gauze soaked in and remoistened every 8 hours with one of five common antiseptics: 5% mafenide acetate, 10% povidone with 1% free iodine (Betadine), 0.25% sodium hypochlorite ("half-strength" Dakin), 3% hydrogen peroxide, and 0.25% acetic acid. Because the gauze was kept continuously moist with the antiseptic solution, any delays in healing would be attributable to the chemical agent as opposed to wound dehydration. Re-epithelialization, angiogenesis, neodermal regeneration, fibroblast proliferation, collagen production, and bacterial colony counts were analyzed at 4 and 7 days after wounding. Interesting to note, wound reepithelialization—the point at which wounds are commonly judged to be clinically healed—was not negatively affected by any of the antiseptic agents, compared with saline controls. In fact, some of the antiseptic agents actually improved angiogenesis and fibroblast proliferation relative to saline controls. This research finding suggests that the effects of antiseptic agents *in vivo* may vary from their effects *in vitro*, where cells are exposed to an environment vastly different from that of the wound tissue. Nevertheless, antiseptics are cytotoxic to all types of cells (bacterial and host cells), and decisions regarding the duration of their use in open wounds should take into account the bacterial status of the wound (e.g., clean versus infected) and the desired outcome.

In general, most skin cleansers are not appropriate wound cleansers because they have been developed for external rather than internal use. What is appropriate for cleansing the skin is not appropriate for open wounds, because an open wound lacks the protection of intact epidermis and provides direct access to internal body structures. For healthy, clean wounds, cleanse with normal saline. For healthy wounds, do not use antimicrobial solutions or skin cleansers.

For infected wounds, cleanse with normal saline or use a 10–14 day cleansing regimen with an antimicrobial solution. For infected wounds, do not use skin cleansers, and do not prolong the use of an antimicrobial solution. Antimicrobial agents may play a minor role in wound cleansing for infected wounds, wounds with large amounts of necrotic debris, or those with large amounts of exudate. Antimicrobial agents should be employed in a manner similar to antibiotics, for short periods of time. Antimicrobial agents used as cleansing agents in the debris-filled wound should be used for 10–14 days and rinsed thoroughly from the wound with saline. Rinsing the wound with saline after cleansing with antimicrobial solutions decreases cytotoxic effects in the wound. Antimicrobial cleansers should be discontinued after the course of therapy (10–14 days) or when the wound is clean and free of debris.

Cleansing Method

There are several methods for cleansing a wound, including soaking, whirlpool therapy, scrubbing, and irrigation. Soaking is a form of hydrotherapy that includes a variety of methods, from the use of a bucket to a Hubbard tank, and may be useful for removing gross contaminants and loosening necrotic tissue. The softening that occurs with soaking helps to ease the separation of necrotic debris from healthy wound tissues. Wound soaking is appropriate only for wounds with large amounts of necrotic debris. Once a wound is clean and proliferating, wound soaking impedes healing and is therefore generally not appropriate.[20,32]

Whirlpool therapy may be useful for more than simply soaking and cleansing, as is the case when using whirlpool therapy to increase perfusion to an area. (See Chapters 26 and 27 for information on pulsatile lavage and whirlpool therapy.) Antimicrobial agents should not be used in either a whirlpool or wound-soaking solution because of wound tissue toxicity. As with soaking, whirlpool therapy is not recommended for wounds that are clean and proliferating.

RESEARCH WISDOM

Use of battery-powered, disposable pulsatile irrigating devices—which irrigate with solutions and simultaneously use suction to remove the irrigation fluid and loosened wound debris—has been shown to be more effective than whirlpool therapy in a study examining the rate of granulation tissue formation.[38] This study found that ulcers cleansed with pulsatile lavage had a rate of granulation tissue formation of 12.2% per week, compared with 4.8% per week for the whirlpool-treated group.

Scrubbing involves use of gauze or sponges applied with mechanical force in direct contact with a wound in order to enhance removal of debris and the efficacy of cleansing solutions.[32] Scrubbing causes microabrasions in the wound, thus delaying healing. Use of a nonionic surfactant cleansing solution limits the damage inflicted with scrubbing, and use of nonabrasive sponges also helps to decrease the damage to the healing wound tissues. The more porous the sponge, the less damage inflicted on the wound surface.[32] Even the use of nonionic surfactant cleansing solutions and nonabrasive porous sponges will injure the fragile wound tissue, however. Therefore, scrubbing is generally not recommended.

CLINICAL WISDOM

Shallow Wound Cleansing Procedure

Cleanse from the center of the wound in a circular motion, working toward the edge of the wound and the surrounding tissues. Do not return to the center of the wound after cleansing at the edge of the wound or the surrounding tissues, because this will recontaminate the clean wound center.

Wound irrigation can be performed using a variety of instruments and equipment. Wound irrigation is particularly appropriate for cleansing deep wounds with undermining or tunneling present. Use a catch basin and towels to absorb and accumulate waste materials and irrigant runoff. Repeat the irrigation procedure at each dressing change. Protect the eyes, face, and clothing of the clinician by using universal precautions. Some newer irrigation devices include a splashguard to help protect the clinician.

The amount of pressure used for irrigation is determined by balancing the desire to preserve healing wound tissues with the need to cleanse a wound effectively. The pressure at which the irrigant is delivered is commonly described as either 'low' or 'high.' Pressure force is more precisely described in pounds per square inch (psi). Pressure force under 4 psi is commonly referred to as low pressure, and can be obtained by use of bulb syringes or just by pouring solution over the wound bed.[32] Pressure force between 4–15 psi is considered high pressure, and can be achieved by using commercial devices, a 35-mL syringe attached to a 19-gauge needle or angiocatheter, pulsatile lavage, or whirlpool therapy.

CLINICAL WISDOM

Deep Wound Cleansing Procedure

Use of a catheter or a syringe to irrigate wounds with undermining and tunneling will not injure the tissues, and can effectively cleanse involved tissues under the skin surface. Flush with copious amounts of irrigant solution, and then gently massage the tissues above the tunneling to express the exudate accumulated in the tunnel. Repeat two or three times until the solution and fluids returned are clear (Figure 9-2). After the wound cleansing, the undermined spaces are usually packed loosely with packing materials, such as roller gauze or alginate rope products, to prevent infection from traveling up the tunnel (Figure 9-3).

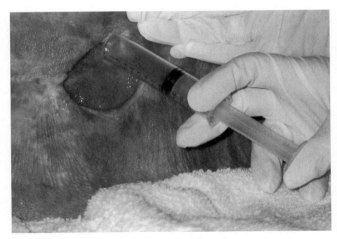

FIGURE 9-2 Irrigation of wound with syringe.

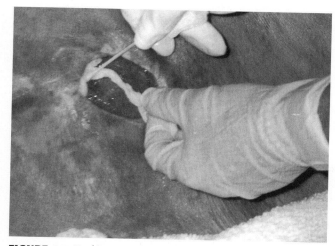

FIGURE 9-3 Packing wound with undermining

High-pressure irrigation using any of these forms is a method of debridement—loosening and softening necrotic tissue for easy separation from healthy tissue. Pressurized irrigation removes bacteria and debris more effectively than do gravity or bulb syringe irrigation. As such, high-pressure irrigation is most effective for wounds with an inflammatory process. Use of high-pressure irrigation is not the method of choice for the healthy, proliferating wound, because fragile blood vessels and new tissue growth can be damaged.

A number of available irrigation devices deliver solutions with too much pressure, thus driving bacteria and irrigant solution deeper into wound tissues. Pressures higher than 15 psi can cause trauma to the wound bed, forcing bacteria deeper into wound tissues. For example, use of a Water Pik at the middle and high settings provides 42 psi and more than 50 psi, respectively, both of which are too high and will drive bacteria farther into the wound tissues. Irrigation pressures between 4 and 15 psi are recommended.

The clinical outcomes of wound cleansing are evaluated by taking account of the original intent of the cleansing and the wound assessment. For predominantly clean wounds with new tissue growth, cleansing is used only to remove dressing residue, and if any additional cleansing is needed, a low-pressure irrigation system should be used. The goals of therapy with low-pressure irrigation are to dislodge wound dressing residue, reduce wound surface contaminants, and protect fragile new tissue growth. For wounds with necrotic tissue or debris, a high-pressure irrigation system should be used. Whirlpool therapy and pulsatile lavage are not always available or appropriate for all patients, and other devices, such as the 35-mL syringe and 19-gauge needle or angiocatheter, may be the best choice. The goals of therapy are to loosen and soften the necrotic debris for easier separation from healthy tissues, reduce the bacterial burden, remove dressing remnants, and prevent undue wound trauma.

Aseptic Technique

One of the continuing debates in wound management is what type of aseptic technique is necessary for wound care in various health-care settings. Asepsis includes activities that prevent infection or break the chain of infection. It is generally divided into two types: surgical asepsis and medical asepsis. Surgical asepsis, or sterile technique, is the method used in surgery in which all instruments and materials used are sterile, and all health-care providers involved wear sterile gloves, caps, masks, and gowns. Medical asepsis, or clean technique, involves procedures to reduce the number of pathogens and decrease the transfer of pathogens. In surgical asepsis, the nurse prepares a sterile field, dons sterile gloves, and follows surgical aseptic techniques in caring for the wound.

There are various viewpoints on which approach is most suitable for wound care patients. Some general guidelines may help to clarify the use of an aseptic technique. Sterile technique is most appropriate in acute-care hospital settings, for patients at high risk for infection (e.g., advanced age, immunocompromised, diabetic) and for certain interventions, such as sharp wound debridement. Clean technique is most appropriate for patients in long-term care settings, home care, and some clinic settings, and for patients who are not at high risk for infection and are receiving routine wound care, such as dressing changes. Further research is needed to determine outcomes with the use of clean technique. Table 9-4 compares general guidelines for clean versus sterile technique for wound-care patients.

Hand Washing and Infection Control

One thing about infection management and wound care that is not under debate is the importance of hand washing by the health-care practitioner. Hand washing is the single most important means for preventing the spread of infection. Use of universal standard precautions and hand washing by the wound care clinician promote health maintenance for patients and caregivers and, as such, are critically important to include when instructing others in wound care programs.

Along with hand washing, caregivers must be instructed in appropriate disposal of infectious waste products, such as used wound dressings, gauze used for wound cleansing, and instruments used in wound care. In institutional settings, such as hospitals and long-term care facilities, there are procedures for disposal of contaminated materials in bags clearly identified as infectious waste (e.g., double-bagging out of isolation rooms, and use of red biohazard trash bags). In the home-care arena, disposal of contaminated waste becomes more problematic, and the clinician must address

TABLE 9-4 Clean versus Sterile Technique General Guidelines

Factor	Sterile Technique	Clean Technique
Settings	Acute care hospitals Clinics in acute care facilities	Home care Long-term care facilities Community clinics Physicians' offices
Procedures	Invasive procedures Sharp debridement	Routine procedures Dressing changes
Patients	Immunocompromised Advanced age or very young age Diabetic	Patients *not* at high risk for infection
Wound dressing procedures	Preparation of a sterile field Clean gloves Decontamination of the wound and surrounding skin Change gloves: sterile gloves Use sterile forceps, scalpel, and scissors Allow only "sterile to sterile" contact of instruments and materials used for the procedure Apply sterile dressing	Preparation of clean field Clean gloves Cleansing of the wound and surrounding skin with an antimicrobial cleanser Change gloves: clean gloves Use sterile forceps, scalpel, and scissors Prevent direct contamination of materials and supplies, but no "sterile to sterile" rules apply Apply clean dressing

disposal based on the area served, local waste collection procedures, and agency protocols. In the home-care setting, education of the caregiver regarding the procedures for waste disposal is essential for maintaining community health.

Topical Antimicrobials

The use of antimicrobials can be an area of confusion for clinicians. Systemic antimicrobial drugs (those agents given orally or intravenously) are often superior to topical agents (ointments, creams, and solutions put directly on the wound surface) in treating invasive tissue infection because of the better penetration of systemic agents into the tissues via the blood supply. However, topical antimicrobials are often effective in limiting surface colonization, so that tissue defenses can clean up without continual reinfection from superficial bacteria. Some superficial infections respond better to topical agents and, in some cases, it is wise to use topical agents to avoid sensitizing the patient or creating resistant microorganisms. Some topical antimicrobials can damage healthy tissues, exacerbating tissue destruction or damaging tissue defenses. The terms *antimicrobial, antibiotic, antibacterial*, and *antiseptic* are often used interchangeably; however, the definitions are slightly different, according to the Food and Drug Administration (FDA). Exhibit 9-2 presents definitions of these terms for easy reference.

The three main classes of antimicrobials used for wounds are antibacterials, antiseptics, and antifungals. Understanding how antimicrobials are prescribed is helpful for wound-care clinicians. The proper use of any antimicrobial requires determination of clinical infection in the wound, correct

identification of the invading organism by culture and Gram stain prior to beginning therapy, and consideration of pharmacology and toxicology when choosing the agent. If an agent must be chosen prior to receiving laboratory results, the decision should be made based on Gram stain smears (either positive or negative), the most likely pathogens involved in the disease process (for example, *E. coli* for a fecally incontinent patient with a sacral pressure sore), and the efficacy of the agent in similar situations.

CLINICAL WISDOM

Factors Altering Response to Topical Antibacterials and Antiseptics

Patient response to antibacterial and antiseptic agents can be altered by age, disease processes (such as diabetes), malignancy, neurologic disorders, immune dysfunction, pregnancy, allergy, and concomitant drug therapy.

Multiple factors influence the transcutaneous penetration of antimicrobial agents, including the physiochemical properties of the drug (polarity, stability, and solubility in base and lipids), nature of the pharmaceutical preparation (drug concentration, composition and properties of the base, and incompatible mixtures), method of application (inert delivery systems, time-released delivery systems, application in conjunction with occlusion, polar compounds to increase absorption, and substances that damage the stratum corneum to improve penetration), and nature of the skin (integrity of the epidermis, variability in skin thickness, and age). Problems associated with topical antimicrobial use in wound care are related to the absorption of chemicals into the body tissues through the wound bed. There are cases in which ab-

EXHIBIT 9-2   Definitions of Antimicrobial Terms

Term	Definition
Antimicrobial	An agent that inhibits or kills microorganisms
Antiseptic	A substance that prevents or arrests the *growth* by preventing multiplication (bacteriostatic) or *action* of microorganisms, either by inhibiting their activity or by destroying or killing them (bactericidal). Applies to substances used on living tissues (e.g., povidone-iodine).
Antibiotic	An organic chemical substance produced by a microorganism that has the capacity in diluted solutions to destroy or inhibit the growth of bacteria and other microorganisms (e.g., penicillin).
Antibacterial	An agent that destroys or stops bacterial growth (e.g., bacitracin).
Antifungal	A wide variety of agents that inhibit or kill fungi (e.g., nystatin).

Adapted with permission from Gilman G, ed. Topical Agents for Open Wounds: Antibacterials, Antiseptics, Antifungals. Reviewed by Rodeheaver G, Cooper JW, Nelson DR, Meehan M. Charleston, SC: Hill-Rom International, 1991.

sorption of certain chemicals contained in an antiseptic through the wound bed has caused systemic health problems. For example, iodine toxicity has occurred as a result of the use of povidone-iodine in open wounds with a large surface area.

Antibacterials

Antibacterial agents are chemicals that eliminate living organisms that are pathogenic to the host or patient. Some examples of antibacterials are bacitracin (Betadine, Cortisporin, Neosporin, and Polysporin), gentamicin (Garamycin), metronidazole gel and cream (MetroGel, MetroCream, Noritate), mupirocin, and silver sulfadiazine (Silvadene, SSD). The use of antibacterials is common for most infections. In the elderly, the primary sites of infection, in order of frequency, are urinary tract, pulmonary system, and wounds.[39,40]

Broad-spectrum antibacterials are useful for mixed infections in which there is more than one pathogen present and quick identification of the organism is difficult. Smaller doses of topical antibacterial agents are appropriate, compared with systemic antibacterials, due to their direct contact with the affected area.[40] The same or better results can be achieved with topical antibacterials, without the risk of toxicity. Systemic agents may be used in combination with topical agents, as in the treatment of impetigo.

Topically administered drugs are in direct contact with organisms, so problems of absorption, distribution, and availability to the infected site are reduced. Frequently, topical agents are used in conjunction with one another to give broader coverage, thereby increasing the rate of bactericidal action against a large spectrum of bacteria.[41]

Topical antibacterials may be used prophylactically. When used properly, they can be effective chemical barriers that impede the entrance of pathogenic organisms and diminish the local or systemic morbidity associated with infected wounds. When using topical antibacterials prophylactically, there is always a danger of overgrowth of resistant organisms; therefore, use of antibacterials for prevention requires good clinical judgment for optimal effectiveness.[41]

CLINICAL WISDOM
Wound Healing and Antimicrobials
No antibacterial agent, whether bactericidal or bacteriostatic, is curative when used in isolation. Attention to nutritional factors, management of underlying pathology, and relief of causative factors are also required.

Topical antibacterials used in a viscous vehicle provide a moist wound-healing environment, facilitating epithelial migration.[42] Topical antibacterials are indicated when the patient has a diagnosed or suspected significant bacterial infection, as well as an indication for prophylactic use, such as underlying disease, increased risk of infection resulting from surgical procedures, viral or metabolic diseases, chemotherapy or radiation therapy, and/or prolonged corticosteroid administration. Contraindications include the excessive use of antibacterials for minor infections and nonbacterial pathogens.[41] Inappropriate use of antibacterials subjects the patient to risk of drug toxicity, allergy, superinfection with resistant organisms, and unnecessary costs.[41,43]

CLINICAL WISDOM
Routine Use of Topical Antibacterials
Routine use of topical antibacterials is strongly discouraged because it frequently leads to the development of resistant organisms. This is particularly true of mupirocin, because it is effective against MRSA. If used inappropriately, however, it will not be effective when most needed.

The base, or vehicle, is the form in which the antibacterial agent is made available. In general, it is best to use a lotion or a paste for application to wet or weeping skin and wounds, and a greasy ointment for application to dry, cracked skin. Creams are convenient because, to some extent, they can be used for wet or dry surfaces and are easier to use. Many ointments contain lanolin or wood alcohols, and patients can readily develop contact sensitivity to these substances. Creams less often contain lanolin, but usually contain a preservative or stabilizer, such as parabens or ethylenediamine dihydrochloride, both of which are known to be occasional sensitizers. Ointments can be confused with creams, particularly with the introduction of synthetic bases that claim to have the properties of both creams and ointments. Lotions are preferable to greasy applications for areas that rub against each other, e.g., groin areas and in between the toes. Lotions are usually less occlusive than ointments.

Antiseptics

Antiseptics are a group of widely differing chemical compounds that possess bactericidal (kills bacteria) or bacteriostatic (prevents bacterial multiplication) properties. Some examples of antiseptics are povidone-iodine, acetic acid, hydrogen peroxide, and hypochlorite. They are employed in medical practice with the objective of preventing or combating bacterial infection of superficial tissues, as well as sterilization of instruments and infected material.

Chemically, antiseptics can be inorganic or organic. Oxidizing disinfectants liberate oxygen when in contact with pus or organic substances. Different bacteria are sensitive to different antiseptics. For example, acetic acid is commonly used against infections caused by *Pseudomonas aeruginosa*. Antiseptic agents are applied directly to tissue to destroy microorganisms or inhibit their reproduction or metabolic activity. It is believed that, by reducing organisms, antiseptics can hasten wound healing and diminish the local or systemic morbidity associated with wound infection.[44]

The major uses of antiseptics are as hand scrubs, cleansers, irrigants, and protective dressings. It is important to remember that the skin cannot be sterilized, and that approximately 20% of the skin's normal resident flora are beyond the reach of antiseptics.[40] Excessive antiseptic use subjects the patient to the risk of allergy, drug toxicity, superinfection, and unnecessary costs, and poses significant public health concerns, due to ecologic pressure favoring the selection of bacteria resistant to antiseptics.[44]

Antiseptic-containing Dressings

Recently, dressings that contain and release antiseptic agents at the wound surface have entered the market. The objective of these dressings is to provide a sustained release of the antiseptic agent at the wound surface in order to provide long-lasting antimicrobial action in combination with the maintenance of a physiologically moist environment for healing.

Iodine has been complexed with a polymeric cadexomer starch vehicle to form a topical gel or paste. The cadexomer moiety provides exudate absorption from the wound, which results in the concomitantly slow release of low concentrations of free iodine from the vehicle. The wound-healing effects of this particular iodophor have been studied in multiple randomized controlled trials. The majority of the studies targeted venous leg ulcers,[45-48] although, diabetic foot ulcers and pressure ulcers were addressed in two of the trials.[49, 50]. Overall, these clinical studies have consistently shown that the cadexomer iodine product is not only effective at reducing bacterial counts in chronic wounds, but also appears to positively affect the healing process when compared with standard treatments (usually gauze and saline) and the cadexomer starch vehicle alone.

Silver has also recently been incorporated into a wide variety of semi-occlusive dressing formats, such as foams, hydrocolloids, alginates, and hydrofibers. All of these products release silver cations into the wound as they absorb or come in contact with wound exudate. No controlled clinical trials of these products in the management of infected chronic wounds are yet available. (Table 9-5 lists some of the antimicrobial dressings that are currently available.)

Antifungals

Fungi comprise five widely differing classes of primitive flora. Thus, antifungal agents include a wide variety of chemical types with a narrow spectrum. Examples of antifungals include nystatin (Mycostatin), ketoconazole (Nizoral), and miconazole nitrate (Monistat-Derm). Not all antifungal agents are fungicidal; many are only fungistatic, and certain of them may owe their efficacy to a keratolytic action.

Broad-spectrum antifungal agents are in general nonselective and are therefore toxic irritants. However, many of these agents have limited absorption through the epidermis, and therefore can be used in dermatologic preparations.[32] An antifungal agent is indicated when a patient has a diagnosed or strongly suspected significant fungal infection, as well as an indication for prophylactic antifungal use, such as underlying disease or an increased risk of fungal infection resulting from invasive procedures or environmental exposure (e.g., diarrhea, diaphoresis, poor hygiene, diabetes). The major contraindication for antifungal use is a known allergy to its ingredients. Antifungals must be used for the entire time prescribed to completely eliminate the infection.

Some areas are more difficult to treat, and some fungi are more difficult to eliminate because of a patient's underlying disease process. External factors can affect the antifungal agent's ability to penetrate the skin, including temperature, ambient water vapor pressure, and drying agents such as powders, which reduce the excess moisture in the skin folds and may aid in the efficacy of antifungals. Non-sporing anaerobes are a significant pathogen in ulcers with a foul smell and exposure to fecal contamination.[40] Metronidazole topical gel (MetroGel) has been shown to be effective in eliminating or decreasing the odor associated with these wounds.[51-54]

RESEARCH WISDOM

Treatment of Malodorous Wounds

Topical metronidazole has been shown to be effective in resolving odor in foul-smelling wounds. Use of a 1% solution or 0.75% gel applied twice daily reduced or eliminated odor in 80%–90% of wounds in 4–7 days. Odor was significantly decreased in 2 days.[51-54]

Topical Dressings for Management of Exudate

Effective management of exudate requires knowledge of the absorptive capacity of dressing materials and attention to fragile wound margins. Excess exudate on the wound edges can lead to maceration and destruction of the critical wound

TABLE 9-5 Antiseptic-Containing Dressings

Dressing Name	Antiseptic ingredient	Dressing Format	Manufacturer
Acticoat	Ionic silver	Wound contact layer	Smith & Nephew
Acticoat absorbent	Ionic silver	Calcium alginate	Smith & Nephew
Actisorb Silver 220	Silver and activated charcoal	Silver impregnated activated charcoal cloth	Johnson & Johnson Wound Management
Arglaes	Ionic silver	Transparent film or powder	Medline Industries
Aquacel AG	Ionic silver	Hydrofiber	Convatec
Contreet H	Ionic silver	Hydrocolloid	Coloplast
Contreet F	Ionic silver	Foam	Coloplast
Iodosorb	Molecular iodine	Gel or paste	HealthPoint Ltd.
Prisma Matrix	Ionic silver	Collagen-oxidized regenerated cellulose	Johnson & Johnson Wound Management
Silvasorb	Ionic silver	Hydrogel sheet or amorphous gel	Medline Industries
Silverlon	Ionic silver	Silver coated nylon cloth	Argentum, LLC.

edge. Use of petrolatum products or other hydrophobic ointments around the wound can provide some protection for the wound edges. Use of a topical dressing that adequately absorbs the wound fluid will also protect the wound edges.

Caution about Petrolatum Around Wound Edges

If petrolatum products are being used and the patient is receiving physical therapy, nurses *must* notify the physical therapist. Petrolatum products can interfere with physical therapy technologies and are difficult to remove from the patient's skin prior to physical therapy interventions.

The choice of a dressing for a wound is, in many cases, dependent on the amount of drainage present in the wound and the expected drainage from the wound. For example, a wound that has been recently debrided of yellow necrotic tissue may have a history of moderate to large amounts of drainage; however, the amount of expected drainage postdebridement is less, usually minimal to moderate amounts. The topical dressing may also become not only the treatment but also the method of determining efficacy. For example, evaluation of the dressing upon removal from the wound allows the clinician to judge what percentage of the dressing material has interacted with wound drainage. Evaluation of the amount of dressing saturated with wound exudate often determines whether treatment will continue with the same dressing or whether a new dressing will be applied. (See *Color Plates 42–47*, reading the dressing, for more information on determining the effectiveness of topical dressings in the management of wound exudate, and how to distinguish exudate from the wound versus material from wound fluid and dressing interaction.)

Table 9-6 presents the generic product categories with notes about the absorptive capability of each dressing type. This information may be useful in choosing dressings for the exudative wound. How to choose a wound dressing to manage exudate is explained in detail in Chapter 11.

The type of wound under treatment also affects the choice of dressing for exudate management. One example is a venous disease ulcer under appropriate management with compression therapy and topical dressings. For a venous disease ulcer in the initial compression therapy stages, the amount of exudate increases as edema in the extremities is managed. Sometimes, the exudate amount remains copious for several weeks as the edema is brought under control. In general, the amount of exudate can be expected to remain significant for 2 weeks.

The presence of large amounts of exudate on a patient should be monitored closely. The skin surrounding the wound can become macerated and, in some cases, a candidiasis or yeast infection can develop around the wound. The continual loss of proteins, fluids, and electrolytes in wound exudate can cause fluid and electrolyte disturbances in severe cases; at a minimum, the loss of proteins and wound healing substrates can slow or impede the wound healing progress. Finally, the presence of a wound with large amounts of draining exudate takes a toll on the patient's daily quality of life, disrupting normal function.

Outcome Measures

Outcome measures are tools used to evaluate the results of therapy. Appropriate characteristics to assess in evaluating the results of exudate management are the amount of exudate in the wound, type of exudate in the wound, and involvement of the wound dressing with the exudate present in the wound. Measurement of exudate is an intermediate outcome measure, and healing is the final outcome.

Amount of Exudate

The amount of exudate should diminish progressively in the wound if therapy is appropriate. The amount of exudate can be measured by using clinical judgment to evaluate the distribution of moisture in the wound and the interaction of ex-

TABLE 9-6 Topical Treatment—Wound Dressings

Wound Dressings: Generic Categories	Not Absorbent	Low to Minimal Absorption	Minimal to Moderate Absorption	Moderate to Large Absorption
Skin sealants	X			
Composite dressings		X	X	
Transparent film dressings	X			
Gauze—woven		X		
Gauze—nonwoven			X	
Gauze—impregnated	X			
Calcium alginates			X	X
Exudate absorbers—beads, pastes, powders, flakes			X	X
Hydrocolloids—regular, thin, pastes, granules		X	X	X (when used with other forms of dressings)
Hydrogels—sheets, wafers, amorphous		X	X	
Lubricating stimulating agents	X			
Foams		X	X	X
Hydrocolloid-hydrogel combinations		X	X	

udate with the wound dressing. A rating scale similar to the following may be used to quantify the amount of exudate:

1 = None = wound tissues dry
2 = Scant = wound tissues moist, no measurable exudate
3 = Small = wound tissues wet, moisture evenly distributed in wound, drainage involved ≤ 25% of wound dressing
4 = Moderate = wound tissues saturated, drainage may or may not be evenly distributed in wound, drainage involved > 25% to < 75% of wound dressing
5 = Large = wound tissues bathed in fluid, drainage freely expressed, may or may not be evenly distributed in wound, drainage involved > 75% of wound dressing

Type of Exudate

The type of exudate should change as the wound improves and heals. As the wound passes through the inflammatory phase of wound healing, serous drainage should become more serosanguineous, then sanguineous in nature. As infection or necrosis is resolved, improvement should be reflected in the exudate type. Foul, purulent drainage should become merely purulent, then seropurulent, and finally serous and serosanguineous in character. Measurement of the type of exudate is best accomplished by the use of a rating scale, such as:

1 = Bloody = thin, bright red
2 = Serosanguineous = thin, watery, pale red to pink
3 = Serous = thin, watery, clear
4 = Purulent = thin or thick, opaque tan to yellow
5 = Foul purulent = thick, opaque yellow to green with offensive odor

Referral Criteria

The determination of whether a patient is a candidate for wound management requires adequate assessment of the patient, with attention to evaluation for possible referral. For example, the following patients would warrant referral to a physician and/or an advanced practice nurse for medical evaluation, immediate intervention, or referral to another health-care professional for consultation.

1. Patients with wound exudate that is copious, malodorous, and prolonged should be evaluated further for infection, cellulitis, abscess, or progressive degeneration. In this case, the advanced practice nurse may choose to manage the patient initially. If the condition worsens or the patient fails to improve over a 2-week time frame, the physician should be consulted.
2. Patients with an elevated temperature or those on a downhill course should be evaluated further. Intervene as in No. 1.
3. Patients with no wound improvement over several weeks should be evaluated further. In this case, the advanced practice nurse may want to consult other health-care practitioners (e.g., physical therapists, dietitians, wound care nurses or enterostomal therapy [ET] nurses, and physicians).

4. Patients with evidence of cellulitis or gross purulence/infection should be evaluated further. Intervene as in No. 1.
5. Patients with impending exposed bone or tendon present in the wound should be evaluated further. Intervene as in No. 3.
6. Patients with evidence of an abscessed area should be evaluated further. Intervene as in No. 3.
7. Patients with extensively undermined areas present in the wound should be evaluated further. Intervene as in No. 3.

Self-Care Teaching Guidelines

Patient and caregiver instruction in self-care must be individualized to the topical therapy care routine, individual patient's wound, individual patient's and caregiver's learning styles and coping mechanisms, and ability of the patient/caregiver to perform procedures. The general self-care teaching guidelines in Exhibit 9-3 provide a model of information to teach, and should be individualized for each patient and caregiver.

EXHIBIT 9-3   Self-Care Teaching Guidelines

Self-Care Guidelines Specific to Exudate and Infection Management	Instructions Given (Date/Initials)	Demonstration *or* Review of Material (Date/Initials)	Return Demonstration *or* Verbalizes Understanding (Date/Initials)
1. Type of wound and reasons for exudate			
2. Significance of exudate and infection			
3. Topical therapy care routine			
a. Clean wound.			
b. Apply absorptive dressing (note appearance of dressing when it interacts with wound drainage and on removal)			
c. Manage wound edges to prevent maceration			
d. Apply secondary or topper dressing, as appropriate			
4. Frequency of dressing changes			
5. Expected change in wound drainage during healing			
6. When to notify the health care provider			
a. Signs and symptoms of infection			
b. Failure to improve			
c. Presence of odor			
d. Pus or purulent drainage			
e. Copious amounts of drainage			
f. Elevated temperature or signs of confusion in the older patient			
7. Universal precautions			
a. Hand washing			
b. Use of gloves during care procedures			
c. Disposal of contaminated materials			
8. Antibiotic regimen			
a. Oral medication use			
b. Topical medication use			
c. Antimicrobial cleanser use			
9. Importance of follow-up with health care provider			

Conclusion

Management of exudate and infection is part of preparing the wound for healing. Differentiation of infection from colonization can be difficult, yet, clinical signs and symptoms of each are similar. Colonization does not usually impair wound healing or invade wound tissues. In contrast, infection invades wound tissues with resultant cellulitis, inflammation, drainage and odor, and impaired wound healing. Correct antimicrobial therapy can assist in both bacterial contamination and infection. Use of antimicrobials should be undertaken with a thoughtful approach in wounds with signs of infection and avoided in wounds that are clean. Advancements in our understanding of wound cleansing, antimicrobial use, and dressings to absorb wound exudate have made obtaining an infection-free, moist but not wet, wound ready for healing more attainable.

REVIEW QUESTIONS

1. Which of the following statements best describes wound colonization?
   a. The presence of proliferating microorganisms in viable wound tissues without a host response
   b. The presence of proliferating microorganisms in viable wound tissues with a host response
   c. The presence of proliferating microorganisms on the wound surface without a host response
   d. The presence of proliferating organisms on the wound surface with a host response
2. A client presents with a clean full-thickness wound. Which of the following solutions would be the best for use in cleansing?
   a. Povidone-iodine
   b. Normal saline
   c. Sodium hypochlorite solution
   d. Hydrogen peroxide
3. Cultures are indicated for which of the following pressure ulcers?
   a. All pressure ulcers involving loss of epidermis and dermis
   b. All full-thickness pressure ulcers
   c. Pressure ulcers with signs and symptoms of localized/systemic infection or bone involvement
   d. Pressure ulcers with necrotic tissue present and surrounding erythema
4. Which of the following provides a safe pressure for use in wound irrigation?
   a. Water Pik on a medium setting
   b. Water Pik on a high setting
   c. 35-mL syringe with 19-gauge angiocatheter attached
   d. Gauze soaked in solution
5. Which of the following reports typically indicates wound infection?
   a. Colony count of more than 1,000 organisms/mL
   b. Colony count of more than 5,000 organisms/mL
   c. Colony count of more than 10,000 organisms/mL
   d. Colony count of more than 100,000 organisms/ mL

REFERENCES

1. Trengove NJ, Bielefeldt-Ohmann H, Stacey MC. Mitogenic activity and cytokine levels in non-healing and healing chronic leg ulcers. *Wound Repair Regen* 2000; 8(1):13–25.
2. Winter GD. Formation of the scab and the rate of reepithelialization of superficial wounds in the skin of the young domestic pig. *Nature.* 1965;193:293–294.
3. Kerstein MD. Moist wound healing: the clinical perspective. *Ostomy/Wound Manage.* 1995;41(suppl 7A):37–45.
4. Stotts NA. Impaired wound healing. In: Carrieri-Kohlman VK, Lindsay AM, West CM, eds. Pathophysiological Phenomenon in Nursing. 2nd ed. Philadelphia: WB Saunders Company, 1993:343–366.
5. Sapico FL, Ginunas VJ, Thornhill-Hyones M, et al. Quantitative microbiology of pressure sores in different stages of healing. *Diagn Biol Infect Dis.* 1986;5:31–38.
6. Xakellis GC, Chrischilles EA. Hydrocolloid versus saline-gauze dressings in treating pressure ulcers: a cost-effectiveness analysis. *Arch Phys Med Rehabil.* 1992;73(5):463–469.
7. Thomas DR, Rodeheaver GT, Bartolucci AA, et al. Pressure ulcer scale for healing: derivation and validation of the PUSH tool. *Adv Wound Care.* 1997;10:(5):96–101.
8. Bates-Jensen BM. A Quantitative Analysis of Wound Characteristics as Early Predictors of Healing in Pressure Sores. Dissertation Abstracts International. Vol. 59, No. 11. Los Angeles: University of California, 1999.
9. Van Rijswijk L, Polansky M. Predictors of time to healing deep pressure ulcers. *Ostomy/Wound Manage.* 1994;40(8):40–50.
10. Cooper DM. The physiology of wound healing: an overview. In: Krasner D, Rodeheaver GT, Sibbald, RG, eds. Chronic Wound Care: A Clinical Source Book for Healthcare Professionals. Wayne, PA: HMP Communications, 2001.
11. Bowler PG. The 10⁵ bacterial growth guideline: reassessing its clinical relevance in wound healing. *Ostomy/Wound Manage.* 2003; 49(1):44–53.
12. Robson, MC. Wound infection: a failure of wound healing caused by an imbalance of bacteria. *Surgical Clinics of North America.* 1997; 77(3):637–650.
13. Thomson PD, Smith DJ. What is infection? *Am J Surg.* 1994;167(suppl 1A):7–11.
14. Pottinger JM. Methicillin-resistant *Staphylococcus aureus* in a sternal wound. In: Soule BM, Larson EL, Preston GA, eds. Infection and Nursing Practice—Prevention and Control. St. Louis, MO: Mosby-Year Book, 1995:240–245.
15. Boyce JM. Methicillin-resistant *Staphylococcus aureus*: detection, epidemiology, and control measures. *Infect Dis Clin North Am.* 1989;3:901–913.
16. Sibbald, RG, Williamson D, Orsted HL, et al. Preparing the wound bed—debridement, bacterial balance, and moisture balance. *Ostomy/Wound Manage.* 2000;45:(11):14–35.
17. Heggers JP. Assessing and controlling wound infection. *Cl in Plastic Surg.* 2003; 30(1):25–35.
18. Gardner SE, Frantz RA, Doebbling BN. The validity of the clinical signs and symptoms used to identify localized chronic wound infection. *Wound Repair Regen.* 2001; 9:178–186.
19. Mosiello GC, Tufaro A, Kerstein MD. Wound healing and complications in the immunosuppressed patient. *Wounds.* 1994;6(3):83–87.
20. Bergstrom N, Bennett MA, Carlson CE, et al. Treatment of Pressure Ulcers. Clinical Practice Guideline No. 15. Agency for Health Care Research and Quality (AHRQ), formerly known as the Agency for Health Care Policy and Research (AHCPR) Publication No. 95-0652. Rockville, MD: AHRQ, U.S. Public Health Service, U.S. Department of Health and Human Services (DHHS); December 1994:15–22.
21. Stotts NA. Determination of bacterial burden in wounds. *Adv Wound Care.* 1995;8:28–52.
22. Robson MC, Heggars JP. Bacterial quantification of open wounds. *Milit Med.* 1969;134:19–24.
23. Wood GL, Gutierrez Y. Diagnostic Pathology of Infectious Diseases. Philadelphia: Lea & Febiger, 1993.
24. Lee P, Turnidge J, McDonald PJ. Fine-needle aspiration biopsy in diagnosis of soft tissue infections. *J Clin Mibrobiol.* 1985;22:80–83.
25. Morrison MJ. A Colour Guide to the Nursing Management of Wounds. Oxford, England: Blackwell Scientific Publications, 1992.
26. Pagana KD, Pagana TJ. Mosby's Diagnostic and Laboratory Test Reference. St. Louis: Mosby-Year Book, 1992.
27. Cuzzell JZ. The right way to culture a wound. *Am Nurs.* 1993;93:48–50.

28. Alvarez O, Rozint J, Meehan M. Principles of moist wound healing: indications for chronic wounds. In: Krasner D, Rodeheaver GT, Sibbald RG, eds. Chronic Wound Care: A Clinical Source Book for Healthcare Professionals. 3rd ed. Wayne, PA: HMP Communications, 2001.

29. Levine NS, Lindberg RB, Mason AD, Pruitt BA. The quantitative swab culture and smear: a quick simple method for determining the number of viable aerobic bacteria on open wounds. *J Trauma.* 1976;16(2):89–94.

30. Georgiade NG, Lucas MC, O'Fallon WM, Osterhout S. A comparison of methods for the quantification of bacteria in burn wounds. *Am J Clin Pathol.* 1970;53:35–39.

31. Duke WF, Robson MC, Krizek TJ. Civilian wounds: their bacterial flora and rate of infection. *Surg Forum.* 1972;23:518–520.

32. Barr JE. Principles of wound cleansing. *Ostomy/Wound Manage.* 1995;41(Suppl 7A):155–225.

33. Lineaweaver W. Cellular and bacterial toxicities of topical antimicrobials. *Plast Reconstr Surg.* 1985;75:394–396.

34. Rodeheaver G. Topical wound management. *Ostomy/Wound Manage.* 1988;20:59–68.

35. Foresman PA, Payne DS, Becker D, et al. A relative toxicity index for wound cleansers. *Wounds.* 1993;5(5):226–231.

36. Hellewell TB, Major DA, Foresman PA, Rodeheaver GT. A cytotoxicity evaluation of antimicrobial and non-antimicrobial wound cleansers. *Wounds.* 1997;9(1):15–20.

37. Bennett LL, Rosenblum RS, Perlov C, et al. An in vivo comparison of topical agents on wound repair. *Plast Reconstr Surg.* 2001;108(3):675–687.

38. Haynes LJ, Brown MH, Handley BC, et al. Comparison of Pulsavac and sterile whirlpool regarding the promotion of tissue granulation. *Arch Phys Med Rehabil.* 1994;74(Suppl 5):54.

39. McConnell ES, Murphy AT. Nursing diagnoses related to physiological alterations: In: Matteson MA, McConnell ES, Linton AD, eds. Gerontological Nursing: Concepts and Practice. 2nd ed. Philadelphia: WB Saunders, 1997.

40. Gilman G, ed. Topical Agents for Open Wounds: Antibacterials, Antiseptics, Antifungals. Reviewed by Rodeheaver G, Cooper JW, Nelson DR, Meehan M. Charleston, SC: Hill-Rom International, 1991.

41. Cooper BW. Antimicrobial chemotherapeutics. In: Soule BM, Larson EL, Preston GA, eds. Infections and Nursing Practice: Prevention and Control. St. Louis: Mosby, 1995.

42. Speight TM. Avery's Drug Treatment: Principles and Practice of Clinical Pharmacology and Therapeutics. 3rd Ed. Baltimore: Williams & Wilkins, 1987.

43. Leaper DJ. Prophylactic and therapeutic role of antibiotics in wound care. *Am J Surg.* 1994;167(Suppl 1A):158S–159S.

44. Crow S, Planchock NY, Hedrick E. Antisepsis, disinfection and sterilization. In: Soule BM, Larson EL, Preston GA, eds. Infections and Nursing Practice: Prevention and Control. St. Louis: Mosby, 1995.

45. Steele K, Irwin G, Dowde N. Cadexomer iodine in the management of venous leg ulcers in general practice. *Practitioner.* 1986;230(1411):63–68.

46. Harcup JW, Saul PA. A study of the effect of cadexomer iodine in the treatment of venous leg ulcers. *Br J Clin Pract.* 1986;40(9):360–364.

47. Ormiston MC, Seymour MT, Venn GE, et al. Controlled trial of Iodosorb in chronic venous ulcers. *Br Med J* (Clin Res Ed) 1985;291(6491):308–310.

48. Skog E, Arnesio B, Troeng T, et al. A randomized trial comparing cadexomer iodine and standard treatment in the outpatient management of chronic venous ulcers. *Br J Dermatol.* 1983;109(1):77–83.

49. Apelqvist J, Ragnarson Tennvall G. Cavity foot ulcers in diabetic patients: a comparative study of cadexomer iodine ointment and standard treatment. An economic analysis alongside a clinical trial. *Acta Derm Venereol.* 1996;76(3):231–235.

50. Moberg S, Hoffman L, Grennart ML, Holst A. A randomized trial of cadexomer iodine in decubitus ulcers. *J Am Geriatr Soc.* 1983;31(8):462.

51. Poteete V. Case study: eliminating odors from wounds. *Decubitus.* 1993;6(4):43–46.

52. McMullen D. Topical metronidazole, part II. *Ostomy/Wound Manage.* 1992;38(3):42–48.

53. Jones P, Willis A, Ferguson I. Treatment of anaerobically infected pressure sores with topical metronidazole. *Lancet.* 1978;1:214.

54. Gomolin I, Brandt J. Topical therapy for pressure sores in geriatric patients. *J Am Geriatr Soc.* 1983;31:710–712.

10

Management of Edema

Evonne Fowler and Stan Carson

CHAPTER OBJECTIVES

At the completion of this chapter, the reader will be able to:

1. Explain the various causes of edema.
2. Describe options for compression therapy.
3. Discuss effective management strategies for various types of edema.

Edema results from fluid accumulation in the interstitial compartment of the extravascular space. Clinical assessment mainly relies on a careful and thorough history and physical examination. In addition, noninvasive duplex vascular ultrasound, computerized tomography, magnetic resonance imaging, and lymphoscintigraphy may be helpful. Without appropriate and timely intervention, the edematous extremity can progress, leading to further tissue damage and functional impairment. Determination of the underlying cause of edema is needed to specifically guide treatment.

Peripheral edema should be classified as unilateral or bilateral (Figure 10-1A and B). Causes of unilateral lower extremity swelling include venous and arterial abnormalities, lymphedema, infection, trauma, and neoplasms. The possible sources of bilateral edema include congestive heart failure, systemic and metabolic abnormalities, endocrine dysfunction, inferior vena cava obstruction by tumor or inflammatory mass, lipedema, and pregnancy.

Treatment helps improve patient comfort and mobility, which in turn can lead to improved patient participation in effective treatment. Successful management of the edematous limb is also closely associated with successful wound healing and a decreased frequency of focal infections.[1–3]

As an illustration of the benefits of controlling edema, studies showing the effectiveness of wound healing in venous ulcers without compression controlling edema are almost nonexistent.[4] Poor epithelialization, decreased oxygenation nutrient diffusion, and decreased immune defense appear to be factors for problems in edematous limbs.[5–7] In many instances, treatment of edema itself may assist in wound healing and prevention.[6–9] In the author's outpatient clinic, during a recent retrospective review of 300 consecutive patients with extremity wounds, 42% of the involved extremities with chronic wounds were associated with edema (unpublished results S.N.C., M.D.). Fully two-thirds of these patients failed to make progress in healing until edema was effectively treated.

Normally, an individual with reasonable circulation and no underlying disorder may have a little lower extremity dependent edema at the end of the day.[10] Significant edema, however, remains a physical sign associated with many different clinical problems and frequently presents as a diagnostic problem. Clinical examination is the primary diagnostic tool. Table 10-1 illustrates physical signs and findings associated with common causes of edema.[10] On the basis of physical exam and history, systemic causes such as drug induced, endocrine, renal, hepatic, cardiac and nutritional causes may be evaluated as outlined in Table 10-2.

The two most common causes of chronic and clinically significant edema worldwide, venous insufficiency and lymphedema, may often be diagnosed based on history and physical exam alone.[1] Also, the type of lymphedema is usually diagnosed by history and physical exam as shown in Table 10-3.[8,11] Note that more than one type of edema may be present in a given situation and additional factors contributing to poor healing may be present. For example, arterial ischemia may coexist with venous disease and the resultant edema and venous disease may also be associated

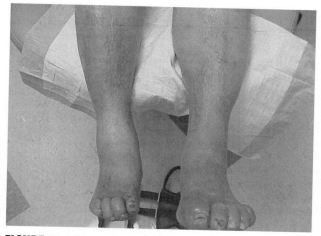
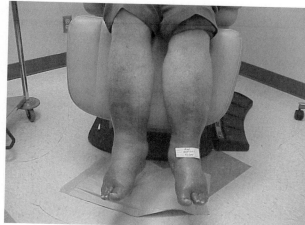

FIGURE 10-1 Determine whether the edema is unilateral or bilateral as shown. (Copyright © Evonne Fowler, RN, CNS, CWOCN)

TABLE 10-1   Physical Signs and Symptoms Seen in Common Causes of Edema

	Lymphedema	Venostasis	Cardiac-Renal-Hepatic Insufficiency	Lipedema
Edema, Consistency	Soft, pitting progressing to spongy and firm	Brawny, pitting	Pitting	Nonpitting
Edema, Distribution	Diffuse, more distal than proximal (from lymph drainage areas)	Ankles and legs, Feet usually spared	Bilateral, greatest distally May appear over back in recumbent patient	Ankles and legs Feet spared
Relief with Elevation	Mild to moderate, over several days	Almost complete in several hours up to 1 day	Almost complete in several hours up to 1 day	Minimal May have associated secondary edema
Bilaterality	As often as not	Occasional	Always	Almost always
Severity of Pain	None or "heaviness"	Ache	Variable, usually none	Usually none
Skin	Eventually thickened Ulceration rare	Atrophic Pigmentation Possible Ulcers	Shiny, no trophic changes	No changes

with lymphedema.[6,10] The authors have observed several patients with malnutrition associated with peripheral edema and arterial and venous disease. Recently, more patients with drug induced or drug exacerbated edema are also being seen (see Table 10-4) and in many wound care clinics in North America, drug induced edema has become the most common cause of edema.

Background Physiology of the Interstitial Space and Edema

The components of the circulatory system that effect edema mainly consist of blood, arteries, arterioles, capillaries, venules, and veins.[12-15] An ultrafiltrate of plasma, the interstitial fluid, occupies the space between cells and the cap-

illaries (*the interstitial space*). Exchanges between blood and cells (i.e., nutrients and oxygen) occur in this space. Understanding interstitial fluid, interstitial space, and circulatory effects on it is key to understanding edema.[11,13] The microcirculation in the interstitial space consists of the lymphatics, capillaries, and interstitial fluid. Tissues contained in this space include collagen along with proteoglycan molecules. Exchange of nutrients, wastes, fluid, electrolytes, and proteins from the vascular system, lymphatic system, and tissue cells occurs through this space.

In general, in the interstitial space fluid, nutrients, and other materials pass to and from the capillaries, go through tissue channels to cells and back, and collect waste products along the way. Pressure in this area may be low and attract fluid into the tissue or be high and force fluid into lym-

TABLE 10-2 Clinical Guide to Lower Extremity Swelling

Condition	Characteristics	Diagnostic Tests	Treatment
Venous Insufficiency	Possible ulcers	Magnetic Resonance Imaging	Cautious compression with active infection
	Pigmentation	Duplex doppler (must be done in proper consistent fashion)	Elastic stockings
	Swelling of extremity usually better after shorter period of elevation	Venous reflux tests with photo or air plethysmography	Elevation Wound care Modified activity Surgery in some cases
Lymphatic Obstruction	History	Lymph isotope study	Lymphedema management program (appropriate massage, exercise, support garments, compression, medications)
	Nodes		Certified lymphedema therapy
	Swelling improves little with elevation		
A-V Fistula	Unilateral Bruit Arterial flow in veins	Arterial study including magnetic resonance angiography or CT angiography	Excision or embolization
Fluid Overload	Renal or cardiac disease Nutritional problem	Central Venous Pressure Intake-output record	Treat cause
	Usually in-hospital complication	Cardiac indices	

TABLE 10-3 Classification of Lymphedema Based on Causes

I. Primary Lymphedema
  A. Congenital (onset before 1 year old)
    1. Nonfamilial
    2. Familial (Milroy's Disease)
  B. Praecox (onset 1–35 years old)
    1. Nonfamilial
    2. Familial
  C. Tarda (onset after 35 years old)
II. Secondary Lymphedema
  A. Filariasis
  B. Lymph node excision +/- irradiation
  C. Tumor invasion
  D. Infection
  E. Trauma
  F. Other

phatics and capillaries.[11] It is in the interstitial fluid space that forces resulting in edema express themselves.

Arteries and Veins

Arteries and veins are the structures that transport blood and its nutrients throughout the body. The arteries transport blood from the heart under high pressure to the tissues. Arteries lead to arterioles, smaller vessels with very muscular walls. Arterioles can shut down completely or increase their diameter several times, thereby increasing or decreasing blood flow to the capillaries.

Capillaries coming off the arterioles are next in line and are thin and permeable, exchanging fluid, nutrients, electrolytes, and other items between the blood and interstitial fluid. Venules collect blood from the capillaries and lead into veins that carry blood back toward the heart. Veins also act as a major reservoir for blood and are greatly distensible, up to nine times their original volume.

Veins have little resistance to blood flow and their average pressure is less than 10 mm Hg greater than the right atrium of the heart. By far the greatest volume of blood at all times is in the veins (about two thirds) while about one-fifth is in the arteries, arterioles, and capillaries.[13]

Hydrostatic pressure in the arteries, arterioles, and the arterial side of the capillaries comes largely from cardiac contraction. Hydrostatic pressure is exerted on blood in the veins, venules, and venous side of the capillaries by gravity and tissue pressures on the venous side of the circulation. The hydrostatic pressure in veins generally increases with distance from the right atrium.

TABLE 10-4 Drugs Contributing to Peripheral Edema

Hormones
- Corticosteroids
- Estrogen
- Progesterone
- Testosterone

Anti-inflammatory Drugs
- Non-steroidal anti-inflammatory drugs
- Cox-2 inhibitors

Antihypertensives
- Hydralazine
- Clonidine
- Reserpine
- Calcium channel blockers (becoming more common, some appear worse than others in this regard)
- Beta-blockers

Monoamine oxidase inhibitors
Multiple infused drugs with high Na content (most are also available with lower sodium content on request)
Thiazolidinediones (i.e., Rosiglitazone™)

The venous system of the lower leg is composed of a superficial system, a connecting perforating system, and a deep system. Blood normally flows from the superficial to the deep system through perforating veins and, at certain areas, at the groin and knee; the superficial system connects directly to the deep system. When intact, valves in the veins are one-way only valves and prevent reflux. The veins connect to large central veins in the abdomen and chest. During muscle contraction, the muscles exert high pressures on the deep veins and pump blood toward the heart.

Venous pressure at the ankle in a standing person is higher than the same pressure taken in a recumbent person whose ankle veins are at about the same level as the right atrium. In a person standing still, the venous pressure at the ankle is about 90 mm Hg. However, when the leg and abdominal muscles are active, they compress the adjacent veins emptying the blood and reducing pressure in the veins (until they fill up again when the muscles are relaxed). The one-way valves in the veins allow blood to flow only toward the heart and in combination with the muscle pumping activity are together known as the venous muscular pump. The most important pump is the calf pump, but the quadriceps in the thigh and the foot pump also play roles in moving venous blood. Clearly the pump does not work without motion, an open unobstructed vein, and the intact valvular mechanisms. When one, two, or all three of these fail, venous pressure can rise dramatically.[13] When this happens in the superficial and deep systems or the deep system alone, edema, prominent varicose veins, and (eventually) venous skin ulcers may occur.[16-18]

Blood flows through the capillaries and its flow is, for the most part, regulated by oxygen needs.[13,16] Exchange between blood via capillaries and the interstitial fluid space occurs by diffusion. Dissolved proteins and salts in the blood and interstitial fluid also exhibit oncotic pressure, or the force to move from a concentrated to a less concentrated area in their surroundings.[13] The interstitial space contains interstitial fluid, which has dissolved proteins and electrolytes and other substances that exert hydrostatic and oncotic forces. Of these, the forces exerted by plasma and interstitial fluid proteins, particularly albumin, seem to be the most important in controlling the respective volumes of both. Therefore, the ability for fluid and substances to filter out of the circulation and back in to it depends not only on the hydrostatic pressures involved, but also on the oncotic pressures of the plasma at the arterial and venous ends of the capillary circulation as well as that of the interstitial space. The permeability of the capillaries and the vascular tone of the blood vessels in the areas involved is an important additional factor as to which substances, how much, and how fast are filtered or taken up.

Lymph System

The lymphatic system consists of lymph, lymphatics, collecting ducts, and lymph nodes. Lymph is derived from and enters from the interstitial space into the smaller initial lymphatics. These lead into larger collecting lymphatics. These, in turn, empty into the lymphatic-venous communications located in the neck and elsewhere. In its passage through lymph nodes, about half of the lymph fluid, but not the proteins, passes directly through to the blood circulation.[11] Lymph is propelled by a combination of various factors. Muscle activity can propel lymph and one-way lymph channels focus the flow. Respiration and arterial pulsations also have an effect on lymph flow. Lymphatics are felt to have intrinsic contractions also promoting propulsion. Regularly, more fluid, and especially more protein, flow into the interstitial space than is returned by the capillaries directly into the blood stream. The lymphatic system picks up the extra fluid and proteins and returns them to the general circulation. The lymphatic fluid is typically rich in protein content. Over a 24 hour period the capillaries may allow 40%–80% of the intravascular protein to enter the interstitial space where it is returned to the circulation by lymphatic transport.[11] In summary, the "proficiency" of the lymphatic system is critical to the body defense mechanism because it transports and filters everything unable to pass from the tissues back into the venous circulation.[13]

Interstitial Space in Action and Causes of Edema

There are four primary forces that determine whether fluid will move out of blood into the interstitial area or in the opposite direction.[17] The rate and direction of water, fluid, and protein movement between blood and tissues is operated by a gradient. Capillary pressure and interstitial fluid pressure, when negative, forces fluid outward through the capillary membrane. Interstitial fluid pressure, when negative forces fluid into the capillaries but in the opposite direction when positive. Capillary oncotic pressure tends to force fluid into the capillaries and interstitial fluid oncotic pressure forces fluid out of the capillaries.

The sum of these forces affected by diffusion, ultrafiltration, and reabsorption control the movement of fluid and dissolved substances. Most solutes (oxygen) and nutrients (protein) tend to diffuse freely across the capillary walls, from areas of higher concentration to areas of lower concentration. The higher concentration of oxygen and nutrients in the capillary plasma promotes diffusion of oxygen and nutrients across the capillaries into tissues where they are constantly consumed. In contrast, the higher concentration of carbon dioxide (CO_2) and waste products in the tissues promotes diffusion of CO_2 and waste products from the tissue back to blood plasma within the veins.

There is a continuous interchange of fluid between blood and tissue at the capillary level. Usually protein attracts water. The high protein content in the plasma of the arterioles and arterial capillary encourages the retention of fluid inside the capillary. The higher blood pressure that is created with each heart beat (hydrostatic pressure) in the arterial end of the capillary (33 mm Hg) lowers pressure in the tissue space (23 mm Hg), thus proteins or water/fluid are driven out into tissue spaces by ultrafiltration. At the venous end, the high pressure in the tissue space (23 mm Hg) lowers pressure in the venous end of the capillary (13 mm Hg) allowing water reabsorption.

In general, hydrostatic forces of increased pressure from the vascular tree seen in heart failure and venous/lymphatic obstruction, decreased oncotic pressure of blood seen in fluid overload/electrolyte imbalance and decreased protein content of serum, injury to capillaries promoting leakage of fluid, and contents such as seen with drugs and sepsis can cause and contribute to edema.[11,13] In most instances, edema occurs outside of cells in the extracellular compartment and the interstitial space. The fluid may leak directly from the lymphatics and venous-arterial system or may represent fluid accumulation in excess of the drainage ability of the tissues.[10,11]

General causes of extracellular edema are unusual leakage of plasma fluid from capillaries into tissue spaces and failure of the lymphatic system to return fluid and proteins into the blood stream. Increased capillary leakage occurs in high venous pressure seen in heart failure, venous blockages from clots or other mechanical blockages, venous obstruction from venous valvular failure and immobility, and excessive renal retention of salts and water. Increased capillary filtration also occurs with decreased arteriolar resistance due to excessive body heat, sympathetic disturbances and local effects seen in sepsis and other toxic events, and increasingly with use of various drugs resulting in vasodilatation.

Increased capillary permeability seen in infections, ischemia, burns, exposure to toxins, vitamin deficiencies, and immune reactions may result in extracellular edema. These are simply causes of increased leakage. Blockage of lymph

return prevents reabsorption of fluids and proteins normally or (in disease conditions) abnormally lost during capillary circulation. Lymph blockages are seen in cancer and after cancer treatments that may obliterate lymph tissue, in infections, in noncancer surgeries, and in the absence and abnormalities of lymph tissues. In general, edema can be caused or worsened by hydrostatic forces of increased pressure from the vascular tree (seen in heart failure and venous/lymphatic obstruction), decreased oncotic pressure of blood (seen in fluid overload/electrolyte imbalance and decreased protein content of serum), and injury to capillaries promoting leakage of fluid and contents (such as seen with drugs and sepsis).[11,13]

Once present, edema may exert oncotic and pressure forces of its own to contribute to the maintenance or increase of edema. Edema may also decrease mobility of the patient due to discomfort and the sensation of heaviness brought about by the swollen limb.[12]

In shock and other instances of compromised cardiac output, decreased oxygen and nutrient supply to the cells result in depression of the cells' metabolic ability to pump excess sodium out: sodium accumulates and draws extra water into the cells. Intracellular edema regularly occurs in inflammation because of the increased permeability induced by inflammatory process.[13]

Pitting edema, edema that leaves a depression in the skin when pressed, occurs mainly in extracellular edema as shown in Figure 10-2. Nonpitting edema occurs in situations where the edema is in the cells or the associated inflammation has been chronic enough to result in excessive protein and fibrinogen deposits in the interstitial space. Occasionally, especially when mixed causes of edema are present and when multiple infections have occurred in an area, both types of edema may be present.[12,13]

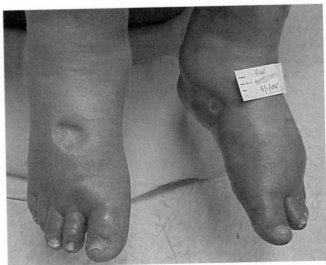

FIGURE 10-2 Pitting edema. (Copyright © Evonne Fowler, RN, CNS, CWOCN)

From the above, it can be noted how these systems can work in concert. For example, obstruction causing elevated venous or lymphatic pressure could decrease the absorption of fluid from the interstitial space and edema may result. Venous back pressure may also cause increased capillary filtration. An increase in interstitial pressure from this fluid accumulation may also increase to the point where lymph flow increases to try to compensate for the increased pressure. Since one of the driving forces in the lymph and venous system is muscle activity, an immobile patient could be expected to have more edema problems than an active patient. A patient with decreased serum proteins from poor nutrition may have edema because the decreased protein content in blood may decrease the oncotic pressure attracting fluid from the interstitial space back into the circulation.

Extracellular edema also occurs with decreased plasma protein content that decreases plasma colloid osmotic pressure, excessive loss of plasma proteins, and lack of ability to adequately produce plasma proteins, which have the same effect. This contributes to and causes edema by decreasing the ability of plasma to reabsorb from the tissues liquids normally lost from the capillaries during circulation.

Assessment

Lower extremity edema is commonly encountered in clinical practice and may be a manifestation of one of many disease processes. Underlying causes of edema should be actively investigated to optimize treatment as well as to diagnose underlying causes.

Evaluation, Diagnosis, History

Type of onset is an important factor in determining the cause of edema. Sudden onset suggests an acute process such as deep vein thrombosis (DVT), trauma, or infection. Gradual onset indicates chronic causes (i.e., venous insufficiency, medications) or a systemic process such as gradual onset of cardiac or renal failure. Waxing and waning edema may occur with focal cellulitis or other soft tissue infection. Pain may be associated with infection or an unrecognized trauma such as fracture or compartment syndrome. Sometimes venous thrombosis is associated with pain and edema although pain is more common with a superficial thrombosis than a deep venous thrombosis. Positional changes associated with changes in edema can help with diagnosis.[1]

Physical Examination

The extremities should be inspected for unilateral or bilateral edema. Focal leg swelling suggests an isolated soft tissue process, such as a hematoma or abscess, muscle injury, and in rarer cases tumor. Lipedema appears as a swollen limb sparing only the foot. Lymphedema fully evolved may involve the entire lower leg and frequently has a dorsal swelling. Edema with warmth, and/or redness and/or pain may represent infection that can be arising *de novo* from a skin break or may be associated with wounds or soft tissue trauma. If crepitus is found in the location, it may represent necrotizing fasciitis, a surgical and medical emergency.

Swelling with heat and tenderness is consistent with an infectious process, most likely cellulitis. Skin changes are commonly associated with chronic inflammation as seen in venous insufficiency, and, occasionally arterial disease or repeat episodes of cellulitis. The latter can be associated with prolonged edema of any type. Note varicose veins and document the presence and absence of arterial pulses.

Adjunctive Tests

Duplex ultrasonography is currently the most reliable and important test associated with diagnosis and management of extremity edema. The test can determine presence or absence of deep vein thrombosis and venous obstruction.[2] This technique is operator-dependent. It should be noted that clinical symptoms and physical findings consistent with deep vein thrombosis are not present in up to 60% of patients with acute deep vein thrombosis. This exam can verify presence or absence of venous valvular insufficiency, a common cause of lower extremity edema.[19,20] Baker's cysts and iliac or popliteal aneurysms can also be detected with duplex ultrasound. Computerized tomography (CT) scanning or magnetic resonance imaging (MRI) are useful diagnostic tools with localized tissue masses.[3,4] The cardiac, renal, hepatic, and (occasionally) endocrine systems should be investigated if systemic abnormalities are suspected. This may require specialty physician consults.

Usually history, physical, and ruling out of other causes will be adequate to diagnose lymphedema. If diagnosis is suspected but uncertain, lymphoscintography is the least invasive and current best diagnostic tool available.

Management and Treatment of Edema

The management of lower leg edema requires an understanding of edema, underlying conditions, as well as therapy options available. Often swelling of the lower legs can be controlled with a combination of compression, leg elevation, exercises, and good skin care. Although the regimen may seen simplistic, adherence to this care plan may be difficult. Successful management depends on patient's ability to cooperate. Often multiple pathologies such as arthritis, obesity, limited mobility, or weakness may be present that complicate management. Lack of caregiver support may also hamper management. For positive outcomes, control of edema requires a commitment of the patient and/or caregiver in time, energy, as well as financial investment. Many times a change in life style is necessary.

Leg Elevation and Exercise

Treatment of leg edema by reducing leg dependency is an extremely important but difficult to achieve objective in the edematous patient. Elevation of the legs facilitates the removal of fluid by gravity, assisting in venous return to the heart.[20,21] The legs should be elevated higher than the heart to reduce swelling. This natural drainage will aid in reducing edema, reducing pain, and healing open wounds. Knees should be positioned above the hips and the ankles above the knees. Elevation of the feet to the hip level does not reduce swelling; however, it will keep the swelling from getting worse. Swelling around the ankle develops because of fluid pooling in the dermis causing heaviness, which is most marked and painful at the end of the day and improves with recumbence. Fluid redistribution occurs as a result of the recumbent position. Elevating the foot of the bed on 6-inch blocks or placing a foam wedge between the mattress and box spring may help reduce the swelling. After long periods of being on one's feet, reclining horizontally on a comfortable surface or bed with both legs elevated 30° above the surface with feet resting against the wall or headboard for 10–15 minutes will aid in reducing edema.

CLINICAL WISDOM

Complete bed rest is discouraged. However, frequent 20–30 minute episodes of elevation throughout the day are recommended. People with cardiovascular conditions may have difficulty breathing when reclining with legs elevated. Those who are obese may have positioning problems with leg elevation. People at risk or who have edematous legs should not sit with legs dependent for long periods of time nor sit with legs crossed at the knees. These positions can slow the circulation and cause pooling of fluids at the ankles and lower legs. For those who sit in wheelchairs for extended times, elevation of foot risers is helpful.

Exercise that results in working the calf muscle pump should be encouraged. During active leg exercises, the calf pump muscles squeeze blood up the veins toward the heart. Ankle exercises should be done on a regular schedule to keep the blood circulating in the feet and legs while standing, sitting, or lying.[22]

CLINICAL WISDOM

Ankle exercises can be done by straightening the legs, then bringing the toes at a right angle toward the head, and holding in place for 5 seconds. Then, point the toes away from the body and hold that position for 5 seconds. Repeat the exercise 30 times every hour. A simple rhyme to remember to do the exercises is "When the clock chimes, exercise your ankle 30 times."

Ankle exercises cause the calf pump to work. To check the action of the calf pump, place the hand on the back of the lower leg at the calf and feel the movement of the muscle during the exercise. The muscle contracts when the toes are forward and relaxes while the toes are back. When it is necessary for the patient to stand for an extended period of time, he or she can do the same exercise by raising up on the toes and holding the position for 5 seconds. Then, lower the feet to a flat position for 5 seconds. When doing "sit down" tasks, attempts should be made to elevate the legs.

For ambulatory people with edema, walking, cycling, and swimming are good exercises. A daily walking program is the simplest, most effective way to improve circulation. Walk at a comfortable pace for 20 minutes, gradually building up walking time and distance. Compression stockings and comfortable shoes with good support should be worn when walking and when up and about. These patients should avoid wearing high heels, as they limit the ability of the calf pump to function. Patients with leg edema should wear compression hosiery when traveling, especially in an airplane or on any long trip involving a prolonged period of sitting. During the trip, periodic walking, stretching, and leg exercises may be helpful.[23,24]

Compression Therapy

Compression is often the key therapy in resolving and controlling edema. Failure to consistently and properly use compression garments is one of the leading causes of failure of edema treatment. Compression improves venous and lymphatic return and counters the effects of ambulatory venous hypertension.[25,26] Compression also helps drain fluid from the tissue, minimizes capillary leakage, and helps reduce discomfort.

Depending on the patient's condition, external wraps can be used for compression or support and applied at high or low compression. Elastic systems offer compression with high pressure at rest and high but less pressure with muscle contraction (multiplayer wraps). A support system is inelastic (relatively rigid) giving very little pressure at rest and high pressure with muscle contraction (paste wraps).[30] The challenge of effective therapy is attaining and sustaining the correct level of compression.

Prior to using compression therapy, the arterial circulation in the lower legs must be assessed. The pulse exam includes locating and grading bilateral femoral, popliteal, dorsalis pedis, and posterior tibial artery pulses. (See Clinical Wisdom in Chapter 7.) When a pulse is diminished or absent, it indicates partial or complete arterial occlusion. If unable to palpate the dorsalis pedis or posterior tibial pulse, a Doppler assessment should be performed. An Ankle/Brachial Index (ABI = Doppler ankle arterial pressure divided by Doppler brachial arterial pressure) is often used to determine the presence and/or severity of peripheral arterial disease. The results of the ABI allow determination of the amount of compression therapy that can be safely applied to reduce lower extremity edema. The ABI can be misleading in cases where the arteries are poorly compressible such as some instances of diabetes and severe atherosclerosis. The latter two will usually give an ABI that is higher than expected. Guidelines for interpretation of ABI:

ABI 0.8–1.0, use high compression
ABI 0.5–0.8, use light compression
ABI 0.5 or below, compression is contraindicated, refer immediately to a vascular specialist for a thorough evaluation of peripheral arterial disease (PAD)

A baseline measurement of the circumference of both lower legs should be taken during the initial assessment and at regular intervals throughout compression therapy. Lower leg edema can be measured by using a measuring tape on the leg circumference at the largest portion of the calf (10 cm below the inferior rim of the patella) and the smallest portion of the ankle (5 cm above the superior rim of the lateral malleolus) as demonstrated in Figure 10-3.

If the edema is pitting, the severity of edema is often graded on a 4 point scale from slight to very severe.

0 to 1/4 inch pitting	= 1+ (mild)
1/4 to 1/2 inch pitting	= 2+ (moderate)
1/2 to 1 inch pitting	= 3+ (severe)
>1 inch pitting	= 4+ (very severe)

Compression therapy works best with exercise to facilitate the movement of excess fluid from the lower extremity. Several options are available for vascular support during compression therapy, depending on need (Table 10-5). The level of compression needed for edema secondary to venous disease, for example, is approximately 40 mm Hg at the ankle, ending with 12–17 mm Hg at the tibial plateau. A lower level of compression may be necessary for a patient with dependent edema who is unable to ambulate as the calf pump interaction is not present.

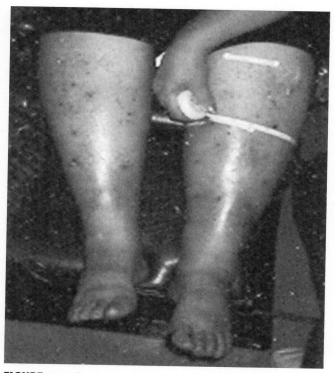

FIGURE 10-3 Correct measurement of an edematous leg. (Copyright © Evonne Fowler, RN, CNS, CWOCN)

The four classes of compression stockings used are as follows:

Class 1: 14–18 mm Hg
Class 2: 18–24 mm Hg
Class 3: 25–35 mm Hg
Class 4: 40–50 mm Hg

Elastic and inelastic systems are therapy options for lower leg edema. Inelastic or short stretch bandages are relatively rigid systems, which provide very little pressure at rest and high pressure with muscle contraction. Inelastic systems such as short stretch bandages and paste wraps provide low compression. These devices provide external support and inhibit swelling of the legs.

Inelastic Systems

Paste bandages, such as the Unna's Boot™, are widely used in the treatment of leg ulcers and control of edema. The boot was developed in the 1880s by a German physician, Paul Gerson Unna, and consists of fine gauze impregnated with zinc oxide, gelatin, and glycerin (some varieties also include calamine). The gauze is applied without tension in a circular fashion from the foot to just below the knee. Paste bandages do not provide compression; however, as the boot dries and stiffens, the leg cannot continue to swell. Application of a compression wrap over the boot or use of a paste bandage with an elastic based cloth bandage will provide mild compression. A paste bandage is routinely changed every 7–10 days.[31]

Other options for inelastic systems are the CircAid™ Compression Bandage System (Coloplast, Marietta, GA) and the Reid Sleeve (Pennisula Medical, Scotts Valley, CA). The CircAid™ Compression Bandage System is a nonelastic, adjustable garment. The system consists of a legging with interlocking, nonelastic bands and Velcro fasteners that surround the leg. By adjusting the bands as the size and shape of the leg changes, it provides constant compression and gradient counter pressure. The garment is washable, easy to put on, take off, and adjust without assistance as shown in Figure 10-4. The Reid Sleeve is a custom-made tubular extremity device with a nylon and Velcro outer shell and a foam insert with a Lycra lining.

Elastic Systems

Multilayered bandages are commonly used for treatment of edematous legs with weepy skin or wounds.[27] Elastic bandages and multilayer wraps are considered moderate to high compression. The multilayer bandages provide graduated, sustained compression through the application of a series of layers, providing protection, padding, and compression. The dressing is removed every 7–14 days. If excessive drainage, strong odor, or clinical signs of infection are present, more frequent change may be necessary. The fit of the wrap must be checked frequently for tightness and slippage. If the wrap feels too tight, if the feet feel numb or tingle, if the toes look cyanotic (blue), or if there is severe discomfort, these symptoms are often due to swelling of the leg from prolonged standing or sitting with the legs dependant.

TABLE 10-5 Vascular Compression Stockings Options

Level of Support	Examples	Recommendations for Use
Light support (8–14 mm Hg)	Fashion hosiery (has limited longevity)	Edema prevention for persons engaged in activity/work that requires standing/sitting with minimal activity
Antiembolism stockings (16–18 mm Hg)	Jobst™, Sigvaris™, or equivalent	Deep vein thrombosis prophylaxis
	TED stockings, prophylaxis only	Nonambulatory clients with edema
Low compression (18–24 mm Hg)	Jobst™, Sigvaris™, Juzo™, or equivalent	Nonambulatory clients with edema failing 16–18 mm Hg stockings
	Elastic wraps Paste bandage	Clients with dependent edema
Low to moderate compression (25–35 mm Hg)	Jobst™, Sigvaris™, Juzo™, or equivalent	Edema secondary to venous insufficiency
	Custom Fit Double reverse elastic wrap Four-layer bandage	Edema in client able to participate in exercise rehab
Moderate compression (30–40 mm Hg)	Jobst™, Sigvaris™, Juzo™, or equivalent	Edema with/without ulceration
	Custom stocking (Jobst™), Sigvaris™, Juzo™, or equivalent)	Edema that persists in spite of lower-level compression options
	Four-layer bandage (i.e., Profore™	Ulcer failing to heal (may be venous or other)
High compression (40–50 mm Hg)	Jobst™, Sigvaris™, or equivalent Custom stockings (Jobst™, Juzo™, Sigvaris™, or equivalent)	Edema secondary to lymphedema

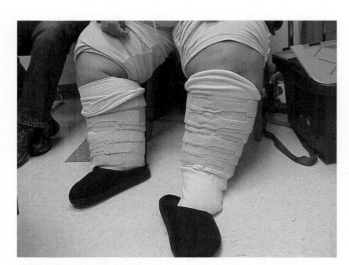

FIGURE 10-4 CircAid™ in place.

Before removing the wrap have the patient lie down and elevate legs above the heart or as high as possible for 30–60 minutes. This should reduce the swelling. Encourage the patient to relax, and if necessary, take pain medication. If the swelling is not relieved, remove the wrap. Remind the patient not to be alarmed if the wrap has a strong odor on removal. The leakage of fluid from the skin may cause staining of the wrap and odor after being in place for an extended time. Dispose of the soiled bandages in an airtight plastic bag and spray the room with air freshener. Wash and dry the leg and foot well (shower or bath). Inspect the legs and feet for signs of change such as decrease in swelling, improvement in the appearance of the skin, or deterioration (more skin irritation, necrotic areas). Place a dressing over the affected area and cover with a compression type bandage (elastic wrap). Continue with the exercise program and leg elevation. Schedule an appointment for evaluation with the health-care provider.

Compression Stockings

Compression stockings provide an external support around the legs, which helps compress the leg muscles, and squeeze the veins to push the blood forward. Compression stockings can also help reduce the diameter of enlarged superficial veins of the legs. In most cases, below the knee graduated compression will provide enough resistance to control the edema. Compression stockings have graduated pressures with the greatest compression at the ankle, gradually decreasing the pressure gradient as the stocking goes up the leg. The squeeze at the ankle is greater than the squeeze at the calf or the thigh. By wearing compression stockings, less blood pools in the legs and swelling (edema) is reduced. For best results in controlling edema and healing open wounds, compression stockings should be put on first thing in the morning shortly after getting out of bed and worn until bedtime. When the edema is reduced and the dermatitis and/or ulcer is healed, compression stockings should be worn regularly to prevent recurrence.

Elastic compression support stockings can be categorized from Class 1–4 and are available in a variety of types, styles, and colors. See table 10-5. This will vary from manufacturer to manufacturer. Choose the stocking to meet the specific therapeutic needs of the patient. Fashion support hosiery provides 8–16 mm Hg support and is indicated for conditions requiring very low compression. Antiembolism stockings provide 16–18 mm Hg and are indicated for DVT prophylaxis and the nonambulatory person. 20–30 mm Hg is the most common compression used in our clinic. Most people can wear below the knee ready-made compression stockings. When measuring for standard size compression stockings, measure the largest circumference of the calf, smallest circumference of the ankle, the length from the bottom of the heel to the bend of the knee, and the foot size. Some patients with large legs or bottle-neck shape legs may need to be fitted with custom-made stockings.

CLINICAL WISDOM

Compression stockings are often difficult for the patient and/or care provider to put on. The health-care professional should demonstrate how to apply the stockings. Turn the stocking inside out to the heel; place both thumbs inside the stocking, and stretch it over the toes. Slip the stocking on the foot and over the heel. Once the stocking is on the foot, begin to pull the top of the stocking over the foot and up the leg. The stocking should fit about 2 finger widths below the crease of the knee. If the stocking is pulled too tight up the leg, there may be an excess of material. Do not turn the top of the stocking on itself, as it might cause constriction. Take the stocking down the leg to the ankle. Begin pulling the stocking up the leg without tension. Smooth out any creases or wrinkles in the stocking.

Compression stockings should be removed at night. Check the manufacturer's suggestion on laundering the stockings. Cleanse and dry the legs and feet, inspect for any skin problems and apply a moisturizing cream to the feet and the legs and rub in well. Patients should have at least two pair of stockings, one to wear and one to wash. Most stockings fit snugly for about 3–6 months. If they seem very easy to put on, the stockings are probably stretched out and need to be replaced.

A helpful tip for compression stockings that are difficult to get on or feel tight is: Encourage the patient or caregiver to be calm and patient while putting on the stockings. It can be frustrating and takes time and practice to learn the easiest technique to put the stockings on. If the patient can put on his or her own stockings, have the patient sit in a comfortable position to best reach the foot. If unable to reach the foot in a sitting position, have the patient stand, leaning against the wall and place the foot on a chair, bringing the hands and feet closer in order to put on the stockings as shown in Figure 10-5A–D. Using a thin silk stocking or liner on the foot before putting the stockings is helpful. Wearing rubber gloves helps to grip the stockings when pulling them on and powdering the foot and leg can aid in putting on the stockings. Figure 10-6 shows a stocking butler that is available to aid in applying the stockings. Compression stockings are often viewed as too difficult to apply and remove, uncomfortable, and too expensive. When the patient cannot or will not wear compression stockings other methods of compression may be implemented.

Elastic bandages (Ace™ Wraps) can provide mild compression when applied properly. They are inexpensive and readily available. Proper application of the bandage can be problematic. Frequent reapplication of the wrap may be necessary due to inconsistent pressure and slippage of the wrap. Compression wraps should be applied within 20 minutes of waking and placing the feet in a dependent position. When applying elastic bandages, manufacturer's guidelines should be followed. Elastic bandages can be applied in spiral fashion or in a figure of eight fashion. Elastic tapered or straight tubular bandages, available in a range of sizes, can also provide light compression (Tubigrip™ Shaped Support Bandage [TSSB]). The tubular dressing provides a consistent pressure to the leg. It is easy to apply and remove and stays in place with movement. It is a low-cost alternative for some patients. To assure proper fit, a tension guide is used to measure the leg. Added compression can be obtained by applying extra layers of the tubular bandages. When the dressing becomes stretched, it is discarded and a new one applied.

Compression Pump Therapy

Sequential compression therapy for the management of lower extremity edema is available. Its use is controversial, however, particularly in lymphedema. The system includes a leg sleeve and a pump. The leg sleeve (either knee-high or thigh-high) is divided into a 3, 5, or 10-chamber style, with peak pressures of 45–60 mm Hg at the ankle. The sleeve inflates first at the ankle, followed 2.5 seconds later at the calf chambers, and 3 seconds later at the thigh chambers. Each successive chamber inflates less, and the total inflation is sustained for approximately 5 seconds, followed by complete deflation. The cycle repeats every 7–8 seconds for the prescribed treatment period, which may range from 1 to 2 hours twice per day. Clients should be encouraged to follow treatment with application of either a fitted stocking or a compression bandage to maintain edema control. Use of compression therapy at night while sleeping is not recom-

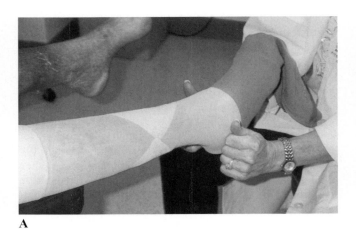

A

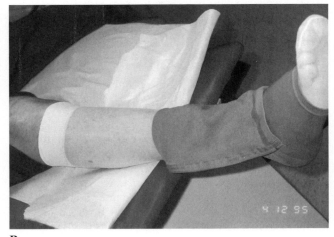

B

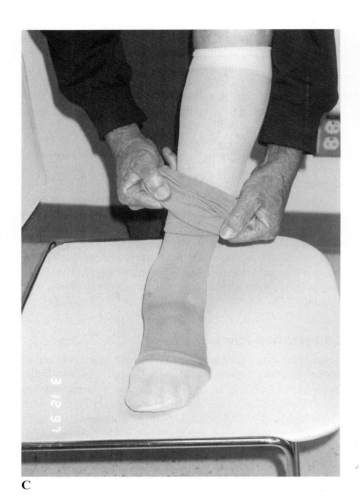

C

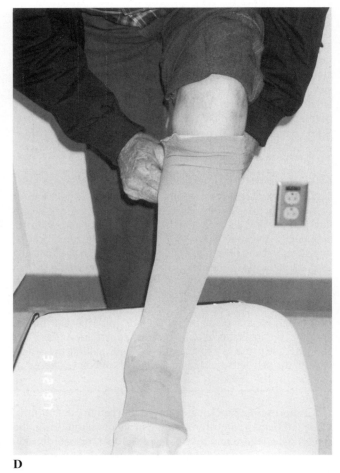

D

FIGURE 10-5 Applying compression stocking. **A.** Turn stocking inside out. A liner makes pulling on stocking easier. (Note dressing under the lining. The liner keeps the dressing positioned correctly.) **B.** Work stocking gradually up leg, smoothing out all wrinkles. (Stockings are available with or without toes.) **C.** Knee-high stockings halfway up showing zipper rear closure. **D.** Stocking extended to below the bend on the knee. Patient is positioning stocking. (Copyright © Evonne Fowler, RN, CNS, CWOCN)

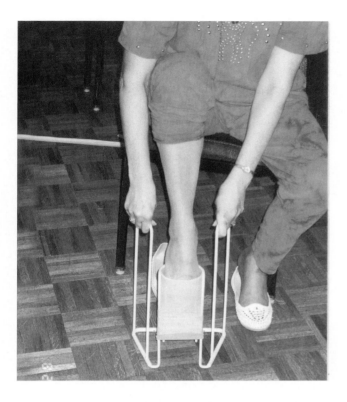

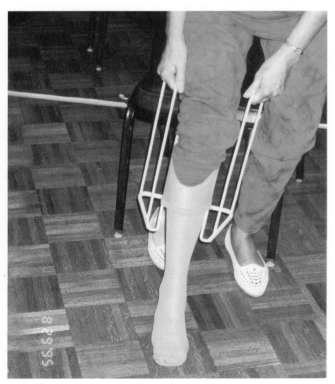

FIGURE 10-6 Using a stocking butler. (Copyright © Evonne Fowler, RN, CNS, CWOCN)

mended. Clients with congestive heart disease should be monitored closely for tolerance of the extra intravascular fluid burden with compression therapy.[31]

Skin Care

Lower leg edema can cause skin problems such as pruritus, dryness, scaling, cracks, fissures, oozing of fluid from under the skin, and open wounds as shown in Figures 10-7A, B. Healthy skin is clean, dry and supple. To keep the skin on the legs and feet soft, wash daily with a mild soap and water, dry, and apply a moisturizing cream. After washing the feet, while the skin is still damp and soft, a coarse emery board can be used to reduce callous formation on the feet. A foot file or emery board can also be used to smooth the nail edges and reduce the nail thickness. Keeping the legs and feet warm can improve circulation. Foot gear should be worn to avoid injury to the feet.

Dry, itching, and scaly skin can be treated using a hot oil treatment to the feet and legs daily for 1 week. Before reclining for the night, bathe or shower. After drying off, rub warm mineral oil thoroughly into the feet and legs. Cover the feet and legs with a plastic wrap (i. e., Saran Wrap) to seal in the oil. Put on a pair of cotton socks. Remove the plastic wrap in the morning, wash and dry the feet well, and apply a thick moisturizing cream on the skin. Fig 10-7 B-C shows the same legs after treatment. If skin maceration occurs discontinue the plastic wrap. If a fungal infection is present, an antifungal cream may be necessary. In severe cases of fungal infection and infection of the nails, an oral antifungal agent may also be employed (see Chapter 20).

Figures 10-8 A and B show severe cases of venous dermatitis. Venous dermatitis may be extremely painful with blistering and weeping skin. Using compression to control swelling can aid in the healing of venous dermatitis and/or ulcers. A paste bandage or multilayer wrap may be applied. The paste bandage has a calamine or zinc oxide base that aids in the healing of the irritated skin by its soothing and drying effect. It can also decrease the itching of the skin. A compression wrap (Coban) or a short stretch bandage should be placed over the paste wrap to provide sustained compression. The multilayer wrap absorbs more fluid and provides sustained compression over a longer period of time. A cream or advanced wound care product can be applied to the irritated skin prior to applying the multilayer wrap.

Venous dermatitis can also be treated with a 1 week course of Domeboro Soaks. Domeboro is an astringent agent made of aluminum acetate and used as a drying agent to decrease weeping, irritated, and itchy skin. The legs and feet should be soaked for 15 minutes twice a day (i.e., morning and evening). A soft foam, cloth, or brush can be used to cleanse the irritated skin. Dry the skin and apply an ointment to the irritated skin and cover with a petroleum type dressing and a compression wrap. Apply a topical antibiotic ointment (Bactroban™) in the morning. Bactroban™ has documented effectiveness against resistant staph and strep and other common organisms found on the skin. Avoid Neosporin and Bacitracin ointment, as they are known skin

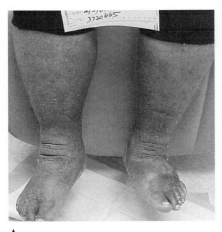

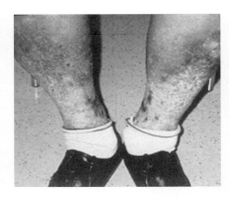

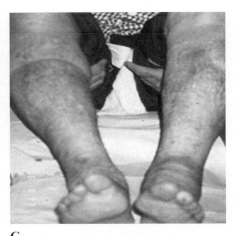

A   B   C

FIGURE 10-7 A. Bilateral edematous legs with dry cracks and fissures. **B.** Edematous legs with dry skin and wounds present. **C.** The same legs as in figure B., 1 week later after using a moisturizing cream and multilayer wraps. (Copyright © Evonne Fowler, RN, CNS, CWOCN)

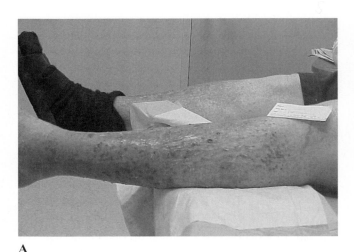

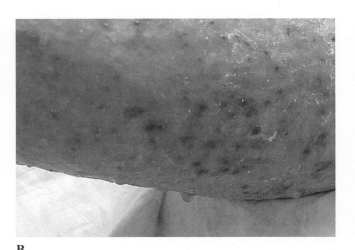

A   B

FIGURE 10-8 A. Venous dermatitis with weeping and oozing. **B.** Close up of oozing/weeping present with venous dermatitis. (Copyright (c) Evonne Fowler, RN, CNS, CWOCN)

sensitizers. After the ointment, apply a petroleum-based dressing (e.g. Adaptic Johnson & Johnson) to keep the ointment in contact with the skin. Cover with a roller gauze and apply a compression wrap (Tubigrip or Ace wrap). In the evening, repeat the same procedure but use a corticosteroid ointment (Lidex ointment or Fluocinonide, Triamcinolone, or over the counter 0.1% hydrocortisone) in place of the antibiotic ointment. Do not apply the corticosteroid to open wounds. A course of oral antibiotics and/or prednisone may also be necessary.[32]

Special Concerns in Lymphedema

Good skin care is essential for persons with lymphedema. The characteristic appearance of the skin of a person with lymphedema often has a woody hardness, and superficial

hyperkeratosis as shown in Figures 10-9A and 10-9B. The skin becomes brown, and may be fissured or have numerous folds in the skin. Mushroom like papules of tissue can be present. Swelling is usually nonpitting and involves the feet as well as the legs. The diameter from the ankle to the knee is almost uniform rather the inverted champagne bottle-like fibrosis seen in long standing venous disease. Swelling of the feet with close apposition of the toes provides an ideal environment for fungal growth. Fissures can act as portals of entry for bacterial infection that can progress to cellulitis.[33]

Use of some or all of the above techniques by themselves have not been shown to be all that beneficial for lymphedema. One of the main problems is that, by the time seen, lymphedema is usually pronounced. Compression, compression garments, exercise, and elevation are helpful. Lym-

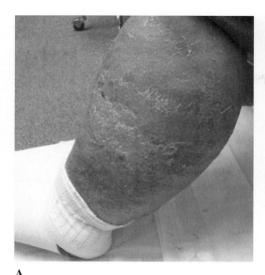 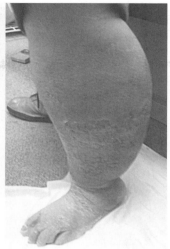

A   B

FIGURE 10-9 A. Lymphedema, woody hardness and superficial hyperkeratosis present. Notice the mushroom-like papules on the lower leg. **B.** Lymphedema. (Copyright © Evonne Fowler, RN, CNS, CWOCN)

phedema is a condition that cannot be cured and requires lifelong treatment to control symptoms that, if left untreated, would progressively worsen. The aim of treatment is to stabilize the edema and empower the patient with the necessary skills to undertake self-care. Four components of treatment are used to achieve this goal: care of the skin, compression and support, lymphatic massage, and exercise.

Massage, complex decongestive physiotherapy, is a particular type and requires a skilled and certified therapist to instruct and administer.[28] It is now the standard of care for lymphedema in this country, and has been the standard in other countries for some time.[29] Usually, a patient with lymphedema will be started on a course of complex decongestive physiotherapy along with temporary short stretch compression bandages. After the course of complex decongestive physiotherapy and bandaging is finished, the patient will be graduated to a compression garment, exercise, and elevation. Massage may be reinstituted for an acute exacerbation.

A condition often misdiagnosed as lymphedema is lipedema. Lipedema is abnormal fatty tissue accumulation in the lower extremities. Usually the dorsum of the foot is spared from edema. Massage and compression techniques used for the management of lymphedema are not useful with this condition (Figure 10-10).

Conclusion

Lower leg edema is a condition that is complex to assess and manage. A clinically relevant history and definitive test must be performed to accurately assess and treat the condition. Choosing the appropriate intervention involves understanding the cause for the edema as well as the different management approaches available. The photo case study in this chapter provides an example of choosing the appropriate intervention by understanding the cause of the edema (Figure 10-11 A, B, C).

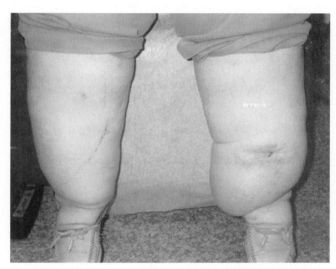

FIGURE 10-10 Lipedema. (Copyright © Evonne Fowler, RN, CNS, CWOCN)

REVIEW QUESTIONS

1. At what level of leg elevation is the client likely to receive edema reduction?
   a. resting on a footstool while watching television
   b. horizontal when in bed (legs neutral to the heart)
   c. elevated 18 cm (7–8 inches) above the level of the heart
   d. watching television in a standard recliner chair
2. A new client has arrived and is determined to have dependent edema and is not ambulatory. What level of compression should you recommend?
   a. Class 4: 40–50 mm Hg
   b. Class 3: 25–35 mm Hg
   c. No level of compression will be tolerated and, therefore, none will be recommended
   d. Class 1 or 2

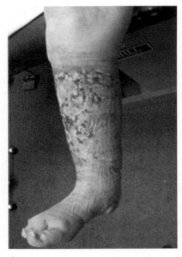

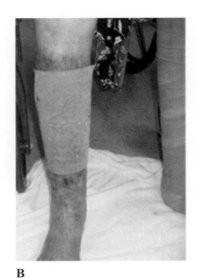

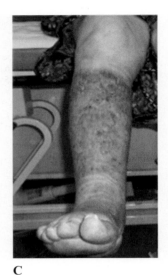

A   B   C

FIGURE 10-11 A. At initial treatment. The patient, a 74-year-old retired surgical nurse was seen and referred to the wound care program with 1) severe mixed venous and lymphatic edema of the legs, 2) history of bilateral deep vein thrombosis following hip surgery 10 years ago, and 3) numerous episodes of wound sepsis and cellulitis legs for the past 10 years. **B.** Silver plated dressings. Following evaluation by the wound care team, the patient was placed in layered compression dressings over silver plated cloth dressings (to control cellulitis and bacterial burden of the wounds). Absorbent cellulose dressings were placed over the silver where exudate was most marked at the beginning of therapy. The patient was also instructed on diet and exercise, and leg elevation. **C.** The healed leg just prior to fitting with an elastic stocking. Subsequently, after 2 months, the leg healed and patient was fitted with 30–40 mm Hg venous compression stockings and instructed on daily use of skin moisturizers. Patient continued her leg elevation and exercise. One year later there have been no recurrent wounds and no episodes of cellulitis.

3. A client has been followed for 4 months and has persistent edema, despite a comprehensive program of leg elevation, exercise, and compression wraps. What is the next plan of action?
   a. Continue to compression wrap
   b. Review client medication profile
   c. Refer to appropriate provider
   d. Advise client that you are unable to help and that he or she will need to see someone else
   e. c, d
   f. a, b, c

REFERENCES

1. Gloviczki P, Calcagno D, Schirger A, et al. Noninvasive evaluation of the swollen extremity. J Vasc Surg 1989;9(5):683–90.
2. Mayberry JC, Moneta GL, Taylor LM Jr, Porter JM. Fifteen-year results of ambulatory compression therapy for chronic venous ulcers. Surgery 1991;109:575–81.
3. Swedborg I. Effects of treatment with an elastic sleeve and intermittent compression. Scand J Rehab Med 1984;16:35–41.
4. Marston WA, Carlin WE, Passman MA et al. Healing rates and cost efficacy of outpatient compression treatment for leg ulcers associated with venous insufficiency. J Vasc Surg 1999;30(3):491–8.
5. Barker WF. In: Bergan, JJ and Yao, JST. *Venous Problems*. Chicago: Mosby Year Book, , 1978, p. 384.
6. Stadelmann WK, Digenis AG, Tobin G. Impediments to wound healing. Amer J Surg. 1998;176(Suppl2A):407.
7. Kawahara A, Yasuoka Y, Kawada H. Regulation of the interstitial fluid volume. Nippon Rinsho 2005;63(1):31–6.
8. Kistner RL. Diagnosis of chronic venous insufficiency. J Vasc Surg 1986;3(1):185–88.
9. Browse NL. The diagnosis and management of primary lymphedema. J Vasc Surg. 1986;3(1):181–4.
10. Fairbairn JF. Clinical manifestations of peripheral vascular disease. In: Juergens, JL et al. *Peripheral Vascular Diseases*. Philadelphia: WB Saunders, 1980, p. 38.
11. Casley-Smith JR. *Modern Treatment for Lymphedema*, 5th ed. Adelaide, Australia: The Lymphedema Association of Australia, Inc., 1997, P. 4–78.
12. O'Donnell TF, Yeager A. In: Haimovici, H. et al. *Haimovici's Vascular Surgery*, East Norwalk: CT Appleton and Lange, 1989, p. 1005–7.
13. Guyton AC, Hall JE. *Textbook of Medical Physiology*. Philadelphia: WB Saunders, 1996, pp. 161–181, 183–197, 308–313, 178, 270.
14. Zierler RE, Strandness DE. Hemodynamics for the vascular surgeon In: Moore WS, *Vascular Surgery* 4th ed. Philadelphia: Saunders, 1993, pp. 179–203.
15. Miller TA. A surgical approach to lymphedema. Am J Surgery 1977 Aug; 134(2):191-195.
16. Allegra C., et al. *Vasomotion and Flowmotion*. Farmington, CT: S Karger Publishers, 1993.
17. Guyton AC. Interstitial fluid pressure. Physiol Rev. 1971;51:527.
18. Alexander House Group. Consensus paper on venous ulcers. Phlebology, 1992;7:48–58.
19. Anderson FA, Spencer FA. Risk factors for venous thromboembolism. Circulation, 2003;107:I9–I16.
20. Clement DL. Management of venous edema: insights from an international task force. Angiology. 2000;51(1):13–7.
21. Xia ZD, Hu D, Wilson JM, et al. How echographic image analysis of venous oedema reveals the benefits of leg elevation. J Wound Care (England), 2004;13(4):25–8.

22. Kan YM, Delis KT. Hemodynamic effects of supervised calf muscle exercise in patients with venous leg ulceration: a prospective controlled study. Arch Surg, 2001;136(12):1364–9.

23. Cesarone MR, Belcaro G, Nicolaides AN, et al. The LONFLIT4-Concorde—Sigvaris Traveno Stockings in long flights (EcoTraS) Study: A randomized trial. Angiology 2003;54(1):1–9.

24. Schobersberger W, Mittermayr M, Innerhofer P, et al. Coagulation changes and edema formation during long-distance bus travel. Blood Coagul Fibrinolysis. 2004;15(5):419–25.

25. Felty CL, Rooke TW. Compression therapy for chronic venous insufficiency. Semin Vasc Surg (United States) 2005;18(1):36–40.

26. Armstrong DG, Nguyen HC. Improvement in healing with aggressive edema reduction after debridement of foot infection in persons with diabetes. Arch Surg, 2000;135(12):1405–9.

27. Browne AC, Coutts P, Sibbald RG. Compression therapies. In: Krasner DL, Rodeheaver GT, Sibbald RG, eds. *Chronic Wound Care: A Clinical Source Book for Healthcare Professionals,* 3rd ed. Wayne, PA: HMP Communications, 2001, pp. 517–524.

28. Wiersema-Bryant L, Kraemer BA. Management of edema. In: Sussman C, Bates-Jensen BM, eds. *Wound Care: A Collaborative Practice Manual for Physical Therapists and Nurses,* 2nd ed. Gaithersburg, MD: Aspen Publishers, 2001, pp. 235–256.

29. Ukat A, Konig M, Vanscheidt W, et al. Short-stretch versus multilayer compression for venous leg ulcers: A comparison of healing rates. J Wound Care (England) 2003;12(4):139–43.

30. Faria D, Fowler E, Carson SN. Understanding edema and managing the edematous lower leg. In: Krasner DL, Rodeheaver GT, Sibbald RG, eds. *Chronic Wound Care: A Clinical Source Book for Healthcare Professionals,* 3rd ed. Wayne, PA: HMP Communications, 2001, pp. 525–540.

31. Sibbald RG, Williamson D, Falanga V, Cherry GW. Venous leg ulcers. In: Krasner DL, Rodeheaver GT, Sibbald RG, eds. *Chronic Wound Care: A Clinical Source Book for Healthcare Professionals,* 3rd ed. Wayne, PA: HMP Communications, 2001, pp. 483–494.

32. Cheville AL, McGarvey CL, Petrek JA, et al. Lymphedema management. Semin Radiat Oncol. 2003;13(3):290–301.

33. Casley-Smith JR. Changes in the microcirculation at the superficial and deeper levels in lymphoedema: The effects and results of massage, compression, exercise and benzopyrenes on these levels during treatment. Clin Hemorheol Microcirc (Netherlands), 2000;23(2–4):335–43.

Management of the Wound Environment with Dressings and Topical Agents

Geoffrey Sussman

CHAPTER OBJECTIVES

At the completion of this chapter, the reader will be able to:

1. Describe the properties of ideal dressings.
2. Explain the differences between inert dressings and interactive dressings
3. List the classifications and uses of the six main dressing product groups.
4. Describe new products on the market.
5. Explain the role of topical antiseptics in wound management.

Introduction to Moist Wound Healing

Traditional theory has always indicated that:

- Wounds should be kept clean and dry so that a scab can form over the wound
- Wounds should be exposed to the air and sunlight as much as possible
- When tissue loss is present, the wound should be packed to prevent surface closure before the cavity is filled
- Wounds should be covered with dry dressings

The clear disadvantage of these principles is that the scab, which is made up of the dehydrated exudate and dead tissue, is a barrier to healing. Scabs delay healing by hindering the movement of epidermal cells, which can lead to poor cosmetic results and scarring. Exposure to air reduces the surface temperature of the wound, further delaying healing. Reduced surface temperature can also result in peripheral vasoconstriction, affecting the flow of blood, oxygen, nutrients, and other factors to the wound. Exposure to air will also increase fluid loss and dry the wound surface. When a wound is packed with dry gauze, the quality of healing is impaired by the adhesion of the gauze to the surface of the wound. This causes the wound to dry out and increases the risk of trauma on removal of the packing.

Wounds managed in a moist environment covered by an occlusive dressing do not form a scab, so epidermal cells are able to move rapidly over the surface of the dermis through the exudate that collects at the wound-dressing in-

terface. The application of a totally occlusive or semipermeable dressing to the wound can also prevent secondary damage as a result of dehydration. Moist wound healing simplifies debridement by assisting in the autolytic debridement of wounds. It facilitates wound cleaning, since wound on-toxi is part of the healing cascade, and has been shown to carry a number of growth factors essential to the healing of wounds. It also protects granulating tissue and encourages epithelialization.

The initial work in understanding the functions of occlusive dressings began in 1948 with the publication by JP Bull of a paper in the *Lancet* entitled, "Experiments with occlusive dressings of a new plastic."[1] Bull's work examined the physical properties of a nylon derivative film. He concluded that the film was an effective barrier against microorganisms and that its physical properties, in particular the water vapor permeability of the film, made it a suitable material for wound dressings. He tested it on human skin to find out whether the film's permeability to water vapor would be sufficient to prevent the skin from becoming soaked. He found that the bacterial flora of healthy skin under the occlusive dressing became modified, *Staphylococcus aureus* disappeared, and the presence of a variety of organisms was reduced.

RSF Schilling studied the use of the nylon derivative film in a specifically industrial setting, conducting a comparative trial with a waterproof dressing in common use at the time.[2] The study concluded that the healing times of wounds treated with the nylon derivative film were significantly shorter. George D. Winter was able to pinpoint specific differences between the healing of wounds left open to the air and those kept under an occlusive dressing in his study "Formation of the scab and the rate of epithelialization of superficial wounds in the skin of young domestic pigs." [3] The experiment showed that wounds healing under moist conditions healed 50% faster than wounds open to the air and healing under dry conditions. Winter's work has since formed the basis of the principles of modern moist wound management.

This work was extended in 1963 by Cameron D. Hinman and others from the Division of Dermatology at the University of California, who published a study on the "Effects of air exposure and occlusion of experimental human skin wounds." [4] In effect, Hinman repeated Winter's work, but this time with healthy adult male volunteers. He again used a sterile polyethylene film in artificially-made wounds that were then either occluded or allowed to heal open to the air. Occluded wounds in Hinman's study showed the same rate of healing as those in Winter's work, confirming the earlier results.

The aim of wound management is to provide the appropriate environment for healing by both direct and indirect methods, together with the prevention of skin breakdown. The history of the development and use of dressings has seen an evolution through many centuries—from inert and passive products, such as gauze, lint, and fiber products, to a dazzling range of modern moist wound dressings.

Inert Wound Dressings

Examining their continued use as described by Turner,[5,6] it is clear that there are a number of drawbacks to the use of passive products, particularly gauze. Being a fibrous material, gauze tends to shed very readily and, as such, will contaminate the wound. Gauze is highly absorbent and, as a primary dressing, will tend to dry the surface of a wound rapidly. Gauze is permeable to bacteria, and moist gauze tends to be an environment that promotes bacterial growth. These bacteria can subsequently penetrate and ultimately contaminate the wound. Gauze is also adherent and will traumatize the wound further on removal, risking pain and damage to granulating tissue. There are now alternatives to gauze swab used both to clean wounds and as primary dressings. Non-woven swabs that do not shed fibers are now available.

In addition to gauze and lint, there are available other simple, modified absorbent pads covered with a perforated plastic film to prevent adherence to a wound, such as Melolin and Telfa, which are used as both primary and secondary dressings. They are used in minor wounds and in those wounds with low exudation. Paraffin (petrolatum) gauze dressings, developed by Lumiere in World War I, were among the earliest modern dressings. Many variations have been developed over the years by changing the loading of paraffin in the base. In general, these dressings produce a waterproof paraffin cover over the wound, which can lead to maceration because paraffin may not allow water vapor and exudate to pass through. These products are permeable to bacteria and are known to adhere to the wound, causing trauma on removal. Their use is limited to simple, clean, superficial wounds and minor burns. They are also used over skin grafts. They need to be changed frequently to avoid drying out, and always require a secondary dressing.[7] One alternative has been an equivalent dressing produced from synthetics fibers tightly meshed and impregnated with an emulsified base, lipid-colloid, or silicone. Examples are Adaptic, Aquaphor gauze, Mepitel, and Urgotul.[8,9,10]

Ideal Dressing

The properties of an ideal dressing have been described as follows:[5]

- Will remove excessive on-toxi from the wound, but will not allow the wound to dry out, maintaining a moist environment
- Will allow gaseous exchange so that oxygen, water vapor, and carbon dioxide can pass into and out of the dressing
- Will be thermally insulating, maintaining the wound core temperature at approximately 37°C
- Will be impermeable to microorganisms, minimizing contamination from outside the wound
- Will be free from either particulate or toxic contamination
- Will be nontraumatic and will not adhere to the wound, so that no damage is done to granulating tissue on removal

In addition, the following properties should be considered when selecting the appropriate dressing:

- Will provide the proper environment for healing
- Will be user-friendly (to ensure compliance)
- Will have ease of application and removal
- Will simplify treatment (minimal changes of dressing)
- Will be cost effective (i.e., total management cost)
- Will be compatible with the wound
- Will have minimal need for secondary dressings
- May be suitable for combined use with compression therapy
- May be used in infected wounds
- Will remain in place

Modern Interactive Wound Dressings

Modern interactive dressings provide the wound environment for healing to take place. The term interactive is used because they are not passive but feature the ability to work actively with wound properties like wound fluid, tissue, cells and growth factors within the wound to enhance healing. Different dressing characteristics are exploited by choosing dressings based on the wound properties to be addressed. For example, interactive dressings vary in their ability to absorb exudates: some have no ability to absorb, some will cope with low levels of exudates and some are able to absorb large volumes of exudate. Each individual dressing type will be discussed with its specific properties to guide the clinician.

Modern interactive dressings are classified in six specific groups each having some different properties. The classification is presented based in the first instance on their relation to wound exudates from products for dry or low exudating wounds to those for low to moderate levels of exudates and those for moderate to high levels. The other group of products are ones that are used to donate moisture in dry or sloughy wounds.

Film Dressings

Film dressings are thin membranes coated with a layer of acrylic adhesive. They are moisture vapor-permeable and oxygen-permeable. These properties vary in only minor ways from brand to brand. One important difference in selecting a dressing is moisture vapour permeability. The moisture vapour permeability is measured with the moisture vapor permeability test.[12] This test is performed under the conditions specified in the *British Pharmacopoeia 1980*. In this test, the cup is either placed upright, so that any loss of fluid occurs by evaporation, or inverted, so that the liquid comes in contact with the membrane. It should be noted that the loss of water vapor from intact skin is 240–1,920 g/m²/24 hours, and the water vapor loss from an open wound is about 4,800 g/m²/24 hours. Table 11-1 lists film dressing products and their vapour permeability. Films are impermeable to microorganisms and moisture. Film dressings are flexible and allow easy assessment of the wound because they are transparent. They do not have the ability to absorb any exudate. The latest films being developed, however, have very high moisture vapor permeability; as such, they can be used on more highly exuding wounds. Film dressings are elastic and extensible.[11,12]

Effects

The effects of film dressings include the following:

- Provide a moist environment
- Enable autolytic debridement
- Provide protection from chemicals, friction, shear, and microbes
- Transmit oxygen into and carbon dioxide and water vapor out of the dressing
- Function as a secondary dressing

Indications for Use

Film dressings are indicated in the management of minor burns and simple injuries (e.g., scalds, abrasions, and lacerations), and as a postoperative dressing over suture lines. They are also used as a protective layer over intravenous catheters, and for the prevention and treatment of superficial pressure areas.[13,14] A film dressing enables autolytic debridement and provides a moist wound healing environment.

TABLE 11-1 **Comparison of Moisture Vapor Permeability of Different Wound Dressings**

Dressing Brand	Cup Upright g/m²/24 hours	Cup Inverted g/m²/24 hours
OpSite	839	862
Bioclusive	547	605
Ensure	436	436
Opraflex	456	477
DermaFilm	422	472
Tegaderm	794	846

Indications for Discontinuation

An increased level of exudation that causes pooling under the dressing can lead to maceration of both the wound and the surrounding skin. Use of the dressing should also be discontinued if the wound becomes clinically infected.

Method of Application

An appropriately sized piece of film should be chosen to cover the wound and provide an overlap of at least 4–5 cm from the edge of the wound. It is important to ensure that the skin around the wound is dry and free from oils or cream, because these may reduce adherence to the skin. The bottom backing paper is removed, and the film dressing is carefully applied over the wound, while maintaining light but firm stretching of the edges of the film to prevent it from sticking to itself. Once the dressing is in place, the upper cover is removed.

Film dressings are also used as a secondary dressing over hydrogels and alginates, as an alternative to tape for holding a dressing in place, and to provide a waterproof covering. In addition to standard film dressings, island versions are now available, comprising a simple absorbent pad covered by the film. These products are able to absorb small amounts of wound exudate and allow their use in wounds with low on-toxi. Simple, small versions of these dressings can also replace plastic first aid strips, with the advantage of not causing the maceration common with plastic strips.

Precautions and Contraindications

Film dressings may remain in place for up to 1 week or even longer. Changing of the dressing will depend on the position, type, and size of the wound. It is important to remove film dressings with care. The dressing should not be pulled back across itself. Care should be exercised in applying film dressings to damaged or frail skin and in those with fine and dry skin. Because of the risks of further damage on removal The film should be carefully pulled away from itself while applying light pressure to the center of the film dressing until it has been entirely removed. Film dressings are not recommended for use over deep cavity wounds, full-thickness burns, and wounds showing signs of clinical infection.

Expected Outcomes

Film dressings provide a transparent, flexible, waterproof, and gas-permeable dressing that protect simple wounds and encourage healing. They can be left in place for 1 week or longer and are cost-effective; only one application of the dressing may be needed to manage the wound. When they are used postsurgically over sutures, they can remain in place until the sutures are removed.

Combination Film Dressings

Ventex combines a vented film dressing and an outer absorbent pad. The vented film is applied directly over the wound, about 2–3 cm greater than the wound size; then the absorbent pad is stuck around the outer edge of the film. The pad remains in place until it is saturated with exudate, after which it is changed for a new pad without removing the vented film covering the wound. Viasorb also combines a vented film and absorbent pad, but they are not separate, so the entire dressing is changed. These dressings are indicated for use in exuding wound ulcers, pressure wounds, abrasions, and minor burns.

Foam Dressings

Foam dressings are produced from polyurethane as soft, open cell sheets, and can be composed of one layer or multiple layers. They are also available impregnated with charcoal and with a waterproof backing.[11] Foam dressings meet many of the standard requirements of the ideal dressing. They absorb exudate, protecting the surrounding skin from maceration, and raise the core temperature of the wound, maintaining a moist environment. There are many polymer products with a similar appearance to foam on-toxic, however these are hydroactive dressings that adsorb moisture into their structure and swell up. They are absorbent dressings, but they are not interchangeable with foam dressings in every situation. Foams are useful as both primary and secondary dressings.

Effects

The effects of foam dressings include the following:

- Provide a moist environment
- Provide high absorbency
- Conform to body shape
- Provide protection and cushioning
- Produce no residue
- Do not adhere to the wound
- Provide thermal insulation
- Transmit moisture vapor out of the dressing
- Require no secondary dressings

Indications for Use

Foams are indicated for a wide range of minor and major wounds, including exuding wounds (both superficial and cavity types), leg ulcers, decubitus ulcers, and sutured wounds. They can be used over skin grafts, donor sites, and minor burns. They also may be used as secondary dressings over amorphous hydrogels. Foams improve the functioning of amorphous hydrogels by removing excess exudate from the wound and raising its core temperature. This assists with autolysis. Foams can also be used around tracheostomy tubes and other drainage tubes and catheters.[15–17] Table 11-2 shows the forms used by different manufacturers.

Indications for Discontinuation

Foam dressings should be discontinued when the level of exudation cannot be absorbed into the dressing in less than a 24-hour period.

Method of Application

The foam dressing is placed over the wound, allowing for a margin at least 3–4 cm greater than the size of the wound. The dressing should be secured in place with one of the following:

- In patients with fine or easily damaged skin:
  1. Lightweight cohesive bandage
  2. Tubular bandage
- In other patients:
  1. Adhesive tape (hypoallergenic)
  2. Tubular or lightweight cohesive bandage

Foam dressings can be used under compression bandaging and as a secondary dressing for amorphous hydrogels and alginates. In the case of a cavity device, select the appropriately sized device to fit comfortably into the cavity and insert it into the wound. It may remain in place for 1–4 days or until saturated with on-toxi. A sheet foam dressing can remain in place for up to 7 days or until the exudate has saturated to the edge of the dressing. Foam dressings can also be cut in shapes to allow better application to specific parts of the body. Foams can be cut in an "L" shape for

TABLE 11-2   Foam Dressings

Dressing Brand	Main Constituent	Forms
Allevyn	Polyurethane	Three layers Film/hydrophilic foam/plastic net
Curafoam	Polyurethane	Single uniform structure
Hydrasorb	Polyurethane	Single uniform structure
Lyofoam	Polyurethane	Two layers hydrophobic foam/ hydrophilic contact layer
Lyofoam Extra	Polyurethane	Three layers film/hydrophobic foam/hydrophilic contact layer

application to fingers or toes. The method is to wind the shaft of the L shape around the finger or toe and secure with tape. The foot of the L is then folded over to complete the dressing and held in place with tape. A square piece of foam can also be cut diagonally to the center and folded within itself to form a cup that can be used over a healing wound.

Precautions

Foam dressings are of little value on dry wounds with a scab or eschar. Cavity dressings similarly should not be used alone in a dry cavity, but they may be used with an amorphous hydrogel. There are no specific contraindications for the use of foam dressings. The author has clinical experience with a local reaction causing erythema, but this may have been due to an allergic reaction or to the increased blood flow caused by the thermal effect of the dressing.

Expected Outcomes

Foam dressings provide a satisfactory primary and secondary dressing for a wide range of wounds. They aid in the removal of exudate, raise the core temperature of the wound, and protect the wound from external irritation. They will also protect the healthy skin around the wound from becoming macerated by the wound on-toxi.

Hydrogels

Hydrogels are a group of complex organic polymers with a high water content, from 30% to 90%. These broad classes of polymers are swollen extensively in water, but they do not dissolve. They are three-dimensional, water-swollen, cross-linked structures formed from hydrophilic homopolymers or copolymers. There are two types of hydrogels: amorphous and fixed. Amorphous hydrogels are nonfixed, three-dimensional macrostructures consisting of hydrophilic polymers or copolymers. The polymers absorb water, progressively decreasing viscosity. They are free-flowing and will easily fill a cavity space. Fixed, three-dimensional macrostructures are usually manufactured in the form of a thin, flexible sheet. These gels swell, increasing in size until the gel is saturated; they do not change their physical form as they absorb fluid. Table 11-3 shows a comparison of the water content of some amorphous hydrogel products.

Effects

Hydrogels provide moisture to dry wounds, but they are also able to absorb fluid. They have the following useful effects:

• Provide a moist environment
• Aid in autolytic debridement
• Conform to body shape
• Do not adhere to the wound
• Provide moisture and absorb moisture
• Relieve pain

Indications for Use

Amorphous hydrogels are generally indicated for dry and sloughy wounds to rehydrate the eschar and enhance rapid

TABLE 11-3 Water Content of Amorphous Hydrogel Products

Dressing Brand	Chemical Type	Water Content
Carrasyn Gel	Triethanolamine, Carbomer 940, Acemannan	95%
DuoDERM Gel	Sodium carboxy-methylcellulose, Pectin, Propylene glycol	81.5%
IntraSite Gel	Modified carboxymethyl-cellulose, Propylene glycol	78%
Purilon Gel	Carboxymethyl-cellulose, Calcium Alginate	90%
Solugel	Propylene Glycol Saline	75%
Saf-Gel	Carbomer Propylene Glycol Sodium/ Calcium Alginate	86%

debridement by autolysis. They are used on leg ulcers, pressure wounds, extravasation injuries, and necrotic wounds. They facilitate granulation and epithelialization by preventing the wound from drying out. They are used on simple-thickness and partial-thickness burns and on pressure wounds. Gels are used to prevent the drying out of such tissue as tendon. Gels are also a useful carrier of topical drugs to be applied to wounds, such as metronidazole and proteolytic enzymes. Hydrogels are suitable for use in infected wounds. Amorphous hydrogels are also used for management of the lesions of chickenpox and shingles.[13,18–21]

Indications for Discontinuation

Use of amorphous hydrogels should be discontinued if on-toxi from a wound is excessive. It is generally thought that the use of sheet hydrogels should be stopped if a wound is clinically infected.

Method of Application

Amorphous hydrogel should be applied to a wound to a minimum thickness of 5 mm and covered with a secondary dressing. The choice of secondary material depends on the type and position of the wound, as well as availability and cost. The author has found that foams are the most satisfactory secondary dressings, by virtue of their properties of exudate absorption, thus maintaining the integrity of the gel for a longer time, protecting the surrounding skin from maceration, and raising the core temperature to aid in autolysis. Other products, such as film dressings, hydrocolloids, and simple nonadherent dressings, may be used. Gauze is also a suitable secondary dressing.

Hydrogels can remain in place for a clean wound for up to 3 days; they should then be removed by irrigation with water or saline. When used for the lesions of chickenpox, they should be applied four or five times a day.

The sheet hydrogels are placed over the wound with at least 3–4 cm coverage greater than the wound. They are held in place with tape or a light cohesive bandage, depending on the skin of the patient. In difficult areas, they should be held in place with a retention sheet, such as Hypafix, Fixomull, or Medipore. The sheet hydrogels do not cause maceration of the surrounding tissue. The sheets are left in place, depending on the wound type and on the amount of exudation, but generally should be removed after 3–4 days. For some superficial burns, they may remain in place for up to 7 days. When removed, they cause no discomfort and leave no residue on the skin.

Precautions and Contraindications

Because of their occlusive nature, sheet hydrogels should not be applied to clinically infected wounds without coverage with systemic antibiotics. Amorphous hydrogels containing propylene glycol should not be used in patients known to be sensitive to propylene glycol. Sheet hydrogels should not be applied over small deep cavity wounds or clinically infected wounds. They should also not be used in heavily exuding wounds.

Expected Outcomes

Hydrogels aid in the rapid removal of necrotic tissue and rehydrate dry wounds, assisting in granulation and reepithelialization. In burns, they reduce heat and pain. The thicker sheet hydrogels, when used in the management of superficial pressure wounds, also reduce pressure by reducing friction and shear forces.

Hydrocolloids

Hydrocolloids are a combination of gel-forming polymers with adhesives held in a fine suspension on a backing of film or foam. Hydrocolloid dressings are composed of a backing of polyurethane foam or film and a mass containing, in most cases, sodium carboxymethyl-cellulose and other gel-forming agents, such as pectin, gelatin, and elastomers. These form a self-adhesive mass.[11] These products are also available as granules, powder, and paste. When placed on a wound, exudate combines with the polymers to form a soft gel mass in the wound.

Hydrocolloids were originally introduced as Stomahesive to protect good skin around ileostomies and colostomies. They vary from being occlusive to being semipermeable.

Hydrocolloids come in a wide range of shapes, sizes, and types. These include regular thickness, thin, bordered, padded, and in combination with alginates, as well as for cavity use as pastes, granules, and powder. When removed, the gel remaining is yellow and malodorous, but not infected. The presence of bacteria under hydrocolloid dressings does not retard healing.

When applied to an exuding wound, the dressing absorbs exudate and forms a gel. This gel will vary in viscosity, depending on the brand of dressing. The dressing does not adhere to the wound itself, only to the intact skin around the wound.

Effects

Hydrocolloids have the following effects:[22,23]

- Provide a moist environment
- Aid in autolytic debridement of wounds
- Conform to body shape
- Protect from microbial contamination
- Provide a waterproof surface
- Require no secondary dressing

Table 11-4 shows a comparison of hydrocolloid products.

Indications for Use

Hydrocolloids are indicated in the management of superficial leg ulcers, burns, donor sites (when hemostasis has been obtained), and pressure wounds. They may be used in small-cavity wounds, in combination with hydrocolloid paste, powder, or granules. Thin versions of these dressings can be used as dressings over sutures after minor and major surgeries.[13,16,24–26]

Indications for Discontinuation

Hydrocolloids should be discontinued on surface granulation of the wound or if hypergranulation occurs.

Method of Application

Hydrocolloids on a superficial wound should be applied to the wound with a margin of at least 3–4 cm greater than the wound size. The skin should be dry to ensure good adhesion, and it is preferable to place one-third of the dressing above the wound and two-thirds below the wound; this will prolong the wear time of the dressing. The dressing may remain in place for 5–7 days or until strikethrough has occurred (i.e., exudate has migrated to the outside edge of the dressing). The dressing should be carefully removed and the

TABLE 11-4   Comparison of Hydrocolloid Dressing Products

Dressing Brand	Main Component	Backing	Forms
Comfeel	Sodium carboxymethyl-cellulose	Polyurethane film	Standard, thin
DuoDERM	Carboxymethyl-cellulose	Polyurethane foam/film	Standard, thin
Tegasorb	Polyisobutylene	Polyurethane film	Standard, thin
Restore		Polyurethane film	Standard, thin

wound irrigated with warm saline before applying a new dressing.

In the case of small-cavity wounds, if relatively moist, the cavity should be filled with hydrocolloid paste, powder, or granules and covered with a sheet of hydrocolloid dressing. With a minimally to moderately exuding cavity, hydrocolloid paste should be inserted carefully and the wound again covered with a sheet of hydrocolloid dressing. The dressing should be changed after 3–4 days by irrigation of the cavity with warm saline and gentle removal of any remaining product before applying the new dressing.

Thin hydrocolloid dressings are applied after surgical wound suturing and, in most cases, can remain in place and be removed at the time of suture, clip, or Steri-Strip removal. These dressings have the advantage of being both flexible and waterproof. They require no secondary dressing, and help to appose wound edges by distributing tension at the suture line across the surface area of the dressing.

Precautions and Contraindications

Care should be taken when using these dressings on patients with thin and fragile skin, because the dressings may cause further damage on removal. There are no absolute contraindications for use of hydrocolloids, but they are not indicated for use in heavily exuding wounds or in clinically infected wounds. They also are not considered suitable for deep-cavity wounds.

Expected Outcomes

Hydrocolloids help to remove necrotic tissue and slough from a wound and encourage angiogenesis and granulation of the wound. The presence of colonized bacteria in a wound does not contraindicate the use of these dressings.

Alginates

Alginates are the calcium or calcium/sodium salts of alginic acid and are composed of mannuronic and guluronic are acids obtained from seaweed, primarily the genus *Laminaria*. When applied to a wound, the sodium ions present in the wound exchange for the calcium ions, producing a hydrophilic gel and providing calcium ions to the wound. This is part of the mechanism by which alginates act as a hemostat.

Alginates are gelling polysaccharides. They are available as either calcium alginate, which is a mixture of sodium and calcium alginate in textile fiber sheets, or as a loose packing ribbon. Alginates combined with activated charcoal are also available. Alginates are combined with some hydrocolloid dressings to aid their fluid-handling properties.

Sodium alginate has the chemical formula $C_6H_7O_6Na$, with a molecular weight in the range of 32,000 to 200,000. Sodium alginate has a complex structure, consisting essentially of two uronic acids, D-mannuronic acid and L-guluronic acid. The ratio of these isomers varies, depending on the species of seaweed from which the alginate is extracted and the method of production. Gels that are rich in mannuronic acid form soft amorphous gels that partially dissolve or disperse in solutions containing sodium ions. Alginates that are rich in guluronic acid tend to swell in the presence of sodium ions, while retaining their basic structure.[11,27]

Effects

Alginates have the following useful effects:

- Provide a moist environment
- Provide a high absorptive capacity
- Conform to body shape
- Protect from microbial contamination
- Provide hemostasis
- Do not adhere to the wound

Table 11-5 shows a comparison of the chemical composition of different alginate products.

Indications for Use

Alginates are used in exuding wounds, such as leg ulcers, cavity wounds, and pressure wounds, and at donor sites (as a hemostat postsurgically) and other bleeding sites. They may be used in infected wounds.[13,17,28–31]

Indications for Discontinuation

Alginates should be discontinued if the amount of exudate is insufficient to cause the fiber to gel. Alginates should not be premoistened with saline before application to a wound.

Method of Application

Sheet alginates should be placed in and conformed to the shape of the wound, and covered with a secondary dressing,

TABLE 11-5   Comparison of Alginate Chemical Composition

Name	Guluronic Acid (%)	Mannuronic Acid (%)	Calcium Alginate (%)	Sodium Alginate (%)
Algoderm	58	42	100	
Curosorb	68	32	100	
Kaltostat	66	34	80	20
CarboFlex	66	34	80	20
Sorbsan	34	63	100	
TegagenHG (discontinued)			100	
Tegagen HI			100	
Cutinova Alginate	70	30	90	10
Calgicare	65	35	80	20

such as a foam, or a nonadherent dressing. Depending on the condition of the patient's skin, the sheets can be held in place with tape or a light cohesive bandage. If the wound is extremely exudative, an additional covering with a simple absorbent pad is appropriate. In the case of a cavity wound, rope or packing alginate material should be placed gently in the cavity, taking care not to pack the material tightly into the space. When used on a donor site, the sheet alginate should be applied to the donor area after skin harvesting and covered with a film dressing or foam. This aids in rapid hemostasis and provides an environment conducive to reepithelialization of the skin. The dressing, in general, should remain in place in clean wounds for no longer than 7 days or when the gel loses its viscosity (this will vary, depending on the level of exudation from the wound). Dressings on clinically infected wounds should be changed daily. The alginate is removed by simple irrigation of the wound or cavity with warm saline. Freeze-dried alginates may be applied not only to the wound but also to cover the periwound skin, because they gel only over the wound, thus protecting the periwound skin from maceration.

Precautions and Contraindications

Dressings on clinically infected wounds should be changed daily, with consideration given to the concurrent use of systemic antibiotics by the prescriber. There are no known contraindications for the use of alginates. They are not suitable for use in dry wounds or in wounds with thick, black eschar.

Expected Outcomes

Alginates absorb exudate and provide a moist environment for granulation. They are suitable for use in infected wounds and are very effective in the management of bleeding, particularly in postnasal surgery, postbiopsy, and when applied to donor sites. They provide a comfortable dressing, and rapid healing of the skin is expected.

Alginate dressings have known hemostatic properties, and factors such as wound type, position, and depth will determine the best dressing to apply over a bleeding wound. One study examined the absorption of blood by moist wound healing dressings and confirmed the action of some alginate dressings.[32]

Combination Alginates

Manufacturers have combined alginates with other products to enhance the effects of each.

Calcium/Sodium Alginate Combination

CarboFlex is a combination of calcium and sodium alginate and Aquacel in a fiber sheet, bonded to a layer of activated charcoal and an outer layer of viscose. This product is a highly absorbent dressing with the ability to absorb odor. It is indicated in infected, malodorous wounds, fungating neoplasms and ulcers, and superficial pressure wounds.

The sheet should be applied to the surface of the wound, ensuring that the white alginate layer is in contact with the

wound, and that the dark charcoal layer is on the outside. The product is covered with a secondary dressing and held in place with tape or a light cohesive bandage. The dressing should be changed every few days, depending on the level of exudate and extent of infection. The use of systemic antibiotics in clinically infected wounds is indicated. The dressing is easily removed, and removal may be assisted by irrigation with warm saline. This dressing, as with other alginates, is of no value in a dry wound with thick, dark eschar.

Alginate/Hydrocolloid Combination

The combining of hydrocolloids and alginates in one dressing, such as in the Curaderm and Comfeel Plus products, enhances the dressings' properties and allows them to be used in more excessively exudative wounds. They are similar in appearance to standard hydrocolloid sheets, and are used in a manner similar to that of hydrocolloids. The combination dressings, however, can remain in place for a longer period of time because of their superior absorptive properties.

Hydroactive Dressings

Hydroactive dressings have some similarities to hydrocolloids, however they are not gel-forming products. They act by absorbing exudate into the structure of the dressing, swelling as the liquid is absorbed. They maintain a moist environment at the interface of the wound.

Hydroactive dressings are multilayered dressings of highly absorbent polymer gel with an adhesive backing. These dressings are composed of an outer polyurethane film membrane, combined with a polyurethane gel and other absorbents (e.g., sodium polyacrylate). They are semipermeable and adhere to the skin. They are available in a number of forms, including cavity fillers, foam-like, and thin types.[11]

Effects

Hydroactive dressings have the following useful effects:

* Provide a moist environment
* Provide high absorbency
* Provide a waterproof surface
* Regain their shape when stretched
* Aid in autolysis
* Leave no residue
* Are semipermeable to moisture vapor

Indications for Use

Hydroactive dressings are indicated for use on exuding wounds, including leg ulcers, pressure wounds, minor burns, and exuding cavity wounds. They are of particular use over joints, such as the elbows, knees, fingers, toes, and ankles, because of their ability to expand and contract without causing constriction.[33–35]

There are foam-like forms of hydroactive dressings. These should not be confused with typical foam dressings, because they react to exudate in a manner different than foams, by adsorbing the exudate into their structure. This can be observed by their change of shape. Hydroactive dressings absorb exudates rapidly, regardless of the amount of exudation.

Indications for Discontinuation

Use of hydroactive dressings should be discontinued for wounds with little or no exudation, or if the dressing is unable to absorb the amount of exudate being produced by the wound.

Method of Application

The method application of hydroactive dressings varies, depending on the type of dressing used. Tielle is placed over the wound so that the central island of dressing completely covers the wound. Allow for a margin 2–3 cm greater than the wound size, and then adhere it to the surrounding skin. Cutinova Hydro is applied directly to the wound, allowing for a margin of 3–4 cm of dressing around the wound. It is preferable to warm the edges of the dressing slightly with the hand to aid adhesion. Allevyn plus Cavity, because of its ability to absorb exudate and expand, should be placed carefully into the cavity, not occupying more than 33% of the space. The outer wound should be covered with a suitable dressing, such as Allevyn Thin or Cutinova Hydro.

These dressings may remain in place for up to 7 days, depending on the amount of exudation. They should be removed carefully from patients with thin or easily damaged skin. When removed, they will leave no residue, however, it may still be necessary to irrigate the wound with warm saline before redressing if there is exudate present on the surface. Biatain and PolyMem are also hydroactive dressings, and are available as both a standard and an adhesive sheet. They are applied in a manner similar to the other hydroactive dressings.

Precautions and Contraindications

Hydroactive dressings are not considered suitable for use on clinically infected wounds or nonexuding wounds. There are no known contraindications, however care should be taken when using these products on fine and easily damaged skin.

Expected Outcomes

Hydroactive dressings absorb on-toxi and provide a moist environment for granulation and epithelialization. They provide a comfortable dressing that will remain in place and have a good wear time.

Miscellaneous Dressings

With research and development in constant progress, new products have entered the market that do not fit into any of the standard groups mentioned. These products have properties resembling those of existing groups but are composed of different materials. Examples are the matrix products that include Promogran™ and Oasis™. Promogran is a freeze-dried matrix composed of collagen and oxidized regenerated cellulose (ORC) formed into a sheet. When applied to a moist wound, it forms a soft biodegradable gel. It binds growth factors and inactivates matrix metalloproteinases (MMPs). Promogran is used in partial-thickness and full-thickness wounds and is applied every 2 to 3 days. Oasis is derived from porcine small intestinal submucosa. It acts as an extracellular matrix and can be used in a range of wound types including ulcers, pressure wounds, and minor burns. It is reapplied at each dressing change on areas no longer covered by the previous application.

Exu-dry is a nonadherent absorbent pad composed of an outer layer of perforated polyethylene-laminated rayon and an inner layer of absorbent rayon/polypropylene blend, with a cellulose backing that wicks wound on-toxi and holds large quantities of fluid. It is indicated in highly exudative wounds, particularly burns.[36] Mepore is a similar nonadherent pad with greater absorbency than simple exudate dressings.

Hydrofibers

Hydrofibers are alginate like in appearance they are fibrous in nature but are composed of the polymer CMC. Hydrofiber dressings are activated by moisture in the wound and they are able, as a polymer, to absorb and trap within their structure the moisture from the wound. While they have a similar ability to absorb exudates as do alginates they do not have the haemostatic property of alginates. There is at this stage only one type of hyrofiber available.

Aquacel is a nonwoven, 100% sodium carboxymethyl-cellulose, spun into fibers and manufactured into sheets and ribbon dressing. This product mirrors the properties and actions of alginate dressings, however it differs in that it rapidly absorbs exudate vertically and will not absorb laterally. It retains fluid within the structure of the fiber. The sodium carboxymethyl-cellulose fibers swell and convert into a gel sheet. This product is indicated in heavily exuding wounds, such as leg ulcers, pressure wounds, cavity wounds, minor burns, and donor sites.

The dressing is applied to the wound, allowing a dressing margin 2–3 cm greater than the wound size or wound cavity. The dressing can remain in place for 1 to 3 days, depending on the on-toxi amount and when the product is saturated. Similar to freeze-dried alginates, hydrofibers can be applied to the periwound skin and the wound without the risk of maceration.

CombiDERM is a multilayer absorbent pad combining a semipermeable hydrocolloid border with absorbent padding of hydrocolloid particles and a nonadherent cover against the wound. This product is highly absorbent and is able to hold the exudate within the dressing, preventing maceration to the surrounding skin. It maintains a moist environment. It is indicated on highly exuding wounds, pressure wounds, leg ulcers, and surgical wounds. It can be used as a secondary dressing over cavity wounds.

Versiva Dressing is a sterile wound dressing consisting of a thin, perforated adhesive layer, a nonwoven fibrous blend layer (with Hydrofiber), and a top polyurethane foam-film layer. The dressing absorbs wound fluid, creates a moist environment, and aids in autolytic debridement.

Alione is a hydrocapillary dressing consisting of a number of fibers combined in the capillaries of the dressing. The capillaries transport the exudate away from the wound, keeping it moist without being wet. The top surface is film, and the core is a hydrocapillary pad; a wound contact layer and either an adhesive hydrocolloid or a microporous skin protection layer complete the dressing.

Silicone

Silicone is a major component of scar-reduction dressings, which are used to reduce hypertrophic and some keloid scars. These dressings (Table 11-6) should be applied as soon as possible after sutures or clips are removed from the incision site. They are removed every 1–3 days, after which the area is washed and the dressing is re-applied. The same piece of dressing may be used for about 7 days, and then a fresh piece is applied. Silicone is also used as the surface layer on a number of dressings, from tulles to foams. The silicone helps maintain adhesion of the dressing onto the skin; however, silicone does not stick and allows atraumatic removal. The dressing also reduces pain at the wound interface and on removal of the dressing.[9,10,37,38]

Topical Antimicrobials

Excessive bioburden on the surface of a wound can retard healing, but difficulties also arise when topical antiseptics are applied that can have a negative effect on wound healing. In recent years, new topical preparations have been developed based on silver and iodine. The following section will discuss use of these topical antiseptics in different forms.

Silver

Silver is one of the oldest elements known to man. It is found naturally and also associated with copper and gold, or as the ore argentite. Metallic silver exists as two isotopes and is inert in this form. In the presence of fluid, silver ions are present as charged ions $Ag+$, $Ag++$, and $Ag+++$, and can form some soluble and mostly insoluble compounds. Silver is used in an elemental form, such as nanocrystalline or foil, in inorganic compounds, such as silver oxide and silver nitrate, and as organic complexes. A number of these forms are used in silver dressings and contrast with silver sulfadiazine, delivered as a cream or tulle. The decreased size of silver particles leads to an increased proportion of surface atoms compared with internal atoms It is believed that the nanocrystalline structure is responsible for the rapid and long-lasting action. The significance of the forms of silver used in dressing products is discussed below.

Silver has been used for many years, and it has proven antimicrobial activity. It is broad spectrum and inactivates almost all known bacteria, including methicillin-resistant *staphylococcus aureus* (MRSA) and vancomycin-resistant enterococci (VRE). No cases of bacterial resistance have been documented. Silver has been used in the treatment of burns as a silver sulfadiazine cream, and this cream has also been applied to some wounds. The difficulty in applying cream to a mucous surface is that it will cause the development of mucilaginous slough. The development of a range of modern silver dressings overcome this difficulty by delivering varying levels of silver directly from the dressing. The base dressings include hydrocolloids, alginates, tulles, hydroactives, foams, gels, and polyethylene mats. The amount of silver and method of action vary greatly between these dressings. Some release silver into the wound, whereas others maintain the silver within the dressing and kill bacteria as they are absorbed into the dressing. Contemporary silver dressings allow for continued release for up to 7 days. The amount of silver contained in the various dressings varies greatly.

In addition to the relationship between silver content and antimicrobial activity, according to Thomas et al, there are other factors that influence the ability of a dressing to kill micro-organisms.[41] These include:

- Distribution of silver in the dressing
- Chemical and physical form (metallic, bound or ionic)
- Dressing's affinity to moisture

The level of silver content contained in dressings varies greatly. The mode of action also varies; that is, some release silver into the wound, others partly release the silver and hold some in the dressing, and others keep the silver within the dressing. Dressings with the silver content concentrated on the surface or those with the silver in ionic form have performed well in tests due to the level of ionic silver released from the dressing.

Indications for Use

Silver dressings are indicated for the reduction of bioburden in surface or cavity wounds in colonized and infected wounds. They may also be used to reduce the risk of infection over skin grafts, burns, and injection sites. The choice of silver dressing will depend on the wound type, level of exudate, and depth.

TABLE 11-6   Silicone Dressings

Brand	Manufacturer	Type
Mepitel	Mölnlycke	Tulle
Mepilex	"	Foam
Mepilex border	"	Combination
Mepilex Transfer	"	Foam
Mepilex Thin	"	Foam
Cica Care	Smith & Nephew	Scar reduction dressing
Mepiform	Mölnlycke	"

Indications for Discontinuation

In general, silver dressings are for short-term use to reduce the bioburden. They are then discontinued to allow other products, depending on the wound, to assist in the healing of the wound.

Method of application
Precautions and Contraindications

See Table 11.7.

Conclusion

The decision whether to use a silver dressing depends on the wound itself, the clear presence of high levels of colonization, and if the wound is clinically infected. Silver should not be the automatic choice in all wounds. Once the decision to use a silver dressing has been made, the product type must reflect the wound environment itself, tissue, depth, and level of exudate.

Topical Antimicrobials—Iodine

Iodine in its various forms has been used as a topical antiseptic since 1840. The newer forms of iodophors have been used since the 1950s. Most of these new forms combine iodine in a complex with a polymer (e.g., Povidone, Cadexomer), which slowly releases the iodine. Iodine is active against bacteria, mycobacteria, fungi, protozoa, and viruses. There is no evidence of resistance to iodine. Povidone iodine comes in many forms, including skin paints, throat gargle, scrub wash, and ointments (Table 11-8).

Cadexomer iodine is the combination of the polysaccharide polymer cadexomer and iodine at low strength. When this product is applied to a wound, the exudate is absorbed into the polymer structure, forming a gel and slowly releasing the iodine at about 0.1% continuously over 72 hours. The product will reduce the level of slough in the wound, absorb on-toxi, is antibacterial, and also stimulates inflammatory growth factors. Iodosorb and Iodoflex are two forms of this product.

Indications for Use

Providone iodine is used as a skin prep pre-procedure in a 10% solution, if applied to a wound it should be diluted to 1% or if used in full strength then applied left in place for 3 to 4 minutes and them washed off. It is also used as a cream at 5% and a gargle diluted to 0.5% by dilution prior to use.

Cadexomer iodine is used on sloughy leg ulcers, pressure wounds, and other nonhealing wounds.

Indications for Discontinuation

Some patients experience pain on initial application of the product. In most cases, this subsides after 1–2 hours. Some patients with a low pain threshold may find it necessary to discontinue use of the product.

Method of Application

Cadexomer iodine is applied directly to the wound as either powder, paste, or dressing. It is covered with a simple nonadherent dressing and left in place for up to 3 days. At dressing changes, the product, initially brown in color, becomes a white, paste-like gel that is washed away, and a fresh application of the product is applied to the wound.

Precautions and Contraindications

Cadexomer iodine should not be used on children younger than 12 years of age, or on patients with a known allergy to iodine. No more than 50 grams as a single dose or 150 grams in a week should be used.

Expected Outcomes

The dressing should reduce odor, level of slough, and pain. The wound should show increased granulation and a decrease in size.[42]

Charcoal

Charcoal is used in combination with a number of dressings, including foam and alginates. It is also available in specific dressings (e.g., Actisorb Plus). The main function of charcoal dressings is to absorb odor.

Collagen

Collagen is a vital structure in wound healing; when crosslinked, it is essential to the tensile strength in a wound. There are dressings composed of a collagen matrix, either bovine collagen or avian collagen. The role of the collagen is to stimulate fibroblast activity and improve the healing cascade. There are many collagen products on the market. Their clinical role has yet to be clarified.

Hyaluronic Acid Derivatives

Hyaluronan is a carbohydrate component of the extracellular matrix that plays an important role in the healing cascade. Forms of hyaluronic acid derivatives are in use clinically, but their role in wound healing is not yet clear. Hyalofill is a hyaluronic acid derivative, Hyaff, and is being used in the management of nonhealing neuropathic ulcers and other chronic wounds. It is made available in the form of a sheet or ribbon. Hyalofill should be applied to the entire surface of the wound, where it will absorb wound exudate and form a hyaluronic acid gel. The dressing is left in place for 3 days.[43]

Enzymes

The body produces a number of enzymes. Proteases are protein-splitting enzymes that have both positive and negative action on wounds. Proteolytic enzymes are applied topically to wounds to aid in the removal of slough and breakdown of nonviable tissue. This method of debridement has been used clinically for many years. The enzymes used in commercial products include papain in Accuzyme and Panafil, and collagenase in Santyl.

TABLE 11-7   Silver Dressings

Product name	Acticoat 3 & 7	Acticoat Absorbent	Contreet-H
Product Type	High-density polyethylene	High-density polyethylene	Hydrocolloid
Manufacturer	Smith & Nephew	Smith & Nephew	Coloplast
Silver Type/Content	Nanocrystalline silver Acticoat 107 mg/100cm2 Acticoat 7 120 mg/100cm2 Held in two layers of polyethylene mesh enclosing a single layer of rayon and polyester; silver is released into the wound. Acticoat-7 has an additional layer of silver-coated polyethylene mesh silver; released silver 24 hr 60 PPM.	Calcium alginate coated with nanocrystalline silver 144 mg/100cm2 Released silver at 24 hr 60 PPM as exudate is absorbed into the dressing; silver is released into the wound.	Silver complex 32 mg/100cm2 30% of the silver is released within 7 days; silver is released into the wound.
Method of Use	Before application, moisten with water (must not be saline, as this will react with the silver). Dressing trimmed to wound size; darker blue surface is placed in contact with the wound. Cover with a secondary dressing depending on the level of exudate.	Applied to moderately to highly exudating surface or cavity wounds; covered with a secondary dressing depending on the level of exudate.	Applied to light to moderately exudating surface wounds.
Frequency of changing	Every 3 days (A-3) Maximum of 7 days (A-7)	Every 3 days	Every 4 to 7 days
Contraindications	Patients with known hypersensitivity	Patients with known hypersensitivity	Patients with known hypersensitivity; use with caution on arterial, diabetic lower leg/foot wounds that need review daily
Warnings	Do not use with oil-based products or topical antimicrobials; if applied to lightly exudating wounds, may need to be re-moistened with water.	Do not use in cavity wounds where sinuses are present.	Potential allergic reaction to adhesive or components; must be removed prior to radiotherapy.
Uses	Partial- and full-thickness wounds, e.g., burns, donor sites, and ulcers covered with a secondary dressing	Partial- and full-thickness, moderate to highly exudating wounds	Partial-thickness wounds, e.g., burns, donor sites, ulcers, pressure sores

Product name	Contreet	Polymem Silver	Aquacel Ag
Product Type	Hydroactive	Hydroactive	Hydrofiber
Manufacturer	Coloplast	Ferris	ConvaTec
Silver Type/Content	Silver complex 47 mg/100cm2 on contact with exudate provides sustained release of the silver; 70% of the silver is released within 7 days. Silver is released into the wound.	Nanocrystalline silver 12.4 mg/100cm2; released silver at 48 hr 50 mcg/100cm2; silver is released into the wound, although mostly held in the dressing.	Sodium Carboxymethylcellulose containing silver 8.3 mg/100cm2 Released silver at 24 hr 20 PPM; silver is released into the wound.
Method of Use	Apply on and around surface wounds and lightly packed into cavity wounds.	Apply to the surface or lightly packed (no more than 80%) into moderate to highly exudating wounds.	Apply to the surface or lightly packed (no more than 80%) into moderate to highly exudating wounds.

(Continued)

TABLE 11-7   Silver Dressings *Continued*

Product name	Contreet	Polymem Silver	Aquacel Ag
Frequency of changing	Up to 7 days	Every 3 days	Depending on the wound, may need to be daily, every third day, or up to 14 days in burns
Contraindications	Patients with known hypersensitivity; should not be used with hydrogen peroxide, hypochlorite solutions, or over exposed muscle or bone	Patients with known hypersensitivity	Patients with known hypersensitivity; little value in lightly exudating or dry wounds
Warnings	May cause transient discoloration of wound bed; should be removed prior to radiation therapy, x-rays, etc.	None provided	Should not be used with other wound care products
Uses	Partial- and full-thickness wounds, e.g., burns, donor sites, ulcers, pressure sores; use in moderately to highly exudating wounds	Partial- thickness or cavity wounds, lightly exudating wounds	Partial- and full-thickness wounds, e.g., burns, donor sites, ulcers, and wounds covered with a secondary dressing, depending on the level of exudate

Product name	Avance	Atrauman Ag	Urgotul SSD
Product Type	Foam	Tulle	Tulle
Manufacturer	SSL	Hartmann	Urgo Lipocolloidal
Silver Type/ Content	Silver zirconium phosphate 1.59 mg/100cm2 Released silver at 24 hr 0 PPM; silver is held in the dressing.	Metallic silver 35 mg/100cm2 Released silver at 48 hr 100mcg/100cm2; silver is released into the wound, although mostly held in the dressing.	Silver sulfadiazine 3.75% = 70 mg/100cm2 SSD is held in a lipido-colloid suspension that absorbs moisture and forms a gel. Released silver 50 mcg/100cm2; silver is released into the wound, although partly held in the dressing.
Method of Use	The foam is applied on and around the surface in lightly to moderately exudating wounds.	Apply to the wound and peri-skin, and cover with a secondary dressing, depending on the level of exudate.	Apply to the wound and peri-skin, and cover with a secondary dressing, depending on the level of exudate.
Frequency of changing	Every 3 days	Every 3–7 days	Every 1–2 days
Contraindications	Patients with known hypersensitivity	Patients with known hypersensitivity	Patients with known hypersensitivity; contraindicated in renal, hepatic insufficiency, pregnancy, and neonates
Warnings	Should not be applied to wounds covered with dry scab or hard black necrotic tissue; do not cover with occlusive film, as this reduces water vapor loss	Should not be used in combination with paraffin-containing dressings or ointments	When used on a large surface area and/or for a prolonged period, consider systemic effects of the SSD; should not be used with any other local treatments
Uses	Partial- and full-thickness wounds, e.g., burns, donor sites, ulcers	Complementary use in infected or contaminated partial-thickness wounds, e.g., burns, donor sites, ulcers	Partial- and full-thickness wounds, e.g., burns, donor sites, ulcers

TABLE 11-7 Silver Dressings *Continued*

Product name	Actisorb Plus	Arglase
Product Type	Silver-impregnated activated charcoal	Impregnated film
Manufacturer	Johnson & Johnson	Unomedical
Silver Type/ Content	Silver 2.43–2.95 mg/100cm2 Released silver 24 hr 0 PPM; silver is held in the dressing	Polymer silver 100 mcg/ 100cm2 Released silver 24 hr 8 PPM.
Method of Use	Apply to the wound and peri-skin, and cover with a secondary dressing, depending on the level of exudate.	The film dressing is applied to the intact skin or to the wound; film is adhesive and will stick to the peri-skin.
Frequency of changing	Up to 7 days	Up to 7 days
Contraindications	Patients with known hypersensitivity and lightly exudating wounds	Patients with known hypersensitivity and greater than lightly exudating wounds
Warnings	Must be used intact; do not cut. Should not be used in conjunction with topical preparations or paraffin-containing products.	Should be used on dry or lightly exudating wounds only.
Uses	Used to reduce bacterial colonization in partial- and full-thickness chronic wounds	Postoperative suture lines, securing IV lines

Reprinted with permission from Sussman G. The Australian silver product tour. *Primary Intention.* 2005;13(4):S23-25.

Hypertonic Saline

Hypergranulation develops when epithelium fails to cover the granulating tissue and continues to grow beyond the surface of the wound. Traditionally this tissue has been reduced by the application of silver nitrate or copper sulphate solutions; however, these are toxic chemicals, and use of a less toxic substance is now recommended. It is important to stop this exuberant tissue growth and encourage new epithelium by the application of hypertonic sodium chloride dressings. These dressings are applied daily until the tissue returns to normal surface depth.

Effects

When hypergranulation tissue is present in a wound, it is essential to reduce this tissue and to encourage new epithelium. One method is to apply a dressing composed of an inert fabric impregnated with sodium chloride. (73) The action of hypertonic saline is to draw fluid from surface cells by setting up an osmotic gradient between the highly concentrated solution in the dressing and the lower concentration of the cells. Examples of hypertonic saline are Mesalt and Curasalt.

Indications for Use

Hypertonic saline is used on hypergranulating and necrotic wounds.

Method of Application

The dressing should be applied only to the wound area, and changed every 24 hours.

Indications for Discontinuation

The dressing should be discontinued if the patient experiences pain on application or if the wound is dry.

Expected Outcomes

Reduction in hypergranulation tissue is expected with use of this dressing.[44]

Chapter 2 has additional information about hypergranulation and the effects of dressings.

TABLE 11-8 Iodine Dressings

Brand	Manufacturer	Type
Betadine Povidone Iodine	MudiPharma Various	Povidone Iodine Solution, Cream, Paint, Gargle
Iodosorb	Smith & Nephew	Cadexomer Iodine Paste/powder
Inadine	Johnson & Johnson	Iodine Tulle

Dressing Choice

Wounds are dynamic and, as such, the choice of dressing will vary and change as the wound changes. That choice should be based on the three major aspects of any wound: *color, depth, and exudate* (Table 11-9). Color will vary from pink (epithelializing), to red (granulating), to yellow (sloughy), to black (necrotic). Depth will include superficial, shallow, and deep cavity. Exudation will be none, minimal, moderate, or high. Other aspects to consider are the presence of infection, the tissue surrounding the wound, the need to add graduated compression, the fragility of the skin, and any medical condition that may have an impact on the dressing choice. For example, a patient who has serosanguineous exudate may benefit from use of an alginate dressing that has hemostatic properties or an infected wound may benefit from a silver or codeximer iodine dressing.

Secondary Dressings

The choice of secondary dressing depends on the nature, position, and level of exudate. In general terms, film dressings and nonadherent dressings are suitable for lightly exuding wounds, but not for high levels of exudation. Foam dressings are useful over amorphous hydrogels and alginates (this does not apply to the foam-like hydroactive dressings). The use of gauze as a secondary dressing is limited, especially over hydrogels or alginates, because it reduces the ability of the dressing to function at its optimum level. The other consideration is the method of dressing retention. If the surrounding skin is good, the dressing can be held in place with high-quality tape. If the skin is poor, a tubular bandage or a lightweight cohesive bandage is suitable.

Use of Antiseptics in Wounds

Antiseptics are an essential part of modern clinical practice. Their value in handwashing prior to an aseptic procedure and in the preparation of a patient's skin prior to surgery is clearly documented. Studies have shown that antiseptics reduce the bacteria on the skin, whether resident or transient, by up to 95%. (51.53). There is not, however, a considerable amount of research on the effects of antiseptics on open wounds. There will always be microorganisms present in a wound, to a greater or lesser extent. One of the most prolific researchers and publishers in the area of antiseptics and healing has claimed that antiseptics for this purpose may, in fact, be harmful, in that they damage healing tissue, thus allowing infection to gain a foothold.[45–49] It was Alexander Fleming in 1919 who said that it is essential in the estimation of the value of an antiseptic to study its effects on the tissues, rather than its effect on bacteria. Unfortunately, Fleming's wise counsel of so many years ago has tended to be ignored in modern practice. It is known that the surface of open wounds does not need to be sterile for healing to take place. There is also no evidence to support the notion that dressing changes performed once or twice a day with antiseptics guarantee protection from invasive infection.

The concern with antiseptics is their toxicity. A number of studies, particularly with hypochlorites, have shown major problems. Brennan and Leaper,[46] in their study of the effects of antiseptics on healing wounds, used a rabbit ear chamber that was irrigated with a number of products. The effect on microcirculation was measured using laser Doppler. This study clearly showed the effects of various antiseptics on microcirculation. In particular, Eusol was shown to occlude microcirculation permanently after a 1-minute exposure, with no change in measured flow after 24 hours.[46]

Apart from wound cell toxicity and the depression of collagen synthesis, hypochlorites can cause localized edema, hypernatremia, hyperthermia, and burns. There have also been reported cases of renal failure associated with topical application of chlorinated solutions to pressure sores. This has been attributed to the release of a toxic lipid from bacteria, causing the bacteremia or endotoxic shock known as Schwartzman's reaction.[50]

Hypochlorites are chemically unstable, have a short shelf-life, are rapidly deactivated by organic material, and are not cost-effective, requiring frequent changes of dressing. After all, sodium hypochlorite is a bleach. A further study by Brennan et al[48] showed that, in particular, hypochlorite retards the deposition of collagen, an essential element in the matrix for the healing of wounds by secondary intention.

The commonly used antiseptics fall into the diguanide. This is a chemical term it is ok group, one example being chlorhexidine, which is a bactericidal agent with activity against both Gram-positive and Gram-negative organisms. It is ineffective against acid-fast bacteria, bacterial spores, fungi, and viruses. Skin sensitivity is reported, and chlorhexidine is incompatible with soap; the presence of blood and organic material also will decrease its activity. Antimicrobial activity is best at neutral or slightly alkaline pH. Chlorhexidine is used most commonly as a hand or skin disinfectant.

The second antiseptic group contains the quaternary ammonium compounds, and there are a number of these, cetrimide being one example. Quaternary ammonium compounds are often used in combination with the chlorhexidine-type preparations, an example of which is Savlon. These are also bactericidal against Gram-positive and Gram-negative organisms. They are relatively ineffective against bacterial spores, viruses, or fungi, and some strains of *Pseudomonas aeruginosa* and *Mycobacterium tuberculosis* are resistant. They can also cause hypersensitivity.

The third most commonly used antiseptic is povidone-iodine, an organic complex of iodine with polymers. It is a polyvinyl-pyrrolidine. It is bactericidal and sporicidal, and is active against fungi and viruses. Local irritation and sensitivity may occur, and it may cause burns if applied to denuded areas. It should not be used on patients with goiter. Its absorption may also interfere with thyroid function tests. It is incompatible with alkalis and is used as a skin preparation and a disinfectant.

TABLE 11-9 Dressing Choice

Wound Type (Color/Exudate)	Aim	Wound Depth	
		Superficial	Cavity
Black/low exudate	Rehydrate and loosen eschar. Surgical debridement is the most effective method of removal of necrotic material. Dressings can enhance autolytic debridement of eschar.	Amorphous hydrogels Hydrocolloid sheets Proteolytic enzymes	
Yellow/high exudate	Remove slough and absorb exudate. Use hydrocolloids, with or without paste or powder, for the deeper wounds. Hydrogels, alginates, and enzymes will aid in the removal of the slough and absorb the exudate.	Hydrocolloid Alginate Enzymes Hydroactive Cadexomer Iodine Silver dressings	Hydrocolloids with paste, granules, or powder Hydrogel Enzymes Alginates Hydroactive cavity Hydrocolloid/alginate Foam cavity dressing Cadexomer iodine Silver dressings
Yellow/minimal exudate	Remove slough, absorb exudate, and maintain a moist environment. Hydrogel, in particular, will rehydrate the slough. Hydrocolloids, films, and enzymes also will aid in autolysis.	Amorphous hydrogels Sheet hydrogels Hydrocolloids Film dressings Cadexomer iodine Silver dressings	Amorphous hydrogels Hydrocolloids with paste Enzymes Hydrocolloid/alginate Cadexomer iodine Silver dressings
Red/large amounts of exudate	Maintain moist environment, absorb exudate, and promote granulation and epithelialization. Foam dressings, alginates, and hydroactive dressings help to control exudate; use hydrocolloids with paste, powder, or granules for deeper areas.	Foam Alginates Hydroactive	Foam cavity dressing Alginates Hydrocolloid/alginate Hydrocolloid with paste, powder or granules Hydroactive cavity
Red/minimal exudate	Maintain moist environment and promote granulation and epithelialization. Hydrocolloids, foams, sheet hydrogels, and film dressings will maintain the environment. It is possible to use a combination of amorphous hydrogels with a foam cavity dressing in deeper wounds.	Hydrocolloids Foams Sheet hydrogels Films In addition, the use of zinc paste bandages in superficial granulating venous ulcers is appropriate.	Hydrocolloids with paste, powder, or granules Amorphous hydrogels Foam cavity dressing
Pink/minimal exudate	Maintain moist environment, protect, and insulate. Foams, thin hydrocolloids, thin hydroactives, film dressings, and simple nonadherent dressings will provide the necessary cover.	Foams Films Hydrocolloids (thin) Hydroactive (thin) Nonadherent dressing In addition, zinc paste bandages may also be used	
Red unbroken skin	To prevent skin breakdown. Hydrocolloids and film dressings provide the best protection.		
Infected wounds	Remove surface debris by washing, debride Slough, eschar Lower bacterial burden	Cadexomer iodine Povidone-iodine Silver dressings	Cadexomer iodine Povidone-iodine Silver dressings

The topical application of an antiseptic will reduce the level of bacteria on the surface of the wound, but will not penetrate into infected tissue.[51] If a wound is clinically infected, the use of systemic antibiotics should be considered as the most appropriate action. Dr. Chris Lawrence considers that antiseptics and, to some extent, certain antibiotics, afford excellent antibacterial prophylaxis in a variety of skin wounds when used wisely. However, unwise use of antibacterial agents—especially antibiotics—can create further problems. Dr. Lawrence and a number of other investigators believe that convincing comparative clinical trials concerning the possible value of antiseptics are lacking. There is, however, sufficient in vitro evidence that would indicate that a problem exists with the prolonged use of antiseptics in chronic wounds.[52]

In general, the use of topical antiseptics in chronic wounds is considered to be of little benefit and may, in fact, be injurious to the tissue. The exceptions are patients with major arterial circulation deficiencies, such as diabetic patients and immunocompromised, neutropenic patients. A decision should be made for the individual patient, taking into account all of the positive benefits and risks. The use of low-strength povidone-iodine or non-toxic cadexomer iodine can be of benefit in some nonhealing chronic wounds.

Antiseptics and Acute Wounds

The use of topical antiseptics and antibiotics for acute wounds is entirely different from that for chronic wounds. In a traumatic wound, the risk of infection from contamination at the time of wounding is very high. Also, in the case of major burns, the presence of necrotic tissue is a focus for infection, and it is mandatory to use topical management. The aim of using antiseptics and antibiotics prophylactically is to reduce the level of bacteria in the wound and allow the body's own mechanisms to destroy the rest. The use of povidone-iodine, chlorhexidine, and chlorhexidine/cetrimide products is appropriate in the early management of acute traumatic wounds. The use of products such as silver sulfadiazine cream (Silvadene, SSD) in burns is part of the early management of this type of wound.

Antibiotics

The use of topical antibiotics in chronic wounds should also be based on the general principle that topical use of antibiotics is not recommended because of the development of resistance and sensitization. However, in surface anaerobic contamination of some wounds, especially fungating wounds, the use of metronidazole gel (MetroGel) is appropriate, and there have been cases of methicillin-resistant *Staphylococcus aureus* in which topical mupirocin (Bactroban) has been used. The other topical antibiotic used in clinical practice is silver sulfadiazine cream in some infected ulcers in which *Pseudomonas* has been found to be present.[53–55]

Wound Cleansing

The approach to cleansing a wound at the time of dressing changes depends on the nature of the wound. In general, if the wound is clean with little or no residue from the dressing, simple irrigation with water or saline is the most appropriate. If there is dressing residue, slough, or dry or scaly tissue, the use of a skin wash with surfactant properties in addition to water or saline will aid in the removal of the debris. It is critical to minimize direct contact with the granulating wound. It is considered best to use the cleansing materials at body temperature, because the application of a cold solution reduces the temperature of the wound and can affect blood flow. The use of antiseptic cleansers is of little value in chronic wounds, however, they are of benefit in the initial cleaning of an acute wound.[56]

Another issue in relation to the use of any skin cleanser is the pH of the product. It is important to maintain an acid pH level of 5–6 in the wound and the periwound skin. It should be noted that most soaps are significantly alkaline and will have a negative effect on the wound and the periwound skin.

Conclusion

Wounds should be cleansed with care health professionals must consider the temperature and the Ph of the products to avoid any unnecessary damage to the wound and the periskin and avoid vigorous cleaning of the wound..

REVIEW QUESTIONS

1. Name two drawbacks to the use of gauze as a primary dressing.
2. Modern dressings are divided into three functional groups. Give an example of each group:
   • Nonabsorbing
   • Absorbing
   • Moisture donating
3. Name two wound types in which the use of topical antiseptics is indicated.
4. Name two dressings that can be used directly over a sutured wound.
5. Name two wound dressings that are suitable for exuding cavity wounds.

REFERENCES

1. Bull JP. Experiments with occlusive dressings of a new plastic. *Lancet.* 1948;213–215.
2. Schilling RSF. Clinical trial of occlusive plastic dressings. *Lancet.* 1950;293–296
3. Winter GD. Formation of the scab and the rate of epithelization of superficial wounds in the skin of the young domestic pig. *Nature.* 1962;193:293–294.
4. Hinman CD. Effect of air exposure and occlusion on experimental human skin wounds. *Nature.* 1963; 200:377–378.
5. Turner TD. Products and their development in wound management. *Plast Surg Dermatol Aspects.* 1979;75–84.

6. Turner TD. Surgical dressings in the drug tariff. *Wound Manage.* 1991;1:4–6.

7. Thomas S. Pain and wound management: Community outlook. *Nurs Times.* 1989;85(Suppl):11–15.

8. Bernard FX, Juchaux F, Laurensou C, Apert L. Stimulation of the proliferation of human dermal fibroblasts in vitro by a lipid colloid dressing. *J Wound Care.* 2005;14:215–220.

9. Bourton F. An evaluation of non-adherent wound contact layers for acute traumatic and surgical wounds. *J Wound Care.* 2004;13:371–373.

10. Terrill PJ, Varughese G. A comparison of three primary non-adherent dressings to hand surgery wounds. *J Wound Care.* 2000;9:359–363.

11. Thomas S. Handbook of Wound Dressings. London: Macmillan, 1994.

12. Thomas S, Loveless P, Hay NP. Comparative review of the properties of six semipermeable film dressings. *Pharm J.* 1988;240:785–788.

13. Golledge CL. Advances in wound management. *Mod Med Aust.* May 1993;42–47.

14. Myers JA. Ease of use of two semi-permeable adhesive membranes compared. *Pharm J.* 1984;233:685–686.

15. Loiterman DA, Byers PH. Effects of a hydrocellular polyurethane dressing on chronic venous ulcer healing. *Wounds.* 1991;3:178–181.

16. Myers JA. LYOfoam: A versatile polyurethane foam surgical dressing. *Pharm J.* 1985;235:270.

17. Foster AVM, Greenhill MT, Edmonds ME. Comparing two dressings in the treatment of diabetic foot ulcers. *J Wound Care.* 1994;3:224–228.

18. Sussman GM. Hydrogels: A review. *Primary Intention.* February 1994;2:6–9.

19. Smith RA, Rusbourne J. The use of Solugel in the closure of wounds by secondary intention. *Primary Intention.* May 1994;2:14–17.

20. Thomas S, Jones H. Clinical experiences with a new hydrogel dressing. *J Wound Care.* 1996;5:132–133.

21. Thomas S. Comparing two dressings for wound debridement. *J Wound Care.* 1993;2:272–274.

22. Thomas S, Loveless P. A comparative study of the properties of six hydrocolloid dressings. *Pharm J.* 1991;247:672–675.

23. Rousseau P, Niecestro RM. Comparison of the physicochemical properties of various hydrocolloid dressings. *Wounds.* 1991;3:43–45.

24. Marshall PJ, Eyers A. The use of a hydrocolloid dressing (Comfeel transparent) as a wound closure dressing following lower bowel surgery. *Primary Intention.* 1994;2:39–40.

25. Banks V, Bale SE, Harding KG. Comparing two dressings for exuding pressure sores in community patients. *J Wound Care.* 1994;3:175–178.

26. Thomas SS, Lawrence JC, Thomas A. Evaluation of hydrocolloids and topical medication in minor burns. *J Wound Care.* 1995;4:218–220.

27. Thomas S. Observations on the fluid handling properties of alginate dressings. *Pharm J.* 1992;248:850–851.

28. Sussman GM. Alginates: a review. *Primary Intention.* 1996;4:33–37.

29. Miller L, Jones V, Bale S. The use of alginate packing in the management of deep sinuses. *J Wound Care.* 1993;2:262–263.

30. Thomas S. Use of a calcium alginate dressing. *Pharm J.* 1985;235:188–190.

31. Thomas S. Alginates: a guide to the properties and uses of the different alginate dressings available today. *J Wound Care.* 1992;1:29–32.

32. Terrill P, Sussman G, Bailey M. Absorption of blood by moist wound healing dressings. *Primary Intention.* 2003;11:7–10,12–17.

33. Williams C. Treating a patient's venous ulcer with a foamed gel dressing. *J Wound Care.* 1993;2:264–265.

34. Achterberg VB, Welling C, Meyer-Ingold W. Hydroactive dressings and serum protein: an in vitro study. *J Wound Care.* 1996;5:79–82.

35. Collier J. A moist odor-free environment. *Prof Nurse.* 1992;7:804–807.

36. Brown-Etris M, Smith JA, Pasceri P, Punchello M. Case studies: considering dressing options. *Ostomy/Wound Manage.* 1994;40:5: 46–52.

37. Dykes PJ, Heggie R, Hill SA. Effects of adhesive dressings on the stratum corneum of the skin. *J Wound Care.* 2001;10:7–10

38. Hollingworth H, Collier M. Nurses' views about pain and trauma at dressing changes: result of a national survey. *J Wound Care.* 2000;9:369–374.

39. Lansdown ABG. Silver1: its antibacterial properties and mechanism of action. *J Wound Care.* 2002;11:125–130.

40. Lansdown ABG. Silver2: toxicity in mammals and how its products aid wound repair. *J Wound Care.* 2002;11:173–177.

41. Thomas S,McCubbin TS. A comparison of the antimicrobial effects of four silver-containing dressings on three organisms. *J Wound Care.* 2003;12:101–107.

42. Sundberg JA. Retrospective review of the use of cadexomer iodine in the treatment of chronic wounds. *Wounds.* 1997;3:68–86.

43. Foster AVM, Edmonds M. Hyalofill: a new product for chronic wound management. *Diabetic Foot.* 2000;3:29–30.

44. Parsons L. Office management of minor burns. *Lippincott's Primary Care Pract.* 1997;1:40–49.

45. Sleigh JW, Linter SPK. Hazards of hydrogen peroxide. *Br Med J.* 1985;291:1706.

46. Brennan SS, Leaper DJ. The effects of antiseptics on the healing wound: a study using the rabbit ear chamber. *Br J Surg.* 1985;72:780–782.

47. Lawrence CJ. Dressings and wound infection. *Am J Surg.* 1994;167(Suppl):21S–24S.

48. Brennan SS, Foster ME, Leaper DJ. Antiseptic toxicity in wounds: healed by secondary intention. *J Hosp Infect.* 1986;8:263–267.

49. Leaper DJ. Antiseptics and their effect on healing tissue. *Nurs Times.* 1986;45–46.

50. Morgan DA. Chlorinated solutions: (E) useful or (e) useless. *Pharm J.* August 1989;243:219–220.

51. Lawrence JC. The development of an in vitro wound model and its application to the use of topical antiseptics. In: Proceedings of the First European Conference on Advances in Wound Management. London: Macmillan; 1992:15–16.

52. Lawrence JC. Wound infection. *J Wound Care.* 1993;2:277–280.

53. Leaper DJ, Brennan SS, Simpson RA, Foster ME. Experimental infection and hydrogel dressings. *J Hosp Infect.* 1984;5:69–73.

54. Young JB, Dobrzanski S. Pressure sores: epidemiology and current management concepts. *Drugs Aging.* 1992;2:42–57.

55. Brown CD, Zitelli JA. A review of topical agents for wounds and methods of wounding. *J Dermatol Surg Oncol.* 1993;19:732–737.

56. Dire JD, Welsh AP. A comparison of wound irrigation solution used in the emergency department. *Ann Emerg Med.* 1990;704–707

57. Product Information from the following companies; Coloplast, Convatec, Ferris, Smith & Nephew, Hartmann, SSL, Johnson & Johnson, Urgo, Unomedical

58. Thomas S, McCubbin P. An in vitro analysis of the antimicrobial properties of 10 silver-containing dressings. *Journal of Wound Care.* 2003;12(8):305-308.

59. Thomas S, McCubbin P, Nielsen PS. Silver dressings: the debate continues. *Journal of Wound Care.* 2003;12(10):420.

60. Lansdown ABG, Thomas S, McCubbin P. Silver-containing dressings: have we got the full picture? A comparison of the antimicrobial effects of four silver-containing dressings on three organisms. *Journal of Wound Care.* 2003;12(3):101-107.

61. Parsons D, Bowler PG, Walker M, Burrell RE. Polishing the information on silver... A scientific perspective on the use of topical silver preparations. *Ostomy/Wound Management.* 2003;49[5A supp]:19-24. 2003;49(8):10-16.

62. Lansdown ABG, Williams A, Chandler S, Benfield S. Silver absorption and antibacterial efficacy of silver dressings. *Journal of Wound Care.* 2005;14(4):155-160.

63. Lansdown ABG. A guide to the properties and uses of silver dressings in wound care *Professional Nurse.* 2005;20(5):41-43.

64. Dowsett C. The use of silver-based dressings in wound care. *Nursing Standard.* 2004;19(7):56-60.

65. Ovington LG. The truth about silver. *Ostomy/Wound Management.* 2004;Supplement: 1S-16S.

66. Lansdown ABG, Thomas S, McCubbin P. Silver-containing dressings: have we got the full picture? A comparison of the antimicrobial effects of four silver-containing dressings on three organisms. *Journal of Wound Care.* 2003;12(3):101-107.

67. Schultz G, Mozingo D, Romanelli M, Claxton K. Wound healing and TIME; new concepts and scientific applications. *Wound Repair & Regeneration.* 2005;13(4):S1-S11.

68. Kingsley A. A proactive approach to wound infection. *Nursing Standard.* 2001;15(30):50-58.

69. Parsons D, Bowler PG, Myles V, Jones S. Silver antimicrobial dressings in wound management: a comparison of antibacterial, physical and chemical characteristics. *Wounds.* 2005;17(8):222-232.

70. Williams C. Arglaes controlled release dressing in the control of bacteria. *Br J Nurs.* 1997;12;6(2):114-115

71. Wright JB, Hansen DL, Burrell RE. The comparative efficiency of two antimicrobial barrier dressings: in vitro examination of two controlled release of silver dressings. *Wounds.* 1998;10(6):179-188.

72. Moore J, Smith P, Steinberg J. A Comprehensive Review of Topical Agents. *Podiatry Today.* 2002;15(7):40-47.

Management of the Wound Environment with Advanced Therapies

*Matthew J. Trovato, Mark S. Granick, Nancy L. Tomaselli,
Barbara M. Bates-Jensen*

CHAPTER OBJECTIVES

At the completion of this chapter, the reader will be able to:
1. Describe criteria for defining a refractory wound.
2. Identify three advanced wound therapies.
3. Compare and contrast advanced wound therapies.
4. Describe and explain indications for each advanced wound therapy.

Advanced wound therapy includes topical wound products and devices. Therapy in this category does not fall into other wound treatment categories and typically costs more than other wound therapies. Examples of advanced wound therapy include living skin equivalents; topical growth factors; devices that directly change the local wound environment, such as negative pressure wound therapy (see Chapter 28 on negative pressure wound therapy) and temperature therapy; and synthetic skin dressings. This chapter will focus on topical growth factors, living skin equivalents, and synthetic skin dressings.

The debate about when the use of advanced wound therapies is appropriate centers around the ability of the clinician to define the appropriate wound candidate. One suggestion is to use advanced therapies only on wounds that fail to heal with standard approaches. Another suggestion is to use them immediately on wounds identified as being potentially harder to heal. Some wound therapies provide specific guidelines for appropriate use, and others provide more general indications. It is accepted that advanced wound therapies are particularly useful for refractory wounds.

Merriam-Webster's Collegiate Dictionary defines *refractory* as "1. Resisting control or authority, stubborn or unmanageable, 2. Resistant to treatment or cure, 3. Unresponsive to stimulus, immune, insusceptible, 4. Difficult to fuse, corrode, or draw out."[1] The term *refractory* is typically used to define wounds that have not healed, despite appropriate treatment. It has come to be used to define difficult-to-heal wounds and wounds that do not progress toward healing.

Wounds may be considered refractory when they present with certain characteristics such as extensive necrosis, undermining, or tunnelling. Some studies have found that undermining present on initial wound assessment was associated with poor wound healing outcomes.[2,3] Others did not find undermining at baseline assessment to be a significant predictor of healing.[4] The presence of necrotic tissue in wounds provides a physical impediment to healing, and, not surprisingly, several have found that healing outcomes in necrotic wounds are fewer than those without necrotic tissue.[5,6] These studies suggest that the presence of necrotic tissue is associated with slower healing times[6] and a decreased proportion of improving ulcers.[5]

Specific comorbidities that are known to compromise wound healing, such as immunosuppression,[7,8] diabetes mellitus,[9,10] vascular disease,[11] or hypovolemia,[12] may determine whether the wound is diagnosed as refractory. There may be an additional significant host burden that impairs healing, such as infection,[13,14] wounds of prolonged duration, or extensive wounds.[5,15–18] Finally, a wound may be diagnosed as refractory when it fails to meet research-based temporal healing expectations. Clean full-thickness pressure ulcers should show signs of wound healing and improvement within 2–4 weeks.[5,18] One retrospective study suggests that pressure ulcers that do not decrease in size and demonstrate overall improvement at 1 week may not progress to healing in a timely fashion.[4] Partial-thickness wounds should show improvement in 1–2 weeks.[19] Exhibit 12-1 presents a proposal for diagnostic criteria for the "refractory" wound to assist clinicians in determining those wounds that may benefit from early use of advanced wound therapy.

Growth Factors

Several growth factors have been identified as regulatory polypeptides that coordinate the complex interaction of cellular and biochemical events that control wound healing. Growth factors participate in the regulation of cell proliferation, differentiation, and organ growth. In the past 10 years, several growth factors, including recombinant human (rh) platelet-derived growth factor (PDGF), epidermal growth factor (EGF), and basic fibroblast growth factor (bFGF) have been produced and are available for use. Only rh-PDGF has been approved by the United States Food and Drug Administration for use in wound therapy.[20]

Platelet-Derived Growth Factor (PDGF)

PDGF and its relative proteins were the first approved proteins for promoting diabetic foot healing and other refractory ulcers. In 1986, Knighton et al reported their successful treatment of chronic ulcers with autologous platelet-derived wound healing formula (PDWHF).[21] In their study, 49 patients with 95 chronic wounds were treated with PDWHF, resulting in a mean time to 100% healing of 10.6 weeks. Patients received 198 weeks of conventional wound care without healing before PDWHF application. Recombinant PDGF was first reported in the treatment of pressure ulcers in a 1992 phase I/II prospective, controlled clinical trial of 20 patients in which 100mcg/dl of topical rhPDGF increased the rate of wound closure compared with other groups.[22] In the phase II follow-up multicenter trial of 45 patients with pressure ulcers, the Mustoe group again reported that topical application of rhPDGF accelerated the rate of wound closure. Ulcers receiving 100mcg/dl of rh-PDGF showed a 71% decrease in area over 28 days and those treated with 300mcg/dl showed a 60% decrease. The report concluded that only a certain dose of growth factors is necessary to facilitate wound healing. Most recently, Rees et al completed a phase II, multicenter, double-blind, parallel group, placebo-controlled trial using rhPDGF-BB (becaplermin) 300mcg/g daily, 100mcg/g twice daily, and

placebo resulting in complete healing in 19%, 23%, and 0%, respectively.[23] Approved by the FDA in 1997, becaplermin is used for pressure, lower extremity diabetic, and neuropathic ulcers.

Description and Effects

Regranex Gel™ is a topical gel that contains the active ingredient becaplermin formulated in an aqueous sodium carboxymethyl-cellulose-based (NaCMC) gel. Each gram of Regranex Gel™ contains 100 micrograms of becaplermin. The biologic activity of becaplermin includes promoting recruiting (chemotaxis) and proliferation (mitosis) of cells involved in wound repair, and enhancing granulation production (synthesis), which is similar to that of endogenous PDGF.

Indications for Use

Regranex Gel™ 0.01% is indicated for use in the treatment of diabetic neuropathic ulcers that extend into the subcutaneous tissue or beyond and have adequate blood supply.[24] When used in conjunction with good wound care, it increases the incidence of complete wound healing. The cornerstones of good wound care include:

• Sharp debridement at all office encounters
• Control of infection
• Off-loading of pressure from the affected area
• Maintenance of a moist, clean wound environment.

The efficacy of becaplermin for the treatment of other types of wounds is currently being evaluated.[23]

Indications for Discontinuation

Regranex™ should be discontinued if the patient has extensive necrosis, untreated active infection, or ischemia. Once the ulcer is debrided, infection is treated, or the area is revascularized, the gel may be used. Continued treatment with becaplermin gel should be reassessed if the ulcer does not decrease in size by approximately 30% after 10 weeks of treatment or if complete healing has not occurred in 20 weeks.[24]

Method of Application

Regranex Gel™ is available in a 15 gram multidose tube as a clear, colorless to straw-color, topical gel. The dosage of gel to be applied will vary, depending on the size of the ulcer area. The formula to calculate the length of gel to be applied daily is length × width divided by 4.[24]

Precautions and Contraindications

Becaplermin gel is for external use only and is contraindicated in patients with known hypersensitivity to any component of the product or known neoplasms at the application site. Erythematous rashes occurred in 2% of patients treated with Regranex Gel™. Wounds that close by primary intention should not be treated with Regranex™ because it is a nonsterile, low-bioburden, preserved product. The effects of becaplermin on exposed joints, tendons, ligaments, and bone have not been established in humans. Carcinogenesis and reproductive toxicity studies have not been conducted. It is not known whether Regranex can cause fetal harm when administered to a pregnant woman, can affect reproductive capacity, or is excreted in human milk. The safety and effectiveness in patients younger than 16 years old has not been established. It is also not known whether Regranex Gel interacts with other topical medications applied to the ulcer site.[24]

Expected Outcomes

When becaplermin gel is used in conjunction with good ulcer care, including regular sharp debridement, pressure relief, and infection control, the gel increases the incidence of complete healing of diabetic ulcers.[25]

Alternative Growth Factor Options

Basic Fibroblast Growth Factor (bFGF)

Basic fibroblast growth factor (bFGF) has also been used in clinical trials to treat chronic ulcers. Robson et al completed randomized, blinded, placebo-controlled human trials of bFGF for pressure sores.[26] Three concentrations of bFGF in five dosing schedules were tested for safety. No toxicity, significant serum absorption, or antibody formation were detected. The slopes of the regression curves of volume decrease with initial pressure sore volume showing a greater healing effect in the bFGF-treated patients. Histologically, bFGF-treated wounds showed an increase in fibroblasts and capillaries. Treatment with bFGF achieved more than 70% wound closure.[24] Fu et al evaluated the safety and efficacy of topical application of recombinant bFGF on the healing of chronic cutaneous wounds resulting from trauma, diabetes mellitus, pressure, and radiation in a prospective, open-label crossover trial.[27] Thirty-three wounds that failed to heal within 4 weeks with conventional therapies were locally treated once daily with 150AU/cm² rbFGF and showed improved healing. Eighteen wounds were completely healed within 2 weeks, four healed within 3 weeks, and another eight completely healed within 4 weeks. The remaining three wounds healed on days 30, 40, and 42 with continued treatment of rbFGF, yielding a 90.9% 4-week efficacy. Histologically, capillary sprouts were more abundant and fibroblasts were more differentiated in wounds treated with rbFGF. No adverse effects were observed. An optimal formulation has not yet been established.

Keratinocyte Growth Factor-2 (KGF-2)

Robson et al conducted a phase II A multicenter, randomized, double-blind, placebo-controlled trial that investigated the effect of KGF-2 on chronic venous stasis ulcers of 3–36 months duration.[28] The 94 study subjects were otherwise treated with standard compression therapy. Compression dressings were changed twice a week, with placebo or 20mcg/cm² or 60mcg/cm² of KGF-2 (repifermin) applied topically during dressing changes. When both active dose groups were pooled, there was a significant improvement in the proportion of wounds that were 75% and 90% healed at 12 weeks. Based on these results, a phase II B trial was undertaken. However, the percentage of patients treated with repifermin who achieved complete wound closure within 20 weeks of treatment was not statistically significant different from the placebo groups, nor were there any favorable trends in the treatment group. As a result, manufacturers have ceased development of repifermin for chronic wound therapy, though Kepivanc was approved in December 2004 for the prevention of chemotherapy-induced mucositis in patients with hematologic malignancies.

Macrophage-Colony Stimulating Factor (M-CSF)

Colony-stimulating factors (CSF) enhance a general wound healing response, working directly on macrophages and monocytes, as opposed to fibroblasts, keratinocytes, or endothelial cells. This is the basis for the rabbit ear chronic wound model study by Wu et al, which hypothesizes that Macrophage-CSF (M-CSF) accelerates healing as a result of generalized macrophage activation, thereby increasing TGF-β transcription and granulation volume.[29]

Marques da Costa et al used compression dressings for a randomized, double-blind, placebo-controlled trial of human granulocyte/macrophage-colony stimulating factor for treatment of venous stasis ulcers.[30] The selected ulcers were less than 30cm² and well-perfused. The ulcers were treated with rhGM-CSF using four equidistant injections near the poles of the target wound. The treatment was placebo or 200mcg or 400mcg of rhGM-CSF, administered once a week for 4 weeks or until wound healing occurred. Using standard wound care, the percentage of ulcers with complete closure at 13 weeks was 61%, 57%, and 19% for 400, 200mcg, and placebo, respectively. Further clinical investigations are necessary for FDA approval.

AutoloGel

Lastly, an autologous, patient-specific topical preparation, AutoloGel™, is available. Platelet-derived wound healing factor (PDWHF) tries to seal the wound with the patient's own blood products, initiates coagulation, and provides growth factors that accelerate the patient's own wound repair cascade. The inflammatory, proliferative, and maturation phases of wound repair are mediated by the autologous tissue coagulum that is applied topically by a physician and redressed after 5 days with an alternative wound dressing for the next 7 days. This is repeated until the wound heals. A recent large retrospective study of PDWHF revealed significantly increased effectiveness for healing diabetic neuropathic ulcers over standard treatment particularly in larger wounds involving deeper structures (e.g., tendon and fascia).[31] No randomized, prospective clinical trial has been able to replicate these results. Since AutoloGel™ is derived from the patient's own blood, its application does not require FDA approval.

■ CASE STUDY

Growth Factor

The patient is a 55-year-old Hispanic female with a 12-year history of type 2 diabetes; a 2-year history of Charcot deformity of the right foot; hypertension; peripheral neuropathy; nonhealing diabetic, neuropathic ulcer on the plantar surface of the right foot for 8 months; and tinea pedis of the toe webs. Figure 12-1 shows the ulcer predebridement, and Figure 12-2 shows the ulcer after debridement and initial application of becaplermin gel. The patient was using a walker and crutches to off-load pressure from the ulcer. Figure 12-3 shows improvement in the ulcer, with a decrease in size from 2.8 × 2.2 × 1.8 cm to 1.8 × 1.1 × 0.7 cm. Figure 12-4 shows further decrease in the ulcer size at 1.1 × 0.6 × 0.4 cm. Figure 12-5 shows complete wound closure, which took 14 weeks after the ulcer was treated with becaplermin gel after weekly debridement. The patient is now in custom-molded shoes with no recurrence of the ulcer. (For basic information on growth factors and physiology of wound healing, see Chapter 2.)

Biological Skin Substitutes

For more than a century, there has been a need for alternatives in the treatment of full-thickness or deep partial-thickness life-threatening burn injuries. Though an invaluable reconstructive tool, there are problems and limitations

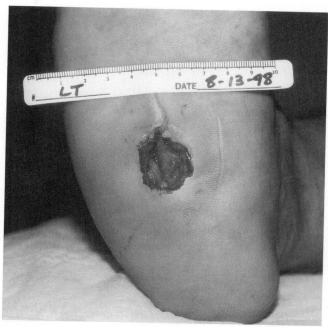

FIGURE 12-2 Ulcer postdebridement, Regranex™ growth factor treatment started. (Copyright © Susie Seaman)

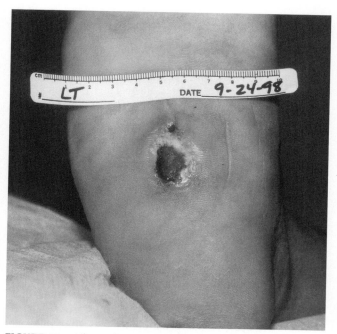

FIGURE 12-3 Ulcer after 6 weeks on Regranex™ growth factor treatment. (Copyright © Susie Seaman)

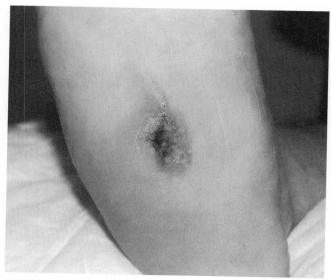

FIGURE 12-1 Ulcer predebridement. (Copyright © Susie Seaman)

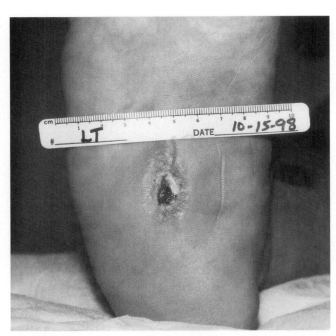

FIGURE 12-4 Ulcer 10 weeks after Regranex growth factor treatment started. (Copyright © Susie Seaman)

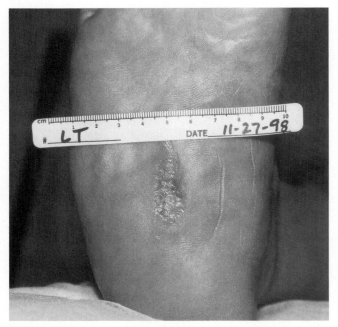

FIGURE 12-5 Complete wound closure. (Copyright © Susie Seaman)

with skin grafting. The donor site can be painful or unsightly. The graft does not always take and heal the wound. In very large wounds or burns, the need for grafts can necessitate the use of reharvested donor sites, unusual donor sites, wide meshing of the grafts, and other creative strategies for obtaining wound coverage. The need for an off-the-shelf skin substitute that can promote healing, eliminate the donor site, be quickly and easily accessible, minimize contracture and scarring, and be immunologically compatible has resulted in the evolution of tissue engineered skin equivalents and skin substitutes. Five tissue engineered skin equivalents are currently approved for use: Biobrane™, Apligraf™, TransCyte™, Integra™, and Dermagraft™ (Table 12-1).[32]

Apligraf

Invented in 1981 at MIT by Eugene Bell as the first medical device containing living cells to receive FDA approval, Apligraf™ (formerly known as Graftskin) is a bilaminar construct consisting of a simulated dermal phase and a simulated epidermal layer.[33] The dermal component is a bovine collagen mesh, seeded with living neonatal fibroblasts. The fibroblasts are a pure cell culture, derived from neonatal foreskin. The epidermal layer is a pure keratinocyte culture, similarly derived from neonatal foreskin. Histologically, it closely resembles normal skin without the rete ridges. The technical difficulties in creating pure cell cultures free of contamination and being able to deliver them to remote sites on demand for clinical use are incredible.

Indications for Use

Apligraf™ was FDA approved in 1998 for venous leg ulcers of greater than 1 month duration that are refractory to conventional therapy, and in 2000 for treating diabetic foot ulcers of greater than 2 weeks duration, without tendon, muscle, capsule, or bone exposure.

Indications for Discontinuation

There are few indications for discontinuation of the product. The presence of infection or allergic reaction would be strong indicators for discontinuing treatment with Apligraf™. Failure of the wound to improve significantly after two applications would be another reason to cease further treatment with the product.

Method of Application

The product arrives in a thermally controlled box. It must be incubated until it is used, which needs to be soon after it is received. The graft is 7.5 cm in diameter. It is packaged on agarose media that is colored with a pH indicator in a petri dish. The graft is gently lifted and placed on the wound with overlapping edges. A compression wrap is used to fix it in place.[34] Apligraf™ is indicated only for use on wounds that are free of infection and necrotic debris so it may be necessary to pretreat the wound with mechanical debridement or topical antibiotics.

CLINICAL WISDOM

During Apligraf use, avoid all cytotoxic substances, such as Dakin's solution, chlorhexidine, or povidone-iodine.

TABLE 12-1   A Guide to Biological Skin Substitutes

Trade Name	Schematic Representation	Layers	FDA approval	Cost
Biobrane		1. Silicone 2. Nylon mesh 3. Collagen	Yes	$
TransCyte		1. Silicone 2. Nylon mesh 3. Collagen seeded with neonatal fibroblasts	Yes	$$$
AlloDerm		1. Acellular de-epithelialized cadaver dermis	n/a	$$
Integra		1. Silicone 2. Collagen and glycosaminoglycan	Yes	$$
Dermagraft		1. Dexon or Vicryl seeded with neonatal fibroblasts	Yes	$$$
Apligraf		1. Neonatal keratinocytes 2. Collagen seeded with neonatal fibroblasts	Yes	$$$$$
CEA (Epicel)		1. Cultured autologous keratinocytes	n/a	$$$$$$
CAK (Laserskin)		1. Cultured autologous keratinocytes 2. Hyaluronic acid with laser perforations	n/a	$$$$$$

Precautions and Contraindications

Apligraf™ is contraindicated in infected wounds or in people who are allergic to bovine collagen or the agarose shipping media.

Expected Outcomes

Initially, the Apligraf™ sticks to a clean wound and looks like a skin graft. After about a week, the material loses its appearance as a graft and takes on a gelatinous look. It is important not to disrupt the "living skin equivalent" (LSE) during the initial 2–3 weeks. Because of these changes, it can be easily washed away. The healing process for the LSE differs significantly from that of a skin graft, despite its initial appearance. The LSE cells are rapidly replaced by the patient's own cells. The wound, typically bearing a chronically indolent, inactive surface, becomes biologically more active as the wound healing cascade is stimulated. The LSE acts as a biologic growth factor factory, as well as a biologic occlusive at the surface. This increased activity continues for 6–8 weeks. With full healing there is minimal contracture, and it achieves a remarkably normal appearance. In fact, the patient's own melanocytes repopulate the healing area to obtain a confluent color. If additional treatment is required, a new LSE may be applied.

■ CASE STUDY

Apligraf™

The patient illustrated in Figures 12-6, 12-7, and 12-8 has chronic venous disease in her leg. She has been treated with chronic compression, with which she has been poorly compliant. Several years ago, she underwent a skin graft that healed an ulcer. She reappeared with a recurrence in the middle of her old skin graft. She was treated with Apligraf. Initially, it had the appearance of a healed skin graft. A gelatinous phase followed. Within 8 weeks the wound healed and has remained so for more thn 1 year.

TransCyte™

TransCyte™ uses human neonatal fibroblasts cultured for 17 days onto the nylon mesh component of Biobrane to secrete extracellular matrix (ECM; fibronectin, type I collagen, proteoglycan, and matrix bound growth factors) into the mesh. The cells are no longer viable in the final product.

Indications for Use

TransCyte™ was FDA approved in March 1997 as a temporary wound covering for surgically excised full-thickness

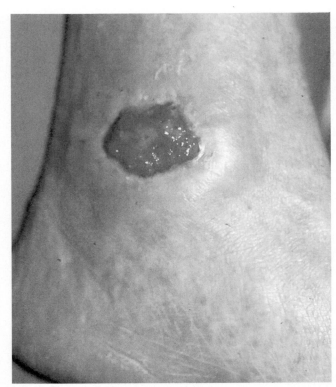

FIGURE 12-6 Recurrent venous ulcer. (Copyright © Mark S. Granick, MD, FACS)

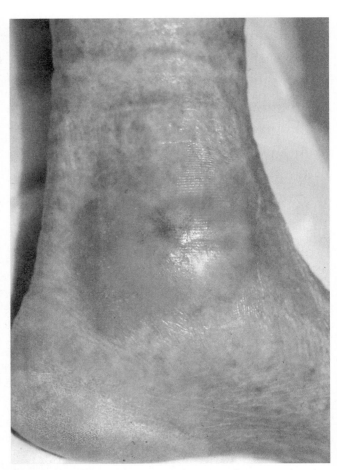

FIGURE 12-8 Complete wound closure within 8 weeks of therapy. The wound has remained healed for over 1 year. (Copyright © Mark S. Granick, MD, FACS)

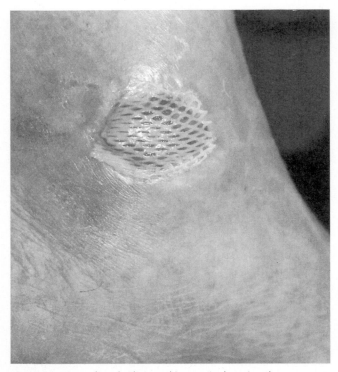

FIGURE 12-7 Apligraf™ living skin equivalent in place. (Copyright © Mark S. Granick, MD, FACS)

and partial-thickness thermal burns in patients requiring coverage prior to autografting. This was based on a 66-patient trial in which comparable full or deep partial-thickness burn sites on each patient were randomized to Trans-Cyte™ or cadaver allograft.[35] The label expanded in October 1997 to include partial-thickness burns mid-dermal to indeterminate depth that may be expected to heal without autografting.

Indications for Discontinuation

The product is applied to a freshly debrided wound. It adheres to the wound and lasts for up to 100 days. If infection or fluid accumulation occurs under the TransCyte, it must be removed.

Method of Application

The product is stored at −70°C. A specific thawing protocol must be followed for TransCyte to work. The product is applied to the wound and placed under a pressure dressing or negative pressure.

TransCyte™ is 3–13 times more expensive than allograft. It is 16 times more expensive than Biobrane and 2–3 times more expensive than Integra. It is also more difficult to store and handle than Biobrane or Integra. It must be stored between -70° and −20°C. When stored correctly, it has a shelf life of 18 months. It is, however, an extremely effective method for treating partial thickness burns or large surface area wounds.

Expected Outcomes

Kumar et al recently showed that, when used in partial-thickness burns in children, TransCyte promotes fastest re-epithelialization and requires fewer overall dressings than Biobrane or Silvazine. Patients who received Silvazine or Biobrane required more autografting than those treated with TransCyte in the study.[36]

Integra

Originally dubbed "Artificial Skin," Integra is a membrane bilayer. The silicone outer layer temporarily provides the sealant properties of the epidermis, and the collagen and chondroitin-6-sulfate layer, after being placed on a wound, is infiltrated by fibroblasts that lay down their own ECM and subsequently remodel the collagen and glycosaminoglycan. Over 3–6 weeks the inner layer takes on the properties of dermis and the synthetic outer layer is then removed and replaced with ultra-thin split-thickness skin grafts (STSG). Retrospective analysis of patients with massive burn injuries at Massachusetts General Hospital over 12 years suggests that the introduction of Integra resulted in improved survival.[37] A postapproval study involving 216 burn injury patients who were treated at 13 burn care facilities in the United States showed that the incidence of invasive infection at Integra treated sites was 3.1% and that of superficial infection 13.2%. The mean take rate of Integra was 76.2%. The mean take rate of epidermal autograft was 87.7%.[38]

Indications for Use

Integra was FDA approved in 1996 for the postexcisional treatment of life-threatening full-thickness or deep partial-thickness thermal injury where sufficient autograft is not available at the time of excision or not desirable due to the physiologic condition of the patient. The label was subsequently expanded based on retrospective uncontrolled studies to include "the management of wounds including: partial and full-thickness wounds, pressure ulcers, venous ulcers, diabetic ulcers, chronic vascular ulcers, surgical wounds (donor sites and grafts, post-Moh's surgery, post-laser surgery, podiatric, wound dehiscence), trauma wounds (abrasions, lacerations, second-degree burns, and skin tears) and draining wounds."

Integra has also been successfully employed for scar reconstruction, including scar resurfacing and keloids. Evaluation of Integra in 89 patients for contracture release (127 procedures) indicated that at 76% of the release sites, range of motion or function was rated as good (significant improvement in range of motion or function) or excellent (maximal range of motion or function possible) by physicians. Responding patients expressed satisfaction with the overall results of treatment at 82% of sites. No recurrence of contracture at 75% of the sites was observed during follow-up monitoring.[39]

Integra benefits the treatment of necrotizing fasciitis by allowing for a height build-up via layering.[40] Several studies have now focused attention on the use of cultured epidermal autografts (instead of STSG) combined with Integra. This use allows for the early physiologic closure of large wounds with decreased donor site morbidity and deals with the challenge of little to no donor site availability.[41,42] Recently, a head and neck full-thickness burn injury was reconstructed with Integra and early implantation of microdissected hair follicles through the silicone epidermis 12 days after the injury resulted in complete re-epithelialization and a hair-bearing scalp without the need for STSG.[43]

Indications for Discontinuation

Infection or lack of adherence to the wound bed is indication for removal.

Method of Application

Standard burn center protocol for topical agents and antibiotics should be employed. Early and complete excision of burn eschar and necrotic and contaminated tissue should be performed, ensuring a viable graft bed, such as white dermis, pure yellow fat, or glistening fascia. Meticulous hemostasis must be achieved to prevent hematoma or seroma formation, and the graft bed should be smooth and flat to ensure good contact with the Integra. The product should be meshed or fenestrated to minimize fluid collection under the graft. If complete excision is not possible, a barrier must be in place to separate Integra from unexcised skin and place an allograft.

The FDA requires physicians to be trained prior to using Integra. In the operating room, Integra may be applied as a sheet or meshed at a 1:1 ratio and fixated with staples or sutures. The meshed product should not be expanded. The advantages of meshing are that it decreases the risk of fluid accumulation and hematoma formation, allows antimicrobials to penetrate the wound bed, and improves conformability. The disadvantages of the meshed Integra are that it does not allow for physiologic closure, is a pathway for bacteria to enter the wound, and may guide granulation tissue to form a mesh pattern.

Postoperatively, compressive elastic net dressing, or negative pressure wound therapy (which promotes good contact of the product with the wound bed, prevents shearing forces, and provides visibility) should be used. An antimicrobial layer that may include moistened Acticoat or burn-roll is necessary over the seams if nonmeshed and over the entire wound surface if meshed. Xeroform or petrolatum products are to be avoided. Compressive Kerlix and Ace wrap are then added for compression. Occupational and physical therapy may begin after 3–5 days.

Integra™ should be monitored daily for infection, seromas, and hematomas. These areas should be aspirated or removed immediately. Otherwise, the elastic net that allows for observation of the operative site should be left intact. Outer dressings may be changed every 4–5 days. Do not allow immersion in water.

Precautions and Contraindications

Integra™ is contraindicated in patients with a known hypersensitivity to bovine collagen or chondroitin materials (the components of the dermal replacement layer). The product is also contraindicated in the presence of wound infection because it is more vulnerable than a standard skin graft and will partially or completely fail.

Expected Outcomes

The silicone layer is removed 14–21 days after application when the deposition of new dermal tissue and resorption of the collagen-glycosaminoglycan matrix has occurred. The neodermis has formed when it blanches under compression, there is separation/wrinkling of the silicone layer, and the color is peachy/pink or yellow. Do not remove the silicone layer until neodermis has formed completely. It should be easy to remove at this point. A thin epidermal graft of 0.003–0.007 inches is harvested. The grafts may be placed as a sheet or a mesh and should be attached per standard protocol.

Integra™ has increasingly shown promising uses in off-label applications because it is well tolerated, does not elicit a rejection reaction,[44] is thought to result in superior cosmesis with reduced donor site morbidity, and is readily available with a shelf life of 2 years at room temperature.

Dermagraft™

Dermagraft™ is a composite of neonatal foreskin fibroblasts cultured onto bioresorbable glycolic acid mesh (polyglactin 910, i.e., Vicryl). The cells deposit ECM (collagens, vitronectin, GAG, and growth factors) prior to cryopreservation at $-70°C$. In contrast to TransCyte™, the cells initially remain metabolically active in Dermagraft™, though they are eventually lost. In this respect, Dermagraft™ is biologically active, stimulating healing through in-growth of fibrovascular tissue.

Indications for Use

Dermagraft™ was FDA approved in September 2001 for use in the treatment of full-thickness diabetic foot ulcers of greater than 6 weeks duration that extend through dermis but without exposed tendon, muscle, joint capsule, or bone. The pivotal study was a 314-patient controlled, randomized clinical trial including Dermagraft™ plus conventional therapy versus conventional therapy alone (sharp debridement, saline-moistened gauze, pressure-reducing footwear) in plantar diabetic foot ulcers. Complete wound closure by week 12 revealed 30% of Dermagraft™ patients healed compared with 18% of control patients.[45] Prior clinical trials had failed to support an FDA approval.[46]

Indications for Discontinuation

If infection occurs or the wound regresses, additional applications should not be placed.

Method of Application

The product is thawed according to protocol and placed directly onto the freshly debrided wound. The overlying dressings keep the Dermagraft™ in place. The dressings should be changed in 5–7 days postapplication.

A second application at 1–2 weeks is usually required.

Precautions and Contraindications

The wounds must be properly debrided prior to each application.

Expected Outcomes

Healing usually takes place within 1 month.

Though dermagraft™ is an excellent wound care product, it's high cost and failure to reach FDA approval for treatment of chronic venous ulcers have caused it to be removed from the market.

REFERENCES

1. Merriam-Webster's Collegiate Dictionary, 10th edition. Springfield, MA: Merriam-Webster; 1993.
2. Allman RM, Walker JM, Hart MK, Laprade CA, Noel LB, Smith CR. Air-fluidized beds or conventional therapy for pressure sores: A randomized trial. Ann Intern Med. 1987;107:641–648.
3. Bates-Jensen BM. The Pressure Sore Status Tool a few thousand assessments later. Adv Wound Care. 1997;10(5):65–73.
4. Bates-Jensen BM. A Quantitative Analysis of Wound Characteristics as Early Predictors of Healing in Pressure Sores. Dissertation Abstracts International, Vol. 59, No. 11, University of California, Los Angeles; 1999.
5. Van Rijswijk L. Full-thickness pressure ulcers: Patient and wound healing characteristics. Decubitus. 1993;6(1):16–30.
6. Xakellis GC, Chrischilles EA. Hydrocolloid versus saline-gauze dressings in treating pressure ulcers: A cost-effective analysis. Arch Phys Med Rehabil. 1992;73(5):463–469.
7. Barbul A, Lazarou SA, Efron DT, Wasserkrug HL, Efron G. Arginine enhances wound healing and lymphocyte immune responses in humans. Surgery. 1990;108(2):331–336.
8. Mosiello GC, Tufaro A, Kerstein M. Wound healing and complications in the immunosuppressed patient. Wounds. 1994;6(3):83–87.
9. Bagdade JD, Root RK, Bulger RJ. Impaired leukocyte function in patients with poorly controlled diabetes. Diabetes. 1974;23(1):9–15.
10. Pecoraro RE, Ahroni JH, Boyko EJ, Stensel VL. Chronology and determinants of tissue repair in diabetic lower extremity ulcers. Diabetes. 1991;40:1305–1313.
11. Coleridge-Smith PD, Thomas P, Scurr JH, Dormandy JA. Causes of venous ulceration: A new hypothesis. Br Med J Clin Res Educ. 1998;296(6638):1726–1727.
12. Hartmann M, Jonsson K, Zederfeldt B. Effect of tissue perfusion and oxygenation on accumulation of collagen in healing wounds. Randomized study in patients after major abdominal operations. Eur J Surg. 1992;158(10):521–526.
13. Sapico FL, Ginunas VJ, Thornhill-Hoynes M, et al. Quantitative microbiology of pressure sores in different stages of healing. Diagn Biol Infect Dis. 1986;5(1):31–38.

14. Robson MC, Stenberg BD, Hegger JP. Wound healing alterations caused by infections. Clin Plast Surg. 1990;17(3):485–492.

15. Allman RM. Pressure ulcers among the elderly. N Engl J Med. 1989;320(13):850–853.

16. Gorse GJ, Messner RL. Improved pressure sore healing with hydrocolloid dressings. Arch Dermatol. 1987;123:766–771.

17. Gentzkow GD, Pollack SV, Kloth LC, Stubbs HA. Improved healing of pressure ulcers using dermapulse, a new electrical stimulation device. Wounds. 1991;3(5):158–169.

18. Van Rijswijk L, Polansky M. Predictors of time to healing deep pressure ulcers. Ostomy/Wound Manage. 1994;40(8):40–50.

19. Ferrell BA, Osterweil D, Christenson P. A randomized trial of low-air-loss beds for treatment of pressure ulcers. JAMA. 1993;269:494–497.

20. Fu X, Li X, Cheng B, Chen W, Sheng Z. Engineered growth factors and cutaneous wound healing: Success and possible questions in the past 10 years. Wound Rep Reg. 2005;13:122–130.

21. Knighton DR, Ciresi KF, Fiegel VD, Austin LL, Butler EL. Classification and treatment of chronic nonhealing wounds. Ann Surg. 1986;204:322–330.

22. Robson MC, Phillips LG, Thomason A. Recombinant human platelet-derived growth factor-BB in the treatment of pressure ulcers. Arch Surg. 1994;129:213–219.

23. Rees R, Robson MC, Smeill JM, Perry BH. Becaplermin gel in the treatment of pressure ulcers: A phase II randomized, double-blind, placebo-controlled study. Wound Repair Regen. 1999;7:141–147.

24. Regranex (becaplermin) Gel 0.01% (product labeling), Raritan, NJ: Ortho-McNeil Pharmaceutical, Inc; 1998.

25. Steed DL, Donohoe D, Webster MW, Lindsley L. The Diabetic Ulcer Group. Effect of extensive debridement and treatment on the healing of diabetic foot ulcers. J Am Coll Surg. 1996;183:61–64.

26. Robson MC, Phillips LG, Lawrence WT, Bishop JB, Youngerman JS, Hayward PG, Broemeling LD, Heggers JP. The safety and effect of topically applied recombinant basic fibroblast growth factor on the healing of chronic pressure sores. Ann Surg. 1992;216:401–406.

27. Fu X, Shen Z, Guo Z, Zhang M, Sheng Z. Healing of chronic cutaneous wounds by topical treatment with basic fibroblast growth factor. Chin Med J. 2002;115:331–335.

28. Robson MC, Phillips TJ, Falanga V, Odenheimer DJ, Parish LC, Jensen JL. Randomized trial of topically applied repifermin (recombinant human keratinocyte growth factor-2) to accelerate wound healing in venous ulcers. Wound Repair Regen. 2001;9:347–352.

29. Wu L, Yu YL, Galiano RD, Roth SI, Mustoe TA. Macrophage colony-stimulating factor accelerates wound healing and upregulates TGF-beta 1 mRNA levels through tissue macrophages. J Surg Res. 1997;72:162–169.

30. Marques da Costa R, Jesus FM, Aniceto C, Mendes M. Double-blind, randomized, placebo-controlled trial of the use of granulocyte-macrophage colony-stimulating factor in chronic leg ulcers. Am J Surg. 1997;173:165–168.

31. Margolis DJ, Kantor J, Santanna J, Strom BL, Berlin JA. Effectiveness to platelet releasate for the treatment of diabetic neuropathic foot ulcers. Diabetes Care. 2001;24:483–488.

32. Jones I, Currie L, Martin R. A guide to biological skin substitutes. Br J Plast Surg. 2002;55:185–193.

33. Falanga V, Sabolinski M. A bilayered living skin construct accelerates complete closure of hard to heal venous ulcers. Wound Rep Regen. 1999;7:201–207.

34. Falanga V. How to use Apligraf to treat venous ulcers. Skin Aging. 1999;Feb:30–36.

35. Purdue GF, Hunt JL, Still JM Jr, Law EJ, Herndon DN, Goldfarb IW, Schiller WR, Hansbrough JF, Hickerson WL, Himel HN, Kealey GP, Twomey J, Missavage AE, Solem LD, Davis M, Totoritis M, Gentzkow GD. A multicenter clinical trial of a biosynthetic skin replacement, Dermagraft-TC, compared with cryopreserved human cadaver skin for temporary coverage of excised burn wounds. J Burn Care Rehabil. 1997 Jan–Feb;18(1Pt1):52–7.

36. Kumar RJ, Kimble RM, Boots R, Pegg SP. Treatment of partial-thickness burns: A prospective, randomized trial using TransCyte. ANZ J Surg. 2004;74:622–626.

37. Tomkins RG. Crit Care Med. 1987;38:107.

38. Heimbach DM, Warden GD, Luterman A, Jordan MH, Ozobia N, Ryan CM, Voigt DW, Hickerson WL, Saffle JR, DeClement FA, Sheridan RL, Dimick AR. Multicenter postapproval clinical trial of Integra dermal regeneration template for burn treatment. J Burn Care Rehabil. 2003 Jan–Feb;24(1):42–8.

39. Frame JD, Still J, Lakhel-LeCoadou A, Carstens MH, Lorenz C, Orlet H, Spence R, Berger AC, Dantzer E, Burd A. Use of dermal regeneration template in contracture release procedures: A multicenter evaluation. Plast Reconstr Surg. 2004 Apr 15;113(5):1330–8.

40. Orgill DP, Strauss FH II, Lee RC. The use of collagen-GAG membranes in reconstructive surgery. Ann NY Acad Sci. 1999;888:233–248.

41. Loss M, Wedker V, Kunzi W, Meuli-Simmen C, Meyer VE. Artificial skin, split-thickness autograft and cultured autologous keratinocytes combined to treat a severe burn injury of 93% TBSA. Burns. 2000;26(7):644–652.

42. Boyce ST, Kagan RJ, Meyer NA, Yakuboff KP, Warden GD. The 1999 clinical research award. Cultured skin substitutes combined with Integra Artificial Skin to replace native skin autograft and allograft for the closure of excised full-thickness burns. J Burn Care Rehabil. 1999;20(6):453–461.

43. Navsaria HA, Ojeh NO, Moiemen N, Griffiths MA, Frame JD. Reepithelialization of a full-thickness burn from stem cells of hair follicles micrografted into a tissue-engineered dermal template (Integra). Plast Reconstr Surg. 2004 Mar;113(3):978–81.

44. Michaeli D, McPherson M. Immunologic study of artificial skin used in the treatment of thermal injuries. J Burn Care Rehabil. 1990 Jan–Feb;11(1):21–6.

45. Marston WA, Hanft J, Norwood P, Pollak R; Dermagraft Diabetic Foot Ulcer Study Group. The efficacy and safety of Dermagraft in improving the healing of chronic diabetic foot ulcers: Results of a prospective randomized trial. Diabetes Care. 2003 Jun;26(6):1701–5.

46. Pollak, RA., Edington, H, Jensen, JL, Kroeker, RO, Gentzkow, GD, et al. A human dermal replacement for the treatment of diabetic foot ulcers. Wounds, 1997;9(1):175–183.

Management of Wound Pain

Carrie Sussman and Barbara Bates-Jensen

CHAPTER OBJECTIVES

At the completion of this chapter, the reader will be able to:

1. Explain the relationship between pain physiology and chronic wound pain.
2. Grasp the consequences of wound pain on wound healing.
3. Characterize wound pain in relation to vascular (venous and arterial), diabetic (neuropathic), pressure ulcers, and postoperativewound etiologies.
4. Use validated tools/methods for assessing wound pain.
5. Choose appropriate wound pain management, including pharmaceutical and nonpharmaceutical strategies.
6. Educate patients and caregivers about pain and wound healing.

The International Association for the Study of Pain (ISAP) has defined pain as, "An unpleasant sensory and emotional experience associated with actual or potential tissue damage or described in terms of such damage."[1] This definition emphasizes that pain involves two components: physical and emotional. These components are present in patients with different wound pain etiologies, whether operative pain associated with surgery or pain from debridement and dressing changes associated with chronic wounds, burns, or cancer. For example, cancer patients who reported high-intensity pain levels also reported correspondingly high levels of frustration and exhaustion.[2]

Pain is described as the patient's reported experience, which may address only the physical component. Pain scales, such as the visual analog, verbal rating scale, and numerical pain scale, are one dimensional and measure only the physical component, intensity of pain.[3] Multidimensional scales, such as the McGill pain questionnaire, that measure both physical and emotional components are used less often. Thus, frequently it is the clinician or caregiver who interprets the patient's pain experience in accordance with his/her own personal perspectives and biases.[4] The result is that a patient's pain experience, especially chronic wound pain, is often marginalized, and pain is poorly controlled.[5, 6] Pain management for all kinds of pain requires highly individualized, skilled care and is very much dependent on the art of the practitioner as well as on medical science. It takes patience and commitment. Pain

management experts are not available in most settings and many clinicians are inadequately prepared to develop pain management plans of care.[5] Historically, the focus of chronic wound management has been on products and strategies to achieve wound healing, and health-care practitioners have neglected consideration of the important patient-related issue of wound pain and the impact of pain on healing and on quality of life.[7]

Pain is not inconsequential. Recent knowledge about the potential to develop chronic/persistent pain problems that can last indefinitely as a result of improper and ineffective wound care strategies highlights the need to raise the level of priority devoted to understanding pain and its management in the scheme of wound caring.[5] Current understanding of wound pain is largely drawn from studies related to the pain associated with other painful conditions like cancer and burns. The burn literature has historically addressed procedural pain at dressing changes and debridement, and what has been learned there is relevant to treatment of other wounds as well.[8] Recent developments suggest that wound pain management is receiving more attention, and there are now observational and descriptive studies looking at the patient and the wound pain problem.[9-11]

Management for all kinds of pain is a requirement. In acute care, the Joint Commission for Accreditation of Health Care Organizations (www.JCAHO.org) considers pain management a quality indicator. The JCAHO pain standards for acute care include appropriate assessment of pain, aggressive and effective pain management, and regular reassessment of pain.[12]

In compliance with JCAHO standards, pain management is used as a measure of the quality of care for most healthcare settings. In long-term care facilities, the minimum data set (MDS) assessment includes items about pain. As one of the MDS quality measures, pain prevalence is reported for all U.S. nursing homes that participate in the Medicare program, and that information is listed on a web site available to consumers (http://www.hhs.gov).

Clinicians need guidelines on management of chronic wound pain and how chronic wound pain differs from other pain problems. The purpose of this chapter is to provide guidelines, beginning with scientific background information about pain physiology and pathophysiology, and the relationship of pain to acute and chronic wounds and wound healing. This will be followed by assessment and interventions to manage or prevent pain and guidelines for referrals and patient self care.

Physiology and Pathophysiology of Wound Pain

The pain experience depends on the interaction and modulation of the biologic and psychosocial characteristics of the individual.[3,13] (Tracy I 2005) Biologic considerations include genetics, sex, and endogenous pain control (e.g., cortisol and endorphins). Psychological characteristics include anxiety, depression, coping skills, behavior, and cognitive status. Pain is also a consequence of the individual's history of disease and present disease status. Environmental factors also are part of the individual's pain responses. Examples of environmental factors are socialization, lifestyle, traumas, and cultural background (expectations, upbringing, and roles).

Understanding and recognizing the nervous system response and adaptation to pain is critical to understanding a patient's pain experiences and selecting appropriate treatment interventions that will address these mechanisms.[14] Clinically, pain management is moving from empiric therapies toward a mechanisms based approach.[3] The following section examines the function of pain, neuroanatomy, and emerging information about the mechanisms of pain. Table 13-1 is a glossary of pain-related terms.

Function of Pain

Pain is an unpleasant, protective bodily function that occurs in response to actual or potential tissue injury.[14] The function of pain can be either beneficial or detrimental. On the beneficial side, pain is protective and serves as a warning sign of imminent or actual danger and triggers an appropriate response within the body to avoid or minimize injury. The pain signal also initiates the release of chemical mediators, as described in Chapter 2, necessary to start the healing cascade. Another benefit of acute pain in inflamed tissues is that pain provokes hypersensitivity of the injured tissues, causing the individual to guard the damaged tissue

while healing occurs.[15] Typically, as healing occurs, pain intensity subsides, as does guarding. Pain can also be a signal of the presence of infection[16,17] calling for action.

On the detrimental side, pain can interfere with the immune response, influence the healing process, and delay wound closure.[5] Pain is not beneficial when it is "out of control" and triggers an emotional response that produces excess release of hormones, such as cortisol and epinephrine, which interfere with healing processes.[18] The effects of cortisol and epinephrine on healing are explained in Chapter 2. Inflammatory mediators and cytokines are helpful following initial injury, but if they are released frequently following repetitive procedures such as sharp or mechanical debridement, or dressing changes, they lower the firing thresholds and decrease the baseline sensitivity of nociceptors in such a way that they begin to respond to normally innocuous thermal and mechanical stimuli, resulting in hyperalgesia.[19] Pain can be both the result of an experienced sensation and a predicted expectation, which illustrates the complex and dynamic interactions that make up the pain experience.[3,13] (Tracy I)

Persistent pain resulting from nerve damage offers no biologic advantage, and causes suffering and distress[19] and is usually irreversible. Another point of view is that persistent pain can be the biologic way of protecting tissues at risk of injury, such as painful joints associated with rheumatoid arthritis and osteoarthritis. In these cases, the pain is protective of further injury.[20] As much as most individuals fear pain and would prefer avoiding the sensation, the inability to feel pain and respond to danger or injury—such as occurs when there is a loss of protective sensation due to neuropathy resulting from diabetes, alcoholism, or chemotherapy, or from nervous system injury or disease like a spinal cord injury or multiple sclerosis—puts the individual at risk for serious bodily harm.

RESEARCH WISDOM

Epidural Anesthesia and Heel Pressure Ulcers

Anesthesia during surgery has both beneficial and detrimental effects. Trauma unrelated to the surgery can occur when pain is absent such as during anesthesia. An example is trauma resulting in heel pressure ulcers in postsurgical patients. For example, case reports and communications in several medical journals discuss the complication of heel pressure ulcers in healthy, young adults after epidural analgesia.[21] Epidural blocks can reduce blood pressure, produce immobility of the lower limbs, and block the nociceptive sensory inputs from the periphery that warn of impending tissue damage.[22]

Neuroanatomy and Mechanisms of Pain

Neuroanatomic organization is used here to look at component structures involved in pain and to review pain physiology. This presentation does not account for the multidimensional aspects of pain; Each section presents information to demonstrate the involvement and interaction

TABLE 13-1 **Glossary of Pain-Related Terminology and Characteristics**

Pain Terminology	Characteristics
Allodynia	Increased sensitivity such that stimulation, which would normally not be perceived as painful, becomes painful
Acute pain	Pain present for 4 weeks or less[21]
A "beta" (Aβ)	Nerve fibers that sense touch and pressure
A "delta" (Aδ)	Large nerve fibers that rapidly transmit sharp acute pain
Afferent	A nerve that conducts a signal from the periphery toward the CNS
Background pain	Persistent pain at rest
Breakthrough pain	Transient exacerbations of pain occurring in the background or continuous pain that is otherwise satisfactorily controlled[112]
C fiber	Small, slow-acting nerve fibers that transmit dull aching pain; unmyelinated
C-nociceptors	Respond to stimuli that are potentially noxious Release a complex mix of pain and inflammatory mediators
Central sensitization (wind up)	Central mechanisms involved in maintaining and generating pain[113]
Chronic wound pain	Pain present for 6 months; usually persistent and occurs without manipulation of tissues such as the throbbing of an abdominal wound when a patient is just lying in bed[43]
Cyclic or episodic acute pain	Is periodic acute wound pain that recurs due to repeated treatments or interventions such as daily dressing changes or turning and repositioning[43]
Disinhibition	Injury to peripheral nerves may reduce the amount of inhibitory control (also called disinhibition) over dorsal horn neurons through various mechanisms
Efferent	A nerve that conducts a signal from the CNS back to the periphery
Hyperalgesia	Exaggerated pain response produced by noxious stimuli[31]
Incident pain	Frequent, predictable pain episodes brought on by certain activities (e.g., wound care procedure); may occur on a background of continuous pain or the patient may otherwise be pain free[112]
Myelin sheath	A fatty sheath that covers the axon nerve fiber, acts like insulation, and assists in rapid transmission of the signal
Neuropathic pain	Damaged nerves cause signals to travel in abnormal pain pathways
Nociceptive pain	Noxious stimuli (chemical, mechanical, and thermal) detected by free nerve endings (nociceptors) perceived as pain
Noncyclic or incident acute pain	A single episode of acute wound pain, for example the pain of surgical debridement or of drain removal[43]
Opioids	Drugs that exert analgesic activity by binding to endogenous (opioid) receptors and that elicit the characteristic stereospecific actions of natural morphine-like ligands[112]
Pain mediators	Activated at time of cell damage. Include: arachidonic acid (Aa), potassium (K+), bradykinin (BK), prostaglandin (PG), histamine (HS)
Peptides (substance P)	Activates the immune system with further release of histamine
Peripheral sensitization	Nociceptors become sensitized and have a lowered firing threshold
Persistent pain	Pain that has been present for more than three months; the pain may be continuous or intermittent[112]
Primary hyperalgesia (wind up)	Increased sensitivity of neurons to repeated stimulus, especially small stimuli that are perceived as painful
	Chemicals released from damaged tissue lowers the firing threshold of nociceptors
Secondary hyperalgesia	May be accompanied by secondary increase in sensitivity in nearby uninjured tissues perceived as painful
Unmyelinated nerve fiber	Nerve fibers that are unsheathed with myelin Slower conductors of neuronal signals

of the components, and where appropriate, how pain mechanisms are affected by wound care interventions and how that may affect healing. The neuroanatomic structures involved are the cerebral cortex, the brain stem, sympathetic nervous system, spinal cord, and peripheral nervous system.[23]

Brain Involvement

Physiologically, the perception of pain is appreciated when nociceptive pain impulses signals arrive at higher centers in the brain that interpret them as "pain". Nociceptive pain impulses reach the brain through spinal nerve tracts ascending through the brainstem, the medulla and the thalamus. The thalamus appears to be the critical relay site for nociceptive input before impulses are transmitted to cortical and subcortical structures.[13,24] How thalamus processing of nociceptive impulses occurs is still relatively poorly understood. The term "pain matrix" is used to describe a set of brain regions involved in processing nociceptive pain. Components commonly associated with the " pain matrix" are the anterior conjugate cortex, insula cortex, somatosensory areas, and possibly the thalamus.[13,24] Activation of areas within this set of "pain matrix" components, by a nociceptive signal, are believed to be sufficient to generate a perception of pain.[13] The pain impulse is modulated by the input from the higher centers of the brain and transmitted via descending inhibitory and facilitory tracts to the dorsal horn of the spinal cord. Changes in the descending pain modulation network have been implicated in central sensitization associated with chronic pain. The dysfunction may be either a dysfunctional descending inhibitory system or an activated and enhanced descending facilitatory system.[13]

Functional magnetic resonance imaging [FMRI] is now used to reveal the regions of the human brain activated by pain and in the future may be an objective method by which to measure pain and the response to treatment.[19,20,24] Over time, injury to the peripheral tissue can not only change the patterns of pain at the spinal cord level but also affect the brain circuitry.[25,15,13] How this pain signal is interpreted depends on many factors. In a normally functioning nervous system, the arrival of an unpleasant stimulus is recognized as pain, and the response, usually withdrawal from the activity, follows. However, the higher brain centers may block or enhance the message completely or partially through behavioral, cognitive, psychological (e.g., anxiety, memory), biologic (e.g., sex hormones), or pharmacologic activities.[3] The result is that individual differences account for different perceptions and responses to the same painful stimulus delivered to the periphery.

All parts of the nervous system can become sensitized to painful stimulation, and there is evidence that the pain states become imprinted in unique central nervous system (CNS) pathways similar to those of memories.[23] The nervous system learns to recognize a sensory experience from the repetitive pairing of environmental cues with sensory stimuli.

The consequence of this imprinting is the same as other learned responses and is retained as a "pain memory." Pain memories are formed when movements or sensation that elicit pain eventually elicit *anticipation* of pain. The patient is usually unaware of these pain memories but responses are different when pain memories are present. This makes extinguishing them very difficult.[23] Work is being done on how to " unlearn" pain memories. Success is reported using patient education about the inappropriate action of the nervous system as being a cause of the problem and by increasing the patient awareness those individuals show increased pain thresholds.[23] Increased or decreased pain intensity *expectations* can powerfully alter the subjective experience of pain since there is evidence that pain expectations *become* the client's reality.[15,26] When there is a *low expectation* of pain intensity, there is a reduction in perceived pain that rivals the effects of an analgesic dose of morphine.[15] Pain-related information is "learned" and stored in brain pain areas of the cerebral cortex such as the somatosensory cortex and the insula area that are now being identified using FMRI.[23,26] The stored information preprograms the CNS pain expectation.[26] These areas can be activated without physical stimulation and thus anticipation of remembered pain from a previous procedure affects the individual's future pain experience for that same procedure (e.g., sharp debridement or dressing change).

Preprogramming of the CNS is demonstrated in an example that many people have experienced: having a childhood injury that was treated with an adhesive bandage and later having the bandage removed, with the pulling of the hair and skin causing noxious pain. Based on this previous experience, whenever an adhesive bandage has to be removed from hairy skin, there is immediate recall of that pain with the anticipation and expectation of intense pain. A common response is both withdrawal and grimacing even before the adhesive bandage is removed. However, if a new adhesive bandage is used that doesn't cause pain when removed, the expectation of pain is changed centrally and anticipation is reduced for the next bandage removal.

Because wound care requires many procedures that can cause pain, preventing or decreasing the pain experience by using less aggressive bandage adhesives or other means of dressing placement can have a powerful effect on patient pain expectations and anxiety about procedures.

Another example of perceived expectations effecting outcomes is the measurement of stress levels in presurgical patients. Patients who worried most about the effects of the surgery before the event had the lowest levels of proinflammatory cytokines and metalloproteinase concentrations in wound fluid after surgery, demonstrating that the expectation of difficulties (e.g., pain) associated with the surgery (stress) produced the reality of an impaired inflammatory stage of wound repair.[18]

Sympathetic Nervous System Involvement

The sympathetic nervous system (SNS) responds to all injuries and pain. Pain perception, as has been stated, is the result of a combination of physiologic, psychological, emotional, cognitive, environmental, and social factors.[3,15] The expectations that individuals have about their wound pain and wound care procedures can greatly influence brain activity and, as a consequence, the SNS and their perception of pain.[15] Following a painful injury, the SNS releases catecholamines, epinephrine, and norepinephrine. Catecholamines increase with fear, anxiety, anger, and frustration and are suppressed and their action ameliorated with relaxation techniques and visual imagery. Apparently the mechanism for abnormal SNS sensitivity results from normal sympathetic secretions that occur in injured nerves and peripheral nociceptor terminals.[20] Techniques to treat the pain mechanisms will be discussed later.

Inputs such as fear, anxiety, and frustration affect the same cluster of neurons in the CNS to create a perceptual experience as do inputs from damaged tissue.[20] Pain generates feelings of powerlessness and dread and creates anxiety, which arouses the SNS with an increase in the amount of cortisol released, increased heart rate, vasoconstriction, enhanced pain perception, and slower wound healing. During a pain experience, heart rate increases in response to the intensity of the pain even if there is no apparent change in affect.[15] Monitoring heart rate during treatment would be useful clinically for monitoring pain but should not be used in lieu of the patient's self report of pain.[27]

Peripheral Nervous System Involvement

Nociceptive Pain. Earlier in this section the processing of a nociceptive impulse in the brain was presented. This section will discuss the initiation of the nociceptive impulse at the peripheral receptors. Nociceptive pain physiology is the easiest to explain and understand. It is a stimulus/response relationship and essential survival mechanism that dominates an individual's attention and drives action. Nociceptive pain originates when there is damage to the sensory nociceptor terminals in the skin, which respond with the release of inflammatory mediators and cytokines.[19] Nociceptors are pain-sensing receptors at the peripheral end of these nerve fibers that respond to these chemical stimuli and relay the pain signals, chemically and electrically, from the peripheral tissues to the CNS. The impulses travel along the axon from the periphery to the dorsal horn of the spinal cord via the sodium channels. Physiologically, transmission of the neural signals is via the large, thinly myelinated Aß and unmyelinated C nerve fibers to the dorsal horn. Aß fibers also transmit sensations, and their malfunction is related to neuropathic pain. From the dorsal horn the sensory information is transmitted to the brain stem and thalamus.[14]

Nociceptors are triggered by different stimuli producing three overlapping nociceptive pain patterns, mechanical, ischemic, and inflammatory, and are usually time limited. Mechanical nociception is triggered by mechanical distortion of the tissues such as during repositioning, pressure, or scar tissue manipulation. Ischemic nociceptive pain occurs when there is interruption of blood flow and resulting alteration of the chemical environment of the tissues. Ischemic tissues become more acidic, are hypoxic, and are rich in no-

ciceptor-sensitizing chemicals: bradykinin, potassium ions, and prostaglandins. An example of ischemic pain is intermittent claudication that occurs during walking and then subsides when the activity ceases. Inflammatory nociceptive pain is related to the inflammatory processes following tissue injury and the chemical mediators involved and will reduce as the tissues heal[20] (see Chapter 2).

Pharmaceutical management of pain transmission via sodium channels is an area of pain research. Two types of sodium channels are found in sensory nerves. The first type is sensitive to tetrodotoxin, a potent puffer-fish toxin, and the second type is insensitive to the same toxin. The channels that are sensitive to the tetrodotoxin are responsible for the initiation of the action potential and exist in all sensory neurons. Drugs that target the tetrodotoxin-*sensitive* channels systemically have widespread effects in the heart and CNS.[3] Those that are *insensitive* to tetrodotoxin are found only on nociceptor sensory neurons and have much slower activation and inactivation kinetics and are implicated in pathologic pain states.[19] This distinction is important because new analgesic medications are being developed that target the sodium channels and in particular the one that is insensitive to tetrodotoxin. If the sodium channels can be blocked peripherally, this will block the pain impulses from reaching the spinal cord and brain levels. One pharmaceutical product that has shown efficacy in blocking the sodium channels insensitive to tetrodotoxin peripherally without adverse effects is Lidocaine patch 5%.[28, 29] The use of lidocaine patch 5% for neuropathic pain will be discussed later. This is an example of how the concept of targeting a specific pain mechanism for treatment instead of using empiric therapies is applied. This is one of the major changes occurring in pain management. [3,30]

Spinal Cord Involvement. Neurons in the dorsal horn of the spinal cord also receive inputs from projection neurons that process and transfer the information about peripheral stimuli to the brain. The firing is not only excitatory but also inhibitory. Inputs are received that can be segmental within the spinal cord or descend from the brain. Injury to peripheral nerves may reduce the amount of inhibitory control (also called disinhibition) over dorsal horn neurons through various mechanisms. Descending nerve input can modulate the incoming pain signals to the spinal cord, but anxiety and depression can inhibit this action. Conversely, increased inhibition will reduce the activity in dorsal horn neurons and act as a spinal "gate." Use of transcutaneous electrical nerve stimulation (TENS) to block pain activates segmental inhibitory pathways.[19] The expected result of the stimulation would be to prevent or manage central sensitization and spread of the pain pattern.

Following acute injury or if nociceptors are in a continuous inflammatory state, such as occurs with repeated procedural traumas like dressing changes, they become sensitized and release a mixture of pain and inflammatory mediators (bradykinin, histamine, and prostaglandins), which lowers the threshold for firing the nociceptor and increases the response to another stimulus when it impacts the nerve endings. This is referred to as *peripheral nerve sensitization,* and the response is called *primary hyperalgesia.*[28] The site of injury is involved in primary hyperalgesia. Hyperalgesias can be classified on the basis of the type of stimulus that provokes a response.

Three types of hyperalgesias are recognized: thermal, mechanical, and chemical. They can occur singularly or in combinations, depending on the nociceptor that has been sensitized.[14] Thermal hyperalgesia is provoked by a slight change in temperature, such as being touched with a cool hand or cool fluid, which is perceived as severe pain. Mechanical hyperalgesias are subdivided into brush evoked (dynamic) and pressure evoked (static) and punctuate (pin prick).[19] As with thermal stimuli, very mild mechanical stimulation such as a gentle breeze is perceived as excruciating pain. The receptors may become sensitized to heat and mechanical stimuli after chemical stimulation.[14]

Hyperalgesia is not confined to peripheral receptors. Neuromas such as occur at the end of an injured nerve (e.g., amputated limb) re-sprout new axons, and these may exhibit exquisite sensitivity to mechanical perturbation because of altered membrane properties of both C and A fiber axons.[19]

A further complication following injury is involvement of the surrounding uninjured tissues. Reaction in the surrounding skin depends on CNS recruitment and is termed secondary hyperalgesia.[14] Secondary hyperalgesia is initiated by a stimulus peripherally and then the sensation is transmitted along the sensory axons centrally to the dorsal horn of the spinal cord. Increased nociceptor drive increases the release of substance P and calcitonin—gene-related peptide, which are normally expressed by nociceptor primary afferent C fibers and Aß fibers during the transmission of impulses from the periphery to the CNS and have been strongly implicated in central sensitization of the dorsal horn neurons.[19] When the input from the A_ fibers reaches the dorsal horn cells, another group of chemical mediators, including N-methyl-D-aspartate (NMDA), which has specific receptors in the dorsal horn of the spinal cord, transmits the signals to other parts of the pain pathway and is involved in the development of central sensitization. NMDA antagonist drugs such as ketamine are now available to block the pain pathway at this point.[21]

With repetitive application of identical non-noxious stimuli to the tissues at a certain rate, there is a progressive build-up in the response at the level of the dorsal horn neurons of the spinal cord. Over time the size of the receptive field within the dorsal horn grows. This is termed "wind up." The result is the progressive increase in the intensity of perceived pain; the physical process is called central sensitization and is a normal response of the undamaged nervous system to repetitive or sustained application of noxious stimuli with any tissue damage.[14] Theoretically, repeated handling of a wound even gently over a prolonged period of time would have the potential to create such a wind-up effect. Gifford and Butler have described patterns suggestive of central sensitization that are clinically useful.[20] These patterns include: on-going pain after expected tissue healing time; unfamiliar anatomic pain patterns; secondary allodynia and hyperalgesia; latency to input; atypical pain behaviors; pain that has "a mind of its own"; pain exacerbated by emotional and physical stress, often significant affective (emotional) and cognitive components; variable responses to passive treatment; and poor response to medication, even opioids.[20] Over time these physiologic conditions will reverse unless there has been significant tissue injury or nerve damage.[14] In a study of patients with chronic low back pain, it was found that there is atrophy of neocortical grey matter (massive loss of brain cells) related to pain duration. Even after nociceptive input ceases some of the brain changes may be irreversible and perhaps explains why the persistant pain condition exists.[13]

The term chronic pain has a negative connotation associated with futility of treatment; it has recently been suggested to change the term to persistent pain to foster a more positive attitude by patients and health-care professionals.[5] This will be the terminology used here.

RESEARCH WISDOM

Increased sensitivity of nociceptors to repetitive stimuli can cause benign sensations to become painful.[14] Patients with chronic wounds experience repetitive stimulation to the wound and the surrounding tissues and are often hypersensitive to handling.

Allodynia refers to the production of pain (including reflex withdrawal) by a stimulus that does not normally provoke pain, such as the breeze described above.[1] Allodynia can occur in two ways:

1. When the large-diameter, low-threshold mechanoreceptors, Aß fibers, are activated following central sensitization produced by C fiber activity. Then the Aß fibers become capable of responding to noxious stimuli and activating CNS pain-signaling neurons, resulting in increased perception of pain from benign stimuli that would not normally be perceived as painful.
2. By a reduction in the threshold of nociceptor terminals in the periphery.[14]

Allodynia is a subclassification of hyperalgesia. It is a common type of pain-associated wound in patients with chronic wounds and may be due to the peripheral sensitization from local wound care procedures. It can last as long as 12 months after the wound is healed.[32]

Pruritus (Itch)

Closely related to pain is the sensation of itch, or pruritus. The evidence does not support that itch is diminutive pain or that it is transmitted by the same C fibers.[30,31] Research of itch pathophysiology is very difficult because the nature of the condition is capricious.[33] Itch can be as severe as or exceed pain in intensity. The question of whether pruritus is nociceptive or neuropathic cannot be answered at this time. What is known is that diffuse itch sensation is induced and transmitted by a specific set of nonmyelinated C fibers that originate in the skin. Nonmyelinated "itch receptors" are presumed to be located in the lower epidermis and possibly at the dermal–epidermal junction. This group of receptors is polymodal and responds to mechanical, thermal, and chemical stimuli. "Itch receptors" can be activated by proinflammatory (pruritogenic) mediators, which stimulate the receptors, and the signals are transmitted via the nonmyelinated C fibers to the dorsal root ganglia, to the dorsal roots, and into the spinal cord where the impulses are sent via spinothalamic tracts to higher centers in the thalamus and hypothalamus by means of the reticular formation.

Peripheral and central mechanisms of itch are not fully understood but are believed to be related to altered peripheral excitation and central disinhibition. The act of scratching is thought to partially restore central inhibition. Endogenous agents are thought to be involved in a causal role, but only histamine has been directly linked as a causative agent. Perhaps it is the repeated release of histamine from trauma during wound care procedures that predisposes these individual to pruritus. Pruritus is reported by patients with underlying medical conditions including chronic renal disease, primary biliary cirrhosis, endocrine disorders (e.g., diabetes), and malignant disease (e.g., lymphoma).[31] Patients with a history of thermal injury often experience severe itching during healing that may last after the wound is completely closed. In elderly patients, dry skin is associated with pruritus. Scratching to relieve the itching contributes to excoriation of the skin. Itch is included in the list of pain quality items evaluated with the neuropathic pain scale.[35] Topical agents like 5% doxepin cream applied after wound closure have been shown to reduce itching,[36] and recently gabapentin has been shown to reduce itching in children recovering from burn wounds.[37] Colloid and oatmeal baths are effective in treating dry skin to relieve itch.

Summary

Multiple components of the nervous system are involved with pain. The action and response is associative and interactive. The nociceptors receive a pain signal, which is the provocation to transmit the signal to other parts of the nervous system, and the reaction is withdrawal from the activity or the brain may perceive a painful experience before it occurs and warn the individual to react. Tissue damage and inflammation increases the sensitivity of the nociceptors that transmit the pain signals. Central sensitization of the spinal neurons occurs when actual tissue damage has ceased and the pain persists after healing as it does in patients who have experienced chronic wounds. Pruritus, while not exactly pain, is a common occurrence in patients with a history of chronic wounds such as venous ulcers or burns. It can be categorized with and is treated similarly to pain.

Persistent (Neuropathic) Pain

Persistent, neuropathic pain is an abnormal functioning of the peripheral or central nerves and may be related to a primary lesion or persistent injury or to neuronal changes associated with disease and can result from a single or multiple pathophysiologies.[19] It is a disease of the nervous system, not a symptom.[25] Persistent pain is defined as pain being present for more than three months and may be continuous or intermittent.[38] An example of persistent pain is background pain which is pain at rest and is often associated with venous ulcers and burns.[39,40] Persistent neuropathic pain causes are heterogeneous and may be inflammatory (e.g., postherpetic neuralgia), metabolic (e.g., diabetes), or ischemic (e.g., arterial insufficiency).[3] Persistent neuropathic pain is divided into two categories: peripheral neuropathic pain that occurs when the lesion or dysfunction affects the PNS and central pain when the lesion or dysfunction affects the CNS.[1,41] Another proposed classification is to divide peripheral neuropathic pain into stimulus-evoked pain or stimulus-independent pain (spontaneous pain).[19] Spontaneous pain arises from spontaneous activity in the spinal cord, brainstem, or thalamic/cortical areas and is less common and may have many mechanisms.[19] Stimulus-evoked pain is a heightened reaction to a painful stimulus, as described previously for hyperalgesia and allodynia, that occurs when the peripheral nerve is damage or altered.[3,19] Initially, these conditions are acute and reversible and the symptoms usually resolve in 12 months,[32] but if there is persistent injury the peripheral nerves can be permanently damaged and the pain becomes constant.

Sensations for acute peripheral neuropathic pain are characteristically independent of a stimulus and the pain can be shooting, lancinating, or burning. Other terms describing acute neuropathic sensations are electric shock, squeezing, throbbing, knife-like, and allodynia. As noted, acute symptoms resolve. Chronic neuropathy symptoms include numbness, tingling, and prickling and do not resolve and may be present continuously or intermittently. The symptoms may be dependent on the activity of the SNS and may be related to SNS dysfunction.[19,32] Persistent pain is different in several ways from acute pain, and it remains after the period of tissue healing, disrupts sleep and normal living, and is no longer providing a protective function.[41] In 99% of persons with persistent pain there is usually some underlying derangement or abnormal function of the nervous system that resulted from an acute incident.[25] For example, a wide area of discomfort surrounding a wound or a stump that healed long ago is the natural consequence of the change in the way that the nervous system responds to signals it receives.[14] Chemicals such as those used to treat cancer or human immunodeficiency virus (HIV) insult the nervous system and cause permanent damage to the nerves.[25] As mentioned earlier, patients with chronic wounds experience significant amounts of repetitive handling and trauma, resulting in sensory stimulation that can be sustained within the CNS due to altered transmissions.

Persistent neuropathic pain can arise from other etiologies, such as spinal compression, spinal stenosis, central poststroke, complex regional pain syndrome (formerly called reflex sympathetic dystrophy), distal polyneuropathy (HIV and diabetes), phantom limb, postherpetic neuralgia, fibromyalgia, multiple sclerosis, and treatment interventions such as chemotherapy or radiation. Chemotherapy- and radiation-associated neuropathies are becoming more common as people are living longer following a cancer diagnosis and many undergo several courses of chemotherapy or radiation with drugs that are toxic to the nervous system.[25]

Many patients with chronic wounds also have other chronic maladies, suggesting that they likely experience mixed pain types. Investigation continues in the development, predictability, and control of neuropathic pain, but as yet these remain important unmet clinical needs and challenges.[19]

Mixed Pain Categories

Many patients have mixed pictures of nociceptive and persistent neuropathic pain. The mixed pain may be caused by both acute injury and secondary effects. Examples of painful conditions found in populations that often have chronic wounds are degenerative joint disease or spinal stenosis pain syndromes, or musculoskeletal problems that overlap nociceptive pain from fracture, surgical wounding, lower extremity arterial insufficiency, or infection. Diffuse pain complaints can mask problems such as a blocked artery that occurred in a resident of a long-term care facility who had multiple areas with musculoskeletal pain and intermittent claudication with walking.[42] When the other pain complaints were addressed and pain was cleared in those areas it became apparent that the cause was visceral and warranted further investigation. It is important for the clinician to distinguish which condition is causing which pain picture and whether the pain is nociceptive or neuropathic or both so they can each be treated effectively.

Chronic Wound Pain Perceptions

Chronic wound pain perceptions are presented in this section. The discussion includes two chronic wound pain models, an international survey of wound care clinicians, and behavioral studies on the effect of pain on wound healing.

The Chronic Wound Pain Experience

Krasner called attention to the chronic wound pain experience in 1995 when she presented an empirically and inductively derived visual schematic model she called the chronic wound pain experience (CWPE) (Figure 13-1).[43] Krasner's model relates the occurrence of pain to time rather than the physiologic or psychosocial aspects of the pain experience. The model does not include psychosocial and behavioral components. From her personal and clinical experience, she pointed out that at different times patients with chronic wounds will experience all three types of pain: noncyclic, cyclic, and chronic. She suggested using the CWPE model to guide wound assessment to plan strategies related to the prevention and relief of wound pain and evaluate the outcomes.[6] The three types of pain are listed below.

1. Noncyclic acute wound pain such as occurs intermittently with sharp debridement or drain removal and is an example of nociceptive pain, The plan of care suggested for pain management includes both pharmacologic and nonpharmacologic interventions such as topical anesthetics, local anesthetics, or anti-anxiety medication prior to debridement. Nonpharmacologic interventions are not listed by Krasner for this pain type.

2. Cyclic acute wound pain, which occurs in a regular time cycle like daily dressing changes or turning or repositioning is also and example of nociceptive pain. The plan of care in addition to the previously listed interventions could include use of nontraumatic dressings, soaking dressings before removal, or timeouts and use of appropriate repositioning devices.

3. Chronic wound pain, which is persistent neuropathic pain, according to Krasner, is felt by the patient all the time (e.g. background pain), even without manipulation The plan of care is as previously suggested for the other pain situations with the addition of nonpharmaceuticals like transcutaneous nerve stimulation or warmth and pharmaceuticals like tricyclic antidepressants.[5, 43]

Additional information about use of the mentioned interventions is presented later in this chapter.

Sibbald Chronic Wound Pain Algorithm

Sibbald developed another empirical scheme for addressing chronic wound pain. This scheme has evolved and currently has been published in three formats.[5,17,44] The basic paradigm is to address three factors related to the treatment of chronic wounds and preparation of the wound bed for healing that contribute to chronic wound pain.[44] The three factors are:

1. Causing Factors (pressure, venous, arterial, surgical, palliative, and diabetic)
2. Local wound factors (debridement, bacterial balance, infection and inflammation, and moisture balance)
3. Patient factors (quality of life and adherence)

Wound Pain Problems at Dressing Changes

An international two-part survey of health-care practitioners from 11 countries explored the understanding of pain and trauma at wound dressing.[7] Part one of the survey looked at causes of wound pain related to dressings and part two was a questionnaire that asked clinicians to rate the patient's pain experience at dressing changes. The answers were ranked by the most perceived painful wound types.

The key findings of the survey related to wound dressings were as follows:

1. Dressing removal is the time of the most pain.
2. Dried-out products and adherent products are most likely to cause pain and trauma at dressing changes.
3. A main consideration at dressing changes is prevention of wound trauma and prevention of pain, infection, and skin damage, in that order.
4. Gauze is most likely to cause pain; new products such as hydrogels, hydrofibers, alginates, and soft silicone dressing are least likely to cause pain (Chapter 11 explains the use of these dressing products).

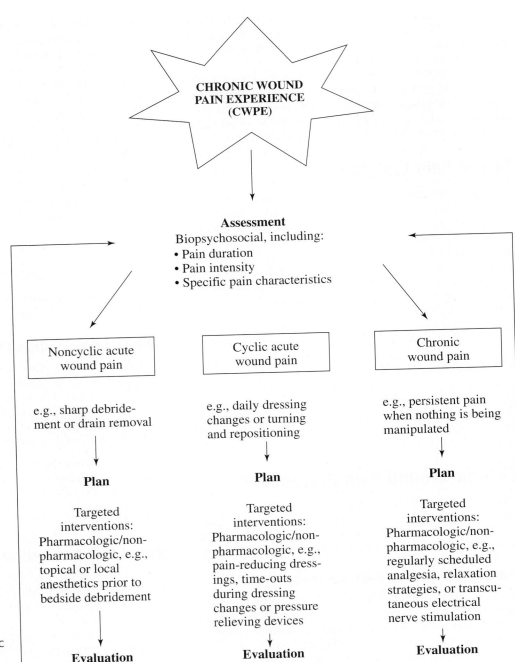

FIGURE 13-1 Krasner chronic wound experience. (Copyright Diane L. Krasner.)

5. Awareness of the products available and the range of and ability to select dressings is highly variable between countries.
6. Use of valid pain assessment tools is considered a low priority in assessment with greater reliance on body language and nonverbal cues.[7]

Wound pain by etiologies were rated by clinicians' perceptions of pain as follows: The most often listed wound pain experience was reported to be leg ulcers, followed by superficial burns, infected wounds, and pressure ulcers.

Other wounds were ranked as less painful. However, the authors caution that this may reflect the practitioner's lack of assessment and experience rather than a true estimate of pain perceived by patients.

Behavioral Studies of Wound-Related Pain

Franks and Moffatt did a qualitative study of the effects of pain on leg ulcer healing and patients' quality of life.[9] They found that the risk of poor healing for venous ulcers can be predicted based on the pain intensity level at baseline. Overall healing rates declined with increasing levels of pain and with daily use of analgesics. Quality of life in the area of wound pain and healing has shown that with effective treatment interventions, levels of pain decrease significantly.[9]

Reddy et al recommend a patient-centered approach to wound pain management.[5] They recognized that pain is related to a multitude of factors that affect an individual's psychological state, which include the attitude, beliefs, and knowledge of the caregiver, the patient, and family. The wound needs to be treated holistically. Dressing changes, for example, need to be viewed not just as a task but also its impact on the patient. To ensure that care is patient centered, the follow adaptation of their recommendations are offered below:

1. Consider all aspects of the patient: physical, psychological, social, familial, and spiritual
2. Enlist the patient in treatment decisions and the process
3. Take time to assess the patient's pain and determine quality-of-life issues
4. Provide pain relief
5. Ensure that the patient's right to pain relief and treatment that minimizes trauma and pain is provided

Wound Etiology

Different wound etiologies are associated with specific nociceptive pain factors that should be considered on an index of suspicion. The limited data that exist are presented for each wound type.

Arterial Ulcers

Peripheral ischemia is responsible for wound pain in patients with arterial insufficiency. Types of arterial insufficiency pain may be nociceptive, that is, positional (increased with elevation and decreased with dependency) or incurred with walking (intermittent claudication relieved with 10 minutes rest), or neuropathic, that is, nocturnal, or at rest without activity or elevated position. The following assessments for indicators of limb ischemia are recommended.[45]

1. Measurements: ankle pressure and toe pressure if there are calcified vessels
   a. Finding of ankle pressure < 40 mm Hg
   b. Finding of toe pressure < 30 mm Hg are signs of critical limb ischemia and ischemic pain
2. Signs/symptoms
   a. Rest pain that requires analgesics
      i. < 2 weeks duration is defined as subcritical limb ischemia
      ii. > 2 weeks duration is defined as critical limb ischemia[45]

Chapter 7 provides more information about these tests and their significance.

3. Intervention: Based on considerable research that exercise is beneficial in reducing claudication pain, exercise is recommended as an intervention for lower extremity arterial disease.[45] Pharmacologic therapy should be included in the treatment regime.

Diabetic Foot Ulcers

Painful diabetic neuropathy is quite common and is a harbinger of loss of sensation. These same symptoms are reported by individuals with other peripheral neuropathy etiologies. A minority of persons with chronic diabetic foot ulcers may experience tingling, burning, stabbing, or shooting sensations related to peripheral neuropathy.[46] Subcritical and critical peripheral ischemia is a complication of diabetes, and ischemic pain is frequently encountered during physical activities such as walking.[47]

Deep compartment infection can cause pain even in persons with severe neuropathy.[46] The typical signs of infection will most likely be blunted or absent in this population, but even mild edema or erythema are signals to pay attention to and take action. If a patient with a previously painless foot reports pain, *urgent* referral is required because it may signal limb-threatening complications of infection.[46] Refer to Table 13-2 for management strategies.

Venous Leg Ulcers

Studies of leg ulcer pain reported in the literature point to a significant prevalence of ulcer pain ranging from 50% to 87%, which until recently has been ignored.[48,49] Pain relief for venous ulcer pain is of concern for most patients but is of greatest concern for those between the ages of 60 and 70 years.[48] It is widely recognized and reported that patients with venous leg ulcers have both nociceptive and neuropathic pain, the latter expressed as constant background pain.[50,51]

Pruritus was reported in 50% of leg ulcer patients.[52] Dermatitis, another complication associated with venous disease, often affects the skin surrounding the ulcer and is a reaction to the use of products that contain allergens and irritants such as topical lubricants, emollients, topical antibiotics, and other wound care products. The complaint is usually in the area of distribution of product use and is usually associated with pruritus and burning sensations.[48] Pain may be constant or intermittent and vary in intensity from severe to mild, with many patients suffering from night pain. Many patients are using analgesics with reported efficacy in most cases.[42,49] The most frequently used medication for management of leg ulcer pain in one study was NSAIDs (70%).[10] The profile of the patient with pain is likely to include the presence of other co-morbid painful conditions, including osteoarthritis or a foot ulcer[49] or a combination of venous and arterial insufficiency. Characteristics that are associated with venous pain include: pitting edema, superficial phlebitis, deep vein thrombosis (DVT), acute lipodermatosclerosis, chronic lipodermatosclerosis, and wound infection. Cellulitis, scarring (atrophie blanche), and acute contact dermatitis are also useful in development

TABLE 13-2   Differential Diagnosis for Diabetic Foot Pain

Diagnosis	Clinical/Investigation	Comments
Ischemia	Pain with walking (claudication) or positional (elevated position relieved with dependency) TcPO₂ ankle pressure < 40 mm Hg Toe pressure < 30 mm Hg	Not a candidate for compression Risk for nonhealing
Neuropathic pain	Sensations Numbness Tingling Burning = nerve irritation Shooting or stabbing = nerve damage Throbbing Paresthesia Electric Shock	Persistent or intermittent Allodynia Hyperalgesia
Deep compartment infection	Sudden onset Mild dermal erythema > 2 cm Mild swelling > 2 cm diameter New wound or increased wound size Temperature increase of 4°F Probes to bone	Needs systemic treatment Refer for medical treatment
Charcot arthropathy	Hot temperature increase of 4 degrees Swollen Very painful foot Biochemical markers of bone formation	Offload (total contact cast or other) Monitor change in temperature; offload until temperature normalizes

Adapted from Sibbald GR, Armstrong DG, and Orsted HI. *Pain in Diabetic Foot Ulcers.* Ostomy Wound Management, Vol 49 Suppl 4A, April 2003.

of differential diagnosis of venous pain.[48] Table 13-3 lists clinical presentation, treatment choices, and comments about the differential diagnosis of venous pain.

Many individuals have lived with venous leg ulcers for more than 10 years.[49,50] Therefore, central and peripheral sensitization are highly probable. Persistent pain in the leg should be evaluated thoroughly. Pain characteristics most frequently reported by patients with leg ulcers are divided into three categories that correspond to the McGill pain questionnaire—sensory, affective, and evaluative. Based on several survey papers, the most frequently reported pain is in the sensory category and includes throbbing, drilling, burning, stabbing, sharp, pressure, aching, sharp, tender, and stinging. These reported sensations are consistent with abnormal nervous system function associated with persistent neuropathic pain. Affective pain descriptors commonly used include nagging, tiring, sickening, troublesome, and unbearable.[10,53,54] Aggravating factors for pain that patients and clinicians listed most frequently include dressing changes, both during and between changes, followed by movement.[54,55] Suggestions for the relief of pain at dressing changes is offered in the section on nonpharmacologic methods of pain relief.

Compression is the current standard of care for treatment of venous leg ulcers, but the relationship of compression to venous leg ulcer pain has been minimally eval-

uated. Nemeth et al reported on the effect of compression on leg ulcer pain and found over a 6-week period that by using compression, there was a trend toward decreased pain scores. (See Chapter 10 for more information about compression.)

CLINICAL WISDOM

Not everyone can tolerate elastic compression because of pain related to the high levels of compression at rest. An alternative treatment plan that may relieve pain is an inelastic support system that does not have high pressure at rest. It is also easier to apply than elastic compression products.[48]

Pressure Ulcer Pain

Pressure ulcer pain has been attributed to pressure, friction/shear, moisture related to incontinence (feces and urine), deep infection, periulcer irritation, poor nutritional status, neuropathy, and muscle spasm. All should be part of the index of suspicion for wounds with this etiology.[56] Dallam et al evaluated stage I and II pressure ulcer pain using a visual analog scale (VAS) or the FACES scale and found that pressure ulcer pain was reported at 4 cm and 3.5 cm on VAS and FACES scales, respectively.[57] Szor and Bourguignon evaluated pressure ulcer pain at rest and during dressing changes in patients with stage II, III, or IV pres-

TABLE 13-3   Differential Diagnosis of Venous Pain

Diagnosis	Clinical/Investigation	Treatment	Comments
Pitting edema	Dull ache at end of day Press thumb into skin and not degree of depression Grade 1+ to 4+	Compression bandaging Support stockings Ambulation, exercise Improve calf muscle pump	Nonelastic stockings or compression bandaging may initially be preferred as they are less likely to cause pain at rest
Superficial phlebitis	Pain and tenderness along affected vein—usually saphenous	Compression Ambulation NSAID therapy	Risk of associated underlying DVT is low, especially if affected area is below the knee
Deep phlebitis (DVT)	Acute, red, tender, swollen calf—almost too painful to touch Doppler necessary to confirm diagnosis	ASA, unfractionated heparin Warfarin Low-molecular weight heparin Bed rest	Suspect a DVT in patients with a sudden increase in calf pain, with risk factors such as im mobilization, recent surgery, oral contraceptives, etc.
Acute lipodermatosclerosis	Diffuse, purple-red, swollen leg resembling cellulitis, aching and tenderness is common	Compression bandaging Support stockings NSAIDs	Usually bilateral, though may be more prominent in one leg Compression therapy essential
Chronic lipodermatosclerosis	Diffuse brown sclerotic pigmentation with widespread chronic pain	Same as with acute lipodermatosclerosis but with topical steroids and lubricants Pentoxifylline	Support stockings may have to be custom made to accommodate for leg shape
Wound infection	Change in pain character associated with other clinical signs of infection	Topical antimicrobial agents and oral antibiotics, if indicated	Maintain bacterial balance, and watch for increase in pain, size, exudates, odor, or granulation tissue as signs of infection
Cellulitis	Diffuse bright red, hot leg, usually unilateral associated with tenderness and often fever	Oral antibiotics, with IV antibiotics needed for severe episodes or with low host resistance	Venous ulcers make individuals more prone to cellulitis
Atrophie blanche	Pain, stellate, white, scar-like areas associated with pain at rest and standing	NSAID therapy Other analgesics	May be seen in association with scars of healed ulcers, or may be an independent clinical feature
Acute contact dermatitis	Itching, burning red areas on leg corresponding to area of use of topical product	Remove the allergen Apply topical steroids	Lanolin, colophony, latex, and neomycin are some of the more likely agents involved

Ryan S, Eager C, Sibbald RG. Venous Leg Ulcer Pain. *Ostomy/Wound Management.* April 2003;49(4A (Suppl)): p. 18.

sure ulcers and found that 18% reported pain at the highest level (e.g., "excruciating"), 84% reported pain at rest, and 42% reported pain both at rest and during dressing changes. Yet, only 6% of those persons reporting pressure ulcer pain received any medication for their pain.[58] Eriksson et al reported that in 186 persons identified with pressure ulcers, 12% reported continuous pain and 54% reported occasional pain or dressing change pain.[59] Roth et al examined persistent pain in patients who received a tissue flap procedure for stage III or IV pressure ulcers or diabetic ulcers and found that 35% of those with stage III or IV pressure ulcers reported pain as compared with 17% of those with stage II pressure ulcers.[60] Manz and colleagues examined pressure ulcer pain in cognitively impaired and nonimpaired nursing home residents with mild to moderate pain. Stage II pressure ulcers were the most painful. Manz also was able to show that both cognitively intact and cognitively impaired persons could differentiate pressure ulcer pain from other pain.[61]

In addition to studies specifically examining pressure ulcer pain, treatment studies often report on pressure ulcer pain. For example, Van Rijswijk in a study of hydrocolloid dressings reported that 21 (37%) ulcers were not all painful and 14 (25%) were very painful during dressing changes.[62] Table 13-4 presents strategies for managing pressure ulcer pain.

TABLE 13-4 **Pressure Ulcer Pain Management Strategies**

Cause of Pain	Definition	Treatment	Comments
Pressure	A force applied to the skin and underlying tissues that inhibits blood flow when it ↓ pressures within the capillary: capillary closing pressure (CCP) = 32 mm Hg (average value)	Special Surface: Pressure Reduction ↓ pressure, but not necessarily below CCP, e.g., high density foam, standard hospital mattresses Synthetic (not sheepskin) heel booties Pressure Relief ↓ pressure below CCP, e.g., dynamic flow beds Turning schedules crucial	Consider: Pressure mapping Wheelchair assessment
Friction	Created by movement of the patient over a surface	Heel booties, e.g., sheepskin booties (do not reduce pressure but may decrease friction) Careful with patient transfers (use turning sheet) Hydrocolloid over bony prominences	On its own, friction doesn't usually cause ulcers. However, friction in addition to pressure greatly ↑ risk of ulcer development.
Shear	Adjacent body surfaces slide across each other (as happens when a patient slides down in bed)	Keep head of bed ≤ 30° tilt seating, rather than recline (may need some recline if slumping is a problem)	Again, more dangerous when combined with pressure
Moisture	Imitation & maceration from sweating, stool, urine, wound drainage	PREVENTION If urine incontinence, bladder training, urinary catheter (in & out rather than permanent, if possible) Change undergarment pads frequently Local wound care to keep surrounding skin from maceration Absorbent surface next to skin TREATMENT Barriers to wound edges (e.g., zinc oxide, petrolatum, occlusive dressing) May need antidiarrhea medications If surrounding dermatitis, may need steroid cream/ointment	Can also use film-forming topical acrylate liquids Watch for secondary yeast, especially in folds
Periulcer irritation	Can be due to dermatitis, maceration, and/or infection (e.g., candida)	To reduce periulcer irritation can apply either Vaseline, zinc oxide; film-forming liquid (e.g., acrylate); occlusive dressings (picture frame technique) and if candida suspected, hydrocortisone in Canesten cream BID	If hydrocortisone in Canesten is being easily wiped off with body positioning and move-movement, then can cover with zinc oxide

Cause of Pain	Definition	Treatment	Comments
Nutrition	Both pain & healing may be exacerbated if a patient has low muscle mass	Major risks: low overall dietary intake, especially protein Consult dietician Consider supplements	No particular evidence than certain vitamins promote healing Check albumin and total lymphocyte count
Deep infection	Infection requiring systemic agents	Probes to bone, osteomyelitis unless proven otherwise; may need long-term antibiotics	Probe ulcer: make sure it doesn't probe to bone & there are no sinus tracts or fistulas
Neuropathic/radicular	Nerve irritation, damage	Consider tricyclic antidepressants (nortriptyline) and convulsants (gabapentin)	Consider referral to anesthesia for nerve blocks
Spasms	Involuntary muscle movement	May need baclofen	Consider referral to psychiatry

Reprinted from Reddy M, Keast D, Fowler E, Sibbald G. *Pain in Pressure Ulcers*. April 2003 Volume 49(4A Suppl), page 32.

CLINICAL WISDOM

Temporary resolution of ischemic pain of a leg or foot may be achieved when the activity is stopped or the legs are placed in a dependent position (e.g., dangling legs down at the edge of the bed). If the cause of the pain has not been evaluated, this would be an indication for referral to a vascular specialist.

Assessment of Wound Pain

Wound pain assessment is not really different from other types of pain assessment, but there are factors related to wounds that are unique and should be considered during the assessment. For example, wound pain may be caused by an as yet undetected infection or it may be related to specific wound care procedures. In all cases, the assessment should focus on the cause of the pain and should lead to development of a pain management plan. Subsequent assessment should focus on the efficacy of that plan. If the plan is not effective and pain is not relieved, a new plan is needed after the cause of the plan failure is determined. Possible causes of plan failure maybe related to a new treatment intervention or to a change in the wound or the host status, or a combination of things.

Elements to include in the initial pain assessment are divided in to the following four categories:[27]

1. Detailed patient history, including pain intensity and character
2. Physical examination, including neurologic component
3. Psychosocial assessment
4. Appropriate diagnostic work-up to determine the cause and type of pain

Patient History

The screening for wound pain begins with a review of the patient's medical history and interviewing the patient. A questionnaire with a body diagram is recommended to speed the interview process and the pain diagnosis. The answers to the questionnaire will help the experienced clinician determine quickly if there is a pain pattern, and develop a diagnosis about the type of pain.[25] Pain scales described below should be part of the assessment process.

Developing a Wound Pain Diagnosis

After the history review, determine if there is a specific pain pattern that can suggest a probable source of the wound pain. Goodman and Snyder suggest that four pain patterns should be considered.[63] The following have been adapted to illustrate relationships to wound-specific pain.

1. Cutaneous (related to the skin). The pain may be superficial or related to subcutaneous tissue. This type of pain pattern often is localized, although skin tenderness may occur in both referred and somatic pain. Infection is an example. If the pain is acute, the intensity should be consistent with the problem, and descriptors used to describe the pain may be sharp or sudden, or intense. If it is persistent neuropathic pain, the pain pattern may be inappropriate and different in character than would be expected, and descriptors used to describe the pain may be burning, throbbing, or shocking.
2. Somatic (emotional). Emotional distress produces physical symptoms that are apparent briefly or that recur, or have multiple manifestations. Some manifestations of distress include anxiety about wound treatment and not keeping clinic appointments. Depression about a wound can manifest as poor acceptance of treatment or result in family issues.
3. Visceral (related to internal organs). Visceral disease may be accompanied by hypersensitivity to touch, pressure, and temperature. Lower extremity ischemic pain, for example, is characterized by burning and boring, and is usually worse at night and relieved in the dependent condition. The patient with an arterial ulcer often will report disturbed sleep.
4. Referred (related to irritation or deep somatic or visceral structures). Referred pain typically occurs in tissues supplied by the same or adjacent nerves as an area of injured

tissue. The patient can usually point to the area that hurts. Pain can be present in adjacent tissue after a wound has healed. This is the type of pain that could characterize secondary hyperalgesia.

Initial Wound Pain Assessment

Pain assessment for wounds, as mentioned, is basically the same as for other types of pain. The difference is the cause or underlying pathology of the pain. Assessment of the fol-

lowing items should be part of the development of the diagnosis of the cause and type of pain. Exhibit 13-1 is a sample pain assessment form that can be used to track the elements.

Onset and temporal pattern: Determine the onset of the wound and the pain problem to focus attention on whether the problem is related to an acute event like a dressing change or to persistent wound pain that is there constantly. For example, wounds of long duration such as

EXHIBIT 13-1   Pain Experience Assessment Form

Do you have pain? _____ Yes _____ No
Location of the pain _____
Intensity of the pain
Pain scale: *Visual Analog (1-10), Numeric Pain Scale, or Faces Pain Scale*
Pain distress scale: _____

Describe the pain

_____ Sharp	_____ Stabbing	_____ Burning
_____ Shooting	_____ Cramping	_____ Dull
_____ Heavy	_____ Aching	_____ Tender
_____ Splitting	_____ Tiring	_____ Exhausting
_____ Throbbing	_____ Difficult to localize	_____ Easily localized

Pain in the legs after walking a short time (claudication)?   _____ Yes _____ No
Pain when legs are hanging down (dependent pain)?   _____ Yes _____ No
Pain when legs are elevated?   _____ Yes _____ No
Pain during the night when you are in bed sleeping?   _____ Yes _____ No
Does the pain wake you up during the night?   _____ Yes _____ No

Duration of the pain

Is the pain constant (continuous)?   _____ Yes _____ No
Is pain intermittent (come and go)?   _____ Yes _____ No
How long does it last?   _____ Minutes _____ Hours _____ Constant
Is the current pain management: _____ Adequate _____ Inadequate

Current Pain Medications:	What Kind	How Much	How Often	Result
_____ Acetaminophen	___	___	___	___
_____ Aspirin	___	___	___	___
_____ NSAIDS/Cox 2	___	___	___	___
_____ Steroids	___	___	___	___
_____ Narcotic (codeine, morphine)	___	___	___	___
_____ Patch	___	___	___	___
_____ Other?	___	___	___	___

Functional Capacity (as affected by pain)

Sleep:	_____ Adequate	_____ Restful	_____ Inadequate	_____ Restless
Appetite	_____ Adequate	_____ Poor		
Bladder continence:	_____ Yes	_____ No		
Bowel continence:	_____ Yes	_____ No		
Toileting	_____ Independent	_____ Assistance	_____ Dependent	
Dressing:	_____ Independent	_____ Assistance	_____ Dependent	
Bathing:	_____ Independent	_____ Assistance	_____ Dependent	
Relationship with others:	_____ Okay	_____ Irritable	_____ Other	
Emotions:	_____ Okay	_____ Irritable	_____ Other	
Work:	_____ Able	_____ Not able		
Drive:	_____ Able	_____ Not able		
Hobbies:	_____ Able	_____ Not able		

Adapted from Fowler E. Plain talk about wound management. *Ostomy Wound Management* November 2005, Volume 51, Issue 11A (Suppl).

venous ulcers are likely to have developed hyperalgesia, and the pain is persistent background pain that is aggravated at dressing changes.

Other comorbidities and wound procedures: Consider the relationship of wound pain to other comorbidities (e.g., peripheral vascular disease, venous insufficiency or diabetic neuropathy, musculoskeletal disease or cancer) and procedures (e.g., surgery, debridement, negative pressure therapy, pulsed lavage) to narrow the index of suspicion as to the etiology of the pain and to differentiate wound pain from other pain sources.

Location and distribution: Critical information needed to make a differential diagnosis of the type of wound pain include the location and distribution of the pain.

Description of the type of pain: Reported sensations like sharp, deep, burning, tingling, light touch help differentiate the type of pain (e.g., local nociceptive, acute hyperalgesia or central sensitization, persistent).

Quality and intensity: Measure the quality and intensity of the pain with validated pain scales. There is agreement that the best assessment of pain is the patient's self report.[27] The self-reporting pain scales presented below are designed to be used with patients with all types of pain etiologies and while subjective, they are validated. Not all patients do well with the same scale, so there are different ones available to meet different needs.

Aggravating and relieving actions: Part of the patient's self report should include aggravating and relieving pain actions. For example, intermittent wound debridement, regular dressing changes, and infection have been identified as aggravating factors, and use of topical analgesics, protective dressings, systemic and local treatment of infection are identified as relieving factors, as well as other methods discussed below.[44]

Associated features or secondary signs and symptoms: Evaluate change in the character of the wound pain associated with signs and symptoms such as increased size of the wound, odor, and cellulitis, which can indicate clinical infection.

Associated factors: Factors like sleep patterns, mood, depression, and anxiety can be related to pain. Pain often varies with stress and activities during the day and from day to day. A pain diary can pinpoint the time of day and the activity associated with pain relief and aggravation. Then the timing for pain relief can be chosen. An example of a pain diary is shown in Exhibit 13-2.

Treatment response: Evaluate medication or nonpharmaceutical treatment for its effect on the pain. Is it effective? For how long? How does it affect activities of daily living? Again, a pain diary is a useful tool to monitor and assess treatment responses.

CLINICAL WISDOM

Invite the patient's significant other to be present during the pain assessment to help identify how and what contributes to the patient's pain, treatment response, and how the pain interferes with daily activities.

Neuropathic Wound Pain Assessment

A simple neurologic physical examination is used to confirm diagnosis and distribution of neuropathic pain.[25,64] The diagnosis of neuropathic pain is made clinically by interpreting the results of negative (e.g., absences of tactile, protective sensation, or diminished reflexes) as well as positive (e.g., report of burning or shocking) findings during the exam along with review of a validated pain questionnaire such as the neuropathic pain scale (NPS). Sophisticated technology tests do not add information needed to diagnose neuropathic pain.[25] Simple clinical tests like testing for protective sensation, vibration testing, and thermal testing as described in Chapters 4 and 19 are appropriate and valid. A simple toolkit is recommended for a quick neurologic exam to confirm diagnosis of neuropathic pain and its distribution.[25,30] Items in the kit include a piece of dry gauze, a reflex hammer, a 5.7 gr monofilament (some come attached to a reflex hammer), and a tuning fork. Directions for using the toolkit, items tested and the associated pain mechanisms and guidelines for conducting a neurologic physical examination and interpreting results are found in Table 13-5.

Pain Scales

Pain scales are or two basic types: unidimensional and multidimensional. It is best to use brief, easy-to-use assessment tools that reliably document pain intensity and pain relief.[24]

EXHIBIT 13-2 Wound Pain Diary

Date	Time	Location	Sensation	Activity	Pain Intensity Rating (0-10)	Medication, Treatment	Results
10/20	1 pm	Lower leg	Burning	Dressing change by nurse	4	None	None
10/20	9 pm	Lower leg	Throbbing	Resting	2	NSAID	Reduced pain to 0 Able to sleep through the night

TABLE 13-5   Assessment of Sensory Symptoms or Signs in Neuropathic Pain[27]

Tool Kit for a Neurologic Exam

A simple tool kit is recommended for performing a quick neurologic exam to confirm diagnosis of neuropathic pain and its distribution.[23,27] Items in the kit include: a piece of dry gauze, a reflex hammer, a 5.7 gr monofilament (some come attached to a reflex hammer), and a tuning fork.

Sensory Symptoms and Signs	Clinical Exam	Mechanism
Negative signs are diminished responses:		
a. touch	Brush skin with gauze	Aβ fibers
b. pin	Poke area of pain with monofilament point	Aδ fibers
c. cold	Place cold tuning fork on painful area	Aδ and C fibers
d. vibration	Strike tuning fork and place on lateral malleolus	Aß fibers
Positive Signs:		
Spontaneous activity		
a. Paresthesia	These are present and graded (from 0–10)	Aß afferents
b. Dysesthesia		C/A δ afferents
c. Superficial burning pain		C nociceptors
d. Deep pain		Joint/muscle nociceptors
Evoked		
Touch: dynamic hyperalgesia	Brush skin with gauze	Central sensitization
Pressure: static hyperalgesia	Gentle mechanical pressure	Central sensitization
Punctate hyperalgesia	Pricking skin with monofilament	Aδ fiber input
Punctate repetitive hyperalgesia (wind up like pain)	Pricking the skin with monofilament 2×/sec for 30 sec	Central sensitization / Central sensitization
After sensation	Time pain duration after stimulation	Aδ fiber input
Cold hyperalgesia	Place cold tuning fork on skin	Central sensitization

Adapted from Jensen TS and Baron R: Translation of symptoms and signs into mechanisms in neuropathic pain. *Pain* 2003;102:1–8.

Examples of tools that meet these criteria are described below.

Unidimensional pain scales: Assessing pain intensity is the most frequently used parameter in clinical practice. While this only captures one aspect of pain it is useful for evaluating pain relief interventions. Pain intensity is commonly measured quantitatively using a numerical rating scale (NRS), verbal descriptor scale (VDS), visual analog scale (VAS), or FACES scale. All provide data about pain intensity and are useful for evaluating the intensity of wound pain. In general, as pain reaches the higher levels on pain intensity scales (such as 7 or 8 out of 10 on an NRS), it interferes with mood, sleep, work, enjoyment of life, and motivates the person to seek help. In contrast, pain felt at lower levels on pain intensity scales (such as 2 or 3 on an NRS) might not be reported by persons as pain at all.[25] Exhibit 13-3A provides examples of two pain scales.

Visual analogue scale: The VAS is a 0 to 100 mm number line with ratio scale properties. It has demonstrated high validity and reliability when used with hospitalized patients.[65,66] Following the instructions for use of the VAS may be difficult for children and frail elders with or without cognitive impairment. A VAS using a color scale has been found to be valid and reliable when tested with cognitively impaired elders.[67] The colored VAS has a visual depiction of pain intensity on one side, which is shown to the patient, and the 0 to 100 mm numerical rating scale on the other side for the clinician.

FACES scale: The FACES scale consists of 5 to 6 cartoon faces ordered from smiling to crying or grimacing and labeled 0 to 5 or 6, respectively.[68] The FACES scale has been used extensively with pediatric populations as well as with adults and cognitively impaired elders.[69,70] When the FACES scale uses oval-shaped faces without tears, the cartoons are more adult-like in appearance. Advantages of the FACES scale are the ease and quickness of administration, simplicity, the correlation with VAS, and little mental energy required by the patient.[71]

Numerical rating scale: NRS uses two number anchors, most typically 0 and 10, in which 0 represents no pain and 10 represents the worst pain imaginable.[72] The NRS is administered verbally, allowing for use over the phone and with those who have visual or physical impairments such that use of other tools is difficult or not possible. NRS have demonstrated sensitivity to treatments that impact pain intensity and is easy to score and use.

EXHIBIT 13-3   A and B Pain Intensity Scales

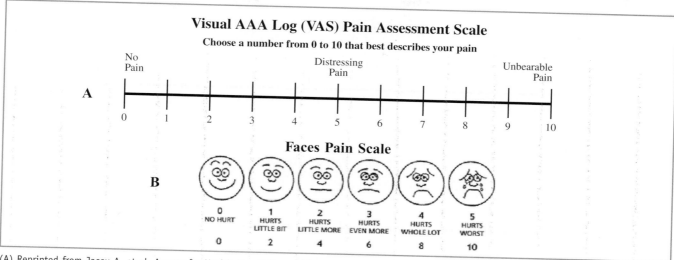

(A) Reprinted from Jacox A, et al. Agency for Health Care Policy and Research (AHCPR), Publication No, 94-0592, 1994, U.S. Department of Health and Human Services, Rockville, Maryland. (B) From Wong DL, Hockenberry-Eaton M, Wilson D, Winkelstein ML, Schwartz P. *Wong's Essentials of Pediatric Nursing*, 6e. St. Louis, 2001, p. 1301. Copyrighted by Mosby, Inc. Reprinted by permission.

Verbal descriptor scale: VDS uses adjectives that reflect extremes of pain and are ranked in order of severity.[61] Each adjective is given a number that constitutes the patient's pain intensity. In general, a VDS is easy to administer and understand. However, the patient must pick one word to describe his or her pain even if no word choice accurately describes it. Furthermore, individuals with limited English and those who are illiterate may have difficulty with this tool.[73]

Pain distress scales: If patients express or exhibit signs of anxiety or other emotional distress during the screening interview, they should be asked to separately rate their emotional distress on pain distress scales that are similar to the pain intensity scales.[27] Three pain distress scales are shown in Exhibit 13-3C.

Use of Pain Scales with Special Populations

Pain assessment for those who cannot communicate verbally, the cognitively impaired, or who have a form of dementia present additional challenges. Mild to moderately impaired elders can respond to simple direct yes/no questions.[65] For those who cannot communicate verbally but who can understand and respond, cue with direct yes/no questions such as, "Do you have wound pain now?" or "Do you have wound pain every day?" Asking the person to identify the location of wound pain using diagrams or body drawings may also be useful. The FACES scale, VAS, or NRS to rate wound pain intensity can also be used with this population. Several studies have demonstrated the ability of elders with mild to moderate levels of cognitive impairment to respond to the FACES scale and VAS.[74,75] Additionally, clinicians should look for behaviors indicating pain such as suggested in the PAINAD scale described below.

Multidimensional Pain Scales

There have been attempts to develop nonverbal pain assessment instruments. One such attempt is the multidimensional PAINAD scale. The PAINAD has been tested in people with advanced Alzheimer disease and other progressive dementias. It requires minimal training and may be useful for detecting wound pain in persons with cognitive impairment. PAINAD rates five behaviors—breathing independent of vocalizations, negative vocalization, facial expression, body language, and consolability—on a 0 to 2 scale, in which 0 indicates normal or none present and 2 indicates the most severe behaviors observed.[76,77] The American Geriatrics Society (AGS) Panel on Persistent Pain in Older Persons recommends looking for the following behaviors[73] that correspond with the items on the PAINAD:

- Facial expressions: frowns, sad frightened face, grimacing, wrinkled forehead, closed or tightened eyes, any distorted expression, rapid blinking
- Verbalizations or vocalizations: sighing, moaning, groaning, calling out, grunting, chanting, noisy breathing, asking for help, verbally abusive
- Body movements: rigid, tense body posture, guarding, fidgeting, increased pacing, rocking, restricted movement, gait or mobility changes
- Changes in interpersonal interactions: aggressive, combative, resisting care, decreased social interactions, socially inappropriate, disruptive, withdrawn
- Changes in activity patterns or routines: refusing food, appetite change, increase in rest periods, sleep, rest pattern changes, sudden cessation of common routines, increased wandering
- Mental status changes: crying or tears, increased confusion, irritability, distress

EXHIBIT 13-3 C Pain distress scales

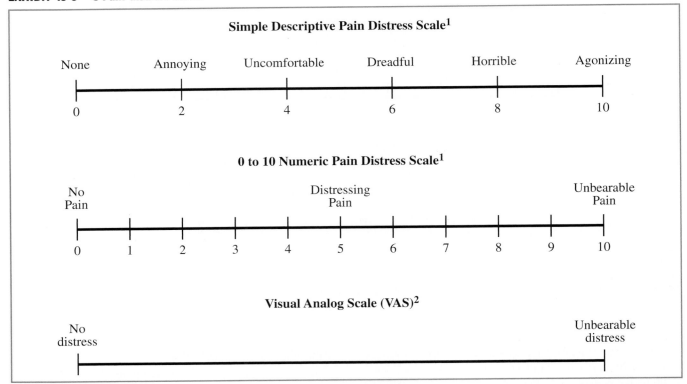

Reprinted from Acute Pain Management Guideline Panel. Acute pain management: operative or medical procedures and trauma. Clinical Practice Guidelines Agency for Health Care Policy and Research (AHCPR), Publication Pub. 92-0032 1992, U.S. Department of Health and Human Services, Rockville, Maryland.

The AGS Persistent Pain Panel cautions that some patients exhibit little or no specific behaviors with pain. The heterogeneity of pain symptoms in the cognitively impaired is what makes pain detection in this population so difficult.

The multidimensional long-form McGill pain questionnaire provides information about pain quality based on 20 descriptor scales.[79] Each scale contains a variable number of words as a list ranked in intensity. The scales are divided into four main dimensions: sensory, affective, evaluative, and miscellaneous. Then the patient is asked to choose one word from any relevant list. The short-form McGill pain questionnaire consists of 11 sensory and 4 affective descriptor scales scores, none, mild, moderate, and severe.[3,79]

Neuropathic Pain Scale

The neuropathic pain scale (NPS) is a multidimensional numeric rating scale for identifying pain intensity related to 10 domains of pain.[28] Each item is rated using a 0 to 10 NRS. Two global measures (intensity and unpleasantness) and eight specific ratings that assess both pain location (deep and surface) and pain quality (sharp, hot, dull, cold, sensitive, and itchy) are scored. Individual item scores and composite scores (determined by summing all items) can be used to determine the overall effects of pain treatments. A subscale (e.g., the NPS-6) specific to the quality of pain

sensation is also useful in evaluating pain relief. The NPS has been shown to be sensitive to changes in pain condition associated with pain treatment, is easy to administer, and reflects both neuropathic and non-neuropathic pain symptoms.[35]

Management of Wound Pain

After the wound pain assessment and the pain diagnosis are made clinically, the next step is to develop a treatment plan to reduce acute pain by treating any underlying conditions such as infection, using wound care procedures that are less painful, and addressing the emotional consequences of having a wound and adequately treating any persistent pain problems the patient may have. The first part of this section focuses primarily on nonpharmaceutical treatment to mitigate pain from wound care procedures and the emotional consequences of having a wound. Nonpharmaceutical options are discussed first because they have great potential to mitigate pain and are minimally invasive and thus have minimal systemic effects and adverse responses. The second part focuses on pharmaceutical options. Either option may be used separately or they can be used together.

As a guideline, severe to moderate pain should be managed primarily with medication (e.g., opioid oral medication for severe pain) and nonpharmacologically as the secondary treatment (e.g., pain-reducing dressings). Low levels of pain may be manageable with nonpharmaceutical methods such as pain reducing wound dressings, relaxation techniques and topical analgesia for procedural pain. Figure 13-2 shows a clinical wound pain decision tree to guide selection of treatment intervention based on the type of wound pain, the pain characteristics, and its causes.

Nonpharmaceutical Options

Positioning

Positioning is a readily available means to help reduce wound pain. Chapters 10 and 17 provide specific suggestions about positioning. The positioning intervention is mentioned here briefly to call attention to the potential for pain relief. For example, offloading of bony prominences will reduce ischemic pain from pressure and traumatic pain from friction and shear, elevation of the legs will reduce edema-related pain in the lower extremities associated with venous insufficiency, and offloading will reduce tissue tension and contact with surgical wounds and reduce pain. For instance, a bed cradle can be used to lift the weight of bedcovers off hypersensitive tissues. Splinting provides immobilization so the painful tissues are not manipulated. Transfer-assist devices are useful to minimize pain when moving a patient in and out of bed or on and off a stretcher. Reposition a patient in bed with lift sheets, not draw sheets, to avoid friction and shear that can lead to painful ulceration.

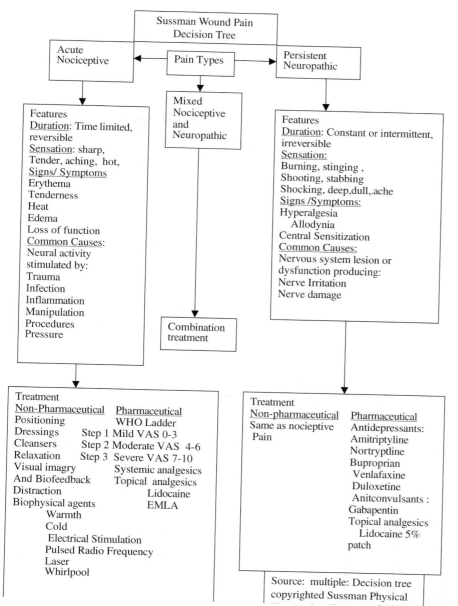

FIGURE 13-2 Wound pain decision tree.

Wound Dressings

Appropriate dressing choice is one of the best nonpharmacologic wound pain treatments. The clinician must be aware of the absorptive capacity, adhesiveness, pain reduction properties, and appropriate use of dressings for specific wound healing goals. Chapter 12 provides information about wound dressings. Here the focus is on selecting the proper dressing to reduce pain. For example, dressings useful for autolytic and enzymatic debridement also retain moisture that bathes exposed nerve endings in moist warm wound fluid, soothing them and reducing pain.

Choose dressings with an adhesive that is aggressive enough to keep the dressing in position but not so aggressive that the surrounding skin or wound bed is traumatized. Self-adhesive dressings have been implicated in aggravating leg ulcers.[80] Use of other methods for dressing placement such as Montgomery straps or nonadhesive netting can help decrease pain related to dressing adhesives. In general, thin film dressings have no absorptive capacity or aggressive adhesive, and they minimize pain by covering exposed nerve endings. Thin film dressings are adherent to the skin surrounding the wound and sometimes the wound itself, making dressing removal more likely to be painful. Thin film dressings have been shown to decrease wound pain when used to dress surgical incisional wounds.[81]

Hydrocolloids, hydrogels, and foam dressings typically have a minimal to moderate absorptive capacity. Hydrocolloid dressings are occlusive and reduce pain by preventing exposure of the wound to air; however, they have aggressive adhesive properties and can cause pain if removed improperly. Foam dressings are moderately absorptive, warmth retentive, which is soothing, and nonadherent, resulting in reduced pain during dressing changes. But they can dry out if the wound is minimally exudative. Hydrogel dressings are cool and soothing and particularly effective in wounds that have a burning sensation. Hydrogel dressings are nonadherent, thus reducing wound pain during dressing changes. Soft silicone dressings absorb minimal amounts of drainage but also are nonadherent and reduce pain associated with dressing changes.

Calcium alginates, alginate collagen dressings, and exudate absorbing beads, flakes, pastes, or powders absorb large amounts of drainage. Dressings with a large absorptive capacity reduce pain related to maceration of surrounding tissues and to pressure caused by excess exudate. Calcium alginates and exudate-absorbing dressings are generally nonadherent and easily removed from the wound during dressing changes. However, similar to gauze and foam dressings, they can dry out if left in the wound for a prolonged time. Thoroughly soak dried dressings, especially the edges, to avoid trauma and pain when they are removed.

Avoid packing wounds too tightly, as this can traumatize tissues and stimulate pain receptors. Granulation tissue can grow into wound-packing materials, and there is minimal benefit reported from soaking to ease removal.[72] For wound pain related to use of negative pressure wound therapy, line the wound with a low-adherent liner to avoid trauma when removing the packing or the sponge used in the therapy, decrease the pressure in-

crementally until pain diminishes, and switch foam types or sponges used in the therapy. (See Chapter 28 for more information on negative pressure wound therapy).

In general, perform dressing changes as infrequently as required depending on the wound characteristics, as this reduces risk of infection by environmental contaminants and trauma from cooling to the cells of repair on dressing removal. Just the provision of a dressing or wrapping may be enough to reduce wound pain without the use of medication.[48] A dressing removes the visible reminder of the wound and the psychological pain as well as reduces the risk of external stimulation such as pressure, friction, and shear.[82] Exhibit 13-4 lists ways to alleviate pain at dressing changes.

CLINICAL WISDOM

Patient-centered Concern:

Patients, with good reason, express fear of dressing changes and debridement procedures. Use gentle hands and acknowledge the patient's pain and fear.[83] Use of pain-reducing wound care strategies including premedication, self removal of wound dressings, and reassurance will reduce anxiety and fear and improve trust and outcomes.

EXHIBIT 13-4 Ways to Alleviate Pain at Dressing Changes

- Maintain moisture balance so nerve endings are bathed in moist wound fluid, which is soothing.
- Thoroughly soak dried dressings, especially the edges, to avoid trauma and pain when they are removed. Alginates as well as gauze and foam products can dry out.
- Protect surrounding skin from wound exudate irritation and maceration with skin sealants, ointment, or barriers to prevent or minimize skin damage and pain.
- Avoid packing wounds too tightly and using dressing products that can traumatize tissues and stimulate pain receptors.
- Line the wound with a low-adherent liner such as safe silicone to avoid trauma when removing the packing or the sponge that accompanies negative pressure therapy.
- Select wound adhesives that are aggressive enough for positioning the dressing but not so aggressive that tissue is damaged when removed.
- Perform dressing changes as infrequently as required depending on the wound characteristics.
- Avoid any unnecessary stimulation to the wound during dressing changes such as a draft from open windows or air conditioning, prodding and poking of the wound or surrounding tissues.
- "Time-outs" and self-dressing changes are recommended to reduce patient anxiety and improve tolerance for the dressing change procedure.
- Position the patient and the wound site so the dressing change can be performed in the most comfortable position for both patient and clinician.
- Premedicate 30 to 90 minutes before dressing changes to reduce anxiety and pain.

Wound Cleansing

Wound cleansing should be gentle, and limited pressure should be applied to limit pain from the procedure. However, enough fluid and pressure should be used to flush out debris and necrotic tissue from the wound to reduce risk of infection. Pressure irrigation such as pulsed lavage with suction (see Chapter 27) can be painful, and premedication and time limits are recommended. If the wound is irrigated, low pressures (e.g., 4–15 psi) should be utilized. Choice of irrigant solution or cleansing agent can affect wound pain. Choose topical agents and wound cleansers that are nontoxic and nonirritating (e.g., hypoallergenic) to wound tissues and surrounding skin. As examples, hydrogen peroxide is caustic to viable tissue cells and surrounding skin, causing a burning sensation; acetic acid, often used to treat *Pseudomonas aeruginosa* wound infection, can cause severe stinging; and silver nitrate sticks used to remove hypergranulation tissue can cause pain.[48,84,85]

Use fluids warmed to at least room temperature when cleansing wound tissues to prevent shocking the cells of repair, startling the patient, and initiating pain. Wound cells interpret the shock as trauma, and cell mitosis is halted for up to 3 hours after dressing change.[86] Further, for patients with hyperesthesia, the shock of a cold fluid can set off a pain cycle. To avoid shocking the patient, always alert the patient before applying the cleansing solution. Even room temperature fluid can startle the patient and set off a destructive SNS response with release of catecholamines, epinephrine, and norepinephrine, all of which interfere with wound healing. Warm cleansing fluids by placing the solution container in a warm water bath while preparing other wound dressing supplies. Always test the temperature of the wound cleansing solution prior to administering to a patient's wound.

Distraction and Reframing

Distraction means turning attention to something other than "the pain." Examples include watching TV or listening to music or the radio. Distraction is useful to temporarily relieve pain such as when it is not yet time for another pain pill or during the time it takes for the medicine to take effect. There is a myth that if the person can be distracted the pain is not severe. This is not necessarily true. It is just one method to temporarily relieve even intense pain. Reframing is a related technique to distraction. Reframing teaches the patient to evaluate negative thoughts and images and replace them with positive or neutral self talk that facilitates coping.[27] A suggestion for coping with wound procedures is for the patient to control the situation with time-outs or helping with dressing removal.

Relaxation, Visual Imagery, and Biofeedback

Relaxation and visual imagery are used to achieve physical and mental relaxation. Relaxation reduces muscle tension that puts stress on the painful tissues around the wound. For some people, relaxing may make them more aware of their wound problems. If this happens, suggest that the patient

talk to someone about those feelings. An individual's ability to relax will change from time to time, and it may take up to two weeks of practice to feel the first results of relaxation. Relaxation can be practiced throughout the day by taking a couple of deep breaths, holding your breath, and then blowing out the air. If the patient has lung problems, check with the doctor before performing deep breathing relaxation. Deep breathing may at first make the patient feel light-headed. If this is a problem, ask the patient to take shallow breaths and/or breath more slowly. Breathing in deeply and slowly will also help bring more oxygen to the lungs and to the tissues that need to heal. Relaxation can be done anyplace, anytime. However, for it to be most successful, it should to be done for 5 for 10 minutes twice a day on a regular schedule in a quiet place in a comfortable position. In the relaxed state, the patient should be asked to visualize something pleasant that will help distract them from pain.

Visual imagery is a powerful method to plant helpful messages deep within the mind and body. During visual imagery the patient is asked to consider directing messages to the body to relax, ease pain, and direct blood flow and healing cells to the tissues for healing. Relaxation with guided imagery has been shown to help postsurgical patients to relax, reduce anxiety levels, and lower cortisol levels and erythema following surgery.[87] In a randomized controlled trial of patients with chronic nonhealing diabetic foot ulcers, biofeedback with muscular relaxation was attributed to promoting significantly increased blood flow and healing in the treatment group as compared with placebo.[88] In a FMRI study of patients who experience phantom limb pain, imagination of moving a phantom hand by upper extremity amputees showed activation in the contralateral primary motor and somatosensory areas of the brain and tracked their ability to reorganize the brain and reduce phantom limb pain.[89]

Psychological Interventions

Psychological interventions are another way to address the emotional component of the pain and the wound. They are used in conjunction with other methods, both nonpharmaceutical and pharmaceutical. As has already been explained, evidence shows that how people think about pain can change their sensitivity to it as well as their feelings and reactions. Psychological interventions include cognitive and/or behavioral techniques. These techniques have been associated with restoring a sense of self control in cancer patients, which is often lost.[27] This strategy can also help the patient coping with a chronic wound and all the associated pain. It can be as simple as holding a patient's hand, offering reassurance, and acknowledging the pain and suffering associated with the wound pain or referral to a health-care professional who is skilled in psychological methods.

Biophysical Agents

Part IV of this book, Chapters 22 through 26 present biophysical agents that are used for wound healing that are also nonpharmaceutical interventions useful for mitigating wound pain, including electrical stimulation, pulsed radio frequency (induced electrical stimulation), laser, and whirlpool. Transcutaneous neuromuscular stimulation (TENS), for example, is recommended to treat wound pain and has the additional benefit of reducing the need for pain-relieving medications but not replacing them.[27,43] The evidence to support the efficacy and utility for pain management of these agents is presented in those chapters. No adverse reactions can be expected using these agents in conjunction with pharmaceutical or other nonpharmaceutical interventions. There is also evidence that supports their use for healing. Biophysical agent interventions are usually provided by physical therapists who have the knowledge and skills needed for successful application and outcomes. Occupational therapists also use biophysical agents and strategies for pain relief and prevention.

Two biophysical agents not discussed in Section IV are the use of topical warmth and cold. These are applied superficially and may act as distractions from the pain and have the benefit that they are interventions that patients or caregivers can use at home. Heat is soothing, induces relaxation, and causes vasodilation and increased blood flow that can help with healing. However, prolonged heating brings more blood to the area, along with the chemical mediators associated with pain, histamine, bradykinins, and prostaglandins. Patients with allodynia may be unable to tolerate even mild heat.

Cold, or cryotherapy may directly or indirectly reduce pain sensations and produce an immediate reduction in pain. Cold applied immediately following a trauma has the ability to reduce capillary permeability and thus block release of substances like histamine and other chemical medicators associated with pain. An example would be to use a cold pack applied to adjacent tissues after a dressing change. Do not apply directly so as not to cool the wound. A 10–15 minute application of a cold pack can control pain for one or more hours.[90] If there is tissue ischemia, cold would be contraindicated because it would further restrict blood flow to the ischemic tissues. As with heat, patients with allodynia probably will find cold intolerable.

Pharmaceutical Interventions

Accurate diagnosis of the pain type is critically important before selecting a pharmaceutical intervention. Recommended treatment for nociceptive pain is usually antiinflammatory or analgesic medications; neuropathic pain is treated with medications that influence neurotransmitters, such as antidepressants and antiepileptic drugs.[91] Recommendations for pharmaceuticals for management of chronic wound pain are not wound pain-specific but are based on evidence about treatment of pain associated with etiologies like cancer, burns, low back pain, fibromyalgia, osteoarthritis, postherpetic neuralgia, and diabetic neuropathy. One such example is the guidelines of the World Health Organization (WHO) analgesic ladder[92] described in this section, which is well validated as an effective method for pain

relief in 90% of cancer patients.[24] Other evidence-based clinical strategies found in the literature are also included.

Guidelines for Analgesic Use

Guidelines for the use of analgesics are provided by the World Health Organization (WHO) analgesic ladder and presented in Table 13-6.[92] The WHO approach is to measure the pain on a pain intensity scale and then match the patient's pain intensity with the potency of analgesic to be prescribed, beginning with non-opioids and progressing to stronger medications if pain is not relieved, adding adjuvants as the ladder is climbed.[93] As an example, mild pain would be indicated by a pain score of 1 to 3 and be treated with nonopioids such as aspirin, acetaminophen, and NSAIDS. Moderate pain would be indicated by a pain score of 4 to 6 and be treated with mild opioids (codeine). In general, it is always better to combine opiods with other analgesic agents such as NSAIDS or acetaminophen. This produces an additive analgesic effect while minimizing the dose of opioids required and thus minimizes undesirable side effects. This "opioid sparing" strategy is the backbone of the WHO "analgesic ladder." Severe pain would be indicated by a pain score of 7 to 10 and be treated with strong opioids such as morphine hydromorphone and transdermal fentanyl. If pain persists or worsens, move to the next level.

NSAIDS are used routinely for common pain complaints like headache, muscular pain, or menstrual cramps, but they are also beneficial following extensive procedures and are more effective than acetaminophen for treatment of inflammatory conditions. However, they are not useful as an analgesic during debridement.[94] Difference of opinion exists about whether NSAIDS are useful as premedication for debridement or if they should be used to control inflammation.[94] Others use the WHO ladder recommended medications, which included NSAIDS 30 to 90 minutes before sharp or mechanical debridement.[56] NSAIDS should not be used for extensive periods because of adverse reactions; they are also contraindicated in patients with gastric ulceration.[95] Caution is needed for NSAID use in the elderly because of the risk of complications such as gastrointestinal bleeding and are best avoided in this patient population.

The effect of NSAIDs on wound healing is controversial. NSAIDS inhibit cyclooxygenase (COX), thus decreasing the synthesis of prostaglandins. NSAIDS also blunt the inflammatory process by deactivation of platelet aggregation, which can impair the wound healing process, depending on how early in the inflammatory phase it is administered.[97-98] Acetaminophen has an advantage in that it does not interfere with platelet function. An explanation of the effects of NSAIDS on wound healing bioactivity is found in Chapter 2 under medications that affect wound healing.

RESEARCH WISDOM

The maximum dose of acetaminophen for patients with normal renal and hepatic function and no history of alcoholism is 4,000 mg per day.[5]

TABLE 13-6   WHO Ladder

WHO Step	Treatment	Pain Mechanism	Advantages	Disadvantages
1 Mild pain 1–3	Nonopioid	Target: the peripheral nerves to block painful impulses	-Useful for mild to moderate pain -Widely available -Low cost -Additive when used with opioids -Patient or caregiver administration	- Ceiling effect to analgesia -Side effects (GI, Renal or Liver) -Caution in elderly
2 Mild to moderate pain 4–6	Opioid for pain ± nonopioid or adjuvant	Target: CNS to alter the perception of pain and peripheral nerves to block painful impulses	-Effective for local and general pain -Ceiling to analgesic effectiveness limited by only by side effects -Patient or caregiver administration -Long acting controlled release forms -Some are low cost	-Prescription is regulated -Side effects limit analgesic effectiveness -Fear of dependency
3 Moderate to severe pain 7–10	Opioid for pain ± adjuvant	Target: CNS to alter the perception of pain	Same as above	- Side effects limit analgesic effectiveness -Withdrawal symptoms likely - Need to taper off dosage gradually -Subject to substance abuse -Psychologic dependence

Opioids are added to the pain management regimen when pain perists or increases. Opiods work on the CNS to alter the perception of pain and nonopioids work on the peripheral nerves to block painful impulses.[93] By combining drugs such as a nonopioid and an opioid, pain relief can be enhanced because they work synergistically. Used together they may decrease the need to progress to higher doses of opioids.[27] Examples are acetaminophen with codeine, acetaminophen with oxycodone, and acetaminophen with dihydrocodeine. The combination of codeine and acetomenophen is recommended for procedure pain relief. However, care is needed when selecting patients to use acetominphen with oxycodone because of serious side effects in individuals with gastrointestinal disease and heart disease. This drug combination needs to be tapered off gradually to avoid withdrawal symptoms. Use of combination drugs is not recommended by all clinicians.[5] Of concern is the fact that combination drugs are often administered in fixed dose combinations that may be limited by the content of acetaminophen or NSAID which may produce dose-related toxicity. If pain is not managed at this level the third step on the WHO ladder is used. At this step separate dosages of the opioid and nonopioid drugs should be used.[27] The guideline for use of combination analgesics is "start low and go slow".[5]

Additional drugs, or adjuvants, should be used if the pain cannot be controlled with the primary drugs.[92] Adjuvants are analgesic drugs that are not a primary analgesic but that research has shown to have independent or additive analgesic properties.[27] Examples are anticonvulsants or tricyclic antidepressants (TCAs). These drugs modulate pain transmission by interacting with specific neurotransmitters and ion channels.[91] A systematic review of the evidence identified significant benefit from the use of TCAs (e.g., amitriptyline, nortriptyline, desipramine, and novel antidepressants bupropion, venlafaxine, and duloxetine) for treatment of both chronic neuropathic and non-neuropathic pain syndromes; this is independent of antidepressant effects.[91] TCAs are tertiary amines that can provide pain relief within 24 hours,[95] are more cost effective as compared with antiepileptic drugs, and have fewer safety concerns for elderly patients.[91]

TCAs in combination with electrical stimulation have shown enhanced efficacy in treatment of neuropathic pain.[87] Antiepileptic drugs are classified into first and second generation. The second-generation group of TCAs has fewer adverse reactions. Adverse effects commonly related to use of these adjuvants include sedation and weight gain; elderly patients should not be treated with tertiary amines because of anticholinergic effects.[91] The second-generation antiepileptic drug gabapentin (Neurontin) has good quality patient-related evidence of efficacy in treatment of diabetic neuropathy and postherpetic neuralgia. In addition to efficacy in treatment of persistent neuropathic pain, TCAs have documented efficacy in treatment of nociceptive pain. TCAs should be considered as a pain adjuvant to promote sleep and alleviate muscle spasm. Successful outcome for pain relief is considered to be a 30 to 50% reduction in pain.[91]

Another adjuvant treatment is the lidocaine patch 5% (Lidoderm), as previously described. The release of lidocaine blocks sodium channels and has been approved for postherpetic neuralgia. Use of lidocaine 5% patch has shown efficacy in reduction of neuropathic pain in both both randomized and open label clinical trials.[29,100] The current accepted use of lidocaine 5% patch is for neuropathic pain. However, it was used in an open label study for nociceptive as well as neuropathic pain with good results.[35] In this study, the lidocaine 5% patches were applied by the patient once daily to cover the area of maximal pain and showed no adverse effects. It was suggested that the patches be applied at the same time each day and be used in conjunction with other analgesic medications.[29] A benefit of using lidocaine 5% patch dermal delivery to the site of pain activity is reduced risks of systemic adverse events and drug interactions.[29,35] Clinical application of lidocaine 5% patch could be useful for control of persistent background pain, promoting function and improving quality of life.

> ### CLINICAL WISDOM
>
> A common problem with opioid analgesia is loss of analgesic effectiveness over time. Use of adjuvants not only can improve analgesia but it may be possible to lower the dosage and reduce adverse opioid reactions such as nausea, vomiting, constipation, pruritus, sedation, and respiratory depression.[95]

Clinical Suggestions

Principles for Using Pain Control Medications. To maintain freedom from pain, drugs should be given "by the clock," that is, every 3-6 hours rather than "on demand." Use the least invasive route for administration first. By starting with low doses, monitoring frequently and titrating as needed, a safe and effective dose can be determined. Be patient, as this process may take 1 to 2 days for short-acting drugs and up to a week for longer-acting drugs.[5] Reassess and adjust the dosage frequently to achieve optimal pain relief, and monitor and manage side effects.[101]

Procedural Medication. Specific medication regimes that are useful for noncyclic and cyclic nociceptive wound pain associated with procedures (e.g., debridement, dressing changes) include providing opioids or benzodiazepines 30 minutes prior to the procedure and afterwards, and administering topical anesthetics, including topical opioids using hydrogels as a transport media. Sequential debridement procedures, such as involved in acute burn care or treatment of chronic wounds, release inflammatory mediators that sensitize the peripheral nociceptors and produce peripheral sensitization and set the stage for central sensitization. Prevention should be given high priority. The following suggestions

have demonstrated efficacy for local anesthesia but have not been studied for prophylactic effects.

Topical analgesics are useful for local anesthesia during local wound treatment. Use of a lidocaine soak (Exhibit 13-5) has been recommended as a quick and efficient way to reduce local wound pain during debridement procedures.[96] Another option is EMLA cream (eutectic mixture of lidocaine 2.5%, prilocaine 2.5%), which reduces debridement pain scores and might have a vasoactive effect cutaneously.[103,104] It should be used only on intact adjacent skin. Apply before sharp or mechanical debridement. Low-dose topical morphine has been used in two small pilot studies to successfully control pressure ulcer-related pain.[105,106]

> ### CLINICAL WISDOM
>
> Clinicians often believe that dead tissue cannot hurt during debridement. Sibbald rates debridement pain severity as follows: surgical and mechanical, ++; and autolytic and enzymatic, +.[5] Wound margins and underlying tissues contain functioning pain receptors that are easily stimulated by a sharp instrument or chemicals used for the debridement procedure.

Procedural sedation and analgesia (PSAA) is used to produce a suppressed level of consciousness adequate for the administration of a painful or unpleasant procedure such as extensive sharp debridement.[107] Medications currently used as first-line agents for PSAA are ketamine for children and Etomidate for adults. Alternatives are fentanyl and midazolam.[107] Benzodiazepines are commonly used in U.S. burn centers, where it is recognized that pain is exacerbated by anxiety, resulting from acute pain triggering SNS activity. Benzodiazepines are used to reduce anxiety while weaning patients from opioids or in combination with a narcotic to control pain in burn patients. Because PSAA suppresses consciousness, the physician must be aware of the potential complications, including the potential for respiratory failure from airway obstruction or hypoventilation. Careful monitoring for respiratory complications is critical because of enhanced respiratory problems over using either drug type separately.[94,107]

EXHIBIT 13-5 Lidocaine Soak Procedure[102]

1. Ask about allergies
2. Lidociane 2%: insert needle and withdraw 5–10 cc of the medication
3. Cleanse the wound after removing the dressing with water, saline, or wound cleanser
4. Place clean dry gauze over the wound
5. Saturate the wound and the periwound skin edges with lidocaine
6. Allow the soaked cause to sit on the wound for 3 to 5 minutes
7. Check if pain sensation and if anesthetized; begin debridement procedure

Adapted from Fowler E. Plain talk about wound pain. *Ostomy* 2005 Vol 51 11A (Suppl) page 6.

Reasons for Referral

If the patient's wound pain is not remitting and is unrelieved, referral for a more complete pain evaluation should be considered. The presence of wound pain that is suggestive of serious complications such as infection, ischemia, or severe tissue tension would warrant an urgent referral to a physician for further evaluation. If the patient is demonstrating weight loss and decreased or absent appetite due to pain, early referral to a dietician or nutritionist in addition to the physician would be indicated.

Self-Care Teaching Guidelines*

The patient self-care teaching guidelines offered here are adapted from materials in Chapter 9, Wound Pain Management, Sussman C Ed., Wound Care Patient Education and Resource Manual Aspen 2002.[110]

Understanding Patients and Caregivers

Many individuals are schooled to believe that "no pain equals no gain," "no pain, no problem," or "no pain, no change." They also have learned stoicism and do not talk about their pain. Misconceptions exist about pain medicine always causing addiction, confusion, or sleepiness. Fear of overmedication may take precedence to the fear of pain. Patients and caregivers are not instructed to use pain medication to PREVENT pain rather than to chase pain. Often they reach for pain medication only when in agony. This perception can lead to inconsistency following a pain management

plan. Other probable causes for lack of consistency include the plan is too difficult to follow, too complicated to understand, difficulty getting the medicine because of cost, unpleasant side effects of treatment, and confusion over medical terminology.[108] The term noncompliance has been overused to describe patients. Lack of adherence to a plan of care may occur for any of the above-mentioned or other reasons. Patients with peripheral neuropathy experience painless wound trauma. They need to be taught to fear the pain that they DO NOT feel and how to care for and protect their feet from trauma (see Chapter 19.)

Collaborative Wound Management: Patient, Caregiver, and Health-care Provider

Wound pain management is a collaborative effort between the patient and their caregiver/family member and the health-care provider. Patients and their caregiver must be active health-care consumers and active participants in their own care. Health-care providers should bring the patient into the process from the beginning by determining the patient's pain problem and the patient's goal for management. Begin by determining the motivation and ability to be part of the process. Empower the individual by letting him/her know that adequate pain relief is a right and that the pain management plan can change if the pain is not under control. The goal is to provide the patient with a feeling of personal control of their pain situation, to dispel myths about pain

---

■ **CASE STUDY**

Protecting Neuropathic Feet

HISTORY

BF was a 69-year-old woman who had a reoccurrence of breast cancer and was treated with several courses of chemotherapy. She was ambulatory and well nourished.

THE REASON FOR REFERRAL

BF developed a pressure ulcer over the 5th metatarsal head that she found when she was putting on her stockings. Skin was black but unpainful. She sought medical care.

TESTS

Tactile sensation was negative and monofilament for protective sensation; findings were negative for 5.7 mg.

DIAGNOSIS AND TREATMENT INTERVENTIONS

Black skin was diagnosed as eschar necrosis and peripheral neuropathy related to her chemotherapy. She was treated with debridement and wound care measures and patient education.
The cause of the ulcer problem: shoes that were too narrow had applied pressure to the soft tissue over the 5th metatarsal head and was undetected due to neuropathy and loss of protective sensation.

OUTCOME OF CARE

Once the diagnosis of pressure ulcer secondary to chemotherapy-related neuropathy was explained to her, the patient replaced her shoes with wider width shoes, learned to examine her feet regularly, and the wound healed uneventfully in 2 weeks. There were no further foot ulcers.

management, and to demonstrate willingness to be equal partners in the process.

Here are some tips to share with patients about communicating wound pain.[109]

1. Remember that you have the RIGHT to adequate pain relief.
2. The relationship between patient and health-care provider is an equal partnership.
3. A pain management plan is a collaborative effort between the health-care provider, the patient, and the caregiver. If the plan isn't working, tell your health-care provider.
4. Get "more mileage" out of a pain pill by taking it on a regular schedule, setting an alarm as a reminder if necessary.
5. Be clear as you can be about your pain when you communicate with your health-care provider. Be specific about where it hurts and when. Draw a picture of a figure and mark the spot(s) where it hurts if that is easier than words.
6. Use a number to indicate the intensity (how much) it hurts. The usual number system rates no pain as 0 and the worst pain as 10. It may not be possible to reach a zero pain level but it does mean getting down to a number that is tolerable.
7. If a number doesn't tell your pain story, make a face about how much it hurts or point to a picture of faces in pain.
8. Use words like sharp, hot, stinging, throbbing, aching, and dull to describe your pain.
9. How does the pain affect your mood? Prickly as a porcupine? Mad as a bear with a thorn in his paw? Helpless? Crabby? Crawling into a shell? Sad?
10. Keep track of what you have done to ease the pain and whether it is effective. A pain diary can help.
11. Communicate your beliefs about showing or talking about pain (Is it a sign of weakness? Or a taboo?)
12. Sudden or increasing pain is often a signal that the wound needs help. Contact your health-care provider right away.
13. Tell your health-care provider about ANY pain that won't go away or gets worse.
14. Medical language is a lot like a foreign language to most people.

Explaining pain management choices to the patient and caregiver is another way to collaborate. Here are some suggestions to use when explaining drug and nondrug treatment of pain.

Drug treatment

- Drug treatment and nondrug treatment can be successful to control and prevent pain. Don't worry about getting "hooked" on pain medicines; this is a rare event unless you already have a problem with drug abuse.
- Pain medicine may be given as a pill or liquid, as a shot or a topical application such as a patch. Do NOT be re-

luctant to take the pain medicine. Take it to PREVENT NOT chase the pain.
* Take action to relieve pain as soon as it starts. It is harder to ease the pain once it starts.
* Pain medicine will take 30–60 minutes to take effect. It will not stop pain immediately. A medication schedule can prevent breakthrough pain. Taking pain medication 30–60 minutes before a wound care procedure (dressing change or debridement) is a good plan.

Nondrug treatment

- Nondrug treatment options include use of warmth, relaxation, music, pastimes that distract you from thinking about the pain, positive thinking, and electrical nerve stimulation. These techniques can be used alone or in conjunction with pain medication.
* Pain at dressing changes is NOT inevitable. Manufacturers have designed dressings and tapes that do not hurt the wound or skin when they are removed.
* Participate in your dressing changes so you can help control the procedure.
* There are lots of pain relief choices; if one isn't working, there is an unlimited number or combinations of pain medicines.

Conclusion

The mnemonic ABCDE summarizes a routine clinical approach to pain assessment and management:[27]*

Ask about pain regularly. Assess pain systematically.
Believe the patient and family in their reports of pain and what relieves it.
Choose pain control options appropriate for the patient, family, and setting.
Deliver interventions in a timely, logical, and coordinated fashion.
Empower patients and their families. Enable them to control their course to the greatest extent possible.

REVIEW QUESTIONS

1. List two probable causes of persistent neuropathic wound pain.
1. Describe five characteristics of persistent neuropathic pain.
2. What are three nonpharmaceutical methods to treat either non-neuropathic or neuropathic pain?
3. What is the effect of past experience on pain expectations? Is this evidence based?
4. What is the WHO ladder and how is it used to treat pain?

---

*Jacox A, Carr DB, Payne R, et al. *Management of Cancer Pain*. Rockville, MD: The Agency for Health Care Policy and Research (AHCPR) now Agency for Health Care Research and Quality (AHRQ); March 1994.

■ **CASE STUDY**_____

MEDICAL HISTORY

Mrs. F, a 65-year-old woman with a history of 3 months of right lower leg edema with weeping skin along the calf and an open ulcer above the medial malleolus was referred to physical therapy for wound pain management because she was experiencing persistent pain in her leg and wound that increases when she moves and at wound dressing changes. She had a medical history of chronic obstructive pulmonary disease, hypertension, and osteoarthritis (OA) of her knees. She had been limiting her mobility (walking) and activities outside the home because of the pain and the weeping skin problems. She was taking NSAIDS for her OA knee pain and wound pain with some efficacy. She was wearing a foam wound dressing with a secondary dressing and netting to hold it in place and then compression bandage wraps over the dressings.

Pain Assessment

Patient Screening
Can you point to where your pain is located?
Can you rate your pain on a scale of 0 = no pain and 10 = maximal pain?
What is your pain level at the low and high times of the day and when is that?

Responses
Pain Location: Pain is from the knee down on the right lower leg and at the knee on the left.
Duration: Persistent but fluctuates in intensity during the day. Pain is worst in the knees in the morning when I get up or after I have been sitting for a while.
Intensity: Patient's VAS rating related to above questions: 3/10 at the low pain time of day, which is in the afternoon and 7/10 at the high period in the morning. Pain increases to 10/10 during dressing changes. She has persistent background pain of 3/10.

Description of Sensation: Can you describe how the pain feels in words?

Response: Pain is throbbing and aching pain and at times it is burning.

Emotional status: Evaluated with the simple descriptive pain distress scale: What word on the line best describes how distressed you feel about your wound or wound care?

Response: Dreadful. She explained that she dreaded coming to her wound care appointments because of her expectation of intense pain during the wound care procedures.

Prior treatment results: What have you done to relieve you pain and what was the result?

Response: Taking NSAID 3 times a day.

Result: Reduced pain level for several hours.

Functional activities: What effect has the wound and pain had on your activities?

Response: I don't walk very much. My knees are very stiff and painful in the morning when I get up and the pain goes all the way to my toes.

FINDINGS AND CLINICAL DECISION MAKING:

1. Pain diagnosis: Based on the reported type of pain sensations: throbbing and aching pain and at times, which are signs of acute pain and it is burning, signs of nerve irritation, with periods of heightened leg pain in the morning and at dressing changes, there appears to be a mixed pain pattern:
   a. Acute wound pain around the venous ulcer. The wound and surrounding tissues have become hyperalgesic.
   b. Cyclic nociceptive pain related to wound care procedures and OA. Patients with OA typically have stiffness and pain in the morning or after a period of inactivity lasting usually less than 30 minutes. Pain and stiffness typically follow periods of inactivity and decreases during the day with activity.[111]
   c. Tissue tension from edema causing pressure on the nociceptors is adding to hyperalgesia.
   d. Psychosomatic pain based on her experience and learned expectation of severe pain with wound procedures causing dread, and so severity of pain (10/10) is probably related to this as well as the nociceptive cyclic pain from the procedure.
2. Evaluation of current plan of care:
   a. Current regime of wound care has probably contributed to her hyperalgesia.
   b. Compression is not effective in controlling tissue congestion, allowing weeping of nonulcered adjacent skin and stimulation of the nociceptors of the leg, adding to the pain problem.
   c. Foam dressings, a nonpharmacological strategy, have not been effective for reducing local wound pain and may be drying out.
   d. Her NSAID pain medication is not controlling the background pain.

(Continued)

CASE STUDY *(Continued)*

PROGNOSIS AND REVISED INTERVENTIONS:

1. Reduce her anxiety and expectation of pain during dressing changes by using a gentle wound dressing.
   a. Selected Intervention: A soft silicone type dressing Mepilex™ border would meet these criteria (Mölnlycke Health Care Ltd. Norcross, GA).
2. Prevent development of central sensitization of her wound pain.
   a. Intervention: Ask her physician about use of a lidocaine 5% patch to control her hyperalgesia and early symptoms of persistent pain along with continued use of NSAIDS for her OA pain.
3. Improve efficacy of compression to control edema, stop weeping, and reduce tissue tension:
   a. Intervention: Evaluate an inelastic compression device instead of the compression wraps since they do not seem adequate to control edema and weeping (see Chapter 10).
4. Improve her mobility, which will help with her edema management and knee stiffness.
   a. Intervention: Instruction in appropriate exercises by a physical therapist. Exercise has been shown to improve OA pain.

OUTCOME OF CARE

After a 7-day trial with the new plan of care, Mrs. F returned to the clinic and was delighted to report that she could now rate her pain as 0 at rest and her pain was 3/10 at that dressing change. Edema was reduced and weeping stopped. She asked to continue treatment with the soft silicone product and inelastic compression. The wound went on to heal in 2 weeks. She continued with her compression regime due to the recurrent nature of her pathology and started a program of physical therapy to improve her mobility. Early intervention with a pain management program probably prevented her pain from progressing to central sensitization and persistent neuropathic pain that is commonly reported in patients with venous ulcers.

REFERENCES

1. IASPTask Force on Taxonomy. Pain Terminology. In: Merskey H BN, ed. *Classification of Chronic Pain.* Seattle, WA: IASP Press ; http://www.iasp-pain.org/terms-p.html#Neuropathic%20pain; 1994:209-214.
2. Sela RA, Bruera E, Conner-Spady B, Cumming C, Walker C. Sensory and affective dimensions of advanced cancer pain. *Psycho-Oncology.* 2002;11(1):23-34.
3. Holdcroft A, Power I. Recent developments: Management of pain. *BMJ.* 2003;326:635-639.
4. Rae C, Gallagher G, Watson S, Kinsella J. An audit of patient perception compared with medical and nursing staff estimation of pain during burn dressing changes. *European Journal of Anaesthesiology.* 2000;17:43-45.
5. Reddy M, Kohr R, Queen D, Keast D, Sibbald R. Practical treatment of wound pain and trauma: A patient-centered approach. An overview. *Ostomy /Wound Management.* April 2003 49(4A(suppl)):2-15.
6. Krasner D. Caring for the Person Experiencing Chronic Wound Pain. In: Krasner D, Rodeheaver G, Sibbald GR, eds. *Chronic Wound Care: A clinical Source Book for healthcare Professionals.* Third ed. Wayne, PA: HMP-Communications; 2001:79-88.
7. Moffatt CJ F, Hollinworth H. Understanding wound pain and trauma: an international perspective. Paper presented at: Pain at Wound Dressing Changes; Spring 2002, Europe.
8. Carrougher GJ PJ, Sharer SR, Wiechman S, Honari S, Paterson DR, Heimbach DM. Comparison of Patient Satisfaction and Self Reports of Pain in Adult Burn-Injured Patients. *J Burn Care Rehabil.* January/February 2003 24(1):1-8.
9. Franks PJ, Moffatt C. Who suffers most from leg ulceration? Paper presented at: Journal of Wound Care; Sept 1998.
10. Goncalves Maristela Lopes, ConceicaodeGouveiSantos Vera Lucia, Andrucioli de Mattos Pimenta Cibele, Suzuki Erica, Komegae Katia Midori. Pain in Chronic Leg Ulcers. *J WOCN.* 2004;31(5):275-283.
11. Fowler Evonne. Wound Pain During Dressing Changes. Paper presented at: How to Decrease Trauma and Pain at Dressing Changes—Satellite Symposium—Symposium For Advanced Wound Care; April 30, 2001, Las Vegas, NV.
12. (JCAHO) JCoAoHO. Pain Management Standards (Standard RI 2.8 and PE 1.4). In: JCAHO, ed. *Comprehensive Accreditation Manual for Hospitals*; 2001.
13. Tracey I. Nociceptive processing in the human brain. *Current Opinion in Neurobiology Sensory systems.* 2005/8 2005;15(4):478-487.
14. Wulf H, Baron R. The Theory of Pain. Paper presented at: European Wound Management Association Position Document; 2002, London, UK.
15. Koyama Tetsuo, McHaffie John G, Laurienti Paul J, Coghill Robert C. The subjective experience of pain: Where expectations become reality. *PNAS.* 2005;102(36):12950-12955.
16. Cutting KF, Harding KG. Criteria to idenify wound infection. *Journal of Wound Care.* 1994;3(4):198-201.
17. Sibbald R, Williamson D, Orsted H. Preparing the wound bed—debridement, bacterial balance, and moisture balance. *Ostomy /Wound Management.* November 2000 46(11):14-35.
18. Broadbent E, Petrie KJ, Alley PG, Booth RJ. Psychological Stress Impairs Early Wound Repair Following Surgery. *Psychosomatic Medicine.* 2003;65:865-869.
19. Woolf CJ. Neuropathic pain: aetiology, symptoms, mechanisms and management. *The Lancet.* June 5, 1999;353:1959-1964.
20. Gifford L, Butler D. The Integration of Pain Sciences into Clinical Practice. *Journal of Hand Therapy.* April-June 1997;10:86-97.
21. Pediani R. What has pain relief to do with acute surgical wound healing? *World Wide Wounds (on line publication).* March 2001.
22. Shah JL. Lesson of the week: postoperative pressure sores after epidural anaesthesia. *BMJ.* 2000;321((7266)):941-942.
23. Hampton T. Pain and the Brain: Researchers Focus on Tackling Pain Memories. *JAMA.* June 15 2005;293(23):2845-2846.
24. Wager TD, Rilling JK, Smith EE, et al. Placebo-Induced Changes in fMRI in the Anticipation and Experience of Pain. *Science.* Feb 20 2004;303(5661):1162-1167.
25. Nicholson BD. Neuropathic Pain: New Strategies to Improve Clinical Outcomes. Paper presented at: The National Initiative on Pain Control; January 2005, online: www.Medscape.com.
26. Raij T, Numminen J, Narvanen S, Hiltunen J, R. H. Brain correlates of subjective reality of physically and psychologically induced pain. *PNAS,* Feb 2005;102(6):2147–2151.
27. Jacox A, Carr DB, Payne R, et al. *Management of Cancer Pain.* Rockville, MD: The Agency for Health Care Policy and Research (AHCPR) now Agency for Health Care Research and Quality (AHRQ); March 1994.
28. Galer B, Sheldon E, Pate N. Development and preliminary validation of a pain measure specific to neuropathic pain: the neuropathic Pain Scale. *Neurology.* 1997;48:332-338.
29. Argoff Charles E, Galer Bradley S, Jensen Mark P, Oleka Napoleon, Gammaitoni Arnold R. Effectiveness of the lidocaine patch 5% on pain quali-

ties inthree chronic pain states:assessment with theNeuropathic Pain Scale. *Current Medical Research and Opinion(r).* 2004;20(Suppl 2):S 21-28.

30. Jensen TS BR. Translation of symptoms and signs into mechanisms in neuropathic pain. *Pain.* 2003 2003;102:1-8.

31. Basbaum AI. Distinct neurochemical features of acute and persistent pain. *PNAS.* July 6, 1999 96(14):7739-7743.

32. Boulton AJM. Management of Diabetic Peripheral Neuropathy. *Clinical Diabetes.* 2005;23(1).

33. Arthur R, Shelley W. The Peripheral Mechanism of Itch in Man. Paper presented at: Pain and Itch: Nervous Mechanisms; March 1959, London.

34. Charlesworth EN, Beltrani S, Vincent S. Pruritic dermatoses: overview of etiology and therapy. *The American Journal of Medicine.* 2002/12/16 113(9, Supplement 1):25-33.

35. Jensen MP DR, Gammaitoni AR, Olaleye DO, Oleka N, Galer BS,. Assessment of Pain Quality in Chronic Neuropathic and Nociceptiv Pain Clinical Trials with the Neuropathic Pain Scale. *The Journal of Pain.* February 2005;6(2):98-106.

36. Demling R, DeSanti L. Topical Doxepin Cream is Effective in Relieving Severe Pruritis Caused by Burn Injury: A preliminary Study. *Wounds : a compendium of clinical research and practice.* June 2001;13(6):210-215.

37. Mendham JE. Gabapentin for the treatment of itching produced by burns and wound healing in children: a pilot study. *Burns.* 2004;30(8):851-853.

38. British Pain Society RCoA, Royal College of General Practitioners, Royal College of Psychiatrists. *Recommendations for the appropriate use of opiods for persistent noncancer pain* March 2004.

39. Meyer III, Walter J, Nichols Ray J, et al. Acetaminophen in the Management of Background Pain in Children Post-Burn. *Journal of Pain and Symptom Management.* 1997;13(1):50–55.\

40. Ryan S. Eager C. Sibbaid RG. Venous Leg Ulcer Pain. *Ostomy/Wound Management.* April 2003;49(4 (Suppl):16–23.

41. Berry PH CC, Covington EC, Dahl JL, Katz JH, Miaskowski C, Mclean MJ. Pain: current Understanding of Assessment, Mangement and Treatments. *American Pain Society* [online]. July 19, 2004. Accessed May 5, 2005.

42. Sliwa JA WS, Novick AK, Charuk G. Concurrent Musculoskeletal Pain in a Patient with Symptomatic Lower Extremity Arterial Insufficiency. *Arch Phys Med Rehabil.* Nov 1989;70:848-850.

43. Krasner D. The Chronic Wound Pain Experience. *Ostomy /Wound Management.* March 1995;41(3):20-27.

44. Sibbald RG. Pain in General. Paper presented at: How to decrease trauma and pain at dressing changes- Satellite Symposium, Symposium for Advanced Wound Care; April 30, 2001, Las Vegas, NV.

45. Bonhsm PA, Flemister BG, Ratliff CR. *Guideline for Management of Wounds in Patients with Lower-Extremity Arterial Disease.* Glenfiew, IL: Wound Ostomy Continence Nurses Society (WOCN); 2002.

46. Sibbald RG, Amstrong D, Orstead H. Pain in Diabetic Foot Ulcers. *Ostomy /Wound Management.* April 2003;49(4A(suppl)):24-29.

47. Miscavige Maria. Considering Patient Priorities When Choosing a Dressing. *Ostom Wound Management.* 2004;50(11):16,18.

48. Ryan S, Eager C, Sibbald RG. Venous Leg Ulcer Pain. *Ostomy /Wound Management.* April 2003;49(4A (Suppl)):16-23.

49. Nemeth Kathleen A, Harrison Margaret B, Graham Ian D, Burke Sharon. Pain in pure and mixed aetiology venous leg ulcers: a three-phase point prevalence study. *J Wound Care.* October 2003;12(9):336-340.

50. Nemeth Kathleen A, Harrison Margaret R, Graham ID, Burke Sharon. Understanding Venous Leg Ulcer Pain: Results of a Longitudinal Study. *Ostom Wound Management.* 2004;50(1):34-46.

51. T S, Kosaka M, Fujishima K. Human thermoregulatory responses during prolonged walking in water at 25, 30 and 35 degrees C. *Eur J Appl Physiol Occup Physiol.* Nov 1998;78(6):473-478.

52. Lindholm C, Bjellerup M, Christianson O, Zederfeldt B. Quality of life in chronic leg ulcer patients. An assessment accordeing to the Nottingham Health Profile. *Acta Derm Venereol.* 1993;73(6):440-443.

53. Nemeth Kathleen A, Harrison Margaret B, Graham Ian D, Burke Sharon. Uneristanding Venous Leg Ulcer Pain: Results of a Longitudinal Study. *Ostom Wound Management.* 2004;50(1):34-46.

54. Shukla Dinesh, Tripathii Anuj Kumar, Agrawal Saurabh, Ansari Mumtaz Ahman, Rastogi Amit, Shukla Vijay Kumar. Pain in Acute and Chronic Wounds: A descriptive study. *Ostom Wound Management.* 2005;51(11):47-51.

55. Moffatt CJ, FranksPJ, Hollinworth H. Understanding wound pain and trauma: an international perspective. Paper presented at: Pain at Wound Dressing Changes; Spring 2002; Europe.

56. Reddy M, Keast D, Fowler E, Sibbald R. Pain in Pressure Ulcers. *Ostomy /Wound Management.* April 2003;49(4A(suppl)):30-35.

57. Dallam L, Symth C, Jackson BS, et al. Pressure ulcer pain: Assessment and quantification. *JWOCN.* 1995;22(5):211-218.

58. SzorJK, Bourguignon C. . Description of pressure ulcer pain at rest and at dressing change. *JOWCN.* 1999;26(3):115-120.

59. Eriksson E, Hietanen H, S. A.-S. Prevalence and characteristics of pressure ulcers: A one-day patient population in a Finnish city. *Clin Nurs Spec.* 2000;14:19-25.

60. Roth RS, LoweryJC, Hamill JB. Assessing persistent pain and its relation to affective distress, depressive symptoms, and pain catastrophizing in patients with chronic wounds A pilot study. *Am J Phys Med Rehabil.* 2004;83:827-834.821.

61. Manz BD, Moser R, Nusser-Gerlach MA, Bergstrom N, Agrawal S. Pain assessment in the cognitively impaired and unimpaired elderly. *Pain Manage Nurs.* 2000;1(4):106-115.

62. vanRijswijk L. Full-thickness pressure ulcers: patient and wound healing characteristics. *Decubitus.* Jan 1993;6(1):16-21.

63. Goodman C, Snyder T. Introduction to Differential Screening in Pysical Therapy. In: Goodman C, Snyder T, eds. *Differential Diagnosis in Physical Therapy.* third ed. Philadelphia: WB Saunders Company; 2000:1-36.

64. Jensen T, Baron R. Translation of symptoms and signs into mechanisms in neuropathic pain. *Pain.* 2003;102:1-8.

65. Scott J, Huskisson EC. Graphic representation of pain. *Pain.* 1976;2:175-184.

66. Wewers ME, Lowe NK. A critical review of visual analogue scales in the measurement of clinical phenomena. . *Res Nurs Health,.* 1990;13:227-236.

67. Freeman K, Smyth C, Dallam L, Jackson B. Pain measurement scales: A comparison of the visual analogue and faces rating scales in measuring pressure ulcer pain. *J Wound Ostomy Continence Nurs.* 2001;28(6):290-296.

68. Wong D, Baker C, . Pain in children: Comparison of assessment scales. *Pediatr Nurs.* 1988;14:9-17.

69. Bieri D, Reeve R, Champion G, Addicoat L, Ziegler J. *The Faces Pain Scale for the self assessment of the severity of pain experienced by children: development, initial validation, and preliminary investigation for ratio scale properties. Pain.* 1990;41:139-150.

70. Simon W, Malabar R, verbally. J Adv Nurs -. Assessing pain in elderly patients who can't respond verbally. *Adv Nurs;* 1995;22(4):663-669.

71. Stuppy DJ. The Faces Pain Scale: Reliability and validity with mature adults. *Appl Nurs Res.* 1998;11:84-89.

72. Paice JA, Cohen FL, Validity of a verbally administered numeric rating scale to measure cancer pain intensity. Validity of a verbally administered numeric rating scale to measure cancer pain intensity. *Cancer Nurs.* 1997;20:88-93.

73. Fink R, Gates R. *Pain assessment in Textbook of Palliative Nursing,* 2nd Edition Ferrell, BR & Coyle, *N (Eds).* New York, New York. Oxford University Press pp 97-127; 2006.

74. TaylorLJ, Herr K, Paice JA. Pain intensity assessment: A comparison of selected pain intensity scales for use in cognitively intact and cognitively impaired African American older adults. *Pain Manage Nurs.* 2003;4:87-95.

75. Galloway S, Turner L. Pain assessment in older adults who are cognitively impaired. *J Gerontol Nurs.* 1999;25:34-39.

76. Lane P, Kuntupis M, MacDonald S, et al. A pain assessment tool for people with Advanced Alzheimer's and other progressive Dementias. *Home Healthcare Nurse,.* 2003;21(1):33-37.

77. Pautex S, Herrmann F, Le Lous P, Fabjan M, Michel JP, Gold G. Feasibility and reliability of four pain self-assessment scales and correlation with an observational rating scale in hospitalized elderly demented patients. *J Gerontol A Biol Sci Med Sci.* 2005;60(4):524-529.

78. AGS Panel on Persistent Pain in Older Persons. The management of persistent pain in older persons. *J Am Geriatr Soc.* 2002;50:S205-S224.

79. Melzack R. The short-form McGill Pain questionnaire. *Pain.* August 1987;30(2):191-197.

80. Karlsmark T, Zillmer R, Agren M, F G. Will self-adhesive dressings cause traum to periwound skin? Paper presented at: The 7th Annual Conference of the Canadian Association of Wound Care; November 2001, London, Ontario, Canada.

81. Briggs M. Surgical wound pain: a trial of two treatments. *J Wound Care.* 1996 1996;5(10):456-460.

82. Briggs M, Torra I, Bou JE. Pain at wound dressing changes: a guide to management. Paper presented at: EWMA Position Document; 2002, London, UK.

83. Krasner D. Caring for the Person Experiencing Chronic Wound Pain. In: Krasner D RG, Sibbald RG,, ed. *Chronic Wound Care: a clinical source book for healthcare professionals.* Third ed. Wayne, PA: HMP Communications; 2001:79-89.

84. Hollinworth H C, M ;. Nurses' view about pain and trauma at dressing changes: results of a national survey. *Journal of wound Care.* Sept 2000;9(8):369-373.

85. Hollinworth H. *Pain and Wound Care.* Ipswich, UK: Wound Care Society; May 2000 2000.

86. Yang Q, Berghe D. Effect of temperature on in vitro proliferative activity of human umbilical vein endothelial cells. *Experientia.* Feb 15, 1995 1995;51(2):126-132.

87. Holden-Lund C. The effects of relaxation with guided imagery on surgical stress and wound healing. *Research in Nursing & Health.* 1988;11(4):235-244.

88. Rice B, Kalker A, Schindler J, Dixon R. Effect of biofeedback-assisted relaxation training on foot ulcer healing. *J Am Podiatr Med Assoc.* March 2001;91(3):132-141.

89. Lotze M, Flor H, Grood W, Larbig W, Birbaumer N. Phantom movements and pain: an FRMI study in upper limb amputees. *Brain.* 2001;1124:2268-2277.

90. Cameron MH. Thermal Agents. In: Cameron MH, ed. *Physical Agents in RehabilitationPhiladelphiaWB Saunders;* 1999:134-135.

91. Maizels M, McCarberg B. Antidepressants and Antiepileptic Drugs for Chronic Non-Cancer Pain. *Am Fam Physician 2005;71:483-90.*

92. Committee WHOE. *World Health Organization. Cancer pain relief and palliaive care.* Geneva, Switzerland: World Health Organization; 1990.

93. Dallam LE, Barkauskas C, Ayello E, Baranoski S. Pain Management and Wounds. In: Baranoski S, Ayello E, eds. *Wound Care Essentials: practice principles.* Philadelphia: Lippincott Williams and Wilkins; 2003:217-236.

94. Kennedy KL, Tritch DL. Debridement. In: Krasner D, Kane D, eds. *Chronic Wound Care: A clinical sourcebook for healthcare professionals.* Wayne, PA: Health Management Publications; 1997:227-235.

95. Goldstein F. Adjuncts to opioid therapy. *J Am Osteopath Assoc.* September 1, 2002;102(9_suppl):15S-.

96. Jones KG, al e. Inhibition of angiogenesis by nonsteroidal antiinflammatory durgs: insight into mechanisms and implications for cancer growth and ulcer healing. *Nat Med.* 1999;5(5):1418-1423.

97. Salcido R. Do Antiinflammatories Have a Role in Wound Healing. Paper presented at: Clinical Symposium on Advances in Skin and Wound Care; October 23-26, 2005, Las Vegas, NV.

98. Schafer AI. Effects of Nonsteroidal Antiinflammatory Drugs on Platelet Function and Systemic Hemostasis . ,. *J Clin Pharmacol.* 1995;35(3)::209-219.

99. Kumar D, Alvaro MS, Julka IS, Marshall HJ. Diabetic Peripheral Neuropathy Effectiveness of electrotherapy and amitriptyline for sympotomatic relief. *Diabetes Care.* August 1998 1998;21(8):1322-1325.

100. Galer B, Jensen M, Ma T, Davies P, Rowbotham M. The lidocaine patch 5% effectively treats all neuropathic pain qualities:results of a randomized, double-blind, vehicle-controlled, 3-week efficacy study with use of the neuropathic pain scale. *Clin J Pain.* Sep-Oct 2002;18(5):297-301.

101. Lawhorne L, Passerini J, Harlan M. *Chronic Pain Management in the Long-Term Care Setting:* American Medical Directors Association; 1999.

102. Fowler E. Plain Talk About Wound Pain. *Ostom Wound Management.* 2005;51(11A (suppl)):4-6.

103. Hafner HM, Thomma SR, Eichner M, Steins A, Junger M. The influence of Emla cream on cutaneous microcirculation. *Clin Hemorrheol Microcirc.* 2003;28:121-128.

104. Cochrane Database Syst. Rev 2003; (1): CD0011177.

105. Zeppetella G, Paul J, Ribeiro M. Analgesic efficacy of morphine applied topically to painful ulcers. *J Pain Symptom Manage.* 2003;25:555-558.

106. Flock P. Pilot study to determine the effectiveness of diamorphine gel to control pressure ulcer pain. *J Pain Symptom Manage.* 2003;25:547-554.

107. Brown T, Lovato L, Parker D. Procedural sedation in the acute care setting. *Am Fam Physician.* January 2005;71(1):85-90.

108. Kohr R. Pain and Wound Trauma, the Ethics of Pain Management. Paper presented at: Decreasing Trauma and Pain at Dressing Changes; November 1-3, 2001, London, Ontario, Canada.

109. Sussman Carrie. Pain Doesn't Have to be a Part of Wound Care. *Ostom Wound Management.* March 2003;49(3):10-12.

110. Sussman C. Wound Pain Management. In: Sussman C, ed. *Wound Care Patient Education and Resource Manual.* Gaithersburg, MD: Aspen; 2002: 9-1:9-46

111. Boissonnault W, Goodman C. Bone, Joint and Soft Tissue Disorders. In: Goodman C, Fuller K, Boissonnault W, eds. *Pathology: Implications for the Ph.ysical Therapist;* 2003.

112. British Pain Society RCoA, Royal College of General Practitioners, Royal College of Psychiatrists. *Recommendations for the appropriate use of opiods for persistent noncancer pain* March 2004.

113. Jensen TS, Baron R. Translation of symptoms and signs into mechanisms in neuropathic pain. *Pain.* 2003;102:1-8.

Management of Scar

R. Scott Ward

CHAPTER OBJECTIVES

At the completion of this chapter, the reader will be able to:
1. Explain the process of scar formation.
2. Identify impairments caused by scar formation.
3. Describe common examination techniques used to assess and document scar tissue.
4. Describe intervention strategies used to treat impairments related to scar formation.

Scar tissue, as a component of wound healing, can lead to functional and cosmetic complications. The hypertrophy associated with keloid or hypertrophic scar formation is disfiguring and is particularly problematic when located at body sites commonly exposed to the public (i.e., face, hands, arms, etc.). Contraction of the forming scar often leads to further disfigurement, as well as restriction of function. Functional deficits occur principally when the scar is situated over joint surfaces, particularly over joints of the extremities. Scarring of the face may also compromise functions such as feeding or speech. Pruritis, some pain, or other annoying paresthesias may also accompany scar formation.

The problems of scar formation have been described as early as the writings of Hippocrates as a torsion resulting from healed burns.[1] Early documentation of surgical correction of scar contractures is included in the writings of Camillo Ferrara (in 1570)[1] and Wilhelm Fabry of Hilden (1560–1634).[1] Fabry of Hilden also described the use of splinting apparatuses to help correct joint deformities secondary to scar contraction. Similar, but certainly more modern, methods of treatment are used today in laboring to control the problems created by active scar formation.

Contemporarily, scar tissue is managed operatively, pharmaceutically, or with conservative measures, including pressure therapy, silicone, exercise, splinting, positioning, and massage. Each of these treatments has demonstrated success that has been documented or is accepted anecdotally because of accounts of clinical success. Further, many of these treatments have been used in combination in an at-tempt to accentuate the expected outcomes of treatment that include improved function and appearance. Common to each of these treatments is the correction of some problem related to the progression of scarring, but it must be understood that none of these interventions cure or stop the process of scarring. Current scientific investigation is uncovering more information about the cause of scarring and may lead to new therapies, such as the use of growth factors that would be aimed more directly at the actual development of scar.

Formation of Scar Tissue

Inflammation occurs following any tissue trauma. Several cell lines are recruited during the inflammatory response to control local infection, debride damaged tissue, nourish surviving and regenerating cells, and release factors that stimulate repair. One cell line that is stimulated to proliferate is fibroblasts. The fibroblast is the cell of origin for scar tissue. Fibroblasts produce elastin and collagen. The secreted elastin becomes elastic fibers that provide normal dermis, or scar, with elasticity and flexibility; however, the ratio of elastic fibers to collagen is less in scar than in normal skin. Collagen secreted by the fibroblasts develops into collagen fibers that are arranged in parallel coils and mainly provide tissue with tensile strength but also afford some flexibility within the normal dermis. The collagen secreted by fibroblasts in scar tissue is laid down in an unorganized, whorl-like pattern. Collagen in both keloid scar and hypertrophic scar is produced at a much greater rate than in normal skin. Ground substance, or extracellular matrix, is comprised of substances including, among others, proteoglycans and glycosaminoglycans. The ground substance provides normal dermis, as well as scar, some cushion, and it allows for the diffusion of oxygen and nutrients in the vicinity. Scar tissue is well vascularized and highly metabolic.

Although scar formation begins with the proliferation and stimulation of fibroblasts during inflammation, the process of scarring continues for weeks, if not months, in most individuals. The growth factors that contribute to the proliferation and activity of fibroblasts in the wound continue to be released through the proliferative and remodeling phases of wound healing. Examples of some of the growth factors that elicit chemotaxis and proliferation of fibroblasts and that are also involved in stimulation of fibroblasts to produce collagen include platelet-derived growth factor (PDGF), tumor necrosis growth factor-ß (TGF-ß), and insulin-like growth factor (IGF). The interaction of these growth factors with other substances in scar tissue is not understood well enough to explain the reason for aberrant scar formation.

Collagen is continually deposited in scar to strengthen the wound site and is also degraded in an attempt to remodel the wound. Some wounds demonstrate an imbalance between the rate of collagen deposition and degradation. If the rate of collagen production exceeds the rate of degradation, a scar that is raised and thick forms.[2,3] Scar may be referred to as *normotrophic, hypertrophic,* or *keloid*. A normotrophic scar is a visible scar that is not raised above the height of the normal skin (see *Color Plate 6*). A hypertrophic scar is raised but does not grow beyond the original wound boundaries (see *Color Plate 48*). A keloid scar is raised and does extend past the original boundaries of the wound (see *Color Plates 49* and *50*). As a scar actively forms, it lacks suppleness, is red and raised. During this "phase" of scarring, the scar is commonly referred to as *immature scar*. As the scar matures in due course, the redness fades, the scar levels out to some degree, and the scar tissue softens (see *Color Plate 51*). It commonly takes 6–18 months for a scar to mature."[4]

There are several clinically observed and documented markers that allow for some prediction of scar formation. The depth of the wound is related to scar formation, in that the deeper the wound, the more likely it is that the wound will scar. The increased chance of scarring is likely due to extended healing time and the associated formation of granulation tissue.[5] In this same light, the length of time it takes for a wound to heal, thereby also implicating the chronicity of inflammation, will also influence scar formation.

Skin with more pigment has been described as being more susceptible to scarring.[3] Skin tension appears to be a contributor to scarring.[3] Microdamage to tissue caused by tension may lead to inflammation that stimulates fibroblasts to create collagen. Young people tend to scar more than elderly people do. This might be due to the "tighter" skin and generally more active lifestyle (causing frequent skin tension) of younger individuals, compared with the "loose" skin and decreased elasticity of the skin in elderly people.

It is generally thought that location of a wound may contribute to the amount of eventual scarring, even though scars have been described on all parts of the body. Keloids most commonly appear somewhere between the ears and the waist or from the elbow to the shoulder.[5] Hypertrophic scarring has been described to occur more likely at the shoulder, upper arm, upper back, dorsal feet, and buttocks.[6] Clinically, keloid scars or hypertrophic scars can form on any body surface. Further, there is probably some genetic predisposition to scar formation.[7]

Complications of Scar Formation

Cosmetic changes are a possible complication of scarring. The location of the scar might be thought to influence it initially. For example, a facial scar is likely to be more a consistent challenge than a scar that is commonly hidden on the body. However, this does not hold true if the person swims or lives in a warm climate that necessitates shorts or other light clothing. Generally, interactions with people beyond health-care providers, family, and friends may be difficult and, therefore, a person may confine himself or herself socially.

Quality of life issues are a concern to patients with scarring, particularly following a trauma such as a burn, and this view also reflects a perceived low level of self-esteem.[8,9] Patients' perceived quality of life may be diminished secondary to the presence of scar because they may hesitate to participate in their normal activities or to commence social relations, thereby losing some of their sense of worth or contribution. Disfigurement can result in a deceased self-esteem for women and men,[9] adolescents,[10] and children.[11] Low self-esteem and quality of life can also be affected by other complications of scarring, such as contraction, changes in sensation, itching, and color variability in the scar.

Hypertrophic scar contracts while it is maturing.[4,12,13,14] Contraction of scar may intensify a cosmetic deformity but can also result in restriction of mobility and potential for chronic soft-tissue length changes. Any scar that is associated with or located over a joint surface has the potential to render fixed contracture. This particular problem is one of the major factors requiring long-term clinical care and follow-up of scars. The types of contracture can most often be predicted, based on the location of the scar. When a scar is forming over a joint or on a particular side of an extremity, the contraction will affect the related motion. For example, a scar located on the anterior surface of the elbow (the antecubital fossa) will be expected to contract the arm into flexion and could lead to limits of extension of the elbow. Scars on the dorsal surface of the toes will "pull" the toes into extension and limit toe flexion. If intervention is not provided and the scar contraction is allowed to progress, it can become a fixed scar contracture. The process of contracture formation also results in the shortening of allied soft tissue, such as muscle, ligament, and joint capsule. The combination of all of these shortened structures makes it an extremely difficult challenge to recover any functional mobility without invasive surgical revision. The regrettable part of surgical revision is the possibility of the very same outcome because of the scarring that results following the revision.

Sensation is affected because of abnormal innervation of scar. Scar is typically less densely innervated than is normal skin. Patients will experience a "dulled" ability to recognize any of the protective sensations normally present in the skin, such as touch, pain, and temperature.[15] Because of these elevated sensory thresholds, a patient may be at risk for trauma to the scar and should be taught to inspect the scar regularly for scrapes, cuts, small burns, or other damage. Interestingly, even though there is a loss of cutaneous temperature sensation, some patients complain of their scar being very sensitive to cold. Patients may describe numbness, tingling, or shooting pain in the scar during cold weather.

Itching or pruritis is also common in maturing scar tissue. Itching may also persist as a chronic problem in some scars. The itching is probably a result of several contributing factors. A low level of inflammation may be present in forming scar, and substances released during inflammation, such as histamine and substance-P, can contribute to itch. The scar also lacks oil-producing glands. The deficiency of skin oils results in a dry surface that may cause itching. It should also be noted that the dry scar is less supple and, therefore, more prone to cracking, which may lead to the development of sores. A patient should be instructed to apply lotion to the scar frequently. If the scar is allowed to stay dry, it may itch more. Patients should also avoid scratching the itch because of the risk of blistering or skin breakdown. Lotion may help to decrease itchiness and prevent the scar from cracking. Perfumed lotions should be avoided because they might cause a rash or skin irritation.

Additional ingredients, such as vitamin E or aloe, are often included in lotions because they are purported to decrease or cure scar. Although neither of these additives will aggravate or worsen a scar, there is also no current evidence that they will improve the appearance of a scar or cure the scar.

CLINICAL WISDOM

If a patient is experiencing a rash or skin irritation, discontinue the soap currently being used for hygiene and body washing and try a mild, nonperfumed lotion. If you are not sure whether it is the soap or lotion that is causing the irritation, have the patient change the soap first for a few days. If the rash has not gone away, try a nonperfumed lotion. If both the soap and lotion are changed to nonperfumed brands and the rash does not go away, consult a physician.

A patient may also notice and report that a scar changes color from time to time. Color changes are probably between varying shades of red, purple, brown, and gray. Posi-

tion often affects the color changes. Generally, the color intensifies if a limb is in a dependent position. Elevation of the same body part should help diminish the amount of color. Extreme ambient environmental temperatures, either hot or cold, might also increase the color of a scar. Color changes associated with position or temperatures are not permanent. However, if a maturing scar is exposed to sunlight, there is a risk that the scar will become permanently hyperpigmented. The mechanism for this hyperpigmentation in scar is not understood at this time, although it may be related to a potential increase in melanocytes and melanin in the scar tissue.[16] A maturing scar *must* be kept protected from sunlight.

CLINICAL WISDOM

Sun Protection

The patient should apply a waterproof sun block or a sunscreen that is at least a sun protection factor (SPF) 30 when planning any outdoor activity. It is also wise to wear light, sun-protective clothing and hats to guard against the rays of the sun. The extra clothing is recommended even when the patient is wearing compression garments. Remember, too, that the harmful rays are also present on cloudy days.

Tests and Measurement

Several characteristics and sequelae of scars can be examined to improve determination of appropriate intervention strategies. Assessment of the scar tissue itself is aimed at determining whether the scar is immature or mature. This is important because a scar that is immature is considered to be more likely to respond to treatment. Specific characteristics of the scar that help in determining maturity and outcome include pigmentation, pliability, height, and texture. Pigmentation may be documented by describing the color of the scar. Generally, immature scars appear hypervascular and, therefore, may be red or violescent. The same scar may turn a deep purple if it is on a body part that is held in a dependent position or is exposed to cold for a period of time. This coloration begins to fade and should generally return to near-normal skin tone through the process of scar maturation. After the scar has matured, it may be either hypo- or hyperpigmented. Patients should understand that variations of the pigment of the scar are probably permanent if they are present following scar maturation.

CLINICAL WISDOM

Cosmetics

Patients with permanent discoloration of scar might benefit from the use of cosmetics. Cosmetics are most useful over areas of visible scarring, such as the hands and face. There are hypoallergenic forms of makeup that can be used to provide a covering for discoloration and minor deformity. Cosmetics with a sunscreen should be selected to protect the scar tissue from the sun.

Palpating the scar and appraising the stiffness of the tissue commonly assess pliability of the scar. Simply pinching the scar may be useful in determining pliability. A scar that is not pliable will be difficult to pinch up between the fingers because of the stiffness of the tissue. Normal pliable skin allows for very localized mobilization of the skin, without much spread to adjacent skin. Also, scar that is not pliable will often move as a unit when mobilized. Mature scars are generally, but not always, more pliable that maturing scars.

Documentation of height provides some indication for the level of hypertrophy of the scar. Height may be difficult to quantify; however, a description that the scar is raised above the plane of the normal adjacent skin demonstrates hypertrophy. The scar will not necessarily flatten as it matures, without some intervention. The texture of the scar may also indicate hypertrophy. As scar tissue is being actively deposited and becomes hypertrophied to any degree, the texture of the scar deviates from that of normal skin. Texture might be described with a variety of adjectives, such as *rough, uneven*, or *bumpy*. Although not necessarily scientific or certainly not quantitative, these terms do relay the presence of an atypical texture, compared with normal skin.

Sequelae of scar that need to be examined are impairments secondary to scar contraction. A decrease in range of motion and associated joint mobility is a major impairment caused by scar contraction. Assessment procedures for examining the loss of range of motion might include standard goniometry, for example. Assessment of functional limitation secondary to contraction, including activities of daily living and instrumental activities of daily living, should be completed. Disfigurement is one of the possible problems associated with contraction. Written description and photography are two assessment methods that can be used to portray the present disfigurement. For example, scarring that occurs on the dorsum of the hand, involving the web spaces of the fingers, may described as "development of web space syndactyly."

Sensation is another impairment that follows scarring.[15] Sensation testing may be performed to assess the degree of sensory ability over a scar. Decreases in sensation may then be documented and used as important information to include in patient education regarding skin protection.

Clinical measurement of scar tissue, including documentation of intervention treatments, historically has been provided simply by objective description of the scar. There are a few documented scar measurement tools that allow some objectification of observed scar traits; however, each of these scales involves observation and some judgment regarding the scar. In 1990, Sullivan and colleagues[17] published the Vancouver Scar Scale as a method for assessing burn-related scars. This scale uses the variables of pigmentation, vascularity, pliability, and height of the scar to describe the current status of the tissue. Scores are assigned based on variances of these variables from normal, with normal being zero. A higher score represents a worse scar. Table 14-1 provides a representation of the scale and the representative values used to score the scar.

Additional scar rating or appearance scales have been described, using photographs of the scar. One such scale uses scar characteristics, including smoothness of scar surface, a depressed scar border, scar thickness, and pigmentation of the scar, which are rated by rating color pictures of

TABLE 14-1   Ratings Used in the Vancouver Scar Scale to Measure Scar Formation

Pigmentation	Vascularity	Pliability	Height	Score
Normal—color that closely resembles the color over the rest of the body	Normal—color that closely resembles the color over the rest of the body	Normal	Normal—flat	0
Hypopigmentation	Pink	Supple: flexible with minimal resistance	Raised < 2 mm	1
Hyperpigmentation	Red	Yielding: giving way to pressure	Raised < 5 mm	2
	Purple	Firm: inflexible, not easily moved, resistant to manual pressure	Raised > 5 mm	3
		Banding: ropelike tissue that blanches with extension of the scar		4
		Contracture: permanent shortening of scar producing deformity or distortion		5

Note: The higher the score reported, the worse the scar.
Reprinted with permission from Sullivan T, Kermode J, McIver E, Courtemanche DJ. Rating the burn scar. *J Burn Care Rehabil.* 1990;11:256–260.

scars.[18] The quality of the photograph and the experience of the evaluator may affect the reliability of this tool; however, if it is used within a particular setting, it may provide useful ways not only of objectifying scar but of documenting it by photograph, as well. Exhibit 14-1 provides a representation of the scale used to assess scar using this method.

Interventions for the Treatment of Scar

Surgical

Surgery is considered in cases where conservative measures of scar control have not completely corrected or controlled scarring. Surgical intervention is indicated to improve specific cosmetic or functional deformities. Results of the surgery depend on location of the scar, timing of the surgery, extent of the deformity, and surgical technique.

Scar at most anatomic locations can be revised; however, areas such as the head and face, neck, and axillae respond more poorly to surgical modification than do other areas.[19] Most scar revisions are performed after the scar tissue has matured. However, individual considerations and the extent of any deformity must be considered when decisions about reconstructive surgery for correction of scar are made. The larger the deformity or scar, the more extensive the surgery will be. A patient's particular needs, goals, and medical history are important matters for deliberation when finalizing any judgment regarding surgery.

Surgical techniques vary, and the type used for any scar revision will be influenced by the factors previously discussed. Small scars can simply be excised and the excision site can then be primarily closed. Larger scars may be excised and a graft placed to cover the wound. The selection of the graft type is important and may lead to further scar formation. Generally, split-thickness meshed skin grafts will scar to some degree, whereas full-thickness skin grafts, skin flaps, or split-thickness sheet grafts are less likely to scar. Of course, there is a risk that a donor site for a skin graft might scar. There is clearly a risk for the donor site of a full-thickness skin graft or a skin flap to scar. Such donor sites will require further skin coverage, either with another split-thickness skin graft or, if the donor site is small enough, primary closure. Another technique used in revising larger scars is serial excision, or segmental scar reduction. This is achieved by excising a central portion of the scar and primarily closing the wound. This procedure is then replicated over a period of several months until the entire scar has been removed.

Realignment of scar tissue may be considered when the scar forms causing abnormally high skin tension lines. This contributes to contracture formation. Z-plasty, Y-V plasty, and local advancement or rotational flaps are surgical techniques used to realign or replace scar and break up tension lines.

Tissue expanders, which are silicone balloons surgically implanted in the subcutaneous fat or under the muscle, are injected with saline and are used to increase the surface area of normal skin adjacent to the scar. This expanded area of skin eventually can be transferred as a flap to cover an excised area of scar. Tissue expansion allows for better matches of skin color, thickness, and texture than do techniques such as grafting.

In any case of scar revision, a patient must be informed that the scar may form again. This would then require continuing treatment to control the new scar.

Pharmaceutical

Some scar tissue responds to injection of cortisone-related medications. Such medications likely are effective because

EXHIBIT 14-1   Ratings Used in a Photographic Scar Scale to Measure Scar Formation

1. Scar Surface

   -1——————— 0——————— -1——————— -2——————— -3——————— 4

   smooth   normal   rough   rough   rough   rough

2. Scar Border Height

   -1——————— 0——————— -1——————— -2——————— -3——————— 4

   depressed   normal   raised   raised   raised   raised

3. Scar Thickness

   -1——————— 0——————— -1——————— -2——————— -3——————— 4

   thinner   normal   thicker   thicker   thicker   thicker

4. Color Differences (between scar and adjacent normal skin)

   -1——————— 0——————— -1——————— -2——————— -3——————— 4

   hypopigment   normal   hyperpigment   hyperpigment   hyperpigment   hyperpigment

Note: The scale ranges from -1 to 4 for each characteristic. Generally, the higher the score reported, the worse the scar.
Reprinted with permission from Yeong EK, Engrav LH, et al. Improved burn scar assessment with use of new scar-rating scale. *J Burn Care Rehabil.* 1997;18:353–355.

of their capability to increase activity of collagenase in breaking down the scar. Injections of this type are recommended only for small scars.

Pressure Therapy

Although previous publications of the effect of pressure on wound healing[20] and scar[21] existed, pressure therapy burgeoned in the 1970s, following the publication of the successful use in treating burn scars.[22] Actual pressures under a pressure garment will vary.[23] It appears, however, that these variable pressures still generally provide an adequate clinical response of controlling scar.[24]

Pressure therapy is typically recommended when a wound takes longer than 14 days to heal. The longer the healing time, the more likely it is that a wound will form scar tissue. It is by and large advised that pressure garments or devices be worn for an average of 23 hours a day while the scar is maturing. Companies manufacture the garments in a variety of colors. Manufacturers also are generally willing to fabricate atypical garments for special circumstances, such as a hand with an amputated finger. The fit of the supports should be checked from time to time because the garments will stretch and wear out. Alterations to existing garments and the fitting of new garments should be carried out as often as necessary to promote the sought-after outcome.

Manufacturers of pressure garments offer garments that fit the face, neck, upper extremity, torso, hand, and lower extremity. Although the different manufacturers may have slightly different methods for measuring each body part for a pressure garment, generally, limb circumferences every 1 inch to 1–1/2 inches are required. Assuring a proper fit of the face, torso, and hands is a bit more complex, and manufacturers' methods for taking measurements of these parts vary to some extent. Specific directions for measurement techniques can be obtained by contacting the manufacturer directly. A list of custom pressure garment suppliers is provided at the end of the chapter.

After a patient bathes or showers, he or she should be instructed to apply some lotion to the scar and to put on a clean pressure garment. The garment previously worn should be washed and dried. The pressure garment can be washed either by hand or on a delicate cycle in a washing machine with mild detergent and warm (not hot) water. If the garment is washed by hand, it should be rinsed thoroughly after washing. The pressure garment should be dried in the air (do not dry in the dryer or by placing the garment on a heater). The garment will dry faster if it is first rolled up in a towel and gently wrung to remove extra water. Pressure garments will not tolerate dry cleaning and should not be ironed. It is recommended that each patient have at least two of each type of garment worn so that a clean one is always available.

Wearing pressure supports might be an issue with some patients. Commonly expressed concerns about the garments include the appearance, the discomfort (tightness), getting the garment on and off, and how hot they make the patient.

Compliance will increase as patients wear the garment for a longer period of time and if they are given a color choice. Education about the benefits and care of the garments will also enhance compliance to treatment.[25]

There may be some difficulty in donning a pressure garment located on the same limb being treated with pressure therapy. Attempting to pull the pressure garment over dressings is difficult and commonly dislodges them. This problem generally can be overcome by pulling on nylon hosiery over the dressed limb, then donning the pressure garment over the nylon hosiery.

Pressure to scar can also be applied through the use of elastic wraps, self-adherent stretch wraps, or elasticized cotton tubular bandages (Figure 14-1). Manufacturers of custom pressure garments also produce noncustom, general fit supports. These less expensive, noncustom options can also be advantageous in treating lymphedema or postwound edema. Early pressure can decrease edema formation and facilitate wound healing. This may also have some effect on eventual scarring because, as mentioned previously, delayed wound healing has been linked to increased scar formation.

Certain areas of the body may be difficult to fit appropriately with a fabric pressure garment. For example, due to the contours of the central portion of the face, palm of the hand, interscapular region, and sternal region, the fabric generally bridges between bony prominences or over anatomic arches. Foam, thermoplastic splinting material, and rubberized compounds can be placed under a pressure garment to conform better to these areas (Figure 14-2). These "inserts" can also be used to augment pressure provided by a well-fitting pressure garment in areas such as the web spaces of the hand (Figure 14-3). Custom-fitted, rigid, transparent, plastic material has also been used successfully to control scarring of the face and could certainly be considered for other areas.[26,27]

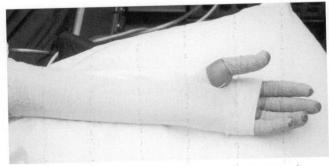

FIGURE 14-1 Self-adherent wrap and cotton elasticized pressure supports may be used to control edema and scarring. Coban™ self-adherent wrap was applied to the fingers in this figure. Tubigrip™ was used to cover the arm and hand in this figure. (Copyright © 2001, R. Scott Ward, PT, PhD)

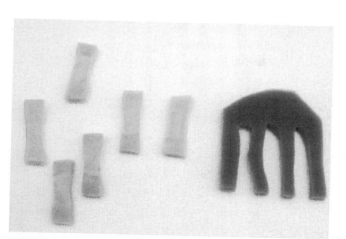

FIGURE 14-2 Examples of how foam was cut for placement in the web spaces of the fingers under a pressure support glove. (Copyright © 2001, R. Scott Ward, PT, PhD)

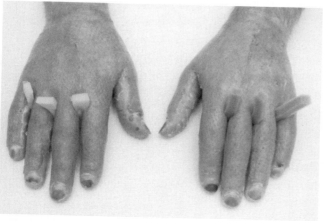

FIGURE 14-3 Application of the foam inserts placed in the web spaces of hands. A pressure support glove is then applied over these inserts. The foam inserts increase the pressure applied to web spaces of fingers and toes and can be used over other areas that may require additional pressure. (Copyright © 2001, R. Scott Ward, PT, PhD)

Massage

Massage has been advocated as a treatment for scar, both to loosen adhesions formed between the scar and adjacent tissue and to prevent or decrease scarring. Evidence for the effectiveness of massage on scar is scarce. The use of some form of friction massage should be useful in mobilizing superficial tissues by loosening the adhesions of scar to the tissue, based on the mechanical effects of the massage. Massage does not appear to decrease scarring or to improve variables of scar formation, such as vascularity, pliability, and height.[28] Although massage does not appear to improve the scar itself, supplementary benefits of massage may include lubrication of the scar to prevent drying and cracking of the skin, a decrease in reported pruritis, and the psychologic benefits of touch. Aggressive massage of early form-

ing scar tissue should be avoided because it may cause blisters or skin breakdown.

Silicone

A silicone polymer gel (the viscosity of silicone used for scar treatment) is produced in sheets or pads that are applied directly over a maturing scar. These manufactured gel pads are commonly offered in several shapes and sizes for application to scars on different areas of the body. Silicone gel has been used successfully in treating scar hypertrophy.[29,30] The mechanism of action behind the success of silicone gel treatment is not known. Silicone gel is most commonly used over small areas, as opposed to large surface areas. It is also used in areas where sufficient pressure cannot be applied to a scar. Reported complications associated with silicone gel application include local rash, skin breakdown, and a lack of durability of some brands of silicone. If a rash develops, the use of the gel product should be suspended temporarily. In general, the rash clears up readily and, because the rash does not predictably reoccur at the same location, the gel may be reapplied, once the site is clear of the rash. Skin breakdown appears to occur in cases where a rash develops and the use of the gel sheet is not interrupted. No systemic complications related to the use of silicone have been reported.

Exercise

Exercise is vital in counteracting the contraction associated with active hypertrophic scar. Directed exercise to prevent deconditioning, functional limitation, and disability is also extremely important. When determining an exercise prescription for a patient with scar, several factors about the scar should be considered; these include location, size (surface area of the scar), and status (phase of wound healing). For example, in some acute situations immediately following a grafting procedure or following tendon repair associated with a skin wound, any type of exercise may be delayed to allow for appropriate healing. Patient variables that also must be considered in the preparation of an exercise prescription include: medical history and current medical status, age, level of cognition, perceived or real level of cooperation, and goals for recovery.

A patient should always be encouraged to put as much stretch on the scar as is safely indicated by the therapist to prevent as much scar contraction as possible. Blanching of the scar is a reasonable clinical indication that the scar is being sufficiently stretched, and the stretch should not exceed the patient's pain tolerance. Stretching of a scar should be done with a slow, sustained elongation of the tissue. Stretching and exercise will also help to prevent other associated soft tissues from shortening.

Types of Applicable Exercise

Active Exercise. Active exercise is the preferred method of exercise in treating scar. This type of exercise allows a patient to control the extent and amount of stretch placed on a scar. Active exercise will also help to overcome any loss of strength or endurance associated with varying levels of muscle disuse sometimes associated with scar formation. An active exercise program should be prescribed and monitored by a therapist.

Active-Assisted Exercise. Active-assisted exercise allows patients who cannot quite achieve full range of motion to be assisted by the therapist. Patients should be encouraged to complete as much of the motion as they can by themselves; then the therapist can apply additional stretch to maximize tissue elongation. Weights may be used to enhance a stretch. The patient may also provide the assistance to active motion by using equipment such as reciprocal pulleys.

Passive Exercise. Passive exercise is effective but does not encourage patient independence. This form of stretching may be necessary if a patient is otherwise unable to stretch a scar because of such problems as weakness or paralysis, or when the patient is otherwise cognitively unable to participate in a prescribed active exercise program. Passive exercise, controlled by the therapist, may also be indicated when a wound is acute enough that a well-intentioned but overzealous patient might compromise healing. The therapist should be cautious not to overstretch the scar or exceed a patient's pain tolerance. Therapists should be aware that overly aggressive stretching might lead to heterotopic ossification.[31] Passive exercise should progress to active-assisted or active exercise as soon as possible.

Strengthening Exercise. There may be variable times of recovery from wounds. As previously mentioned, delayed wound healing also is associated with increased scar formation. Any reason for a decrease in normal use of a muscle (or muscle group) can lead to a decrease in strength of that muscle. Strength testing should be a part of any physical examination associated with scarring. If strength deficits are found, a prescribed series of resistance exercises should be provided to regain lost strength. Strengthening exercises will also assist with any decreases in endurance or conditioning.

Directed Functional Exercise. Scar contraction can also lead to an inability to strengthen a muscle through its normal range of motion. These scar contraction-related impairments of strength or range of motion can lead to functional limitations. Age-appropriate functional exercises should be instituted to improve motor skills, enhance confidence in daily activities, and allow the patient to resume his or her expected daily role in society.

Splinting

Splints are generally indicated for the positioning of a scar to avoid deformation or to maintain or increase the stretch on a scar. The therapist can fabricate splints and some effective prefabricated splints are available. Thermoplastic material is the most common item used by therapists to fabricate custom splints. It is common that these splints, when

used for scar, are fabricated as *conforming splints*. A conforming splint is one that is custom-fit to a patient and matches the patient's anatomic shape. A custom-fit, conforming splint decreases the likelihood of a poorly fitted splint and might also apply some pressure to the scar, therefore assisting in controlling scar formation.

Splints may also be referred to as *static splints, dynamic splints,* or *serial splints.* A static splint has a fixed shape and maintains a position through immobilization of the splinted part.[32] Static splints are commonly used in the early phases of scar formation. They are generally molded and applied following an exercise treatment to maintain the elongation of the scar achieved during the session. They may be left on for an extended period of time to preserve range of motion gains. Dynamic splints apply a force, or a stretch, to a body part or allow resistance to movement for exercise.[29] This type of splint can be used to continue a gentle force to scar, thus providing an extended period of stretching. Serial splints are basically static splints that are remolded to a newly achieved position of a body part. Serial splints (or casts) might be used if a scar is particularly difficult to stretch. A maximal tissue stretch is completed, then the splint is reformed to the new stretched position. This procedure is followed serially until full range of motion is realized.

Splinting should be discontinued if there is any associated pain, sensory disturbance (numbness, tingling, etc.), or skin breakdown.

Positioning

Positioning may be used to sustain tissue elongation to counter scar contraction.[33] General positions of preference are listed in Table 14-2. Custom-made or prefabricated splints may be used as "positioning" devices. However, positioning devices need not be sophisticated or expensive. For example, pillows may be used to position the hips or shoulders, and high-top tennis shoes make a reasonable positioning device for the foot and ankle.

Physical Agents

Thermal agents are the common therapeutic modalities used to treat scar or the sequelae of scarring. Warming the scar, in particular, may have the most effect on the tissue because of the high concentration of collagen in scar. Gersten[34] demonstrated that collagen extensibility could be increased with therapeutic applications of ultrasound. The combined work of Gersten and others groups also provided the strong advocation that collagen tissue is most effectively stretched when a blend of heat and gentle stretch are provided.[35,36] Superficial forms of heat may also provide the most effective method of heating surface scar and allowing enhanced elongation of the tissue; however, very little research exists to support the efficacy of superficial heat on integumentary scarring.

Because scars are also normally hypesthetic, caution must be taken when applying thermal agents to the scar tis-

TABLE 14-2   Preferred Anticontracture Positions for Major Joints

Joint/Joint Complex	Preferred Position
Neck	Hyperextension, no rotation
Shoulder	Abduction (90°), slight horizontal flexion
Elbow	Extension, supination
Wrist/Hand	Slight wrist extension, slight MCP flexion, PIP/DIP extension, thumb abduction
Trunk	Straight postural alignment
Hip	Extension, abduction (20°), no rotation
Knee	Full extension
Ankle/Foot	Neutral ankle (no plantar flexion), neutral toes

sue. A sensory examination should be completed, and tissue should be inspected frequently to ensure that no tissue damage is occurring secondary to the heat or coupling media.

Patient Education and Self-Care

Patients and their families or other caregivers should be trained to apply and assess scar control techniques. This includes care of the scar, pressure supports, silicon gel, exercise, splints, and positioning. Sufficient time for observation of the techniques, followed by opportunities to practice the techniques while supervised, will enhance the confidence of the patients/caregivers in their abilities. Providing written or pictorial supplemental materials can be useful additions to an education program. Having a patient/caregiver demonstrate the appropriate application of interventions is a logical discharge goal for patients with actively forming scar.

Patients/caregivers must be educated about the reasons for treatments being used and the goals of the interventions. An increased understanding will lead to more "buy-in" of the treatment. Patients are more likely to take some personal responsibility regarding their care if they truly buy in to the plan.[37] Reassurance that you will be willing to provide further assistance and advice, should it be needed, will also quell some concerns they might have about forgetting a component of the intervention or asking questions that arise concerning the progression of the scar. The supplemental material provided might be sufficient for some, but a contact phone number with an invitation to call can also be reassuring.

Conclusion

When considering treatment for a scar, all aspects of the scarring process must be deliberated. This includes the appearance of the scar and the limitations that result from the contraction of the scar. It is important to remember that scarring is a process and that it commonly takes several months for a scar to mature. Therefore, much of what is done to treat scar cannot be employed on a short-term basis only. This requires high-quality patient education and follow-up to monitor the progression of the scarring properly for the best possible clinical outcome.

■ CASE STUDY

B.G. is a 34-year-old Caucasian female with healed full-thickness burns to the dorsum of her left hand and the dorsal surface of all left fingers. She is 3 weeks post–split-thickness autografting to the hand wound. Her burn injury included partial-thickness burns to her left arm that have fully healed. She is otherwise healthy, with no significant past medical history.

On examination, there is no evidence of scarring on the left arm over the site of the partial-thickness burns. The skin-grafted areas of the left hand are showing signs of scarring. The tissue is red, has a mildly decreased pliability, and is slightly raised and uneven. Range of motion measurements demonstrated the following limitations: the left wrist is 0–80° extension, 0–65° flexion; an average loss of 20° of motion in the left MCPs of the fingers; an average loss of 25° in the PIP joints of the fingers; an average loss of 15° in the DIP joints of the fingers; a loss of 20° in thumb abduction; and a 10° loss of the thumb MCP and IP flexion. The patient is also concerned about the appearance of the scar.

Therapy interventions for the problem at its current level include:

• Passive stretch of all joints affected by decreased range of motion. These stretches will be taught to the patient and should be performed six or more times daily.

• Active range of motion exercises, including encouraging full use of the hand in normal daily functional activities. The active motion exercises should be performed following each session of passive stretches. The hand should be used actively for all normal activities.

• Measurement and application of a custom-fit, antiscar support glove. The patient will be educated on the application and care of the pressure garment. One to two additional gloves will be ordered.

• Application of moisturizer to the scar, as needed, for itching and discomfort. The patient will be educated in the indication for application of moisturizer, including itching, discomfort, and "scaliness."

All of these interventions will continue through to maturation of the scar, which may be 6–18 months. The frequency of the stretching and range of motion exercises may be decreased, depending on the level of ongoing limitation and impairment.

The discharge outcome for this patient would be a scar that closely matches normal skin pigment, is relatively pliable, is smooth, and does not limit mobility and function of the hand.

REVIEW QUESTIONS

1. How is scar tissue formed and what are predictors for scar formation?
2. Describe the characteristics of scar and impairments related to scar contraction.
3. What interventions may be useful in treating the disfigurement of a scar that is immature and hypertrophic?
4. What interventions may be useful in treating range of motion impairment secondary to scar contraction?

RESOURCES

Custom Pressure Garment Manufacturers

Barton-Carey Medical Products
26963 Eckel Road, Suite 303
Perrysburg, OH 43551
(800) 421-0444

Bio-Concepts, Inc.
2424 East University Drive
Phoenix, AZ 85034-6911
(800) 421-5647
www.bio-con.com

Gottfried Medical, Inc
4105 West Alexis Road
Toledo, OH 43623
(800) 537-1968
www.gottfriedmedical.com

Juzo
P.O. Box 1088
Cuyahoga Falls, OH 44223
(216) 923-4999
www.juzousa.com

Torbot Group, Inc.
Jobskin Division
653 Miami Street
Toledo, OH 43605
(800) 207-1074
www.torbotgarments.com

Medical Z
6800 Alamo Downs Parkway
San Antonio, TX 78238
Phone: (800) 368-7478
www.gottfriedmedical.com

REFERENCES

1. Thomsen M. It all began with Aristotle-the history of the treatment of burns. *Burns Incl Therm Inj* 14(Suppl): S1-S8, 1988.
2. Ketchum L. Hypertrophic scars and keloids. *Clin Plast Surg* 4: 301-310, 1977.
3. Rockwell WB, Cohen IK, Erlich HP. Keloids and hypertrophic scars: A comprehensive review. *Plast Reconstr Surg* 84: 827-837, 1989.
4. Hunt T. Disorders of wound healing. *World J Surg* 4: 289-295, 1980.
5. Cohen IK, McCoy BJ. The biology and control of surface overhealing. *World J Surg* 4: 289-195, 1980.
6. Deitch EA, Wheelahan TN, Rose MP, et al. Hypertrophic burn scars: Analysis of variables. *J Trauma* 23: 895-898, 1983.
7. Lewis WHP, Sun KKY. Hypertrophic scar: A genetic hypothesis. *Burns* 16: 176-178, 1990.
8. Blumenfield M, Reddish PM. Identification of psychologic impairment in patients with mild-moderate thermal injury: Small burn, big problem. *Gen Hosp Psychiatry* 9: 142-146, 1987.
9. Cobb N, Maxwell G, Silverstein P. 1990;11:330-333. Patient perception of quality of life after burn injury: Results of an eleven-year study. *J Burn Care Rehabil* 11: 330-333, 1990.
10. Robert R, Meyer W, Bishop S, Rosenberg L, Murphy L and Blakeney P. Disfiguring burn scars and adolescent self-esteem. *Burns* 25: 581-585, 1999.
11. Abdullah A, Blakeney P, Hunt R, Broemeling L, Phillips L, Herndon DN and Robson MC. Visible scars and self-esteem in pediatric patients with burns. *The Journal of burn care & rehabilitation.* 15: 164-168, 1994.
12. Clark JA, Cheng JCY, Leung KS, Leung PC. Mechanical characterization of human postburn skin during compression therapy. *J Biomech* 20: 397-406, 1987.
13. McHugh A, Fowlkes B, Maevsky E, Smith D, Jr., Rodriguez J and Garner W. Biomechanical alterations in normal skin and hypertrophic scar after thermal injury. *Journal of Burn Care & Rehabilitation* 18: 104-108, 1997.
14. Steed DL. Wound-healing trajectories. *The Surgical clinics of North America.* 83: 547, 2003.
15. Ward RS, Tuckett RP. Quantitative threshold changes in cutaneous sensation of patients with burns. *J Burn Care Rehabil*: 569-575, 1991.
16. Sowemimo GO, Naim J, Harrison HN and Lee JC. Repigmentation after burn injury in the guinea-pig. *Burns, including thermal injury.* 8: 345-357, 1982.
17. Sullivan T, Smith J, Kermode J, McIver E, Courtemanche DJ. Rating the burn scar. *J Burn Care Rehabil* 11: 256-260, 1990.
18. Yeong EK, Mann R, Engrav LH, et al. Improved burn scar assessment with use of new scar-rating scale. *J Burn Care Rehabil* 18: 353-355, 1997.
19. Kraemer MD, Jones T, Deitch EA. Burn contractures: Incidence, predisposing factors, and results of surgical therapy. *J Burn Care Rehabil* 9: 261-265, 1988.
20. Blair VP. The influence of mechanical pressure on wound healing. *Ill. Med J* 46: 249-252, 1924.
21. Cronin T. The use of a molded splint to prevent contracture after split skin grafting on the neck. *Plast Reconstr Surg* 27: 7-18, 1961.
22. Larson DL, Abston S, Evans EB, Dobrkovsky M, Linares HA. Techniques for decreasing scar formation and contractures in the burned patient. *J Trauma* 11: 807-823, 1971.
23. Mann R, Yeong EK, Moore M, Colescott D, Engrav LH. Do customfitted pressure garments provide adequate pressure? *J Burn Care Rehabil* 18: 247-249, 1997.
24. Cheng JCY, Evans JH, Leung KS, Clark JA, Choy TTC, Leung PC. Pressure therapy in the treatment of post-burn hypertrophic scar: A critical look into its usefulness and fallacies by pressure monitoring. *Burns Incl Therm Inj* 10: 154-163, 1984.
25. Rosser P. Adherence to pressure garment therapy of post traumatic burn injury. *J Burn Care Rehabil* 21 (Part 2): S178, 2000.
26. Rivers E, Strate RG, Solem LD. The transparent face mask. *Am J Occup Ther* 33: 11-113, 1979.
27. Shons AR, Rivers E, Solem LD. A rigid transparent face mask for control of scar hypertrophy. *Ann Plast Surg* 6: 245-248, 1981.
28. Patino O, Novak C, Merlo A, Benaim F. Massage in hypertrophic scars. *J Burn Care Rehabil* 19: 268-271, 1998.
29. Gold H. A controlled clinical trial of topical silicone gel sheeting in the treatment of hypertrophic scars and keloids. *J Am Acad Dermatol* 30: 506-507, 1994.
30. Sang TA, Monafo WW, Mustoe TA. Topical silicone gel: A new treatment for hypertrophic scars. *Surgery* 106: 781-787, 1989.
31. Van Laeken N, Snelling CFT, Meek RN, Warren RJ, Foley B. Heterotopic bone formation in the patient with burn injuries: A retrospective assessment of contributing factors and methods of investigation. *J Burn Care Rehabil* 10: 331-335, 1989.
32. Duncan R. Basic principles of splinting the hand. *Phys Ther* 69: 1104-1116, 1989.
33. Rudolf R. Construction and the control of contraction. *World J Surg* 4: 279-287, 1980.
34. Gersten J. Effect of ultrasound on tendon extensibility. *Am J Phys Med* 34: 362-369, 1955.
35. LaBan M. Collagen tissue: Implications of its response to stress in vitro. *Arch Phys Med Rehabil* 43: 461, 1962.
36. Warren CG, Lehmann JF, Koblanski JN. Elongation of rat tail tendon: Effect of load and temperature. *Arch Phys Med Rehabil* 57: 122-126, 1976.
37. Peloquin S. Linking purpose to procedure during interactions with patients *Am J Occup Ther.* 42: 775-781, 1988.

PART

III

Management by Wound Etiology

Barbara M. Bates-Jensen

Determining the cause or etiology of a wound is a critical element in creating a comprehensive treatment plan for patients with wounds. The chapters in Part III focus on management by wound etiology, including specific information on acute surgical wounds, pressure ulcers, vascular ulcers, and neuropathic ulcers. Emphasis is placed on understanding the pathophysiology involved in the wound type, assessment methods, and prevention and management of specific wound types. Improving and expanding knowledge of wound etiology empowers clinicians to provide quality comprehensive care in clinical practice.

Chapter 15 presents management of the acute surgical wound. The chapter begins by defining acute versus chronic wounds. When does an acute wound become a chronic wound? A better understanding of acute wounds improves a clinician's ability to monitor and treat all wounds. Types of surgical wound healing—primary intention, secondary intention, and tertiary intention—are presented. Extrinsic factors that affect wound healing during the preoperative, intraoperative, and postoperative time periods are described. Surgical wound classifications are presented and reviewed. Interventions for managing hypovolemia, thermoregulation strategies, and methods of optimizing tissue oxygen perfusion are described.

Intrinsic factors that affect healing of the acute surgical wound, such as age, concurrent conditions, nutritional status, and oxygenation and tissue perfusion are all discussed, with special attention to the patient with diabetes. Examination of the surgical incision includes evaluation of wound characteristics, such as incision location and length, presence of healing ridge, type and amount of exudate, type of wound closure materials, and approximation of wound edges. The incisional examination forms the basis of acute surgical wound assessment and is presented by phase of wound healing (inflammatory, proliferative, and remodeling).

The discussion includes types of dressings used for primary and secondary dressings. Wound healing in secondary intention and tertiary intention wounds is explained and contrasted with primary intention incisions.

Outcome measures for evaluating healing in incisional wounds following the phases of wound healing are presented and described, with examples of appropriate documentation of the healing incision. The chapter concludes with a case study for review of material and self-care teaching guidelines for use with other health-care providers, family caregivers, and patients.

Chapters 16 and 17 describe issues related to the management of pressure ulcers. Chapter 16 is focused on pathophysiology and prevention of pressure ulcers. It begins with a definition of pressure ulcers and an extensive review of the pathophysiology of pressure ulcer development. The relationship between time and pressure in the development of pressure ulcers is explained, as well as the clinical presentation of pressure ulceration and the most prevalent locations for pressure ulcer development. Specific information is included on assessment of darkly pigmented skin for risk of pressure ulceration.

The history of staging systems and the current system recommended by the Agency for Healthcare Research and Quality (AHRQ, formerly the Agency for Health Care Research and Policy) and the National Pressure Ulcer Advisory Panel are described. Pressure ulcer assessment and the use and misuse of staging classification systems are subjects of debate and controversy. Pressure ulcer development does not necessarily progress from one stage to the next, and there can be different etiologic factors for various stages. Discussion of deep tissue injury as part of the staging system is also reviewed in Chapter 16.

A discussion of pressure ulcer pathophysiology and etiology would not be complete without considering other interacting factors. Factors that contribute to pressure ulcer development by force over a bony prominence and those that affect the tolerance of the tissues to pressure are presented and described. Particular attention is given to immobility or severely restricted mobility because it is the most important risk factor for all populations and a necessary condition for the development of pressure ulcers. The most common risk assessment tools are presented and explained.

Appropriate prevention interventions can be focused on eliminating specific risk factors. Thus, early intervention for pressure ulcers is risk factor-specific and prophylactic in nature. The prevention strategies are presented by risk factors, beginning with general information and ending with specific strategies for a particular risk factor. Chapter 16 includes specific information on the use of support surfaces, with definitions of pressure-reducing and pressure-relieving devices, pillow bridging, and passive repositioning. Extensive information on nutrition interventions and management of incontinence is included. Skin hygiene and maintenance interventions round out the prevention strategies. Chapter 16 concludes with outcome measures for evaluating the success of a pressure ulcer prevention program and extensive self-care teaching guidelines for other health-care providers, family caregivers, and patients.

In Chapter 17, Rappl continues the discussion of support surfaces that began in Chapter 16 and looks at therapeutic positioning for pressure ulcer prevention. Individuals who become sitting-dependent more than ambulatory and those who use the lying-down or the sitting position for the majority of their days are at high risk for skin breakdown. Also, for a patient with an existing pressure ulcer, proper positioning in the most active and functional position possible, both in sitting and in recumbent positions, improves the healing rate of the ulcer and minimizes the likelihood of developing new ulcers. Chapter 17 provides an overview of therapeutic positioning knowledge and describes the areas clinicians should examine to determine the need for intervention. This chapter covers the basics of therapeutic positioning and how it affects body system impairments. The chapter includes a table on functional diagnosis and its relationship to prognosis, interventions, and outcomes related to therapeutic positioning. The ideal sitting position is described, and basic seating principles related to pelvic control, thigh control, seat depth, and footrest are discussed. Finally, specific information on positioning a patient with an existing ulcer, both in sitting and recumbent positions, are described. An extensive discussion of the methods of determining appropriate wheelchairs and sitting positions, as well as procedures for recumbent positioning for patients, is presented.

Chapter 18 provides an in-depth analysis of the diagnosis and management of vascular ulcers. The chapter begins with a review of general anatomy and physiology of the circulatory system and pathophysiology related to lower extremity ulcers. A thorough history and physical assessment is essential for patients with lower leg ulcers. Information for each ulcer type, as well as risk factors for arterial/ischemic, venous, and diabetic ulcers, are discussed. The presentation and assessment of common findings related to lower leg ulcers, such as intermittent claudication, rest pain, altered ankle-brachial index, edema, and tissue changes, are described, including associated diagnostic tests for the lower leg.

Differential diagnosis for leg ulcers is a key factor in determining appropriate treatment. For example, an intervention that is appropriate for a venous ulcer can be contraindicated for an arterial/ischemic ulcer. The presenting clinical manifestations, diagnostic tests, and differential wound assessments are presented for each lower leg ulcer type. Medical and surgical management related to arterial/ischemic, venous disease, and diabetic ulcers is described. Special attention is given to diagnosing osteomyelitis in the patient with diabetes and describing the pathophysiology of edema related to venous disease, with indications for clinical management.

Chapter 19 opens with Elftman's discussion of the necessity of interdisciplinary collaboration in the management of neuropathic ulcers. These patients often have dysvascular components that must be addressed by a medical team, rather than by one specialty. The trineuropathy assessment, with attention to sensory, motor, and autonomic neuropathy, is explained. Gradual and sudden-onset peripheral neuropathy are compared for simple differential diagnosis. Diabetic neuropathy is the focal point of Chapter 19. Common infections and dermatologic changes are presented. The definitions of wet and dry gangrene are presented, and the two conditions are compared. Footwear assessment guidelines and interventions, based on the Wagner ulcer grade, are explained. Chapter 19 also includes in-depth explanations of sensory, pressure, vibratory, and foot deformity evaluation. Charcot's deformity is explained and the method of assessment described. Management with orthotic devices is explained. Specific instructions for procedures, such as how to make a foam toe separator, are included. Interventions to decrease pressure, such as total-contact casting, use of splints and inserts, and neurowalkers, are discussed. (Chapter XX on care of the skin and nails of the neuropathic foot by Conlan contains practical detailed instructions.) The chapter concludes with self-care teaching guidelines for use with patients and family caregivers, as well as documentation requirements for neuropathic ulcers.

Chapter 20 continues the examination of lower extremities with a focus on the skin and nails of the foot. Kelechi provides vivid photographs to help clinicians with diagnosis of common foot problems in the older adult. The chapter presents the underlying pathology, differential diagnosis, treatment, and plan for evaluation for three common foot problems: tinea pedis, onychomycosis, and plantar fasciitis. Tinea pedis is the most common form of dermatophytoses, or fungal infection, of the feet. Commonly known as athlete's foot, tinea pedis is a disorder that can be classified into three categories: interdigital infections, scaling hyperkeratotic moccasin-type infections of the plantar surface, and highly inflammatory vesiculobullous eruptions. Diagnosis and treatment of each is presented and discussed.

Plantar fasciitis is the most common form of heel pain. It is due to inflammation, microruptures, hemorrhages, and collagen degeneration of the plantar fascia. The major underlying factor is overuse injury to soft tissue involving repetitive, excessive loading impact on heel strike over time. Interventions include treatment of pain, restoring flexibility to the ankle and arch, strengthening the muscles in and around the foot, and gradual resumption of activities. Conservative approaches are presented.

Onychomycosis (tinea unguium) is an infection of the toenails in which fungal organisms invade the nail unit via the nail bed or nail plate, causing insidious, progressive destruction of the nail plate if left untreated. Treatment measures are presented, including topical nail reduction using urea compound (20%–40%) in petrolatum under thin film dressing and topical antifungal agents. This chapter concludes with a brief discussion of miscellaneous conditions of the foot.

The final chapter in this part, Chapter 21, presents management of malignant wounds and fistulas. Palliative care and the role of wound care clinicians when faced with wounds with little or no healing potential, are emphasized in this chapter. Malignant wounds and fistulas are often complex and difficult to manage. Clinicians must use creativity and sensitivity in treating patients who present with malignant wounds or fistulas. The basic goals of therapy are presented with attention to reducing symptoms. Techniques are described and discussed on pain management, odor control, management of bleeding, and pouching for fistula output. Several techniques are illustrated, with step-by-step photographs to complement the text. This chapter provides a thoughtful, caring framework for clinicians managing malignant wounds and fistulas.

Although similarities exist in the treatment of any wound, the treatment approach varies depending on wound etiology. The chapters in Part III form a foundation on knowledge of wounds of various etiologies. This foundation should provide clinicians with a stronger and more individualized approach to the patient with a wound.

Acute Surgical Wound Management

Barbara M. Bates-Jensen and Nina Woolfolk

CHAPTER OBJECTIVES

At the completion of this chapter, the reader will be able to:
1. Define key characteristics of the acute surgical wound.
2. Describe assessment factors for the acute surgical wound.
3. Identify factors that affect wound healing in the acute surgical wound during the preoperative, intraoperative, and postoperative periods.
4. Explain the relationship between tissue perfusion and oxygenation and wound healing.

Acute Surgical Wound Definition

Acute wounds are defined as disruptions in the integrity of the skin and underlying tissues that progress through the healing process in a timely and uneventful manner. The acute elective surgical wound is an example of a healthy wound in which healing can be maximized. However, not all surgical wounds are uncomplicated, with maximal healing potential or the possibility of uneventful healing. For example, acute surgical wounds can occur in unhealthy tissues, in a compromised host, or as a result of unexpected or significant trauma.

Surgical wounds can be allowed to heal by one of three methods: primary intention, secondary intention, and tertiary intention (Table 15-1). Wounds that heal by primary intention are wounds with edges that are approximated and closed. Secondary wounds are wounds left open after surgery. Secondary intention healing involves scar tissue replacement in the tissue defect. Tertiary intention healing, or delayed primary closure, involves aspects of both primary and secondary wound healing. In tertiary intention healing, the wound is left open initially; after a short period of time, the edges are approximated, and the wound is closed. Wound healing by secondary intention or dehisced wounds may not follow a timely and uneventful healing course. Thus, they may be considered "chronic" wounds by some clinicians.[1]

When does an acute wound become a chronic wound? The simplest and perhaps least controversial defining characteristic of an acute wound that becomes a chronic wound is failure to follow the normal wound healing temporal sequence. In general, an acute surgical wound should complete the proliferative phase of wound healing in 4 weeks; that is, it should have filled with granulation tissue and be resurfaced with epithelial tissue. Acute surgical wounds that progress at a slower pace or fail to progress are considered chronic.

A surgical incision healing by primary intention could be described as the ideal wound for healing. The wound is controlled with attention to tissue handling and proper use of surgical instruments by the surgeon, and the wound edges are apposed and aligned immediately to decrease the risk of infection. The acute surgical incision wound healing by primary intention is the focus of this chapter.

Factors Affecting Healing in Acute Wounds

Healing in acute surgical wounds involves the interaction of extrinsic and intrinsic factors. Extrinsic factors relate to those agents outside the person, whereas intrinsic factors are those influencing the person internally or systemically.

Extrinsic Factors

The physical environment before and during surgery, surgical preparation, surgical techniques, and types of sutures are all examples of extrinsic factors that can affect acute wound healing. Thus, for the surgical wound, evaluation of the perioperative period is important, because it plays a role in the

TABLE 15-1   Types of Surgical Wound Healing

Wound Healing Type	Definition
Primary intention	Wound edges approximated and closed at time of surgery
Secondary intention	Wound left open after surgery and allowed to heal with scar tissue replacing the tissue defect
Tertiary or delayed primary closure	After surgery, wound left open initially; after short period of time, wound edges are approximated, and wound is closed

wound outcome. Wound infection is the major cause of surgical wounds failing to progress through the healing process in a timely and uneventful manner. Operating room protocols, attention to instrumentation, and appropriate surgical technique are all means of decreasing the risk of infection and ensuring optimal healing from the outset for the surgical wound.

Preoperative Period

The length of time a patient spends in the hospital prior to surgery influences the rate of surgical wound infection. As the length of hospital time increases prior to surgery, the risk of wound infection increases.[2] Preparation of the operative site also influences the risk of wound infection. The use of a systems approach for preoperative skin preparation has been found to decrease surgical site infection rates by sustaining a greater and longer reduction of contaminating microflora as compared with a single approach alone.[3] Showering immediately prior to surgery, using a hexachlorophene soap, has been shown to result in a decrease in infection rate as compared with not showering.[2] Use of a preoperative shower should occur 24 hours prior to surgery, followed by a preoperative skin preparation with a chemistry compatible with that of the soap product to reduce skin irritation.[3] Shaving the operative area and the method used to shave the area have also been implicated in surgical wound infection,[2] because shaving causes skin aberrations that can become infected by proliferating microorganisms.[4]

RESEARCH WISDOM

Operative Site Preparation

Use of depilatory creams, electric razors, or clippers is associated with reduced wound infection rates when compared with the use of nonelectric razors to shave the operative area.[4] Despite the research, however, most operative site preparations still include nonelectric shaving, most commonly performed in the operating room. The poor implementation of the research may be due to the absence of electric razors and clippers in the operating room. Hair removal performed the morning of surgery is also associated with reduced risk of infection compared with hair removal the evening before surgery.[4]

Intraoperative Period

Limiting the infection rate intraoperatively is largely under the control of the surgeon. Sometimes, infection control is

difficult to achieve. For example, the surgeon has limited power over the nature of the problem for which the surgery is performed, the operative site, and the general condition of the patient; all are more complicated factors that are not easily controlled. The type of surgical procedure also influences the risk of infection. Surgical procedures are classified according to the risk of infection.[5] Table 15-2 presents wound classifications for surgery. Clean wounds are those nontraumatic injuries in which no inflammation is encountered during the procedure, and there is no break in sterile technique. Clean-contaminated wounds are procedures wherein the gastrointestinal or respiratory tract is entered without significant contamination. A contaminated wound is one in which a major break in sterile technique or gross spillage from the gastrointestinal tract occurs. Procedures in which acute bacterial inflammation or pus is encountered with devitalized tissue or contamination are classified as dirty or infected wounds.

The National Nosocomial Infections Surveillance (NNIS) System Basic Surgical Site Infections (SSI) Risk Index is another method for determining the risk of infection. The NNIS system scores surgical procedures by including the American Society of Anesthesiologists (ASA) classification perioperatively, whether the procedure is contaminated or dirty-infected, and the duration of the surgical procedure.[6] The NNIS Basic SSI Index is a multivariate index for wound classification that compensates for the limitation of the traditional wound classification system, which does not take into account a patient's intrinsic risk of developing a surgical wound infection.[6] The degree of wound classification, ASA score, and duration of the surgical procedure have each been found to be independently associated with surgical wound infections.[7] Increased duration of the operative procedure increases the risk for wound infection significantly. One study found that the infection rate doubled each hour that the surgical procedure continued.[2] Strict adherence by operating room personnel to an infection control protocol has also resulted in decreased wound infection rates.[8]

Some degree of mechanical stress on tissue during surgery is inevitable; however, excess trauma can lead to a prolonged inflammatory phase of healing, decreased tensile strength, and increased risk of infection.[9] Surgeons must be concerned with wound tension, vascular supply, and proper surgical technique. If the wound cannot be closed without a significant amount of tension or if the vascular supply is

TABLE 15-2 Surgical Wound Classifications

Wound Classification	Surgical Label	Definition	Procedure Types
I	Clean	• Nontraumatic injuries • No inflammation found during procedure • No break in sterile technique	Exploratory laparotomy Mastectomy Total hip replacement Vascular surgeries
II	Clean-contaminated	• Procedures involving GI or respiratory tract • No significant contamination	• Bronchoscopy • Small bowel resection • Whipple pancreatico-duodenectomy
III	Contaminated	• Major break in sterile technique • Gross spillage from GI tract	• Appendectomy for inflamed appendicitis • Bile spillage during cholecystectomy • Diverticulitis
IV	Dirty or infected	• Acute bacterial inflammation found • Pus encountered • Devitalized tissue encountered	• Excision and drainage of abscess • Perforated bowel • Peritonitis

poor, there is increased risk of dehiscence, necrosis, and infection.[10] Suturing technique can assist with optimal wound healing outcomes. Use of buried sutures can improve primary wound healing by decreasing the potential for hematoma formation in dead space under the incision, giving tensile support in the first 2 to 4 months while the wound is still weak[10] to decrease tension on the apposed wound edges.[11] Surface sutures can negatively impact optimal healing because they provide additional "wounds" to heal alongside the incision.

Postoperative Period

The stress response associated with surgery has also been shown to impair wound healing. The stress of surgery stimulates the sympathetic nervous system, with a resultant sympathetic nervous system-mediated vasoconstriction. High levels of circulating catecholamines in the immediate postoperative period cause the resulting vasoconstriction, with factors that trigger the sympathetic nervous system, including hypoxia, hypothermia, pain, and hypovolemia.[12] In the immediate postoperative period, measures of subcutaneous tissue/wound oxygenation are lower after major operations and correlate with extensive, more complex surgical procedures.[12] Attempts to restore tissue and wound oxygen deficits minimize the risks of hypothermia, pain, hypovolemia, and hypoxia simultaneously in the immediate postoperative period.

CLINICAL WISDOM

Maximizing Wound Healing

Critical measures to maximize wound healing in the immediate postoperative period include keeping the patient:

• Warm
• Well hydrated, intravenously or orally
• Pain-free by use of patient-controlled analgesia, if possible
• Well oxygenated by use of supplemental oxygen, if needed

Thermoregulatory responses are diminished in surgical patients because of their prolonged exposure to the cold operating room environment. Patients treated with active rewarming by use of heated blankets during the recovery period experience a faster return of normal tissue/wound oxygen levels than do those allowed to return to normothermia without rewarming interventions.[12] The routine use of measures to actively warm the patient during the surgical procedure, such as warming blankets and warmed intravenous fluids, along with active monitoring during surgery, help to prevent thermoregulatory problems. It is easier to prevent thermoregulatory problems than to remedy them.

Correcting hypovolemia with adequate fluid infusion prevents the continuing vasoconstriction caused by hypovolemia. Fluid replacement occurs simultaneously with rewarming efforts. Assessment and management of pain and tissue perfusion are also recommended to ensure optimal wound healing.[12]

Additional factors that are crucial to optimal surgical wound healing in the postoperative period are intrinsic factors, which can be controlled.

Intrinsic Factors

Intrinsic factors that affect healing of the acute surgical wound are those that influence the patient systemically. Intrinsic factors include age, concurrent conditions, nutritional status, and oxygenation and tissue perfusion.

Age

The physiologic changes that occur with aging place the older individual at higher risk for poor wound healing outcomes.[13-15] Aging causes skin changes, including decreased elastin in the skin with thinning of the dermoepidermal junction and decreased collagen and elastin content of the skin.[16] Cellular changes occur as well. Neutrophils and macrophages demonstrate decreased growth factor production, migration, and phagocytosis.[17] Growth factors are less responsive, and their amounts are decreased.[17] A decreased rate of migration by keratinocytes affects the rate of wound healing and, in particular, reepithelialization of the skin.[18] Finally, older adults demonstrate decreased ability to replace collagen after abdominal surgery.[19]

Several aging-related changes have been shown to be reversible. Estrogen hormone replacement therapy increased healing capacity in test wounds with normal older adult volunteers.[20] The provision of low-dose growth hormone resulted in increased healing capacity in older men with age-related growth factor deficiency.[21]

CLINICAL WISDOM

Risk of Delayed Wound Resurfacing in the Older Adult

Delays in wound resurfacing put older patients at risk for wound infection. Daily wound assessments and use of topical dressings for protection are required for a longer period of time than is necessary for younger patients. However, clinicians can expect the final outcome to be consistent with that of younger individuals despite the age-related changes in older adults.[13,14]

Immune system function declines with age, which may account for the increased risk of infection in older adults. The diminished immune response allows microorganisms to proliferate in the wound before they can be removed. Older adults present with chronic diseases, circulatory changes, and nutritional problems, all of which increase the risk for poor or delayed wound healing. Decreased motor coordination and diminished sensory function increase the potential for injury, wound complications, and repeated wounding at the same site.[14]

Concurrent Conditions

The presence of certain diseases, conditions, and treatments can influence wound healing outcomes. Diabetes mellitus is one condition that interferes with wound healing. Diabetes is associated with small vessel disease, neuropathy, and problems specific to glucose control—all of which predispose the individual to impaired wound healing. Diabetic wound healing problems include increased risk of infection, delayed epithelialization, impaired or delayed collagen synthesis, and slowed wound contraction and closure.[8] Hyperglycemia can affect the cellular response to wounding. There may be a delayed response or impaired functioning of the leukocyte and fibroblast cells, both of which are essential for wound repair.[22]

The effect of surgery on diabetic patients can be dramatic. Patients with diabetes respond to the stress of surgery by releasing a series of hormones: epinephrine, glucagon, cortisol, and growth hormone. These stress hormones reduce the amount of circulating insulin while increasing circulating glucose. Elevated glucose levels can reduce the effectiveness of neutrophils' phagocytotic function and alter the deposition of collagen by fibroblasts, leading

to a decrease in wound tensile strength.[22] Elevated glucose levels can also lead to cellular malnutrition, because insulin is the key for allowing nutrient use in cells. When glucose cannot be used as energy, proteins and fats are used as fuel, depleting the necessary substrates for wound healing. Controlling the glucose level during the postoperative period is likely advantageous for positive wound healing outcomes in diabetic patients. Maintaining glycemic control during the postoperative period with serum glucose levels of 120–180 mg/dL is recommended for patients with diabetes to decrease their risk for wound infection.[23] In the immediate postoperative period, close monitoring of blood glucose and insulin supplements, as indicated, is required for adequate wound healing. Careful attention to blood glucose levels can assist significantly in positive outcomes and prevent an acute surgical wound from becoming a chronic wound.

Other conditions also affect wound healing. Cardiovascular disease presents risks for wound healing because of the associated perfusion alterations, impaired blood flow, and vascular disease. Atherosclerosis is a common cause of inadequate perfusion of wounds.[24] Immunocompromised patients are an additional group at risk for poor healing outcomes. The immune system plays a significant role in wound healing, and any impairment (e.g., aging, malnutrition, and cancer) can result in serious sequelae for wound patients.

Treatments that affect wound healing include steroids, antiinflammatory drugs, antimitotic drugs, and radiation therapy. Steroids inhibit all phases of wound healing, affecting phagocytosis, collagen synthesis, and angiogenesis. The effects of steroids can be diminished with the use of topical vitamin A; when applied directly to a wound, it acts as an inflammatory agent. Vitamin A is appropriate to apply to open wound beds. However, wounds healing by primary intention that are closed with well-approximated edges may not be appropriate candidates for topical vitamin A.

CLINICAL WISDOM

Vitamin A Use for Wounds

The usual dose of topical vitamin A is 1,000 U applied three times a day to the open wound bed for 7–10 days.

Other antiinflammatory drugs also inhibit wound healing, with effects seen predominantly during the inflammatory phase. Cancer therapies, antimitotic medications, and radiation therapy impede the normal cell cycle in rapidly dividing cells. The antimitotic activity interferes with new tissue generation in wounds. In addition, radiation therapy has both acute effects on cellular function and long-term sequelae for healing. Its long-term effects are caused by hypoperfusion of tissues in the irradiated field due to damage, deterioration, and fibrosis of the vasculature.[5]

Nutritional Status

Adequate nutrition is essential for wound healing. In healthy surgical patients, malnutrition may not be an issue. However, with the population aging and more procedures being performed on older adults, nutritional status is a concern for wound healing. Adequate amounts of calories, proteins, fats, carbohydrates, vitamins, and minerals are all required for wound repair. Inadequate amounts of any nutrients negatively influence wound healing.[25]

Proteins are needed for neovascularization, fibroblast proliferation, collagen synthesis, and wound remodeling. Amino acids, which are the structural components of proteins, are essential parts of deoxyribonucleic acid (DNA) and ribonucleic acid (RNA). DNA and RNA provide the pattern for cell mitosis and enzymes required for tissue generation. Protein malnutrition results in the loss of body stores of amino acids and insufficient substrates for wound repair and new tissue growth.

Carbohydrates and fats provide the energy required for cellular function. When there are inadequate amounts of carbohydrates and fats (calorie malnutrition), the body uses catabolism to break down proteins in order to meet energy requirements. Glucose balance and available essential fatty acids are essential substrates for wound healing.

Vitamins and minerals play an important role in wound healing. Several vitamins and minerals have specific functions for wound healing. Vitamin A is a fat-soluble vitamin that is responsible for supporting epithelialization, angiogenesis, and collagen formation. It is also important for the inflammatory phase of wound healing. The water-soluble B vitamins are cofactors in enzymatic reactions. Vitamin C has been associated with wound healing and is essential for angiogenesis and collagen synthesis. Vitamin C also supports fibroblast function and is critical for leukocyte function. For patients with wounds, infection, or significant injury, supplemental vitamin C is often provided at the recommended daily allowance to assist in meeting the increased metabolic and wound healing needs. Supplemental megadoses of vitamin C have not been proven beneficial. Vitamin C use and elimination increase with exercise, stress, injury, increases in metabolic rate, and smoking. Vitamin D is required for bone healing and absorption of calcium, which is important in enzyme systems. Vitamin K is necessary for coagulation and hemostasis. Vitamin E is used for fat metabolism; excess amounts are not beneficial to wound healing.

Minerals also play a role in wound healing, particularly zinc and iron. Zinc plays an essential role in enzyme systems and immune system function, and is a cofactor for collagen synthesis. The highest demand for zinc occurs from the time of injury through the beginning of the inflammatory phase of wound healing.[26] Zinc deficiency contributes to disruption in granulation tissue formation, diminished tensile strength, dehiscence, and evisceration.[25] Low levels of zinc are found in older adults and low-income patients, with losses associated with diarrhea, renal failure, diuretic and laxative use, and parenteral and enteral nutrition.[27] Iron is a cofactor in collagen synthesis and acts to transport oxygen. Iron deficiency can be present in those individuals with changes in eating habits, intestinal damage, and increased metabolic needs.

Oxygenation and Perfusion

Adequate wound oxygenation is essential for wound healing. The initial injury causes hypoxia, and the resultant growth factor release supports initial capillary budding. Oxygen is influential in angiogenesis, fibroblast function, epithelialization, and resistance to infection.[28-32] Tissue perfusion is intertwined with tissue oxygenation; that is, satisfactory tissue perfusion is essential for oxygenation. Ample circulating blood volume carries oxygen-rich hemoglobin to the tissues. Tissue perfusion alone, however, does not guarantee wound oxygenation.

Problems related to tissue perfusion and oxygenation can be due to cardiovascular disease, pulmonary disease, and other conditions such as hypovolemia. Thus, maintaining vascular volume is critical for ensuring adequate tissue perfusion. Clinicians must balance fluid replacement to prevent both underhydration and overhydration. Excess hydration can lead to hypervolemia and edema, which can decrease tissue oxygenation. To optimize oxygenation in the presence of adequate tissue perfusion, use of pulmonary hygiene interventions, assessment and monitoring of tissue oxygen levels, and low-flow supplemental oxygen may be warranted.[32] Pulmonary hygiene, including incentive spirometry, deep breathing and coughing, and postural drainage, improves the pulmonary toilet and increases the likelihood of adequate oxygenation of the wound. Low-flow oxygen can saturate hemoglobin so that the supply to the tissue is ample. Promoting activity, such as repositioning and early ambulation, can also be beneficial for peripheral tissue perfusion and oxygenation.[32] Oxygenation and perfusion are vital to wound healing, and postoperative interventions to improve the circulatory and oxygen-carrying capacity of the tissues and blood (the oxygen saturation of tissues) can enhance wound healing.

Assessment of the Acute Surgical Wound

Assessment of the acute surgical wound involves physical examination of the wound site and surrounding wound tissues in relation to the wound healing process (Figure 15-1). This examination includes measurement of the incision; observation of the wound tissues, with attention paid to epithelial resurfacing, wound closure, wound exudate, and surrounding wound tissues; and palpation of the incision, with attention paid to collagen deposition and surrounding tissues. The linear measurement of the length of the incision

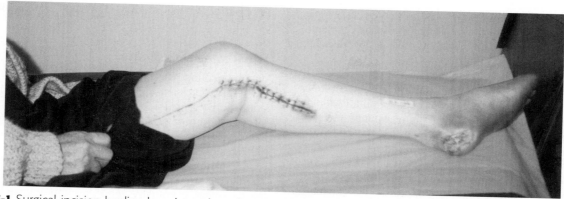

FIGURE 15-1 Surgical incision healing by primary intention. Note the lack of wound edge approximation and absence of a healing ridge at the posterior half of the incision. Sutures remain present along the posterior incision. (Courtesy of Evonne Fowler, MN, RN, CETN, Banning, California.)

(in centimeters) and anatomic location of the incision provide a baseline measure.

Observation and palpation of the incision line provide insight into the healing process that occurs in the underlying tissues. Healing proceeds in the surgical incision as it does in other wounds with inflammation—proliferation of new tissues and remodeling. In the surgical incision, the wound healing processes are not always visible. Thus, the standard for assessment of healing may be best based on time since the surgical injury. It is important for clinicians to track the postoperative time, because the healing progress of the wound can be measured against the standard time expectations for acute wound repair.

Knowledge of the wound healing process provides a critical foundation for assessment of the acute surgical incision. During the inflammatory process, assessment focuses on identification of signs and symptoms of inflammation, evaluation of wound closure materials and wound dressings, and appraisal of epithelial resurfacing. The central point during the proliferation phase of wound healing is evaluation of collagen deposition, wound exudate, and tissues surrounding the incision. Assessment during the remodeling phase is directed toward examination of collagen remodeling at the incision site.

The Inflammatory Phase

The major assessment finding in the first 4 postoperative days is the identification of inflammation. The surgical incision may feel warm to the touch, and there may be surrounding erythema and edema at the incision site. Signs of inflammation are expected and normal during the first 4 postoperative days.

CLINICAL WISDOM

Signs of Inflammation

It is normal to observe signs of inflammation, such as warmth, erythema or discoloration, pain, and edema, at the incisional wound site during the first few days after surgery.

Patients who are immunocompromised as a result of age, disease, or therapy (such as steroid treatments) may not be able to mount an effective inflammatory process; thus, the signs of inflammation at the incision are not visible. In fact, lack of inflammation at the incision site is an indication of immune system compromise. Thus, an incision with no indication of inflammation is an abnormal finding during the first 4 days after surgery. The process of epithelial resurfacing also occurs during the inflammatory phase of wound healing.

In the acute surgical incision, new epidermal tissues are generated quickly because of the presence of intact hair follicles and sebaceous and sweat glands, as well as the short distance the epithelial cells must travel to resurface the incision. The surgical incision is resurfaced with epithelium within 72 hours postsurgery. The new epidermis provides a barrier to bacterial organisms and, to a small degree, external trauma. The tensile strength of the incision is relatively weak, and the incision is not able to withstand force.

Astute clinicians can observe changes in the new incision that indicate the presence of new epithelial tissue. The incision is evaluated for close approximation of the wound edges and color of the incision line. Wound edges should appear well aligned, with no tension observed.

CLINICAL WISDOM

Incisional Color Changes

As new epithelial tissue migrates across the incision, the color of the incision can change from bright red to pink; although this change is not observed in all patients, it is a useful clinical sign that demonstrates maturing epithelial tissue.

Once epithelial resurfacing has occurred, a wound dressing is no longer necessary to prevent bacterial contamination of the incision. However, wound dressings provide other benefits at this stage. Some clinicians suggest that the presence of a dressing at this point can be a reminder of the wound's presence and the need to use care in the wound area. The dressing provides a physical barrier to rough edges of clothing to limit local irritation, and it can help patients include the wound in their new body image by allowing gradual viewing of the wound.

Wound closure materials are assessed for the reaction of the surrounding incisional tissues. The use of sutures of any type to approximate the wound edges creates small wounds alongside the incision wound. The suture wounds increase inflammation at the wound site and can cause ischemia if the sutures are pulled taut with increased tension, either from poor technique or postoperative wound edema. The continued presence of sutures or staples provides additional tensile strength for the wound, but sutures can also increase the risk of infection and potential for wound ischemia. Use of Steri-Strip tapes for wound closure or early removal of sutures with Steri-Strip tape replacement can decrease the problems associated with sutures. Removal of the wound sutures or staples in a timely manner is a proactive healing intervention. Removal of sutures in healthy surgical patients in 7 to 10 days postoperatively can be used as a general guideline, depending on surgical site.

The Proliferative Phase

Palpation of the surgical incision reveals the underlying process of collagen deposition. New collagen tissues can be palpated as a firmness along the incision, extending 1 cm on either side of the incision.[8] This firmness to the tissues, caused by new collagen deposition in the wound area, is called the *healing ridge*. The healing ridge should be palpable along the entire length of the incision between day 5 and day 9 postoperatively; if it is not palpable in this time frame, the wound is at risk for dehiscence or infection.[8]

Evaluation of surgical incisional wound exudate requires knowledge of the expected characteristics of wound exudate during the course of healing. The character and amount of exudate changes as wound healing progresses. The wound exudate immediately after surgery is bloody. Within 48 hours, the wound drainage becomes serosanguineous in nature and, finally, the exudate is serous. The amount of wound exudate should gradually decrease throughout the healing period. An increase in wound exudate usually indicates compromised wound healing caused by infection. New drainage from a previously healed incision heralds wound dehiscence, infection, and, in some cases, fistula formation.

The tissues immediately surrounding the incision should be observed and palpated for the presence of edema and induration, and for color changes. The presence of edema retards the wound healing process because excess fluid in the tissues provides an obstacle to angiogenesis and increases the potential for wound ischemia. Skin color changes can indicate the presence of bruising or hematoma formation caused by surgery. The skin color will appear dark red or purple. Skin color changes can also indicate impending infection. Signs of erythema, warmth, and edema, as well as increased pain at the incision wound, are indicators of possible wound infection. Evaluation of the healing ridge, wound exudate, and surrounding incisional tissues provides

information on the progress of wound healing during the proliferative phase.

The Remodeling Phase

The remodeling phase of wound healing is best assessed in the surgical incision by evaluation of the color of the incision. As the scar tissue is remodeled and organized structurally, the color of the tissue changes. The remodeling phase of wound healing can last 1 to 2 years. The color of the incision changes throughout the first year, gradually changing from bright red or pink to a silvery gray or white. The tensile strength of the wound gradually increases over the first year, eventually achieving approximately 80% of the original strength of the tissues. The focus of interventions at this stage is to limit force and tension on the wound site, including teaching the patient to avoid heavy lifting, bending, and straining at the site.

Management of the Acute Surgical Wound

Management of the surgical incision includes attention to factors that affect wound healing, as addressed earlier, as well as dressing care. The surgical dressing includes the primary and secondary dressings. The primary, or first, surgical dressing is the dressing that is in direct contact with the wound. The direct wound contact requires that the primary dressing be nontraumatic to the wound. The primary dressing absorbs drainage, maintains a sterile wound environment, and serves as a physical barrier to further wound trauma. The primary dressing should be nonadherent to the wound site. A traditional gauze dressing adheres to the new incision and, upon removal, can cause new tissue injury. Use of nonadherent, absorptive dressings can facilitate wound healing because their nonharmful nature allows wound healing to proceed.

The primary dressing absorbs wound exudate and wicks it away from the wound site, allowing the exudate to be absorbed into the secondary dressing. Secondary wound dressings provide increased absorptive capacity or hold the primary dressing in place. Secondary wound dressings are applied on top of the primary dressing and can be composed of the same materials as the primary dressing. The secondary dressing is important when increased amounts of wound exudate are anticipated, because it absorbs drainage from the primary dressing and wicks the exudate away from the wound bed and into the absorbent material of the dressing.

CLINICAL WISDOM

Surgical Incisional Dressings

The majority of primary intention surgical wound dressings continue to be gauze. Conversion to moist wound healing in the immediate postoperative period can facilitate wound healing and provide for patient comfort during dressing changes. Education of surgeons on "better" primary wound dressings is helpful. ■

Tape is usually used to secure wound dressings. Premature and frequent dressing changes can damage the tissues surrounding the incisional wound and negatively affect wound healing. Use of Montgomery straps, skin sealants, or hydrocolloid frames around the wound and underneath the tape can eliminate skin stripping around the incisional wound from frequent dressing changes. Frequent dressing changes are more likely to be a problem with wounds that are healing by secondary intention or tertiary intention, and with draining wounds. (See Chapter 11 for more information about wound dressings.)

Secondary and Tertiary Intention Wound Healing

Surgical wounds that are left open to heal by secondary or tertiary intention have a reparative trajectory similar to that of chronic wounds. Secondary intention healing is allowing wounds to heal without surgical closure; instead, they heal by scar tissue replacement. The tissue defect at the wound site must fill with new collagen tissue during the proliferative phase of wound healing. The inflammatory phase of wound healing may be prolonged because of the contaminated nature of the wound (see Chapter 2).

Tertiary intention is a combination of primary and secondary intention wound healing. The wound is allowed to heal secondarily, and then primarily closed for final healing.[11] Tertiary wound healing is designed for specialized wounds in which primary intention is preferred but not possible at the time of wounding. The delay in primary closure can be allowed to clear infection, allow for some wound contracture, or create a healthy granulation base for a graft.[11]

Most surgical wounds that are left to heal by secondary or tertiary intention are those in which the risk of infection is increased or the tissue loss is such that the wound edges cannot be approximated without unacceptable tension on the incision. Reversal of both conditions—infection and extensive tissue loss—can be maximized in the early weeks following surgery. The administration of systemic antibiotics, when appropriate, and careful wound observation and care can lessen the infection risk. The process of wound contraction and proliferation of granulation tissue occurs as the healing response attempts to decrease the total surface area of the wound[5] and decrease tissue loss.

The primary wound dressing becomes critically important in wounds that are healing by secondary or tertiary intention. Nonadherent, absorptive dressings optimize healing in these wounds. Assessment of the wound for signs and symptoms of infection includes evaluation of the character and amount of wound exudate, and examination of the wound and surrounding tissues for erythema, edema, induration, heat, and pain. Wounds healing by secondary or tertiary intention should be evaluated using the same parameters that are used for chronic wounds. Evaluate the wound size and depth, presence or absence of necrotic tissue, characteristics and amount of exudate, condition of the surrounding tissues, and presence of the healing characteristics of granulation and epithelialization.

Outcome Measures

Outcome measures for acute surgical incisions relate to healing progress according to time frame since injury, as described below.

Postoperative Day 1 through Day 4

The following signs and symptoms represent measures of positive outcomes for acute surgical incision wounds. During the first 4 days after surgery, the presence of an inflammatory response, including erythema or skin discoloration, edema, pain, and increased temperature at the incision site, is a sign of normal healing. The lack of inflammation at a new surgical incision is a negative outcome. Wound exudate should be bloody in character initially; toward day 3 and day 4, it should change to serosanguineous in nature. The amount of wound exudate should gradually decrease from a moderate amount to scant exudate by day 4. Many surgical wounds have no exudate past days 2 or 3, especially facial wounds. Failure of the wound exudate to decrease in amount and to change in character from bloody to serosanguineous is a negative indicator for healing. Epithelial resurfacing should be complete by day 4. The incision will appear bright pink, as opposed to its initial red color. The lack of epithelial resurfacing of the surgical incision indicates delayed healing and less than optimal outcomes.

One negative outcome that can occur at any time during the postoperative course of the patient is the development of a hematoma (swelling or mass of blood, usually clotted, confined in the tissues and caused by a break in a blood vessel). External evidence of hematoma formation includes swelling or edema at the site; a soft or boggy feel to the tissues initially, which may be followed by induration at the site; and color change of the skin (similar to bruising).

Postoperative Day 5 through Day 9

The major healing outcome in the surgical incision on days 5 through 9 is the presence of a healing ridge along the entire length of the incision. A healing ridge indicates new collagen deposition in the wound site. Lack of development or incomplete development of a healing ridge can be prodromal to wound dehiscence and wound infection. A deficient or nonexistent healing ridge is a negative outcome measure for wound healing.

Wound exudate character should change from serosanguineous to serous and gradually disappear over days 4 to 6. The exudate amount should diminish from a minimal amount to none present. Any increase in the amount of wound exudate during days 5 to 9 is considered a negative outcome and heralds probable wound infection.

Suture materials should begin to be removed from the incisional site during days 5 through 9. Adhesive tape strips or steri-strips can be used to provide additional wound tensile strength. Failure to remove any of the wound suture materials during days 5–9 can indicate a negative outcome for the wound.

Continued signs of inflammation at the incision site during days 5–9 are indicative of delayed wound healing. Signs of erythema or edema, extensive pain, and increased temperature at the incision wound during this time frame indicate that wound healing is not normal. Prolonged inflammation can occur as a result of underlying infection, immunocompromise, and continued trauma at the wound site. Documentation of all characteristics of the incision and healing are important for continuity of care throughout the wound recovery period, but especially during this time frame, because the patient will likely be changing healthcare settings. For example, surgical patients are often discharged from an acute care hospital to the home setting very soon after surgery.

Postoperative Day 10 through Day 14

The major outcome measure for day 10 through day 14 is the removal of external incision suture materials. Internal or "buried" sutures remain in place. Failure to remove external suture materials during this time frame will prolong incision healing. Healing is delayed by increasing the risk of infection from the suture microwounds and the continued insult to the tissues by the presence of the foreign objects (the suture materials), prolonging the inflammatory response.

Postoperative Day 15 through 1–2 Years

During the end of the proliferative phase of wound healing and throughout the remodeling phase, attention is directed toward changes in the incisional scar tissue. The collagen deposited alongside the incision is gradually realigned, restructured, and strengthened. The outcome measure for this time period is predominantly based on changes in the color of the incisional scar tissue. The color of the incision changes from a bright pink after the initial epithelial resurfacing, gradually fading to pink and, eventually, turning a pearly gray or silvery white color. In addition, the noticeable induration and firmness associated with the healing ridge gradually softens during this time frame. Negative outcomes include reinjury of the incisional line, such as herniation of the wound site, and complications associated with scarring, such as keloid formation and hypertrophic scarring. Functional ability with the scar tissue becomes a key outcome measure for many surgical incisional wounds during this time frame.

A positive outcome measure at year 1 for the incisional wound includes lack of significant hypertrophic scarring and wound herniation, maximal functional ability with the new scar, and acceptable cosmetic results of healing, with a silvery white or gray scar line. Tables 15-3 and 15-4 present the positive and negative outcome measures for time frames from the point of surgery to the end of remodeling. Chapter 13 discusses management of scars.

■ CASE STUDY

Lack of Inflammatory Response Postoperatively

M.J., a 71-year-old Caucasian woman, was admitted for bowel surgery with resection of the descending colon and low anterior anastomosis. M.J.'s history included long-term steroid therapy for rheumatoid arthritis. On postoperative day 1, her midline incision primary dressing showed evidence of bright red bleeding. The wound edges were well approximated, with staples as the closure material. Assessment of the incision on postoperative days 2 and 3 revealed no evidence of edema, warmth, erythema, or discoloration at the incision site. Exudate was moderate and serosanguineous to seropurulent in nature. By postoperative day 4, the incision was not fully resurfaced with new epithelial tissue. Signs of inflammation, although now present, were diminished, and the exudate remained seropurulent and moderate in amount. M.J. showed signs of confusion and agitation (signs of infection in older adults), and lab tests confirmed the presence of wound infection. In this case, the absent signs of inflammation were early warning signs of impaired healing and wound infection.

CLINICAL WISDOM

Documentation of Incisional Wound Healing

Documentation should include all of the following:

- Time since surgery in days
- Location
- Size in centimeters
- Closure materials present
- Color of the incision
- Type and amount of exudate
- Presence or absence of epithelial resurfacing
- Presence or absence of collagen deposition or healing ridge
- Actions taken for follow-up or referral, as necessary
- Primary and secondary dressings, as appropriate

Example: *Postop day 6 for a 12-cm midline abdominal incision with Steri-Strips present. Incision is completely re-epithelialized, with no exudate present. Incision is bright pink, with healing ridge palpable along anterior 10 cm of incision. Posterior 2 cm of incision is soft and boggy to touch, with no healing ridge palpable and erythema present. Physician notified of possible impaired healing. Dry gauze 2 × 2-inch dressing applied to posterior aspect of incision for protection of site.*

Conclusion

There are many strategies that clinicians use to optimize wound healing in the acute surgical incision. Astute and attentive clinicians can diminish risk of complications, identify delayed or impaired healing, and provide for a supportive healing environment. The key to successful intervention for the patient with an acute surgical incision is knowledge of normal healing mechanisms and temporal expectations, knowledge of factors that impair wound heal-

TABLE 15-3 Positive Outcome Measures for Incisional Wound Healing

Outcome Measure	Days 1–4: Inflammatory Phase	Days 5–9: Proliferative Phase	Days 10–14: Proliferative Phase	Day 15—Years 1–2: Proliferative/ Remodeling Phase
Incision color	Red, edges approximated	Red, progressing to bright pink	Bright pink	Pale pink, progressing to white or silver in light-skinned patients; pale pink, progressing to darker than normal skin color in darkly pigmented skin
Surrounding tissue inflammation	Edema, erythema, or skin discoloration; warmth, pain	None present	None present	None present
Exudate type	Bloody or sanguineous, progressing to serosanguineous and serous	None present	None present	None present
Exudate amount	Moderate to minimal	None present	None present	None present
Closure materials	Present, may be sutures or staples	Beginning to remove external sutures/ staples	Sutures/staples removed, Steri-Strips or tape strips may be present	None present
Epithelial resurfacing	Present by day 4 along entire incision	Present along entire incision	Present	Present
Collagen deposition (healing ridge)	None present	Present by day 9 along entire incision	Present	Present along entire incision

ing, and vigilant attention to both. The case study presented helps to demonstrate the interaction between knowledge of normal healing and the time sequence associated with wound healing, and factors that interfere with normal healing

Referral Criteria

Watchful assessment of the patient with an acute surgical incision can trigger prompt referral to a physician or advanced practice nurse for evaluation and intervention for complications of wound healing. The following criteria are helpful guidelines for referral of patients to another level of health care and to other specialty providers for their expertise:

- Patients with markedly increased bloody drainage during the immediate postoperative period may be at risk of hemorrhage from undetected leaking blood vessels in the surgical field.
- Patients with exudate that changes from bloody or serosanguineous to purulent should be evaluated for wound infection or abscess formation and treated with appropriate antimicrobial therapy.

- Any increase in the amount of exudate after postoperative day 4 is indicative of wound infection or abscess formation; this situation requires evaluation by the primary-care provider and appropriate antimicrobial therapy.
- The absence of a healing ridge along the entire length of an incision wound by postoperative day 9 indicates impaired healing and, often, abscess formation. Prompt referral to the primary-care provider usually results in drainage of the abscess area, antimicrobial therapy, and a wound left to heal by secondary intention.
- Patients with signs and symptoms of wound infection, including erythema, edema, elevated temperature, and increased pain along the incision after day 4, *and/or* signs of systemic infection, including elevated temperature, elevated white blood cell count, and confusion in the older adult, require evaluation. These signs and symptoms suggest a wound infection, and the primary-care provider should evaluate and treat the patient appropriately.
- Patients with frank wound dehiscence or fistula formation require evaluation by the primary-care provider, usually the surgeon, and may warrant a referral to a certified wound nurse (a nurse specializing in management of draining wounds) for management.

TABLE 15-4 **Negative Outcome Measures for Incisional Wound Healing**

Outcome Measure	Days 1–4: Inflammatory Phase	Days 5–9: Proliferative Phase	Days 10–14: Proliferative Phase	Day 15—Years 1–2: Proliferative/ Remodeling Phase
Incision	Red, edges approximated, but tension evident on incision line	Red, edges may not be well approximated; tension on incision line evident	May remain red, progressing to bright pink	Prolonged epithelial resurfacing, keloid or hypertrophic scar formation
Surrounding tissue inflammation	No signs of inflammation present: *no* edema, *no* erythema or skin discoloration, *no* warmth, and minimal pain at incision site; hematoma formation	Edema, erythema, or skin discoloration; warmth, pain at incision site; hematoma formation	Prolonged inflammatory response with edema, erythema, or skin discoloration; warmth and pain; hematoma formation	If healing by secondary intention, may be stalled at a plateau (chronic inflammation or proliferation), with no evidence of healing and continued signs of inflammation
Exudate type	Bloody or sanguineous, progressing to serosanguineous and serous	Serosanguineous and serous to seropurulent	Any type of exudate present	Any type of exudate present
Exudate amount	Moderate to minimal	Moderate to minimal	Any amount present	Any amount present
Closure materials	Present, may be sutures or staples	No removal of any external sutures/ staples	Sutures/staples still present	For secondary intention-healing, failure of wound contraction or edges not approximated
Epithelial resurfacing	Present by day 4 along entire incision	Not present along entire incision	Not present along entire incision; dehiscence evident	Not present or abnormal epithelialization, such as keloid or hypertrophic scarring
Collagen deposition (healing ridge)	None present	Not present along entire incision	Not present along entire incision; dehiscence evident	Abscess formation with wound left open to heal by secondary intention

Self-Care Teaching Guidelines

Every patient's and caregiver's instruction in self-care must be individualized to the type of surgical incision and the patient's wound, the specific incisional dressing management routine, the individual patient's learning style and coping mechanisms, and the ability of the patient/caregiver to perform procedures. The general self-care teaching guidelines in Exhibit 15-1 must be individualized for each patient and caregiver.

REVIEW QUESTIONS

1. Which of the following provides the best example of the acute surgical wound?
   a. Surgical wound healing by secondary intention
   b. Dehisced surgical wound
   c. Pressure ulcer
   d. Surgical incision
2. Which of the following statements best describes the effects of age as an intrinsic factor affecting wound healing?
   a. Aging decreases elastin in the skin; affects collagen replacement; decreases the rate of replacement of cells, delaying reepithelialization; and causes a decline in immune function.
   b. Aging decreases protein synthesis, causes lower levels of serum albumin, and causes a decline in immune function.
   c. Aging causes collagen weakness, leading to poor binding with ground substances, and causes a decrease in fibroblast function and poor white blood cell function.
   d. Aging increases blood glucose levels, leading to poor leukocyte function and inadequate protein synthesis.
3. Factors affecting wound healing in the immediate postoperative period include which of the following?
   a. hydration, pain management, and protein intake
   b. tissue perfusion, pain management, and temperature
   c. tissue perfusion, protein intake, age, and concurrent conditions
   d. volume status, pain management, tissue perfusion, and temperature

EXHIBIT 15-1   Self-Care Teaching Guidelines

Self-Care Guidelines Specific to Acute Surgical Incisions	Instructions Given (Date and Initials)	Demonstration *or* Review of Material (Date and Initials)	Return Demonstration *or* States Understanding (Date and Initials)
1. Type of incisional wound and specific cautions required			
a. No heavy lifting and other measures to prevent hernia formation			
b. Showering or bathing area			
c. Importance of adequate nutrition for wound healing			
2. Significance of wound exudate, incision wound tissue color, surrounding tissue condition, and presence of healing ridge			
3. Wound dressing care routine			
a. Wash hands and then remove old dressing and discard			
b. Clean wound with normal saline			
c. Apply primary dressing to wound			
d. Apply secondary dressing, if appropriate			
e. Secure dressing with tape			
f. Universal precautions and dressing disposal			
g. Frequency of dressing changes			
4. Expected change in wound appearance during healing process			
a. Scheduled removal of closure materials			
b. Incision color change as wound heals (bright red or pink to pale pink and finally to silvery white or gray)			
5. When to notify the health-care provider			
a. Signs and symptoms of wound infection (erythema, edema, pain, elevated temperature, change in exudate character or amount, discoloration in tissues surrounding incision wound)			
b. Absent or incomplete healing ridge along incision after postoperative day 9			
6. Importance of follow-up with health-care provider			

4. A clinician assessing a client's abdomen 3 days post abdominal-perineal resection surgery notes erythema, slight edema, and a slight increase in temperature at the incision site. These findings are most consistent with which of the following?
   a. These are normal signs of the inflammatory phase of wound healing.
   b. The wound is exhibiting early signs of impending infection.
   c. The wound is in the proliferative phase of wound healing.
   d. The wound is exhibiting signs of abscess formation.

5. A clinician is evaluating a client's status post abdominal surgery on postoperative day 8. In assessing the midline abdominal incision, the clinician should be aware of which of the following?
   a. Signs of inflammation, including redness, warmth, pain, and edema are expected signs of normal healing at this time.
   b. A moderate amount of serous to serosanguineous drainage is expected during this phase of healing.
   c. A healing ridge or collagen matrix deposition should be palpable along the incision line.
   d. The wound edges should begin to show signs of approximation by this time

■ **CASE STUDY**

Incisional Wound Healing

P.L., a 78-year-old African American man, was admitted for radical prostatectomy surgery for prostate cancer. P.L. has a history of diabetes mellitus, hypertension, obesity, and peripheral vascular disease. His diabetes is managed with oral hypoglycemic agents and an 1800-calorie diabetic diet (with which he is noncompliant). P.L. lives alone on a small pension and fixed income. He is a smoker. He was admitted with a random blood sugar of 198 mg/dL.

PREOPERATIVELY

Assessment of P.L. revealed several risk factors for impaired healing: uncontrolled diabetes mellitus, obesity, advanced age, hypertension, and peripheral vascular disease. Control of blood sugar level was identified as a goal in the preoperative period, and P.L. was started on sliding-scale insulin therapy with blood glucose monitoring. P.L.'s history of hypertension and peripheral vascular disease put him at risk for poor tissue perfusion; thus, in the immediate postoperative period (days 1 and 2) he was put on supplemental oxygen by nasal cannula to optimize tissue oxygenation. Obesity is a risk factor for excess incision wound tension, which increases the potential for poor perfusion of the incision wound due to the presence of excess subcutaneous fat.

POSTOPERATIVE DAY 4

P.L.'s 15-cm midline abdominal incision showed evidence of inflammation with edema, skin discoloration, and warmth at the site. There was evidence of epithelial resurfacing, and the incision line was bright pink. There was a continued minimal amount of serous drainage, and staples remained in place. The primary gauze dressing was changed daily. Blood sugars ranged from 110–132 mg/dL on insulin therapy. Oxygen was administered the first 2 days postoperatively at 2 L by nasal cannula.

POSTOPERATIVE DAY 9

P.L. was discharged from the hospital to his home with home-health nursing follow-up. Upon discharge from the hospital, P.L.'s incision was bright pink with no exudate present. The incision was completely resurfaced with new epithelial tissue present along the entire incision, and half of the staples had been removed. A healing ridge was palpable along the anterior 13 cm of the wound, but not palpable at the posterior aspect of the wound.

POSTOPERATIVE DAY 10

The home-health nurse evaluated P.L.'s incision and found surrounding skin discoloration, increased pain, and edema present at the posterior aspect of the wound. No healing ridge was palpable at the posterior aspect of the wound, although collagen deposition was evident along the anterior 13 cm of the wound. Half of the original staples were still present in the incision line. The physician was notified, and P.L. was referred to the physician's office for evaluation of the incision.

POSTOPERATIVE DAY 12

The physician removed the remaining staples, performed an incision and drainage (I&D) of the posterior aspect of the incision in the office, started P.L. on systemic antibiotics, and left the posterior aspect of the wound open to heal by secondary intention, using moist saline gauze dressings.

POSTOPERATIVE DAY 15

P.L.'s posterior incision is 75% filled with granulation tissue, and there is minimal serous exudate present. The anterior aspect of the incision is well healed and pale pink. P.L.'s incision wound went on to heal uneventfully by secondary intention over the next 10 days.

REFERENCES

1. Lazarus GS, Cooper DM, Knighton DR, et al. Definitions and guidelines for assessment of wounds and evaluation of healing. *Arch Dermatol.* 1994;130:489–493.
2. Cruse PJE, Foord F. The epidemiology of wound infection: A ten-year prospective study of 62,939 wounds. *Surg Clin North Am.* 1980;60:27–40.
3. Seal LA, Paul Cheadle, D. A systems approach to preoperative surgical patient skin preparation. *American Journal of Infection Control.* 2003;32:57-62.
4. Kjonniksen I, Andersen BM, Sondenaa VG, Segadal L. Preoperative hair removal—a systemic literature review. *Association of Perioperative Registered Nurses.* 2002;75:928-940.
5. Burns JL, Mancoll JS, Phillips LG. Impairments to wound healing. *Clinics in Plastic Surgery.* 2003;30(1):47-56.
6. Gaynes RP, Culver DH, Horan TC, et al, and the National Nosocomial Infection Surveillance System. *Clinical Infectious Diseases.* 2001;33:69-77.
7. Narong MN, Thongpiyapoom S, Thaikul N, et al. Surgical site infections in patients undergoing major operations in a university hospital: Using standardized infection ratio as a benchmarking tool. *American Journal of Infection Control.* 2003;31:274-279.
8. Cooper DM. Acute surgical wounds. In: Bryant RA, ed. *Acute and Chronic Wounds: Nursing Management.* St. Louis, MO: Mosby-Year Book, 1992:91–104.
9. Phillips SJ. Physiology of wound healing and surgical wound care. *American Society of Artificial Internal Organ Journal.* 2000;46:S2-S5.
10. Shelton RM. Repair of large and difficult to close wounds. *Dermatologic Clinics.* 2001;19.
11. Moy LS. Management of acute wounds. *Dermatol Clin.* 1993;11:759–766.

12. Whitney JD, Heitkemper MM. Modifying perfusion, nutrition, and stress to promote wound healing in patients with acute wounds. *Heart Lung.* 1999;28(2):123-33.

13. Gerstein AD, Phillips TJ, Rogers GS, Gilchrest BA. Wound healing and aging. *Dermatol Clin.* 1993;11:749–757.

14. Gosain A, DiPietro LA. Aging and wound healing. *World Journal of Surgery.* 2004;28:321-326.

15. Stotts NA, Hopf HW. Facilitating positive outcomes in older adults with wounds. *Nurs Clin of North Am.* 2005;40:267-279.

16. Kurban RS, Bhawan J. Histologic changes in skin associated with aging. *J Dermatol Surg Oncol.* 1990;16: 908-914

17. Ashcroft GS, Horan MA, Ferguson MW. Aging is associated with reduced deposition of specific extracellular matrix components, an upregulation of angiogenesis, and altered inflammatory response in a murin incisional wound healing model. *J Invest Dermatol.* 1997;108:430-437.

18. Xia YP, Zhao Y, Tyrone JW, et al. Differential activation of migration by hypoxia in keratinocytes isolated from donors of increasing age: implications for chronic wounds in the elderly. *J Invest Dermatol.* 2001;116:50-56.

19. Lenhardt R, Hopf HW, Marker E., et al. Perioperative collagen deposition in elderly and young men and women. *Arch Surg.* 2000;135:71-74.

20. Ashcroft GS, Mills SJ, Ashworth JJ. Aging and wound healing. *Biogerontology.* 2002;3:337-345.

21. Papadakis MA, Hamon G, Stotts N, et al. Effect of growth hormone replacement on wound healing in healthy older men. *Wound Repair Regen.* 1996;4:421-425.

22. Greenhalgh DG. Wound healing and diabetes mellitus. *Clinics in Plastic Surgery.* 2003;30:37-45.

23. Hoogwerf BJ. Postoperative medical complications: Postoperative management of the diabetic patient. *Medical Clinics of North America.* 2001;85.

24. Weingarten MS. Obstacles to wound healing. *Wounds.* 1993;5:238–244.

25. Williams JZ, Barbul A. Nutrition and wound healing. *Surg Clin North Am.* 2003;83(3): 571-596.

26. MacKay D, Miller AL. Nutritional support for wound healing. *Alternative Medicine Review.* 2003;8:359-377.

27. Wagner PA. Zinc nutriture in the elderly. *Geriatrics.* 1985;40(3):111–125.

28. Jonsson K, Jensen JA, Goodson WH, Hunt TK. Wound healing in subcutaneous tissue of surgical patients in relation to oxygen availability. *Surg Forum.* 1986;37:86–89.

29. Pai MP, Hunt TK. Effect of varying oxygen tensions on healing of open wounds. *Surg Gynecol Obstet.* 1972;135:756–758.

30. Knighton DR, Silver IA, Hunt TK. Regulation of wound-healing angiogenesis: Effect of oxygen gradients and inspired oxygen concentration. *Surgery.* 1981;90:262–269.

31. Tandara AA, Mustoe TA. Oxygen in wound healing—more than a nutrient. *World Journal of Surgery.* 2004;28:294-300.

32. Gottrup F. Oxygen in wound healing and infection. *World Journal of Surgery.* 2004;28:312-315.

16

Pressure Ulcers: Pathophysiology and Prevention

Barbara M. Bates-Jensen

CHAPTER OBJECTIVES

At the completion of this chapter, the reader will be able to:

1. Define each stage in the pressure ulcer classification system, according to the National Pressure Ulcer Advisory Panel.
2. Explain frequency of risk assessment for home care, long-term care, and acute care.
3. Describe the Braden Scale for Predicting Pressure Sore Risk.
4. Identify and explain three interventions for preventing pressure ulcers.
5. Define prevalence and incidence.

Pressure Ulcer Definition

Pressure ulcers are areas of local tissue trauma, usually developing where soft tissues are compressed between bony prominences and any external surface for prolonged time periods.[1] A pressure ulcer is a sign of local tissue necrosis and death. Pressure ulcers are most commonly found over bony prominences subject to external pressure. Pressure exerts the greatest force at the bony tissue interface; therefore, there may be significant muscle and subcutaneous fat tissue destruction underneath intact skin.

Pressure Ulcer Significance

The incidence and prevalence of pressure ulcers are high in all health-care settings. Among hospitalized elders of all ages, the prevalence of pressure ulcers has been estimated at 15%.[2] Pressure ulcers represent a significant health concern for those in long-term care facilities, rehabilitation systems, and for special populations. The incidence of new lesions varies widely by clinical situation: the highest rates are found among orthopedic populations (9–19% incidence)[3,4] and quadriplegics (33–60% incidence).[5,6] Among nursing homes, prevalence estimates vary from 2% to 24%.[6,7] Incidence in long-term care is equally diverse, with reports as low as 3.1% in Veteran's Administration nursing homes[8] to a high of 73.5% in a study of a single nursing home.[9] One study found that 11% of nursing home residents had pressure ulcers on admission; 13%

of the remaining residents developed an ulcer during the next year, and 22% within two years.[10] To get a better understanding of whether or not there have been improvements in pressure ulcer care, Berlowitz and colleagues[8] examined the temporal trends in pressure ulcer development from 1991 to 1995 in a chain of 100 private, for-profit nursing homes. Pressure ulcers were measured using the Minimum Data Set, and risk-adjusted rates demonstrated a 25% decrease in pressure ulcer development over the 5-year period.

In home health-care settings, the prevalence of pressure ulcers has been estimated to be 6%–9%.[6,11,12] In outpatient settings, the prevalence of pressure ulcers is estimated to be 1.6%.[13] African Americans demonstrate a higher incidence of pressure ulcers compared to Caucasians in long-term care facilities with incidence rates reported as 0.56 per person year compared to 0.35 per person year for Caucasians in nursing homes.[14]

Rehabilitation facilities present special concerns related to pressure ulcer development because patients in rehabilitation facilities have conditions that limit mobility, such as spinal cord injury, traumatic brain injury, cerebral vascular accident, burns, multiple trauma, or chronic neurologic disorders. Prevalence rates are reported between 11%–12%[15,16] and 25%.[17] Incidence rates over 2 months have been reported at 4%.[18] Individuals with spinal cord injury are at higher risk for pressure ulcer development, with incidence rates reported at 20% for those undergoing spinal surgery[19] to 31% over 1 year's time.[20] Prevalence rates are reported at

10%, based on physical examination during the first annual exam at Model Spinal Cord Injury Centers.[21]

Although, in some cases, it appears that pressure ulcer care has improved, there are many problems with methodology in studies on pressure ulcer incidence and prevalence, including database use versus clinical site data, sampling issues, and calculation issues. These areas of concern make it difficult to draw firm conclusions about the status of pressure ulcers and the significance of the problem. The reality is that pressure ulcers occur in all health-care settings and cost health-care systems in terms of actual dollars spent in care and time and labor spent in caregiving.

Pressure ulcers have become a quality issue for all areas of health care. Pressure ulcer incidence and severity are used as markers of quality care by regulators in long-term care facilities and in home care agencies and acute care hospitals. This emphasis on pressure ulcers across the spectrum of health-care settings highlights the importance of the condition for clinicians. As a result of these potential risks for pressure ulcers, the Department of Health and Human Services' health goals for the nation, *Healthy People 2010*,[22] has identified a 50% decrease in the prevalence of pressure ulcers in nursing homes as a part of the nation's health agenda. Pressure ulcers have also received attention in the courtroom. Organizations have been prosecuted for negligence related to pressure ulcer care and development, and, in a landmark case, a care-home operator was found guilty of manslaughter for a resident's death related to improper care for her pressure ulcers.[23] Clearly, pressure ulcers are a significant problem for all clinicians.

Pressure Ulcer Pathophysiology

Pressure ulcers are the result of mechanical injury to the skin and underlying tissues. The primary forces involved are pressure and shear.[24–28] Pressure is the perpendicular force or load exerted on a specific area, causing ischemia and hypoxia of the tissues. High-pressure areas in the supine position are the occiput, sacrum, and heels. In the sitting position, the ischial tuberosities exert the highest pressure, and the trochanters are affected in the side-lying position.[25,29]

As the amount of soft tissue available for compression decreases, the pressure gradient increases. Likewise, as the tissue available for compression increases, the pressure gradient decreases; thus, most pressure ulcers occur over bony prominences where there is less tissue for compression and the pressure gradient within the vascular network is altered.[29] Figure 16-1 demonstrates this relationship.

The changes in the vascular network allow an increase in the interstitial fluid pressure, which exceeds the venous flow. This results in an additional increase in the pressure and impedes arteriolar circulation. The capillary vessels collapse, and thrombosis occurs. Increased capillary arteriole pressure leads to fluid loss through the capillaries, tissue edema, and subsequent autolysis. Lymphatic flow is decreased, allowing further tissue edema and contributing to the tissue necrosis.[26,28,30–32]

Pressure, over time, occludes blood and lymphatic circulation, causing deficient tissue nutrition and buildup of waste products, due to ischemia. If pressure is relieved before a critical time period is reached, a normal compensatory mechanism, reactive hyperemia, restores tissue nutrition and compensates for compromised circulation. If pressure is not relieved before the critical time period, the blood vessels collapse and thrombose. The tissues are deprived of oxygen, nutrients, and waste removal. In the absence of oxygen, cells use anaerobic pathways for metabolism and produce toxic byproducts. The toxic byproducts lead to tissue acidosis, increased cell membrane permeability, edema, and eventual cell death.[26,30]

Tissue damage may also be due to reperfusion and reoxygenation of the ischemic tissues or postischemic injury.[33,34] Oxygen is reintroduced into tissues during reperfusion following ischemia. This triggers oxygen-free radicals known as *superoxide anion*, hydroxyl radicals, and hydrogen peroxide, which induce endothelial damage and decrease microvascular integrity.

Time and Pressure

Ischemia and hypoxia of body tissues are produced when capillary blood flow is obstructed by localized pressure. How much pressure and what amount of time is necessary for ulceration to occur has been a subject of study for many years. In 1930, Landis,[35] using single-capillary microinjection techniques, determined normal hydrostatic pressure to be 32 mm Hg at the arteriole end and 15 mm Hg at the venule end. His work has been the criterion for measuring occlusion of capillary blood flow. Generally, a range from 25 to 32 mm Hg is considered normal capillary blood flow and is used as the marker for adequate relief of pressure on the tissues.

Pressure is the greatest at the bony prominence and soft tissue interface and gradually lessens in a cone-shaped gradient to the periphery.[25,36,37] Thus, although tissue damage apparent on the skin surface may be minimal, the damage to the deeper structures can be severe. In addition, subcutaneous fat and muscle are more sensitive than the skin to ischemia. Muscle and fat tissues are more metabolically active and, thus, more vulnerable to hypoxia with increased susceptibility to pressure damage. The vulnerability of muscle and fat tissues to pressure forces explains pressure ulcers where large areas of muscle and fat tissue are damaged with undermining due to necrosis, yet the skin opening is relatively small.[31]

Intensity and Duration of Pressure

There is a relationship between intensity and duration of pressure in pressure ulcer development. Low pressures over a long period of time are as capable of producing tissue damage as are high pressures for a short period of time.[25] Tissues can tolerate higher cyclic pressures versus constant pressure.[38] Pressures differ in various body positions. Pressures are highest (70 mm Hg) on the buttocks in the lying

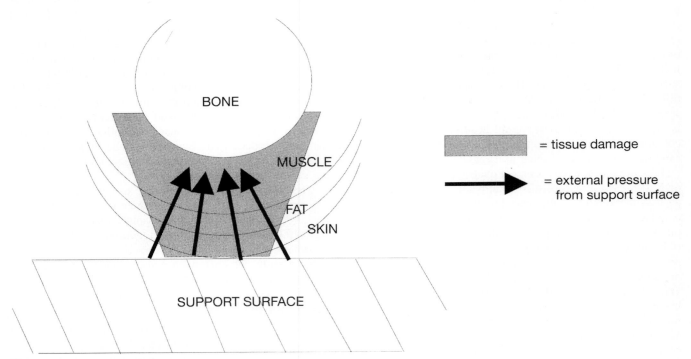

FIGURE 16-1 Pressure gradient at the bony prominence. (Courtesy of Barbara Bates-Jensen.)

position, and in the sitting position can be as high as 300 mm Hg over the ischial tuberosities.[25,29] These levels are well above the normal capillary closing pressure and are capable of causing tissue ischemia. When tissues have been compressed for prolonged periods of time, tissue damage continues to occur, even after the pressure is relieved.[36] This continued tissue damage relates to changes at the cellular level that lead to difficulties with restoration of perfusion.

Figure 16-2 shows the relationship between time, pressure, and tissue destruction.

Four levels of skin breakdown occur, depending on the amount of time exposed to unrelieved pressure.[39] Hyperemia can be observed within 30 minutes or less; it is manifested as redness of the skin and dissipates within 1 hour after pressure is relieved. Ischemia occurs after 2–6 hours of continuous pressure; the erythema is deeper in color and may take 36 hours or more to disappear after pressure is relieved. Necrosis is the third level and occurs after 6 hours of continuous pressure. The skin may take on a blue or gray color and become indurated. Damage that has progressed to this level disappears on an individual basis. Ulceration is the fourth and final level and may occur within 2 weeks after necrosis with potential infection; it resolves on an individual basis.

In dark-skinned patients, it is often difficult to discern redness or erythema of the skin. Redness and erythema may appear as a deepening of normal ethnic color or as a purple hue to the skin.[40,41] (See *Color Plate 21.*) Other manifestations in dark-skinned patients are local changes in skin temperature and skin texture. The immediate response of inflammation of the tissues can be seen by an increase in skin temperature. As the tissues become more disturbed, the temperature decreases, signaling underlying tissue damage. Skin texture may feel hard and indurated, and observation of the skin may reveal heightened skin features or an orange-peel appearance.[40,41] (See Chapter 4 for more information on assessment of the dark-skinned patient.)

Clinical Presentation of Pressure Ulcers

The clinical presentation of a pressure ulcer has been described as a predictable cutaneous chain of events. The first clinical sign of pressure ulcer formation—blanchable erythema—presents as discoloration of a patch or flat, nonraised area of the skin larger than 1 cm. This discoloration presents as redness or erythema that varies in intensity from pink to bright red in light-skinned patients (see *Color Plates 14–15*). In dark-skinned patients, the discoloration appears as deeper normal ethnic pigmentation; a purple or blue-gray hue to the skin (see *Color Plate 19*). Other characteristics include slight edema and increased temperature of the area. In light-skinned patients, the severity of the tissue insult can be evaluated by testing for blanchability of tissues. After finger pressure is applied to the area, complete blanching occurs, followed by quick return of redness, once the finger is removed. In dark-skinned patients, it is difficult to dis-

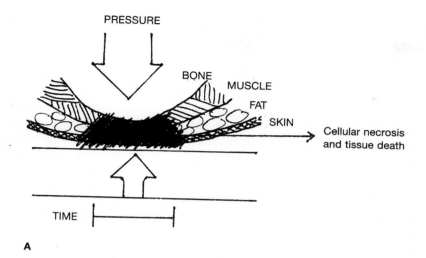

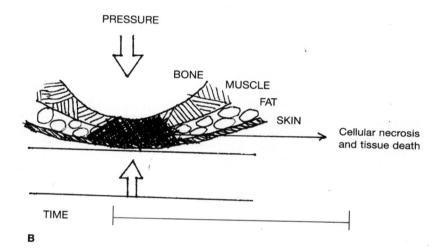

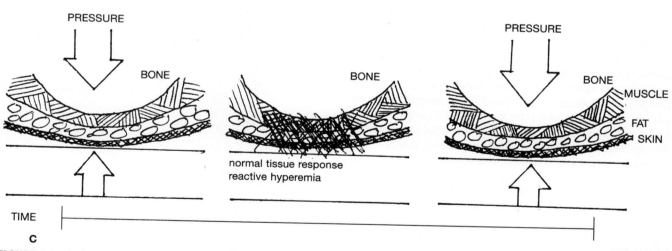

FIGURE 16-2 Relationship of time versus pressure. **A.** High pressure over a short period of time. **B.** Low pressure over a long period of time. **C.** Intermittent pressure. (Courtesy of Barbara Bates-Jensen.)

cern blanching. Use of temperature is a more valuable assessment of the severity of tissue damage in the dark-skinned patient. Initial skin trauma and discoloration exhibit an elevated skin temperature, as compared with that of healthy tissues. The beginning clinical indicators of pressure ulceration all relate to the signs of inflammation in the tissues. At this beginning stage of damage, if the pressure is relieved, the skin can return to normal in 24 hours.[42] If pressure is not relieved, the damage progresses.

Nonblanchable erythema involves more severe damage and is commonly the first stage of pressure ulceration (see *Color Plate 15*). The color of the skin is more intense. It varies from dark red to purple or cyanotic in both light- and dark-skinned patients. Dark-skinned patients exhibit deepening of normal skin color, a purple or gray hue to the skin, and changes in skin texture, with induration and an orange-peel appearance.[40,41] Skin temperature is now cool, compared with healthy tissues, and the area may feel indurated. In light-skinned patients, nonblanchable erythema is detected by testing for blanching of tissues. The damage to tissues is more severe and is indicated by the inability of the tissues to blanch. This stage of tissue destruction is also reversible, although tissues may take 1–3 weeks to return to normal.[42]

The result of further deterioration in the tissues is evidenced as the epidermis is disrupted with subepidermal blisters, crusts, or scaling. If properly treated, the situation may resolve in 2–4 weeks.[42] The early pressure ulcer reflects continued tissue insult and progressive injury. The early ulcer is superficial, with indistinct margins and a red, shiny base (see *Color Plate 14*). It is usually surrounded by nonblanchable erythema. If not dealt with aggressively, progression to a chronic, deep ulcer is inevitable. Superficial ulcers begin at the skin surface and progress to deeper layers. Deep ulcers do not originate at the skin surface; they begin at the bony prominence–soft tissue interface and spread to involve the skin structures (see *Color Plates 19–20*).

The chronic deep ulcer usually has a dusky red wound base and does not bleed easily (see *Color Plate 36*). It is surrounded by blanchable or nonblanchable erythema or deepening of normal ethnic tone, induration, and warmth, and possibly is mottled. Undermining and tunneling may be present with a large necrotic cavity (see *Color Plates 28 and 30*). Eschar formation may be a result of larger vessel damage below the skin surface from shearing forces.[42] Eschar is the formation of an acellular dehydrated compressed area of necrosis, usually surrounded by an outer rind of blanchable erythema. Eschar formation indicates a full-thickness loss of skin (see *Color Plates 20–21, 25,* and *29*).

Location

More than 95% of all pressure ulcers develop over five classic locations: sacral/coccygeal area, greater trochanter, ischial tuberosity, heel, and lateral malleolus (see *Color Plates 3, 11, 24, 35,* and *52–54*).[1] Common pressure ulcer sites occur over bony prominences and depend on the patient's po-

sition; areas with large amounts of soft tissue between bone and skin are least susceptible to breakdown.[39] Several multisite prevalence surveys of pressure ulcers in hospitals have found the sacrum the most common location of pressure ulcers, followed by heels, and the trochanter the location of the most severe ulcers.[6,43,44]

Correct anatomic terminology is important in identification of the true location of the pressure ulcer. For example, many clinicians often document pressure ulcers as being located on the patient's hip. The hip, or iliac crest, is actually an uncommon location for pressure ulceration. The iliac crest is located on the front of the patient's body and is rarely subject to pressure forces. The area that most clinicians are referring to is correctly termed the *greater trochanter*. The greater trochanter is the bony prominence located on the side of the body, just above the proximal, lateral aspect of the thigh or "saddle-bag" area. The majority of pressure ulcers occur on the lower half of the body. The location of the pressure ulcer may have an impact on clinical interventions. For example, the patient with a pressure ulcer on the sacral/coccygeal area with concomitant urinary incontinence will require treatments that address the incontinence problem (see *Color Plate 16*). Ulcers in the sacral/coccygeal area are also more at risk for friction and shearing damage, due to the location of the wound. Figure 16-3 presents the usual locations of pressure ulcer development with correct anatomic terminology.

Pressure ulcers commonly occur over bony prominences, but ulcers can develop at any site where tissues have been

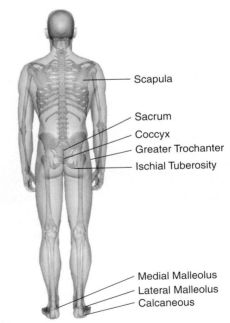

FIGURE 16-3 Correct anatomical names and locations of common pressure ulcer sites. (Courtesy of LifeART image copyright © 2006 Lippincott Williams & Wilkins. All rights reserved.)

compressed, causing tissue ischemia and hypoxia. Patients with contractures are at special risk for pressure ulcer development because of the internal pressure of the bony prominence and the abnormal alignment of the body and its extremities. (Refer to Chapter 17 on therapeutic positioning.)

CLINICAL WISDOM

Contractures and Pressure Ulcer Formation

The compression of tissues may be greater in the presence of contractures, and the management of the contracture must be considered when assessing the patient for risk of pressure ulcer development.[45]

Pressure Ulcer Staging

Pressure ulcers are commonly classified according to grading or staging systems based on the depth of tissue destruction. The stage is determined on initial assessment by noting the deepest layer of tissue involved. The ulcer is not restaged unless deeper layers of tissue become exposed. Historically, one problem in assessment was the lack of a universal staging system for classifying the severity of pressure ulcers. Many of the staging systems available are based on Shea's initial 1975 article[46] describing a method of classifying pressure sores. Shea believed that a pathology-based classification system would simplify communication for health-care professionals, provide a mechanism for identification of pressure ulcers, and suggest a broad guide for determining whether operative care was needed. Shea defined each grade of pressure ulceration by the anatomic limit of soft tissue damage that could be observed. His numeric classification system suggested an orderly evolution of pressure ulceration. However, we now know that pressure ulcers may not heal or deteriorate in a linear fashion. The National Pressure Ulcer Advisory Panel (NPUAP)[47] and the Agency for Health Care Research and Quality (AHRQ), formerly

known as the Agency for Health Care Policy and Research (AHCPR),[48] recommend use of a universal four-stage classification system to describe depth of tissue damage. The recommended system is similar to Shea's original system, with the major exception being that of defining stage I lesions. Exhibit 16-1 shows the staging system recommended by the NPUAP.

The issue of pressure ulcer assessment and the use and misuse of staging classification systems is a subject of debate and controversy. Pressure ulcer development does not necessarily occur from one stage to the next in a logical and linear fashion, and there may be different etiologic factors for various stages. Ulcers do not heal by reverse staging. Staging systems measure only one characteristic of the wound, should not be viewed as a complete assessment independent of other indicators, and should not be the sole criterion in determining treatment plans (see Chapter 4 on wound assessment). Staging classification systems do not assess for criteria in the healing process and hinder tracking of progress because of inability to demonstrate change over time. Staging systems do not allow for movement within and between stages.[49] Many clinicians use the staging system as a measure of healing, despite the inherent difficulties associated with back-staging or downstaging (use of the stages in reverse order, e.g., a wound moving from stage IV to stage II). Determining the stage of the pressure ulcer is a diagnostic tool for evaluating the level of tissues exposed. Once the stage of destruction is determined, the stage should not change, even as the wound heals. In a full-thickness pressure ulcer (stage III or IV), the wound defect is filled with granulation tissue as the wound heals. The granulation tissue does not replace the structural layers of muscle, fat, and dermis that were present in the original tissues. Back-staging of pressure ulcers does not reflect physiologic healing phenomena.[49]

Pressure induced skin damage that manifests as purple, blue, or black areas of intact skin may represent deep tissue

---

EXHIBIT 16-1   Pressure Ulcer Staging Criteria

Pressure Ulcer Stage	Definition
Stage I	An observable pressure-related alteration of intact skin whose indicators, as compared with the adjacent or opposite area on the body, may include changes in one or more of the following: skin temperature (warmth or coolness), tissue consistency (firm or boggy feel), and/or sensation (pain, itching). The ulcer appears as a defined area of persistent redness in lightly pigmented skin, whereas, in darker skin tones, the ulcer may appear with persistent red, blue, or purple hues. (See *Color Plates 14–15*.)
Stage II	Partial-thickness skin loss involving epidermis or dermis, or both. The ulcer is superficial and presents clinically as an abrasion, blister, or shallow crater. (See *Color Plate 17*.)
Stage III	Full-thickness skin loss involving damage or necrosis of subcutaneous tissue, which may extend down to but not through underlying fascia. The ulcer presents clinically as a deep crater, with or without undermining of adjacent tissue. (See *Color Plate 45*.)
Stage IV	Full-thickness skin loss with extensive destruction, tissue necrosis, or damage to muscle bone or supporting structures (such as tendon, joint capsule). (See *Color Plates 1, 3, 7, 37, and 39*.)

injury (DTI).[50] These lesions commonly occur on heels and the sacrum and signal more severe tissue damage below the skin surface. DTI lesions reflect tissue damage at the bony tissue interface and may progress rapidly to large tissue defects.

The terms *partial thickness* and *full thickness* are commonly used to describe wounds of various skin depths that heal by either regeneration or scar formation. Partial-thickness wounds involve only the epidermis and dermis. Full-thickness wounds involve complete destruction of the epidermis and dermis, and extend into deeper tissues.

Superficial lesions involving the epidermis and dermis generally heal in days to weeks. Deeper lesions involving the subcutaneous tissues and muscle may require weeks to months to heal.[51] Tissue trauma extending to bone or joint structures may result in osteomyelitis and further prolong healing time. Ulcers involving the subcutaneous tissue layers may be obscured by necrosis or eschar and additionally may present as areas of both partial- and full-thickness tissue losses. Chapter 2 also discusses the anatomy of the skin.

Pressure Ulcer Prediction: Risk Factor Assessment

Discussion of pressure ulcer pathophysiology and etiology would not be complete without mention of other interacting factors. Pressure ulcers are physical evidence of multiple causative influences. Factors that contribute to pressure ulcer development can be thought of as those that affect the pressure force over the bony prominence and those that affect the tolerance of the tissues to pressure. The conceptual schema of Braden and Bergstrom[52] divides factors into categories according to the role played in eventual pressure ulcer development. Figure 16-4 illustrates Braden and Bergstrom's conceptual framework for pressure ulcer development.

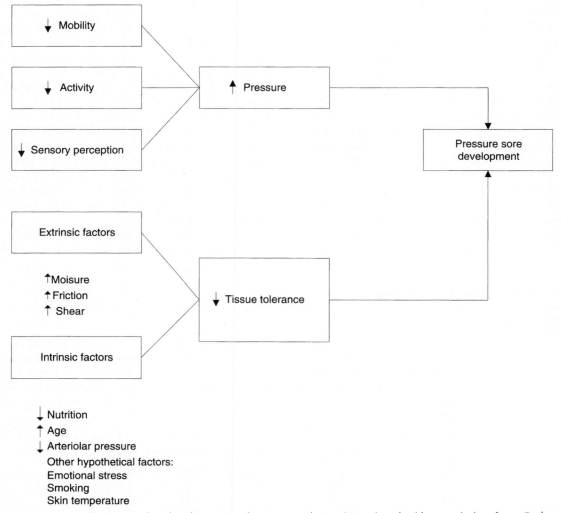

FIGURE 16-4 Factors contributing to the development of pressure ulcers. (Reprinted with permission from Barbara Braden, PhD, RN, FAAN. Reprinted from *Rehabilitation Nursing*, 12(1), 9, Association of Rehabilitation Nurses, 4700 W. Lake Avenue, Glenview, IL 60025–1485. Copyright © 1987. Association of Rehabilitation Nurses.)

Mobility, sensory loss, and activity level are related to the concept of increasing pressure. Extrinsic factors (shear, friction, and moisture) and intrinsic factors (nutrition, age, and arteriolar pressure) relate to the concept of tissue tolerance. Several additional areas may influence pressure ulcer development: emotional stress, temperature, smoking, and interstitial fluid flow.[53]

Pressure Factors

Immobility, inactivity, and decreased sensory perception all affect the duration and intensity of the pressure over the bony prominence. Immobility or severely restricted mobility is the most important risk factor for all populations and a necessary condition for the development of pressure ulcers. Mobility is the state of being movable. Thus, the immobile patient cannot move, and facility or ease of movement is impaired. Exton-Smith and Sherwin[54] demonstrated that 90% of individuals with 20 or fewer spontaneous nocturnal body movements developed a pressure ulcer, whereas none of the persons with greater than 50 movements per night developed a pressure ulcer. Closely related to immobility is limited activity level.

RESEARCH WISDOM

Immobility

Immobility or severely restricted mobility is the most important risk factor for all populations and a necessary condition for the development of pressure ulcers.

Activity is the production of energy or motion and implies an action. Activity is often clinically described by the ability of the individual to ambulate and move about. Those persons who are bed- or chair-bound and, thus, inactive, are more at risk for pressure ulcer development.[48,55] A sudden change in activity level may signal significant change in health status and increased potential for pressure ulcer development.

Sensory loss places patients at risk for compression of tissues and pressure ulcer development because the normal mechanism for translating pain messages from the tissues is dysfunctional. Patients with intact nervous system pathways feel continuous local pressure, become uncomfortable, and change their position before tissue ischemia occurs. Patients with spinal cord injury have a higher incidence and prevalence of pressure ulcers.[56,57] Patients with paraplegia or quadriplegia are unable to sense increased pressure, and if their body weight is not shifted, pressure ulceration develops. Likewise, patients with changes in mental status functioning are at increased risk for pressure ulcer formation. They may not feel the discomfort from pressure, not be alert enough to move spontaneously, not remember to move, be too confused to respond to commands to move, or be physically unable to move.

Extrinsic Factors

Shear

Extrinsic risk factors are those forces that make the tissues less tolerant of pressure. Extrinsic forces include shear, friction, and moisture. Shear is a parallel force. Whereas pressure acts perpendicularly to cause ischemia, shear causes ischemia by displacing blood vessels laterally and, thus, impeding blood flow to tissues.[58–60] Figure 16-5 shows the effect of shearing on the tissues.

Shear is caused by the interplay of gravity and friction. Shear is a parallel force that acts to stretch and twist tissues and blood vessels at the bony tissue interface and, as such, shear affects the deep blood vessels and deeper tissue structures. The most common circumstance for shear occurs in the bed patient in a semi-Fowler's position (semisitting position with knees flexed and supported by pillows on the bed or by elevation of the head of the bed; Figure 16-6). The patient's skeleton slides down toward the foot of the bed, but the sacral skin stays in place (with the help of friction against the bed linen). This produces stretching, pinching, and occlusion of the underlying vessels, resulting in ulcers with large areas of internal tissue damage and less damage at the skin surface.

CLINICAL WISDOM

Shear Injury

Shear is the reason many pressure ulcers are much larger than the bony prominence over which they occur. In clinical practice, this explains, in part, pressure ulcers with large undermined areas.

Friction

Friction and moisture, although not direct factors in pressure ulcer development, have been identified as contributing to the problem by reducing tolerance of tissues to pressure.[60] Friction occurs when two surfaces move across one another (see Figure 16-5). Friction acts on the tissue tolerance to pressure by abrading and damaging the epidermal and upper dermal layers of the skin. Additionally, friction acts with gravity to cause shear. Friction abrades the epidermis, which may lead to pressure ulcer development by increasing the skin's susceptibility to pressure injury. Pressure combined with friction produces ulcerations at lower pressures than does pressure alone.[60] Friction acts in conjunction with shear to contribute to development of sacral/coccygeal pressure ulcers on patients in the semi-Fowler's position.

Moisture

Moisture contributes to pressure ulcer development by removing oils on the skin, making it more friable, as well as interacting with body support surface friction. Constant moisture on the skin leads to maceration of the tissues. The waterlogged tissues lead to softening of the skin's connective tissues. Macerated tissues are more prone to

Bony Prominence
without Pressure

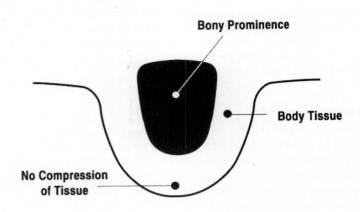

Bony Prominence
with Pressure

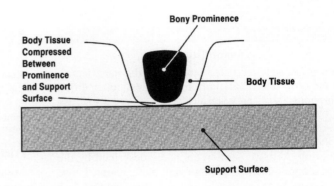

Bony Prominence
with Pressure plus Shear

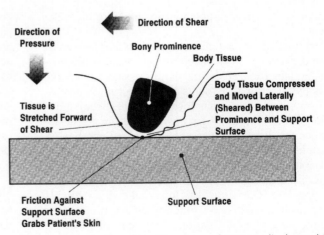

FIGURE 16-5 Effects of shearing and friction in conjunction with pressure on the skin. (Courtesy of RIK Medical, Boulder, Colorado.)

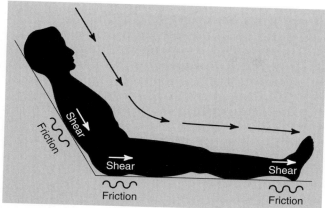

FIGURE 16-6 Shear effect of raising the head of the bed. Mechanical forces contribute to pressure ulcer development. As the person slides down or is improperly pulled up in bed, friction resists this movement. Shear occurs when one layer of tissue slides over another, disrupting microcirculation of skin and subcutaneous tissue. (Reprinted with permission from SC Smeltzer, BG Bare. Brunnar & Suddarth's Textbook of Medical-Surgical Nursing, 9th ed. Philadelphia: Lippincott Williams & Wilkins 2000.)

erosion, and, once the epidermis is eroded, there is increased likelihood of further tissue breakdown.[61] Moisture alters the resiliency of the epidermis to external forces. Both shearing force and friction increase in the presence of mild to moderate moisture. Excess moisture may be due to wound drainage, diaphoresis, and fecal or urinary incontinence.

Urinary and fecal incontinence are common risk factors associated with pressure ulcer development. Incontinence contributes to pressure ulcer formation by creating excess moisture on the skin and by chemical damage to the skin. Fecal incontinence has an added detrimental effect: the presence of bacteria in the stool, which can contribute to infection as well as to skin breakdown. Fecal incontinence is more significant as a risk factor for pressure ulceration because of the bacteria and enzymes in stool and the subsequent effects on the skin.[62] In the presence of both urinary and fecal incontinence, the pH in the perineal area is increased by the fecal enzymes' conversion of urea to ammonia. The elevated pH increases the activity of proteases and lipases found in stool, which, in turn, cause increased permeability of the skin, leading to irritation by other agents, such as bile salts.[63–65] Inadequately managed incontinence poses a significant risk factor for pressure ulcer development, and fecal incontinence is highly correlated with pressure ulcer development.[55,66]

Intrinsic Risk Factors
Nutrition

There is some disagreement on the major intrinsic risk factors affecting tissue tolerance to pressure. However, most studies identify nutritional status as playing a role in pressure ulcer development. Hypoalbuminemia, weight loss, cachexia, and malnutrition are all commonly identified as risk factors predisposing patients to pressure ulcer development.[67–69] Malnutrition is associated with pressure ulcer development.[67,69] Individuals with low serum albumin levels are associated with both having a pressure ulcer and developing a pressure ulcer.

Age

Age itself may be a risk factor for pressure ulcer development, with age-related changes in the skin and wound healing increasing the risk of pressure ulcer development.[70] The skin and support structures undergo changes in the aging process. There is a loss of muscle, a decrease in serum albumin levels, diminished inflammatory response, decreased elasticity, and reduced cohesion between the dermis and epidermis.[70,71] These changes combine with other changes related to aging to make the skin less tolerant of pressure forces, shear, and friction.[71]

Medical Conditions and Psychologic Factors

Certain medical conditions or disease states are also associated with pressure ulcer development. Orthopaedic injuries, altered mental status, and spinal cord injury are such conditions.[56,57,70,72] Others have examined psychologic factors that may effect risk for pressure ulcer development.[73–75] Self-concept, depression, and chronic emotional stress have been cited as factors in pressure ulcer development.

Risk Assessment Tools

For practitioners to intervene cost-effectively, a method of screening for risk factors is necessary. There are several risk assessment instruments available to clinicians. Screening tools assist in prevention by distinguishing those persons who are at risk for pressure ulcer development from those who are not. The only purpose in identifying patients at risk for pressure ulcer development is to allow for appropriate use of resources for prevention. The use of a risk assessment tool allows for targeting of interventions to specific risk factors for individual patients. Selection of which risk assessment instrument to use is determined by reliability of the tool for the intended raters, predictive validity of the tool for the population, sensitivity and specificity of the instrument under consideration, and ease of use and time required for completion. The most common risk assessment tools are the Norton Scale,[76] Gosnell's Scale,[78] and the Braden Scale for Predicting Pressure Sore Risk.[80]

The Norton Scale

The Norton Scale is the oldest risk assessment instrument. Developed in 1961, it consists of five subscales: physical condition, mental state, activity, mobility, and incontinence.[76] Each parameter is rated on a scale of 1–4, with the sum of the ratings for all five parameters yielding a total score, ranging from 5 to 20. Lower scores indicate increased risk, with a score of 13 to 16 indicating "onset of risk" and scores 12 and below indicating high risk for pressure ulcer formation.[77] Others, such as the Gosnell tool, have revised the Norton tool and developed additional tools for assessing risk.

Gosnell's Scale

Gosnell based her scale on further refinement of the Norton Scale. Gosnell kept the original categories on the Norton Scale, changed the general condition category to nutrition, and renamed the incontinence category to *continence*.[78,79] She added skin appearance, medication, diet and fluid balance, and intervention categories to the tool, along with detailed instructions for use. Gosnell reversed the numerical scaling so that the higher score would indicate the higher the risk of pressure ulcer development, so a Gosnell score of 5 is the lowest risk, and a score of 20 is the highest risk (see Exhibit 16-2).

The Braden Scale for Predicting Pressure Sore Risk

The Braden Scale was developed in 1987 and is composed of six subscales that conceptually reflect degrees of sensory perception, moisture, activity, mobility, nutrition, and friction and shear.[52,53] All subscales are rated from 1 to 4, except for friction and shear, which is rated from 1 to 3. The subscales may be summed for a total score, with a range from 6 to 23 (see Exhibit 16-3).

Lower scores indicate lower function and higher risk for developing a pressure ulcer. The cutoff score for hospitalized adults is considered to be 16, with scores of 16 and below indicating at-risk status.[53] In older patients, some have found cutoff scores of 17 or 18 to be better predictors of risk status.[69,80] Levels of risk are based on the predictive value of a positive test. Scores of 15–16 indicate mild risk, with a 50–60% chance of developing a stage I pressure ulcer; scores of 12–14 indicate moderate risk, with a 65–90% chance of developing a stage I or II lesion; and scores below 12 indicate high risk, with a 90–100% chance of developing a stage II or deeper pressure ulcer.[69,80] The Braden Scale has been tested in acute care and long-term care settings with several levels of nurse raters and demonstrates high interrater reliability with registered nurses. Validity has been established by expert opinion, and predictive validity has been studied in several acute care settings, with good sensitivity and specificity demonstrated.[53,69] The Braden Scale has a firm evidence base and solid research as a foundation for use.

CLINICAL WISDOM

Quick Risk Assessment Screening

The Braden Scale activity subscale can be used as a quick screening tool. Those patients who receive a score of 1 (indicating patients who are ambulatory) may be considered at low or no risk, and no further assessment is required. All other patients should receive the full Braden Scale assessment, and prevention interventions should be instituted specific to level of risk and individual risk factors present.

Evidence-Based Practice: Does Risk Assessment Matter?

Bergstrom and colleagues[81] examined the incidence of pressure ulcers and the relationship to risk level, demographic characteristics, diagnoses, and prescription of preventive interventions. This study involved two skilled nursing homes, two university-operated tertiary care hospitals, and two Veterans' Administration Medical Centers (VAMCs). Over a four-week period, Bergstrom and colleagues found the following pressure ulcer incidence rates:

- 8.5% in the tertiary care facilities
- 7.4% in the VAMCs
- 23.9% in the nursing homes

The results indicated that scores from the Braden Scale were predictive of pressure ulcer development, and were prescriptive for preventive interventions for turning and pressure reduction. Further, those individuals who did not have a risk assessment completed were less likely to have written orders for preventive measures. Additional evidence supports risk assessment use in each health-care setting.

Hospital Studies on Risk Assessment. Bergstrom and colleagues' findings are similar to a report of three cross-sectional surveys in a teaching hospital in Switzerland. Perneger[82] and colleagues reported increased risk for pressure ulcer development with increased age and Norton Scale score and that Norton Scale scores were significantly associated with preventive device use. Three cohort studies conducted outside the United States provide evidence in support of conducting risk assessment on admission (and at various frequencies thereafter) to a hospital. Schoonhoven and colleagues conducted a prospective cohort study to evaluate whether risk assessment scales can be used to identify patients who are likely to get pressure ulcers. Researchers studied 1,229 patients admitted to two large hospitals in the Netherlands.[83] The investigators evaluated the Norton, Braden, and Waterlow scales, all validated risk assessment instruments, which were administered to adult patients without existing pressure ulcers within 48 hours of admission to the hospitals. During the four weeks after admission, 135 persons developed pressure ulcers. Area under the receiver operating curves was used to evaluate the three scales with 0.56, 0.55, and 0.61 area for the Norton, Braden, and Waterlow scales respectively. The authors conclude that risk assessment scales predict the occurrence of pressure ulcers although the conclusions are tempered by the low positive predictive values demonstrated for each of the scales in this population.[83]

Perneger and colleagues provide stronger evidence related to frequency of risk assessment in a hospital setting in Switzerland.[84] This prospective study to derive a new pressure ulcer risk assessment scale evaluated pressure ulcer incidence among 1,190 consecutive hospitalized adult patients. They demonstrated the majority of pressure ulcers developed within the first 5 days of hospitalization. Further, the predictive ability of two standardized risk assessment scales (e.g., Norton and Braden scales) decays over time

EXHIBIT 16-2   Gosnell's Tool

GOSNELL SCALE—PRESSURE SORE RISK ASSESSMENT

I.D. _____

Age_____

Height:_____ Sex_____

Weight: _____

Date of Admission _____

Date of Discharge_____

Medical Diagnosis: _____

Primary _____

Secondary_____

Nursing Diagnosis:_____

_____

_____

Instructions: Complete all categories within 24 hours of admission and every other day thereafter. Refer to the accompanying guidelines for specific rating details.

DATE	Mental Status	Continence	Mobility	Activity	Nutrition	TOTAL SCORE
	1. Alert 2. Apathetic 3. Confused 4. Stuporous 5. Unconscious	1. Fully Controlled 2. Usually Controlled 3. Minimally Controlled 4. Absence of Control	1. Full 2. Slightly Limited 3. Very Limited 4. Immobile	1. Ambulatory 2. Walks with Assistance 3. Chairfast 4. Bedfast	1. Good 2. Fair 3. Poor	

GENERAL SKIN APPEARANCE

Date	Vital Signs	24-Hours Fluid Balance	Color	Moisture	Temperature	Texture	Interventions No Yes Describe
			1. Pallor 2. Mottled 3. Pink 4. Ashen 5. Ruddy 6. Cyanotic 7. Jaundice 8. Other	1. Dry 2. Damp 3. Oily 4. Other	1. Cold 2. Cool 3. Warm 4. Hot	1. Smooth 2. Rough 3. Thin/Transp 4. Scaly 5. Crusty 6. Other	

PRESSURE SORE RISK ASSESSMENT MEDICATION PROFILE

Medication	Dosage	Frequency	Route	Date Begun	Date Discon.

GOSNELL SCALE—GUIDELINES FOR NUMERICAL RATING OF THE DEFINED CATEGORIES

Rating:	1	2	3	4	5
Mental Status: An assessment of one's level of response to the environment.	**Alert:** Oriented to time, place, and person. Responsive to all stimuli, and understands explanations.	**Apathetic:** Lethargic, forgetful, drowsy, passive, and dull. Sluggish, depressed. Able to obey simple commands. Possibly disoriented to time.	**Confused:** Partial and/or intermittent disorientation to TPP. Purposeless response to stimuli. Restless, aggressive, irritable, anxious, and may require tranquilizers or sedatives.	**Stuporous:** Total disorientation. Does not respond to name, simple commands, or verbal stimuli.	**Unconscious:** Nonresponsive to painful stimuli.

(Continued)

EXHIBIT 16-2 *(Continued)*

Rating:	1	2	3	4	5
Continence: The amount of bodily control of urination and defecation.	**Fully Controlled:** Total control of urine and feces.	**Usually Controlled:** Incontinent of urine and/or feces not more often than once q 48 hrs OR has Foley catheter and is incontinent of feces.	**Minimally Controlled:** Incontinent of urine or feces at least once q 24 hrs.	**Absence of Control:** Consistently incontinent of both urine and feces.	
Mobility: The amount and control of movement of one's body.	**Full:** Able to control and move all extremities at will. May require the use of a device but turns, lifts, pulls, balances, and attains sitting position at will.	**Slightly Limited:** Able to control and move all extremities but a degree of limitation is present. Requires assistance of another person to turn, pull, balance, and/or attain a sitting position at will but self-initiates movement or request for help to move.	**Very Limited:** Can assist another person who must initiate movement via turning, lifting, pulling, balancing, and/or attaining a sitting position (contractures, paralysis may be present).	**Immobile:** Does not assist self in any way to change position. Is unable to change position without assistance. Is completely dependent on others for movement.	
Activity: The ability of an individual to ambulate.	**Ambulatory:** Is able to walk unassisted. Rises from bed unassisted. With the use of a device such as cane or walker is able to ambulate without the assistance of another person.	**Walks with Help:** Able to ambulate with assistance of another person, braces, or crutches. May have limitation of stairs.	**Chairfast:** Ambulates only to a chair, requires assistance to do so OR is confined to a wheelchair.	**Bedfast:** Is confined to bed during entire 24 hours of the day.	
Nutrition: The process of food intake.	Eats some food from each basic food category every day and the majority of each meal served OR is on tube feeding.	Occasionally refuses a meal or frequently leaves at least half of a meal.	Seldom eats a complete meal and only a few bites of food at a meal.		

Vital Signs:	The temperature, pulse, respiration, and blood pressure to be taken and recorded at the time of every assessment rating.
Skin Appearance:	A description of observed skin characteristics: color, moisture, temperature, and texture.
Diet:	Record the specific diet order.
24-hour Fluid Balance:	The amount of fluid intake and output during the previous 24-hour period should be recorded.
Interventions:	List all devices, measures, and/or nursing care activity being used for the purpose of pressure sore prevention.
Medications:	List name, dosage, frequency, and route for all prescribed medications. If a PRN order, list the pattern for the period since last assessment.
Comments:	Use this space to add explanation or further detail regarding any of the previously recorded data, patient condition, etc. OR Describe anything which you believe to be of importance but not accounted for previously.

EXHIBIT 16-3   Braden Scale for Predicting Pressure Sore Risk

Patient's Name_____ Evaluator's Name_____				Date of Assessment	
SENSORY PERCEPTION ability to respond meaningfully to pressure-related discount	**1. Completely Limited:** Unresponsive (does not moan, flinch, or grasp) to painful stimuli, due to diminished level of consciousness or sedation. OR Limited ability to feel pain over most of body surface.	**2. Very Limited:** Responds only to painful stimuli. Cannot communicate discomfort except by moaning or restlessness. OR Has a sensory impairment that limits the ability to feel pain or discomfort over 1/2 of body.	**3. Slightly Limited:** Responds to verbal commands, but cannot always communicate discomfort or need to be turned. OR Has some sensory impairment that limits ability to feel pain or discomfort in 1 or 2 extremities.	**4. No Impairment:** Responds to verbal commands. Has no sensory deficit which would limit ability to feel or voice pain or discomfort.	
MOISTURE degree to which skin is exposed to moisture	**1. Constantly Moist:** Skin is kept moist almost constantly by perspiration, urine, etc. Dampness is detected every time patient is moved or turned.	**2. Very Moist:** Skin is often, but not always moist. Linen must be changed at least once a shift.	**3. Occasionally Moist:** Skin is occasionally moist, requiring an extra linen change approximately once a day.	**4. Rarely Moist:** Skin is usually dry, linen only requires changing at routine intervals.	
ACTIVITY degree of physical activity	**1. Bedfast:** Confined to bed.	**2. Chairfast:** Ability to walk severely limited or nonexistent. Cannot bear own weight and/or must be assisted into chair or wheelchair.	**3. Walks Occasionally:** Walks occasionally during day, but for very short distances, with or without assistance. Spends majority of each shift in bed or chair.	**4. Walks Frequently:** Walks outside the room at least twice a day and inside room at least once every 2 hours during waking hours.	
MOBILITY ability to change and control body position	**1. Completely Immobile:** Does not make even slight changes in body or extremity position without assistance.	**2. Very Limited:** Makes occasional slight changes in body or extremity position but unable to make frequent or significant changes independently.	**3. Slightly Limited:** Makes frequent though slight changes in body or extremity position independently.	**4. No Limitations:** Makes major and frequent changes in position without assistance.	

(Continued)

EXHIBIT 16-3 *(Continued)*

	1. Very Poor:	2. Probably Inadequate:	3. Adequate:	4. Excellent:	
NUTRITION *usual* food intake pattern	Never eats a complete meal. Rarely eats more than 1/3 of any food offered. Eats 2 servings or less of protein (meat or dairy products) per day. Takes fluids poorly. Does not take a liquid dietary supplement. OR Is NPO and/or maintained on clear liquids or IVs for more than 5 days.	Rarely eats a complete meal and generally eats only about 1/2 of any food offered. Protein intake includes only 3 servings of meat or dairy products per day. Occasionally will take a dietary supplement. OR Receives less than optimum amount of liquid diet or tube feeding.	Eats over half of most meals. Eats a total of 4 servings of protein (meat, dairy products) each day. Occasionally will refuse a meal, but will usually take a supplement if offered. OR Is on a tube feeding or TPN regimen which probably meets most of nutritional needs.	Eats most of every meal. Never refuses a meal. Usually eats a total of 4 or more servings of meat and dairy products. Occasionally eats between meals. Does not require supplementation.	
	1. Problem:	2. Potential Problem:	3. No Apparent Problem:		
FRICTION AND SHEAR	Requires moderate to maximum assistance in moving. Complete lifting without sliding against sheets is impossible. Frequently slides down in bed or chair, requiring frequent repositioning with maximum assistance. Spasticity, contractures, or agitation leads to almost constant friction.	Moves feebly or requires minimum assistance. During a move skin probably slides to some extent against sheets, chair, restraints, or other devices. Maintains relatively good position in chair or bed most of the time but occasionally slides down.	Moves in bed and in chair independently and has sufficient muscle strength to lift up completely during move. Maintains good position in bed or chair at all times.		**Total Score**

such that risk assessment should be repeated at frequent intervals in the hospital setting.[84]

The third study from outside the United States provides limited evidence tying risk assessment to improved pressure ulcer outcomes. Gunningberg and colleagues[85] report a significant reduction in pressure ulcer incidence among patients admitted to the hospital for hip fracture, from 55% in 1997 prior to the intervention to 29% in 1999 following intervention ($\chi^2 = 4.5$, $P = 0.05$). The multifaceted intervention included risk assessment on admission to the hospital and continuing risk assessment on the orthopedic ward thereafter. Because of the multifaceted nature of the inter-

vention it is difficult to attribute the decline in pressure ulcer incidence to use of risk assessment alone.[85]

In the United States, Fife and colleagues had similar findings in another high risk population, neurologic intensive care unit patients. Fife et al followed 186 patients admitted to a neurologic intensive care and intermediate unit in a level I trauma center. All patients were evaluated for pressure ulcer risk within 12 hours of admission using the Braden Scale and every 4 days after admission. They report an incidence rate of 12% (stage II and greater pressure ulcers), 68% of which developed within the first 7 days of admission to the neurologic intensive care unit, and a strong predictive relationship between pressure ulcer development and Braden Scale score. Further, risk for developing a stage II pressure ulcer increased significantly with Braden Scale scores of 13 or below and with low body mass index at admission.[86]

Finally, Lewicki and colleagues evaluated risk assessment using the Braden Scale in cardiac surgery patients and specifically recommended repeating risk assessments on postoperative day 1, 3, and 5 along with use of different cutoff scores for each of these time points (13, 14, and 20 respectively).[87] In Lewicki et al's study of 337 pressure ulcer-free patients undergoing cardiac surgery, Braden Scale scores with lower cutoff scores correctly classified patients on each of these days: 67% pressure ulcer-positive patients on postoperative day 1, 57% on postoperative day 3 and 50% on postoperative day 5.[87]

Frantz and Baranoski in a review of studies of pressure ulcer prevention programs suggest that such programs that generally include risk assessment, reduction of pressure, and staff education result in a decrease in incidence for hospitals ranging from 11% to 16%.[88] While none of the above studies provides definitive evidence linking risk assessment directly with pressure ulcer prevention, taken as a whole they provide supportive evidence suggesting a tie between conducting risk assessment and initiating preventive interventions leading to decreased pressure ulcer incidence. Clinical guidelines as well as experts in the field provide more specificity related to frequency of risk assessment in the hospital setting. Persons admitted to general medical-surgical units of hospitals should have risk assessment conducted on admission and if risk assessment indicates "at risk," every 48 hours after admission. Those persons admitted to intensive or critical care units should have risk assessment conducted on admission and if risk assessment indicates "at risk," daily thereafter.[89]

Nursing Home Studies on Risk Assessment. In a quasi-experimental study in two nursing homes Lyder and colleagues[91] demonstrated a decrease in pressure ulcer incidence after implementation of risk assessment followed by preventive interventions based on risk level. This pre/post design study used both retrospective and prospective data to evaluate the effects of risk assessment using the Braden Scale and preventive interventions specific to individual risk levels. The retrospective data showed a 5-month cumulative incidence rate of 43% for both homes combined and this reduced to 28.5% cumulative incidence rate for the 5 months after implementation of the prevention program. Individual facilities had decreases in their pressure ulcer incidence of 87% (pressure ulcer incidence August 1999 of 13.2% dropped to 1.7% in December 1999) and 76% (pressure ulcer incidence August 1999 of 15% dropped to 3.5% in December 1999).[90]

Bergstrom and Braden prospectively evaluated pressure ulcer risk among nursing home residents. This cohort study evaluated 200 newly admitted residents to a 250-bed nursing home in the Midwest. Skin assessment, Braden Scale score, blood pressure, body temperature, anthropometrics, and dietary intake were studied weekly. Stage I pressure ulcers developed in 35% (n = 70) of the residents, and stage II pressure ulcers or worse developed in 38.5% (n = 77) of the residents. The best predictors of pressure ulcer formation were the Braden Scale score, diastolic blood pressure, temperature, dietary protein intake, and age.[69]

Two studies have examined the rate of pressure ulcer formation in nursing home residents that informs how often risk assessment should be conducted. One study found a 23.9% incidence of pressure ulcers over a 4-week period[81] while the other study found that almost three-quarters of newly admitted nursing home residents (73.5%) developed pressure ulcers after admission.[69]

Xakellis and colleagues evaluated implementation of preventive interventions based on risk assessment with the Braden Scale in a 77-bed nursing home over 6 months.[92] They stratified preventive interventions according to intensity of risk determined by the Braden Scale score. Xakellis et al reported a significant decrease in pressure ulcer incidence over 6 months (from 23% preintervention to 5% postintervention) and a significant increase in the mean number of ulcer-free days (146.4 days preintervention to 157.5 days postintervention; log rank = 8.63, P = .003).[92]

Bates-Jensen and colleagues' cross-sectional descriptive evaluation of pressure ulcer care processes in eight nursing homes supports the need for formal risk assessment as a stimulus to initiate preventive interventions.[93] They reviewed 93 medical records of residents who were admitted within 12 months of data collection and whose medical record documented as "at risk" according to the Minimum Data Set assessment. They found only 62% had a risk assessment conducted on admission to the facility. Additionally, a significant difference occurred between those "at risk" residents who had an admission risk assessment and "at risk" residents without a risk assessment on documentation of pressure ulcer preventive interventions. Seventy-six percent of "at risk" residents with an admission risk assessment also had chart documentation of three preventive interventions compared to 14% of "at risk" residents without risk assessment ($?^2 = 29.779$, $P < .001$).[93]

Defloor and Grypdonck also reported the importance of formal risk assessment compared to nursing judgement (informal risk assessment) in their prospective cohort study. They observed 1,772 residents of 11 long-term care facilities in Belgium over 4 weeks. Residents were randomly selected and then assigned to a "turning" versus a "nonturning" group. Risk assessment was formally conducted by research staff with both the Braden Scale and the Norton Scale and staff nurses used clinical judgment and experience to judge risk on all residents twice a week during the study. The sensitivity and specificity for each risk assessment scale were 79.8 and 64.6 for the Braden Scale and 62.3 and 71.8 for the Norton Scale. Nurses using their judgment predicted those residents at risk for pressure ulcer development less well than either the Braden or the Norton Scale.[94]

Thus there is evidence to recommend performing pressure ulcer risk assessment on admission to the nursing home and if the risk assessment score indicates "at risk" then weekly for 4 weeks, and for all residents quarterly or whenever a change in status occurs.[89]

Home Health-Care Studies on Risk Assessment. Bergquist and Frantz report a secondary analysis of data from a retrospective cohort study of risk factors for pressure ulcer development in 1,696 nonhospice, pressure ulcer-free older adults with Braden Scale scores who were receiving home health care.[95] Patient medical records were followed forward chronologically until one of the following: a pressure ulcer developed, home health services were complete, death, institutionalization, or end of the study period. Incidence of pressure ulcer development during the home health-care period was 6.3%. They report that 20% of the pressure ulcers developed in the first week after admission and the incidence increased 10% each week through week 4. Of those who developed a pressure ulcer, 50% developed the ulcer within 24 days after admission. Patients who developed pressure ulcers had significantly lower Braden Scale scores compared to those without pressure ulcers. The study authors recommend risk assessment on admission to home health care, weekly for the first 4 weeks, and every other week reassessments thereafter until day 62 depending on patient condition and frequency of home visits.[95]

Ferrell and colleagues evaluated pressure ulcers in a cross-sectional survey of 3,048 patients admitted to home health-care agencies in 14 states.[96] They report a pressure ulcer prevalence of 9.2% with 30% of persons admitted to home health at risk for developing a pressure ulcer based on Braden Scale scores. Pressure ulcers were more likely to occur with lower Braden Scale scores.[96] These two studies and a variety of expert panels and groups recommend performing pressure ulcer risk assessment on admission to home health-care agencies and if the risk assessment score indicates "at risk" then weekly for 4 weeks, and every other week thereafter or whenever a change in status occurs.[89]

Of course, regardless of health-care setting, risk assessment should be performed whenever a significant change occurs in the patient's general health and status. A registered nurse should perform risk assessment. However, in many instances, a registered nurse will need input from the direct-care provider, such as a family member or a nursing attendant.

Specific prevention strategies should be targeted to risk factors identified in individual patients. In those persons in whom prevention is not successful, the continued monitoring of risk status may prevent further tissue trauma at the wound site and development of additional wound sites. The prevention interventions presented in the remainder of the chapter are based on the Braden Scale Risk Assessment instrument items. Exhibit 16-4 presents a flow diagram for determining prevention strategies based on risk factor assessment.

Risk Stratification and Risk Adjustment

Risk stratification is arranging data related to quantifiable outcomes, resource utilization, or other phenomena associated with pressure ulcer prevention or treatment by level of risk to facilitate analysis and to reflect more accurately ef-

---

EXHIBIT 16-4 Flow Diagram for Determining Prevention Strategies Based on Risk Factor Assessment

Presence of tissue trauma over bony prominence? **(usual locations: sacral/coccygeal, trochanter, ischial tuberosity, malleolus, heel)**					
NO			YES, provide for wound assessment and treatment plus prevention strategies		
Patient NOT chair- or bed-bound and thus at no or low risk? **(patient scores a 1 or 2 on Braden Scale activity subscale)**					
NO, complete full risk assessment				YES, do not need further risk assessment	
Pressure ulcer risk factors present?					
Immobility	Inactivity	Decreased Sensory Perception	Nutrition	Friction and Shear	Moisture Urinary and Fecal Incontinence
Prevention interventions by risk factors:					
Immobility, Inactivity, and Decreased Sensory Perception			Malnutrition	Friction and Shear	Moisture Incontinence
passive repositioning, pillow bridging, pressure-reducing/ relieving support surfaces			provide nutrition supplement: protein, calorie, vitamin C, zinc, iron	cornstarch, lubricants, pad protectors, transparent film, thin hydrocolloid dressings, turning, and draw sheets	absorbent products, diagnosis of incontinence, general skin care

fect of case mix. For example, using the Braden Scale for Risk Assessment instrument, patients can be stratified or grouped according to their levels of risk, as follows:

- Mild Risk = 15–18 Braden Score
- Moderate Risk = 13–14 Braden Score
- High Risk = 10–12 Braden Score
- Very High Risk ≤ 9 Braden Score

Risk adjustment or stratification can give a more realistic picture of the progress in prevention as acuity levels wax and wane. Risk adjustment supplies a more realistic comparison between one institution's outcomes and those of other agencies or facilities. Risk stratification can also provide a tool to see where strengths and weaknesses in the program of prevention might exist.

CLINICAL WISDOM

Risk adjustment or stratification can also be used with pressure ulcer assessment data. For example, the Bates-Jensen Wound Assessment Tool (BWAT, formerly the Pressure Sore Status Tool) can be a useful instrument to determine severity levels of pressure ulcers as follows:

- Minimal severity = 13–20 BWAT Total Score
- Mild severity = 21–30 BWAT Total Score
- Moderate severity = 31–40 BWAT Total Score
- Critical severity = 41–65 BWAT Total Score

Pressure Ulcer Prevention: Early Interventions

Prevention strategies are targeted at reducing risk factors present. Appropriate prevention interventions can focus on eliminating specific risk factors. Thus, early intervention for pressure ulcers is risk factor-specific. The prevention strategies are presented by risk factors, beginning with general information and ending with specific strategies for a particular risk factor. The Braden Scale is the basis for these prevention interventions. Prevention interventions should be instituted that are appropriate to the patient's level of risk and specific to individual risk factors.[48] For example, the risk factor of immobility is managed very differently for the comatose patient versus the spinal cord-injured patient. The comatose patient requires caregiver education and caregiver-dependent repositioning. The spinal cord-injured patient requires self-care education and may be able to perform self-repositioning. Thus, the intervention for the risk factor of immobility is very different for these two patients.

Immobility, Inactivity, and Sensory Loss

Patients with impaired ability to reposition and who cannot independently change body positions must have local pressure alleviated by any of the following interventions.[48,97]

- Passive repositioning by the caregiver
- Pillow bridging
- Use of pressure-relief or pressure-reduction support surfaces for chair and bed

In addition, measures to increase mobility and activity and to decrease friction and shear should be instituted. Overhead bed frames with trapeze bars are helpful for patients with paraplegia, stroke patients with upper body strength, and obese patients, and may increase mobility and independence with body repositioning. Wheelchair-bound patients with upper body strength can be taught and encouraged to do wheelchair pushups to relieve pressure and allow for reperfusion of the tissues in the ischial tuberosity region. For patients who are weak from prolonged inactivity, providing support and assistance for reconditioning and increasing strength and endurance will help to prevent future debility. Mobility plans for each patient should be individualized, with the goal of attaining the highest level of mobility and activity individually possible. Mobility plans are the responsibility of nurses and physical therapists working together in all health-care settings. It is essential that health-care professionals train and observe home caregivers in the mobility plan and, in particular, passive repositioning techniques. Caregivers in the home are often left to fend for themselves for prevention interventions and may be frail and have health problems themselves. A return demonstration of a repositioning procedure can be very informative to the health-care provider. The health-care provider may need to coach, improvise, and think of creative strategies for caregivers to use in the home setting in order to meet the patient's need for movement and tissue reperfusion.

Passive Repositioning by Caregiver

Turning schedules and passive repositioning by caregivers is the normal response for patients with immobility risk factors. Typically, turning schedules are based on time or event. If time based, turning schedules are usually every 2 hours for full-body change of position and more often for small shifts in position. Event-based schedules relate to typical events during the day, e.g., turning the patient after each meal. Full body change of position involves turning the patient to a new lying position, e.g., turning the patient from the right side-lying position to the left side-lying position or the supine position. When the side-lying position is used in bed, avoidance of direct pressure on the trochanter is essential. To avoid placing pressure on the trochanter, position the patient in a 30° laterally inclined position instead of the commonly used 90° side-lying position, which increases tissue compression over the trochanter.[98] The 30° laterally inclined position allows for distribution of pressure over a greater area (see Figure 16-7). Use of diagrams with clock faces and body position of patient are helpful in reminding staff when and how to position the patient[99] (see Figure 16-8).

Small shifts in position involve moving the patient but keeping the same lying position,[100] e.g., changing the angle of the right side-lying position or changing the lower extremity position in the right side-lying position. Both strategies are helpful in achieving reperfusion of compressed tissues, but *only full body change of position completely relieves pressure.*

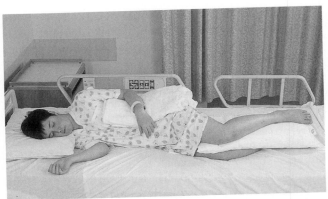

FIGURE 16-7 Lateral side-lying position. Note the pillow between the knees. Pillows can also be placed between the ankles to alleviate pressure. One pillow is placed behind the back for the patient to lean back against, leaving the patient in a 30° side-lying position. (Reprinted with permission from SC Smeltzer, BG Bare. Brunnar & Suddarth's Textbook of Medical-Surgical Nursing, 9th ed. Philadelphia: Lippincott Williams & Wilkins 2000.)

There are techniques to make turning patients easier and less time-consuming. Turning sheets, draw sheets, and pillows are essential for passive movement of patients in bed. Turning sheets are useful in repositioning the patient to a side-lying position, and draw sheets are used for pulling the patient up in bed and help to prevent dragging the patient's skin over the bed surface. Two-person repositioning is a simple task with the turning sheet and can be accomplished in a very small amount of time with little risk of dragging the patient's skin across the bed linens:

1. Position one person on each side of the bed.
2. Bend the patient's knees and fold the patient's arms across the chest.
3. Roll up the draw sheet next to the patient's body and grasp firmly.
4. On a prearranged verbal cue, both persons lift and move the patient up in bed.
5. Next, one person pulls on the turn sheet to roll the patient passively toward the side.
6. The person on the other side of the bed immediately places pillows behind the patient's back for support.
7. Additional pillows are then used for easing pressure on other bony prominences.

The recommended time interval for full change of position turning is every 2 hours, depending on the individual patient profile and the use of support surfaces. Defloor and colleagues[101] conducted a controlled clinical trial evaluating the effects of different turn intervals in conjunction with support surface use. They investigated four different turn intervals: 2 hours on a standard mattress (2 hrs), 3 hours on a standard mattress (3 hrs), 4 hours on a pressure-reducing surface (4 hrs), 6 hours on a pressure-reducing surface (6 hrs) and a control group with usual care (no turns). Over 4 weeks, 838 geriatric nursing home residents were evaluated. Stage II pressure ulcer incidence was significantly decreased in the 4 hrs group compared to all other groups (3% compared to 20%—no turns, 14.3%—2 hrs, 24.1%—3 hrs, and 15.9%—6 hrs; $P = .002$).[101] They provide convincing evidence to support use of repositioning schedules in conjunction with support surfaces to reduce the incidence of pressure ulcers in persons at risk for pressure ulcers.

Similar approaches are useful for patients in chairs. Full-body change of position involves standing the patient and resitting him or her in the chair. Small shifts in position for those in chairs might be changing lower extremity position. For the chair-bound patient, it is also helpful to use a footstool to help reduce the pressure on the ischial tuberosities and to distribute the pressure over a wider surface. Attention to proper alignment and posture is essential. Individuals at risk for pressure ulcer development should avoid uninterrupted sitting in chairs and should be repositioned every hour. The rationale behind the shorter time frame is the extremely high pressure generated on the ischial tuberosities in the seated position.[1] Those patients with upper body strength should be taught to shift weight every 15 minutes to allow for tissue reperfusion. Again, pillows may be used to help position the patient in proper body alignment. Physical therapy and occupational therapy can assist in body alignment strategies with even the most contracted patient. (See Chapter 17 for further discussion on orthotic devices and seating therapeutics.)

Pillow Bridging

Pillow bridging involves the use of pillows to position patients with minimal tissue compression. The use of pillows can help to prevent pressure ulcers from occurring on the medial knees, the medial malleolus, and the heels. Pillows should be placed between the knees, between the ankles, and under the heels.

CLINICAL WISDOM

Positioning Pillows

Five pillows can overcome repositioning pressure point difficulties. Use the pillows in the following positions:

Pillow 1: under legs to elevate the heels
Pillow 2: between the ankles
Pillow 3: between the knees
Pillow 4: behind the back
Pillow 5: under the head

(Use a small pillow for comfort under the arm in side-lying position.)

Pillow use is especially important for reducing risk of development of heel ulcers, regardless of the support surface in use. The best prevention strategy for eliminating pressure ulcers on the heels is to keep the heels off the surface of the bed. Use of pillows under the lower extremities will keep the heel from making contact with the support surface of the bed. Pillows help to redistribute the pressure

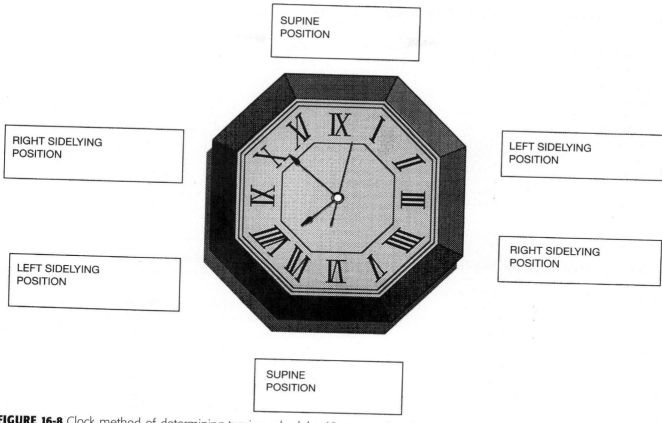

SUPINE
POSITION

RIGHT SIDELYING
POSITION

LEFT SIDELYING
POSITION

LEFT SIDELYING
POSITION

RIGHT SIDELYING
POSITION

SUPINE
POSITION

FIGURE 16-8 Clock method of determining turning schedule. (Courtesy of Barbara Bates-Jensen.)

over a larger area, thus reducing high pressure in one specific area. Some specialized heel pressure-reducing devices are effective in reducing pressure on heels. Look for devices that are easy to apply and remove to assure compliance.

RESEARCH WISDOM
Donut Pillow Devices

One type of pillow device is not recommended for use. Use of a donut type or ring cushion device is contraindicated. Donut ring cushions cause venous congestion and edema, and actually increase pressure to the area of concern.[48]

Use of Pressure-Relief or Pressure-Reduction Support Surfaces

There are specific guidelines for the use of support surfaces to prevent and manage pressure ulcers.[1] Regardless of the type of support surface in use with the patient, the need for written repositioning and turning schedules remains essential. The support surface serves as an adjunct to strategies for positioning and careful monitoring of patients. The type of support surface chosen is based on a multitude of factors, including clinical condition of the patient, type of care setting, ease of use, maintenance, cost, and characteristics of the support surface. The primary concern should be the therapeutic benefit associated with the surface. Table 16-1 cate-gorizes the types of support surfaces available and their general performance characteristics;[1] Exhibit 16-5 presents ideal support surface characteristics. Table 16-1 and Exhibit 16-5 are presented as an overview to the remainder of this section. The information on support surfaces is organized in the following manner: First, information on tissue interface pressure is presented; second, information on pressure-reducing and pressure-relieving support surfaces is presented; finally, this section ends with information and guidelines on how to determine the appropriate surface for specific patients.

Tissue Interface Pressures. Tissue interface pressures are commonly evaluated by using capillary closing pressure (generally considered to be 12–32 mm Hg) as an indirect measure to label effectiveness of support surfaces. The use of capillary closing pressures implies that skin surface interface pressure is equal to capillary closing pressures. Further, as tissue interface (skin surface) pressures approach capillary closing pressures (12–32 mm Hg), the support surface is more effective and less likely to occlude blood vessels (less likely to cause pressure ulcer formation). One of the difficulties with the use of capillary closing pressures is the assumption that capillary closing pressures are absolute values. Capillary closing pressures may be more individualized than absolute values imply. Capillary closing pressures assume that skin interface pressures reflect pressure at

TABLE 16-1 Selected Characteristics for Classes of Support Surfaces

Performance Characteristics	Air Fluidized (High Air Loss)	Low Air Loss	Alternating Air (Dynamic)	Static Flotation (Air or Water)	Foam	Standard Hospital Mattress
Increased support area	Yes	Yes	Yes	Yes	Yes	No
Low moisture retention	Yes	Yes	No	No	No	No
Reduced heat accumulation	Yes	Yes	No	No	No	No
Shear reduction	Yes	?	Yes	Yes	No	No
Pressure reduction	Yes	Yes	Yes	Yes	Yes	No
Dynamic	Yes	Yes	Yes	No	No	No
Cost per day	High	High	Moderate	Low	Low	Low

Reprinted with permission from N. Bergstrom, M.A. Bennett, C.E. Carlson, et al., *Treatment of Pressure Ulcers*, Clinical Practice Guideline No. 15, December, 1994, U.S. Department of Health and Human Services, Public Health Service, Agency for Health Care Policy and Research, AHCPR Publication No. 95–0652.

EXHIBIT 16-5 Ideal Support Surface Characteristics

- Reduces/relieves pressure under bony prominences
- Controls pressure gradient in tissue
- Provides stability
- No interference with weight shifts
- No interference with transfers
- Controls temperature at interface
- Controls moisture at skin surface
- Lightweight
- Low cost
- Durable

Reprinted with permission from J. McLean, Pressure reduction or pressure relief: making the right choice, *Journal of ET Nursing*, Vol. 20, No. 5, pp. 211–215, © 1993, Mosby Year-Book, Inc.

the bony tissue interface. Some suggest that pressure on subcutaneous tissues may be three to five times higher than skin interface pressure. Interface pressure is a measurement obtained by placing a sensor between the skin and the resting support surface. It is usually obtained with some type of electropneumatic pressure sensor connected to an inflation system and gauge. Typically, three or more readings are obtained, and the average of the readings is used as the reported value. Instrumentation (size of sensor, shape of sensor, and position of sensor) greatly affects values of pressure readings, so it is difficult, if not impossible, to make comparisons between studies.

Pressure-Reducing Support Surfaces. Pressure-reduction devices lower tissue interface pressures but do not *consistently* maintain interface pressures below capillary closing pressures in all positions, on all body locations.[102] These devices are also called low end surfaces, or Group 1 devices. Pressure-reducing support surfaces are indicated for patients who are assessed to be at risk for pressure ulcer development, who can be turned, and who have skin breakdown involving *only one sleep surface*.[48] Patients with an existing pressure ulcer who are determined to be still at risk for development of further skin breakdown should be man-

aged on a pressure-reducing support surface. Pressure-reduction devices can be classified as static or dynamic devices.

Static devices do not move; they reduce pressure by spreading the load over a larger area. The easy definition of a static support surface is a device that does not require electricity to function, usually a mattress overlay (lies on top of the standard hospital mattress). Examples of static devices are foam, air, or gel mattress overlays and water-filled mattresses. When considering the foam mattress overlays, the health-care provider should consider stiffness of the foam and the density and thickness of the foam. Indentation load deflection (ILD) is a measure of the stiffness of the foam; generally, the ILD should be 25% for 30 pounds. The density and thickness of the foam relate to the foam's ability to deflect the pressure and redistribute the pressure over a wider area. Typically, the density and thickness of a foam product should be 1.3 pounds per cubic foot and 3–4 inches, respectively.[1] Foam devices have difficulties with retaining moisture and heat, and not reducing shear. Air and water static devices also have difficulties associated with retaining moisture and heat.

Dynamic support surfaces move. The easy definition of dynamic support surfaces is that they require a motor or pump and electricity to operate. Examples are alternating pressure air mattresses. Most of these devices use an electric pump alternately to inflate and deflate air cells or air columns, thus the term *alternating* pressure air mattress. The key to determination of effectiveness is the length of time that cycles of inflation and deflation occur. Dynamic support surfaces may also have difficulties with moisture retention and heat accumulation.[1]

Pressure-reduction devices can also be categorized as overlays or replacement mattresses. Mattress overlays are devices that are applied on top of the standard mattress. Most overlays are pressure-reduction devices and require a onetime charge, setup fee, daily rental fee, or a combination of fees. Most are single-use items and may present environmental issues for disposal. When using mattress overlays, the height of the bed is increased, so transfers and linen fit may be complicated. Mattress overlays may be static or dynamic. Some provide air movement to reduce moisture buildup. Some examples include foam, gel, water, or air-filled mattresses, alternating pressure pads, and low-air-loss overlays.

RESEARCH WISDOM

Evaluating Studies Using Tissue Interface Pressures

- Look for interface pressures stated as a percentage against a standard surface, usually a hospital mattress. Standard hospital mattress interface pressures for sacrum = 36 to 48 mm Hg and for trochanter = 62 to 97 mm Hg.[103] For example, a support surface that reports tissue interface pressure readings of 25 mm Hg for the sacrum has approximately 30% lower pressures than the standard hospital mattress pressures for the sacrum (25 mm Hg/36 mm Hg × 100 = 69.44; 100–70 = 30% of hospital mattress pressures).
- Look for standard deviations (SD) reported in the study—95% of measurements lie within 2 SD of the mean (average). So, the larger the standard deviation, the less reproducible the pressure measurements and the more variable the results with the product.[83,84] For example, a study reports mean tissue interface pressures of 25 mm Hg with standard deviation of 8.2. So, 95% of all the measurements were between 8.6 and 41.4 mm Hg. This is not so bad at the 8.6 end, but what about the 41.4 mm Hg? That figure is far higher than capillary closing pressure of 32 mm Hg.
- To interpret the study results, consider these issues:[83]

  1. Range and number of pressure readings obtained for each site. How was site placement determined? (The bony prominence is usually larger than the pressure probe. Was it placed in the center of the bony prominence? Was the site marked so subsequent readings were taken at the same location?)
  2. Procedure used to acquire the pressure readings should be described as well as the training procedures for those conducting the testing.
  3. Who were tested and how do they compare with the patients you care for?
  4. How were they tested?
  5. How often was equipment recalibrated? (The equipment is fragile and subject to malfunction.)

One additional concern when using mattress overlays is the bottoming out phenomenon. Bottoming out occurs when the patient's body sinks down, the support surface is compressed beyond function, and the patient's body lies directly on the hospital mattress. When bottoming out occurs, there is no pressure reduction for the bony prominence of concern. Bottoming out typically happens when the patient is placed on a static air mattress overlay that is not appropriately filled with air or when the patient has been on a foam mattress for extended periods of time. The health-care provider can monitor for bottoming out by inserting a flat, outstretched hand between the overlay and the patient's body part at risk. If the caregiver feels less than an inch of support material, the patient has bottomed out. It is important

to check for bottoming out when the patient is in various body positions and to check at various body sites. For example, when the patient is lying supine, check the sacral/coccygeal area and the heels; when the patient is side-lying, check the trochanter and lateral malleolus.[1] Use of a static support surface is warranted if the patient can turn off of the pressure ulcer site without bottoming out.

Replacement mattresses are designed to reduce interface pressures and replace the standard hospital mattress. Most are made of foam and gel combinations. Some are air-filled chambers and foam structures. All are covered with a bacteriostatic cover that can be maintained with standard cleaning. These mattresses involve an initial significant expense, and there are minimal data on long-term effectiveness.

Pressure-Relieving Support Surfaces. Pressure relief devices *consistently* reduce tissue interface pressures to a level below capillary closing pressure, in any position and in most body locations. These devices may also be called high end or high tech devices, and Group 2 or 3 devices. Pressure-relief devices are indicated for patients who are assessed to be at high risk for pressure ulcer development and who cannot turn independently or those who have skin breakdown involving more than one body surface. Most commonly, pressure-relief devices are grouped into low-air-loss therapy (e.g., high tech devices or Group 2 devices) or fluidized air or high-air-loss therapy, and kinetic therapy (e.g., all high end devices or Group 3 devices).

Low-air-loss therapy is a bed frame with a series of connected air-filled pillows with surface fabrics of low-friction material. The amount of pressure in each pillow can be controlled and can be calibrated to provide maximum pressure relief for the individual patient. They provide pressure relief in any position, and most models have built-in scales.

Fluidized air or high-air-loss therapy consists of a bed frame containing silicone-coated glass beads and incorporates both air and fluid support. The beads become fluid when air is pumped through, making them behave as a liquid. High-air-loss therapy has bactericidal properties because of the alkalinity of the beads (pH 10), the temperature, and entrapment of microorganisms by the beads. High-air-loss therapy relieves pressure and reduces friction, shear, and moisture (due to the drying effect of the bed). It is difficult to transfer patients in these devices because of the bed frame. There is increased air flow, which can increase evaporative fluid loss, leading to dehydration. Finally, if the patient is able to sit up, a foam wedge may be required, thus limiting the beneficial effects of the bed on the upper back of the patient.

Kinetic therapy beds are designed to counter the effects of immobility by continuous passive motion. Kinetic therapy is believed to improve respiratory function and oxygenation, prevent urinary stasis, and reduce venous stasis. Multiple body systems are involved in the therapy, and, generally, the patient must have a stable spine. The beds usually are of two types: Either the bed frame itself moves or the air cushions inflate or deflate, rotating the patient from side to side or pulsating. Pressure relief and low-friction surfaces are provided with repositioning. Most models include built-in scales. Conscious patients may not tolerate the movement of the bed.

The last category of support surfaces includes bariatric devices. These support surfaces are designed to provide pressure reduction for the severely obese patient and can accommodate extreme loading, as is the case with the obese patient. Bariatric devices have features similar to the other support surfaces described. Generally, the bed frame is larger and many include the capability of raising the patient to a standing position while positioned in the bed. There are also chair devices for the obese patient.

Support Surface Selection. Determining which support surface is best for individual patients can be confusing. The primary concern must always be the effectiveness of the surface for the individual patient's needs. The original AHCPR guidelines on prevention and prediction of pressure ulcers recommend the following criteria for determining how to manage tissue loading and support surface selection.[48]

- Assess the patient with existing pressure ulcers to determine the risk for developing additional pressure ulcers. If the patient remains at risk, use a pressure-reducing surface.
- Use a static support surface if the patient can assume a variety of positions without bearing weight on an existing pressure ulcer and without bottoming out.
- Use a dynamic support surface if the patient cannot assume a variety of positions without bearing weight on an existing pressure ulcer, if the patient fully compresses the static support surface, or if the pressure ulcer does not show evidence of healing.
- If a patient has large stage III or stage IV pressure ulcers on multiple turning surfaces, a low-air-loss bed or a fluidized air (high-air-loss) bed may be indicated.
- When excess moisture on intact skin is a potential source of maceration and skin breakdown, a support surface that provides airflow can be important in drying the skin and preventing additional pressure ulcers.
- Any individual assessed to be at risk for developing pressure ulcers should be placed on a static or dynamic pressure-reducing support surface.

Use of an algorithm can also be helpful in making clinical decisions. There are multiple decision trees and algorithms available. The algorithm recommended by the AHCPR guidelines (Figure 16-9) is offered as one example of a clinical decision-making tree or treatment algorithm.[1]

There are additional concerns in choosing a support surface. Criteria for choosing support surfaces can be classified as intrinsic and extrinsic. Intrinsic criteria include wound burden (tissue history—previous ulcers, surgical repair, stress, duration of pressure ulcer, number of pressure ulcers present), body build (obese, thin, contractures present), and the magnitude and distribution of interface pressures (location of highest pressures, etc.). The following case examples help to illustrate how intrinsic criteria are used for determination of support surface: Patients who undergo specific surgical operative repair of the pressure ulcer may need to be placed on high-air-loss or fluidized air therapy postoperatively. Patients with multiple ulcers involving more than one turning surface also need to be placed on pressure-relieving devices, such as low-air-loss therapy or high-air-loss therapy. Patients with severe contractures may not require a support surface that has good heel pressure readings (with contraction of the legs, the heels do not reach the bottom of the mattress). If the bony prominence of concern is the greater trochanter, the support surface chosen must adequately reduce pressure over the trochanter. Although an algorithm is a helpful tool in choosing a support surface, as these case examples illustrate, the clinician must also evaluate the individual patient's needs.

Extrinsic criteria include all of the following:

- The number of hours spent on the support surface daily (Will product be needed for short- or long-term use?)
- Shear and friction effects
- Environmental factors (temperature, humidity, continence, and moisture)
- Living arrangements (Will patient be in acute care, long-term care, or home care setting?)
- Self-care deficits (Is the risk of pressure ulcer development likely to increase or decrease?)
- Ease of transition and weaning to other products or other health-care settings
- Ease of use and manageability
- Cost—reimbursement level
- Service and warranty
- Availability of product
- Scientific validity

Evaluation of extrinsic criteria requires the clinician to review the goals for therapy. For example, the patient who uses the support surface only at night and spends most of the day in the chair will require an aggressive approach to seating support surfaces, and a lesser support surface can be chosen for the bed. If the patient spends most of the day in bed, the support surface chosen will be different. A support surface's ability to handle shearing and friction may be critical for agitated patients (particularly those with continual body motions), and good choices may involve evaluation of the support surface covering. The external environment is also essential to include in choosing a support surface. If the patient is at home, with no air conditioning, is incontinent of urine, and lives in a humid environment, the ability of the support surface to breathe and the ability to handle moisture are essential to positive outcomes. Likewise, evaluation of the patient's prognosis is helpful in support surface choice. Is the patient expected to recover and improve? If so, a pressure-reduction or lower-end support surface device may be appropriate. However, if the patient is expected to decline in function, choosing a support surface that will meet future, as well as present, skin care needs may be pru-

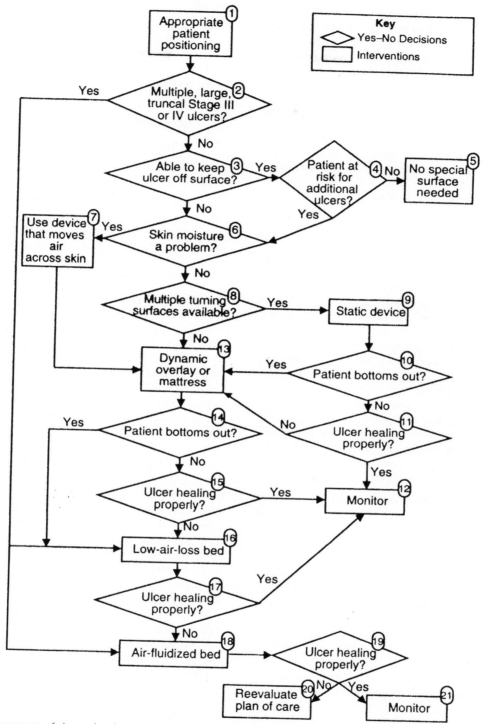

FIGURE 16-9 Management of tissue loads. (Reprinted with permission from N. Bergstrom, MA Bennett, CE Carlson, et al. *Treatment of Pressure Ulcers.* Clinical Practice Guideline No. 15, December, 1994, U.S. Department of Health and Human Services, Public Health Service, Agency for Health Care Policy and Research, AHCPR Publication No. 95–0652.)

dent. Throughout the decision-making process one thought should prevail: it is important to promote patient independence, not patient dependent behavior. Encouraging patient movement out of bed and, thus, off of the support surface is important for those patients who are able, and this must be considered by the clinician.

CLINICAL WISDOM
Reimbursement of Support Surfaces

Support surfaces are reimbursed in home care under Medicare Part B benefits. Medicare requirements for reimbursement include the following:
- Must be stage III or IV pressure sore
- Must have pressure sore located on trunk of body
- Must have current Medicare Part B coverage
- Must be in permanent residence (own home, long-term care facility, etc.)

Seating Support Surfaces. Support surfaces for chairs and wheelchairs can be categorized as for the support surfaces for beds. In general, providing adequate pressure relief for chair-bound or wheelchair-bound patients is critical, because the patient at risk for pressure ulcer formation is at increased risk in the seated position because of the high pressures across the ischial tuberosities. Most pressure-reducing devices for chairs are static overlays, such as those made out of foam, gel, air, or some combination. Positioning chair-bound or wheelchair-bound individuals must include consideration of individual anatomy and body contours, postural alignment, distribution of weight, and balance and stability, in addition to pressure relief. Chapter 17 provides additional information on therapeutic positioning.

Evaluating Outcomes of Support Surfaces. To evaluate outcomes from the support surfaces chosen for a particular health-care setting, *baseline data must be available on the prevalence and incidence* of the condition in the setting. *Prevalence is the number of all persons with the condition at one particular point in time.* Prevalence includes both facility-acquired cases and those admitted with the condition. Prevalence studies can be done on one day (one point in time) and require a team to review all medical records and perform skin inspections of all patients in the organization on that day. *Incidence is the number of new cases developing over a period of time.* Incidence includes only facility-acquired conditions and, as such, reflects the effectiveness of the prevention program in the organization. Incidence studies are done over a period of time (a month, a quarter, a year) and require evaluation of all new patients with the condition (medical record review and skin inspection). The evaluation team reviews all patients (but counts only those with new conditions) at periodic intervals over the time period, e.g., once a week for 4 weeks to determine monthly incidence. Many times, prevalence and incidence studies are combined. The team performs a prevalence study on one day, then continues to evaluate the population over a period of time to evaluate the incidence also. Incidence is the most

valuable of the two baseline studies because it reflects actual occurrence of pressure ulcer development in the facility. Over time, with an effective prevention program, including availability of the appropriate support surfaces, the incidence of pressure ulcer development in the facility should decline, assuming there are no changes in the patient population.

CLINICAL WISDOM
Teaching Wheelchair-Bound Patients

Wheelchair-bound patients with upper body strength can be taught and encouraged to do wheelchair pushups every 15 minutes to relieve pressure and allow for reperfusion of the tissues in the ischial tuberosity region. Use of a watch with a timer device may be a helpful reminder. The use of a chair support surface can help lessen the burden of wheelchair pushups, but does not eliminate the need for reperfusion of the tissues.

Choosing support surfaces for clients based on algorithms (see Figure 16-9) and predetermined criteria (factors chosen by the clinician, such as the support surface's ability to handle friction, cost, service, etc), use of a multidisciplinary team to finalize selections, and periodic reevaluation of products and patient/institution needs, based on baseline prevalence and incidence data, are the keys to effective support surface use. These steps are critical as limited evidence exists to support use of one specific device versus another in the same category.

Evidence-Based Practice: Which Support Surface Is Best?

There is one comprehensive systematic review of support surface research. This review by Cullum and colleagues as part of the Cochrane Collaboration covered 41 randomized controlled clinical trials of pressure reduction support surfaces published up to January 2004 and provides a recent thorough review of the evidence in this area.[104] Eight randomized controlled trials of pressure reducing support surfaces provide convincing evidence supporting lower pressure ulcer incidence for persons placed on pressure reduction surfaces compared to standard mattresses. A meta analysis, using a random effects model, of five trials comparing foam alternatives to standard mattresses yielded a pooled relative risk of 0.40 (confidence interval [CI] 0.21–0.74) or a relative reduction in pressure ulcer incidence of 60%. One large study comparing alternating pressure surfaces to standard mattresses yielded a relative risk (RR) of 0.32 (CI 0.14–0.74).[104]

Thirteen trials report a head to head comparison of low tech surfaces (also called pressure reduction devices, Group 1 devices) and an additional 11 trials report either a head to head comparison of high tech surfaces (also called pressure relief devices, or Group 2 and 3 devices) or a comparison of low tech to high tech surfaces.[104] However, no clear evidence exists to support the use of one specific support surface (e.g., low tech versus high tech or any low/high tech versus any other low/high tech) over another for pressure ulcer prevention. At this time support surfaces may be considered functionally equivalent.

Four randomized controlled trials have evaluated methods to reduce pressure in the operating room. One trial compared a visco-elastic polymer surface with standard operating table and found a relative reduction in incidence of postoperative pressure ulcers of 47% for those persons undergoing elective major general, gynecological, or vascular surgery (RR 0.53, CI 0.33–0.85).[104] Two other trials compared a high tech alternating surface used during surgery and postoperatively with standard care (gel pad during surgery and standard mattress postoperatively); Cullum and colleagues[104] report a pooled relative risk of 0.21 (CI 0.06–0.7). The fourth trial reported increased skin changes postoperatively with use of a foam overlay on the operating table (six stage II pressure ulcers in the intervention group compared to three stage II pressure ulcers in the control group). These findings are difficult to interpret because the product is unnamed, postoperative skin care is not described, and details on stage of pressure ulcers that developed postoperatively by group are not given.[104] These findings suggest that use of pressure reduction surfaces in the operating room and postoperatively can reduce the incidence of postoperative pressure ulcers although some evidence exists that certain overlays may result in some skin changes postoperatively.

Since the systematic review by the Cochrane group, Theaker and colleagues[105] have reported a controlled trial comparing two high tech support surfaces for pressure ulcer prevention in intensive care. Sixty-two intensive care patients identified as at high risk for pressure ulcers but pressure ulcer-free were randomly assigned to either an alternating pressure surface or a low-air-loss bed. Subjects were evaluated every 8 hours for presence of pressure ulceration during the intensive care stay and for an additional 2 weeks when discharged from the ICU. There were no statistically significant differences in pressure ulcer incidence between the two devices. This study has some power issues related to a relatively small sample size and low frequency of pressure ulcer incidence. These findings support the conclusion by the Cochrane review that head to head comparisons of high tech surfaces have not demonstrated that one device is superior to any other.

In the Cochrane review, Cullum and colleagues[104] describe a recent study of 297 orthopedic patients comparing Australian medical sheepskin to standard mattress yielding a relative risk for pressure ulcer development of 0.30 (CI 0.17–0.52). These findings are confirmed in a study by Jolley and colleagues.[106] They report on 441 low to moderate risk general adult hospital patients randomly assigned to receive the sheepskin versus standard mattress. They report a cumulative incidence of pressure ulcers of 9.6% (CI 6.1%–14.3%) in the sheepskin group compared to 16.6% (CI 12.0%–22.1%) in the standard mattress group and relative risk of 0.42 (CI 0.26–0.67) findings of lower pressure ulcer incidence. Thus, the risk of developing a pressure ul-

cer in the sheepskin group was 40% less than for those on standard mattresses in a low to moderate risk general adult hospital population.[106]

Two randomized controlled trials evaluated wheelchair surfaces. Rosenthal and colleagues[107] compared a generic total contact seat surface with low air loss bed surfaces in healing stage III and IV pressure ulcers in 207 residents of long-term care facilities over 4 weeks. At 4 weeks, ratings of pressure ulcer status were better for those pressure ulcers treated with the generic total contact seat surface than the low air loss surface (P<.001). One of the important findings from Rosenthal and colleagues is that individuals with existing pressure ulcers can still be up in a chair without impairing healing (and in the case of this study, healing actually improved in the group allowed to sit up on the generic total contact seat).[107] The second pilot study by Geyer et al[108] compared incidence of pressure ulcers among 32 elderly nursing home wheelchair users randomly assigned to prescribed pressure reducing cushions or foam wheelchair surfaces. In this study, no differences were noted between pressure ulcer incidence in the two groups (overall incidence 50%), however, the prescribed pressure reducing cushion group had a lower incidence in sitting-acquired (e.g., ischial) pressure ulcers (0 versus 8 in the foam wheelchair surface group, P<.005).[108] The findings indicate that use of pressure reducing cushions in wheelchair users may decrease the incidence of sitting-acquired (ischial) ulcers.

Two studies provide evidence for the use of pressure reduction surfaces to improve pressure ulcer healing.[109,110] Two randomized controlled clinical trials reported improved clinical outcomes with improved reduction in pressure ulcer surface area; however, neither of the studies reported a significant difference in ulcer healing. In a randomized, controlled study of 84 nursing home residents with stage II to IV pressure ulcers, Ferrell and colleagues evaluated pressure ulcer response to low-air-loss beds versus a 4-inch convoluted foam overlay.[109] Wounds treated with low-air-loss beds were more likely to show a decrease in surface area for both deep (P = 0.004) and superficial ulcers (P = 0.02). However, there was no significant difference in the percentage of ulcers that healed completely. Pressure ulcers on the low-air-loss beds were 2.5 times more likely to heal than those on the foam overlays (P = 0.004). Yet when deep and superficial ulcer data were analyzed separately, the improved odds of healing were significant only for the superficial ulcers. Although the likelihood of deep pressure ulcer healing on the low-air-loss beds was increased over the foam overlay, this difference was not statistically significant (P = 0.18).[109] Mulder and colleagues also examined pressure ulcer response to low-air-loss beds and foam in a sample of 42 nursing home residents with stage III to IV pressure ulcers.[110] Similar to Ferrell's group, Mulder's study demonstrated a decrease in ulcer surface area and volume for those on the low-air-loss beds, yet found no statistically significant difference in the number of ulcers healed in the low-air-loss group versus the foam overlay group.[110]

One retrospective multisite comparison study by Ochs and colleagues[111] reports faster healing of existing pressure ulcers when persons are placed on high end support surfaces (e.g., air fluidized therapy). They report a mean healing rate of 5.2cm^2/week for the air fluidized surface group compared to 1.5cm^2/week for the low tech group and 1.8cm^2/week for the high tech group ($P = .007$).[111] This relatively recent comparison study (compares high end surfaces to low tech and high tech surfaces) confirms findings from studies in the late 1980s on increased rate of pressure ulcer healing when persons are placed on air fluidized therapy surfaces.

Together these studies and clinical practice guidelines provide compelling support for use of pressure reduction support surfaces instead of standard mattresses for persons at risk for pressure ulcers with relative reduction in pressure ulcer incidence of 60%. Moderate evidence exists to support use of support surfaces in the operating room to reduce postoperative pressure ulcer incidence (two pooled trials relative risk = 0.21, 95% confidence interval [CI] 0.06–0.7). However, the relative merits of high tech surfaces versus low tech (e.g., constant low pressure such as contoured foam, static air, gel-filled, and bead-filled support surfaces) surfaces are not clear. More limited evidence exists for use of high end (group 3 air fluidized therapy support) surfaces to improve pressure ulcer healing, use of scheduled repositioning programs in conjunction with support surfaces, and use of Australian medical sheepskin to reduce incidence of pressure ulcers.

Friction and Shear

Measures to reduce friction and shear relate to passive or active movement of the patient. To reduce friction, several interventions are appropriate. Providing topical preparations to eliminate or reduce the surface tension between the skin and the bed linen or support surface will assist in reducing friction-related injury. Use of appropriate techniques when moving patients so that skin is never dragged across linens will lessen friction-induced skin breakdown. Patients who exhibit voluntary or involuntary repetitive body movements (particularly of the heels or elbows) require stronger interventions. Use of a protective film, such as a transparent film dressing or a skin sealant; a protective dressing, such as a thin hydrocolloid; or protective padding will help to eliminate the surface contact of the area and decrease the friction between the skin and the linens.[40] Even though heel, ankle, and elbow protectors do nothing to reduce or relieve pressure, they can be effective aids against friction.

CLINICAL WISDOM

Reducing Friction

Sprinkling cornstarch on the bed linen or use of skin lubricants is helpful in reducing overall friction.

Most shear injury can be eliminated by proper positioning, such as avoidance of the semi-Fowler's position and limiting use of the upright position (positions over 30° inclined). Avoidance of positions greater than 30° inclined may prevent sliding and shear-related injury. Use of footboards and knee gatches (or pillows under the lower leg) to prevent sliding and to maintain position, are also helpful in reducing shear effects on the skin when in bed. Observation of the patient when sitting is also important, because the patient who slides out of the chair is at equally high risk for shear injury. Use of footstools and the foot pedals on wheelchairs and appropriate 90° flexion of the hip (may be achieved with pillows, special seat cushions, or orthotic devices) can help in preventing chair sliding.

Nutrition

Nutrition is an important element in maintaining healthy skin and tissues. There is a strong relationship between nutrition and pressure ulcer development.[112] The severity of pressure ulceration is also correlated with severity of nutritional deficits, especially low protein intake or low serum albumin levels.[112–115] The nutritional assessment is key in determining the appropriate interventions for the patient. A short nutritional assessment should be performed on all patients determined to be at risk for pressure ulcer formation at routine intervals. See Chapter 3 for more information on assessment of nutrition.

Malnutrition can be diagnosed if serum albumin levels are below 3.5 mg/dL, total lymphocyte count is less than 1,800 mm,[24] or body weight decreases by more than 15%.[1] Exhibit 16-6 provides an example of a nutritional screening tool. Malnutrition impairs the immune system, and total lymphocyte counts are a reflection of immune competence. If the patient is diagnosed as malnourished, nutritional supplementation may be indicated to help achieve a positive nitrogen balance. Examples of appropriate oral supplements are assisted oral feedings and dietary supplements. The goal of care is to provide approximately 30–35 kcal/kg of weight per day and 1.25–1.5 g of protein per kg of weight per day.[1] Patients should be encouraged to improve their own dietary habits, and education should focus on healthy nutrition with adequate caloric and protein intake. It may be difficult for a pressure ulcer patient or an at-risk patient to ingest enough protein and calories necessary to maintain skin and tissue health. Oral supplements can be very helpful in boosting calorie and protein intake. Liquid nutritional supplements are designed to be used as an adjunct to regular oral feedings. Monitoring nutritional indexes is essential to determine effectiveness of the care plan. Serum albumin, protein markers, body weight, dietary intake, and nutritional assessment should be performed at least every 3 months to monitor for changes in nutritional status.

Hypoalbuminemia (serum albumin levels below 3.5 mg/dL) may be associated with pressure ulceration,[112,115] although some have found no relationship and little prognostic value for pressure ulcer healing.[116–118] When protein intake is insufficient, the serum albumin decreases. Serum albumin contributes to the amino acid pool, and amino acids are essential building blocks for new tissue development.

EXHIBIT 16-6   Example of Nutritional Assessment Guide for Patients with Pressure Ulcers

Patient Name: _____ Date: _____ Time: _____

To be filled out for all patients at risk on initial evaluation and every 12 weeks thereafter, as indicated. Trends will document the efficacy of nutritional support therapy.

Protein Compartments

Somatic:
Current Weight (kg) _____
Previous Weight (kg) _____ (_____ date)
Percent Change in Weight _____

Height (cm) _____
Height/Weight _____
Current Body Mass Index (BMI) _____ (wt(ht)²]
Previous BMI _____ (_____ date)
Percent Change in BMI _____

Visceral:
Serum Albumin _____
(Normal (≥3.5 mg/dL)
Total Lymphocyte Count (TLC) _____ (optional)
   (White Blood Cell count × percent Lymphocytes/100)
Guide to TLC:
• Immune competence   ❑ 1,800 mm³
• Immunity partly impaired   < 1,800 but ❑ 900 mm³
• Anergy   < 900 mm³

State of Hydration

24-Hour Intake _____ mL   24-Hour Output _____ mL

Note: Thirst, tongue dryness in nonmouth breathers, and tenting of cervical skin may indicate dehydration. Jugular vein distention may indicate overhydration.

Estimated Nutritional Requirement

Estimated Nonprotein Calories (NPC)   _____/kg   Estimated Protein _____ (g/kg)
Actual NPC   _____/kg   Actual Protein _____ (g/kg)

Recommendations/Plan

1.
2.
3.
4.

Reprinted with permission from N. Bergstrom, M.A. Bennett, C.E. Carlson, et al., *Treatment of Pressure Ulcers*, Clinical Practice Guideline No. 15, December, 1994, U.S. Department of Health and Human Services, Public Health Service, Agency for Health Care Policy and Research, AHCPR Publication No. 95–0652.

Serum albumin also maintains oncotic pressures within the vascular fluid compartment. Colloidal oncotic pressure is the total influence of proteins on the osmotic activity of plasma. When albumin levels decrease, there is a decrease in the oncotic pressure (fewer proteins in the plasma, leading to increased osmotic activity from the vascular bed as the blood vessels attempt to maintain homeostasis by allowing osmosis of water out of the vessels and into surrounding tissues), which leads to edema, further compromising tissue perfusion. Ensuring adequate protein intake is a critical element in nutritional interventions for pressure ulcer patients and those at risk for pressure ulceration.

Evidence-Based Practice: Research on Nutrition and Pressure Ulcers

While multiple studies have demonstrated a relationship between different markers of malnutrition (e.g., serum albumin level, dietary protein intake, inability to feed self, and weight loss) and pressure ulcer formation and severity, defining a causal relationship between malnutrition and pressure ulcer development, something that seems so logical, has proven difficult. Data supporting a prophylactic effect of nutritional supplements on pressure ulcer development is not so clear.

The most compelling data in support of providing nutrition supplementation to persons at risk for pressure ulcers are the systematic review by Langer and colleagues as part of The Cochrane Collaboration[119] and Stratton et al's meta-analysis of the same studies in the Cochrane Review.[120] Langer and colleagues[119] reviewed eight randomized controlled clinical trials of nutritional supplementation for pressure ulcer prevention and healing published up to June 2003 and provided a recent thorough review of the evidence in this area. Four randomized controlled trials of nutritional supplements as an intervention to prevent pressure ulcer development are reviewed. Three studies evaluated pressure ulcer development in patients with hip fracture; one study was of questionable value due to methodological flaws and omitted information. In the largest study, Bourdel-Marchasson and colleagues[121] conducted a randomized controlled trial with 672 critically ill hospitalized older adults for 15 days with a follow-up of 70%. Those patients in the intervention group received two oral nutritional supplements per day in addition to the normal diet and the control group received the normal diet alone. At 15 days, the cumulative incidence of pressure ulcers of all stages was 40% in the intervention group compared to 48% in the control group[121] (relative risk = 0.83, CI 95% 0.70–0.99[119]). In multivariate analysis, patients receiving the intervention were less likely to develop a pressure ulcer.[119]

Hartgrink and colleagues[122] evaluated 140 patients with fracture of the hip and an increased pressure ulcer risk over 2 weeks in a hospital. The intervention group was treated with standard hospital diet plus additional nasogastric tube feeding that was administered via feeding pump overnight. The control group received standard diet alone. After 2 weeks, there was no difference in the pressure ulcer incidence between the groups with 25 of the 48 remaining patients in the intervention group (52%) and 30 of the 53 patients in the control group (56%) developing pressure ulcers of stage II or greater (relative risk = 0.92; CI 95% 0.64–1.32; $P = 0.6$). It should be noted that only 16 patients tolerated the intervention tube feeding for the 2 weeks of the study.

Houwing et al[123] evaluated use of one supplement daily with a normal hospital diet in 103 hip fracture patients with a follow-up time of 28 days. After 2 weeks there was no significant difference in pressure ulcer incidence between the two groups (55% versus 59%, rr = 0.92, CI 95% 0.65–1.3). The incidence of stage II pressure ulcers, while not statistically significant, was lower in the intervention group (18% versus 28%, rr = 0.6; CI 95% 0.3–1.6). The study was severely underpowered.

In the systematic review and meta-analysis by Stratton and colleagues, they pooled the four randomized controlled trials of nutritional supplements compared to normal, standard diet and yielded an odds ratio of 0.75 (CI 95% 0.62–0.89).[120] It should be noted that the Cochrane Review

did not conduct a meta-analysis as they believed the studies were too disparate to pool.[119]

The strongest evidence for providing nutrition supplementation for healing existing pressure ulcers is Chernoff and colleagues'[124] small enteral feeding randomized trial with 12 patients followed for 12 weeks. Intervention subjects received very high protein (25% calories from protein or 1.8g/kg protein) supplements and the control group received high protein (17% calories from protein or 1.2g/kg) supplements. Those pressure ulcers in the intervention group had a 73% improvement in ulcer surface area compared to 43% improved ulcer surface area in the control group even though the intervention group started the study with larger pressure ulcer surface areas.[124] Breslow and colleagues[125] found similar findings with those persons receiving 24% protein nutrition supplementation demonstrating greater decrease in truncal pressure ulcer surface area compared to those receiving the 14% protein nutritional supplementation. While the evidence is not overwhelming, there is a suggestion of improved pressure ulcer healing with increased high protein nutritional supplementation.

Langer and colleagues' systematic review discusses two trials of ascorbic acid as nutritional supplementation to increase pressure ulcer healing. Their review showed at best, unclear results from the two trials and no strong evidence to support provision of vitamin C supplements to improve pressure ulcer healing. There is no data to support nutrition supplementation of other vitamins or minerals to promote ulcer healing.[119]

These studies, federal guidelines, and all clinical practice guidelines and expert panels provide modest evidence to support providing nutritional support for those persons at risk for pressure ulcers with relative reduction in pressure ulcer incidence of 25% (odds ratio 0.75, 95% CI 0.62–0.89). More limited evidence exists for use of high protein nutritional supplements and improved pressure ulcer healing with two small, methodologically flawed, disparate trials showing persons who received high protein (24%–25% protein) diets healed their pressure ulcers at a greater rate than those on a standard diet (e.g., 14%–17% protein). The relative merits of providing nutritional supplementation by tube-feeding to persons with pressure ulcers are controversial and generally not supported by data, thus use of tube feedings in persons with pressure ulcers is not recommended.[126–128] No evidence exists for use of supplemental vitamins or minerals (e.g., vitamin A, E, C, and zinc) in persons with pressure ulcers and no coexisting specific vitamin/mineral deficiency to improve pressure ulcer healing.

CLINICAL WISDOM

When to Consult the Dietitian

General parameters for consultation with the dietitian for a thorough nutritional assessment are:

- Inadequate dietary intake (e.g., less than 50% of most meals consumed)
- Drop in body weight of 5%, *or*
- Serum albumin level below 3.5 mg/dL

Moisture

The preventive interventions related to moisture include general skin care, accurate diagnosis of incontinence type, and appropriate incontinence management.

General Skin Care

General skin care involves routine skin assessment, incontinence assessment and management, skin hygiene interventions, and measures to maintain skin health. Routine skin assessment involves observation of the patient's skin, with particular attention to bony prominences. Reddened areas should not be massaged. Massage can further impair the perfusion to the tissues.[129] The skin should be evaluated for dryness and cracking. Older adults are at higher risk for dry skin, and dry skin may decrease tissue tolerance to external forces. Lack of moisture in the air may contribute to dry skin and can be counteracted by use of a humidifier in the room.[130] Attention should also be focused on gentle handling to prevent skin tears in older patients. The epidermis and dermis junction is lessened with age, making older patients at higher risk for skin tears. Other factors to include in a skin assessment include temperature, sensory ability, turgor, and texture.[131] Skin normally should be warm to touch. The dorsal aspect of the hand is more sensitive to temperature changes than the palm of the hand; thus, clinicians should use the dorsal aspect of the hand to judge skin temperature. Two-point discrimination is used to evaluate skin sensation. Normally, the patient should be able to distinguish sharp, dull, or pressure sensations against the skin surface. Diminished sensation may be generalized or localized to a specific area, such as the lower extremities. Skin tone should be smooth and elastic. Edema causes the skin to appear taut and shiny, and dehydration is present if the skin is dry, wrinkled, and withered. Observing the skin surface for texture and moisture may reveal signs of excessive moisture or dryness. Most factors in a skin assessment can be reviewed through observation and palpation skills. The information gathered through the simple act of inspection can form a basis for general skin care interventions and for pressure ulcer prevention interventions.

Incontinence Assessment and Management

Specifically related to moisture, the skin should be assessed for signs of perineal dermatitis. Evaluating perineal dermatitis requires understanding of the concepts of tissue tolerance, perineal environment, and toileting ability. (See *Color Plates 14* and *16*.) Objective signs of perineal dermatitis include erythema, swelling, vesication, oozing, crusting, and scaling, with subjective symptoms of tingling, itching, burning, and pain.[132] The perineal region is broadly defined as the perineum (area between the vulva or scrotum and anus), buttocks, perianal area, coccyx, and upper/inner thigh regions.

The clinical presentation is variable and may be dependent on the frequency of incontinence episode, rapidity and efficacy of postepisode hygiene, and duration of incontinence. Acute and chronic clinical manifestations of skin reactions in elderly nursing home patients have been described based on clinical experience.[133]

Skin reactions can be divided into acute reactions and chronic changes. Perineal dermatitis may present with acute episode characteristics or with more long-standing chronic skin changes apparent. In acute episodes, the skin characteristics most predominant are erythema, papulovesicular reaction, frank erosions and abrasions, and, in some cases, evidence of monilial infection, due to the moist warm environment. In general, a diffuse blanchable erythema is present involving buttock areas, coccyx area, perineum, perianal area, and upper/inner thighs. The extent of the erythema varies, and the intensity of the reaction may be muted in immunocompromised and some elderly patients. A papulovesicular rash is particularly evident in the groin and perineum areas (upper/inner thigh, vulva/scrotal area). Secondary skin changes include crusting and scaling, and are usually evident at the fringes of the reaction. Erosions and frank denudation of the skin may be more common with incontinence associated with feces. The distribution of the dermatitis differs in men and women, as might be expected. Typically, the more severe damage in male patients occurs on the posterior aspect of the penile shaft and the anterior aspect of the scrotum. More damage is seen in the lower perineal regions, such as the inner thighs and low buttocks, than in the higher perineal regions, such as the sacral/coccygeal area or groin. In women, the skin damage usually involves the vulva and groin areas, and spreads distally from those sites.

Chronic skin changes in elderly patients with long-standing incontinence include a thickened appearance of skin where moisture is allowed to maintain skin contact, and increased evidence of scaling and crusting. The thickened appearance of the skin is similar to the changes seen in peristomal skin of patients with urinary diversions or ileostomies who have pouches with too large an aperture, allowing the urine or fecal effluent to pool around the stoma. This skin is overhydrated and easily abraded, with minimal friction. The reaction is notable at the coccyx, scrotum, and vulva. In a cognitively impaired nursing home sample,[134] there was also evidence of excoriation from patients' scratching at the affected sites. This provides early clinical validation of the symptom of itching in perineal dermatitis.

In many cases, partial-thickness ulcers are present over the sacral/coccygeal area and medial buttocks region, close to the gluteal fold. Although these lesions present in a typical pressure ulcer location, the underlying etiology may be the effects of incontinence on the skin. There are some characteristics of these partial-thickness ulcers that assist in differentiating them from true pressure-induced skin trauma. First, the lesions tend to be multiple. The ulcers are almost always partial-thickness lesions. The lesions may or may not be directly over a bony prominence, and, finally, the lesions are typically surrounded by other characteristics of perineal dermatitis (e.g., diffuse blanchable erythema). When caring for patients who are incontinent of urine and feces, healthcare providers are faced with the challenge of preventing perineal dermatitis and pressure ulceration as a result of the decreased tissue tolerance to trauma. True pressure ulcers result from compression of the soft tissue between the bony prominence and the external surface. When moisture, urine, and feces have caused maceration and overhydration of the epidermis, the skin and tissues are less tolerant of the pressure force. Stage II pressure ulcers and partial-thickness skin lesions, such as abrasions, are most commonly attributed to friction and shearing forces. It is likely that incontinence plays a critical role in the development of stage II pressure ulcers.[61]

Volumes have been written about various incontinence management techniques. This discussion is meant to serve as a stepping stone to those resources available to clinicians on management of the incontinent patient. Therefore, the discussion, by necessity, is noninclusive of all management strategies and only briefly addresses several strategies most pertinent to the patient at high risk of developing a pressure ulcer and measures to protect the skin from wetness and irritants. Management of incontinence is dependent on assessment and diagnosis of the problem.

Incontinence Assessment. Assessment parameters to be addressed include history, physical examination, environmental assessment, voiding/defecation diary, laboratory studies, and other diagnostic studies. The history is critical to assessing the problem accurately. History taking should elicit information on patterns of urinary/fecal elimination and past/current management program, patterns of incontinence, characteristics of the urinary stream/fecal mass, sensation of bladder/rectal filling, and a focused review of systems and medical-surgical history.[135] The physical examination is designed to gather specific information related to bladder/rectal functioning and, thus, is limited in scope. A limited neurologic examination should provide data on the mental status and motivation of the patient/caregiver, specific motor skills, and back and lower extremities. The genitalia and perineal skin are assessed for signs of estrogenization, pelvic descent, perineal skin lesions, perineal sensation, and bulbocavernosus response in women, and penis/scrotal contents, rectal and prostate, and bulbocavernosus response in men.

The environmental assessment should include inspection of the patient's home or nursing home facility to evaluate for the presence of environmental barriers to continence. The voiding/defecation diary is the real tool for management of continence in patients without cognitive impairment. The diary provides baseline data on the problem and so provides a mechanism for determining therapy effectiveness for the future. The diary may provide valuable information for diagnostic purposes. In cognitively impaired patients, the caregiver may complete the diary, and management strategies again can be identified from the baseline data.

Laboratory tests help to rule out infections and other pathology responsible for the incontinence. Some specialized studies are helpful in further evaluation of the condition. Urodynamic studies for urinary incontinence provide valuable data related to the pathology. Even in nursing home populations, simple bedside urodynamics can be a useful clinical tool to elicit more specific data on urinary function. Management strategies for incontinence are grouped into three main areas for this discussion: behavioral management, containment strategies, and skin protection guidelines.

Incontinence Management Strategies. Patients at risk for pressure ulcer development are not candidates for all methods of behavioral management. The most successful behavioral management strategies for the frail, cognitively impaired patient typically at risk of pressure ulcer development include prompted voiding and scheduled toileting programs. Both strategies are caregiver dependent and require a motivated caregiver to be successful. Scheduled intake of fluid is an important underlying factor for both strategies.

Scheduled toileting or habit training is toileting on a planned basis. The goal is to keep the person dry by assisting him or her to void at regular intervals. There can be attempts to match the interval to the individual patient's natural voiding schedule. There is no systematic effort to motivate patients to delay voiding or to resist the urge to void. Scheduled toileting may be based on the clock (toilet the patient every 2 hours) or based on activities (toilet the patient after meals and before transferring to bed). Several studies have demonstrated improvement in continence status in some patients.[136]

Prompted voiding has been shown to be effective in dependent and cognitively impaired nursing home incontinent patients.[137,138] Prompted voiding involves use of a toileting schedule (every 2 hours) similar to habit training or scheduled toileting. Prompted voiding supplements the routine with teaching the incontinent patient to discriminate their continence status and to request toileting assistance. The three major elements in prompted voiding include monitoring the incontinent patient routinely, prompting the patient to use the toilet, and praising the patient for maintenance of continence. Prompted voiding results in 40–50% reduction in frequency of daytime incontinence, and between 25% and 33% of urinary incontinent patients in nursing homes respond to the therapy.[99,100] Both of these behavioral management strategies have the added benefit of moving the patient at routine intervals, which should relieve pressure over bony prominences and reduce the risk of pressure ulcer development by allowing reperfusion of the tissues.

Underpads and briefs may be used to protect the skin of patients who are incontinent of urine or stool. These products are designed to absorb moisture, wick the wetness away from the skin, and maintain a quick-drying interface with the skin. Studies with both infants and adults demonstrate that products designed to present a quick-drying surface to the skin and to absorb moisture do keep the skin drier and are associated with a lower incidence of dermatitis. It is important to note that the critical feature is the ability to absorb moisture and present a quick-drying surface, not whether the product is disposable or reusable. Regardless of the product chosen, containment strategies imply the need for a check and change schedule for the incontinent patient so that wet linens and pads may be removed in a timely manner. Underpads are not as tight or constricting as briefs. Kemp[61] suggests alternating the use of underpads and briefs if the skin irritation is thought to be related to the occlusive nature of the brief. Her recommendations echo the early work of Willis[139] on warm water immersion syndrome, who found that the effects of water on the skin could be reversed and tempered by simply allowing the skin to dry out between wet periods. Use of briefs when the patient is up in a chair, ambulating, or visiting another department and use of underpads when the patient is in bed is one suggestion for combining the strengths of both products.

External collection devices may be more effective with male patients. External catheters or condom catheters are devices applied to the shaft of the penis to direct the urine away from the body to a collection device. Newer models of external catheters are self-adhesive and easy to apply. A key concern with use of external collection devices is routine removal of the product and inspection and hygiene of the skin.

There are special containment devices for fecal incontinence, as well. Fecal incontinence collectors consist of a self-adhesive skin barrier attached to a drainable pouch. Application of the device is somewhat dependent on the skill of the clinician, and the patient should be put on a routine for changing the pouch prior to leakage to facilitate success. The skin barrier provides a physical obstacle to the stool on the skin and helps to prevent dermatitis and associated skin problems. In fact, skin barrier wafers without an attached pouch can be useful in protecting the skin from feces or urine.

Use of moisturizers for dry skin and use of lubricants for reduction in friction injuries is recommended in clinical practice guidelines and by expert panels. Moisture barriers protect the skin from the effects of moisture. Although the recommendation is made to use products to provide a moisture barrier, the reader is cautioned that the recommendation is derived from usual practice and professional standards, and it is not research based. The success of the particular product is linked to how it is formulated and the hydrophobic properties of the product.[61] Generally, pastes are thicker and more repellent of moisture than are ointments. A quick evaluation is the ease with which the product can be removed with water during routine cleansing. If the product comes off the skin with just routine cleansing, it probably is not an effective barrier to moisture. Use of mineral oil for cleansing some of the heavier barrier products, such as zinc oxide paste, will ease removal from the skin.

The role of incontinence as a risk factor in predicting pressure ulcer formation is somewhat unclear. From a pathophysiologic perspective, creating a skin environment favorable to friction and abrasion makes incontinence a key risk

factor for those persons with additional risk for pressure ulcer development. When caring for the incontinent patient, health-care providers must address prevention by assessment and treatment of transient causes of the condition. Systematic assessment is the key to defining management strategies. Assessment includes the parameters of patient history, physical examination, environment, voiding/defecation diary, laboratory studies, and other diagnostic studies. Measures to manage incontinence include caregiver-dependent behavioral management therapies of scheduled toileting and prompted voiding, containment devices and products, and skin protection using barriers.

Skin Hygiene Interventions. Skin hygiene interventions involve daily skin hygiene and skin cleansing after fecal or urinary incontinent episodes. The older adult's skin is less tolerant of the drying effects of soap and hot water. Use of warm water and a mild soap (if any soap at all) can limit skin drying. Daily bathing is not necessary for skin health in older adults. Use of a schedule of twice weekly or every other day bathing or showering is sufficient for older adults. Daily cleansing of the feet, axilla, and perineal areas is appropriate, but daily showers or baths can be damaging to the skin. Use of solutions designed for incontinence care cleansing can be protective of the skin and can decrease the time and energy involved in postincontinent episode cleansing. These commercially available cleansers include surfactants as ingredients. The surfactants make the removal of urine and stool residue easier, with less abrasiveness. Every attempt should be made to cleanse the perineal skin immediately after an incontinent episode to limit the amount of contact time between the urine or stool and the skin.

Skin Maintenance Interventions. Skin maintenance interventions involve actions to prevent skin breakdown and actions to promote healthy skin. Maintaining skin lubrication is an important skin maintenance intervention. Use of moisturizers on a routine basis can prevent skin drying and cracking. Application of moisturizers immediately after bathing or showering helps to remoisturize and lubricate the skin. There are three main types of moisturizers—lotions, creams, and ointments. Lotions have the highest water content and, therefore, must be reapplied more frequently to be effective. Creams are mixtures of oil and water and, for best results, should be applied 4 times a day. Ointments (generally lanolin or petrolatum bases) have the lowest water content, are the most occlusive, and have the longest duration of moisturizing action. Special attention to moisturizing the lower legs and feet is often needed to compensate for decreased perfusion and diminished skin health in these areas.

Outcome Measures

The most appropriate outcome measures to evaluate the effectiveness of prevention programs are incidence and prevalence rates. When a prevention program is successful, the organization's incidence of pressure ulcer development should decrease (if appropriate) or remain at a low level.

Incidence and prevalence data should be risk-adjusted by using risk-stratification techniques when gathering data. This will allow comparison of data with other health-care facilities for benchmarking and adequate evaluation of prevention programs as case-mix of the organization varies over time. If a patient already has a pressure ulcer, a successful outcome for pressure ulcer prevention is no further areas of skin breakdown. Again, risk-stratification techniques should be used so that data can be compared with other facilities and so that severity of pressure ulcers can be evaluated accurately.

Referral Criteria

Referral criteria for pressure ulcer prevention programs relate to the need for an interdisciplinary approach to prevention of pressure ulcers. Referrals assist with appropriate management of particular risk factors for developing pressure ulcers. Use referral in the following circumstances:

- Nutritional consultation for patients determined at risk for malnutrition or with nutritional concerns
- Enterostomal therapy or continence nurse (or clinical specialist in this area) consultation for patients with urinary or fecal incontinence
- Physical therapy for assistance with correct positioning in seated individuals

Self-Care Teaching Guidelines

Patient's and caregiver's instruction in self care must be individualized to specific pressure ulcer development risk factors, the individual patient's learning style and coping mechanisms, and the ability of the patient/caregiver to perform procedures. These general self-care teaching guidelines must be individualized for each patient and caregiver. In teaching prevention guidelines to caregivers, it is particularly important to use return demonstration by the caregiver as evaluation of learning. Observing the caregiver performing turning maneuvers, repositioning, managing incontinence, and providing general skin care can be enlightening and provides the context in which the clinician provides support and follow-up education. Exhibit 16-7 provides general self-care teaching guidelines.

REVIEW QUESTIONS

1. According to the available evidence, when should risk assessment for pressure ulcers be conducted in the nursing home setting? The home care setting? The acute care setting?
2. Which of the following extrinsic risk factors decrease the tissue tolerance to pressure?
   a. shear, friction, and moisture
   b. nutrition, age, psychologic issues, and temperature
   c. immobility, inactivity, and loss of sensation
   d. time of pressure, duration of pressure, and compression force

3. Which of the following statements best defines prevalence?
   a. The number of new and old cases at any given point in time requires only one observation with one specific population.
   b. Determination of the rate at which cases develop requires repeated observations on one specific population.
   c. The number of new cases observed over a period of time on one specific population.
   d. The number of old cases at any given point in time requires only one observation with one specific population.
4. A stage II pressure ulcer is best defined as which of the following?
   a. nonblanchable erythema of intact skin
   b. lesions involving only the epidermis and dermis
   c. lesions involving the epidermis, dermis, and subcutaneous tissue extending down to, but not through, the fascia
   d. lesions involving the epidermis, dermis, subcutaneous tissue, and extending to muscle, bone, joint, and tendon
5. The clinician is asked to recommend a support surface for P.L., who has three pressure sores: one on the sacral/coccygeal area, one on the left greater trochanter, and one on the right ischial tuberosity. The ulcers range in severity from clean, healing stage II on the sacral/coccygeal area to necrotic stage III on the left trochanter and clean stage IV on the right ischial tuberosity. Which of the following is the MOST appropriate support surface choice?
   a. a foam gel combination mattress
   b. an alternating air mattress
   c. a mattress replacement
   d. a low-air-loss bed
6. Friction causes what type of skin damage?
   a. superficial abrasion and damage to the epidermis
   b. full-thickness skin loss
   c. skin tears with dermal involvement
   d. stage III pressure ulceration

RESOURCES

National Pressure Ulcer Advisory Panel
http://www.npuap.org

Wound Ostomy Continence Society
http://www.wocn.org

Centers for Medicare and Medicaid Services
Tag F314 Guidance to Surveyors: Pressure Ulcers. Interpretive guidelines: Pressure ulcers. CMS Manual System, Pub 100–07 State Operations, Provider Certification. Centers for Medicare & Medicaid Services, Nov. 12, 2004. On-line: www.cms.hhs.gov/manuals/pm_trans/R4SOM.pdf

EXHIBIT 16-7   Self-Care Teaching Guidelines

Self-Care Guidelines Specific to Pressure Ulcer Prevention	Instructions Given (Date/Initials)	Demonstration *or* Review of Material (Date/Initials)	Return Demonstration *or* States Understanding (Date/Initials)
1. Identification of specific risk factors for pressure ulcer development			

2. Immobility, inactivity, and decreased sensory perception strategies
  a. Passive repositioning
    (1) Demonstrates one-person turning			

(2) Demonstrates two-person turning			
(3) Frequency of turning/repositioning			
(4) Full shifts in position versus small shifts in position			
(5) Avoidance of 90° side-lying position, demonstrates 30° side-lying position			
(6) Passive range of motion exercises and frequency			
b. Pillow bridging (1) Use of pillows to protect heels			
(2) Pillows between bony prominences			
c. Pressure-reducing/relieving support surface (1) Management of support surface in use			
(2) Devices for sitting			
(3) Up in chair for _____ hour(s), _____ time(s) per day			

3. Nutrition strategies
  a. Provide adequate nutrition
    (1) Small frequent (six meals a day) high-calorie/high-protein meals			

(2) Nutritional supplements provided. Give ___oz of _____ supplement ___ times per day.			
b. Provide adequate hydration (1) Eight 8-oz glasses of noncaffeine fluids per day unless contraindicated			
c. Provide general multivitamin as needed			
4. Friction and shear strategies a. Use of turning and draw sheets			
b. Use of cornstarch, lubricants, pad protectors, thin film dressings, or hydrocolloid dressings over friction risk sites			
c. General skin care (1) Skin cleansing			
(2) Skin moisturizing (use _____ product on _____ areas of skin, _____ times a day)			

(Continued)

EXHIBIT 16-7 *(Continued)*

Self-Care Guidelines Specific to Pressure Ulcer Prevention	Instructions Given (Date/Initials)	Demonstration *or* Review of Material (Date/Initials)	Return Demonstration *or* States Understanding (Date/Initials)
5. Moisture-incontinence management strategies a. Use of absorbent products (1) Pad when lying in bed			
(2) Brief or panty pad when up in chair or walking			
b. Use of ointments, creams, and skin barriers prophylactically in perineal and perianal areas (use _____ product on perineal/perianal areas of skin, _____ times a day)			
c. Use of behavioral management strategies for incontinence (1) Scheduled toileting: toilet every _____ hours			
(2) Prompted voiding			
d. General skin care (1) Skin cleansing			
(a) Cleanser: _____			
(b) Soap: _____			
(c) Frequency: _____			
(2) Skin moisturizing (use _____ product(s) on _____ areas of skin, _____ times a day)			
(3) Skin inspection daily			
6. Importance of follow-up with health-care provider			

Comprehensive Listing of Clinical Practice Guidelines and Quality Indicators:

- Preventing Pressure Ulcers. Patient Guide No. 3. U.S. Department of Health and Human Services. Public Health Service. AHCPR. AHCPR Publication No. 92–0048. May 1992.
- Pressure Ulcers in Adults: Prediction and Prevention. Quick Reference Guide for Clinicians No. 3. U.S. Department of Health and Human Services. Public Health Service. AHCPR. AHCPR Publication No. 92–0050.
- Pressure Ulcers in Adults: Prediction and Prevention. Clinical Practice Guideline No. 3. U.S. Department of Health and Human Services. Public Health Service. AHCPR. AHCPR Publication No. 92–0047. May 1992.
- Bergstrom, NA, Bennett, MA, Carlson, CE, et al. Treatment of Pressure Ulcers. Clinical Practice Guideline. U.S. Department of Health and Human Services. AHCPR. AHCPR Publication No. 95–0652, 1994.
- Statement on Pressure Ulcer Prevention, 1992. National Pressure Ulcer Advisory Panel (NPUAP). www.npuap.org
- NPUAP Statement on Reverse Staging of Pressure Ulcers 2000. National Pressure Ulcer Advisory Panel. www.npuap.org
- Minimum Data Set-2 (MDS-2) & Skin Ulcer Assessment. National Pressure Ulcer Advisory Panel. www.npuap.org

- Stage I Assessment in Darkly Pigmented Skin, 1998. National Pressure Ulcer Advisory Panel. www.npuap.org
- Laouri, Mittman, et al., Developing Quality and Utilization Review Criteria for Pressure Ulcers in Adults: Phase II Final Report, March 1995. RAND. PM–403–AHCPR.
- American Medical Directors Association. Pressure Ulcers. Clinical Practice Guideline. 1996.
- American Medical Directors Association (AMDA). Pressure Ulcer Therapy Companion. Clinical Practice Guideline. 1999.
- Registered Nurses Association of Ontario. Risk Assessment & Prevention of Pressure Ulcers. Nursing Best Practice Guideline. 2002 Jan.
- Registered Nurses Association of Ontario. Assessment & Management of Stage I to IV Pressure Ulcers. Nursing Best Practice Guideline. 2002 Aug.
- Folkedahl, B, Frantz, R, Goode, C. Treatment of Pressure ulcers. The University of Iowa's Gerontology Nursing Interventions Research Center; 2002 Aug. (Evidence-Based Protocol).
- Folkedahl, B, Frantz, R, and Goode, C. Prevention of Pressure Ulcers. The University of Iowa Gerontological Nursing Interventions Research Center, Research Development and Dissemination Core, 1997.

- National Pressure Ulcer Advisory Panel. Cuddigan, J, Ayello, E, Sussman, C (Eds). 2001. Pressure Ulcers in America: Prevalence, Incidence, and Implications for the Future. Reston, VA: NPUAP.
- Consortium for Spinal Cord Medicine. Pressure Ulcer Prevention and Treatment following Spinal Cord Injury: A Clinical Practice Guideline for Health Care Professionals. 2000; Paralyzed Veterans of America, Consortium for Spinal Cord Medicine.

REFERENCES

1. Bergstrom N, Bennett MA, Carlson CE, et al. Treatment of pressure ulcers. Clinical Practice Guideline No. 15. Agency for Health Care Research and Quality (AHRQ), formerly known as the Agency for Health Care Policy and Research (AHCPR) Publication No. 95–0652. Rockville, MD: AHRQ, U.S. Public Health Service (PHS), U.S. Department of Health and Human Services (DHHS); December 1994.
2. Whittington KT, Briones R. National prevalence and incidence study: 6-year sequential acute care data. Adv Skin Wound Care. 2004;17(9):490–4.
3. Stotts NA, Deosaransingh K, Roll FJ, Newman J. Underutilization of pressure ulcer risk assessment in hip fracture patients. Adv Wound Care 1998;11(1):32–83273.
4. Baumgarten M, Margolis D, Berlin JA, Strom BL, Garino J, et al. Risk factors for pressure ulcers among elderly hip fracture patients. Wound Repair Regen 2003;11(2):96–103.
5. Fuhrer MJ, Garber SL, Rintala DH, et al. Pressure ulcers in community-resident persons with spinal cord injury: Prevalence and risk factors. Arch Phys Med Rehabil 1993;74:1172–7.
6. National Pressure Ulcer Advisory Panel. Cuddigan J, Ayello E, Sussman C, eds. Pressure Ulcers in America: Prevalence, Incidence, and Implications for the Future. Reston, VA: NPUAP, 2001.
7. Coleman EA, Martau JM, Lin MK, Kramer AM. Pressure ulcer prevalence in long-term nursing home residents since the implementation of OBRA '87. J Am Geriatr Soc 2002;50:728–732.
8. Berlowitz DR, Bezerra HQ, Brandeis GH, Kader B, Anderson JJ. Are we improving the quality of nursing home care: The case of pressure ulcers. J Am Geriatr Soc 2000;48(1):59–62.
9. Bergstrom N, Braden B. A prospective study of pressure sore risk among institutionalized elderly. J Am Geriatr Soc 1992;40(8):747–758.
10. Spoelhof GD, Ide K. Pressure ulcers in nursing home patients. Amer Fam Phys 1993;47:1207–1215.
11. Ferrell BA, Josephson K, Vorvid P, Alcorn H. Pressure ulcers among patients admitted to home care. J Am Geriatr Soc 2000;48:1042–1047.
12. Bergquist S. Pressure ulcer prediction in older adults receiving home health care: Implications for use with the OASIS. Adv Wound Care 2003;16–132–9.
13. Margolis DJ, Knauss J, Bilker W, Baumgarten M. Medical conditions as risk factors for pressure ulcers in an outpatient setting. Age Ageing 2003;32(3):259–64.
14. Baumgarten M, Margolis D, van Doorn C, Gruber-Baldini AL, Hebel JR, Zimmerman S, Magaziner J. Black/White differences in pressure ulcer incidence in nursing home residents. J Am Geriatr Soc 2004;52(8):1293–8.
15. Hunter SM, Langemo DK, Olson B, et al. The effectiveness of skin care protocols for pressure ulcers. Rehabil Nurs 1995;20(5):250–255.
16. Schue RM, Langemo DK. Pressure ulcer prevalence and incidence and a modification of the Braden Scale for a rehabilitation unit. J Wound Ostomy Continence Nurs 1998;25(1):36–43.
17. Hunter SM, Cathcart Silberberg T, Langemo DK, et al. Pressure ulcer prevalence and incidence in a rehabilitation hospital. Rehabil Nurs 1992;17(5):239–242.
18. Baggerly J, DiBlasi M. Pressure sores and pressure sore prevention in a rehabilitation setting: Building information for improving outcomes and allocating resources. Rehabil Nurs 1996;21(6):321–325.
19. Waters RL, Meyer PR Jr, Adkins RH, Felton D. Emergency, acute, and surgical management of spine trauma. Arch Phys Med Rehabil 1999;80(11):1383–1390.
20. Garber SL, Rintala DH, Hart KA, Fuhrer MJ. Pressure ulcer risk in spinal cord injury: Predictors of ulcer status over 3 years. Arch Phys Med Rehabil 2000;81(4):465–471.
21. Eastwood EA, Hagglund KJ, Ragnarsson KT, Gordon WA, Marino RJ. Medical rehabilitation length of stay and outcomes for persons with traumatic spinal cord injury 1990–1997. Arch Phys Med Rehabil 1999;80(11):1457–1463.
22. Department of Health and Human Services. Objective 1–16. In: Healthy People 2010. Washington, DC: DHHS, 2000.
23. Waite D. Caregiver guilty in fatal neglect of patient's bedsores. The Honolulu Advertiser, Saturday, October 28, 2000.
24. Daniel RK, Priest DL, Wheatley DC. Etiologic factors in pressure sores: An experimental model. Arch Phys Med Rehabil 1981;62(10):492–498.
25. Kosiak M. Etiology and pathology of ischemic ulcers. Arch Phys Med Rehabil 1959;40:62–69.
26. Reuler JB, Cooney TG. The pressure sore: Pathophysiology and principles of management. Ann Intern Med 1981;94:661.
27. Seiler WD, Stahelin HB. Recent findings on decubitus ulcer pathology: Implications for care. Geriatrics 1986;41:47–60.
28. Witkowski JA, Parish LC. Histopathology of the decubitus ulcer. J Am Acad Dermatol 1982;6:1014–1021.
29. Lindan O, Greenway RM, Piazza JM. Pressure distributor on the surface of the human body. Arch Phys Med Rehabil 1965;46:378.
30. Scales JT. Pressure on the patient. In: Kenedi RN, Cowden JM, eds. Bedsore Biomechanics. Baltimore: University Park Press, 1976.
31. Parish LC, Witkowski JA, Crissey JT. The Decubitus Ulcer. New York: Masson Publishing, 1983.
32. Slater H. Pressure Ulcers in the Elderly. Pittsburgh, PA: Synapse Publications, 1985.
33. Walker PM. Ischemial reperfusion injury in skeletal muscle. Ann Vasc Surg 1991;5(4):399–402.
34. Hernandez-Maldonado JJ, Teehan E, Franco CD, Duran WN, Hobson RW. Superoxide anion production by leukocytes exposed to post-ischemic skeletal muscle. J Cardiovasc Surg 1992;33:695–699.
35. Landis EM. Micro-injection studies of capillary blood pressure in human skin. Heart 1930;15:209.
36. Husain T. An experimental study of some pressure effects on tissues, with reference to the bedsore problem. J Pathol Bacterio 1953;66:347–358.
37. Salcido R, et al. Histopathology of decubitus ulcers as a result of sequential pressure sessions in a computer-controlled fuzzy rat model. Adv Wound Care 1993;7(5):40.
38. Kosiak M, Kubicek WG, Olsen M, Danz JN, Kottke FJ. Evaluation of pressure as a factor in the production of ischial ulcers. Arch Phys Med Rehabil 1958;39:623.
39. Edberg EL, Cerny K, Stauffer ES. Prevention and treatment of pressure sores. Phys Ther 1973;53:246–252.
40. Bennett MA. Report of the task force on the implications for darkly pigmented intact skin in the prediction and prevention of pressure ulcers. Adv Wound Care 1995;8(6):34–35.
41. Graves DJ. Stage I in ebony complexion. Decubitus Letter to the Editor 1990;3(4):4.
42. Parish LC, Witkowski JA, Crissey JT, eds. The Decubitis Ulcer in Clinical Practice. Berlin, Germany: Springer-Verlag, 1997.
43. Whittington K, Patrick M, Roberts JL. A national study of pressure ulcer prevalence and incidence in acute care hospitals. J WOCN 2000;27(4):209–215.
44. Barczak CA, Barnett RI, Childs EJ, Bosley LM. Fourth national pressure ulcer prevalence survey. Adv Wound Care 1997;10(4):18–26.
45. Knight DB, Scott H. Contracture and pressure necrosis. Ostomy/Wound Manage 1990;26(1):60–67.
46. Shea JD. Pressures sores: Classification and management. Clin Orthop 1975;112:89–100.
47. NPUAP Staging Report. 11/2003. National Pressure Ulcer Advisory Panel (NPUAP). www.npuap.org. http://www.npuap.org/positn6.html. Accessed 12-20-05.
48. Panel for the Prediction and Prevention of Pressure Ulcers. Pressure Ulcers in Adults: Prediction and Prevention. Clinical Practice Guideline No. 3. AHRQ Publication No. 92–0047. Rockville, MD: AHRQ, PHS, DHHS; 1992.
49. Maklebust J. Pressure ulcer staging systems: NPUAP Conference Proceedings. Adv Wound Care 1995;8(4):28–11–28–14.

50. Ankrom MA, Bennett RG, Sprigle S, Langemo D, Black JM, Berlowitz DR, Lyder CH; National Pressure Ulcer Advisory Panel. Pressure-related deep tissue injury under intact skin and the current pressure ulcer staging systems. Adv Skin Wound Care 2005 Jan–Feb;18(1):35–42.

51. Allman RM. Pressure ulcers among the elderly. N Engl J Med 1989;320:850.

52. Braden BJ, Bergstrom N. A conceptual schema for the study of etiology of pressure sores. Rehabil Nurs 1987;12(1):8–12.

53. Bergstrom N, Demuth PJ, Braden BJ. A clinical trial of the Braden Scale for predicting pressure sore risk. Nurs Clin North Am 1987;22:417–428.

54. Exton-Smith AN, Sherwin RW. The prevention of pressure sores: Significance of spontaneous bodily movements. Lancet 1961;2:1124–1126.

55. Allman RM, Goode PS, Patrick MM, et al. Pressure ulcer risk factors among hospitalized patients with activity limitations. JAMA 1995;273:865–870.

56. Curry K, Casady L. The relationship between extended periods of immobility and decubitus ulcer formation in the acutely spinal cord injured individual. J Neurosci Nurs 1992;24:185–189.

57. Hammond MC, Bozzacco VA, Stiens SA, et al. Pressure ulcer incidence on a spinal cord injury unit. Adv Wound Care 1994;7(6):57–60.

58. Reichel SM. Shearing force as a factor in decubitus ulcers in paraplegics. JAMA 1958;166:762–763.

59. Bennett L, Kavner D, Lee BY, Trainor FS. Skin stress and blood flow in sitting paraplegic patients. Arch Phys Med Rehabil 1984;65(4):186–190.

60. Dinsdale JM. Decubitus ulcers: Role of pressure and friction in causation. Arch Phys Med Rehabil 1974;55:147–153.

61. Kemp MG. Protecting the skin from moisture and associated irritants. J Gerontol Nurs 1994;20(9):8–14.

62. Bates-Jensen B. Incontinence management. In: Parish LC, Witkowski JA, Crissey JT, eds. The Decubitus Ulcer in Clinical Practice. Berlin, Germany: Springer-Verlag, 1997, pp. 189–199.

63. Berg RW, Milligan MC, Sarbaugh FC. Association of skin wetness and pH with diaper dermatitis. Pediatr Dermatol 1994;11:18–20.

64. Zimmerer RE, Lawson KD, Calvert CJ. The effects of wearing diapers on skin. Pediatr Dermatol 1986;3:95–101.

65. Buckingham KW, Berg RW. Etiologic factors in diaper dermatitis: The role of feces. Pediatr Dermatol 1986;3:107–112.

66. Maklebust J, Magnan MA. Risk factors associated with having a pressure ulcer: A secondary data analysis. Adv Wound Care 1994;7(6):25–42.

67. Pinchcovsky-Devin G, Kaminsky MV Jr. Correlation of pressure sores and nutritional status. J Am Geriatr Soc 1986;34:435–440.

68. Bobel LM. Nutritional implications in the patient with pressure sores. Nurs Clin North Am 1987;22:379–390.

69. Bergstrom N, Braden B. A prospective study of pressure sore risk among institutionalized elderly. J Am Geriatr Soc 1992;40:747–758.

70. Allman RM, Laprade CA, Noel LB, et al. Pressure sores among hospitalized patients. Ann Intern Med 1986;105:337–342.

71. Jones PL, Millman A. Wound healing and the aged patient. Nurs Clin North Am 1990;25:263–277.

72. Eaglestein WH. Wound healing and aging. Clin Geriatr Med 1989;5:183.

73. Versluysen M. Pressure sores in elderly patients: The epidemiology related to hip operations. J Bone Joint Surg Br 1985;67:10–13.

74. Anderson TP, Andberg MM. Psychosocial factors associated with pressure sores. Arch Phys Med Rehabil 1979;60:341–346.

75. Vidal J, Sarrias M. An analysis of the diverse factors concerned with the development of pressure sores in spinal cord patients. Paraplegia 1991;29:261–267.

76. Norton D, McLaren R, Exton-Smith NA. An Investigation of Geriatric Nursing Problems in Hospitals. Edinburgh, Scotland: Churchill-Livingstone, 1962.

77. Norton D. Calculating the risk: Reflections on the Norton Scale. Decubitus 1989;2(3):24–31.

78. Gosnell DJ. Pressure sore risk assessment: A critique. I: The Gosnell Scale. Decubitus 1989;2(3):32–39.

79. Gosnell DJ. Pressure sore risk assessment: A critique. II. Analysis of risk factors. Decubitus 1989;2(3):40–43.

80. Braden B, Bergstrom N. Clinical utility of the Braden Scale for predicting pressure sore risk. Decubitus 1989;2(3):44–51.

81. Bergstrom N, Braden B, Kemp M, Champagne M, Ruby, E. Multi-site study of incidence of pressure ulcers and the relationship between risk level, demographic characteristics, diagnoses, and prescription of preventive interventions. J Am Geriatr Soc 1996;44(1):22–30.

82. Perneger TV, Heliot C, Rae AC, et al. Hospital-acquired pressure ulcers: Risk factors and use of preventive devices. Arch Int Med 1998;158:1940–1945.

83. Schoonhoven L, Haalboom JR, Bousema MT, Algra A, Grobbee DE, et al. Prospective cohort study of routine use of risk assessment scales for prediction of pressure ulcers. BMJ 2002;325(7368):797.

84. Perneger TV, Rae AC, Gaspoz JM, Borst F, et al. Screening for pressure ulcer risk in an acute care hospital: Development of a brief bedside scale. J Clin Epidemiol 2002;55(5):498–504.

85. Gunningberg L, Lindholm C, Carlsson M, Sjoden PO. Reduced incidence of pressure ulcers in patients with hip fractures: A 2-year follow-up of quality indicators. International Soc for Quality in Health Care 2001;13(5):399–407.

86. Fife C, Otto G, Capsuto EG, et al, Incidence of pressure ulcers in a neurologic intensive care unit. Crit Care Med 2001;29(2):283–290.

87. Lewicki LJ, Mion LC, Secic M. Sensitivity and specificity of the Braden Scale in the cardiac surgical population. J WOCN 2000;27(1):36–41.

88. Frantz R, Baranoski S Pressure ulcer prevention programs in various settings: What works? What doesn't. In: National Pressure Ulcer Advisory Panel. Cuddigan J, Ayello EA, Sussman C, eds. Pressure Ulcers in America: Prevalence, Incidence, and Implications for the Future. Reston, VA: NPUAP, 2001.

89. Ayello EA, Braden BJ How and why to do pressure ulcer risk assessment. Adv Skin Wd Care 2002;15(3):125–131.

90. Ayello EA, Preventing pressure ulcers and skin tears. In: Mezey M, Fulmer T, Abraham I, Zwicker, DA, eds. Geriatric Nursing Protocols for Best Practice. New York: Springer Publishing Company, 2003, pp. 165–184.

91. Lyder CH, Shannon R, Empleo-Frazier O, McGeHee D, White CA. A comprehensive program to prevent pressure ulcers in long term care: Exploring costs and outcomes. Ostomy Wound Manage 2002;48(4):52–62.

92. Xakellis GC, Frantz RA, Lewis A, Harvey P. Cost-effectiveness of an intensive pressure ulcer prevention protocol in long-term care. Adv Wd Care 1998;11(1): 22–29.

93. Bates-Jensen BM, Cadogan M, Jorge J, Schnelle JF. Standardized quality-assessment system to evaluate pressure ulcer care in the nursing home. J Am Geriatr Soc 2003;51:1195–1202.

94. Defloor T, Grypdonck MF. Pressure ulcers: Validation of two risk assessment scales. J Clin Nurs 2005;14(3):373–82.

95. Bergquist S. Frantz RA. Braden scale: Validity in community-based older adults receiving home health care. Appl Nurs Re 2001;14(1):36–43.

96. Ferrell BA, Josephson K, Norvid P, Alcorn H. Pressure ulcers among patients admitted to home care. J Am Geriatr Soc 2000;48(9):1042–7.

97. Bergstrom N, Braden BJ, Boynton P, Bruch S. Using a research-based assessment scale in clinical practice. Nurs Clin North Am 1995;30:539.

98. Seiler WO, Allen S, Stahelin HB. Influence of the 30 degrees laterally inclined position and the "super soft" 3-piece mattress on skin oxygen tension on areas of maximum pressure: Implications for pressure sores prevention. Gerontology 1986;32:158–166.

99. Lowthian PT. Practical nursing: Turning clock system to prevent pressure sores. Nurs Mirror 1979;148(21):30–31.

100. Smith AM, Malone JA. Preventing pressure ulcers in institutionalized elders: Assessing the effects of small, unscheduled shifts in body position. Decubitus 1990;3(4):20–24.

101. Defloor T, DeBacquer D, Grydonck MH. The effects of various combinations of turning and pressure reducing devices on the incidence of pressure ulcers. Int J Nurs Stud 2005;42(1):37–46.

102. Wound Ostomy Continence Nurses Society (WOCNS). Guidelines for prevention and management of pressure ulcers. WOCN Clinical Practice Guideline Series, 2003.

103. Krouskop TA, Garber SL. Interface pressure confusion. Decubitus 1989;2:8.

104. Cullum N, McInnes E, Bell-Syer SE, Legood R. Support surfaces for pressure ulcer prevention. Cochrane Database Syst Rev 2004;(3):CD001735.

105. Theaker C, Kuper M, Soni N. Pressure ulcer prevention in intensive care—a randomised control trial of two pressure-relieving devices. Anaesthesia 2005;60(4) 395–9.

106. Jolley DJ, Wright R, McGowan S, Hickey MG, et al. Preventing pressure ulcers with the Australian Medical Sheepskin: An open-label randomised controlled trial. Med J Aust 2004;180(7):324–7.

107. Rosenthal MJ, Felton RM, Nastasi AE, Naliboff BD, et al. Healing of advanced pressure ulcers by a generic total contact seat: 2 randomized comparisons with low air loss bed treatments. Arch Phys Med Rehabil 2003;84(12):1733–42.

108. Geyer MJ, Brienza DM, Karg P, Trefler E, Kelsey S. A randomized control trial to evaluate pressure-reducing seat cushions for elderly wheelchair users. Adv Skin Wound Care 2001;14(3):120-9.

109. Ferrell BA, Osterweil D & Christenson P. A randomized trial of low-air-loss beds for treatment of pressure ulcers. JAMA 1993;269:494–497.

110. Mulder GD, Tara N, Seeley JE, Andrews. A study of pressure ulcer response to low air loss beds vs. conventional treatment. J Geriatr Dermatol 1993;2:87.

111. Ochs RF, Horn SD, van Rijswijk L, Pietsch C, Smout RJ. Comparison of air-fluidized therapy with other support surfaces used to treat pressure ulcers in nursing home residents. Ostomy Wound Manage 2005;51(2):38–68.

112. Pinchcovsky-Devin G, Kaminsky MV Jr. Correlation of pressure sores and nutritional status. J Am Geriatr Soc 1986;34:435–440.

113. Bobel LM. Nutritional implications in the patient with pressure sores. Nurs Clin North Am 1987;22:379–390.

114. Bergstrom N, Braden B. A prospective study of pressure sore risk among institutionalized elderly. J Am Geriatr Soc 1992;40:747–758.

115. Allman RM, Laprade CA, Noel LB, et al. Pressure sores among hospitalized patients. Ann Intern Med 1986;105:337–342.

116. Berlowitz D, Wilking S. The short term outcome of pressure sores. J Am Geriatr Soc 1990;38:748–752.

117. Hill DP, Cooper DM, Robson MC. Serum albumin is a poor prognostic factor for pressure ulcer healing in controlled clinical trials. Wounds 1994;6(5):174–178.

118. Stotts N. Nutritional parameters at hospital admission as predictors of pressure ulcer development in elective surgery. J Parenter Enter Nutr 1987;11:298–301.

119. Langer G, Schloemer G, Knerr A, Kuss O, Behrens J. Nutritional interventions for preventing and treating pressure ulcers. Cochrane Database Syst Rev 2003;(4):CD003216.

120. Stratton RJ, Ek AC, Engfer M, et al, Enteral nutritional support in prevention and treatment of pressure ulcers: A systematic review and meta-analysis. Ageing Res Rev 2005;4(3):422–450.

121. Bourdel-Marchasson I, Barateau M, Rondeau V, Dequae-Merchadou L, et al. A multi-center trial of the effects of oral nutritional supplementation in critically ill older inpatients. GAGE Group. Groupe Aquitain Geriatrique d'Evaluation. Nutrition 2000;16(1):1–5.

122. Hartgrink HH, Wille J, Konig P, et al. Pressure sores and tube feeding in patients with a fracture of the hip: A randomized clinical trial. Clin Nutrition 1998;17(6):287–292.

123. Houwing RH, Rozendaal M, Wouters-Wesseling W, et al, A randomized, double-blind assessment of the effect of nutritional supplementation on the prevention of pressure ulcers in hip-fracture patients. Clin Nutrition 2003;22(4):401–405.

124. Chernoff RS, Milton KY, Lipschitz DA. The effect of very high-protein liquid formula on decubitus ulcers healing in long-term tube fed institutionalized patients. J Am Diet Assoc 1990;90:A–130.

125. Breslow RA, Hallfrisch J, Guy DG, et al. The importance of dietary protein in healing pressure ulcers. J Am Geriatr Soc 1993;41(4):357–62.

126. Thomas DR. Issues and dilemmas in the prevention and treatment of pressure ulcers: A review. J Gerontol Medical Sciences 2001a;56A(6):M328–M340.

127. Thomas DR. Improving the outcome of pressure ulcers with nutritional interventions: A review of the evidence. Nutrition 2001b;17(2):121–125.

128. Finucane TE. Malnutrition, tube feeding and pressure sores: Data are incomplete. J Am Geriatr Soc 1995;43(4):447–451.

129. Olson B. The effects of massage for prevention of pressure ulcers. Decubitus 1989;2(4):32–37.

130. Franz RA, Gardner S. Clinical concerns: management of dry skin. Gerontol Nurs 1994;20(9):15–18,45.

131. Gosnell DJ. Assessment and evaluation of pressure sores. Nurs Clin North Am 1987;22:399–416.

132. Brown DS, Sears M. Perineal dermatitis: A conceptual framework. Ostomy/Wound Manage 1993;39(7):20–25.

133. Brown DS. Perineal dermatitis: Can we measure it? Ostomy/Wound Manage 1993;39(7):28–31.

134. Schnelle JF, Adamson GM, Cruise PA, et al. Skin disorders and moisture in incontinent nursing home residents: Intervention implications. J Am Geriatr Soc 1997;45(10):1182–1188.

135. Urinary Incontinence Guideline Panel. Urinary Incontinence in Adults: Clinical Practice Guidelines. AHRQ Publication No. 92–0038. Rockville, MD: AHRQ, PHS, DHHS, March 1992.

136. Schnelle JF, Newman DR, Fogarty T. Management of patient continence in long-term care nursing facilities. Gerontologist 1990;30:373–376.

137. Schnelle JF. Treatment of urinary incontinence in nursing home patients by prompted voiding. J Am Geriatr Soc 1990;38:356–360.

138. Ouslander JG, Schnelle JF, Uman G, et al. Predictors of successful prompted voiding among incontinent nursing home residents. JAMA 1995;273:1366–1370.

139. Willis I. The effects of prolonged water exposure on human skin. J Invest Dermatol 1973;60:166–171.

Management of Pressure by Therapeutic Positioning

Laurie M. Rappl

CHAPTER OBJECTIVES

At the completion of this chapter, the reader will be able to:

1. Explain the effect of body alignment in the sitting and recumbent positions on pressure distribution over at-risk skin sites.
2. Initiate and complete an examination and evaluation of a client with limited mobility in the sitting and recumbent positions.
3. Prescribe the best positioning device options for both sitting and recumbent situations.
4. Evaluate seating and mattress or support surface products for their benefits to client treatment.
5. Explain the potential healing benefits of proper therapeutic positioning interventions.

Therapeutic positioning is a dynamic and necessary part of the wound care prevention and management program for disabled clients. Without properly positioning a client in bed or in a sitting position, skin management care plans can be devastated by inappropriately high carrying loads on vulnerable tissues overlying bony prominences. Clients who are more sitting-dependent then ambulatory and/or who use the recumbent and sitting positions for the majority of the day are at high risk for tissue breakdown. For clients with existing pressure ulcers, proper positioning in the most active and functional positions possible, both sitting and recumbent, improves healing rates of the ulcers and helps to minimize the likelihood of recurrence.

Advances in equipment have elevated therapeutic positioning to a specialty among therapists and technology suppliers. The huge variety of equipment available and the individual needs of clients requiring specialized equipment make this a complex specialty. Although it is beyond the scope of this chapter to cover all seating and positioning topics thoroughly, it provides information on the following topics:

- Overview of the areas that the clinician should examine to determine the need for intervention
- Basics of therapeutic positioning
- How therapeutic positioning affects body system impairments
- Specifics in positioning clients with existing ulcers, both sitting and recumbent

Need for Therapeutic Positioning

Just as pressure ulcers affect patients of all ages – from pediatric to young adult, to middle-aged and elderly – the need for therapeutic positioning is necessary for all age groups.

Although the incidence rates of ulcers overlying specific bony prominences vary, it is conservative to estimate that 50% of all tissue breakdown occurs on the sacrum and the ischial tuberosities (IT's).[1,2] Sacral wounds are most often associated with the recumbent position, whereas ischial ulcers, which are located on the major weight-bearing surfaces of the sitting-dependent client, are associated with the sitting position.[3] It has been estimated that 75% of the sitting-dependent population will develop pressure ulcers. Of these, 75% will have a recurrence of that same breakdown.[4–6] Literature reports the failure rates for flap surgeries at 76%–91%.[4,5] In addition, it is standard procedure for plastic surgeons to plan for five more flap donor sites on a client before doing the first one, which confirms what is already known: Treating the symptom does not cure the problem. Therapeutic positioning, using correctly chosen equipment, plays a direct and critical role in reducing these staggering numbers.

Proper positioning has been identified as important for good health in non-wheelchair using populations. Significant amounts of resources and attention are paid to correctly position and support people who sit in their jobs even part-time, such as office workers, automobile drivers and computer users. It is reasonable to conclude, then, that disabled part-time and full-time wheelchair users and bed-bound clients are also in great need of proper support.

The human body requires support for proper postural alignment in order to perform functional activities and protect tissues from harm, both in the sitting and recumbent positions. Any disabled client who is sitting-dependent for any part of the day or night should be evaluated by a therapist experienced in positioning to ensure that the optimal position is being attained. The same is true for individuals who are recumbent with limited mobility. The more sitting-dependent and/or bed-dependent the client is, the more critical the need for proper positioning interventions. Although full-time wheelchair users are often considered the only candidates for therapeutic positioning, part-time wheelchair users who sit for relatively shorter periods of time each day are also candidates.

Reevaluation should occur when there is a significant change in condition, such as the development of a deformity, significant weight gain or loss, occurrence of tissue breakdown, or change in the client's mobility status, such as increased weakness that inhibits mobility. Reevaluation may also be necessary if current equipment breaks or is in disrepair making equipment replacement necessary, or warranties expire

Applying the Diagnostic Process to Therapeutic Positioning

The diagnostic process, which is outlined in Chapter 1, begins with the reason for referral. The clinician determines the reason for referral, medical history, and systems to review. The clinician then performs a review of systems and determines the possible related impairments, which suggest the examination strategy. After the examination, the clinician analyzes the information gathered to determine a functional diagnosis related to the need for therapeutic positioning, which guides selection of the equipment and positioning interventions required. Prognosis and expected outcome complete the process.

Reason for Referral

The reason for referral is the statement that explains why the client is seeking therapy services. This includes the medical diagnosis, pertinent medical history, and social history. The data collection process usually includes an initial interview or questionnaire that elicits information about the reason for referral, which then sets the stage for the rest of the diagnostic process.

The reason for referral gives the clinician the first clue about the positioning needs of the client. The reason may come from the referring provider and may or may not coincide with the reason the family, caregiver, or client provides for seeking positioning assistance. However, the reasons of the family, caregiver, and client should take priority. For example, the goal of the caregiver may be comfort in recum-

bent positions for an uncommunicative client, whereas the clinician may want to pursue an aggressive program to reverse contractures. The clinician's goal may be viable, but if the caregiver cannot devote the time, interest, or financial resources to an aggressive program, the clinician will have to consider less aggressive positioning goals. Reasons for therapeutic positioning can include the following:

- Decrease pain
- Increase a specific functional ability
- Increase independent mobility
- Increase ease of care for the caregiver
- Decrease risk of tissue breakdown
- Assist in healing existing tissue breakdown

The reason for referral can also be reevaluation of positioning and/or equipment due to a change in the client's condition. Examples include surgery that changes anatomical alignment such as scoliosis, weight gain or loss that changes the fit of the wheelchair, and tissue breakdown that can be caused in part by poor positioning with excessive weight bearing on one bony prominence such as the ischium.

Part of the interview process includes the social situation of the client. For example, it is necessary to consider factors such as the living situation and the client's level of independence. These factors are important for selecting the appropriate examinations and the level of complexity of equipment. For example, a client in a solid, supportive home environment with a limited number of consistent caregivers may be able to handle more complicated equipment than an individual in a group living situation with multiple caregivers. The number of hours spent sitting or lying down will indicate the risk of breakdown. Generally, long time periods in sitting or recumbent positions indicates a high risk of breakdown and the need for more care in equipment selection and training.

Medical History

The past and current medical history should be reviewed for information that would affect appropriate positioning. Comorbidities should be noted, as they will affect the choice of systems to review related to appropriate positioning. For example, pulmonary and cardiac pathologies may necessitate special positioning that provides for optimal breathing function as well as prevention or healing of pressure ulcers.

Medications also affect positioning choices. For example, antispasmodic medications would indicate that spasticity and/or abnormal movement synergies have been a problem and need to be addressed.. Other classes of medications affect cognition and alertness.

Any past surgeries or conditions that would limit the ability of the client to achieve the "ideal" sitting position or require accommodation to help the client maintain that position would be of interest, such as orthopedic procedures that affect skeletal movement. For example, spinal fixation can limit range of motion in the spine and pelvis; this could necessitate equipment that does not force the body to sit in level planes, but instead accommodates and supports a tilted pelvis or curved back posture. Another example of significant surgical history is a report of any flap or graft surgeries on the seating surface that would raise awareness of scar tissue in the area and predisposition of the tissue to ulcer recurrence.

Systems Review and Examinations

A review of systems is used to identify pathologies and system impairments that can potentially be addressed with therapeutic positioning. Pathologies and impairments that will potentially benefit from therapeutic positioning occur in the neuromuscular system, musculoskeletal system, cardiopulmonary and vascular systems, integumentary system, and psychosocial/cognitive system. Positioning can be used to compensate for changes or to promote improved function in the bed or chair. Some of these system impairments have been included in a lengthy list called the *hazards of immobility* and are well known. They include respiratory dysfunction, range of motion limitation or contractures, muscular weakness, slowing of the digestive system, and cognitive changes. Systems review also guides the choice of systems examinations that would be used. Examples of each are discussed in the following sections:

Neuromuscular System Review

Pathology of the central or peripheral nervous system leads to many impairments that affect positioning and the development of pressure ulcers. If sensation is diminished, the skin and soft tissues over bony prominences in the insensate areas of the body that are weight bearing will have an undue susceptibility to pressure ulceration. Equipment selection and positioning must protect and redistribute pressure on tissue over bony prominences in the impaired areas as much as possible. In sitting, these prominences are the ischials, sacrum, and coccyx. Bed-restricted individuals and those with poor self-repositioning abilities often develop tissue breakdown over several bony prominences, including occiput, scapula, sacrum, heels, malleoli (ankles), and trochanters (hips). The choice of a support surface or seating system, as well as instruction in proper positioning, are critical in protecting these individuals

If a client has suffered an insult to the central nervous system, such as a stroke, brain injury, or spinal cord injury, or disease of the central nervous system, such as Parkinson disease, the damage can cause spasticity and/or abnormal movement synergies, both of which can lead to impaired postural alignment. The equipment must support the body so as to distribute pressure and provide safe, secure seating and bed positioning. Proper equipment gives the client the ability to maintain postural alignment that will reduce predisposition to pressure problems while facilitating visual perception, swallowing, and social interaction. Appropriate therapeutic positioning in the chair and bed can prevent the development of irreversible muscle and joint contractures, which impair functional activities.

Individuals with degenerative diseases of the central nervous system, such as multiple sclerosis, have different needs. These persons may benefit from therapeutic positioning for postural support of weak muscles, which will prolong functional activities, conserve energy, prevent contractures, and increase comfort and safety. Equipment needs can be expected to change over time.

Most of the attention paid to individuals with diabetic neuropathy is focused on protecting the feet from injury, but diabetic neuropathy also affects positioning decisions if the individual is bed-bound or wheelchair-bound because of risk of trauma to areas that are insensate, such as the feet and hands. Also, many individuals in this group are amputees who have special support surface needs due to weight concentration over smaller body areas.

Neurologic Examination. Central nervous system damage can result in problems of motor control that involve components of the neuromuscular system. Motor control problems can include the inability to sequence movements, recruit muscles in the proper sequence, scale the activities, and adapt motor responses to changing task conditions. Impairments of neuromuscular components required for motor control should be identified by the therapist using specific tests. Areas to evaluate can include: hyperactive reflexes, abnormal muscle tone, and movement synergies. The neurologic examination identifies the impairments that can be influenced by positioning. It is beyond the scope of this book to provide examination strategies for all of these impairments, however, some examples are presented here. Additional resource information is provided at the end of the chapter.

One component commonly seen in central nervous system pathologies is hyperactive reflexes that affect postural control, for example, the asymmetric tonic neck reflex (ATNR). This reflex causes the individual to extend the extremities on the face side and flex the extremities on the occiput side when the head is rotated. Such a reflex can interfere with motor control of the upper extremities when performing functional activities. For example, this reflex can cause the client driving a motorized wheelchair with a side-mounted joystick to have difficulty controlling the device. A center-mounted joystick may solve this problem. A strong dominant ATNR will make maintaining a side-lying position very difficult, since it involves not only the upper extremities, but the trunk and lower extremities as well. The trunk and uppermost side of the body will need to be positioned to avoid triggering this hyperactive reflex. Positioning the client so that he or she can see when someone approaches without having to turn the face to look over the uppermost shoulder will also help to compensate.

Another common hyperactive reflex is symmetric tonic neck reflex (STNR), which is also influenced by head position. When the neck is flexed, the arms flex and the legs extend. When the neck is extended, the arms extend and the legs flex. The STNR must be accommodated by limiting the movement of the head so that voluntary control of the body is maintained.

Extensor thrust, which is described as uncontrolled extension of the trunk, hips, and knees, can be the result of extensor spasticity, an associated reaction, or an extensor synergy. It can be triggered by common activities, such as talking or reaching. The neurologic examination is used to determine the underlying problem and trigger for this response. Then, the clinician can assess what is needed for the client to maintain as close to a 90—95° hip angle as possible. This may be with seat and back equipment, hip belts, and lap trays that will help the client maintain a functional sitting posture. Contact of the ball of the foot on the footrest or floor can trigger a spastic reaction known as clonus. Positioning of the foot to avoid contact with the ball of the foot on the footres can decrease this uncontrolled movement.

In the supine position, another reflex, the tonic labyrinthine reflex (TLR), can be hyperactive. In this position, extensor posture is activated. This posture increases the risk of breakdown on the occiput and heels, and its presence indicates the need for repositioning so that there is flexion of the hips and knees. Usually, pillows are not stable enough to do this; an investment may have to be made in foam positioning aids specifically designed for certain positions and body parts. These products may seem more expensive than pillows, but their effectiveness outweighs the cost. Positioning devices designed for controlling the body position are described later in this chapter.

CLINICAL WISDOM

Position the individual with a strong ATNR so that he or she can visualize the entrance to the room with ease from a frontal position rather than needing to rotate the head.. This simple act will eliminate much fear and agitation. Caregivers should be instructed to approach from the noninvolved side first, and then to move to the involved side as the client learns to visually track to and beyond the midline.

Sensory Examination. Sensation can be partially or completely impaired by a central nervous system insult. For example, in a complete spinal cord lesion, there can be a complete loss of sensation below the lesion. However, if the lesion is due to a cerebral vascular accident or traumatic brain injury, the result can be an incomplete loss of sensation. A sensory examination is useful to determine the extent and type of sensory loss.

In the context of prevention and treatment of pressure ulcers with therapeutic positioning, the sense of particular interest is the ability to detect both light and deep pressure and pain on all areas of the body that are weight bearing or may come into contact with equipment. The inability to detect pain or pressure can lead to tissue breakdown because the client does not know when to shift weight to relieve pressure. For the insensate client, great care must be taken to search for and prescribe equipment that not only positions the body, but also protects insensate skin (see the section on seat cushion categories). Chapter 4 includes information on performing sensory testing, and Chapter 13 discusses pain testing.

Another important sensory loss is vision. Those clients with a visual loss on one side of the body can neglect one side, and attention must be paid to protecting the involved limbs and positioning the client to provide for maximum environmental interaction..

Musculoskeletal System Review

The musculoskeletal system is responsible for skeletal support and motor function.. Impairments of the musculoskeletal system include impairments in range of motion and muscle strength. Impairment of the musculoskeletal system can change body positions and biomechanics, resulting in the impaired ability to perform movement including activities of daily living (ADLs). Other consequences of poor postural alignment are risk to soft tissue and skeletal structures.

Equipment that accommodates for postural deformities is different than that used for clients with more intact musculoskeletal systems. Correct positioning to ensure proper body alignment and skin safety is important in sitting and recumbent positions. Impairments in range of motion and/or muscle strength directly affect the ability of the body to maintain the ideal position and shift weight to relieve pressure on the sitting area, which increase the risk of tissue breakdown. For example, a client who cannot reach 90° of hip flexion will "sacral sit" on a flexed lumber spine, putting excessive pressure on the sacrum, coccyx, and lumbar spinous processes. Equipment must be chosen that accommodates for the limitations in range by supporting the body at the angle available at the hip with a supportive cushion, possibly an angled seat, and a back rest that can be fixed to open the seat-to-back angle to match achievable hip flexion. This is called an angle-adjustable back or an open seat-back angle. Another example is a client who eats sitting up in bed or seated in a mobility base; the positioning system must support upright posture for functional use of the upper extremities, safe swallowing, and social interaction.

Muscle weakness that impairs movement is identified by a manual muscle test and mobility assessment. Weakness and poor movement abilities affect a client's ability to self-position, be mobile, and maintain correct postures. The degree and location of muscular weakness also have an impact on the choice of mobility base (such as wheelchair, scooter, recliner chair, tilt-in-space, etc.). Powered bases may be required for those clients with considerable weakness. Mobility bases are discussed more fully later in this chapter. A firm support surface is used to enhance mobility and facilitate independent repositioning of the client with weakness, thus enhancing the safety of the skin.

Clients who have had a cerebrovascular accident resulting in a hemiparesis or hemiplegia have patterns of muscle weakness on one side of the body. This imbalance predisposes the client to sit unevenly, thus overweighting one ischium and the overlying soft tissue. Spinal and pelvic malalignment also add to overload in that location. Uncorrected, spinal joint impairments such as scoliosis can ensue.

Skeletal deformities can have different etiologies, such as a traumatic deformity resulting from an accident, or an intentional deformity as a consequence of surgery. Skeletal deformities are either fixed or flexible. A flexible deformity is an impairment that can potentially be corrected by therapy and/or the selection of the proper positioning equipment. A fixed deformity, however, is a disability that is immovable and must be accommodated by the equipment. A curved leg resulting from a traumatic break to the tibia is an example of inflexible deformity that requires accommodation with equipment to compensate. Accommodation would be necessary if the curved lower leg made the level of the knees and lap uneven, causing the leg to push against the leg rest and cause pressure.

An example of a surgical deformity is a unilateral ischiectomy, which can result in an asymmetric pelvis (pelvic obliquity) and change the biomechanics of the spine from erect alignment to a curvature of the spinal structures. Seating for this client requires careful clinical decision making. The ischiectomy causes the pelvis to sit unevenly on a cushion, which requires weighting the ischials and can lead to spinal curvature or tissue breakdown on the sitting surface of the lower side, i.e., the remaining ischium A cushion that depends on femoral weight bearing may accommodate this client better than a cushion that uses ischial weight bearing If the ischiectomy resulted in a fixed pelvic obliquity, the cushion may need to be raised on one side to accommodate the tilt of the pelvis. Rather than attempting to correct the problem associated with a fixed deformity, the equipment must conform to the deformity and help to hold the client in the best functional position as close to "ideal" as possible.

Evaluation or reevaluation for seating needs should be done when there are changes in the patient condition, such as significant weight loss, which can make bony prominences that were once fairly protected much more vulnerable to the effects of pressure and shear. Significant weight gain will result in poorly fitting equipment, possibly limiting mobility and transfers, and putting skin at increased risk.

Musculoskeletal Impairments. Examinations of joint range of motion (ROM) and muscle strength should be performed to determine the contribution of each to the motor coordination problem affecting postural control. Musculoskeletal problems often develop as secondary complications following neurological lesions associated with reduced mobility or immobility. For example, a client with a recent neurologic insult can benefit from positioning to prevent the development of contractures if muscle weakness or spasticity are identified early as impairments. For the individual who has a less recent neurologic insult, the ROM and/or muscular strength component that contributes to the problem can be identified and a positioning plan developed for secondary prevention or worsening of contractures.

ROM and strength impairments are also found in patients who have impaired mobility or reduced cognitive

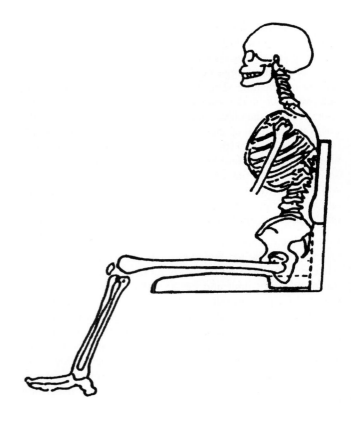

FIGURE 17-1 Ideal sitting position is approximately 95° at hip and knee, and 90°-95° at the ankle. This is a reference point only; therapists should work to position clients as close to this position as possible. (Courtesy of Span-America Medical Systems, Greenville, South Carolina.)

functions. For example, elderly patients or those with progressive neurologic diseases who have identified muscle weakness can be given support for improved postural alignment while sitting that reduces the risk of tissue breakdown by relief of pressure, shear and friction, and improves swallowing and nutrition, as well as respiratory and digestive function.

Range of Motion Examination. ROM evaluation should include the spine and pelvis, as well as the extremities. Examine the spinal curves for proper alignment in sitting, as shown in Figure 17-1. Deviations from the normal can include:

1. Limitations in the range of motion of the spine that affect the client's ability to sit upright easily. These problems should be noted as *fixed*, i.e., immovable, or *flexible*, i.e., movable or correctable. Fixed problems need to be accommodated for as a disability, whereas flexible problems should be noted as those for which the proper equipment or positioning can help To correct.
2. Limitations in movement and position of the pelvis should be evaluated for range of motion in anterior and

posterior tilt, and lateral rotation. The anterior/posterior tilt is assessed from the side. The anterior superior iliac spines (ASIS) should be roughly level with the posterior superior iliac spines (PSIS). A posterior tilt in which the PSIS are lower than the ASIS will flatten and flex the lumbar spine, decrease hip flexion, and cause the body to attain a "slouched" position. In this case, weight will be concentrated on the ITs. The thoracic spine will also flex. To stand up or to shift weight off of the ITs, the individual must be able to shift the weight of the upper body forward by tilting the pelvis forward, extending the lumbar and then the thoracic spine, and raising the neck and head. Inability to perform this motion puts the tissue over the ITs at risk for high pressure and tissue breakdown. Pelvic rotation, a twist about a vertical axis, is noted if one iliac crest sits in front of the other. A tilt to left or right in the frontal plane is termed a *pelvic obliquity*. See Exhibit 17-1 for a method of testing for pelvic obliquity.

3. Lack of ROM of hip flexion to 90° that affects the client's ability to be accommodated in a chair with a 90° seat-to-back angle. Accommodations will be needed, such as a backrest that is angled back in relation to the seat to open the seat-to-back angle, and a seat cushion that provides enough pelvic stability to keep the hips from sliding forward. A seat that tilts up in front may be helpful if used with a reclining backrest as described.

4. Knee flexion fixed at less than 90° from straight or more than 90° from straight. In either case, the legs will tend to pull the body forward from the back of the seat and out of position. Footrests that support the foot and allow the hip and knee to achieve approximately 90° flexion or the specific client's range will help to position the lower body.

5. Limitations in ankle dorsiflexion or plantarflexion or inversion/eversion ROM that affect the support of the lower extremity on the footrest. If the ankle cannot be maintained in a neutral (right angle) position with 0° of inversion/eversion, a footrest that can change angulation is necessary to accommodate the position of the foot as closely to ideal as possible.

6. Decreased or imbalanced muscular strength of the trunk and upper extremitiesWeakness of the trunk contributes to postural instability and an inability to shift weight off of the ischial on the weak side. A hypotonic or weak arm can also affect positioning, because it lacks the ability to provide support from that side.

//Mobility Examination – Recumbent. Activities performed in bed should be evaluated for movement impairments that can become the focus of the positioning intervention. Movement impairments to consider include motor coordination, motor planning, and strategies for movement in the recumbent position. Tasks to evaluate include the following: rolling right or left from supine; shifting the body from side to side; moving from sitting to supine, supine to sitting, sitting to standing (get out of bed), and standing to sitting (get into

---

EXHIBIT 17-1 Pelvic Obliquity Evaluation

Pelvic obliquity should be assessed as *fixed* or *flexible*. Examination steps follow:

1. Place the client on a firm seat with knees at 90° and feet supported.
2. Note whether one iliac crest is higher than the other.
3. Note the presence of a lateral curvature of the trunk, both with and without upper extremity support.
4. Place a support under the ischium on the lower side of the pelvis to even the iliac crests.
5. If the trunk curvature remains, and the client becomes more unstable when the arms are raised, the obliquity is fixed.
6. The fixed obliquity should then be accommodated for by building up the cushion under the higher ischium to maintain the pelvic obliquity.
7. If the trunk curvature decreases, and the client is more stable, the obliquity is flexible.
8. The flexible obliquity can be accommodated for in one of two ways:
   a. Putting the client on a firm cushion with both ischials unsupported and both femurs fully supported and at the same height, inducing a level pelvis
   b. Building up the cushion under the lower, supported ischium to even the iliac crests

---

bed); moving the body toward head of bed, and moving body toward foot of bed.

Assess for the ability and the strategy used by the client to perform transfers independently, dependently, or assisted in many combinations: bed to chair, chair to bed, commode to bed, bed to commode, and sit to stand. This will impact the choice of support surface for the client. Firm, stable support surfaces that do not move under the client make bed mobility much easier to perform for all clients.

For clients with pressure ulcers, functional mobility occasionally may be compromised in favor of a less stable surface for improved tissue load management, but this compromise is usually not necessary. Consider support surfaces that offer the preferred pressure distribution therapy, such as alternating pressure for pressure-related wounds, low-air-loss for patient with excessive perspiration, high air loss for patients with both needs, and static pressure redistribution for patients who can utilize a variety of positions. Once the pressure ulcer is closed, a non-moving support surface can be evaluated for the functional mobility of the client on the surface and its efficacy in managing tissue load through pressure redistribution.

Mobility Examination – Sitting. The purpose of the sitting evaluation is to determine the best mobility base and seating system to meet the needs of the patient for postural stability, mobility, and for safety. Many factors go into the decision regarding choice of mobility systems. Some of these include the motor status of the individual; ability to function at the speed afforded by a motorized wheelchair, including such factors as cognition and visual spatial capabilities; required mobility status; cardiovascular status; strength and endurance status; functional goals of the client or family; and method that will be used to relieve pressure on the seating surface. Other considerations in choosing the mobility base are the dependent versus independent mobility status of the individual, which includes what is easiest and safest for him or her to use. If the client does not have the physical, cognitive, or visual perceptive abilities to be safely independently mobile in a manual or power chair, other sitting equipment should be considered.

Some of the considerations in selecting a mobility base include:

- Recliner Geri-chairs are commonly used in long-term care settings, but they do not provide good support for postural alignment and are not safe for soft tissues without significant extra padding.
- If a client can self-propel, the therapist has a choice of a variety of manual chairs, depending on what limbs the client can use for mobility.
- Clients who need one or both feet to propel may best be fitted with a hemi-height wheelchair, which has a lower-than-standard seat-from-floor height. This allows clients to contact the ground firmly with the propelling foot (feet), without having to scoot the pelvis forward on the chair, which can cause shear and friction to the skin over the IT's as the client pulls the body forward with the leg. The most efficient foot propulsion can be accomplished if the client can achieve a heel-toe pattern in forward propulsion.
- A client who has the functional use of only one arm may be a good candidate for a one-arm-drive chair. However, this equipment is heavy and difficult for some weak individuals to operate.
- A client who is strong and can use both arms but not the feet to propel a wheelchair is a good candidate for a standard-height wheelchair with footrests.
- If a client has cognitive and perceptive skills, but not physical skills, a powered base, either a power wheelchair or a scooter style, may best meet mobility needs.

Shear and Friction Examination. Friction and shear are two causes of tissue breakdown that commonly occur during wheelchair propulsion, when postural changes occur while the client is seated and during transfers. Proper equipment and positioning can control trunk and pelvic movement in order to limit friction and shearing during these activities. Observe the method of transfer and movement in the wheelchair for potential risk of shear and friction. The best and safest transfer method that reduces risk factors for shear and friction should be determined, and then seating equipment should be selected to meet those requirements. For example, removable or swing-away hardware and positioning pieces can markedly facilitate transfers without shear and friction.

Signs of friction stresses are identified on the skin by elongated, reddened areas on weight-bearing surfaces, such as the sacrum or ischials. This is in contrast to signs of high pressure, which are evidenced by rounded areas over bony prominences or the shape of the object that caused the pressure. Shear causes injury to deep tissues that results in undermining of pressure ulcers or the formation of pockets of fluid or tissue damage deep to the skin.

CLINICAL WISDOM

Transfer Technique

Poor transfer technique is a major contributor to tissue breakdown, because the skin is dragged across surfaces or subjected to sudden overload when the client is set down suddenly.

Activities of Daily Living Evaluation ADLs are evaluated to determine how they affect movement that puts the client at risk for tissue breakdown. The more ADLs done in the wheelchair, such as dressing, bathing, eating, and toileting, the more the equipment will need to accommodate beyond simple positioning. For example, noncontoured seating can assist caregivers with dressing and bathing because the client can be placed in different positions to pull clothing on and off and to bathe the various body parts. Clothing is easier to pull up using noncontoured seating.

A client who is able to transfer independently and does so while performing ADLs such as toileting needs a clear path in which to move, so consider the best way based on the findings to minimize the number of extra devices, such as medial and lateral thigh supports used for positioning. These devices tend to get in the way of independent transfers and are cumbersome for caregivers in dependent transfers.

Interface Pressure Examination. Interface pressures are the pressures between the body and the support surface, measured by single-cell devices or larger, multiple-cell devices that map an entire seat or mattress surface simultaneously. Mapping devices give pictorial readouts of the pressure recorded by each cell, reported either numerically or with colors that correspond to various pressure intervals. These devices are also programmed to give the viewer information such as the total number of cells activated (possibly the amount of immersion or partial sinking of the body into the support surface), the cell with the peak pressure, and many other data points that enhance reading and use of pressure mapping. Color Plates 88 and 89 show mapping devices for sitting and recumbent applications.[CPR]

In a study conducted by the University of Pittsburgh, higher interface pressures were directly associated with a higher incidence of pressure ulcers on the sitting surfaces of the body 7 The goal of pressure reading is to determine the location and value of peak pressures on a particular client on a particular cushion. High pressures on the most vulnerable prominences (ischial, coccyx, sites of previous or current breakdown) can indicate that the cushion and client are not an appropriate match. Reducing or eliminating pressure on the ischials and coccyx is the goal of most seat cushion interventions. Reducing pressure by equalizing pressure over the entire sitting surface may be enough intervention for some clients. Other clients may require that the areas of highest risk (i.e., ischials and coccyx) record lower pressures than those at lower risk, such as the femurs; structurally, the femurs tolerate more load and can, therefore, tolerate higher pressures and carry more weight than the vulnerable ischials and coccyx.

Interface pressures are taken outside the surface of the body, and the absolute values do not equate to capillary closure pressures in the subdermal tissues. Using a finite element modeling approach, Ragan et al found interface pressures to be good indicators of subcutaneous stress8 Peak pressures and average pressures over the sitting surface typically do not vary significantly between cushions in a category, but these are the numbers that inexperienced viewers often focus on when reading mapping. Looking instead at the distribution of pressure off of bony prominences and across the entire surface, while somewhat subjective, is the most effective way to use mapping in a clinical setting. In laboratory settings, such measurements as dispersion index, contact area, percent of force in the ischial region, peak pressure index, and frequency analysis are being tested to determine if any or all can be used to objectify differences between cushions and aid in the selection process. 9, 10

Intuitively, the better product choice would be the one with the lower peak pressure. However, peak pressure can be recorded by a single, small, aberrant cell that folded or one that recorded a clothing seam rather than a true peak pressure point. Some professionals within the international pressure mapping community have begun to average the readings of the peak pressure cell and the 8 cells around it to get a more accurate picture of the pressures in that small area.

Pressure measurements can be taken with single-cell, hand-held devices or larger, multiple-cell, computerized mapping devices. The hand-held, single-cell monitors are more portable and less expensive, but the single cell has a tendency to move during the inflation/deflation cycle. It also gives the reading over one small area, and the peak pressure may be far removed from the placement of the cell. The multiple-cell device gives a better overall picture of the pressures on the entire seating surface simultaneously and prints those pressures out in numeric or pictorial form on a computer screen. These larger, computerized mapping devices are much more expensive and less portable, but they are valuable because the entire sitting surface is read at the same time, rather than just a single site.

Single-cell meters operate in one of two ways: inflate-placement-deflate-read or deflate-placement-inflate-read. Accurate readings depend heavily on proper placement of the cell under the bony prominence while the client is sitting upright and stable. After taking the first reading, most clinicians remove the cell, replace it, and repeat the reading two times to get at least three readings per bony prominence. Some manufacturers recommend taking three readings and averaging the results. Make sure that the cell is not wrinkled during use and that it is placed in the same spot each time. Multiple-cell, or pressure mapping devices, should also be used according to manufacturer directions, including frequent calibration, no wrinkles, use of incontinent covers, and no hammocking over the sitting surface. The sitting surface should be used according to manufacturer's directions for inflation or support, placement on the chair, and use of extra pieces, such as a solid base, a cover, medial or lateral thigh support, or obliquity wedges. The surface of the cushion should be smooth and free of wrinkles and excessive layers of padding.

With the advent of sophisticated interface pressure mapping devices, many facilities and clinicians are using these measurements as the major factor in determining seat selection. Although pressure is one of the factors that causes breakdown, it is only one of several. The clinician should consider shearing, friction, heat/moisture buildup, and sitting instability as equally important, even though they are more difficult to measure than interface pressure. Other practical considerations include ease of maintenance and ease of transfers and ADLs with a particular cushion, factors that are subjective and require assessment with the client and the caregiver. The clinician must use interface pressure measurements carefully and in conjunction with the total picture of the client and equipment.

Cardiopulmonary and Vascular Systems

Pathology of the cardiopulmonary and vascular systems directly affects the ability of the blood to carry oxygen and nutrients to the integumentary system. Medical diagnoses such as chronic obstructive pulmonary disease, emphysema, cardiomyopathy, arteriosclerotic vascular disease, and hypertension indicate pathology that affects these systems.

Inactivity and extended bed rest have several negative effects on these systems. Without an active muscle pump or the effects of gravity on the upright body, blood flow and blood diffusion is slowed throughout the body and, therefore, to any wound sites. Increased resting heart rate and decreased maximum oxygen consumption (VO_2max) are also potential problems. Immobility promotes fluid stasis in the kidneys, which can lead to kidney stones and infection.11 Inactivity and bedrest can impair nutrition intake by reducing the appetite. Recumbence also inhibits safe swallowing and facilitates aspiration of food, which can lead to pneumonia. Swallowing occurs 24 hours per day, not just at mealtime. The correct head and neck positions conducive to safe swallowing should be identified and attained in the chair and the bed; consultation with a speech/language pathologist may be necessary for success in this area.

Proper upright positioning allows greater diaphragmatic expansion and facilitates breathing, thus improving oxygenation of the blood as well as pulmonary function through better movement of pulmonary secretions.11, 12 Upright positioning in a functional and comfortable position will improve general circulation by encouraging activity and movement. Cardiac function is also improved in the upright position.

The Dangers of Bedrest

Although sitting-related pressure ulcers can be totally relieved of pressure through bedrest, the hazards of immobility, the increased risk for breakdown on other bony prominences, and the psychological ramifications of an enforced sedentary lifestyle make bedrest a radical treatment recommendation that should be made with great caution, forethought, and patient preparation.

Integumentary System Review and Evaluation

Skin is more susceptible to breakdown if it is dry, flaky, friable, aged, insensate, prone to excessive sweating, or subjected to incontinence, friction, or shear. Positioning can affect the integumentary system by protecting the skin over bony prominences on weight-bearing surfaces and through correct use of the proper equipment to maintain safe postures and reduce tissue loads on those bony prominences. For some people, an equalization of pressure is sufficient to protect skin from breakdown. For others, positioning options need to be considered that reduce a maximal amount of pressure because their combination of risk factors makes them highly susceptible to pressure ulcers. For example, the skin over the coccyx is prone to breakdown because of the shape of the bone, lack of padding over the coccyx, and frequent use as a weight-bearing surface. Equipment that takes pressure off the coccyx in the sitting position, when used correctly, can help to avoid or treat this breakdown.

Check the skin and soft tissues over bony prominences for signs of injury, for example, a change in color (red, blue, purple) from the adjacent skin color. If trauma is identified, consider the anatomic locations of each area of trauma and its relationship to positioning. Note areas of previous breakdown and any previous surgeries to repair skin, because these areas are at high risk of reopening and must be protected at all costs. Chapter 4 provides information about skin and wound assessment.

Even if there is no current tissue breakdown, soft tissues covering bony prominences on weight-bearing surfaces can be at risk. Palpation and observation will identify those at highest risk by showing which ones are most prominent, least protected, and bear the most weight. For example, muscle atrophy of the gluteals and significant weight loss make the ischium or sacrum more prominent than usual and can make protection from breakdown a primary need in the selection of seat cushions and bed positioning devices.

Clients who had pelvic irradiation prior to 1980 are at very high risk for tissue breakdown over the sacrum, coccyx, and buttocks, due to tissue changes caused by the irradiation used at that time.

Psychosocial/Cognitive System

The treatment program for skin ulcers, whether pressure ulcers or vascular ulcers, often entails a decrease in mobility. This can be as minor as occasional periods of time elevating the feet higher than the heart to assist blood/lymph flow.

It can be as drastic as 24/7 bedrest for an ischial ulcer on a sitting-dependent client. Extended unnatural periods of immobility can lead to many physical and psychological impairments, which are often referred to as *hazards of immobility*. These hazards include affective complications such as subjective sensory distortions after as little as 2.75 hours in bed; this condition persists for a period of time equal to the period of confinement. Other complications cited are intellectual and perceptual disorders, depression, anxiety, hostility, embarrassment, helplessness, and "learned helplessness."13 Extended bed rest or loss of mobility leads to cognitive dysfunction in both intellectual and perceptual functions. The recumbent position induces mental and physical lethargy. Often, a client who refuses to follow prescribed treatments, including extended bed rest, is labeled "noncompliant." In many cases, however, he or she may simply be issuing a cry for help in changing the wound management program, because bed rest can be considered as radical as imprisonment. If such behavioral signs are observed, the patient should be referred to psychosocial services for help, and the team caring for the client should be advised as well.

The client with impaired cognitive abilities can be unsafe for self-mobility or the ability to maintain safe postures independently. The equipment for someone with cognitive impairments will likely need to be more supportive than that for a client with full abilities to reposition or request assistance in maintaining safe postures.

Summary

Tables 17-1 and 17-2 list examples of medical and functional diagnoses relating to the need for therapeutic positioning, prognosis, related interventions, and expected functional outcomes for sitting and recumbent clients.

Based on functional diagnosis, clinicians establish the prognosis and select interventions, with a targeted outcome for each intervention. Interventions include analysis of the most effective forms of equipment required, selection of appropriate equipment to achieve correct therapeutic position, analysis of the client using the selected equipment, and education of the client and caregivers in correct use. Therapeutic exercise often is another important component of the total therapy plan of care.

Intervention in the Sitting Position

Sitting can be regarded as either a cause of tissue breakdown or a part of the solution. In a proactive environment in which educated clinicians have access to the proper equipment and are skilled in the techniques of therapeutic positioning, sitting can and should be part of a prevention program that can improve the quality of life for clients and assist in the healing of tissue breakdown if it occurs. In addition, sitting can decrease medical costs over the course of time. In a study of 30 long-term care residents, Trefler et al showed that individually fitted wheelchair systems were

TABLE 17-1 Functional Diagnosis–Sitting Position

Medical Diagnosis—Functional Diagnosis	Prognosis	Intervention	Outcome
Kyphosis—Client cannot maintain 90° hip flexion or keep face vertical due to thoracic kyphosis	Client will sit upright with face vertical and as close to 90° hip flexion as possible	Open seat-to-back angle adjustable backrest with stabilizing seat cushion; may need antitippers	Client able to sit stabilized as close to 90° back-to-seat angle as possible with face vertical
Scoliosis (fixed)—Client cannot sit with shoulders and hips level due to fixed asymmetric spine or pelvis	Client will maintain sitting position with shoulders and hips as level as possible	Cushion with buildup under higher ischium to accommodate asymmetry; back support to assist in comfortable trunk positioning	Client able to maintain upright sitting with shoulders and hips as close to level as possible
Scoliosis (flexible)—Client sits asymmetrically with one shoulder and hip elevated and opposite shoulder and hip depressed, but has potential to sit with shoulders and hips level	Client will maintain upright sitting position with level shoulders and hips without strain	Cushion with pressure elimination at ischials and full femur support or cushion with buildup under lower ischium to raise that side of pelvis; three lateral trunk supports: apex of the curve, and the hip and upper trunk on the contralateral side	Client able to maintain upright sitting with shoulders and hips level and spine straight
<90° Hip flexion—Client cannot achieve the 90° seat-to-back angle built into the majority of standard wheelchairs	Cient will maintain correct sitting position with hips on back of seat	Positioning cushion to stabilize pelvis, with open seat-to-back angle adjustable backrest; angle of recline approximates maximum hip flexion allowed by range of motion limitations	Client will maintain upright sitting as close to 90° as is allowed by range limitations
<90° Knee Flexion available—Client unable to bend knee to 90° to reach standard footrests for support	Provide equipment that supports lower extremity at available range so that client can maintain proper sitting position	Hanger with calf and foot support; angle set at maximum angle allowed at knee	Client will maintain upright sitting with hips on back of seat and lower extremities maintained at allowed knee flexion
>90° Knee Flexion available – Client cannot achieve 90° knee flexion	Provide equipment that supports lower extremity at available range so that client can maintain proper sitting position	Angle adjustable foot/leg support to hold lower leg at comfortable position	Client will maintain upright sitting with hips on back of seat and lower extremities maintained at allowed knee flexion
Foot propeller—Client requires use of feet to mobilize chair; unable to reach floor to propel	Provide equipment that allows efficient heel strike on the floor	Hemi-height chair with cushion or drop seat and cushion, so that total seat-to-floor height is equal to height from bottom of shoe to back of knee of propelling leg; involved leg requires 60° or 70° hangar with thigh supported by wedge	Client will be self-mobile via foot propulsion while maintaining proper seating posture
One-arm driver—Client can use only one arm for self-mobility	Provide equipment designed for propulsion with one arm	One-arm-drive wheelchair	Client will be self-mobile using one arm while maintaining proper seating posture

(Continued)

TABLE 17-1 *(Continued)*

Medical Diagnosis—Functional Diagnosis	Prognosis	Intervention	Outcome
Above the knee amputee—Client has limited femur length to support body weight; difficult to maintain posture in sitting; may lead to tissue breakdown on ischials due to increased weight on ischials	Provide firm, flat support for femurs and protection for ischials	Stabilizing seat cushion; amputee adapters to move rear wheel axle backward from normal position; antitippers	Client will maintain upright sitting with full protection of ischials and full femur support
tissue breakdown on sitting surfaces (ischials, sacrum, or coccyx)—Client cannot sit without pressure eliminated at ulcer site	Pressure elimination on ulcer while maintaining correct postural alignment	Cushion with selective pressure elimination	Client will maintain sitting schedule with pressure elimination provided at the site of breakdown
Asymmetric tonic neck reflex (ATNR) influence—Client has difficulty controlling direction of chair with side-mounted joystick when head moves	Change placement of joystick to midline to decrease influence of ATNR	Position joystick in center of lap tray	Client will drive safely and in control despite movement of head
Hip fracture—Client cannot sit with full 90° hip flexion; may lead to skin breakdown due to ischial and coccyx weight bearing	Provide seating arrangement that allows <90° hip flexion with skin protection	Seat cushion that provides ischial/coccyx pressure reduction or elimination with positioning and can be customized with unilateral sloping to accommodate the lack of hip flexion on the involved side; open seat-to-back angle adjustable backrest with sacral protection; solid seat beneath cushion, may require cutout in board.	Client will maintain upright sitting with maximum allowed hip flexion and no pressure on coccyx
Trunk/hip hyperactive extensor tone—Client cannot maintain hips in proper position on seat due to uncontrolled hip extension; may lead to tissue breakdown due to shearing	Provide seating arrangement that best positions the client as close to 90° hip flexion as possible; antithrust seat assembly with pre-ischial block	Increase trunk/lower extremity angle past 90°; firm contoured back support; 90° positioning belt	Client will maintain proper seated posture with hips on back of seat and trunk upright

Copyright © Laurie Rappl.

beneficial in terms of independent mobility, functional reach, quality of life, and satisfaction with an individual's assistive technology.14 Once equipment is prescribed, follow-up to ensure adequacy of equipment and proper usage is essential. In a study of 42 long-term care residents who used wheelchairs and equipment purchased by Medicaid, 27 were found to have inadequate seat frames, and 24 had inadequate seat cushions. The authors hypothesize that lack of follow up may have contributed to the frequency of problems discovered.15

When the sitting skeleton is viewed from the side, it is apparent that the ischial tuberosities (ITs) extend approximately 1.5 inches past the femurs, making the ITs the major weight-bearing points on the sitting surface (see Figure 17-1). The skin over these points is also the most vulnerable to tissue breakdown because of their conical shape and poor natural padding. As a client becomes less mobile and more sitting-dependent, muscle atrophy of the gluteal muscles causes the minimal natural padding to deteriorate, making that client even more vulnerable to tissue breakdown. The ITs are the fulcrum, or pivot,

TABLE 17-2   Functional Diagnostic Process—Recumbent Position

Functional Diagnosis	Prognosis	Intervention	Outcome
Cardiorespiratory or gastrointestinal pathologies requiring elevation of the head of the bed	Client will assume Fowler position with proper positioning and skin protection devices to protect heels and sacrum	Hip aligned at gatch or bend of bed; sacrum protected by lifting under one hip with pillow or foam support; heel protection devices employed; frequent turning/repositioning schedule. Do not substitute elevated head of bed for upright sitting in a supportive chair. Alternately, gatch the knees so that the hips and knees are flexed to 90 degrees and heels are off loaded. Monitor sacrococcygeal area for pressure.	Client will tolerate head of bed elevated without sliding down on the bed causing shear and friction on the sacrococcygeal areas
Less than full hip or knee extension allowed due to joint ROM impairment at the knees; undue susceptibility to pressure ulcers due to potential exposure of heel and sacrum to pressure	Client will assume supine position with foam support devices in place to accommodate hip/knee flexion requirements, and with protection of occiput, heels, and sacrum	Foam positioning devices to protect occiput and heels, and to elevate lower extremities to accommodate flexion contractures; one side of pelvis elevated slightly with towel roll or foam to protect sacrum	Client will maintain supine position with support devices correctly placed
Influence of the asymmetric tonic neck reflex (ATNR) causes involuntary movements into trunk extension and inability to maintain side-lying position	Client will be positioned with strong side down and trunk and upper limbs fully supported OR Client will be positioned with strong side up, body fully supported along full trunk, and the bed situated so that client is not required to turn the face up to view the room	Position with stronger side down and trunk fully supported from shoulder to pelvis; bed is placed so that need for cervical movement is minimized, e.g., against far wall, facing door of the room	30° foam wedge fully supporting trunk, pelvis, shoulders, and uppermost arm and leg supported away from midline in abduction; head supported in midline in both frontal and sagittal planes
Venous ulcers on lower extremity with edema	Client will maintain supine or side-lying positions with lower extremity elevated to reduce swelling, and with ulcer and heels pressure-free	Foam device to support leg above the level of the heart in supine position and in 30° side-lying position	Client will maintain safe postures with limb elevated and sacrum protected

points for the pelvis. When bearing weight, they cause the pelvis to rock about a horizontal axis through the frontal plane that leads to anterior or posterior pelvic tilt. Most often, people tend to sit in a posterior tilt, or a slouched position. The act of moving into the slouch causes shearing forces on the ITs, and sacral sitting can lead to the formation of pressure ulcers on the sacrum and coccyx, by causing those bones to be weight bearing The goal in seating a client is to help maintain a position that is as close to ideal as possible. Orthopedic or neu-

rologic limitations can prevent achievement of the ideal position as a realistic goal, but it is the benchmark position.

Ideal is the position that the body could be in if range of motion, muscle and soft tissue flexibility, neurological integrity, and physical capabilities allowed it to be anatomically aligned for muscle balance; to achieve proper alignment of the bones and joints according to their design; to take advantage of the most load-tolerant areas of the body in handling pressure to keep the skin safe from breakdown; and to maximize safe and functional mobility. "90/90/90" is an old positioning mantra that has been dispelled over time. This referred to 90° angles at the hip, knee, and ankle. This is uncomfortable for long-term-sitting, and has been softened to approximately 95° at the hip and knee, and 90°—95° at the ankle (see Figure 17-1 for an approximation of this position). Each individual must be evaluated for their ability to achieve the "ideal" position described below, and should be positioned as close to that ideal position as possible.16-22

In the "ideal" position, the ear should be in line with the acromion process and hip. The thigh should be parallel to the ground so that the hip and knee are in line with one another. The spine should be supported in its natural curves in the cervical, thoracic, and lumbar regions. The face should be vertical Viewed from the front, the trunk and head should be comfortably upright with the shoulders and hips (pelvic crests) level, thighs in neutral position (i.e., not internally or externally rotated), feet flat on the footrests and pointed straight ahead, and arms supported so that the shoulders are not elevated or depressed when the elbows rest on the armrests. Dignity issues clearly indicate the need for women to be positioned with their legs together, rather than separated.

Sitting Posture Examination and Evaluation

Knowledge of the ideal sitting position enables clinicians to evaluate clients to determine how closely they can come to achieving the ideal position comfortably, what impairments prevent them from attaining that position, and then what equipment interventions can assist them in maintaining a position as close to ideal as is possible or functional. This evaluation has been discussed under the Systems Review sections earlier in this chapter.

Intervention Using the Principles of Seating

Therapeutic positioning requires skill in evaluation and interpretation of clients' needs and in the matching of equipment to clients. 16-22 Therapeutic positioning has traditionally been considered the realm of physical therapy and/or occupational therapy practice. Many physical therapists and occupational therapists who are highly skilled and specialized in therapeutic positioning work in seating clinics for clients with all types of positioning needs. Unfortunately, many clinicians and clients do not have ready access to the skilled intervention of such knowledgeable PTs and OTs. However, proper seating and positioning must be a priority for all clinicians and caregivers. Knowledge and application of the basic principles of seating will benefit the majority of clients.

Basic principles of proper positioning can be learned and applied in the home setting, skilled nursing facility, and rehabilitation facility, by all clinical staff (Exhibit 17-2). Of course, some clients need more intervention than just these basic principles. Clinicians and caregivers need to identify when the basic seating principles will not or cannot help the client, or when equipment needs to accommodate a position that varies from these basic principles, and seek a referral to a skilled outside source.

EXHIBIT 17-2 Basic Seating Principles

Basic seating principles include the following:

- Level the cushion and seat upholstery (base of support) to keep thighs horizontal to the ground; knees and hips should be even.
- Support the feet so that the knees are even with the hips.
- Support the back so that natural spinal curves are maintained; the ear, shoulder, and hip should be in alignment.
- When the pelvis is properly positioned on the seat, the seat cushion ends 1.5—2 inches from the back of the knee.

Additional Seating Concepts

Pelvic control. Pelvic control is the cornerstone of seating. If the pelvis rolls out of position, the entire sitting posture is difficult to control. Therefore, stabilizing the pelvis is the foundation for stabilizing the entire body. However, the basis of this cornerstone, the ischials, are also the most vulnerable areas for tissue breakdown and the pivot points for pelvic rotation. Most cushions, in equalizing pressure across the sitting surface, maintain pressure on the ischials and address pelvic stability by padding all around the ischials. An alternative way to keep the pelvis in place is to stop the fulcrum action of the ischials by eliminating pressure on them. The pelvis can then be stabilized through the stabilization of the femurs. 22-27

The femurs are joined to the pelvis at the hips and work together with the pelvis to stabilize the body. Transferring weight onto the femurs unloads the ischials and provides a larger surface area for the cushion to control. The cushion must match the posterior surface of the femurs with firm, flat support, especially the proximal femur closest to the pelvis. Stabilizing here controls rotation of the entire femur and holds the pelvis on the back of the seat. Movement of the pelvis is contained within the pressure elimination area (Figure 17–2), and the ischials are free of contact. This type of cushion design is contraindicated in patients with unstable hip joints, severe fixed pelvic obliquity, and hip disarticulations.

Any chosen cushion requires the assistance of a back support. The top of the back of the pelvis must be supported with a back support so that it cannot rock backward. The back support also fills in the lumbar curve for more supported and comfortable sitting and relieves stresses related to back pain by improving the seating ergonomics. Seat cushions are discussed in more detail below.

Thigh Control. Except for clients with a strong anterior pelvic tilt, the thighs should be positioned so that they are parallel to the ground. The seat should be flat, with the hips and knees horizontally aligned. If the knees are lower than the hips, the weight of the legs pulls the body forward on the seat and pulls the pelvis into a posterior pelvic tilt, which clinicians work to avoid, and the client slouches. This

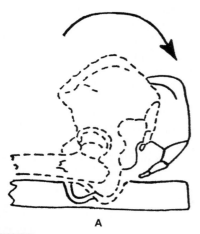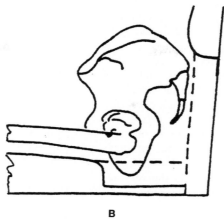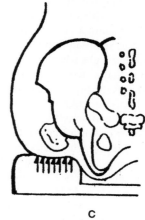

A   B   C

FIGURE 17-2 Pressure equalizing versus pressure eliminating. **A.** Side view of pressure equalizing cushion; loads the ischium, which allows pelvic tilt. **B.** Side view of pressure-eliminating cushion. Note pre-ischial bar limiting forward ischial movement. **C.** Rear view of pressure-eliminating cushion. Note pressure distribution across full width of femur to support the load of the body. (Courtesy of Span-America Medical Systems, Greenville, South Carolina.)

is the position most commonly seen in settings where generic chairs are used with footrests that are lengthened as much as possible or have been lost.

Conversely, if the knees are higher than the hips, as in the use of a wedge cushion, the natural curve of the lumbar lordosis is lost; the proximal femur, along with the sacrum, coccyx, and ischials, bear an inordinate amount of weight, and the client is put at high risk of tissue breakdown and back pain. These wedge-type cushions are typically used in an attempt to keep the client from sliding out of the seat. Wedge cushions cause so many problems that they should be prescribed with extreme caution. These problems can include tissue breakdown on the sacrum and spine due to excessive body weight being forced on those prominences, discomfort in a flexed lumbar spine, difficulties in transferring, and loss of mobility and ADL skills.

Postural Control and Stability. In order for products to help the client as much as possible, they must provide for sitting stability and comfort. The client must be supported in as close to an upright and aligned posture as possible. This will keep pressure on bony surfaces that can tolerate it (femurs) and off of surfaces that are less tolerant (ischials, coccyx, sacrum, and spinous processes). Stability and comfort also make clients as functional as possible and help to prevent further complications, such as contractures and internal organ compression.

CLINICAL WISDOM

Simple Tools

A simple toolbox is a necessity and a relatively inexpensive investment when working with seating equipment. This should include a variety of screwdrivers, wrenches, and a lubrication agent. For example, a simple wrench is usually all that is needed to change the height of a footrest so that it is the proper height for full foot support.

Wheelchairs or Mobility Bases

The major piece of equipment in seating, which carries the highest price tag and serves as the basis for the rest of the seating system, is the chair, sometimes referred to as the *mobility base*. Figure 17-3 is an algorithm to guide the clinician through the decision-making process to determine mobility needs.

The appropriate mobility base must be determined along with the seating system. It is often impossible to make any seating system, even the appropriate one for the client, work on an inappropriate seating base. For example, many people move their chair by propelling with their feet. If the wheelchair seat is too high to allow the feet to reach the ground, any seat cushion will put the client even higher and further reduce mobility. "Quick fixes," such as a drop seat, are often only fair compromises, at best.

In the same way, using a seating system on a base for which it is not designed will compromise the effect of the system. Reclining geriatric or Geri-chairs offer little to no support and are not designed to accept most seating systems. However, these chairs are sometimes the only available alternative to bed rest; therefore, it is necessary to adapt even these chairs to fit the individual's needs by utilizing the appropriate seat and back cushions, head supports, lateral trunk or hip guides, and lower extremity support.

The standard wheelchair—a folding frame style with adjustable or fixed armrests, a seat 18 inches wide by 16 inches deep, and elevating or adjustable footrests—is created more for temporary transportation than for mobility and positioning usage all day, every day. The vast majority of users require more support than these chairs can give. There is a multitude of variations on the standard frame:

- Hemi-height wheelchair —The axle for the back wheel is fixed higher on the frame than on standard chairs, thereby lowering the height of the seat and allowing clients who propel with their feet to reach the floor and propel the chair using a heel-toe pattern. Also used for shorter people to facilitate transfers.

- Lightweight wheelchairs—These chairs are useful for individuals such as the frail elderly because they take less energy to propel than standard chairs. Conserving these clients' energy gives them more overall endurance for functional activities.
- Sport or Ultra-lightweight – These chairs are for the very active user who needs the lightest frame possible for transporting and maximum mobility.
- Rigid—This is a nonfolding frame style for the very active user; it is less prone to breaking and loosening, and increases stroke propulsion efficiency.
- Pediatric-sized—These chairs are for the child or the child-sized adult.
- Tilt-in-Space – Rather than reclining just the backrest and opening up the seat-to-back angle, tilt-in-space maintains the seat-to-back angle of upright sitting and tilts or reclines the entire seat system. Tilt-in-space is favored over reclining back chairs.

- Reclining back chairs—These are adjusted by manual releases, hydraulic releases, ratchet-style fixation, or power. The seat-to-back angle can be changed to accommodate the client who cannot attain upright sitting or who needs to recline for some time during the day, but not necessarily out of the chair. Similarly, upholstered recliners, such as Geri-chairs or living room reclining chairs allow the body to slouch from upright. These chairs cause many positioning problems; for the most part, they have been replaced by tilt-in-space chairs.
- Power chairs—These are available in wheelchair style or as scooters.

Wheelchair Measurement

Comfortable and functional wheelchair seating requires that the seat-to-back angle accommodate the client in approximately a 95° hip flexion angle, or as close to that angle as the body will allow. Proper measurements for a wheelchair include seat depth, as described below; back height from seat cushion to the point on the back that gives needed support without hindering function; width from hip to hip and shoulder to shoulder, kept as close as is comfortable so that

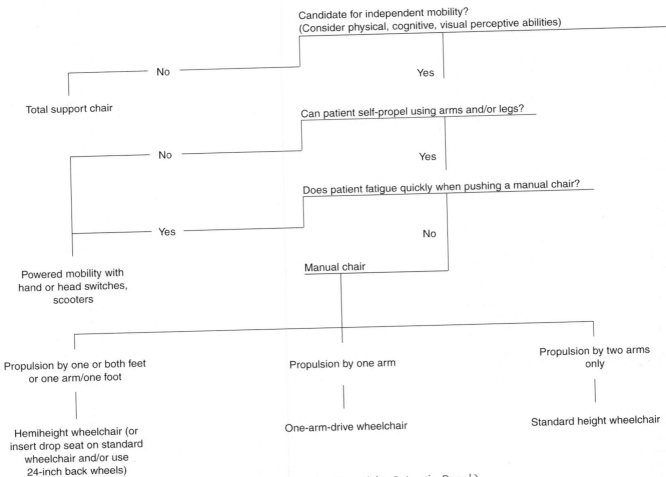

FIGURE 17-3 Algorithm for determining mobility base needs. (Copyright © Laurie Rappl.)

the overall chair is as small as possible; and the footrest adjusted so that the knee is even with the hip and the foot is flat on the flootrest.. This foot support measurement will be the floor-to-seat height in hemi-style chairs, or the footrest selection and setting in a manual or power-propelled chair.

Measurements must include the cushion when measuring the backrest height, seat-to-floor height, and footrest length (Figure 17-4). Otherwise, the cushion and chair will not work together to position the client successfully.

The client's needs and the features of the product are assessed by the clinician. When choosing equipment, match the needs of the client with the features of a product. Don't rely strictly on history or manufacturers' claims to determine what products to use; predetermine what features the product should have to fulfill the client's needs and use clinical decision making skills, including common sense, to make the product selection with the most benefits for the client.

Seat Depth. The seat depth, i.e., the length of the seat cushion from the backrest to the front edge of the seat upholstery, should be about 11/2–2 inches shorter than the distance from the seat back to the back of the knee. Seats with less depth than this do not take advantage of the weight bearing or support that the posterior femur can give; seats with greater depth than this will pull the body forward on the chair and out of position. Many fleet or institution chairs have very short seat depths, so people tend to slide about on their chairs and slide out of position. Large recliner-style chairs have seat depths that are too deep, causing pressure on the back of the lower legs and pulling the body forward on the seat.

Seat Cushions

Seat cushions are commonly considered to be the primary intervention in positioning clients.23-25 Products should be evaluated for how well they control physical and physiologic factors that cause skin and seating problems. These factors are pressure, shear, heat and moisture buildup, and postural control and stability (see Exhibit 17-3).

Pressure. Pressure causes ischemia or loss of circulation to the cells that are under pressure. Pressure is considered the major causative factor of tissue breakdown on the body's sitting surfaces, with the greatest effect over bony prominences, where high forces are generated on small areas. Large, flat surfaces, such as the posterior femurs, seldom

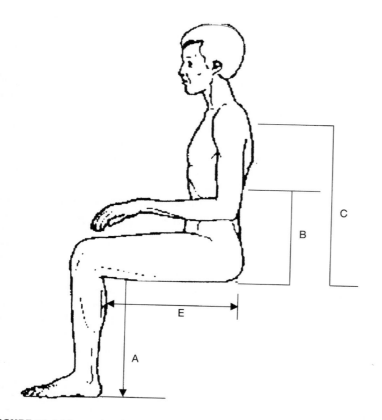
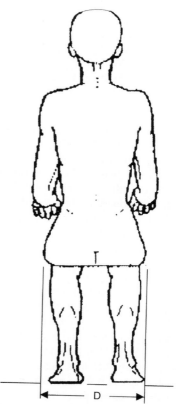

FIGURE 17-4 Measuring for a wheelchair. **A.** Seat-to-foot support height. **B.** Seat to top of sacrum for placement of lumbar support. **C.** Height of backrest needed for back support. **D.** Seat width. **E**. Seat depth, measured from backrest to popliteal fossa less 1.5 inches. (Courtesy of Span-America Medical Systems, Greenville, SC.)

EXHIBIT 17-3   Seat Cushions Are Not Mattresses in Miniature

It is important to understand that the seat cushion is not a mattress in miniature. Consider that a mattress has the advantage of the entire weight-bearing surface of the body over which to spread the load. Because there is more tissue in contact with the bed, the goal of a mattress can be tissue support, i.e., equalizing pressure across the bony prominences and plateaus such that pressures are not high enough to cause breakdown on any one point. Compare this with the seat cushion, which must bear 75% of the body weight on a small area, average size 18 × 16 inches.

In seating, that body weight is concentrated on two prominences, the ischials, which are the lowermost skeletal points on the sitting surface. The ischials are small, pointed, and unprotected; therefore, they are less load tolerant than the large, flat, padded femurs. With this disparity in load tolerance in mind, it is imperative that the seat cushion be examined for the skeletal support it can provide to protect the skin over these at-risk areas. Then, shift the support to the load-tolerant areas. This is not equalization, but load distribution consistent with tolerances. Equalizing the pressure over the sitting surface causes low-tolerance, high-risk prominences (the ischials) to bear the same weight as the high-tolerance, low-risk areas (the femurs). The skin management principle that dictates removal of pressure at pressure ulcer sites infers that the ischials—on which breakdown occurs most frequently—should bear less weight than the femurs and should not bear any weight in the presence of tissue breakdown. This is also true for those individuals who are identified as being at high risk for tissue breakdown.

break down because they distribute forces over a larger area. Conversely, the ischials are a common site for tissue breakdown; they are small and pointed, concentrating pressure over the peak of the bony prominence.

It is generally acknowledged that the ischials can safely tolerate only one-third to one-half of the amount of pressure that the femurs can tolderate.26-27 Any cushion being considered for a client must be assessed for its abilities to reduce pressure under the ischials. This can be done with either a pressure-mapping device, single-celled, hand-held pressure meter, or by palpation. To palpate, the clinician places the seat cushion on the seat and positions the client appropriately on the cushion. The clinician inserts a hand, palm up, between the bottom of the seat cushion and the upholstery of the chair, and under the ischium. There should be at least 1 inch of soft support material (e.g., foam, gel, or rubber and air) between the ischium and the seat upholstery to protect the skin from pressure. Remember that muscle tissue is affected by pressure before skin is, which explains why pressure ulcers often show deep tissue destruction well before indications on the skin surface appear. "A little bit of breakdown" can be the tip of the iceberg.

Many people believe that a cushion must be 4 in (10 cm) thick to be effective. However, the effectiveness of a cushion depends on many more dimensions than simply thickness. Foams have a wide range of qualities and are specified by industry measurements such as the 25% indentation load deflection (ILD), 65% ILD, and the modulus. None of these specifications has been correlated to cushion effectiveness. Ragan et al found that subcutaneous pressures and stresses decreased with thicker cushions, but almost all of the reduction was obtained with a cushion 8 cm thick; reduction was negligible after this height was reached.8 The specifications of the foam cushions used in the study were not discussed.

Shear. Shear is the distortion force applied to soft tissues when bone movement pulls the skin one way and the surface pulls the skin the opposite way. The result is a tearing or occlusion of the capillaries, interruption of blood flow, stress in soft tissues, and tissue destruction. Shearing magnifies the effects of pressure, causes increased soft tissue damage and undermining, and makes it more difficult to keep ulcer dressings in place. At this time, shear cannot be measured, nor is there a benchmark for determining "too much shear." Many clinicians suspect that shear is underappreciated and even more dangerous to tissues than pressure.

To address shear, the seat cushion must eliminate one of the two opposing forces at work on the skin (i.e., the force coming from the surface onto the pressure-sensitive prominences) or provide inherent movement with significant amplitude in individual cells that can shift with the body and decrease drag on the skin.

Heat and Moisture. Dispersion of heat and elimination of moisture should be prime considerations when selecting seat cushions. The combination of heat and moisture leads to maceration or softening of the skin. In this state, the skin is more susceptible to damage from increased friction between the skin and the surface material, which results in shear stresses to the subcutaneous tissues and puts them at risk for pressure damage.

Heated tissues can handle less pressure than cooler tissues because heating of the skin increases metabolic demand 6%—13% per degree Celsius rise in temperature.28,29 Increased metabolic demands require increased blood perfusion and oxygenation . Higher metabolism will produce more metabolites that need to be removed by the blood stream. At a certain pressure, perfusion is hampered as vessels are compressed. Cooling the tissues decreases metabolic demand so that decreased perfusion and blood supply are required for oxygenation. At lower tissue temperature, there is reduced metabolic demand by the tissues so that under even higher pressures, tissues can handle more compression without damage.

In an integrative review using simple graphical techniques, Lachenbruch estimated that an 8°C reduction in skin temperature would be equivalent to a 29% reduction in interface pressure, and that a 3°C temperature reduction would be equivalent to a 14% reduction in interface pressure.30

This is significant when choosing a seat cushion because sitting on cushions that depend on immersion or enveloping of the buttocks into the cushion to equalize pressure can allow sweat and heat to be contained around the ischials. This buildup causes maceration of the skin, which puts the skin at risk of breaking down.

Another complication of heat and moisture is loosening of dressing adhesives that keep dressings in place. When this happens, the clinician can be tempted to choose dressings with aggressive adhesives that can be dangerous to fragile skin. One way of mitigating the heat and moisture problem is to choose cotton or air-exchange covers. These covers help, but they cannot combat total contact around the ischium. The most desirable cushion should provide full ventilation of the ischial area with no contact.

Types of Cushions. Cushions can be divided into groups according to their features and abilities to meet various levels of client need for positioning, tissue breakdown risk, and treatment. In 2004, the Centers for Medicare and Medicaid Services (CMS) categorized cushions into six groups:

1. General use
2. Positioning
3. Skin protection
4. Skin protection and positioning
5. Adjustable
6. Custom.

Each group has specific client criteria that must be met in order for the client to qualify for a cushion from that group.31 Each group is given two codes, one for cushions less than 22 in wide, and one for cushions greater than 22 in wide. The groups are named for either a function or a use, but the criteria for inclusion of a product into a group is based on physical characteristics of the product; these characteristics are not meant to imply endorsement of effectiveness, but are measurable characteristics that can enhance effectiveness for the intended target client group.

In this text, cushions are divided into four groups based on their design philosophy for addressing tissue breakdown:

1. Pressure reduction or equalization (redistribution)
2. Generically contoured or precontoured
3. Selective pressure elimination
4. Fully customized contouring.

A list of product examples for each group are listed at the end of this chapter. Figure 17-5 shows examples of three of these cushions.

Pressure-reduction or equalization (redistribution) cushions decrease pressure on the ischials and coccyx (compared with no cushion at all) and attempt to equalize or redistribute that pressure across the entire sitting surface (Figure 17-5A). This group comprises a wide range of cushions made from flat, noncontoured foam, gel, single- or multiple-cell air bladders, and plastic matrix hon-

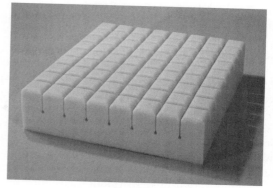

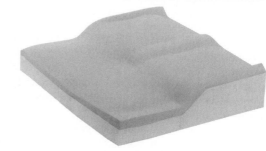

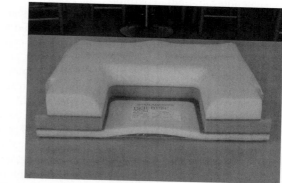

FIGURE 17-5 Examples of seat cushions. **A**. Pressure reduction/equalization/redistribution cushion. **B**. A generically-contoured or precontoured cushion **C**. Selective pressure elimination. (Courtesy of Span-America Medical Systems, Greenville, SC.)

eycomb products. The amount of pressure reduction off bony prominences, pressure equalization across the surface, or pressure redistribution depends on the amount of immersion of the body into the surface, the resulting shaping of the cushion around the body, and the prevention of bottoming out. Most of these equalizing cushions do little to address shearing forces, and they may address heat/moisture via cover materials only. These cushions are appropriate for clients at risk for tissue breakdown. For many clients, redistributing or equalizing pressure is enough to allow healing.

There are many cushions at many price levels that satisfy these basic requirements. The clinician must assess the risk level of the client for tissue breakdown and the pressure-redistributing capabilities of the cushion without regard to price, and balance the capabilities of the product with the cost and acuity of the client's needs. The comparable CMS category would be the General Use Seat Cushions, and the Adjustable Skin Protection cushions that are air-filled cushions that equalize pressure, but do not offer positioning features.

Generically contoured or precontoured cushions are shaped with a bucketed area under the pelvis to assist with pelvic placement and channels under the femurs to assist in neutral alignment or optimal lower extremity positioning (Figure 17-5B). These cushions are more sophisticated than pressure equalization or redistribution cushions because they have some means of actively molding to or mirroring the shape of the body's sitting surfaces to equalize pressure across the ischials and femurs (via air cells, gel or viscous fluids, viscoelastic foam, etc.), while offering contouring for body support. These products are appropriate for clients who are at moderate risk for tissue breakdown and/or require more assistance with positioning than a noncontoured cushion can provide.

It is important to note that the generic contour base is shaped to a muscled bottom, not to the atrophied bottom of a sitting-dependent patient. Therefore, they often do not hold the pelvis as securely as cushions more specifically contoured to fit individual bone structure. Many manufacturers have added the flexibility of providing optional components, such as medial thigh supports, lateral thigh supports, hip guides, and obliquity wedges that can customize the cushion to control lower extremity positioning even further. Generically contoured cushions offer better stability to the user when tested during reaching tasks than air-filled or flat foam, simple pressure reduction cushions.[32] These cushions are distributed through four CMS categories: skin protection, positioning, skin protection and positioning, and adjustable, depending on the depth of immersion of the ischials allowed by the cushion and the height of the positioning features of the cushion.

A feasibility study published by the University of Pittsburgh compared the efficacy of generically contoured cushions with simple foam slab cushions. Although no statistically significant differences were seen between the groups for overall pressure ulcer incidence, the generically contoured cushions were more effective in preventing ischial pressure ulcers specifically.[7]

Selective pressure elimination cushions (Figure 17-5C) are identified by an area that eliminates pressure on the ischials via a pocket that is sized to the user's ischial span—the measurement from the center point of one ischium to the center point of the other. They also offer flat support to the full length and width of the posterior femurs, thereby supporting the body on the femurs, not in the elimination area (see Figures 17-2B and C). This not only protects the skin over the ischials, but also protects the femurs by pressure distribution. Although appropriate for the moderate-risk client as well, these products are often used for high-needs clients, who may be characterized by some of the

following: sitting-dependent; minimally ambulatory, if at all; insensate; limited abilities to reposition themselves to relieve pressure; existing or recurrent breakdown on the bony prominences of the sitting surfaces (ischials, sacrum, or coccyx); currently in the granulation or remodeling phases of wound healing; and history of tissue breakdown on those sitting surfaces. Selective pressure elimination at the ischials, shearing elimination, and maximum ventilation puts the skin over the ischials in the healthiest possible environment. These requirements mirror and follow basic medical protocol for pressure ulcer treatment.[6,33-37] The benefits of pressure elimination to prevent and treat tissue breakdown have been well documented.[16, 22-27, 38-42] These cushions are in the CMS category of skin protection and positioning.

This time-tested, fitted cushion design should never be confused with the donut design, which is specifically recommended against by the Agency for Health Care Research and Quality (AHRQ) — formerly known as the Agency for Health Care Policy and Research (AHCPR) — guidelines.[43] Unlike a true selective pressure elimination cushion, which involves a full seating surface with a small relief area fitted to the user's bone structure, a donut cushion is simply a closed ring of material that cuts off circulation by inducing the tourniquet effect. In addition, the ring forces weight bearing on the area around the ischials, rather than on the femurs, which are the anatomically load-tolerant areas. For these reasons, the donut cushion should never be used, especially by clients with existing breakdown or at high risk for breakdown.

As with any sitting-dependent client, especially those with tissue breakdown, maintenance of the properly seated position is essential to enhance function and endurance, and to protect the skin under other areas of the sitting surface from breaking down. The pressure elimination cushion positions the pelvis in three ways. First, the ischials are unweighted and cannot act as pivot points for pelvic rotation. Second, the body is controlled by fully supporting the femurs (both length and width) in a nonrotated position such that they are even with each other in the horizontal plane. This keeps the pelvis and the trunk level (rather than obliquely inclined), keeps the pelvis toward the back of the seat, and prevents the pelvis from falling into the cutout area. Third, the walls of the elimination area confine movement of the pelvis to a defined area and keep the ischials from sliding forward with an effective pre-ischial block. As with any cushion, the top of the back of the pelvis must also be supported with a back support so that it cannot rock backward. The back support also fills in the lumbar curve for more supported and comfortable sitting.

Fully customized contouring cushions are unique cushions fashioned specifically for individual clients. These are usually prescribed for users with severe structural deformities that cannot be accommodated by off-the-shelf products or for clients with excessive trunk and lower extremity tone that pulls them out of position on other cushions. The CMS category "custom" covers these cushions.

Other features to consider when evaluating cushions include urine-proof surface, stability of the sitting surface, washability, weight for portability, leak-proof surface, low maintenance, ease of correct use, cosmesis, durability, and slip resistance. A representative listing of manufacturing sources for these categories of seat cushion is found at the end of this chapter.

The algorithm in Figure 17-6 can help clinicians make appropriate seat cushion choices.

Back Supports

A seat cushion is only one part of the seating system. To support a body adequately, the proper back support must also be prescribed. Most wheelchairs have a material back that allows the chair to fold. Unfortunately, this material bows in the opposite direction that the back requires. Therefore, almost every client sitting in a standard folding wheelchair requires an accessory back support to accommodate the lumbar and thoracic curves. The complexity and expense of the back support depends on the needs of the client and the number of roles that the back support must fill. The algorithm shown in Figure 17-7 can help clinicians choose the appropriate back support for a client.

A relatively new development in back upholstery is the tension-adjustable back. A series of horizontal Velcro straps between the seat back uprights and under the fold-over upholstery can be tightened or loosened to conform the back to the individual user's body. These backs are not as firm as solid back supports, but weigh less, are easily changed, and can be sufficient for some individuals. .

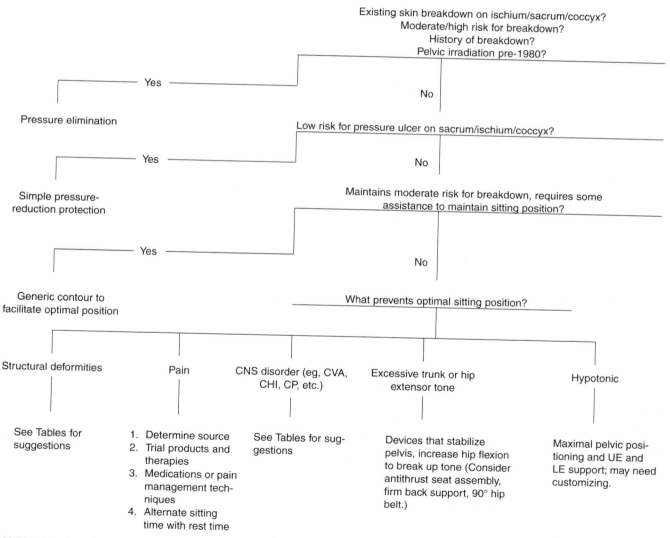

FIGURE 17-6 Algorithm for determining sitting surface. The surface must work with the mobility base to achieve optimal sitting height. CNS = central nervous system; CHI = closed head injury; CP = cerebral palsy; UE = upper extremity; LE = lower extremity. (Copyright © Laurie Rappl.)

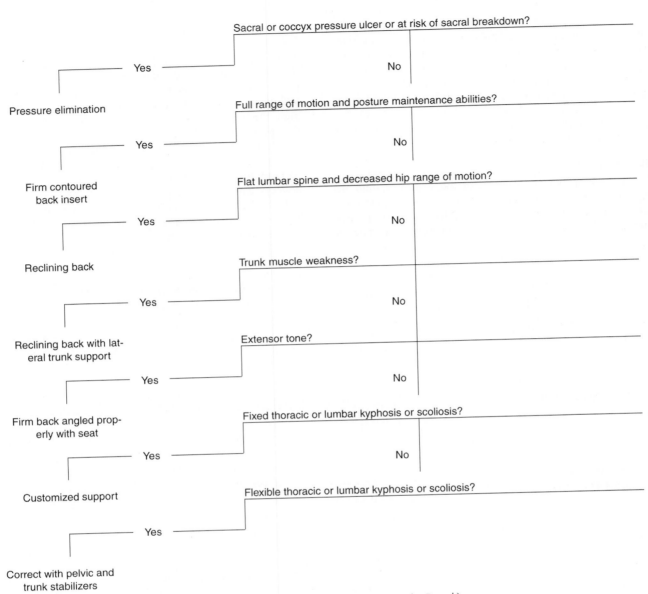

Sacral or coccyx pressure ulcer or at risk of sacral breakdown?

Yes — No

Pressure elimination

Full range of motion and posture maintenance abilities?

Yes — No

Firm contoured back insert

Flat lumbar spine and decreased hip range of motion?

Yes — No

Reclining back

Trunk muscle weakness?

Yes — No

Reclining back with lateral trunk support

Extensor tone?

Yes — No

Firm back angled properly with seat

Fixed thoracic or lumbar kyphosis or scoliosis?

Yes — No

Customized support

Flexible thoracic or lumbar kyphosis or scoliosis?

Yes

Correct with pelvic and trunk stabilizers

FIGURE 17-7 Algorithm for determining back support needs. (Copyright © Laurie Rappl.)

tissue breakdown on the sacrum is a deciding factor in selecting a back support. tissue breakdown requires that the back support remove pressure from and ventilate the area. Postural support in an upright sitting position can require support on natural spinal curves, accommodation for fixed deformities, or correction of flexible deformities. None of these needs can be overlooked when positioning a client with sacral tissue breakdown in a sitting position. When treating sacral tissue breakdown, look for a commercially available device that is designed to meet all of these goals for the client.

Clients who can maintain the upright ideal position with little or no assistance may require only minimal back support, perhaps a firm, contoured back that can be slid into the chair with an attachment to the upholstery.

If the lumbar spine is flattened and hip range of motion is compromised so that it is less than 90°, a chair fixed at a 90° seat-to-back angle is inappropriate. This combination of physical factors, often found in the older adult population, can be accommodated by a backrest that can be adjusted back to open the seat-to-back angle. This allows the client to be positioned with the hips all the way back on the seat for full support; the back can be supported at the appropriate degree of recline to facilitate safe swallowing and maximize mobility and function for the client.

Clients who have little inherent trunk support abilities can benefit from back supports that have the flexibility of lateral supports to help maintain the trunk in an upright position. A flexible thoracic or lumbar kyphosis or scoliosis can be handled by correcting the position of the pelvis and possibly using lateral supports on the trunk. Back supports can also be fully customized to fit the unique contours of an individual. Such a support is indicated for clients with fixed trunk deformities or severe trunk weakness.

Footrests

Footrests should support the leg so that the thigh is parallel to the ground. If the footrest is too high, the weight is unevenly distributed across the femur; if it is too low, the weight of the poorly supported leg pulls the body out of position. To keep the thighs parallel to the ground, simply adjust the height of the footrests of the wheelchair. Care should be taken to ensure that individuals wear the appropriate supportive footwear to protect the feet from trauma, evenly distribute pressures across the entire foot, and assist in decreasing dependent fluid buildup in the feet.

Accessories

The seat, back, and mobility base are the three key elements in a seating system. Many clients require the extra assistance of accessory products, such as head supports, solid seat bases, ,, armrests, angle adjustable footrests, footrest plates, back and front wheels, and ancillary devices.

Head Supports. Head supports come in a variety of models, depending on the amount of support needed and the ability of the backrest to support the headrest. Models include flat (attached to the seat back uprights of manually reclining chairs), molded around the neck and occipital regions, adjustable in height and angle, and fixed.

Solid seat base Seat cushions have been discussed above. When cushions are placed on sagged seat upholstery, many of the positioning effects are negated. The seat support can be stiffened by adding a solid seat or board to the chair or by adding a drop seat that drops the seat pan beneath the level of the seat rails and lowers the client closer to the floor. Consider adding a cutout seat board under the seat cushion to eliminate the sling of the upholstery and distribute interface pressure away from the ischial tuberosities. Be aware that, when a solid seat is added, this can increase the interface pressure over the ischial tuberosities if the cushion is inadequate in pressure distribution over time; in other words, if the cushion bottoms out, the ischial tuberosities will press into a solid, unforgiving surface that could then contribute to the formation of a pressure ulcer.

Armrests. Armrests generally come in two styles: tubular with padding or standard with flat metal or plastic skirt guards. Either can be attached to the chair in a fixed position or can swing away or be removed for ease of transfer. Standard armrests come in full length, shortened desk length (allows the chair to be pulled up closer to a table or desk), and height adjustable to accommodate the needs of a wide range of client heights.

Angle –adjustable footrests and footrest plates. Footrests are critical pieces of the seating system. As a general rule, footrests are adjusted so that the knees are even with the hips. Most footrests are adjustable in height, and some allow adjustment in the sagittal plane to change the angle of the ankle. The pedal or platform of the footrest can be ordered in various sizes to support as much of the foot as possible. Elevating-height footrests, although thought not effective, don't raise the foot higher than the heart useful for edema, can actually pull the body out of position and extend the turning radius of the chair, thus limiting mobility. The elevation has little effect on edema, because the extremity must be positioned above the level of the heart for passive edema control.

Back Wheels. The back wheels of standard wheelchairs are usually 24or 26 inches in diameter and come in a variety of widths. Tilt-in-space chairs have 12—24 inch wheels, and hemi-height chairs also have smaller diameter wheels. The major choice to make is whether to order solid or inflated tires and treaded or nontreaded tires. For everyday, general use, most people use inflatable tires with moderate tread. Solid tires made with treads are now available for individuals who want to avoid the possibility of flat tires. For mainly indoor use, consider a minimal tread. There are also various tread patterns to benefit various terrains, such as indoor tile, outdoor pavement, and outdoor rough ground. Hint: The height of the seat from the floor—a critical factor in the client's mobility—can be affected by changing the diameter of the back wheel

Front Wheels. The front wheels of wheelchairs (also called "casters") come in almost as many varieties as the back wheels—solid or inflatable, in various widths and diameters. The standard caster is 8 inches in diameter, solid rubber, and minimally treaded, if at all. Sport-type chairs are often seen with casters as small as roller blade wheels for increased turning abilities. Outdoor chairs have more substantial casters with larger diameters and widths (and often treads). Larger diameters are better over rough terrain, whereas smaller diameters are more adaptable to indoor needs.

Ancillary Devices. Ancillary devices include the following:
- Lap belts, seat belts, and anterior pelvic belts—usually placed at a 45° angle to the seat-to-back angle, but often more effective when secured to the seat side rail, a few inches in front of the seat-to-back junction and crossing the proximal femur at a 90° angle, just below the trunk/leg crease.
- Lap trays—full or partial, clear or solid, padded or unpadded to assist with upper extremity support. These should not be used as a restraint, but as an assist to ADLs, including communication, for support to a flaccid arm, and to help provide a point of stability for hypertonic extremities. Lap trays can also provide trunk support for clients who fatigue over time.
- Antitippers—small wheels that attach to the back of the wheelchair to keep it from tipping over backward, usually used as a safety factor. In everyday life, it is necessary to tip wheelchairs backward in order to lift the front of the

chair over small bumps and curbs, so antitippers can limit mobility while providing safety for the client. They can be removable.

- Amputee axle adapters—allow the rear wheels to be moved posterior to the seat back upright to keep the user safe from tipping over backward. Amputees have less weight on the front of the chair, so moving the wheels back provides counterbalance and stability.
- Residual limb support—holds the residual limb of the below-the-knee amputee.
- Chest straps—provide anterior support for the chest and upper trunk.

Working with Suppliers

Suppliers are important resources on the wound care team. A good supplier will help clinicians match equipment to individual needs, and help clinicians keep abreast of new technology and new items on the market. Do not work with a supplier who limits access to equipment, for example, by offering only one or two lines of chairs and seating equipment. Look for suppliers who carry multiple lines and are proactive in assisting with this critical part of client care—equipment selection. Ultimate accountability for decision making resides with the clinician working with the client and the physician, who ultimately prescribes the equipment.

Intervention in the Recumbent Position

The average client spends about one-third of his or her life in bed. Clients who cannot maintain standing or sitting positions for typical amounts of time spend increasing time in the recumbent position. Just as with sitting, choosing the proper support surface and correctly positioning the client on the surface are necessary parts of humane and holistic treatment. The human body requires support for proper alignment in the recumbent position. Technically, any client who depends on the recumbent position for any part of the day or night should be evaluated to ensure that the optimal positions are being attained. The more time spent in bed, the more need there is for positioning intervention. Certainly, clients who have musculoskeletal or neurologic insults that limit self-mobility also have impaired sensation to detect the need for position change. Disuse atrophy can make their bony prominences more prominent and, therefore, at higher risk of breakdown. These clients require therapeutic positioning. 44-48

Bed rest puts the tissue over many bony prominences of the body at risk for tissue breakdown, including the occiput, shoulders, elbows, trochanters, sacrum, heels, and malleoli. For this reason, there are many "support surfaces" used to protect the body in this relatively dangerous but necessary environment. Statistics show that the sacrum and heels are the most likely areas to break down. Oot-Giromini 1 reported incidence rates of up to 48% and 14%, respectively, while Cuddigan and Young reported prevalence rates of 28.3% and 24.1%, respectively.49

Proper utilization of support surfaces, including proper choice and correct and consistent positioning on the sur-

face, can minimize contractures, minimize the effects of hyperactive reflexes and muscle synergies that affect the integrity of the skin, provide restful sleep, and maximize a client's independence in self-mobility. Mattresses either equalize pressure by passive or powered redistribution or by alternately removing pressure from areas at even intervals ("alternating pressure"). The clinician chooses the appropriate surface, determines the therapeutic positions for the client, chooses the equipment to attain those positions, and instructs caregivers on use of the equipment.

Effects on Pressure Ulcer Formation

No matter how conforming the surface of the bed, when the many contours of the body are placed on a relatively flat bed, tissues over bony prominences are likely to endure high pressures that lead to tissue breakdown. These tissues—at the occiput, shoulder, elbow, lateral trochanter, sacrum/coccyx, fibular head, malleoli, and heels—must be protected when they are on the weight-bearing surface of the client. The positioning goals are to support the body, position the major joints in good alignment, and achieve muscular relaxation.

In the supine position, the head and neck should be centered, with the cervical and lumbar curves supported. The trunk should be aligned and straight. Anatomically, the resting position for the hips and knees is not fully extended or straight, but bent or flexed 25°–30°.44 Maintaining this slight flexion for the hips in the supine position can put increased pressure on the sacrum and heels. Therefore, these prominences must be watched carefully and provided with extra protection if the surface itself is not adequate.

Protection for the sacrum can take the form of lifting one side of the pelvis so that the sacrum is not directly bearing weight. The heels can be protected by elevating them with a firm pillow under the calves or with heel protection devices on the feet or under the lower leg (Figures 17-8A and B). Devices should be chosen that take all weight off of the heel to eliminate pressure, rather than simply putting a layer of padding under the heel.50 The ankles should be maintained close to 90° (a right angle) if bedrest will be prolonged to prevent the development of foot drop or contractures in the plantar flexors.

In the supine position, the lower extremities should be maintained in a neutral position, with the knees and toes pointing straight up to the ceiling and about shoulder-width apart. Protection in the form of pressure-reducing surfaces or ancillary positioners may be required for the at-risk areas of the occiput, thoracic spinous processes, and elbows.

Many people consider side-lying to consist of turning the body so that it is at a 90° angle from supine. However, this is documented to put the greater trochanter at tremendous risk of breakdown, and documentation advocates the use of a 30° incline, rather than a 90° incline.43,51 This position takes direct pressure off the pointed lateral trochanter and distributes weight across flatter areas of the posterolateral femur. In this position, the head and neck should be centrally aligned, with the cervical curve supported. Support is

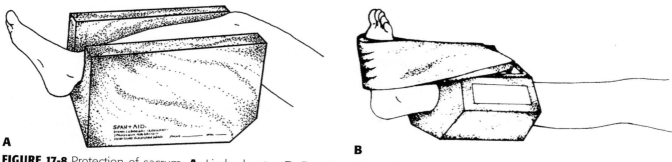

FIGURE 17-8 Protection of sacrum. **A.** Limb elevator. **B.** Foot Drop Stop. (Courtesy of Span-America Medical Systems, Greenville, South Carolina.)

needed behind the entire trunk and pelvis to maintain the 30° position as shown in Chapter 16. CS The uppermost leg tends to adduct and rest on the bed, but should be elevated with pillows or foam positioners so that it is aligned with the trunk and maintained in a neutral rotation, with slight hip and knee flexion for comfort. The lowermost leg must be protected from pressure from the uppermost leg so that tissue breakdown on the medial knee, malleolus, and foot can be avoided. Protection in the form of pressure-reducing surfaces or ancillary positioners may be required for the at-risk areas of the lowermost ear, shoulder, greater trochanter, lateral knee, lateral malleolus, and fifth metatarsal head, and the uppermost medial knee and medial malleolus. The uppermost arm must be given support as close to the open-pack or resting position of the shoulder (55° abduction with 30° horizontal adduction48) as can be achieved comfortably, so that it does not fall forward across the body or fall backward, pulling the trunk into a twisted position.

The prone position requires full range of motion of the cervical, thoracic, and lumbar spine and is not well tolerated by most clients. This position requires full extension at the hip and knee, and full external rotation of the shoulders. The trunk should be centrally aligned, with the head turned to the side. The hips should be in neutral rotation and slight abduction, and the ankles plantarflexed. The bony prominences at risk are the ears, patellas, and dorsum of the feet. Not only does the prone position put the shoulder into its most stressful position of full external rotation with abduction, but it can also encourage footdrop, due to the ankle position. However, it takes all weight off of sitting weight-bearing surfaces, and is used to stretch the hips and back into extension, the opposite of their sitting position.

Choosing Equipment

Many factors go into choosing bed support surfaces,. Here, surfaces are presented in categories. Each of these categories offers positive and negative features for maintaining position and maximizing mobility.

In 2001, the National Pressure Ulcer Advisory Panel (NPUAP) initiated the Support Surfaces Standards Initiative (S3I), a workgroup tasked with developing uniform terminology and test methods, and reporting standards for support surfaces. The resulting guidelines will be an objective means for evaluating and comparing support surface characteristics. At of the time of this writing, their work is incomplete. Progress and output of this workgroup can be found at the NPUAP website, www.npuap.org.

Overlays

The term "overlay" is often misused to include any mattress other than a standard hospital or consumer mattress. In fact, overlays are designed to be used on top of mattresses. They are usually thinner than a mattress, approximately 1–4 inches thick. Whether powered alternating surfaces, cut foam, water or gel-filled, all overlays raise the level of the bed surface. This can make the sit-to-stand movement easier; however, moving from standing to sitting and sitting on the edge of a bed are safer to accomplish when the height of the surface of the bed is equal to the distance from the back of the knee to the bottom of the foot. Overlays tend to raise this level, making ingress and egress more dangerous. However, overlays are inexpensive, and foam overlays with individual, undercut and cross-cut cells (e.g., Geo-Matt) are extremely effective pressure distributors.52 If the level of the height of the bed can be changed or if ingress and egress are not issues, an overlay can be a cost-effective and appropriate choice.

For the most part, overlays are used for prevention of tissue breakdown in clients who are at-risk. They are seldom recommended for treatment, as they are, of necessity, too thin to prevent the client from bottoming out onto the very surface they are being protected from.

Mattress Replacements

Most clinicians prefer a mattress replacement with a stable bolster edge for client safety when sitting on the edge of the bed. A trapeze setup can help clients lift their bodies to move, rather than sliding across a surface. This helps to limit shearing forces.

Static Mattress Replacements. Static mattress replacements come in a variety of mediums: all foam, foam/air, foam/water, and foam/gel. They are not powered, i.e., they do not have a motor or plug into the wall. These surfaces replace standard mattresses and offer better redistribution of pressures than standard mattresses. They eliminate the extra height that an overlay entails and are often purchased as permanent equipment for the client, rather than as a rental

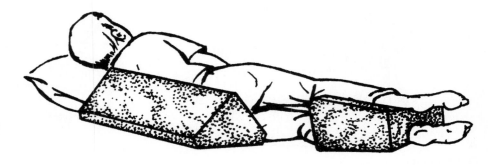

FIGURE 17-9 30° Wedge for body alignment in side-lying. (Courtesy of Span-America Medical Systems, Greenville, South Carolina.)

item. However, they are more expensive than an overlay. Static surfaces generally offer a more stable surface to accomplish bed mobility, ingress, and egress than do alternating pressure or low-air-loss mattresses.

Static mattress replacements are sometimes called "Group I" products, as this is the name for the group of static mattresses that is reimbursable under Medicare for prevention and first-level ulcer treatment intervention.

Powered Dynamic 397 Mattress Replacements. This group of mattresses is commonly paid for by Medicare and insurance companies during the treatment of tissue breakdown. Since a client should not be positioned on the ulcer, the effect of these surfaces in actually affecting healing is questionable. At the very least, they prevent breakdown on the weightbearing surfaces of the body by directly affecting the tissues through pressure changes or moisture removal.

Powered dynamic mattresses entail some means of moving air through the mattress using electrically powered motors. One technology, low-air-loss, uses a porous fabric to wick heat and moisture down into the mattress system and a blower to move the air, heat, and moisture out of the system. This decrease in maceration of the skin makes it less susceptible to pressure. Using graphical techniques and documented changes in oxygenation over the sacral skin with cooling, Lachenbruch estimated that a 3°C drop in skin temperature might equate to a 14% reduction in interface pressure.[30] Another technology that cyclically moves air through chambers in the mattress to alternately put pressure on and take pressure off of each area of the body at regular intervals is called "alternating pressure." This technology does not remove moisture as the low-air-loss mattresses do.

Powered surfaces are often referred to as "Group II" surfaces, as this is the name for the group of mattresses that is reimbursable under Medicare for the treatment of pressure ulcers, given certain conditions.

Nonpowered Dynamic Mattress Replacements. This category of mattresses offers the stability of the static mattress replacement for maintaining or changing position, along with the skin protection of a dynamic mattress. Some accomplish this by dynamic air movement for self-adjustment to bony prominences accomplished by interconnected elasticized reservoirs that accept air from and release air into the support tubes (e.g., PressureGuard CFT).[53] Others accomplish this with gel/fluid bladders that conform to the

body and reduce shearing (e.g., RIK Mattress). Still others use self-adjusting air valves that maintain air pressures within the air cylinders for pressure redistribution.

Air-Fluidized Surfaces. These surfaces are considered to be the best surfaces for equalizing pressures across the entire body and reducing soft tissue shearing, heat, and moisture on the skin. In a large retrospective study, Ochs et al found that ulcers on air-fluidized surfaces had significantly faster healing rates for all ulcer stages, particularly stage III and IV pressure ulcers, than did ulcers on powered surfaces referred to as Group II surfaces.[54] However, air-fluidized surfaces are extremely difficult to maintain therapeutic positions on, and independent ingress or egress is nearly impossible; maximal assist is usually required.

Reports in the literature have been inconclusive regarding whether any one of these methods of pressure redistribution is superior to the other in healing tissue breakdown. Many clinicians feel that powered surfaces are safer for the skin than are static surfaces, due to the constant changes in pressure, temperature, and moisture on any one body part. In a large literature review of randomized controlled trials, Cullum et al found that the benefits of alternating pressure and low-air-loss for ulcer prevention were unclear.[55] One significant disadvantage of powered mattresses is that the movement in the surface makes maintaining or changing a position more of a challenge than on a static surface. Surfaces that alternate under the client can make transfers and edge-of-bed sitting more dangerous because the bed surface is constantly shifting beneath the client.

Positioning Supplies

Since the resting position of major joints such as the hips, knees, and shoulders is slightly flexed, and bony prominences such as the trochanters require positioning in the 30° side-lying position, it is safe to say that all clients require the use of positioning devices to help maintain therapeutic and anatomic body alignment and protect bony prominences. Pillows are an inexpensive support, but they are only minimally effective. They are puffy rectangles that do not naturally conform to body contours, have a tendency to slide on the surface when body pressure is applied, and are often not readily available for positioning. Foam positioners are available that are shaped for supporting specific body contours, do not shift on the surface when pressure is applied, and are less likely to be confiscated for other purposes. These devices are often inexpensive to purchase, and they afford the client quality of alignment, positioning, and protection. Table 17-3 describes the use and expected outcomes for commonly used and available positioning supplies.

CLINICAL WISDOM
Photographs

Photograph a client in position with all appropriate positioning devices, and display the photo in a place easily seen by caregivers. This can be the most helpful way to describe positions and use of devices to all caregivers, so that devices are used consistently and appropriately.

Self-Care Treatment Guidelines

Clients and caregivers must be taught as much as possible about the equipment that has been prescribed, including why each piece was chosen, how to use it properly, where

it was ordered (for warranty repair), and how to care for it. Some clients may need to be "weaned" onto a schedule because new equipment can sit the client differently or put loads on the skin in patterns different from those of the old equipment. A sample of such a schedule follows:

Day 1: 1 hour in morning and afternoon; assess skin response after each session.

Day 2: 1.5 hours in morning and afternoon; assess skin response after each session.

Day 3: 2 hours in morning and afternoon; assess skin response after each session.

Increase the sitting time gradually until a full day of sitting is achieved.

Similarly, some patients can spend a full night in one position, with no adverse effects to their skin or tissues. This should be determined carefully, with a gradual increase in time between position changes, and a careful inspection of the skin on the wieghtbearing surfaces for redness that does not blanch or disappear within an hour or so.

TABLE 17-3 Positioning Supplies for Recumbent Position

Device	Function	Action/Outcome
Abduction pillow	Maintains lower extremities in slight abduction, neutral rotation, and knee extension	Supine—maintains lower extremities (LEs) in neutral positions Side-lying—maintains separation of LEs to protect medial knee and malleolus of upper leg
30° Incline wedge (See Figure 17-9)	Supports trunk and pelvis in 30° side-lying position	Side-lying—protects lower greater trochanter by maintaining 30° incline position
Cradle Boot or Heel Protector	Keeps heel elevated off surface while maintaining right angle or neutral ankle dorsiflexion	Supine—Protects heel from breakdown by suspending off surface Should also protect malleoli, fifth metatarsal heads, and Achilles tendon Side-lying—suspends lower malleoli and fifth metatarsal head
Limb elevator (See Figure 17-8A)	Uses wedge with leg trough to put LE in slight hip/knee flexion with ankle elevated above knee	Supine—maintains neutral hip position with slight hip/knee flexion and foot elevation Side-lying—is used with trough side down to cup the lower leg and maintain leg separation for skin protection
Flexion/abduction pillow	Maintains slight knee flexion with separation of medial knee surfaces	Supine—maintains hip/knee flexion while breaking up adduction tone
Cervical pillow	Shaped to support cervical curve while cradling occiput	Maintains cervical curve in supine or side-lying positions
Occipital pillow, head-neck cushion, Occi-Dish	Cradles posterior surface of skull to reduce or eliminate pressure on occiput.	Supine—protects occiput by pressure removal, supports cervical curve, in hibits tonic lab reflex Side-lying—protects lower ear and supports cervical curve

Conclusion

Positioning in the seated and recumbent positions requires constant learning, creativity, and patience. It is up to the responsible clinician to begin and continue the learning process by evaluating new technology as it is developed, determining client needs, assessing features of new products, and matching needs with features to optimally benefit clients. Because positioning is a dynamic process, a reassessment date should be set so that the therapist can monitor the fit and functioning of the equipment and modify it to match the client's needs.

CASE STUDY

Therapeutic Positioning for Pressure Ulcer Healing

HISTORY

The client is a long-term resident of a skilled nursing facility. Past medical history includes surgical removal of a benign brain tumor 10 years prior to current therapy intervention. She has paralysis of the lower extremities and significant cognitive deficits (see Figures 17-10A and B). She sits in a wheelchair for 6 hours, two times per day, for a total of 12 hours daily, and is totally dependent for changing position in bed and sitting. She requires a two-person assist for all transfers. She is totally dependent in all ADLs (feeding, wheelchair propulsion, dental hygiene, dressing)

REASONS FOR REFERRAL

- Right ischial tuberosity pressure ulcer, stage III, increasing in length, width, and depth
- Hyperactive reflexes, extensor synergy in trunk and hip musculature with mild flexion contractures in knees that make positioning in bed and pressure relief in wheelchair difficult.

EXAMINATIONS

Neuromuscular

Reflex exam shows hyperactive reflexes of the trunk and hip present in recumbent and sitting positions.

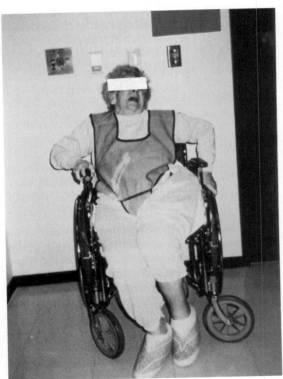 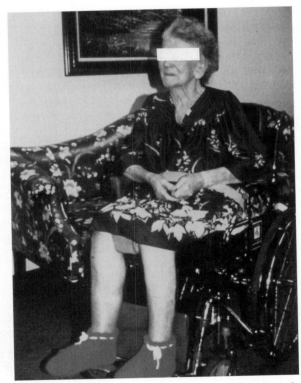

FIGURE 17-10 Therapeutic positioning for pressure ulcer healing. **A**. Before therapeutic positioning. Note cervical and trunk hyperextension, pelvis/chest restraint, right pelvic obliquity, hips forward on seat, lower extremities unsupported. **B**. After therapeutic positioning. Note that head, neck, and trunk are in good postural alignment and are in a safe and functional position. Shoulders are relaxed and equal, and hands are in client's lap. She is facing forward and able to make eye contact. The knees are level and lower extremities are supported. (Courtesy of Debby Hagler, PT, Cheyenne Mountain Rehabilitation.)

■ CASE STUDY *(Continued)*

Musculoskeletal

Muscle Strength Exam. Trunk strength is poor, and upper extremity strength is fair but not functional. The client has no volitional movement in lower extremities.

Range of Motion Exam. All joint ranges of motion are within functional limits with the exception of knee flexion contractures, which measure 20° bilaterally. There is a flexible right pelvic obliquity, 2 inches lower on the right than on the left.

Postural Exam. The client prefers full fetal position with flexion of all major joints in side-lying when recumbent; in supine recumbent position, head and neck are hyperextended into the pillow, and extensor posture dominates at all other major jointsIn sitting, she demonstrates trunk, hip, and knee extension with pelvis sliding forward on the seat and into posterior tilt, and the cervical spine is in hyperextension. She is bearing weight on her hands and right hip. The right side of the pelvis is rotated and tilted posteriorly. The right hip is externally rotated, and the left hip is internally rotated. Both knees are flexed (see figure 17- 10A).

ADL. The client is unable to move or change positions volitionally in the bed or wheelchair. She is dependent in all transfers, requiring total assistance of two-person transfer. She is dependent for all ADLs, including feeding, hygiene, dressing, and wheelchair propulsion.

Sensory

The client is unable to detect deep or surface pressure on sitting surfaces and lower extremities.

Integumentary

The client has a Braden Scale pressure ulcer risk assessment score of 12, which is considered high risk.

She presents with a stage III pressure ulcer on the right ischial tuberosity, measuring 3 cm × 3 cm × 1 cm deep. The pressure ulcer is 50% yellow slough and 50% granulation tissue. The surrounding skin is pale, and the perimeter is macerated. Drainage is serosanguineous. No undermining or tunneling is present.

Interface pressures over the sacrum, trochanter, heels, and shoulders in the supine and side-lying positions in bed were considered unsafe, as they ranged from 70 mm Hg to greater than 100 mm Hg and were higher than the flat surfaces of the body. Interface pressures over the right ischial tuberosity and coccyx in the sitting position in the wheelchair were also considered unsafe, as they were greater than 100 mm Hg and higher than the flatter areas of the sitting surface.

EVALUATION

Muscle weakness and joint impairment contribute to her inability to weight shift in the sitting and recumbent positions. She has a learned disuse of her arms and does not demonstrate postural movement strategies to change her position. Her sitting posture puts her at a biomechanical disadvantage to use her weakened muscles, which prevents functional movement. The stage III pressure ulcer over the right ischial tuberosity is a consequence of her inability to weight shift off of the bony prominence of the ischial. Maceration around the wound site is probably a combination of factors that disrupt the moisture balance in the area, including heat and moisture build up around her seat cushion, the 6-hour period of time she is seated in her wheelchair twice daily, and possible wound exudate and/or incontinence. Her sensory impairments on the seating surface and impaired cognition contribute to her tissue breakdown.

FUNCTIONAL DIAGNOSIS

• Patient is disabled and unable to fulfill functional roles due to her lack of mobility, putting her at risk for pressure ulcers on bony prominences

NEED FOR PHYSICAL THERAPIST SERVICES

The client needs intervention by a physical therapist to achieve the following goals:

1. Healing the pressure ulcer
2. Correct postural alignment, including ability to shift weight and redistribute pressures on the seating surface off of bony prominences to tolerant areas
3. Retrain functional movement for weight shifting and use of upper extremities
4. Reduce risk of additional ulcerations

PROGNOSIS

1. The ulcer will heal.
2. The risk of further pressure ulceration will be reduced by positioning intervention to allow restoration of functional mobility.
3. Adaptive support surface and positioning equipment will aid in restoration of function.
4. The client will sit in a functional upright position in wheelchair with a 90° hip-to-back angle with a side-to-side wedged, pressure-eliminating seat cushion and a firm back cushion, with lower extremities supported and protected.
5. In the functional upright position, she will be retrained to use her upper extremities for self-care.
4. The sitting schedule will be changed to 2 hours, three times per day, for a total sitting time of 6 hours; the time up in the wheelchair will be coordinated with the meal schedule to facilitate safe swallowing, improved nutritional intake, and environmental stimulation. Sitting time will be increased gradually according to a prescribed sitting schedule.
5. The client will be positioned in functional positions in supine and 30° side-lying positions on a prescribed support surface in bed, with safe interface pressure readings on all bony prominences in all positions.
6. Staff will demonstrate correct use of all equipment supplied and therapeutic positioning of this client at all times, whether in bed or in the wheelchair.

(Continued)

CASE STUDY *(Continued)*

INTERVENTION: THERAPEUTIC POSITIONING

Recommendations for adaptive seating equipment.

1. Wedged seat assembly with 5 in on one side, decreasing to 3 in on the other, with full pressure-relief pocket at ischials and coccyx, sized to distribute pressure fully over posterior trochanter and thighs
2. Firm back support to maintain an 85° seat-to-back angle to prevent extensor synergy
3. A positioning hip belt secured midway down the seat rail to fasten at a 90° angle to the thigh to assist in keeping the pelvis and lower extremities in appropriate position
4. Padded lap tray to provide upper extremity and trunk support
5. Footrests, calf support, and protective footwear to protect and support lower extremities and facilitate appropriate positioning
6. Hip abduction wedge to inhibit adductors and extensors and to facilitate positioning and pressure distribution on the seat assembly
7. Analysis of client using adaptive equipment for appropriateness and safety
8. Instruction of caregivers in correct use of positioning devices

Recommendations for Therapeutic Positioning in Bed:

1. A self-adjusting, dynamic air/foam mattress replacement to encourage mobility and allow skin protection
2. Positioning in a 30° side-lying position to distribute interface pressure away from the trochanter and shoulder
3. Wedges and a pillow placed between the knees to maintain the side-lying position
4. In supine, use of a leg-elevating positioning cushion to facilitate reduction in hip extensor muscle hyperactivity, accommodate for the knee flexion contractures, and position heels off the bed
5. Head-positioning cushion to provide occipital and cervical spine support and prevent excessive cervical extension in supine
6. Over-the-bed trapeze and side rails, and encouragement in their use to assist client in self-mobility

Assessment of client using recumbent positioning and pressure-relief devices for safety and proper pressure relief

Staff instruction:

1. Instruction in appropriate use of all seating and bed-positioning supplies and equipment
2. Instruction in safe and effective position changes, transfers, and positioning in the bed and wheelchair
3. Provide instruction for two shifts of nursing personnel because of projected sitting schedule of 2 hours, three times per day, coordinated with the meal schedule
4. Provide instruction about monitoring strength, endurance for sitting, and skin tolerance under the new prescribed schedule
5. Follow-up assessment of staff for appropriate and safe use of devices and components of the devices

FUNCTIONAL OUTCOMES

1. The client is able to sit in a functional and safe position for a total of 9 hours per 24-hour period (3 hours, three times per day).
2. Interface pressure is eliminated on the ischial tuberosities and coccyx, and pelvic alignment obliquity is corrected.
3. With corrected postural alignment, movement has been facilitated, and she has learned improved motor control and better use of her weakened muscles in the neck, trunk, hips, and abdomen. She has recovered functional use of her arms and is now using her arms to feed herself and propel the wheelchair.
4. The client is positioned in a safe and functional position in bed on a nonpowered dynamic air/foam mattress replacement with safe interface pressure on all bony prominences in all positions; in side-lying, using a wedge cushion behind the back, a wedge cushion under the bottom leg, and a pillow between the knees; and in supine, using a leg-positioning cushion and head-positioning cushion.
5. The client is able to assist in repositioning self from side to side, using the trapeze and side rails. No additional ulcers have developed,. The risk assessment score is reduced to 16.
6. The pressure ulcer on the ischial tuberosity is healed.

Note: Case study and photographs provided by Debby Hagler, PT, Cheyenne Mountain Rehabilitation.

REVIEW QUESTIONS

1. What are the most vulnerable bony prominences for tissue breakdown in the seated position? In the recumbent position?
2. What are the skin signs of shear and friction? Where are they most likely to occur?
3. It has been noted that bed is the most dangerous place for a client to be. Discuss the negative effects of prolonged bedrest, and the sites on the body most likely to break down from lying in bed.
4. Describe the ideal sitting position.
5. What are the five measurements that must be taken on the body when measuring a client for a new wheelchair? Why is each measurement important to the fit of the wheelchair?

RESOURCES

Motor Control Theory

Shumway-Cook A, Wollacott MH. Motor Control: Theory and Practical Applications. 2nd Edition. Baltimore: Lippincott Williams & Wilkins, 2001.

The following is a representative listing of manufacturing sources for the categories of seat cushion products discussed in the text. Some manufacturers have products in multiple categories.

Pressure Reduction
AliMed
Ken McRight Supplies - Bye-bye Decubiti
Maddak
Skil-Care
Span-America Medical - Geo-Matt

Generic Contour
Cascade Designs - Varilite
Crown Therapeutics - Roho family
Jay Medical - Jay basic, Jay2
Span-America Medical - Geo-Matt Contour, EZ-Dish
Supracor

Selective Pressure Elimination
Span-America Medical; ISCH-DISH
Ride Designs

Customized Contour
Freedom Designs
Invacare – Contour-U
Otto Bock Shape System
Signature 2000
Ride Designs

SCI Clinical Practice Guidelines
Paralyzed Veterans of America

Wheelchair Seating Standards
International Standards Organization Working Group–II

Support Surface Standards
Support Surface Standards Initiative (S3I); supported by the National Pressure Ulcer Advisory Panel (NPUAP) found at www.npuap.org.

REFERENCES

1. Oot-Giromini B. Pressure ulcer prevalence, incidence and associated risk factors in the community. *Decubitus.* 1993;6(5):24–32.
2. Maklebust J, Sieggreen M. *Pressure Ulcers: Guidelines for Prevention and Nursing Management.* West Dundee, IL: S-N Publications, 1991.
3. Pompeo M, Baxter C. Sacral and ischial pressure ulcers: Evaluation, treatment, and differentiation. *Ostomy/Wound Manage.* 2000;46(1):18–23.
4. Disa J, Carlton J, Goldberg N. Efficacy of operative care in pressure sore clients. *Plast Reconstr Surg.* 1992;89:272–278.
5. Evans G, Dufresene CR, Manson PN. Surgical correction of pressure ulcers in an urban center: Is it efficacious? *Adv Wound Care.* 1994;7(1):40–46.
6. Curtin I. Wound management care and cost: An overview. *Nurse Manage.* 1984;15(2):22.
7. Geyer M, et al. A randomized clinical trial to evaluate pressure reducing seat cushions for at-risk, elderly nursing home residents. *Adv Wound Care.* 2001;14(3):120-9; quiz 131-2.
8. Ragan R, Kernozek TW, Bidar M, Metheson JW. Seat-interface pressures on various thicknesses of foam wheelchair cushions: a finite modelling approach. *Arch Phys Med Rehabil.* 2002;83(6):872-5.
9. Sprigle S, Dunlop W, Press L. Reliability of bench tests of interface pressure. *Assist Technol.* 2003;15(1):49-57.
10. Eitzen I. Pressure mapping in seating: a frequency analysis approach. *Arch Phys Med Rehabil.* 2004;85(7):1136-40
11. Ross J, Dean E. Integrating physiological principles into the comprehensive management of cardiopulmonary dysfunction. *Phys Ther.* 1989;69:255–259.
12. Gerhart K, Weitzenkamp D, Charlifue S. The old get older: Changes over three years in aging SCI survivors. Report from Rehabilitation Research and Training Center on Aging with an SCI, Craig Hospital. *New Mobility.* June 1996;18–21.
13. Norton L, Sibbald G. Is bed rest an effective treatment modality for pressure ulcers? *Ostomy/Wound Manage.* 2004;50(10):40-52.
14. Trefler E, Fitzgerald SG, Hobson DA, et al. Outcomes of wheelchair systems intervention with residents of long-term care facilities. *Assist Technol.* 2004;16(1):18-27.
15. Fuchs RH, Gromak PA. Wheelchair use by residents of nursing homes: effectiveness in meeting positioning and mobility needs. *Assist Technol.* 2003;15(2):151-63.
16. Mooney V, Einbund MJ, Rogers JE, Stauffer ES. Comparison of pressure distribution qualities in seat cushions. *Bull Prosthet Res.* 1971;10(15):129–143.
17. Engstrom B. *Seating for Independence: Manual of Principles.* Waukesha, WI: ETAC USA, 1993.
18. Kreutz D. Seating and positioning for the newly injured. *Rehab Manage.* 1993;6:67–75.
19. Manser S, Boeker C. Seating considerations: Spinal cord injury. *PT Magazine.* December 1993;47–51.
20. Presperin J. Postural considerations for seating the client with spinal cord injury. In: *Proceedings from RESNA Seating Conference;* June 6–11, 1992; Vancouver, BC, Canada.
21. Walpin LA. Posture—The process of body use: Principles and determinants. In: Gelb H, ed. *New Concepts in Craniomandibular and Chronic Pain Management.* St. Louis, MO: Mosby-Year Book, 1994:13–76.
22. Zacharkow D. *Wheelchair Posture and Pressure Sores.* Springfield, IL: Charles C Thomas, 1984.
23. Rappl L. A conservative treatment for pressure ulcers. *Ostomy/Wound Manage.* 1993;39(6):46–48, 50–55.
24. Garber S. Wheelchair cushions for spinal cord injured individuals. *Am J Occup Ther.* 1985;39:722–725.
25. Ferguson-Pell M. Seat cushion selection. *J Rehabil Res Dev.* 1990;(Suppl 2):49–73.
26. Key AG, Manley MT. Pressure redistribution in wheelchair cushion for paraplegics: Its application and evaluation. *Paraplegia.* 1978–1979;16:403–412.
27. Peterson M, Adkins H. Measurement and redistribution of excessive pressures during wheelchair sitting. *Phys Ther.* 1982;62:990–994.
28. DuBois EF. Basil Metabolism in Health and Disease. 3rd Ed. Philadelphia: Lea and Febiger, 1936.
29. Ruch RC, Patton HD, eds. Physiology and Biophysics. 19th Ed. Philadelphia: WB Saunders, 1965:1030-1049.
30. Lachenbruch C. Skin cooling surfaces: estimating the importance of limiting skin temperature. *Ostomy/Wound Mgmt.* 2005;51(2):70-79.
31. Local Coverage Determination for Wheelchair Seating, Palmetto GBA Medicare Region C, L15887. Medical Criteria for Seat Cushions, Original effective date 07/01/2004. http://www.palmettogba.com/palmetto/lmrps_dmerc.nsf/final/202772596F05D33285256F51006A855D?OpenDocument.
32. Aissaoui R, Boucher C, Bourbonnais D, et al. Effect of seat cushion on dynamic stability in sitting during a reaching task in wheelchair users with paraplegia. *Arch Phys Med Rehabil.* 2001;82(2):274-81.
33. Knight A. Medical management of pressure sores. *J Fam Pract.* 1988;27:95–100.
34. National Pressure Ulcer Advisory Panel. Pressure ulcers—Prevalence, cost, and risk assessment: Consensus development conference statement. *Decubitus.* 1989;2(2):24–28.
35. Noble PC. The prevention of pressure sores in clients with spinal cord injuries. In: *International Exchange of Information in Rehabilitation.* New York: World Rehabilitation Fund, 1981.
36. Stotts N. The physiology of wound healing. In: Stotts N, Cuzzell J, eds. *Proceedings from the AACCN National Teaching Institute.* Kansas City, MO: Marion Laboratories, 1988.
37. van Rijswijk L. Full thickness pressure ulcers: Client wound healing characteristics. *Decubitus.* 1991;6(1):16–21.
38. Ferguson-Pell MW, Wilkie IC, Reswick JB, Barbenel JC. Pressure sore prevention for the wheelchair-bound spinal injury client. *Paraplegia.* 1980;18:42–51.

39. Perkash I, O'Neill H, Politi-Meeks D, Beets CL. Development and evaluation of a universal contoured cushion. *Paraplegia.* 1984;22:358–365.

40. Reswick JB, Rogers JE. Experience at Rancho Los Amigos Hospital with devices and techniques to prevent pressure sores. In: Kenedi RM, Cowden JM, Scales JT, eds. *Bedsore Biomechanics.* Baltimore: University Park Press, 1976:301–310.

41. Rogers J, Wilson L. Preventing recurrent tissue breakdowns after "pressure sore" closures. *Plast Reconstr Surg.* 1975;56:419–422.

42. Rappl L. Seating for skin and wound management. In: *Proceedings from Thirteenth International Seating Symposium.* Pittsburgh, PA: January 23–25, 1997.

43. Pressure Ulcers in Adults: Prediction and Prevention Clinical Practice Guideline Number 3, AHCPR Pub. No. 92-0047: May 1992 . http://www.ahrq.gov/clinic/cpgonline.htm

44. Metzler D, Harr J. Positioning your client properly. *Am J Nurs.* 1996;96:33–37.

45. Plautz R. Positioning can make the difference. *Nurs Homes Long Term Care Manage.* 1992;41:30–34.

46. Cantin JE. Proper positioning eliminates client injury. *Today's OR Nurse.* 1989;11:18–21.

47. Kozier B. *Fundamentals of Nursing: Concepts, Process and Practice.* 4th ed. Redwood City, CA: Addison-Wesley Publishing, 1991.

48. Magee D. *Orthopedic Physical Assessment.* Philadelphia: WB Saunders, 1992.

49. Cuddigan J, Young J. Trends in pressure ulcer prevalence; 1989-2004. Platform presentation at Wound Ostomy Continence Nurse 2005 Annual Conference, June, 2005, Las Vegas, NV.

50. Pinzur M, et al. Preventing heel ulcers: A comparison of prophylactic body-support systems. *Arch Phys Med Rehabil.* 1991;72:508–510.

51. Seiler WO, Stahelin HB. Decubitus ulcers: preventive techniques for the elderly client. Geriatrics 1985;40(7):53.

52. Day A, Leonard F. Seeking quality care for clients with pressure ulcers. *Decubitus.* 1993;6(1):32-43.

53. Branom R, Rappl L. 'Constant force technology' vs. low-air-loss in the treatment of wounds. *Ostomy/Wound Management.* 2001;47(9):38-46.

54. Ochs R, Horn S, van Rijswijk L, et al. Comparison of air-fluidized therapy with other support surfaces used to treat pressure ulcers in nursing home residents. *Ostomy/Wound Management.* 2005;51(2):38-68.

55. Cullum N, McInnes E, Bell-Syer SE, Legood R. Support surfaces for pressure ulcer prevention. Cochrane Database Syst Rev. Issue 3, pages CD001735.

Diagnosis and Management of Vascular Ulcers

Roland A. Palmquist, Lilly Shimahara, Carlos E. Donayre

CHAPTER OBJECTIVES

At the completion of this chapter, the reader will be able to:

1. Describe the vascular anatomy of the lower extremity and its relationship to peripheral vascular disease.
2. Identify signs and symptoms of peripheral vascular disease.
3. Analyze ulcer risk factors for patients with arterial occlusive disease.
4. Review the pathogenesis of diabetes and foot ulceration.
5. Describe the pathophysiology of venous stasis ulcers.
6. Explain the differential diagnosis of venous stasis ulcers.
7. Describe medical treatment and classification of venous stasis ulcers.
8. Describe the anatomy of the lymphatic circulation.
9. Describe the features and causes of atypical, nonatherosclerotic ulcers.

Homeostasis, or the ability of a living system to maintain itself within a physiologic range compatible with life, is a key concept in physiology. A functional living system will repair itself if it is able. If a living system is unable to maintain homeostasis, wounds can develop, and ultimately death will ensue. There are three primary reasons why wounds do not heal:

1. Inadequate vascular support (arterial, venous, or lymphatic flow)
2. Excessive pressure (biomechanical, weight, or sheer pressure)
3. Inadequate nutritional support to grow new tissue

When a clinician is faced with a wound that is not healing sufficiently, the above factors should be reviewed. All effort should be made to minimize the detrimental effects of these factors. Numerous approaches to wound management have been proposed, all of which can be considered subsets of the above three factors. For example, infection or increased bioburden amplifies local oxygen consumption, thereby increasing vascular demand and inducing local ischemia, which inhibits wound healing. If there is inadequate vascular supply to support the healing tissue, no form of advanced wound dressing will heal the wound. However, advanced wound dressings can aid in supporting the vascula-

ture, decreasing pressure, and improving local tissue nutrition to achieve healing in severely compromised patients. The purpose of this chapter is to review the assessment and treatment of the vascular system in patients with acute and chronic wounds.

When one considers the tasks that feet routinely accomplish, it is not difficult to understand why they develop so many problems. A man of average weight (160–180 pounds) walks 7.5 miles on an average day. This requires that each foot carry more than 500 tons a day! Women's lighter bodies place fewer demands on the feet than do the usually heavier men's bodies, but fashionable footwear nullifies this weight advantage. High-heeled shoes put 75% more pressure on the balls of the feet than does walking barefoot. The constant wear and tear that feet submit to daily takes its toll, and as individuals age, it is more likely they will develop foot problems. At one time or another, 85% of all Americans experience foot problems serious enough to require professional attention. In patients in long-term care facilities, this figure rises to nearly 100%.[1]

Most people afflicted with foot ailments fail to seek professional help promptly, relying instead on self-diagnosis and treatment. The causes of foot problems are rarely obvious, and delays in correcting them give the underlying disorder more time to develop and worsen. Furthermore, when a serious disease is misdiagnosed as a minor foot malady, results are often drastic and costly. Therefore, patient education regarding the potential complications and associated treatment of foot problems is critical to preventing and minimizing sequelae. Dry skin, brittle nails, numbness, discoloration, and coolness are usually minor signs and symptoms of foot ailments, but they can also be the first indication of vascular insufficiency or diabetes (see Chapter 19).

Vascular Anatomy of the Lower Extremities

To clearly understand the effects of altered circulation on the feet, a basic knowledge of vascular anatomy is needed. Neither the vascular system of the lower extremities nor the tasks it performs is terribly complicated. The vascular supply of the body is composed of three subsystems, the arterial, venous, and lymphatic systems. The main role of arteries is to provide a pulsatile flow of oxygen and nutrient-rich blood to the tissues. The role of the venous system is to return the oxygen-depleted and toxin-laden blood back to the heart for restoration to the arterial system. The role of the lymphatic system in the lower extremities is to collect lymph fluid from the interstitial spaces and maintain normal fluid balance through protein transport; perform immune surveillance and trap bacteria and foreign material in lymph nodes; and return the lymph from the lower extremities to the venous circulation via left subclavian vein.

Arterial System

The aorta, the largest blood vessel in the body, divides into two large branches, the right and left common iliac arteries, at the level of the umbilicus (Figure 18-1). Each of these branches divides again into external and internal iliac arteries. The internal iliac artery, also known as the *hypogastric artery*, supplies the pelvis via a variety of branches. The external iliac artery travels distally and becomes the common femoral artery when it crosses the inguinal ligament. This vessel again divides and gives rise to the superficial femoral and deep femoral arteries. The deep femoral artery, or profunda femoris, supplies the muscles of the thigh and is truly the workhorse of the leg. This vessel becomes a major collateral pathway to the lower extremity when the superficial femoral artery becomes occluded (e.g., due to atherosclerotic disease). The superficial femoral artery becomes the popliteal artery when it crosses the adductor canal, which is formed by the tendon of the adductor magnus muscle. This is the most common site of atherosclerotic disease in the lower extremity and may be related to local vessel trauma caused by the constant pulsation of the superficial femoral artery against this hard, tendinous structure.

The popliteal artery courses medially and divides below the knee to give rise to its first branch, the anterior tibial artery and tibioperoneal trunk. This trunk divides into the peroneal and posterior tibial arteries (Figure 18-2). The peroneal artery terminates at the ankle; only the

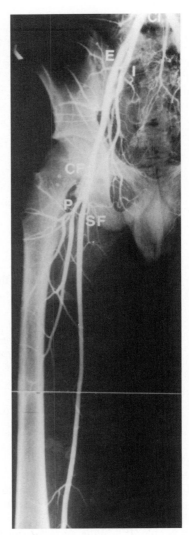

FIGURE 18-1 Normal arterial anatomy in the pelvic region. An angiogram demonstrates the usual course of the right iliac vessels: common iliac (CI), external iliac (E), and internal iliac (I) arteries. The external iliac artery becomes the common femoral artery (CF) when it crosses the inguinal ligament and gives rise to the profunda femoris artery (P) and superficial femoral artery (SF).

anterior and posterior tibial arteries travel into the foot. The region of the arterial tree where the popliteal artery branches to form the peroneal, anterior tibial, and posterior tibial branches is known commonly as the trifurcation. The anterior tibial artery continues in the foot as the dorsalis pedis artery, but it is absent or terminates early in 2% of individuals. When this occurs, the perforating branch of the peroneal artery functions as the dorsalis pedis artery. In up to 5% of individuals, the posterior tibial artery is either absent or terminates early. In this situation, the communicating branch of the peroneal artery gives rise to the plantar arches.[2] The plantar arch is formed

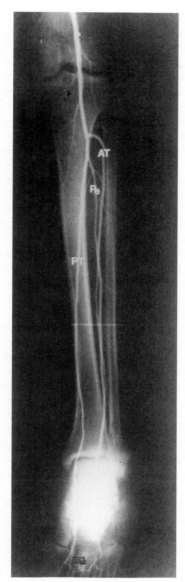

FIGURE 18-2 Normal arterial anatomy in the lower extremity. An angiogram of the left lower extremity demonstrates the usual course of the vessels. The superficial femoral artery traverses the adductor magnus canal to become the popliteal artery (P), which bifurcates into the anterior tibial artery (AT) and a tibioperoneal trunk. The tibioperoneal trunk also bifurcates to give rise to the posterior tibial (PT) and peroneal (Pe) arteries. The peroneal artery terminates at the ankle; only the anterior and posterior tibial arteries travel into the foot. The anterior tibial artery continues in the foot as the dorsalis pedis artery, and the posterior tibial artery bifurcates into the medial and lateral plantar arteries.

by the lateral plantar artery from the posterior tibial artery and the deep plantar arch from the dorsalis pedis artery. The predominant blood supply to the plantar arch originates from the dorsalis pedis artery. In most individuals, the dorsalis pedis artery and deep plantar arch give

rise to the dorsal and plantar metatarsal arteries, which go on to supply the toes.

Venous System

The venous system of the lower extremity is, in a sense, more complex to describe than the arterial system because of the numerous vessels involved and the great number of anatomic variants. A short description will suffice to provide an adequate background for the following discussion of chronic venous insufficiency.

The veins of the lower extremity are divided into superficial, deep, and perforating veins (Figure 18-3). The superficial veins are located in the subcutaneous tissues, superficial to the fascial envelope of the thigh and calf muscles. The deep veins accompany the above-mentioned arteries and lie deep to the fasciae and muscles. The perforating veins penetrate the deep fascial envelope to connect the superficial and deep venous systems. Venous flow normally occurs from the superficial to the deep veins and is directed by a system of one-way bicuspid valves, which are present in all three venous groups. These valves are more numerous in the deep venous system and distal veins.[3]

There is an important fact about venous nomenclature with regard to the superficial femoral vein: This vein begins at the adductor hiatus as a continuation of the popliteal vein. It is joined by the deep femoral vein just below the inguinal ligament to form the common femoral vein, which receives the venous drainage from the longest vein of the body, the greater saphenous vein. The superficial femoral vein is *not* a superficial vein, and any evidence of thrombosis or reflux in this vessel must not be ignored.

Lymphatic System

The lymphatic system of the lower extremity comprises a series of blind-ending vessels that return lymph to the venous system. The lymph system roughly parallels the venous system. The anatomy is highly variable, and the lymph vessels commonly form a plexus about the venous system. The blind-ending vessels originate in the interstitial spaces where the arterial-venous capillary exchange occurs. The lymphatic capillaries lack smooth muscles and thus are highly permeable to large macromolecules, such as proteins. If macromolecules are not adequately removed from interstitial tissues, lymphedema will result. The lymphatic capillaries become collecting lymphatic vessels, which have a thin layer of smooth muscle. The smooth muscle acts as a pump that propels the lymph forward through a series of unidirectional valves. The lymphatic vessels have thinner walls, more valves, and relatively larger lumens then veins. The lymphatic vessels transport the lymph fluid to lymph nodes, which filter out bacteria and foreign material, and enrich the lymph with lymphocytes. The lymphatic vessels of the lower extremity ultimately form the thoracic duct, which drains into the left subclavian vein. It is interesting to note that the final valve in the thoracic duct is reversed to prevent blood from entering the lymphatic system.[4]

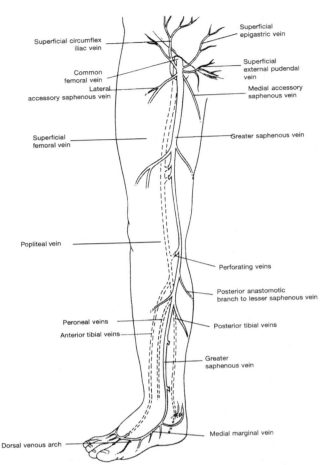

FIGURE 18-3 Normal venous anatomy. The veins of the lower extremity are divided into superficial, deep, and perforating veins.

Occlusive Peripheral Vascular Disease

Conditions of the lower extremities can usually be diagnosed accurately by obtaining a careful history and performing a detailed physical examination.

Intermittent Claudication

Intermittent claudication is the most common presenting complaint in patients with chronic arterial occlusion of the lower extremities. Charcot described the first case of intermittent claudication in humans in 1858. The word *claudication* comes from the Latin word *claudus*, which means lame or to limp. However, patients with claudication do not limp; they stop to rest. The pain from intermittent claudication is characterized by a cramping or aching sensation that occurs most often in the calf. It is associated with walking and relieved by stopping without the need to sit down. Intermittent claudication most commonly occurs as pain in the calf area; however, higher vascular obstruction, such as aortic or iliac occlusion, can cause pain in the buttocks and upper thigh, and is frequently accompanied by impotence in

men. This is known as *Leriche syndrome* or *aortoiliac occlusive disease*. If the occlusion occurs in the ankle or foot region, the patient may complain of cramping in the arch or foot.

The symptoms of intermittent claudication depend on the degree of ischemia to which the muscles in the legs are submitted. The distance a person can walk varies from patient to patient, and intermittent claudication can occur after only a short distance if the individual is walking up a hill, on a hard surface, or at a fast pace. The distance a person can walk will be longer if he or she walks more slowly and avoids inclines or hills. Over time, people with progressive intermittent claudication develop discomfort at shorter and shorter walking distances. If intermittent claudication is progressive, the patient should be promptly referred for vascular evaluation.

Examination of the patient with intermittent claudication involving the calf muscle can reveal both femoral and pedal pulses, but no popliteal pulse. In these patients, the foot will become pale and pulseless after a brisk walk because the blood flow bypasses the skin of the foot and tends to flow to the skeletal muscles of the calf instead. Intermittent claudication usually results from a single arterial blockage, which can be predicted accurately by a carefully performed pulse examination. If a femoral pulse is present, but a popliteal pulse is diminished or absent, a stenosis or occlusion likely exists in the superficial femoral artery at the adductor canal. Intact pedal pulses in the absence of a popliteal pulse imply disease of the infrapopliteal vessels or trifurcation disease. Physical findings, such as lack of hair growth on the dorsum of the foot, thickening of toenails, and delayed capillary filling, are signs of chronic arterial insufficiency.

Another part of the physical examination that should routinely be performed on patients with suspected vascular insufficiency is the resting ankle-brachial pressure measurement or index. With the patient placed in a supine position, bilateral brachial and ankle (posterior tibial and dorsalis pedis arteries) pressures are measured by obliterating blood flow with a standard, adult-sized sphygmomanometer (blood pressure) cuff. The exact pressure at which there is cessation of arterial blood flow, as determined by the use of a continuous-wave Doppler instrument placed over the area of maximum audible flow, is recorded. The systemic blood pressure can vary in patients; therefore, absolute ankle pressure is usually normalized by expressing it as a ratio of the highest obtainable brachial pressure, or ankle-brachial index (ABI).[5]

In a healthy patient, the ankle pressure is usually greater than or equal to the brachial artery pressure, with an ABI slightly greater than 1.0 mm Hg. An ABI equal to or less than 0.9 mm Hg almost always represents some degree of arterial insufficiency. For each major arterial blockage that is present, the ABI is usually reduced by 0.3 mm Hg. Thus, in patients with intermittent claudication, the resting ABI will vary between 0.5–0.8 mm Hg. In the presence of arterial sclerosis, the vessel walls are not compressible, and the ABI is artificially elevated. If the ABI is greater than 1.1 mm Hg, arterial sclerosis should be suspected (Exhibit 18-1).

Characteristic clinical signs of arterial insufficiency are *dependent rubor* and *pallor on elevation*. Dependent rubor occurs when an ischemic limb is placed in a dependent position. Gravity-assisted arterial blood flow brings oxygen-depleted blood to an area, causing vasodilation and a reddish appearance. Elevation of the extremity results in inadequate blood perfusion, which produces a pale appearance to the limb or *pallor on elevation*.

Nocturnal Pain

Nocturnal pain is a form of ischemic neuritis that usually precedes rest pain. It occurs at night, because during sleep, blood essentially circulates around the core of the body, with little perfusion to the lower extremities. The pain is classically described as occurring in the toes, across the base of the metatarsals, and in the plantar arches. Ischemic neuritis becomes intense at night or when resting and disrupts sleep. Patients gain relief by standing up, dangling their feet over the edge of the bed, or, on occasion, walking a few steps. As the occlusive disease progresses, the pain starts to occur during waking hours, which is known as rest pain. Nocturnal pain interferes with normal sleep patterns, causing patients to wake up and move their limbs, which increases blood pressure and improves peripheral perfusion.

Rest Pain

Rest pain is caused by increased nerve ischemia as a result of arterial insufficiency. The pain is persistent in nature with peaks of increasing intensity. It is worse at night and usually requires the use of narcotics for pain control. Rest pain is decreased by dependency of the lower extremities, but is aggravated by heat, elevation, and exercise. Because dependence provides relief, patients with rest pain often sleep in chairs; consequently, leg edema is secondary to constant dependence. This increases cardiac output, which leads to improved perfusion of the lower extremities and relief of the ischemic neuritis. Thus, patients with rest pain commonly display chronically edematous, erythematous feet and ankles, and may rely on a dependent position for relief of symptoms.

Rest pain usually indicates the presence of at least two hemodynamically significant arterial blocks. The ABI is re-

duced by 0.6 mm Hg with two arterial blockages, and these patients usually have an ABI of less than 0.5 mm Hg. If the lesions that produce nocturnal and rest pain are not corrected by vascular surgery, tissue necrosis and gangrene typically develops, necessitating amputation. Long-lasting local anesthetic blocks can provide short-term relief until perfusion can be restored.

Ulceration and Gangrene

Ulceration and gangrene of the lower extremities represent the most advanced complications of arterial occlusive disease and are generally associated with diffuse, severe, multilevel arterial obstruction (Figure 18-4). Ischemic ulcers generally occur on the distal portion of the foot, toe, or heel and are particularly painful. These commonly result from inadequately fitted shoes, positional pressure, or sheering in hemodynamically or medically compromised patients. These ulcers generally do not bleed and often have a necrotic rim or crater. The associated pain can be relieved by depen-

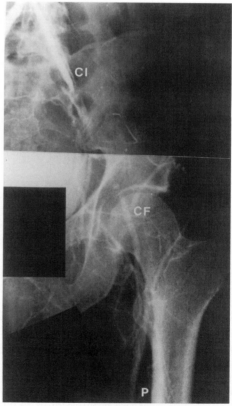

FIGURE 18-4 An angiogram reveals occlusion of left common iliac artery (CI), reconstitution of the common femoral (CF) and profunda femoris (P) arteries via collateral pathways, and occlusion of the superficial femoral artery. Multilevel atherosclerotic disease is consistent with failure of tissue healing and a decreased ABI. (See *Color Plate 55* for photos of the ulcer on this same patient.)

EXHIBIT 18-1   Noninvasive Evaluation of Arterial Insufficiency: Ankle-Brachial Index

Index	Clinical Description
> 1.1 mmHg	Calcified, noncompressible vessels must be suspected
0.9–1.1 mmHg	Normal vessels
0.5–0.8 mmHg	Intermittent claudication
< 0.5 mmHg	Rest pain, ulceration, and tissue loss

dence. As in patients with rest pain, the ABI is usually less than 0.5 mm Hg. Arterial reconstruction, if feasible, must be undertaken in patients with ulceration to prevent limb loss.

Risk Factors

The importance of risk factors in patients with arterial occlusive disease and their order of appearance or development vary widely from patient to patient. Genetic factors are extremely important risk factors; for example, premature atherosclerosis is frequently seen in family groups, with an age of onset of 40 years or older. However, it is not rare to find significant peripheral vascular disease (PVD) before the age of 40 in diabetic patients.

Smoking is another important risk factor. Clinical experience strongly confirms that patients who smoke and have chronic occlusive arterial disease affecting the extremities have a poor prognosis.[6] Among patients under the age of 50 years who quit smoking after they developed intermittent claudication, none progressed to rest pain, as opposed to those who continued to smoke. Smoking causes decreased blood flow to the extremities and a decrease in the skin temperature of the digits. A single cigarette can cause spasms of the arteries and reduction of blood flow that can last 1 hour or longer.

The mechanism by which smoking is atherogenic is unknown, but it may be related to intimal injury, which is caused by increased levels of carboxyhemoglobin. Or, it may be caused by an effect on platelet function and an increased tendency toward thrombus formation.[7] Another effect of smoking is the influence it exerts on prostacyclin, an important prostaglandin produced by the endothelium of blood vessels, which prevents platelet aggregation and promotes vasodilation. Recent work has shown that cigarette smoking inhibits prostacyclin formation.[8]

Hypertension is another extremely important risk factor in the development of PVD. In the Framingham Study,[9] hypertension imposed a threefold increased risk of developing intermittent claudication during a follow-up period of 26 years. The frequency of hypercholesterolemia and hypertriglyceridemia has also been found to be significant in most clinical diseases of the peripheral vascular system. It has been suggested that a high level of high-density lipoprotein (HDL) cholesterol does not protect patients if their low-density lipoprotein (LDL) is also inordinately high. It is probably the ratio of HDL to LDL that determines the risk factor, rather than the absolute level of each.

Patients presenting with signs and symptoms of arterial insufficiency should be counseled and educated about risk factor modification if disease progression is to be avoided.

Diabetes and Foot Ulceration

Ulceration and other complications of the foot associated with diabetes are increasing problems of significant epidemiologic proportions. Greater than 60% of nontraumatic amputations in the United States occur as a complication of diabetes.[10] Seven percent or 20.8 million people in the United States had diabetes in 2005.[10] Each year, 150,000 patients are admitted for limb amputation due to diabetes or peripheral vascular disease, at an estimated cost of $4.3 billion (1996 dollars).[11] This figure does not include the cost of loss of time from work, loss of jobs, or public assistance payments.

The amputation rate in people with diabetes is 15 times that of the nondiabetic population. The initial lesion in most of these cases is painless trauma that occurs in a neuropathic, insensate foot. It is the presence of PVD, however, that prevents these lesions from healing. Impaired circulation is a major contributor to infection, because the delivery of leukocytes and antibiotic agents is compromised by the lack of sufficient blood flow. The decreased delivery of oxygen to infected tissues further promotes the growth of highly destructive anaerobes. Studies have demonstrated that oxygen is necessary for macrophage mobility in wound debridement and the ingrowth of granulation tissue during wound healing.[12]

The function of some tissue growth factors is oxygen-dependent. Furthermore, some antibiotics, principally the aminoglycosides, depend on oxygen for their function. The triopathy of neuropathy, vascular insufficiency, and an altered response to infection makes diabetic patients uniquely susceptible to pedal complications. Not surprisingly, foot problems remain the most common indication for hospitalization in patients with diabetes mellitus.

Approximately 8% of non–insulin-dependent (type II) diabetic patients exhibit evidence of PVD at the time of diagnosis. The incidence of PVD rapidly increases with age and the duration of diabetes. Nearly 45% of patients with diabetes over 20-year duration have evidence of PVD, and this percentage is much higher in those patients who smoke. Vascular disease affecting the lower extremities of diabetic patients is similar to that found in nondiabetic patients. Changes in the vessel wall, in both the media and intima (i.e., deposits of platelets, smooth muscle cells, lipids, cholesterol, and calcium), are qualitatively the same in both groups, although these changes are quantitatively greater in patients with diabetes. There are, however, some important differences. The atherosclerotic process is more commonly seen in diabetic patients than in nondiabetic patients. It occurs at an earlier age, advances more rapidly, and is almost as common in women as in men. Differences also exist with regard to the vessels that are involved and the extent of the involvement. The femoral, iliac, and aortic vessels appear to experience a similar degree of atherosclerotic changes in diabetic and nondiabetic patients. The profunda femoris artery is affected with greater frequency and extent in diabetics, but the vessels most frequently involved in diabetes are those below the knee—the tibial and peroneal arteries and their smaller branches. In diabetic patients, multi-segment occlusions can be seen with diffused mural changes proximally and distally, whereas, in nondiabetic subjects, occlusions most often involve a single segment with a normal adjacent arterial tree. Once the process begins in diabetic patients, both lower extremities are usually involved; in nondiabetic patients, the lesions are more likely to be unilateral. A summary of 485 patients in five studies showed that, following the initial limb amputation, 42% of diabetics in the first 3 years and 56% in 3–5 years required a contralateral amputation (greater than 10% per year).[13]

Diabetes poses a unique risk because diabetic individuals tend to have severely diffuse vascular disease. Diabetic patients must pay particular attention to foot care to ward off ulceration and infection, which mandate an increase in blood flow that their vascular systems cannot supply. A major risk factor that has always been considered important in the development of diabetic vascular disease is the control of blood sugar.[14] The Diabetes Control and Complications Trial Research Group in 1993 published a study of 1,444 patients followed for 6.5 years to assess the progression of retinopathy, nephropathy, and neuropathy. Clinical neuropathy was defined as abnormal neurologic examination findings consistent with peripheral neuropathy, plus either an abnormal nerve conduction test result in at least two peripheral nerves or unequivocal autonomic nerve testing. In this multicenter study, patients were randomly assigned to standard insulin control or an intensive therapy administered by external insulin pump or three or more daily injections of insulin, guided by frequent blood sugar monitoring. The developments of neuropathy and nephropathy were each significantly reduced by the strict monitoring of insulin levels. In patients assigned to an intensive management group, the incidence of retinopathy was reduced by 76%, compared with that in patients receiving the usual twice-daily insulin injections. Equally impressive, a 69% reduction in the onset of neuropathy was reported. The findings represent the 3% incidence of neuropathy in those patients with intensive insulin management versus 10% development in those with the usual insulin management during this 5-year study. The results support the theory that more stringent insulin management will reduce the onset and progression of neuropathy. The study did note, however, that there was a twofold to threefold increase in severe hypoglycemic reactions in the strict control group, which required management.. No fatalities or serious complications were reported, despite this complication.

This and other studies support the need for optimum insulin control in diabetic patients. A therapy regimen designed to maintain blood glucose values as close to the normal range as possible would seem to prevent the onset and progression of diabetic complications. Thus, such monitoring should be part of optimum diabetic foot care.

In summary, the risk for developing PVD in diabetic patients stems from a combination of factors. Heredity, age, and the duration of diabetes are factors that cannot be controlled. Nevertheless, the blood sugar level should be well controlled – but balanced against the risk of hypoglycemia. Although each risk factor can have a variable degree of importance by itself, a combination of these factors can become very significant. Therefore, it is extremely important to control hypertension and reduce cholesterol and triglyceride levels. Needless to say, one of the strongest risk factors discussed above is smoking. It is critically important that diabetic patients and certainly all patients who have PVD do not smoke.

A common complaint of patients with peripheral vascular insufficiency is cold feet. It is the discomfort of cold feet that prompts many diabetic patients to use hot water bottles, heating pads, and hot water soaks. These practices can result in severe burns to feet that have become insensitive to heat because of peripheral neuropathy. At an ambient foot temperature of approximately 70°F, a patient requires 1 ml of blood flow per 100 g of tissue per minute. A patient with even moderate PVD can manage this. Soaking the foot in hot water can quickly raise the skin temperature to 104°F, which requires an increase of 10 times the flow of blood. A patient with PVD cannot achieve this. This results in blistering, ulceration, infection, and gangrene, which can lead to amputation.

Diabetic patients also complain of rest pain. However, in these patients, rest and nocturnal pain can be absent, despite severe ischemia, because neuropathy has destroyed sensory perception. This fact emphasizes the need for careful examination of these patients for vascular sufficiency at every visit.

All of the modern advances in medicine, including sophistication of microbiologic analyses, new and more potent antibiotics with improved antimicrobial activity, advances in radiologic imaging of the foot and leg, and better education and understanding on the part of health-care professionals and patients about the etiology and therapy of diabetic foot infections, should have significantly reduced the major amputation rate for diabetic patients. Unfortunately, that is not the case. The triopathy of neuropathy, vascular insufficiency, and an altered response to infection makes the diabetic patient uniquely susceptible to foot problems. Diabetics live quite normally with all of these complications until minor trauma results in cutaneous ulceration and the development of an acute infection that can lead to hospitalization and limb loss. Neuropathy probably represents the greatest risk for ulcer development. Diminished or absent proprioception and sensation quite often delay early recognition and treatment of a seemingly benign problem. Autonomic nerve dysfunction, characterized by dry skin, absent sweating, and increased capillary refill secondary to arteriovenous shunting, leads to fissure, cracking, and a false sense of security about circulation. Motor neuropathy leads to denervation of the intrinsic skeletal muscles of the foot and leg. This results in progressive contractures and bony deformities, which place excessive pressure on skin structures, producing calluses, which can lead to the development of the classic diabetic neuropathic ulcer. Another related problem is the development of Charcot neuroarthropathy. In this condition, loss of proprioception and pain leads to the development of progressive bone collapse and loss of normal skeletal architecture.

Ischemia can complicate up to one-half of diabetic foot ulcers; 40% of diabetic patients presenting with gangrene or severe limb-threatening infections have palpable popliteal pulses. Aggressive vascular evaluation and treatment are essential for healing ischemic ulceration and must be considered for chronic ulcers that fail to respond to treatment. Diabetic patients tolerate infection poorly. Defects in the host defense include altered leukocyte function and wound repair. Most important is the fact that systemic signs and symptoms of a septic process often occur late, making unexplained and uncontrollable hyperglycemia the only reliable sign of a potentially serious limb-threatening and/or life-threatening infection. Less than one-third of patients with pedal osteomyelitis have elevated temperature or white blood cell count. The lack of blood flow reduces oxygen to the afflicted tissue and contributes to the development of foot sepsis. Studies have demonstrated that oxygen is necessary for macrophage mobility in wound debridement and the ingrowth of granulation tissue during wound healing.[12]

Another type of diabetic ischemic complication occurs when there is acute blockage of a blood vessel, leading to necrosis of a muscular compartment or avascular necrosis of bone. This is termed a pedal vascular accident (PVA) and is related to liquefactive necrosis of a compartment or Charcot-type changes within a bone or joint. If this condition is diagnosed in the early stages, intraoperative deep cultures will be negative because this is a sterile abscess. Bone pathology will show avascular necrosis of the bone. The underlying pathology of PVA is similar to, but must be carefully distinguished from, osteomyelitis and Charcot bone. Pathology will generally be reported initially as osteomyelitis; however, upon closer review, the absence of bacteria will be noted with variable amounts of inflammation as the body reacts to the presence of necrotic tissue. Treatment is supportive. Infection must be prevented or cellulitis, wet gangrene, and/or osteomyelitis can ensue.

Restoration of blood flow with increased oxygen levels to ischemic tissue is of the utmost importance for limb salvage.[15] The extent and severity of the infected diabetic foot ulcer determines the course of treatment. To determine the severity, one must perform a careful initial inspection of the wound. Because of neuropathy, this examination can usually be done at the bedside. Sterile forceps, a probe, scissors, and a good light are all that are needed. Sterile technique should be used to avoid inoculation of infection into dysvascular tissue. Deep wound cultures should be considered.

The severity of tissue destruction and sepsis may not be totally apparent from simply looking at the ulcer or infected callus, especially in those patients who continue to bear weight on a painless area or who do not have the visual acuity to recognize a problem. The clinician should unroof all encrusted areas and, using a probe, inspect the wound to determine deep-tissue destruction and possible bone and joint involvement. A determination can be made regarding whether the ulcer is superficial and treatment can be done at home, or whether there is limb-threatening potential that requires immediate hospital admission. Patients with superficial ulceration and minimal (less than 2 cm) cellulitis can be treated at home initially if there is no evidence of systemic toxicity, the patient is compliant and reliable, and the patient has an adequate support system. Mechanical stress on the wound must be reduced to a level compatible with healing. Non-weight bearing is preferred, but is difficult to comply with due to the length of time required for healing.

Contact casting and other immobilization endeavors are highly effective, but must be closely monitored by experienced practitioners. The wound specimen is cultured at initial debridement, and broad-spectrum oral antibiotics are begun (when indicated), with changes made based on sensitivity reports and the response of the wound. Simple dressings appear to work best, so that the patient can comply with recommended treatment. Wet-to-dry dressings of saline or diluted antiseptic solutions applied one to three times per day, depending on the size and area being treated, work well to debride necrotic tissue. Dry, scaly skin is best treated with lubricated creams, and cracks and fissures are best managed with antibiotic ointment or creams. Patients must be examined every 24–48 hours; if there is no improvement, hospitalization is recommended.

Once healing is ensured, weight bearing is progressed in modified footwear to protect high-risk areas. Allowing the patient to return to full activity or weight bearing can result in acute Charcot's foot or recurrent breakdown. Shoe modification and periodic follow-up are essential to all patients at risk.

Patients with limb-threatening infections are managed with hospitalization. Again, inspection is essential, because one cannot rely on systemic signs and symptoms to ascertain severity. Indications for hospitalization include deep ulcers with bone or joint involvement, cellulitis greater than 2 cm, lymphangitis, and systemic toxicity. Initial management includes immediate hospitalization, medical stabilization, control of blood sugar, and complete bed rest.

With regard to the treatment of diabetic infection, there is probably no greater controversy at this time than the proper diagnosis and treatment of osteomyelitis. One thing is known for certain: inadequate diagnosis and treatment of osteomyelitis increase the risk for major amputation. Methods to diagnose osteomyelitis include plain radiographs, bone scans, leukocyte scans, computed tomography scans, magnetic resonance imaging, bone biopsy, bone culture, and clinical evaluation. Proponents of each radiologic test quote acceptable sensitivity and specificity, but largely without confirmation by microbiologic or histopathologic proof. Whatever test one uses, it should not delay urgent or emergent surgical intervention.

With fixed reimbursement the norm, cost is now also an important consideration, and these tests are costly. Thus, the use of a sterile probe to examine the wound is very cost-effective. If a sterile probe taps the bone or joint, there is excellent sensitivity and specificity that the area is involved with osteomyelitis. A plain radiograph should be obtained, with or without magnification views, to look for gas, foreign bodies, associated fractures, and other bony abnormalities. Antibiotics are an adjunct to proper surgical debridement and management. At the time of debridement, deep culture specimens are obtained, and bone or biopsy of deep tissue is taken whenever possible to ensure a reliable specimen.

The majority of cultures from patients with limb-threatening disease grow Gram-positive bacteria, 50% grow Gram-negative enteric bacteria, and 50%–70% of these patients also grow anaerobes. Therefore, antibiotic selection must take this into account, and broad-spectrum intravenous antibiotics or combination therapy are recommended to ensure maximum delivery to the infected site. Antibiotic changes are made on the basis of sensitivity reports, the response of the wound, and the medical condition of the patient.

Except in rare circumstances, antibiotics do not cure osteomyelitis. In general, studies supporting the use of antibiotics alone for curing osteomyelitis lack histopathologic or microbiologic proof and accept a major amputation rate of almost 30% after treatment.[16] Opponents also note that bacteremia, open wounds after treatment, gangrene, and ischemia are associated with poor outcomes. Courses of antibiotics of 6 weeks or longer are also costly, even when delivered on an outpatient basis.

Infected limb-threatening ulcers are a surgical emergency. Surgical debridement and drainage of the infection should be carried out as expeditiously as possible. In a medically compromised patient, local or regional anaesthesia can be used to reduce the physiologic strain induced by general anesthesia. Also, long-acting local anesthesia has a vasodilatory effect on the local blood supply postoperatively and helps to control postoperative pain. Diabetics do not tolerate undrained sepsis, and patients with systemic toxicity will not improve until drainage is completed. A good monitor of accuracy of debridement is to follow blood sugar levels and management, which should improve dramatically as infection is controlled. Incisions are carefully placed, ensuring adequate debridement and conserving as much healthy tissue as possible, such as small skin flaps that can later be used in reconstruction. Any viable area should be left and protected, even if this requires multiple trips to the operating room for infection control. Most of the debridement can be done with little or no anesthesia because of the presence of neuropathy.

The location of the ulcer, extent of the infection and its control, and adequacy of circulation will determine the final result. In an ischemic, non-reconstructible foot infection, all dissection must be avoided; the only chance for salvage is a guillotine amputation proximal to the infection, followed by immediate application of moist wound healing principles. A neuropathic foot with excellent circulation is managed differently than the same infection in an ischemic foot. Once sepsis is controlled, evaluation and treatment of the ischemia are the most important factors. The overwhelming success of surgical revascularization, even to the pedal vessels, supports an aggressive approach. Once circulation is reestablished, revisions or more definitive local

surgical procedures can be performed. It is important to try to save as much of the weight-bearing part of the foot as possible, especially the first toe and its metatarsal head. With aggressive control of diabetic sepsis, aggressive wound care, extensive patient education and compliance, restoration of foot pulses by revascularization, and a multidisciplinary team approach, the amputation rate in this challenging group of patients can be reduced (see Chapter 18).

CLINICAL WISDOM

Blood sugar levels should fall as infection is controlled.

Venous Stasis Ulcers

Despite decades of clinical and laboratory research, the exact mechanisms by which patients develop venous stasis ulcers remain uncertain. There is little doubt that sustained venous hypertension remains the underlying etiologic factor common to all patients with venous stasis ulcers. Venous hypertension can occur primarily in the deep venous system or can be isolated to the superficial saphenous veins. These entities can also occur in combination. This has been associated with congenital or acquired valvular dysfunction within the deep veins and with valvular incompetence at the saphenofemoral junction or via incompetent perforators below the knee. Clearly, the underlying pathologic process must be determined in each individual patient prior to initiating a specific treatment plan.

The Swollen Leg

One of the first complaints of patients with venous insufficiency is swelling of the legs, which is sometimes accompanied by discomfort and a heavy feeling in the lower extremities. Contrary to similar complaints in patients with arterial insufficiency, this complaint is readily relieved by leg elevation in patients with venous disease. A basic understanding of the function and structure of the venous system is necessary to comprehend the pathophysiologic derangements that are responsible for the development of lower extremity edema.

The main and foremost task of the venous system is to return blood from the periphery to the heart. It also serves as a storage network that is intimately involved in blood volume regulation and facilitates the exchange of substances between tissue and blood in the capillary region. To carry out these functions and maintain a vigorous flow of blood in a low-pressure system, the venous vessels must rely on the elastic components of their walls (see *Color Plate 56*). The walls of veins consist of an intact endothelium that coats a thin basal membrane. An adjoining layer of fibrous connective tissue with strands of collagenous and muscle fibers helps to stabilize the walls of the veins and, in conjunction with a delicate system of valves, is responsible for the return of venous blood to the heart. The slightly helical structure of muscle fibers and collagenous strands enables healthy veins to return to their original position after undergoing distention of length and girth from increased blood volumes. Failure of this collagenous and muscular infrastructure results in veins that become wider, longer, and convoluted, giving rise to the formation of tortuous varices. Progressive venous dilation can lead to valvular incompetence by interfering with the delicate apposition of venous valve leaflets, which is required for transport of blood up the leg and into the central circulation. Thus, the failure of proper venous valve closure can be the result—and not the primary cause—of blood vessel widening.

Venous congestion can also alter the delicate balance that exists between arterioles, venules, and capillaries. About 20 L of fluid are filtered into the interstitial space by this complex system each day, with 18 L (90%) being reabsorbed by the venous branches of the capillary system. The remaining 2 L (10%) return to the circulatory system through lymph drainage. Hydrostatic and colloidal-osmotic forces work together in capillary filtration and reabsorption. Intracapillary pressure drops from 35 mm Hg in the arterial branches to 15 mm Hg in the venous branches. Higher pressure in the arterial side leads to outward filtration, which is counteracted on the venous side by a continuous reabsorption, driven by colloidal and osmotic forces. A delicate balance is maintained as long as the amounts of filtered and reabsorbed fluid remain equal. Altered venous return due to increased venous dilation and valvular deficiency results in perceptible increases in capillary hydrostatic pressure and permeability of the capillary endothelium. These two factors lead to the enhanced filtration of fluid into the interstitial space and the classic appearance of the signs and symptoms of peripheral edema.

The lymphatic system can also be involved in chronic venous insufficiency. Both the lymphatic and venous systems share an early embryologic development and an intimate anatomic relationship. The lymphatic channels course along the pathway of the lesser and greater saphenous veins to drain into the superficial inguinal lymph nodes. The deep lymphatic vessels of the lower extremity likewise accompany the deep vessels of the leg to the popliteal lymph nodes, and then continue along the femoral vessels to reach the deep inguinal lymph nodes.

Congenital or acquired insufficiency of the lymphatic transport system results in lymph stasis and the accumulation of protein-rich interstitial fluid. Chronic lymphedema, however, develops only if the collateral lymphatic circulation is inadequate or tissue macrophages (which aid in the removal of macromolecules from the interstitial space) are overwhelmed. Impaired lymphatic drainage results in significant structural changes in the lymphatic vessels themselves and the subcutaneous tissues they serve. This leads to fibroblast proliferation, sclerosis of the subcutaneous tissues, and increased vascularity—changes that are usually associated with chronic inflammation.[17] Secondary changes in lymph vessels due to lymph stasis include fibrosis of the wall with loss of permeability and lymph-concentrating ability. Furthermore, just as in the venous system, lymphatic valves can also fibrose or become incompetent as a result of

proximal lymphatic obstruction and distal vessel dilation. The lymph vessel wall loses its intrinsic contractility, and the muscle pump is rendered ineffective. Lymph stasis favors the development of obstructive lymphangitis, with further destruction of the main and collateral lymphatic channels.

Chronic venous insufficiency can lead to recurrent attacks of skin cellulitis, which can result in increased destruction of cutaneous lymphatic channels and subsequent obstructive lymphatic patterns.[18] This phenomenon is strongly suggested by lymphoscintigraphy, a noninvasive imaging modality used to interpret the morphologic and functional alterations that occur in the lymphatic system. Lymphoscintigraphy has shown that the lymphatic system is often impaired in patients with chronic venous insufficiency. This impairment is reflected by the development of anatomic changes in lymphatic vessels and presence of a delayed lymphatic flow. These changes ultimately may interfere with the absorption of interstitial fluid in the extremities of patients with chronic venous insufficiency, thereby contributing to increased clinical swelling.

Pathophysiology of Venous Ulceration

The literature describes several mechanisms for the pathophysiologic events leading to skin ulceration. Browse and Burnand initially described the concept of fibrin cuffs developing at the capillary level in 1982.[19] These authors suggested that sustained venous hypertension is transmitted to the superficial veins in the subcutaneous tissue and overlying skin. This, in turn, causes widening of the capillary pores and allows the escape of large macromolecules (including fibrinogen) into the interstitial space. Owing to associated defects in the fibrinolytic process, fibrin accumulates around these capillaries, forming a mechanical barrier to the transfer of oxygen and other nutrients. Ultimately, this leads to cellular dysfunction, which, in turn, leads to cell death and skin ulceration. Unfortunately, there is no published evidence that fibrin provides a barrier to oxygen diffusion.

In more recent years, additional physiologic changes have been noted in the microcirculation of patients with chronic venous hypertension, specifically, an altered inflammatory mechanism. These changes have been linked to the accumulation of white blood cells at the capillary level, which has been termed the *white blood cell-trapping hypothesis*.[20, 21] Transient elevations in venous pressures have been shown to decrease capillary blood flow, resulting in trapping of white blood cells at the capillary level. This occurs to a much greater extent in patients with long-standing venous hypertension and liposclerotic skin. These marginated white blood cells, in turn, plug capillary loops, resulting in areas of localized ischemia. These cells can also become activated at this level, causing the release of various proteolytic enzymes, superoxide free radicals, and chemotactic substances. These substances ultimately lead to direct tissue damage and, thus, to ulceration[22] (see Chapter 2 for a more comprehensive discussion of the mechanisms of ischemia reperfusion injury).

Medical Treatment of Venous Stasis Ulcers

Definitive treatment of venous stasis ulcers depends on the operative repair of the underlying cause of venous incompetence in the affected extremity. This is seldom possible, however, and long-term success is rarely achieved. Excision and grafting of the ulcerated area and surrounding scar tissue, even when accompanied by local and regional subfascial ligation of perforating vessels, does not uniformly result in the return of long-term skin integrity. Therefore, there remain a great many patients whose venous stasis ulcers need to be managed nonoperatively.[23]

Before attempting medical management of a venous stasis ulcer, the diagnosis must be assured. Noninvasive measurements must eliminate a significant ischemic component to that etiology. The ABI must be at least greater than 0.5 mm Hg and, preferably, greater than 0.75 mm Hg. If transcutaneous oxygen measurements are performed, the foot's dorsal pressures should exceed 30 mm Hg. (see Chapter 7). Hemoglobin electrophoresis should eliminate sickle cell disease and, if suspected, a biopsy should eliminate vasculitis as the cause of the ulcer.

To allow the ulcer to heal by secondary intention, the wound must be in bacterial balance and contain 10^5 or fewer bacteria per gram of tissue; it must not harbor beta-hemolytic streptococci. If a biopsy shows the wound to be infected, bacterial balance is best reestablished by a topical antimicrobial agent. Systemically administered antibiotics do not lower the bacterial count in granulation tissue. However, systemic antibiotics are effective and indicated if the ulcer has an area of surrounding cellulitis. Another method of reestablishing bacterial balance is with the use of temporary biologic dressings, such as allograft skin. Once the ulcer is in bacterial balance, it can heal by secondary intention. The process of epithelialization is more important than the process of contraction for these ulcers.

CLINICAL WISDOM

To achieve bacterial balance:

1. Apply topical antibiotics/disinfectants if wound shows signs of infection.
2. Administer systemic antibiotics if periwound skin shows signs of cellulitis.

Compression therapy is the cornerstone of effective nonoperative treatment of venous stasis ulcers. Many combination dressings, such as the time-honoured Unna boot, have been reported to provide adequate compression if good patient compliance is achieved.[24] The U.S. Food and Drug Administration currently considers compression therapy to be the standard of care for venous stasis ulcers. *Color Plate 57* shows a patient with venous stasis ulceration, and *Color Plate 58* shows an ulcer with associated signs of chronic venous insufficiency. Chapter 10 describes the management of edema associated with venous stasis ulcers, and Chapter 12 explains the use of bioengineered skin, a recent addition to

the therapeutic agents for venous stasis ulcers of long duration and/or large size.

Recently, a variety of growth factors have been introduced for the treatment of venous stasis ulcers. A trial with transforming growth factor-β (TGF-β) in a collagen sponge delivery system has given the most encouraging data of those trials that have been completed.[25] The topical antimicrobial silver sulfadiazine (Silvadene, SSD) has also shown beneficial results. It is thought that the base of this compound contains properties that stimulate wound epithelialization. Contrary to previous experience, many patients who have healed during carefully controlled clinical trials have remained healed, as long as they comply with compression therapy. Because the underlying etiology of the ulcer is not treated with medical therapy, such treatment can be considered only palliative. However, as more is learned about modulating the wound healing process, palliation may be extended for the life of the patient.

To evaluate properly the many therapeutic modalities that are being applied in the treatment of chronic venous disease, the Ad Hoc Committee on Reporting Standards in Venous Disease of the Society of Vascular Surgery and the North American Chapter of the International Society for Cardiovascular Surgery have recommended the use of a classification designed to allow such comparisons.[26] Limbs with chronic venous disease should be classified according to clinical signs (C), etiology (E), anatomic distribution (A), and pathophysiologic condition (P) (Exhibit 18-2).

Any limb with possible chronic venous disease is first placed into one of seven clinical classes (C_{0-6}) according to objective clinical signs. It is further characterized as being asymptomatic ($C_{0-6,A}$) or symptomatic ($C_{0-6,S}$). Because therapy can alter the clinical category of chronic venous disease, limbs should be reclassified after any form of medical or surgical treatment. The venous dysfunction is then classified according to one of three mutually exclusive categories: congenital (E_C), primary (E_P), or secondary (E_S). Next, the anatomic site or sites affected with venous disease are described as involving the superficial (A_S), deep (A_D), or perforating (A_P) veins. Finally, the pathophysiologic reason for the development of signs and symptoms of chronic venous disease is determined as being the result of reflux (P_R), obstruction (P_O), or both ($P_{R,O}$). Observance of this classification system in the clinical arena can lead to an improvement in communications in the field of venous disorders and help in the evaluation and proper application of therapeutic regimens.

Differential Diagnosis of Venous Stasis Ulcers

All ulcers are not venous in origin. The common feature of all leg ulcers is an underlying systemic or local problem that complicates the healing of wounds that are inevitably traumatic in origin. Those ulcerations that are not venous but can mimic or be confused with venous ulcers are to be differentiated on the basis of a different historical evolution, the presence of other systemic or local disease processes, and often subtle but important different physical findings (Exhibit 18-3).

EXHIBIT 18-2   Classifications of Chronic Lower Extremity

CLINICAL CLASSIFICATION

Class	Clinical Description
0	No visible signs of venous disease
1	Telangiectasias, reticular veins, malleolar flare
2	Varicose veins
3	Edema without skin changes
4	Skin changes ascribed to venous disease (e.g., pigmentation, venous eczema, lipodermatosclerosis
5	Skin changes as defined above with healed ulceration
6	Skin changes as defined above with active ulceration

ETIOLOGIC CLASSIFICATION

Etiology	Description
Congenital	Cause of chronic venous disease present since birth
Primary	Chronic venous disease of undetermined cause
Secondary	Chronic venous disease with an associated known cause (postthrombotic, posttraumatic, other)

ANATOMIC CLASSIFICATION

Veins Involved	Description
Superficial	Telangiectasias/reticular veins and greater saphenous veins; lesser saphenous veins and nonsaphenous veins
Deep	Inferior vena cava, iliac, pelvis, gonadal, femoral, popliteal, tibial, and muscular veins
Perforating	Thigh and calf

PATHOPHYSIOLOGIC CLASSIFICATION

Type	Description
R	Reflex
O	Obstruction
R,O	Reflux and obstruction

Adapted with permission from Porter JM, Moneta GL, International Consensus Committee on Chronic Venous Disease. Reporting standards in venous disease: An update. *J Vasc Surg*. 1995;21:635–645.

EXHIBIT 18-3   Differential Diagnosis of Lower Extremity Ulcers

	Ischemic	Venous Stasis	Neuropathic
Etiology	Arterial insufficiency	Chronic venous insufficiency	Diabetes
Usual location	Distal to medial malleolus; dorsum of foot or toes	Proximal to medial malleolus; lateral lower leg	Along pressure points; plantar aspect of metatarsal heads (first or fifth)
Pain	Severe; nocturnal, relieved by dependency	Mild; relieved by elevation	None
Bleeding	Little or none	Venous ooze	Can be brisk
Lesion characteristics	Irregular edge; poor granulation tissue	Shallow, irregular shape; granulating base with rounded edges	Punched-out; callous edges with deep sinus
Associated findings	Trophic skin changes (dry skin, brittle nails, alopecia); absent pulses	Stasis dermatitis; hyperpigmentation; palpable pulses	Neuropathy; warm skin; pulses may be present or absent

Modified with permission from Rutherford RB. The vascular consultation. In: Rutherford RB, ed. *Vascular Surgery*. Fourth Ed. Philadelphia: W.B. Saunders Company, 1995, p. 9.

Atypical Nonatherosclerotic Ulcers [27]

There are numerous skin ulcerations that are less common in clinical practice, including vasculitis, hypercoagulable states, microemboli, cryoglobulinemia, Raynaud's phenomenon, thromboangiitis obliterans, sickle cell disease, and calciphylaxis. The common feature of these ulcers is ischemia related to occlusive arterial or venous disease. As such, these lesions are classically severely painful, unless they occur in the presence of neuropathy (e.g., diabetic neuropathy). These diseases, which are also known as thrombophilias, are associated with hypercoagulable states. These states include inherited and acquired defects in coagulation, which increases the risk of thrombotic events, especially venous thrombosis. Thrombosis within the dermal vessels can lead to tissue necrosis and ulceration.

Systemic diseases associated with atypical ulcers include:

• Systemic lupus erythematosus
• Collagen vascular diseases
• Antiphospholipid syndrome (APS)
• Protein C deficiency
• Protein S deficiency
• Factor V Leiden
• Antithrombin deficiency
• Prothrombin gene mutation G20210A
• Increased levels of factor VII, VIII, IX, XI, von Willebrand factor
• Cryoglobulinemias
• Hepatitis C virus
• Rheumatoid arthritis

The clinical appearance of these ulcerations is similar, due to related underlying pathology. Clinicians should have a high index of suspicion when evaluating wounds that have not responded to prior treatment. Common associated cutaneous manifestations include extremely painful necrotic ulcers, livedo reticularis, necrotizing purpura, digital cyanosis or gangrene, Raynaud's phenomenon, and possible coexisting chronic venous insufficiency (Figure 18-5A-D).

Laboratory studies to evaluate atypical ulceration can include a CBC with differential, PT, aPTT, RA factor, BUN, creatine, antiphospholipid antibodies, anticardiolipin antibodies (IgG, IgM, IgA), lupus anticoagulants, anti-β2GP1(if above are normal), Factor V Leiden, prothrombin gene mutation G20210A, antithrombin, Protein C, and Protein S.[28]

Dermatopathology is recommended for atypical or unresponsive wounds. A biopsy should include the ulcer bed, wound margins, and junctional tissue at any associated rash margin. This can be obtained by dermal ellipse or multiple punch biopsies. Pathology can demonstrate noninflammatory thrombosis of small dermal vessels, capillary proliferation, dermal hemorrhage, and hemosiderin deposition.

Treatments for atypical ulcerations are based on the underlying medical conditions causing the ischemic pathology. Figure 18-6 presents an algorithm for determining the etiology of atypical ulcers. Surgical revascularization is usually not possible for these conditions. Anticoagulation, plasmapheresis, and immunosuppression therapy may be required for some medical conditions, whereas prostacyclin analogues may decrease pain in other conditions. Amputation may be required to treat infection or recalcitrant pain. Cessation of smoking is, however, the one common treatment for all atypical ulcerations.

Local wound care and dressing choice should be directed at prevention of infection, supporting ischemic tissue and maintenance of moist wound healing principles. All necrotic tissue must be debrided from the wound to decrease oxygen demand and control infection risk. Associated chronic venous insufficiency must be controlled. Usually the patient will not tolerate compression therapy, so elevation can be utilized. If the patient complains of increased pain with elevation, it is usually due to ischemia, and a dependent position is required for perfusion. Protect the patient from cold. Gentle warming will increase vasodilation, but excess temperature will increase oxygen demand and ischemia.

When the clinician encounters a wound that is morphologically unusual or fails to respond as expected, consider an atypical ischemic ulceration. These patients are often labeled as noncompliant because of the unusual nature of the underlying pathology.

REVIEW QUESTIONS

1. Name the major arteries and veins of the lower extremity.
2. Describe the three signs and symptoms of occlusive PVD and their significance.
3. List four risk factors for development of arterial ulcers.
4. What clinical signs are reliable indicators of systemic infection in diabetic patients?
5. How do the venous and lymphatic systems relate to the "swollen leg"?
6. What steps must be performed before attempting medical management of venous stasis ulcers?
7. Name five types of atypical ischemic ulcers.
8. What is the most common dermal finding associated with atypical ischemic ulcerations?

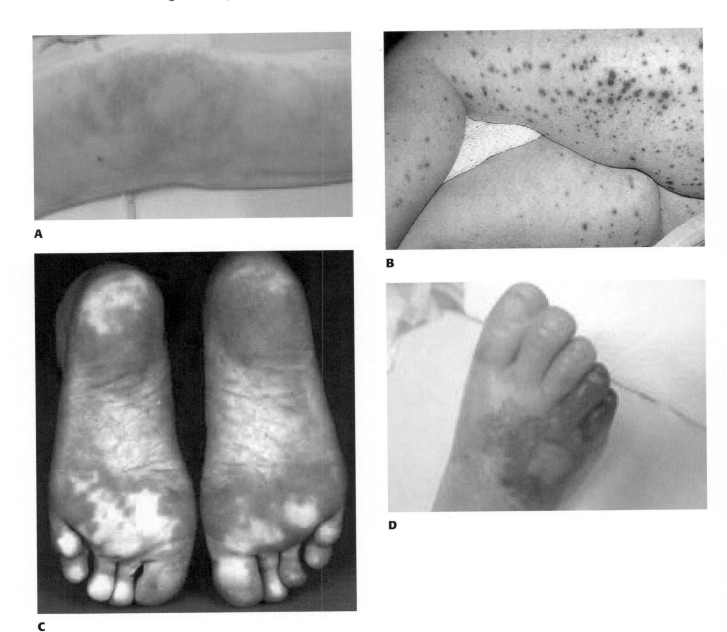

FIGURE 18-5 Common associated cutaneous manifestations for atypical ulcers. **A.** Livedo reticularis. This condition can lead to more severe conditions with small ulcerations and purpura due to clogging of the small cutaneous vessels. Smoking exacerbates this process. (Reprinted with permission from Barankin, Benjamin M.D., Dr. Barankin Dermatology Collection, WK Health, image provided by Stedman's.) **B.** Necrotizing purpura. (Copyright Current Medicine Group, Ltd. www.nephrohus.org/uz/vascularites_renal.) **C.** Raynaud's phenomenon on the feet. (Source: www.dermnetnz.org.) **D.** Digital cyanosis and early gangrene. (Reprinted with permission from Barankin, Benjamin M.D., Dr. Barankin Dermatology Collection, WK Health, image provided by Stedman's.)

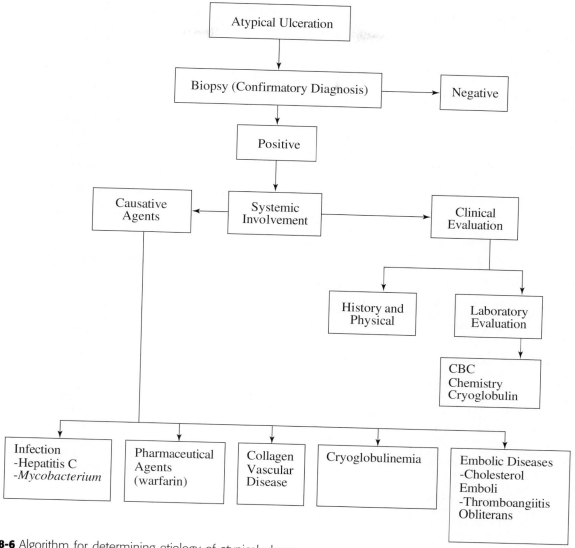

FIGURE 18-6 Algorithm for determining etiology of atypical ulcers.

REFERENCES

1. McGann MM, Robinson LR. *The Doctor's Sore Foot Book*. Avenel, NJ: Wing Books, 1994.
2. Kadir S. Arterial anatomy of the lower extremity. In: Kadir S, ed. *Atlas of Normal and Variant Angiographic Anatomy*. Philadelphia: WB Saunders, 1991:123–160.
3. Lundell C, Kadir S. Lower extremities and pelvis. In: Kadir S, ed. *Atlas of Normal and Variant Angiographic Anatomy*. Philadelphia: W.B. Saunders Company, 1991:203–225.
4. Karpanen T, Makinen T, Regulation of lymphangiogenesis—From cell fate determination to vessel remodeling. *Exp Cell Res*. 2005 Dec 9. PMID: 16343484.
5. Strandness DE Jr, Summer DS. Application of ultrasound to the study of arteriosclerosis obliterans. *Angiology*. 1975;26:187–189.
6. Jonason T, Rinquist I. Factors of prognostic importance for subsequent rest pain in patients with intermittent claudication. *Acta Med Scand*. 1985;218:27–36.
7. Couch NP. On the arterial consequences of smoking. *J Vasc Surg*. 1986;3:807–812.
8. Hillis LD, Hirsch PD, Campbell WB, et al. Interaction of the arterial wall, plaque, and platelets in myocardial infarction. *Cardiovasc Clin*. 1983;14:31–44.
9. Kannel WB, McGee DL. Update on some epidemiologic features of intermittent claudication: The Framingham Study. *J Am Geriatr Soc*. 1985;33:13–21.
10. National Institute of Diabetes and Digestive and Kidney Diseases. National Diabetes Statistics Fact Sheet: General Information and National Estimates on Diabetes in the United States. Bethesda, MD: U.S. Department of Health and Human Services, National Institute of Health, 2005.
11. Dillingham TR, Pezzin LE, Shore AD. Reamputation, mortality, and health care costs among persons with dysvascular lower-limb amputations. *Arch Phys Med Rehabil*. 2005;86(3):480-6. PMID: 15759232.
12. Vogelberg KH, Konig M. Hypoxia of diabetic feet with abnormal arterial blood flow. *Clin Invest*. 1993;71:466–470.
13. Kucan JO, Robson MC. Diabetic foot infections: Fate of the contralateral foot. *Plast Reconstr Surg*. 1986;77:439–441.
14. McDermott JE. *The Diabetic Foot*. Rosemont, IL: American Academy of Orthopaedic Surgeons, 1995.
15. LoGerfo FW, Gibbons GW, Pomposelli FB, et al. Evolving trends in management of the diabetic foot. *Arch Surg*. 1992;127:618–621.
16. Bamberger DM, Daus GP, Gerding DN, et al. Osteomyelitis in the feet of diabetic patients: Long-term results, prognostic factors and the role of antimicrobial therapy and surgical therapy. *Am J Med*. 1987;83(4):653–660.
17. Olszewski W. Pathophysiology and clinical observations of obstructive lymphedema of the limbs. In: Clodius L, ed. *Lymphedema*. Stuggart, Germany: Georg Thieme Verlag, 1977:79–102.
18. Hammond SL, Gomez ER, Coffey JA, et al. Involvement of the lymphatic system in chronic venous insufficiency. In: Bergan JJ, Yao JST, eds. *Venous Disorders*. Philadelphia: WB Saunders, 1991:333–343.
19. Browse NL, Burnand KG. The cause of venous ulceration. *Lancet*. 1982;2:243–245.
20. Thomas PRS, Nash GB, Dormandy JA. White cell accumulation in the dependent legs of patients with venous hypertension: A possible mechanism for trophic changes in the skin. *Br Med J*. 1988;296:1693–1695.
21. Butler CM, Coleridge-Smith PD. Microcirculatory aspects of venous ulceration. *Dermatol Surg Oncol*. 1994;20:474–480.
22. Coleridge-Smith PD, Thomas P, Scurr JH, et al. Causes of venous ulceration: A new hypothesis. *Br Med J*. 1988;296:1826–1872.
23. Robson MC. Medical treatment of venous stasis ulcers. Presented at American College of Surgeons Postgraduate Course 13: *Current Treatment of Venous Stasis Ulcers*. October 22–27, 1995; New Orleans, LA.
24. Villavicencio JL, Rich NM, Salander JM, et al. Leg ulcers of venous origin. In: Cameron JL, ed. *Current Surgical Therapy*. Toronto, Canada: BC Becker; 1989:610–618.
25. Bishop JB, Phillips LG, Mustoe TA, et al. A prospective randomized evaluator-blinded trial of two potential wound healing agents for the treatment of venous stasis ulcers. *J Vasc Surg*. 1992;8:251–257.
26. Porter JM, Moneta GL, International Consensus Committee on Chronic Venous Disease. Reporting standards in venous disease: An update. *J Vasc Surg*. 1995;21:635–645.
27. Kirsner RS, Seaman S. Atypical Wounds: Nonatherosclerotic Ischemic Ulcers. SAWC Session 26. Audio recordings 2004.
28. Buchanan GS, Rodgers GM, Branch DW. The inherited thrombophilias: genetics, epidemiology, and laboratory evaluation. *Best Pract Res Clin Obstet Gynaecol* 2003;18:397-411.

SUGGESTED READING

1. Beitz JM, Burton CS. Kerstein MD, et al. Venous Leg Ulcer Guidelines. Philadelphia: University of Pennsylvania, 1997. Print copies and video available from the University of Pennsylvania School of Medicine, Attn: Maryanne McGuckin, MD, 605A Stellar Chance Bldg., 422 Curie Blvd., Philadelphia, PA 19104–6021. Telephone: (215) 573–3066 or (215) 898–4969; fax (215) 573–0826. Summary available at National Guideline Clearinghouse. http://www.guideline.gov/index.asp
2. Bick BL. Antiphospholipid thrombosis syndromes. *Hematol Oncol Clin N Am*. 2003;18:115-147.
3. Browne AC, Sibbald RG. The Diabetic neuropathic ulcer: An overview. *Ostomy/Wound Manage*. 1999;45(Suppl. 1A):6S–20S.
4. Buchanan GS, Rodgers GM, Branch DW. The inherited thrombophilias: genetics, epidemiology, and laboratory evaluation. *Best Pract Res Clin Obstet Gynaecol*. 2003;18:397-411.
5. Davis M, Su W. Cryoglobulinemia: resent findings in cutaneous and extracutaneous manifestations. *Int J Dermatol*. 1996;35:240-248.
6. Falanga V. Care of venous ulcers. *Ostomy/Wound Manage*. 1999;45(Suppl. 1A):33S–43S.
7. Falanga V, Fine MJ, Kapoor WN. The cutaneous manifestations of cholesterol crystal embolization. *Arch Dermatol*. 1986;122:1194-1198.
8. Klucan J. Lower Extremity Ulceration Guidelines. American Society of Plastic and Reconstructive Surgeons (ASPRS); 1998. Print copies available: 444 E. Algonquin Rd, Arlington Heights, IL. Outline available at National Guideline Clearinghouse. http://www.guideline.gov/index.asp.
9. Mills J. Burger's disease in the 21st century: diagnosis, clinical features and therapy. *Semin Vasc Surg*. 2003;16:189-189.
10. Perry SL, Ortel TL. Clinical and laboratory evaluation of thrombophilia. *Clin Chest Med*. 2003;24:153-180.
11. Seaman S. Considerations for the global assessment and treatment of patients with recalcitrant wounds. *Ostomy/Wound Manage*. 2000;46(suppl 1A):10S-29S.

Management of the Neuropathic Foot

Nancy Elftman and Joan E. Conlan

CHAPTER OBJECTIVES

At the completion of this chapter, the reader will be able to:

1. Identify patients at risk for foot ulceration due to lack of protective sensation.
2. Explain the relationship between surface temperature and inflammation.
3. Implement off-loading techniques with wound care protocol.

Medical research has provided advancements in medication and technology that now extend the lives of patients with previously fatal diseases: The prognosis has changed from fatality to chronic complications.[1] The chronic disease complication addressed in this chapter is neuropathy. The objective of management of the problem is to control progression and reduce amputations conservatively.

The patient with neuropathy often has dysvascular components that must be addressed by a medical team, rather than one specialty (see Chapter 18). With the team approach, the limb can be evaluated, treated, and monitored through follow-up to provide continued ambulation for the patient.[2] The team goal is the prevention or delay of amputation and/or limb salvage of lower extremities. In the formation of clinical teams, there has been a trend to include practitioners of several disciplines, including the wound care, advanced practice, or enterostomal therapy (ET) nurse; diabetologist/endocrinologist; vascular surgeon; physical therapist; orthotist/pedorthist; orthopaedic surgeon/podiatrist; and dermatologist.

The multidisciplinary approach to treating foot problems is an optimum intervention for prevention of amputations. The disciplines playing the most important roles are nurse educators, who encourage high-risk patients to modify their behavior; orthotists, for recommendation of suitable footwear, stockings, and orthoses; and primary-care providers, to remove calluses, treat minor trauma, and provide health care. Physical therapists will play a role in all of these aspects of care. Referrals should be available to vascular surgeons and other specialists when specified by a physician.[3]

The multidisciplinary clinic requires special training in treatment of chronic disabilities. Although the individual training programs of professionals include normal foot anatomy and biomechanics, few describe the neuropathic foot and associated complications, leading to inadequate medical advice or treatment.[4] In the clinical setting, no initial problem is too small to address. The clinical team is important and must treat minor trauma immediately to prevent deterioration of the condition. There is a destructive chain of trauma surrounding the neuropathic foot, as follows:

1. Trauma
2. Inflammation
3. Ulceration
4. Infection
5. Absorption
6. Deformity
7. Disability

This chain can be broken with proper objective measurement, treatment, and patient education.[2]

The patient with neuropathy requires a consistent follow-up schedule relating to level of insensitivity, history of complications, and general physical condition. A patient with loss of protective sensation (10 g of force) and no history of ulceration will require less frequent follow-up than will the patient with a chronic breakdown history. Records should reflect as many objective measurements as possible and a method of classification of patient types. Management of the neuropathic and dysvascular limb is a process of continuing evaluation. The process of history, examination, and charting details cannot be overemphasized. All clinical findings should be charted and relayed to the patient's primary care provider.[5]

Although neuropathy exists in many disease processes, there are concerns about the growing number requiring management. When breakdown occurs in one neuropathic limb, the contralateral limb is commonly involved within 18 to 36 months, so prophylactic measures are especially important. Many considerations must be addressed by the team treating the neuropathic and dysvascular limb before a treatment plan is developed. Once the plan is in place, it is imperative to educate and involve the patient in the plan.

Pathogenesis

The neuropathic process is poorly understood, and there are many theories regarding its etiology. When evaluating the neuropathic patient, the medical team encounters the following obstacles:

- Lack of clear definition of diabetic neuropathy
- Absence of single, repeatable tests of neuropathy that are not dependent on either expensive technology or subjective clinical judgment
- Varied manifestations of neuropathy: distal symmetric, mononeuropathies, autonomic neuropathies
- Separation of diabetes from other potential etiologies of neuropathy

The neuropathic foot is affected by a trineuropathy, which consists of three phases that occur simultaneously; manifestations of two of these phases are shown in Figure 19-1.

1. Sensory neuropathy—loss of sensation, leaving patient incapable of sensing pain and pressure. The patient has no sense of identity with the feet.
2. Motor neuropathy—loss of intrinsic muscles, resulting in clawed toes (Figure 19-2) and eventual foot drop. The ankle jerk reflex is absent.[6]
3. Autonomic neuropathy—loss of autonomic system function, resulting in the absence of sweat and oil production, leaving skin dry and nonelastic.

Until recently, all forms of neuropathy were lumped together. It is now clear that there are different types, which develop differently. Peripheral neuropathy can be broken down into two major groups:

1. Gradual onset—those that develop gradually and are usually painless. The exact cause is unknown but may be related to duration of diabetes and level of blood sugar control. Symptoms may include numbness, tingling, burning, and a pins-and-needles sensation.
2. Sudden onset and disappearance—those that develop suddenly (or acutely) and are almost always painful; then the pain disappears, leaving sensory loss.

Many believe that neuropathy is caused by hyperglycemia—high levels of glucose in the blood. Tight control may be the best prevention of severe neuropathy.[7]

Medical History

The medical history is a useful way to identify potential neuropathy that may be present in many disease processes.

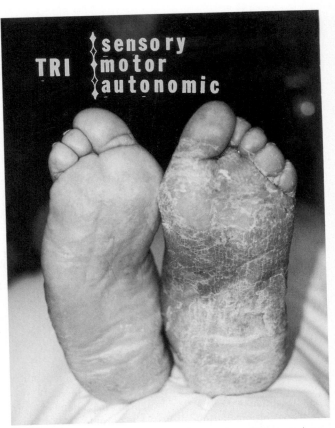

FIGURE 19-1 Feet of a patient with sensory, motor, and autonomic neuropathies. Manifestations of motor neuropathy (deformity, clawed toes, toe amputation, foot imbalance needing immediate intervention) and autonomic neuropathy (dry, cracked skin) are evident. Note the difference in trophic changes between the feet. (Reprinted with permission from N. Elftman, Clinical Management of the Neuropathic Limb, *Journal of Prosthetics and Orthotics.* Vol. 4, No. 1. pp. 1–12. Copyright © American Academy of Orthotists and Prosthetists.)

The neuropathy may be isolated (nerve damage or entrapment) but, for most chronic disease processes, the effect is peripheral. The most common disease processes resulting in peripheral neuropathy are the following:

- Diabetes
- Spina bifida
- Hansen's disease
- Systemic erythematosus lupus
- Acquired immune deficiency syndrome (AIDS), human immunodeficiency virus (HIV) infection, AIDS-related complex
- Cancer
- Vitamin B deficiency
- Multiple sclerosis
- Uremia
- Vascular disease
- Charcot-Marie-Tooth muscle disease

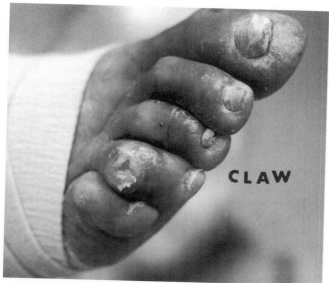

FIGURE 19-2 Clawed toes. Note the corn on the fourth toe, caused by rubbing from the top of the shoe.

Toxins and toxic syndromes can also cause insensitivity in the limbs, including those related to overuse of or exposure to alcohol, arsenic, lead, steroids, gold, and isoniazid.

Many other chronic complications may result in neuropathy, but the above list indicates why all patients must be evaluated for neuropathy, regardless of reported history. Congenital sensory loss, as in spina bifida, is important to the examiner because the patient has never experienced normal sensation and cannot evaluate his or her own sensory status.[8–10]

Diabetic Neuropathy

The most common disease process seen in neuropathy is diabetes, which results in true peripheral neuropathy. Statistics on diabetes are growing, and the medical cost related to diabetes in the United States is currently $14 billion per year. Included in this cost are 54,000 lower extremity amputations per year, of which 50%–70% could have been prevented by team management. It is estimated that 50%–84% of the lower extremity amputations were preceded by a foot ulcer. More than 14 million Americans have diabetes (half are undiagnosed), with 700,000 cases diagnosed per year. In the general population, 1 in 20 has diabetes. Many diabetics are diagnosed when they present a nonhealing foot ulcer.[11–16] Of major concern is the mortality rate after amputation, which is 50% within 3–5 years. The rate of contralateral amputation is 50% within 4 years.[17] The World Health Organization has estimated that the number of diabetics will climb to 366 million by 2030.[18]

Although there are several different divisions of diabetes, the two main categories are insulin-dependent diabetes mellitus (IDDM), or type I, and non-insulin-dependent diabetes mellitus (NIDDM), or type II. In IDDM, the insulin defi-ciency is due to pancreas islet cell loss. It occurs at any age but is common in youth. NIDDM is more frequent in adults but occurs at any age. The majority of patients with NIDDM are overweight.[19]

The dysvascular patient may also be diabetic, which leads to impaired healing of a limb that cannot deliver antibiotics sufficiently to combat extremity infection (see Chapter 17). One limb may be severely insensitive while the other is mildly affected (see Figure 19-1). The loss of vascularity caused by calcified arteries or a disease process is first referred to the vascular surgeon for possible correction or improvement.

The four types of stress that lead to ulceration and destruction of tissue in the neuropathic limb are as follows:

1. Ischemic necrosis is usually seen on the lateral side of the fifth metatarsal head and is due to wearing a shoe that is too narrow. The ischemia is caused by a very low level of pressure (2–3 psi) over a long period of time, causing death of the tissue.
2. Mechanical disruption occurs when a direct injury caused by high pressure (600+ psi) inflicts immediate damage to tissue. This also can be caused by heat or chemicals that damage the skin. Such injuries commonly occur by stepping on a foreign object.
3. Inflammatory destruction occurs with repetitive moderate pressures (40–60 psi). Inflammation develops and weakens the tissue, leading to callus formation and ulceration from thousands of repetitions per day.
4. Osteomyelitis (and other sepsis) destruction is the result of a moderate force in the presence of infection. Infection is spread as forces are applied by intermittent pressure.[20]

The highest incidence of ulceration occurs at sites of previous ulceration. The history should be reviewed carefully for previous ulcers or infection.[21] A newly healed ulcer is covered by thin skin that is likely to tear. In completely healed ulcer areas, scar tissue may adhere to underlying structures. The healed areas are composed of tissues of different density and, therefore, compress uniquely, causing shear between opposing tissue durometers.[22,23]

The progression of breakdown continues at the metatarsal heads, due to migration of fat pads, leaving bone and skin to absorb shock. The neuropathic limb has lost heat and cold sensation and reflex response. The incidence of ulceration is 71% on the forefoot, with the third metatarsal head most commonly affected, followed by the great toe and first and fifth metatarsal heads. Once breakdown has begun on the foot, 53% of the contralateral limbs follow the progression of breakdown within 4 years.[23] Newly healed wounds need time to mature and become strong, yet there will always be a potential for breakdown in a previous area of ulceration. Scar compresses at a different rate than does other tissue, and the area of adherence will be prone to shear stresses.[24]

Of all amputations, 86% could have been prevented by patient education and appropriate footwear.[3] The aging process alone will produce changes in appearance and alterations in sensitivity, joint motion, and muscle-force production, any of which can lead to dysfunction.[25] Improper nutrition can also delay healing.[26] The majority of amputations are due to gangrene (90%), followed by infection (71%), and nonhealing ulcers (65%).[27] The dry, dark ulcers of gangrene are usually found on toes or bony parts of the foot. Neuropathic ulcers are usually moist and draining.[15] Diabetic neuropathic ulcers occur in a foot with severe sensory impairment, yet they typically have adequate blood supply for healing.[25,28]

There are two types of gangrene: wet and dry. Dry gangrene is due to loss of nourishment to a part, followed by mummification. The area is dry, black, and shriveled, and results in a well-defined line of demarcation with specific localization and self-amputation (autoamputation; Figure 19-3A). Wet gangrene is the necrosis of tissue, followed by destruction caused by excessive moisture. Bacterial gases accumulate in the tissue. The line of demarcation is ill defined, and the limb is painful, purple, and swollen. Wet gangrene is common when infection exists.[29,30] Figure 19-3B shows wet gangrene of the fifth toe. *Do not* debride. The patient needs immediate referral to a surgeon.

Systems Review and Examination

A multisystems review and examination for the patient with neuropathy is required to determine the coimpairments that will affect wound healing and require management. Four systems to review for this patient population are the neuromuscular system, the vascular system, the musculoskeletal system, and the integumentary system.

Neuromuscular System

A foot with neuropathy is dry, with small fissures; has toes that are clawed; and is incapable of sensing trauma. The rigid anesthetic foot is more likely to break down than is a flexible anesthetic foot.[31] The insensitive foot should be evaluated carefully and bilaterally. Any form of peripheral neuropathy can produce the discomfort of paresthesia: prickling, burning, and jabbing sensations.[32,33] The length of this period of discomfort is unknown; it varies among patients. Neuromuscular system examinations to assess for neurologic changes are the focus of the foot screening process and are described in detail later.

RESEARCH WISDOM

Interventions for Paresthesia

Paresthesia may be helped by use of a transcutaneous electronic nerve stimulator (TENS) unit, which generates small pulses of electricity similar to an electric massage. Another method of controlling the discomfort is with topical creams.[34,35] See Chapter 21 for more information.

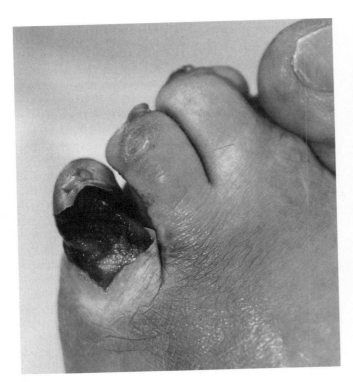

A

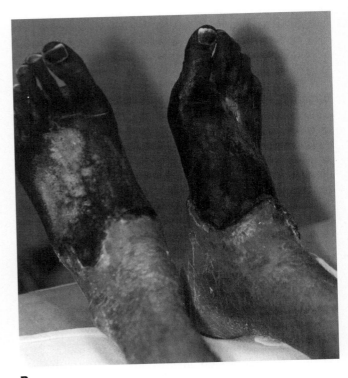

B

FIGURE 19-3 A. Dry gangrene. Such a lesion needs immediate referral to a surgeon. It should not be debrided. **B.** Wet gangrene. Such a lesion needs immediate referral to a surgeon. There is probable infection.

Vascular System

Peripheral vascular disease (PVD) is a serious complication affecting millions of Americans. Of the 500,000 vascular-related ulcerations, 10% are arterial and 70% are venous ulcerations; some individuals have both venous and arterial diseases.[16] Many patients with neuropathy also have PVD. Therefore, it is critical to review the vascular history (to identify strategies that are being used to manage vascular problems) before planning any intervention. Some of the related circulatory system diseases that usually accompany neuropathy and management recommendations are described here. Chapter 18 describes the pathogenesis and management of vascular problems in more detail. Chapter 7 discusses noninvasive vascular testing for patients with diabetes.

Atherosclerosis is also known as hardening of the arteries. The interior wall of arteries is usually smooth but with atherosclerosis platelets, calcium, and connective tissue deposit on the walls. In early stages, the patient may experience intermittent claudication or cramping in the lower limb, which goes away with rest. As the disease progresses, symptoms appear when the patient is not walking (rest pain).[16] Arterial compromise can be noted by the loss of hair growth, shiny skin, atrophy, and cool skin over the toes.[36] Atherosclerosis leads to impaired circulation in the legs and is one of the most important causes of gangrene, leading to amputation.[37] Arterial ulcers are located on tips of (or between) toes, on heels, on metatarsal heads, on sides or soles of foot, and above the lateral malleoli. The ulcer will look punched out, with well-demarcated edges, and be nonbleeding (see *Color Plate 54*). The ulcer base may be deep and pale or black and necrotic. Treatment involves vascular reconstruction, bed rest, and immobilization. Arterial ulcers have a poor prognosis. Misdiagnosis of an arterial ulcer as a venous ulcer can lead to serious complications.

The venous stasis ulceration has a better prognosis for healing than does the arterial ischemic ulceration. Veins are less elastic than are arteries. The valves within veins no longer function to return blood to the heart against gravity, leaving blood to pool in the lower limb. The pooling does not allow new oxygenated blood into the area, and the cell walls of the veins begin to break down. The waste blood products begin to weep through the lower limb. Venous stasis ulcerations are commonly located in the anteromedial malleolus and pretibial areas. The ulcerations are irregular in shape, surrounded by bluish, brown skin. These ulcers are exudative and show evidence of bleeding.

Treatment of venous stasis ulcerations begins with leg elevation.[38] The limb must be treated with compression bandages or an Unna boot. The Unna boot is a semirigid dressing of gelatin and zinc oxide. Its application protects vulnerable skin from the weeping exudate, especially below the ulcer site. The Unna boot is applied wet. When it dries, it forms a nonelastic, nonexpandable, nonshrinkable, porous mold that sticks to the skin. This treatment has been used on venous ulcers for 100 years. It is a means of controlling edema when it is applied across a joint. The motion of the joint generates a pumping action.[1]

The chronic venous stasis lower limb without an open ulceration will show signs of edema that must be controlled. The presence of small water blisters or weeping will be a sign that compression should begin (see *Color Plates 59 and 60*). This limb should be treated with pressure-gradiated stockings as daily prevention; an Unna boot with Ace bandage wrap is required for severe edema or periods of breakdown. Pressure-gradiated stockings have a graduated pressure to facilitate pumping action and assist the venous system in removing fluids from the lower limb. Antiembolism stockings are not designed for the ambulatory patient and do not supply the pumping action required. Antiembolism compression is for the recumbent hospitalized patient.

Compression can be ordered to begin at the metatarsal heads and decrease pressure in the calf (neuropathic compression stocking; Figure 19-4) as a further assist to the venous system. Most patients do well with compression in the range of 30–40 mm Hg at the foot and ankle. When using these stockings for the neuropathic/dysvascular patient, remember to avoid seams around bony prominences, and never place a zipper over the malleoli.

When venous stasis ulceration occurs on one limb, begin compression therapy on the contralateral side. The appearance of small water blisters or weeping is a sign that compression should begin. The prosthetic shrinker sock (Figure 19-5) should be used following a major limb amputation to reduce edema and shape the residual limb. The prosthetic shrinker applies both circumferential and vertical (distal to proximal) compression.[39] Chapter 10 describes procedures for management of edema.

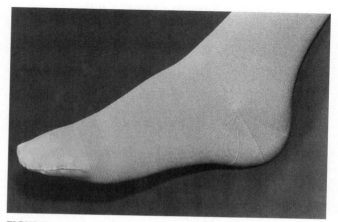

FIGURE 19-4 The full foot compression stocking begins compression at the metatarsal heads and decreases compression above the ankle to assist in the venous pumping mechanics. (Courtesy of Juzo-Julius Zorn, Inc., Cuyahoga Falls, Ohio.)

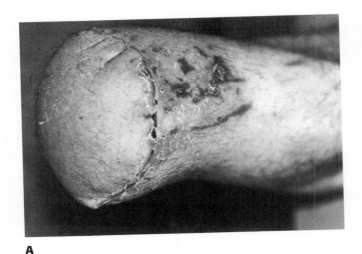

A

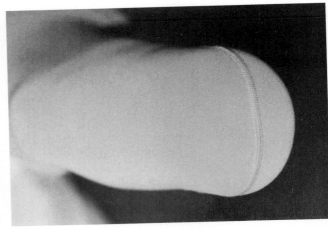

B

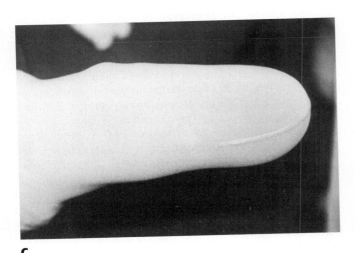

C

FIGURE 19-5 The prosthetic shrinker assists in shaping the limb following major amputation surgery. **A.** Postop bulbous residual limb of below knee (transtibial) amputee. **B.** Application of prosthetic shrinker. **C.** Final residual limb shape for prosthetic application. (*B and C:* Courtesy of Juzo-Julius Zorn, Inc., Cuyahoga Falls, Ohio.)

Musculoskeletal System Examination

The musculoskeletal system examination includes examination of joint integrity, range of motion, skeletal deformity, and muscle strength. Motor neuropathy will distort skeletal alignment, and Charcot joint will leave a foot deformed, as will be shown later in this chapter. An analysis of abnormal gait should also be included. Beginning with the joint range of motion review, it is important that the foot has a dorsiflexion range of at least 10° to allow ambulation without harm to the great toe.[40] The forces on the plantar surface can peak to 275% of body weight when running and 80% when walking.[41] With limited motion in the joints, the trauma can result in ulceration. It is important to test range of motion, as well as to perform manual muscle testing.[2,42] There is an absence of the ankle jerk reflex when neuropathy is advanced to glove-and-stocking distribution.[43]

Leg length discrepancy affects 70%–80% of the population and often does not cause pain or deformity. A discrepancy can relate to chronic complications, such as hammertoes, hallux valgus, and referred joint disruption of the ankle, knee, hip, and lower back. A 2-cm discrepancy is sufficient to cause symptoms and requires shoe lifts with physical therapy. Any lift over 1/4 inch should be placed on the sole of the shoe and added gradually to allow the body to respond to changes as the pelvis levels.[44]

There is a constant concern with toe deformities that may result in ulceration. In the case of claw toe deformity, the toes are dorsiflexed at the metatarsal-phalangeal joints, with flexion at the interphalangeal joints.[45] The great toe should be examined for deformity. A fibrous proximal joint can cause ulceration that is especially difficult to relieve. Great toe extension can be seen when weight bearing, because the patient will thrust the toe into extension when ambulating, causing calluses and discoloration on the distal tip near the nail from contacting the shoe. Great toe pronation is seen on the medial/plantar surface of the great toe. Hallux rigidus refers to limited range of motion in the proximal great toe metatarsal-phalangeal joint and requires a rigid rocker-bottom shoe to allow ambulation without excessive pressure on the great toe. Hallux valgus (bunion) is the increased valgus angle of the great toe in relation to the metatarsal, requiring a shoe that can be modified and molded to conform to the medial bunion formation.

Toe amputations may be required for single or multiple toes (see Figure 19-1). The amputation may be a disarticulation or a resection (metatarsal shaft is removed). The distal end of the amputation site must be followed carefully and protected from trauma.

Common complications must be addressed with the neuropathic limb. Bursa formation over the navicular prominence is due to the constant high forces and must be provided with an area of pressure relief before ulceration occurs. A sinus tract formation will result when previous areas of ulceration heal over a pocket of bacteria instead of healing from internal to external tissues. The small pocket of bacteria will be moved anteriorly through the tissues, causing infection to spread.

A common complication of the neuropathic patient is severe foot deformity following neuropathic fractures or Charcot arthropathy (discussed later in this chapter), including joint subluxation or dislocation. The presence of severe foot deformity has been shown to be predictive of prolonged healing time for patients treated with total-contact casting (TCC). Sinacore et al[46] found that fixed foot deformity prolonged healing of ulcers with TCC when located in the midfoot and rearfoot. Ulcers located in the midfoot healed in 73 ± 29 days, and rearfoot ulcers healed in 90 ± 19 days. Individuals without fixed deformities with chronic diabetes mellitus and those with forefoot ulcers healed in 41 days. Therefore, early detection during the musculoskeletal examination of a fixed foot deformity in a patient with an ulcer located in the midfoot or rearfoot can be used to determine a prognosis that healing time will be significantly longer when a TCC is used as the treatment intervention.

Motor neuropathy produces common abnormal gait characteristics in the neuropathic population. The shoes are worn on the lateral side of the sole because of a varus deformity (see Figure 19-6). This weakness often causes ankle injuries. After further deterioration, foot drop can occur. The stiffness in the complex joint structures leads to abnormal motion in the foot's function. Muscle atrophy, imbalances, and deformity lead to abnormal concentration of forces and shear forces that are precursors to wound formation.[47]

CLINICAL WISDOM

Modification of a Standard-Depth Shoe

To compensate for varus gait abnormalities, shoes need to be modified. The modifications required are (1) a full, lateral-flare sole, as shown in Figure 19-6, (2) a strong counter to support the heel, and (3) a high top to support the ankle. A standard-depth shoe can be modified by an orthotist, or a shoe repairperson may be able to do the job, if guided. Although not all orthotists will agree to modify an existing shoe, others will. This will save the patient money.

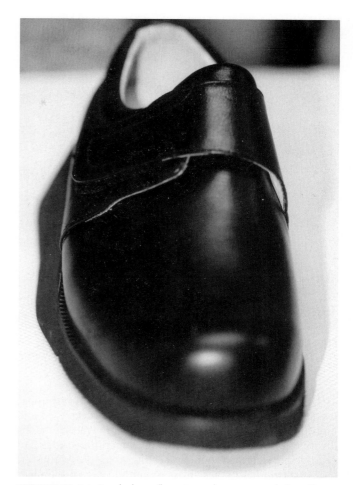

FIGURE 19-6 Lateral shoe flare to reduce varus deformity progression due to motor neuropathy. (Courtesy of Nancy Elftman.)

Integumentary System Examination

Integumentary system examination of the foot includes the toenails. Toenail deformities are commonly seen in the neuropathic foot. Hypertrophic nails are caused by onychomycosis (fungus) infection (Figure 19-7) and are common in the diabetic population. The nails tear shoe lining and create areas of rough surface to abrade the toes. Nail care for fungus, ingrown toenails, and trimming must be performed by trained medical personnel to ensure that injury is not inflicted. Soft corns are hyperkeratotic lesions found between toes (usually between the fourth and fifth toes), due to pressure of an opposing toe in a region that is moist.[30] Injury and maceration of the toes is commonly controlled by the use of lamb's wool between the toes or tube foam to space toes and prevent friction (Figure 19-8A, B, and C, Exhibit 19-1). Buildup of callus is indicative of high pressures and stress of an isolated area that must be relieved. The thickening of the skin in the area of a callus is preceded by abnormal pressure or friction.[30,48] Areas of excess pressure require pressure redistribution in the clinic setting, rather than scheduling additional appointments.

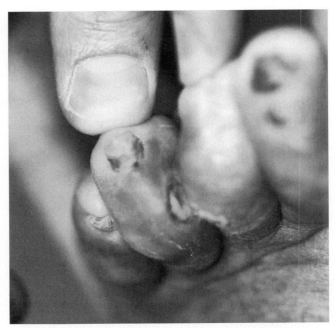

FIGURE 19-7 This foot has soft corns between toes, thickened toenails, and onychomycosis (fungal) infection.

Dryness of the skin is the result of autonomic neuropathy in which the sweat and oil production is decreased and moisture must be replaced. Loss of hair growth may be indicative of vascular impairment. Ulcerations that are necrotic are debrided to allow healing to progress from internal to external tissues for optimum closure of the ulcer site.

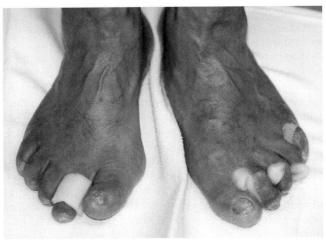

A

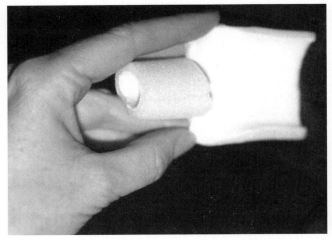

B

CLINICAL WISDOM

Tube Foam and Lamb's Wool for Quick Relief of Pressure on Toes

Claw toes, hammer toes, calluses, corns, and small ulcerations can be relieved of pressure by inserts and shoe modifications and spaced with tube foam or lamb's wool separators to allow air flow. Separators prevent maceration and skin breakdown; they should be removed before and replaced after bathing. In addition, the custom tube foam separator serves as a toe separator, reduces shear from the shoe, cushions metatarsal heads, and can be used as a positioner for overlapping toes. Figure 19-8A shows lamb's wool pieces placed between toes. Figure 19-8B shows a tube foam toe separator in place. Figure 19-8C and Exhibit 19-1 illustrate and describe the diagram of steps to create a tube foam separator. The tube foam is available from podiatric supply companies.

Another common occurrence is burns, due to either heat or chemicals, such as over-the-counter remedies. Soaking the foot in hot water is a specific cause of burns. A common wisdom is that neuropathic patients should *never* soak their feet. The insensitive foot cannot produce the warning signals necessary to prevent severe burns (see Chapter 5).

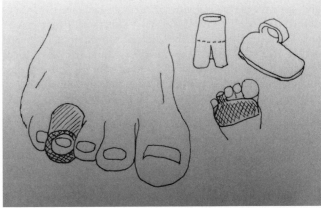

C

FIGURE 19-8 A. To keep the web space open and dry, use tube foam or lamb's wool. **B.** The tube foam should be cut to allow a "tail" under the foot. This extension will deter migration of the pad. **C.** Diagram of construction of a tube foam separator. *(A and B: Courtesy of Nancy Elftman.)*

EXHIBIT 19-1   Instructions for Making a Foam Toe Separator

> **Make a custom foam toe separator (Figures 19-8B and 19-8C) by the following steps:**
>
> 1. Select a size of tube foam with a diameter that will not constrict the toe.
> 2. Cut a 21/2–3-inch piece of the foam.
> 3. To make the toe cuff:
>   a. Measure back 1/2 to 3/4 inch from one end of the tube foam and mark.
>   b. Cut across the diameter of the tube three fourths of the way through.
>   c. Slit up the tube to the marking on the side that is cut to the diameter cut (see diagram).
>   d. The foam will flatten out (see diagram).
>   e. The tube will slip over the toe and the flat section will be located on the plantar surface of the foot.

Dermatologic conditions can affect treatment programs until they are resolved. Necrobiosis lipoidica diabeticorum may be seen on the shin (along tibia) as a dermatologic condition in diabetic patients (Figure 19-9). The condition manifests as irregular patches of degenerated collagen with reduced numbers of fibrocytes. The dry, scaly areas have been infiltrated with chronic inflammatory cells.[49] Necrobiosis can be confused with venous stasis disease but does not require or respond to extensive treatment. The round, firm plaques of reddish brown to yellow are seen three times more often in women than in men.[50,51] These ulcerations are common along the tibia and require only protective dressings.

The callus (or tyloma) is a yellowish-gray lesion that may be flat or raised and spread over a large area. The callus is caused by friction (shear), irritation, and/or pressure. There is hyperemia and thickening of the skin. The skin is compressed, and superficial layers of callus are laid down. The callus may be reduced mechanically with tools and the forces to the area reduced. Many facilities use sanding tools and callus reducers to break the chain of callus buildup. The pumice stone is used as a wet tool on wet skin. The callus reducer debrides dry callus with a dry tool (Figure 19-10).[52]

Keratoderma plantaris, characterized by keratin cracks and ulcerations, is caused by the loss of sweat and oil elasticity in the skin (autonomic neuropathy). As keratin builds up, it creates small fissures that allow entrance of bacteria, and infection begins. The entire sole around the margin of the heel will undergo diffuse thickening and develop painful fissures if the foot is sensate or will go undetected if insensate (see Figure 19-11). Prevention includes reduction of keratin buildup and retention of skin moisture.[30] There are many forms of rashes and dermatologic conditions that must be evaluated and treated in the neuropathic limb. These are usually discovered by inspection, rather than patient dis-

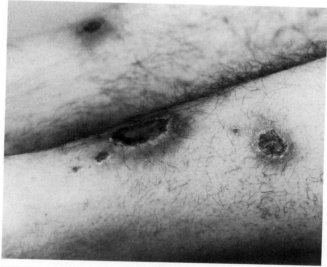

FIGURE 19-9 Necrobiosis lipoidica diabeticorum: a dermatologic condition often present in the diabetic, neuropathic limb.

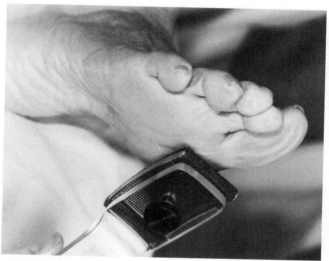

FIGURE 19-10 Callus reducer: a tool used dry on dry callus to remove buildup and reduce the superficial layers.

comfort. Typical skin conditions in the diabetic population include shin spots and diabetic bullae (with less frequency than necrobiosis).[52]

Infections are commonly seen in the neuropathic foot, including *Pseudomonas* infection, which is bacterial growth that occurs within a moist environment. Signs and symptoms of infection are usually absent in the neuropathic foot, even though the infection is present and virulent, due to impaired circulation and immunosuppression. Both are other common coimpairments of neuropathy. The problems of infection are identified during the integumentary system review. See Chapter 9 for strategies to assess and treat infection.

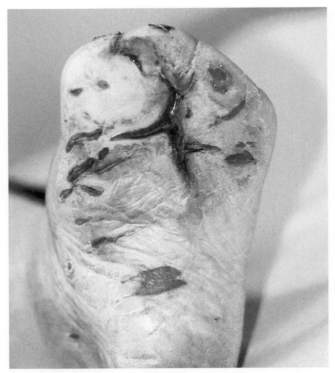

FIGURE 19-11 Typical neuropathic foot with keratoderma plantaris. Note the dry, cracked skin, dirt imbedded in the skin, open wounds, and the absence of dressing, due to lack of awareness of the condition.

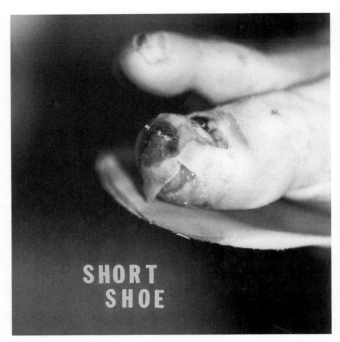

FIGURE 19-12 Short shoe. The toe extends to the end of the insole. (Reprinted with permission from N. Elftman, Clinical Management of the Neuropathic Limb, *Journal of Prosthetics and Orthotics*, Vol. 4, No. 1, pp. 1–12, Copyright © American Academy of Orthotists and Prosthetists.)

Dry gangrene is another finding that may be discovered during the integumentary system review. When dry gangrene is present, there is a line of demarcation at which the body will auto-amputate the affected area. This process of autoamputation could take weeks to months;[45] it is nature's way of protecting the body from infection and should not be disturbed. Figure 19-3A (Wagner grade 5, discussed below) is a photograph of a foot with dry gangrene. A patient with dry gangrene needs immediate referral to the surgeon.

Further Visual and Physical Assessments

Examination of the neuropathic limb includes further visual and physical examination to avoid future complications. The patient is never asked for his or her own foot evaluation. The shoes are removed to allow the practitioner to examine the foot. The neuropathic patient will not limp, even with a foot ulceration (see Figures 19-11 and 19-12). Inspection should be both weight bearing and nonweight bearing.

Footwear Assessment

The footwear must be examined for wear of orthosis and sock patterns indicating excessive pressure. The ends of the toes should be examined for injury caused by a short shoe. Figure 19-12 shows a toe wound caused by a short shoe. Notice that the toe extends to the end of the shoe insole. Alignment is required when fitting a shoe for proper weight distribution and length measurement, and will be discussed later in this chapter. The interventions section of this chapter describes orthotics and adaptive equipment and includes instructions in footwear interventions. Shoes should show a normal wear pattern on the lateral heel of the sole, as contrasted with the pattern in Figure 19-6A. Shoes should be resoled on a regular basis to keep sides from wearing down. Inserts are replaced as required when relief modifications are no longer sufficient and shock absorption is decreased.

Wound Assessment

The Wagner scale[53] for grading neuropathic ulcers classifies ulcer severity in six grades, based on the depth of the ulcer and the presence of infection or necrosis. Ulcer grading is useful for prognosis and for selection of treatment intervention. In addition, the Wagner ulcer grading system is a uniform system that is used by health-care practitioners of different disciplines to describe ulcers in neuropathic limbs. Ulcers with low grades are managed by conservative measures, whereas ulcers with higher grades are a direct threat to limb loss and require surgical management. The neuropathic limb often suffers from dysvascularity, as well; therefore, the system is often used for both populations. The

Wagner ulcer classification system differs from other grading systems by including a grade of zero, which describes preulcerative skin, healed ulcers, and the presence of a bony deformity where the skin is intact (Figure 19-13A). Preulcerative areas include calluses located under the metatarsal heads or areas of weight bearing.[54] For continuity of documentation and communication, the team must understand the Wagner scale of ulcer grading and use it consistently. Exhibit 19-2 shows the six Wagner ulcer grades. The preferred conservative method of treatment is guided by the Wagner grade. Exhibit 19-3 shows how the different grades dictate different treatment strategies.[55]

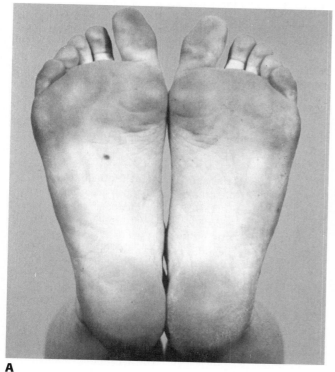

A

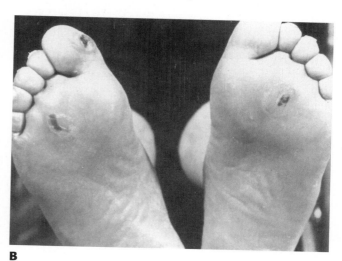

B

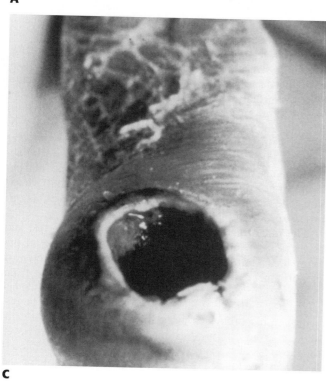

C

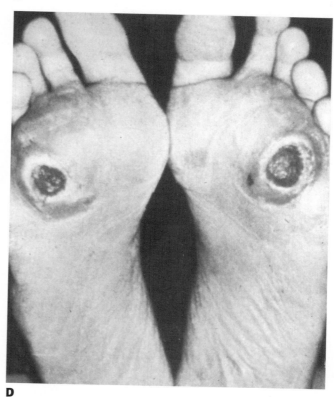

D

FIGURE 19-13 A. Skin intact, Wagner grade 0. **B.** Superficial ulcer, Wagner grade 1. **C.** Deeper ulcer to tendon or bone, Wagner grade 2. **D.** Ulcer has abscess or osteomyelitis, Wagner grade 3.

(Continued)

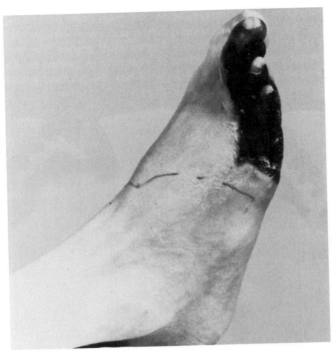

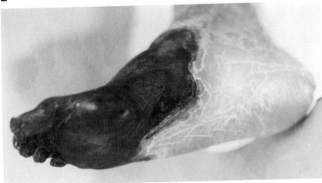

E

F

FIGURE 19-13   *(Continued)*
E. Gangrene on forefoot, Wagner grade 4. **F.** Gangrene over major portion of foot, Wagner grade 5.

Sensation Testing

When evaluated for insensitivity, most patients who had hypoesthesia could sense pinprick and cotton wisp applications. Patients with foot ulcers were observed to have less *pressure sensation* than did those without foot ulcers.[56] In 1898, von Frey attempted to standardize the stimuli for testing the subjective sense of light touch by using a series of horse hairs of varying thicknesses and stiffness. Wienstein used nylon monofilaments mounted on Lucite rods as substitutes for the hairs.[57] The Semmes-Wienstein monofilaments can be obtained commercially in elaborate sets for precise measurement, but research at Carville Hansen's Disease Center in Carville, Louisiana, has consolidated the testing to three sizes of monofilaments for grading the in-

EXHIBIT 19-2   Wagner Scale

Grade	Description
Grade 0	Skin intact (Figure 19-13A)
Grade 1	Superficial ulcer (Figure 19-13B)
Grade 2	Deeper ulcer to tendon or bone (Figure 19-13C)
Grade 3	Ulcer has abscess or osteomyelitis (Figure 19-13D)
Grade 4	Gangrene on forefoot (Figure 19-13E)
Grade 5	Gangrene over major portion of foot (Figure 19-13F)

Reprinted with permission from F.E.W. Wagner, The Dysvascular Foot: A System for Diagnosis and Treatment, *Foot and Ankle*, 2:64–122, © 1981, American Orthopaedic Foot and Ankle Society.

EXHIBIT 19-3   Conservative Management by Wagner Ulcer Grade

Wagner Ulcer Grade and Treatment Protocol	
Grade 0	Depth shoes and shock-absorbing insert.
Grade 1	Cast, ODS splint, or wound care shoe to reduce weight at ulceration site; antibiotic intervention as required.
Grade 2	Debridement and cast, ODS splint or wound care shoe for weight distribution; antibiotics as required.
Grade 3	Remove infected tissue, cast and antibiotic intervention.

sensitive foot (Exhibit 19-4).[58] The 4.17 monofilament supplies 1 g of force and is indicative of normal sensation. If the patient cannot feel the next monofilament (5.07), he or she does not have the protective sensation level of 10 g and cannot sense trauma to the foot to cease weight bearing. Failure to sense the 10-g monofilament is used as the determining factor for use of protective footwear and accommodative orthotics. No patient with protective sensation can ambulate on an ulcerated foot. A large percentage of patients do not feel the largest monofilament (6.10), which indicates a loss of sensation at 75 g. This largest-diameter monofilament indicates an insensate foot that must be accommodated and followed closely. Use of the monofilament is not to be confused with the testing for sharp/dull sensation. The sharp/dull test stimulates multiple nerves, as opposed to a single-point perception test.

The monofilament is a single-point perception test and requires the examiner to place the monofilament on the skin, press until the monofilament bends (diameter of monofilament controls point of bend), and remove it from the skin surface. The monofilaments are tested and determined to be reliable at the 95% confidence level.[58] The patient is to respond when he or she feels the pressure sensation. To avoid errors in testing, the monofilament is never used in areas of scarring, calluses, or necrotic tissue. The bilateral testing for sensation is especially important for the

EXHIBIT 19-4   Screening Form for Diabetes Foot Disease

Name: _____ Date: _____ ID#: _____

I. Medical History (Check all that apply.)
____ Peripheral neuropathy
____ Retinopathy
____ Cardiovascular disease
____ Nephropathy
____ Peripheral vascular disease

(For Sections II & III, fill in the blanks with an "R," "L," or "B" for positive findings on the right, left, or both feet.)

II. Current History
1. Any change in the foot since the last evaluation? Y ____ N ____
2. Current ulcer or history of a foot ulcer? Y _____ N _____
3. Is there pain in the calf muscles when walking that is relieved by rest? Y _____ N _____

III. Foot Exam
1. Are the nails thick, too long, ingrown, infected with fungal disease? Y _____ N _____
2. Note foot deformities
____ Toe deformities
____ Bunions (hallus valgus)
____ Charcot foot
____ Foot drop
____ Prominent metatarsal heads
Amputation (Specify date, side, and level.)

3. Pedal Pulses (Fill in the blanks with a "P" or an "A" to indicate present or absent.)

Posterior tibial:
Left ____ Right____
Dorsalis pedis:
Left ____ Right ____

4. Skin Condition (Measure, draw in, and label the patient's skin condition, using the key and the foot diagram below.)

C = Callus
U = Ulcer
R = Redness
W = Warmth
M = Maceration
PU = Preulcerative lesion
F = Fissure
S = Swelling
D = Dryness

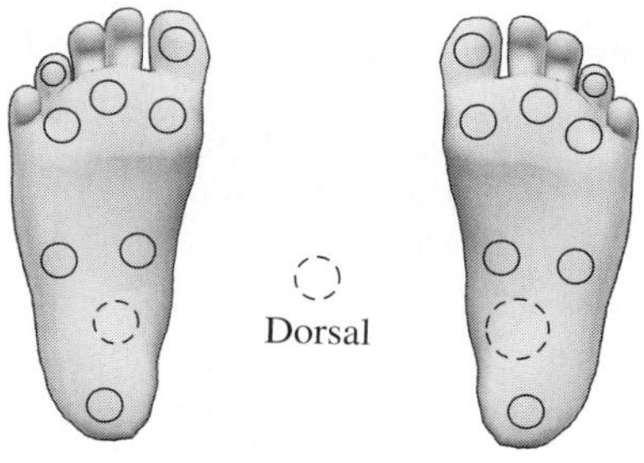

Dorsal

Right Foot   Left Foot

IV. Sensory Foot Exam (Label sensory level with a "+" in the five circled areas of each foot if the patient can feel the 5.07 Semmes-Wienstein (10-g) nylon filament and "-" if the patient cannot feel the filament.)

V. Risk Categorization (Check appropriate box.)
____ Low-Risk Patient

All of the following:
____ Intact protective sensation
____ Pedal pulses present
____ No severe deformity
____ No prior foot ulcer
____ No amputation
____ High-Risk Patient

One or more of the following:
____ Loss of protective sensation
____ Absent pedal pulses

____ Severe foot deformity
____ History of foot ulcer
____ Prior amputation

VI. Footwear Assessment (Fill in the blanks.)
Does the patient wear appropriate shoes? Y ____ N ____
Does the patient need inserts? Y ____ N ____
Should therapeutic footwear be prescribed? Y ____ N ____

VII. Education (Fill in the blanks.)
Has the patient had prior foot care education? Y ____ N ____
Can the patient demonstrate appropriate self-care?
Y ____ N ____

VIII. Management Plan
(Check all that apply.)
____ Provide patient education for preventive foot care.
Date: _____

Diagnostic studies:
____ Vascular laboratory
____ Other: _____
____ Schedule follow-up visit.

Footwear recommendations:
____ None
____ Athletic shoes

____ Accommodative inserts
____ Custom shoes
____ Depth shoes
Refer to:
____ Primary care provider
____ Diabetes educator
____ Orthopaedic foot surgeon

____ RN foot specialist
____ Orthotist
____ Podiatrist
____ Pedorthist
____ Endocrinologist
____ Rehab specialist
____ Vascular surgeon
____ Other: _____

Date: _____   _____
                                    Provider Signature
NOTES:

Reprinted from *Feet Can Last a Lifetime: A Health Care Provider's Guide to Preventing Diabetic Foot Problems,* Institute of Diabetics and Digestive and Kidney Diseases, U.S. Department of Health and Human Services, National Institutes of Health, Bethesda, MD.

unilateral and bilateral amputee to determine areas of insensitivity and progression of the neuropathy. Figure 19-14 shows the proper method for the monofilament testing procedure. Note the bend of the monofilament. This must occur to measure correct pressure sensation.

At Hansen's Disease Center, Birke[59] developed a risk classification system based on the loss of protective sensation. Loss of protective sensation, history of prior ulceration, and reduced circulatory perfusion are important factors in development of foot ulcers. A risk classification system based on these factors is useful in identifying patients who would benefit from different levels of intervention (see Exhibit 19-3). Risk is classified by four grades: 0, no loss of protective sensation; 1, loss of protective sensation (no deformity or history of plantar ulceration); 2, loss of protective sensation and deformity or abnormal blood flow without history of plantar ulcer; and 3, history of plantar ulcer. Three interventions have proven effective in reducing risk of ulceration: protective footwear, patient education, and frequent clinic follow-up. For example, when a patient's ulcer is grade 0, preulceration, and the patient can sense the 10-g monofilament (has protective sensation), he or she will sense pain before damage occurs to the feet. Pa-

tients in this category usually do well with a standard shoe of correct sizing and a simple shock-absorbing pad.

The patient without protective sensation will not cease ambulating when damage begins to tissues. Patients with feet such as those in Figure 19-11 who walk into the clinic are insensate. They require extra-depth shoes with a total-contact accommodative insert to distribute pressure and reduce forces on areas of potential breakdown. The insert may be molded to the patient or fabricated on a cast. The cast does not have corrective forces added, only accommodation.

The accommodative insert does not apply correction; it fills only the spaces between the flat shoe and the foot contours. Any force added will receive full weight bearing, and breakdown will occur. If the addition of metatarsal head (MTH) pads or scaphoid pads is requested, these pads must be of a soft durometer. Rigid pad additions will cause excess pressure and ulcerations. The MTH pads are placed proximal to the MTHs to redistribute the weight from the heads to the metatarsal shafts (Figure 19-15).

Testing for vibratory sensation may be accomplished by using the bioesthesiometer. This instrument is essentially an electrical tuning fork that uses repetitive mechanical indentation of skin delivered at a prescribed frequency and amplitude.[60] The simple graduated tuning fork is a rapid means of sensory testing.[61,62] The purpose of all sensory testing equipment is to identify those at risk.[63]

Upper and lower extremity peripheral neuropathy is present when sensation testing reveals that the level of sensation loss is symmetric and equidistant from the spine in both arms and legs. The hands of these patients should be considered in the evaluation process. Physical signs of upper extremity involvement include cheiroarthropathy (motor

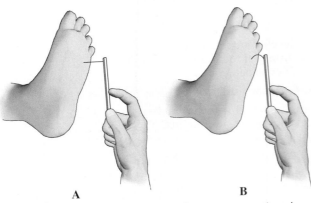

A   **B**

FIGURE 19-14 Sensory Foot Exam. The sensory testing device is a 10-g (5.07 Semmes-Wienstein) nylon filament mounted on a holder that has been standardized to deliver a 10-g force when properly applied. Research has shown that a person who can feel the 10-g filament in the selected sites is at reduced risk for developing ulcers. (1) The sensory exam should be done in a quiet and relaxed setting. The patient must not watch while the examiner applies the filament. (2) Test the monofilament on the patient's hand so he or she knows what to anticipate. (3) The five sites to be tested on each foot are indicated on the screening form. (4) Apply the monofilament perpendicular to the skin's surface (part A of figure). (Reprinted with permission from *Feet Can Last a Lifetime: A Health Care Provider's Guide to Preventing Diabetic Foot Problems,* Institute of Diabetes and Digestive and Kidney Diseases, U.S. Department of Health and Human Services, National Institute of Health, Bethesda, MD.)

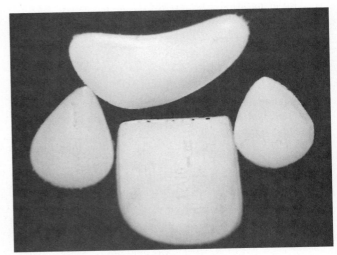

FIGURE 19-15 Metatarsal pads made of soft durometer to aid in pressure relief of metatarsal heads and increase transverse arch of foot. (Courtesy of UCO International, Inc., Wheeling, Illinois.)

neuropathy in upper extremity), when the patient cannot touch the palms together in the prayer position. Another physical sign is atrophy of the web space between the thumb and first finger. This is the first sign of motor neuropathy in the hand. Consideration of the hand deficit must be taken into account for donning, doffing, and choice of closures for orthotics and footwear.[42] Little attention has been paid to the diabetic hand syndrome, or limited joint mobility (LJM), in which the joints of the fingers and wrists become limited. This condition occurs in 30%–50% of people who have had type I diabetes for more than 15 years. One test for LJM is performed by having the patient place the hands flat on a table. Patients with severe LJM will not be able to flatten the fingers onto the table. The skin will also be thick and can be tented on the back of the metacarpophalangeal (MCP) joint[64] (Figure 19-16).

Body Temperature Testing

Since the time of Hippocrates, physicians have known that body temperature variations offer important clues for diagnosing disease. Diagnostic tools convert infrared radiation and display it on monitors with the use of thermography.[62] There are many methods of acquiring surface temperatures. The objectives and procedure for doing so are listed in the box below.

Thermistors or thermocouples are accurate recording devices that, when touched to the skin for 10 seconds, give a numeric display of temperature.[65] Wound temperature depends on the vascularity of the area and can be measured by thermography. In a study of vascular wounds, vascularity was measured indirectly by measuring skin temperatures. The subject surgical site was measured prior to surgery and postoperatively for 8 days at a specified time. The first- through third-day temperatures increased at the surgical wound and a wide surrounding area. Days 4 through 8 had lower temperatures, and the zones of warm surrounding area became narrower. The stitches were removed at day 7, and, by day 8, the area assumed preoperative temperatures, except in the very narrow incisional site. Documentation noted that the persistence of a wider zone of increased temperatures after day 4 predicts wound infection and disturbed healing.[66] The infrared scanner thermometer unit (Figure 19-17A and B) allows accurate, immediate spot temperature reading and the feature of scanning the foot quickly. A recent study evaluated the effectiveness of at-home infrared temperature monitoring as a preventive tool in diabetics at high risk for lower extremity ulceration and amputation. The study group measured temperatures in the morning and evening and were instructed to reduce their activity and contact the study nurse when temperatures increased. This group had significantly fewer foot complications due to early warning of inflammation and tissue injury.[67]

The use of temperature is valuable as an objective measurement of tissue damage and inflammation produced by repeated mechanical (pressure) trauma.[68] When evaluating the limb, the most distal aspects of extremities are cool. Muscular areas with good blood supply are warmer than bony regions. Arches are several degrees warmer than heels or toes.[65] Excessive heat in an area of the foot is a vascular response to trauma. The trauma may be due to external forces, infection, Charcot joint, or other internal complications. The examiner can feel the increased heat manually and determine where complications may reside, but without instrumentation to record actual numbers, there will not be objective documentation for follow-up and comparison. Using a surface-sensing temperature device (thermocouple or infrared), temperatures are recorded in predetermined areas, usually those related to common areas of breakdown. When there is one definite area whose temperature is 3° F higher than that of adjacent areas, it can be assumed to be an area of high pressure or stress. If there is no current breakdown, this area must be relieved of pressure and the pressure distributed over the remaining weight-bearing surfaces. Upon follow-up of this same patient, the temperature differentiation should decrease as healing of tissue progresses. In a comparison of contralateral limbs, vascular impairment should be suspected when one limb is significantly colder or distal portions of the foot show an extreme drop in temperature. A chronic hot spot points to the fact that there is a chronic stress or an underlying bone or joint problem. Increased temperature tells that there is a problem and where it is—not what it is![22]

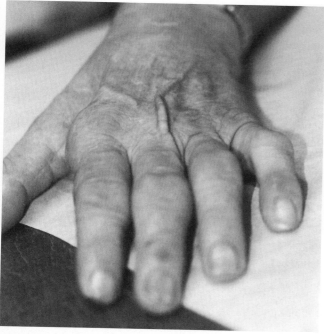

FIGURE 19-16 Neuropathic hand. Motor neuropathy testing reveals tenting on the back of the MCP joint, clawing of the fingers, and atrophy of the web space between the thumb and the first finger.

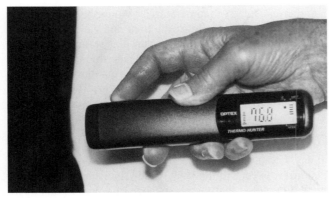

A

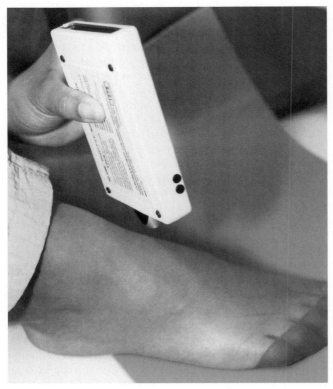

B

FIGURE 19-17 A. Measurements, Inc. infrared thermometer. **B.** Deltatrak infrared thermometer. (Courtesy of Measurements, LLC, New Orleans, Louisiana.)

Objectives and Procedure for Taking Temperature

Objectives for taking temperature:

- To evaluate baseline temperature at sites of high incidence of ulceration
- To determine presence of inflammation
- To evaluate sites of baseline elevated temperature for decrease in temperature after intervention to relieve pressure

Procedure for taking and recording temperature:

1. Expose the bare skin of the foot to the room temperature for 5–10 minutes before recording any temperature.
2. Take temperature at 10 locations on the sole of foot and toes (shown by circles on foot evaluation form Exhibit 19-4).
3. Follow steps for measuring temperature.
4. Record readings in degrees at each location on foot evaluation form and date.
5. Record readings at each location on successive evaluations below the initial reading and date.

Procedure for Use of an Infrared Scanner Thermometer*

Follow these steps in measuring temperature with an infrared scanner thermometer:

1. Temperature testing may be done with or without contact of skin.
2. Read the first number seen.
3. Avoid pressure against the skin that causes ischemia.

Pressure Testing

A rubber mat was developed by R.I. Harris that would print light foot pressures in large, light squares (formed by tall grid ridges) and heavier pressures in darker, smaller squares (deep ridges).[2] The Harris mat will give a grid analysis of pressure distribution at a relatively low cost per patient. The Harris mat can be used for static and dynamic assessment and can provide permanent records. Figure 19-18 shows an imprint on a Harris mat. The darker areas are areas of high pressure.

Force plates have given us valuable information regarding peak pressures during ambulation but represent a single step on the plate. Attempts to place sensors in the shoes have been unreliable because of the sensor structure and attachment within the shoe.[69] The new age of computer-aided documentation provides color replicas of three-dimensional pressure recordings and illustrations that can be used for static or dynamic documentation. Although costs of the computer-aided devices are high, technology is advancing to provide unrestricted data collection.[70] Progress is also being made to produce live scanning of the foot in order to provide a positive mold for orthotics, as well as for custom shoes.[71] Using computed three-dimensional, digital computer graphics, a plastic sock may be molded to the patient and converted to a shoe cast.[72]

Charcot Joint Examination

Charcot joint (Charcot arthropathy) is a relatively painless, progressive, and degenerative arthropathy of single or multiple joints, caused by underlying neuropathy. The neuropa-

---

*Courtesy of Measurements, LLC, New Orleans, Louisiana. (See Figures 19-17A and 19-17B.)

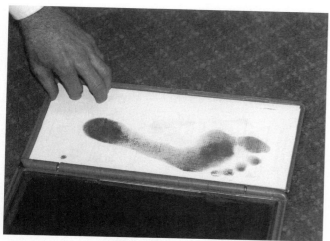

FIGURE 19-18 Harris mat pressure testing record. Darker areas represent higher pressure.

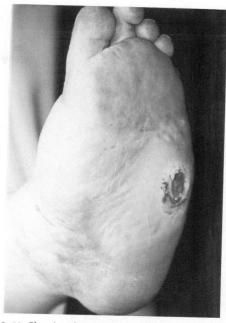

FIGURE 19-19 Classic Charcot rocker bottom foot deformity. Note ulceration over bony deformity surrounded by callus formation.

thy may be periosteal and not cutaneous. There are several theories behind the causes of Charcot joint, as follows:

- Multiple microtraumas to the joints cause microfractures. These fractures lead to relaxation of the ligaments and joint destruction.[73]
- There is increased blood flow (osteolysis) and bone reabsorption. Patients with Charcot joints have bounding pulses.
- Changes in the spinal cord lead to trophic changes in bones and joints.
- Osteoporosis is accompanied by an abnormal brittleness of the bones, leading to spontaneous fracture.[74]

In clinical observations, the limb is usually painless, swollen, and red. Unhealed painless fractures are often radiographically present. In advanced Charcot disease, there are multiple fractures, accompanied by extensive bone demineralization and reabsorption. Later stages reveal architectural distortion of the foot, with shortening and widening of the joint.[51] The foot joints most commonly affected are the following:

- tarsometatarsal (30%)
- metatarsophalangeal (30%)
- tarsus (24%)
- interphalangeal (4%)

Charcot joint is frequently misdiagnosed and mistreated, leaving the patient with deformities that require further medical intervention and/or expensive footwear (see Figure 19-19). The acute stage will show a foot that is 5–10° hotter than the contralateral limb in the same area. The red, hot, swollen foot will usually not have a skin opening or ulceration. Laboratory tests, including radiographs, may not show changes in the acute stage to differentiate Charcot disease from other diagnoses.

The duration of the catastrophic destruction, dissociation, and eventual recalcification found with Charcot joint will vary with the individual, but the average healing time in a cast for the hindfoot is 12 months; for the midfoot, 9 months; and for the forefoot, 6 months. By evaluating with comparative temperature measurements of the contralateral foot, the stages can usually be verified by radiograph. As the involved foot temperature increases, the destruction and dissociation are taking place. The temperature gradually decreases as recalcification is in progress. A radiograph shows that recalcification is complete when temperatures bilaterally are within 3° F.

The treatment plan for acute Charcot joint is the TCC. The cast must be changed in 1 week to accommodate volume changes. Following the period of volume changes, the cast should be changed every 2–3 weeks. When the temperature is equal to that of the other limb, the patient may be weaned gradually from the cast to a splint, then to shoes. Follow-up should continue to ensure that there is no recurrence of an episode of Charcot joint.

Osteomyelitis Examination

The clinical observations for Charcot joint and osteomyelitis are very similar, and the patient should be monitored closely to verify the diagnosis. Laboratory tests will also be similar. The only exception would be the presence of an opening in the skin to allow an entrance for bacteria to infect the bone (see Figure 19-20A). Take the temperature over the best surrounding skin. Refer for immediate medical management. The recalcification would not occur radiographically as in Charcot disease (Figure 19-20B.) Verification may be made for osteomyelitis with a three-phase bone scan or biopsy (Figure 19-20C).[21]

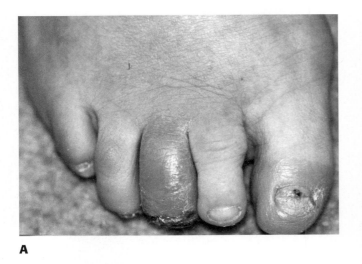

A

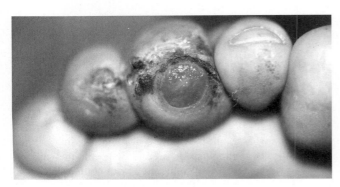

B

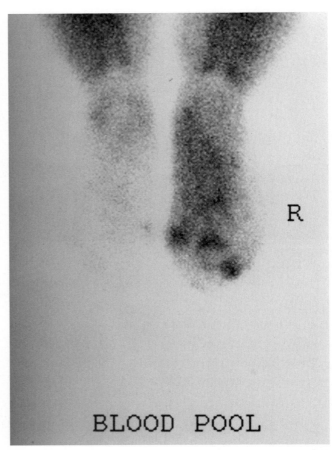

C

FIGURE 19-20 A. Red, hot, swollen toe: infection suspected. **B.** Distal tip of inflamed toe. **C.** Blood pooling of inflamed toe: infection confirmed. (Courtesy of Nancy Elftman.)

Diabetic patients with foot ulcers that expose bone should be treated for osteomyelitis, even if there is no evidence of inflammation.[75]

Interventions

Orthotics and Adaptive Equipment

Treatment of the neuropathic foot requires accommodation, relief of pressure/shear forces, and shock absorption. Regardless of materials used for accommodative inserts, the combination of materials must be compressible by one-half of original thickness to accommodate for pressure relief through the gait cycle.[22] It is important to evaluate the materials you will be utilizing in the manufacture of inserts. Cellular polyethylene foams, such as Aliplast, Plastazote, and Pelite, are composed of a mass of bubbles in a plastic and gas phase. The bubbles are cells with lines of intersection called *ribs* or *strands*, and the walls are called *windows*. In closed-cell materials the gases do not pass freely; open-cell material has no windows, leaving many cells interconnected so that gas may pass between cells. Cell walls are not totally impermeable to the flow of gases. Under a sustained load (especially the heavy patient), gases are squeezed out; when the load is removed, gases are drawn back into the cells.[76] These materials will bottom out from compaction of the materials as cells fracture under repetitive stress. The advantages are low-temperature molding, nontoxicity, water resistance, and washability without absorbency of fluid.[77] Plastazote has a limited effective period of about 2 days; Poron remains effective for 6–9 months. The two materials can be combined for their attributes and perform well as a single unit.[78,79] There are different types of inserts, as follows:

- Soft: cushioning/accommodation, improves shock absorption
- Semirigid: some cushion/accommodation; affords pressure relief
- Rigid: hard, single layer of plastic; it controls abnormal foot and leg motion[80]

The Aliplast/Plastazote insert is an immediate preparation and can be provided within a clinic setting, but it has a relatively short life of compressibility (6–8 months).

■ CASE STUDY

Charcot Arthropathy

The patient was a 44-year-old woman with a 15-year history of non-insulin-dependent diabetes mellitus (NIDDM). She had neuropathic extremities to mid-calf bilaterally, loss of sensation, and motor function demonstrated by bilateral foot drop. She had a right foot Charcot arthropathy 4 years ago. The extremity was treated with a series of total-contact casts for 11 months and gradually weaned to ankle-foot orthotics with shoes. The contralateral side used ankle-foot orthosis to control foot drop.

The patient came to the clinic for an emergency check-up due to a weekend traumatic injury to the left foot. She recalls twisting the left ankle and slight discomfort. Within an hour, there was swelling so she went to a local emergency department. The patient was told that she had possibly torn a ligament and was put in a precautionary plaster cast with a rubber walking pad.

When the patient came to the clinic 2 days later, she was in a great deal of discomfort and the plaster cast seemed to have absorbed exudate. The toes were left exposed in the cast and had swollen beyond the confines of the distal cast edge. When the cast was removed, it was observed that the walking pad had been forced through the plaster on the plantar surface and traumatized the entire plantar midfoot. The patient had Charcot arthropathy of the midfoot that was further destroyed by the nonreinforced walking pad. The edges of the plaster caused open abrasions to the exposed toes, leading to infection.

The patient was treated for abrasions and put into a total-contact cast. After 16 months, the Charcot episode was over but the foot was left with deformities that could not be accommodated in a standard shoe. A custom shoe was ordered for the left foot deformity.

KEY POINTS

1. Immediate total-contact casting could have reduced the deformities and length of treatment.
2. A total-contact cast differs from a standard short leg cast and should be applied by a skilled technician.

Plastazote is a closed-cell polyethylene foam that can be heated to 280° F and molded directly onto the patient's foot.[23] Care must be taken never to mold the toes or create ridges that the toes will ride over as the patient ambulates. By combining materials over a cast model of the foot, the composite type of insert can achieve all goals of the accommodative insert and provide a minimum life of 1 year.

An insert with a Plastazote surface in contact with the foot can be used as an excellent diagnostic tool for future follow-up. The self-molding properties of Plastazote reveal deep sock prints in areas of high pressure. These high-pressure areas should be noted and relieved in future insert designs for the patient. By using temperature as a tool for evaluation, the areas of high trauma will be noted as increased temperature locations. After the patient has worn accommodative inserts, the temperature differentiation will decrease if the proper accommodation has been achieved. If the temperature has not decreased in the area, the relief may require enhancement, or there may be other underlying complications to be investigated. All relief areas are applied on the underlying surface in contact with the shoe, never in contact with the foot. The surface in contact with the foot is always a solid, uninterrupted surface that will not apply edges for the foot to receive shear forces. Figure 19-21 shows the several different layers that make up an accommodative insert.

Shoes for the insensitive foot should be of soft leather that will conform to abnormalities on the dorsal surface and allow for the depth of an accommodative insert. Figure 19-22 shows modifications of the depth shoe appropriate for the insensitive foot.

Leather gradually adapts to the slope of the foot and will retain shape between wearings. The leather will breathe and absorb perspiration.[77] The patient should not depend on the "feel" of a shoe for correct size. The shoe must be full width and girth and allow 1/2 to 3/4 inches of space beyond the longest toe to prevent distal shoe contact

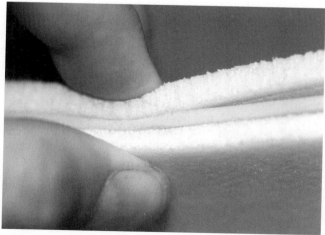

FIGURE 19-21 Accomodative inserts require multiple layers of varied durometer materials. Compression should reduce thickness by half. (Courtesy of Nancy Elftman.)

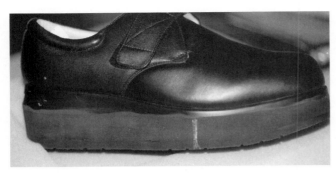

A

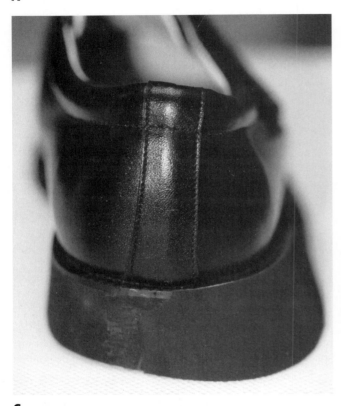

C

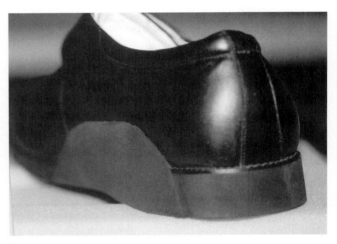

B

D

FIGURE 19-22 Common shoe modifications for the neuropathic foot. **A.** Rocker sole for limited great toe motion and forefoot complications. **B.** Heel wrap to widen heel contact surface and increase stability. **C.** Lateral flare for varus deformity. **D.** Bolster for midfoot medial support. (Courtesy of Nancy Elftman.)

through the gait cycle. Standard modifications of extra-depth shoes for the neuropathic patient include stretching of the soft toe box for clawed toes, flared lateral soles to discourage varus instability, and shank/rocker bottom for a partial foot, hallux rigidus, or decreased motion at the metatarsal heads. A rocker bottom should be added to the shoe when metatarsophalangeal extension is to be avoided.[23] When properly fit, the instep leather should not be taut. There are three tests to determine the proper fit of shoes (see Figure 19-23):

1. *Length:* Allow 1/2 to 3/4 inch of space in front of longest toe.

2. *Ball width:* With the patient weight bearing, grasp the vamp of the shoe and pinch the upper material; if leather cannot be pinched, it is too narrow. The ball should be in the widest part of the shoe.[81]

3. *Heel to ball length:* Measure the distance from the patient's heel to the first and fifth metatarsal heads. Bend the shoe to determine toe break, and repeat measurements on the shoe. They should be close to the same measurements.[82]

The simple addition of shoes instead of walking barefoot may correct many deformities.[83] Laced shoes will give the best control, but they must be broken in slowly, beginning

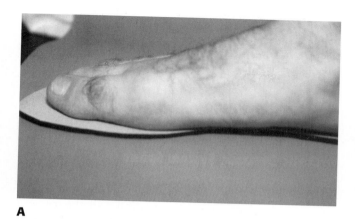
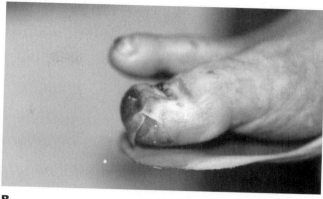

FIGURE 19-23 A. The neuropathic foot requires shoes that have a space of 1/2–3/4 inch of space beyond the longest toe. **B.** The wound on the distal end of the great toe due to a short shoe. (Courtesy of Nancy Elftman.)

with 2 hours per day and slowly adding time.[23] Caution should be taken with cutout sandals for the possibility of irritation along the borders of the sandal and straps.[84] To evaluate pressures within a shoe, there is a pressure-sensitive sock that is coated with dye-filled wax capsules. The capsules fracture when a certain pressure threshold is exceeded, leaving dye stains in areas of high pressure.[77] To protect a healing area in which dressings will be applied, a healing shoe lined with Plastazote will allow greater circumference and volume adjustability.

Socks for the neuropathic limb should have no mended areas or seams over bony prominences. A cotton/acrylic blend will assist in the wicking of perspiration away from the foot.[85] The sock should be fully cushioned and have a nonrestrictive top. The partial foot requires a sock that will conform to the shape without distal prominent seams or excess material at the distal end. For the active patient, socks can be obtained with silicone over high-stress areas to prevent shear for full or partial feet.

The partial foot may require a block within the shoe for the area of amputation. The purpose of a block is to reduce migration of the partial foot and medial/lateral shear for the toe amputation. No block or "prosthetic toe" is to be used for a central digit amputation. The low pressures applied by a block to central digits cause ischemic ulcerations on opposing surfaces. Medial or lateral amputations (first and fifth toes) may require a block to hold the foot in the correct position within the shoe. The forefoot block holds the shoe leather away from the distal end of the foot and discourages distal migration of the foot. All forms of blocks must have space from the amputation site and be an integral part of the insert, not added to an existing orthotic. Forefoot blocks require a rigid rocker sole to prevent ulceration to distal end.

By utilizing state-of-the-art foams and room temperature vulcanized (RTV) silicone elastomers, shear can be reduced in areas of skin grafts, chronic ulcerations, and calcanectomies within more rigid orthotics. The viscoelastomer gel is a two-part gel that can be adjusted for durometer desired.

The mixture can be used for shock absorption and shear reduction. Scar-adherent areas can benefit from a medium durometer mixture. The disadvantage is weight, so it should be used in small areas. Low-density foams can be designed into orthotics, such as toe breaks and forefoot blocks and reliefs. Reliefs for heel pain can be designed into the insert or shoe sole as a Sach heel. Sach heels use soft and medium durometer soling to simulate plantar flexion and provide shock absorption at heel strike.

Total-Contact Casting

The TCC method provides decreased plantar pressures by increasing weight bearing over the entire lower leg. It has been successful as a treatment for plantar ulcerations but requires careful application, close follow-up, and patient compliance with scheduled appointments to minimize complications.[86] Brand introduced the total-contact cast to the United States in the 1950s to redistribute walking pressures, prevent direct trauma to the wound, reduce edema, and provide immobilization to joints and soft tissue. The average healing time for ulcerations treated with the healing cast was 6 weeks.[84] This method has been used for patients with and without evidence of severe peripheral vascular disease.[87] The cast spreads weight evenly over the lower limb so that no part of the foot takes more than 5 psi. There is never a window cut in the cast or there may be localized swelling, shear stresses, and, eventually, a secondary wound (see Figure 19-24).[23]

Application methods of the total-contact healing cast vary by institution. The healing cast was originally designed with minimal padding, but padded variations are utilized. Although the steps for application of the Carville type TCC are given, remember that it is most important to have the cast applied by a skilled technician, because harm can occur from improper application. Following are steps for fabrication of the Carville-type TCC:

1. The ulcer is covered with a thin layer of gauze.
2. Cotton is placed between the toes to prevent maceration.

3. A stockinette is applied.
4. A 1/4-inch piece of felt is placed over the malleoli and anterior tibia.
5. Foam padding is placed around toes.
6. A total-contact plaster shell is molded.
7. The shell is reinforced with plaster splints.
8. A walking heel is attached.
9. A fiberglass roll is applied around the plaster.

The patient is instructed to ambulate only 33% of usual activity. The cast is removed in 5–7 days and reapplied. New casts are applied every 2–3 weeks.[86] To allow thorough drying, the patient should not stand or walk on the cast for 24 hours.[84]

While not as effective as total contact, a posterior splint covers the posterior lower leg and plantar foot surface, and is held in place with elastic wrap. The splint acts to protect the plantar surface. This casting procedure may be chosen for the patient with a limb compromised by poor circulation or when the patient cannot tolerate the confinement of a cast.[88]

There have also been attempts to heal ulcers by using a healing cast shoe molded of plaster. This healing cast shoe must be changed in 3 days, then reapplied every 10 days. Results have reported healing of plantar ulcers in 39 days.[89] Contraindications for the use of a healing cast shoe include infection (redness, swelling, warmth, fever) and hypotrophic skin (thin, shiny appearance, marked dependent edema).[84]

Orthotic Dynamic System Splint

The orthotic dynamic system (ODS) splint was developed to take advantage of the casting method of a TCC with the inclusion of a custom-molded insert that could be removed and reliefs modified. With all of the advantages of the TCC, the advantages that were added with the ODS splint included the possibilities for daily inspection, regular cleaning/dressings/debridement, and adjustments to areas of excessive pressure and/or friction (Figure 19-25).

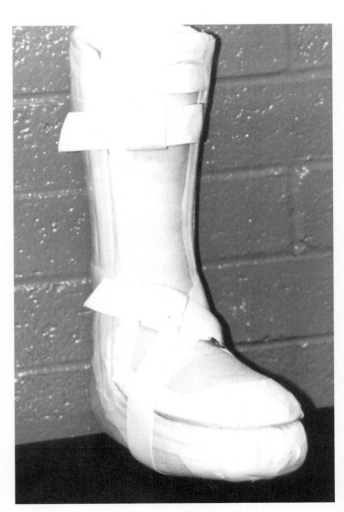

FIGURE 19-25 The ODS splint will be fit with a cast shoe for ambulation. (Courtesy of Nancy Elftman.)

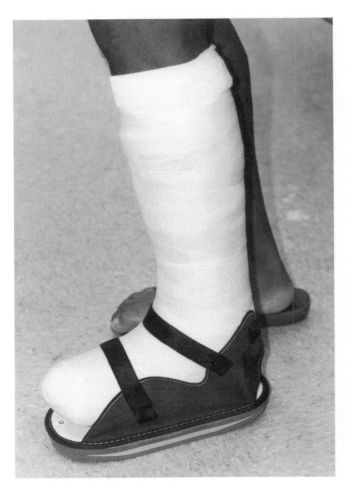

FIGURE 19-24 Total-contact cast.

Bathing While Wearing a TCC Is Simplified by Wearing a Seal Tight Cast and Bandage Protector

This heavyweight plastic vinyl bag slips over the cast and forms a seal that is watertight. The product is convenient to use, durable, and has a sueded sole to minimize slippage in the shower.

The Plastazote/Aliplast insert is first molded to the patient's foot and trimmed to follow the plantar surface, with 1/4-inch of length added beyond toes. A stockinette is placed on the leg, the insert is positioned, and another stockinette is applied to hold the insert in place. A padded TCC is applied, using Fiberglas only. The cast is bivalved; straps are added; edges are finished; and the insert is removed, relieved, and replaced to unweight the area of ulceration. After insert modification, it is replaced within the splint, and the patient may ambulate with a rocker-bottom cast shoe under the splint. The patient is instructed on volume control with sock thickness.

The disadvantage will lie with compliance of the patient. The splint design allows donning and doffing by the patient, therefore allowing him or her to remove the cast. The total contact of a healing cast cannot be compared in its superiority, but the clinical experience of the author has found the daily inspection and relief adjustability to be a great asset in the treatment protocol.

Neuropathic Walker

The neuropathic walker is a combination of an ankle-foot orthosis (AFO) and a boot that is custom-designed to be total contact for weight distribution (Figure 19-26). The ankle is locked to reduce force through the Lisfranc joint and/or ankle. The design is indicated for the patient with changes of Charcot joint in the tarsal and ankle joints, chronic recurrence of Charcot disease, and chronic ulcerations. The orthosis is easily donned and doffed, and is fabricated of a copolymer plastic with a closed-cell lining. The removable insert may be adjusted to reassign weight-bearing areas on the plantar surface. The insert may also be formed over chronic breakdown areas, such as the malleoli, posterior heel, and bunions, to reduce pressure. The rocker sole allows for easy ambulation, but the contralateral shoe must be adjusted for height.

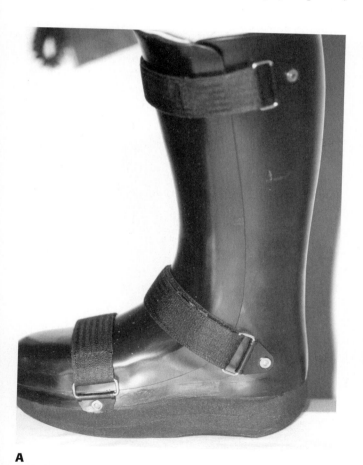

A

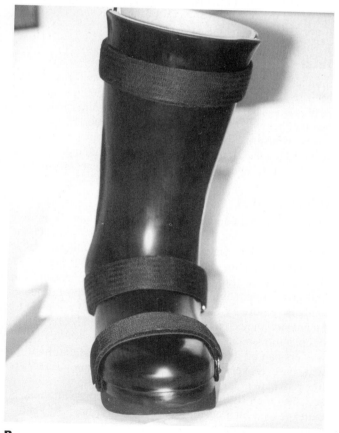

B

FIGURE 19-26 A. The custom neuropathic walker has a rocker sole and provides total contact for the high-risk foot. **B.** The orthosis fits the individual and supports deformity. (Courtesy of Nancy Elftman.)

When casting for the neuropathic walker, the patient's limb is wrapped and placed on a soft foam block until the plaster is set. The plantar surface will accommodate without excessive pressures on bony prominences. Modifications of the positive model include smoothing the plantar surface but never removing plaster. Any area that has had plaster removed during modification will be an area of excess pressure in the finished orthosis. The distal end is built up at the medial and lateral metatarsal areas and the length is extended 1/2 inch to allow room for the toes and to decrease the chances of maceration.

Fabrication is completed on the modified positive cast. The insert is first fabricated, finished, and placed in position. The posterior Plastazote lining is pulled over the insert, followed by the copolymer (plastic) vacuum-formed shell. The entire posterior section is finished and trimmed. The anterior Plastazote is positioned, and the copolymer shell is applied over the entire posterior. There should be a 1/2- to 1-inch overlap of copolymer on the finished orthosis. The Velcro straps and rocker bottom are attached (apex of rocker proximal to MTH).

The patient must be instructed to check skin for redness and possible breakdown. The patient should be followed and temperatures of the plantar surface recorded for possible adjustment of insert pressures. Sock management will be very important to continue a snug fit of the orthosis and volume control.

Total-Contact Ankle-Foot Orthosis

Similar to the neuropathic walker, the total-contact AFO is utilized for the patient who has an area of trauma in the mid- or hindfoot. The orthosis includes a custom, removable insert and is lined with Plastazote. This orthosis must be fit within a shoe, which may be difficult in standard shoes. The casting procedure is the same as that for the neuropathic walker. The toes are open, and the anterior shell terminates at midfoot.

Other Devices

Short leg walkers and orthopaedic walkers have been used by some clinics, but they compromise the total-contact feature. The walkers have become popular as alternatives to cast immobilization but the indications for their use are for foot and ankle fractures, sprains, acute ligament/muscle, and postsurgical immobilization. Although prefabricated walkers (Figure 19-27) are not custom-made to provide total contact, they contain some features that may assist in reducing movement of the limb within the walker.[90] The walkers can be improved in function with the addition of a wide base, rocker sole, and custom off-loading insert.[91] The low risk patient does well in the orthosis with a custom insert. The high risk patient with sensory neuropathy may be better served by a custom total contact orthosis.[92] Patellar tendon-bearing (axial resist) designs are intended to decrease forces on the plantar weight-bearing surface of the foot. With this design as a casting procedure, there have been attempts at its use in place of plaster cast immobi-

lizations.[93] The design transmitted considerable axial forces from the knee region onto the cast, but it did not offer rotary stability. The results offered very little effectiveness in reducing the load off the lower leg.[94] The patellar tendon-bearing design AFO has been used successfully for calcanectomy, plantar skin graft, and heel ulceration. This orthosis is contraindicated in the patient with vascular impairment because of the excess restriction in the popliteal area of arterial flow.

The prosthesis has been the orthotic replacement when the amputation case is complicated and the patient is not a candidate for prosthetic management. The prosthesis becomes a useful device for transfers and limb protection. This is always a creative design, with no two the same, unique to the individual and his or her needs.

The nonambulatory patient must be examined carefully for pressure ulceration due to positioning. Heel ulcers are particularly difficult to off-load in the recumbent position (Figure 19-28A). The prefabricated soft ankle foot orthosis (soft AFO) is constructed of a soft foam over a semirigid posterior/plantar support. The device allows decreased pressure at the posterior, medial/lateral, and plantar areas of the heel (Figure 19-28B). The soft outer construction decreases trauma to the contralateral leg.[90]

Off-Loading of Foot Ulcerations

In the treatment of foot ulcerations, there must be wound care protocol with debridement/cleansing and simultaneous

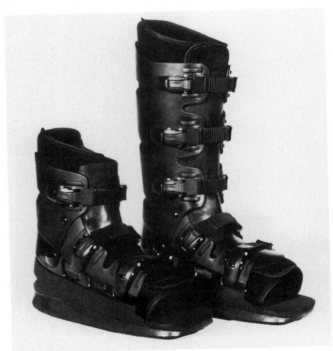

FIGURE 19-27 Prefabricated walker to assist in reducing motion at the ankle. (Courtesy of Darco International, Huntington, West Virginia.)

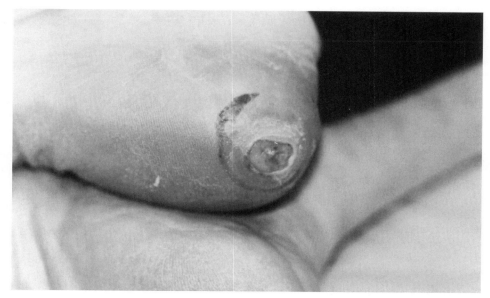

A

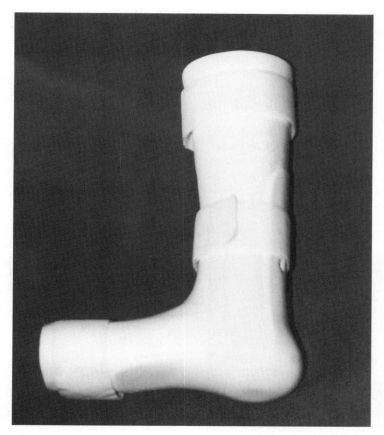

B

FIGURE 19-28 A. Common heel ulceration; **B.** Soft AFO for the recumbent patient to off-load heel ulceration and prevent trauma to contralateral limb. (Courtesy of Boston Brace International, Avon, Massachusetts.)

off-loading of the affected area. This combination has shown optimal results in the healing of wounds. There are prefabricated, as well as custom applications that the team must consider for each individual patient. Many patients are given crutches, walker, or wheelchair but they must have the upper body strength, cardiovascular reserves, and/or motivation to use assistive devices.[90] Bed rest eliminates the pressures on the foot but promotes deconditioning of the patient.[91]

Plastazote Healing Sandals

The custom Plastazote sandal contains a molded foot bed and has a rigid rocker sole (Figure 19-29). The device is lightweight but requires considerable time and experience to fabricate.[90] The Carville sandal has been used as a successful off-loading shoe and interim device following the TCC and before definitive shoewear.[95]

Prefabricated Off-Loading Alternatives

There are inexpensive alternatives for off-loading ulcerations with wound care protocol. For optimal healing, the wound must be off-loaded in conjunction with moist healing methods.[96] Over a third of the patients seen by home care practitioners have wounds. There is a low use of specialty dressings in home care, and the methods are usually clean instead of sterile.[97] Introduction of off-loading devices enhances the home care protocol. The following prefabricated products are improved in function by the addition of a customized, accommodative off-loading insert. The area of off-loading can be designed using the patient's floor reaction imprint (Harris mat) as a pattern. Follow-up appointments should include temperature measurements to ensure proper off-loading. If the temperatures have increased, the off-loading area must be increased; if the temperature differential is lower, there is an indication of decreased inflammation, and healing is occurring.[98]

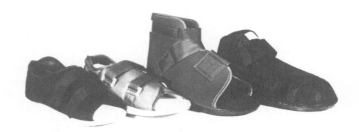

FIGURE 19-30 Post op/med surg/cast shoes: An inexpensive alternative to off-loading a wound on the plantar foot surface when plantar insert is supplied. (Courtesy of Darco International, Huntington, West Virginia.)

Post Op/Med Surg/Cast Shoe

An inexpensive alternative for wound off-loading would be the postoperative (rigid sole) and cast shoes (roller sole) to contain the ulcerated foot and off-loading insert (Figure 19-30). These shoes adjust for bandage volume but do not offer an intimate fit to control foot motion.[92] These shoes usually require extensions to Velcro straps and minor modifications. Use of the shoes as off-loading devices requires careful monitoring of the patient.

Wedged Shoe

The wedged shoe (Figure 19-31) has full contact with the plantar surface of the foot but reduces load forces applied from the ground. The sole angle is designed to shift weight bearing away from the ulcerated area. The wedge shoe is contraindicated when the patient does not have the range of motion to accompany the shoe angle. A patient with poor proprioception may not be able to ambulate without assistive devices.

Half Shoes

Many clinics use the half shoe (Figure 19-32) to suspend the ulcerated area, providing complete off-loading of the ulcerated area. The forefoot half shoe provides a pressure-free area for the forefoot, especially for the common ulcerations of the hallux. The heel relief shoe suspends the heel for non-

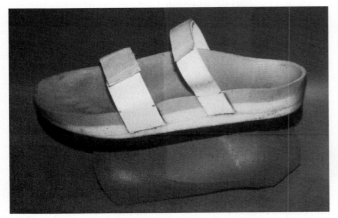

FIGURE 19-29 Plastazote Healing Sandal developed at Carville to provide a molded foot bed and rigid rocker sole. (Courtesy of the Department of Health and Human Services, Division of National Hansen's Disease Program.)

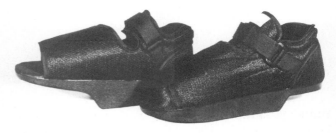

FIGURE 19-31 Wedged shoe reduces floor reaction forces to healing plantar surfaces. (Courtesy of Darco International, Huntington, West Virginia.)

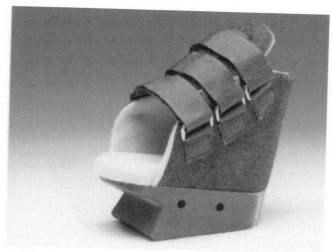

FIGURE 19-32 Half shoes suspend ulcerated area to eliminate external pressure. (Courtesy of Bauerfeind USA, Inc, Kennesaw, GA.)

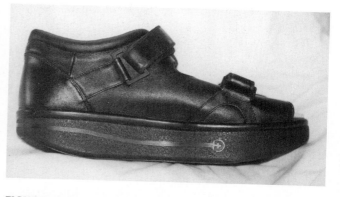

FIGURE 19-33 The wound healing system provides optimal environment for wound care protocol and simultaneous off-loading to encourage healing. (Courtesy of Darco International, Huntington, West Virginia.)

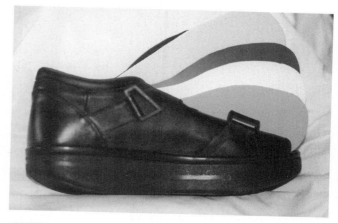

FIGURE 19-34 The wound shoe system allows off-loading of plantar, as well as dorsal wounds.

contact. These devices may be contraindicated for the patient with limited ankle motion or balance problems associated with proprioception. Assistive devices may be required to reduce incidence of falls.[90,91]

Wound Healing System

The wound healing system (Figure 19-33) was designed for the practitioner who does not have casting facilities or available support to off-load ulcerations by TCC or ODS splint. The wound care provider can supply off-loading properties in conjunction with the wound care protocol to deliver optimal healing of ulcerations in any environment. The basic wound shoe provides a base that allows relief of pressure for the dorsum, medial, lateral, and posterior ulceration. The plantar contact system (Figure 19-34) enables the practitioner to off-load plantar ulcerations with four layers (multiple durometer) of material (Figure 19-35A). The system is to be worn until the ulceration has healed. On final closure of the wound, a long-term material layer is added, and the wound shoe becomes the casual slipper to be worn at all times when definitive off-loading footwear is not being used (Figure 19-35B). A previous ulceration site is susceptible to breakdown repeatedly, and the wound shoe used as a casual slipper ensures that pressure relief is achieved at all times. The patient must never walk barefooted.

The floor reaction imprint (Harris mat, Figure 19-36) is helpful as a pattern for the off-loading position but is not necessary. The top layer to contact the foot is always a solid interface that will mold to the foot contours. There are two layers of higher durometer that will be relieved using available tools (scissors, scalpel, blade). The lower grades (Wagner 0 and 1) will utilize one off-load layer (Figure 19-35C), whereas the higher grades will have two off-loading layers available (Figure 19-35D). On wound closure, a shock-absorbing layer is to be added to prolong use of the system as a slipper (Figure 19-35E).

For the ulcerations that are not weight bearing (not plantar surface), the double-layer upper construction can be trimmed to off-load pressure areas without allowing window edema to occur (Figure 19-37A, B). The Velcro system is adjustable for bandage volume. The off-loading system allows for minimal dressings, which will usually add excess pressure areas when the patient is weight bearing. The goal of the wound healing system is to allow partial weight bearing while off-loading the high-risk foot with ulcerations. The combination of state-of-the-art wound care preparations and off-loading delivers optimal outcomes, as well as unlimited adjustments to forces applied.

Surgical Management

The most conservative treatment of foot infections will be utilized to rehabilitate, but antibiotic therapy alone is

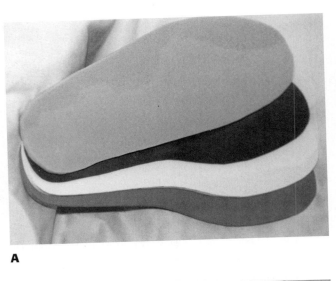

A

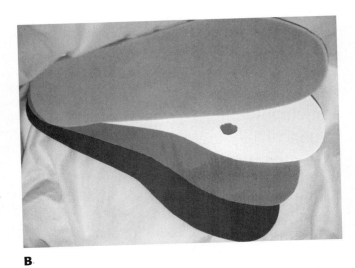

B.

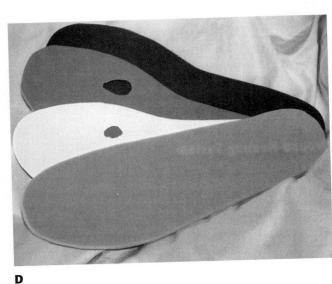

C

D

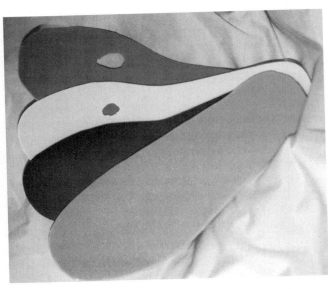

E

FIGURE 19-35 A. Plantar layers provide immediate in-clinic off-loading of wounds using four color-coded materials of varying durometers. **B.** Upon the healing of the ulceration, the material order is changed to utilize the shoe as an off-loading house shoe. **C.** Superficial wounds (Wagner grade 0 +1) use one off-loading modified layer. **D.** Wagner grade 2+ ulcerations will require two off-loading layers. **E.** Upon healing of the superficial layer, the order of the materials is changed to provide an off-loading shoe for home ambulation.

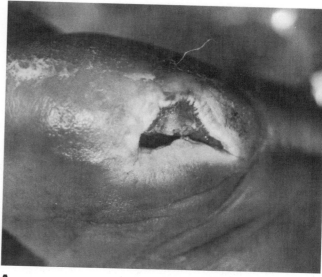

A

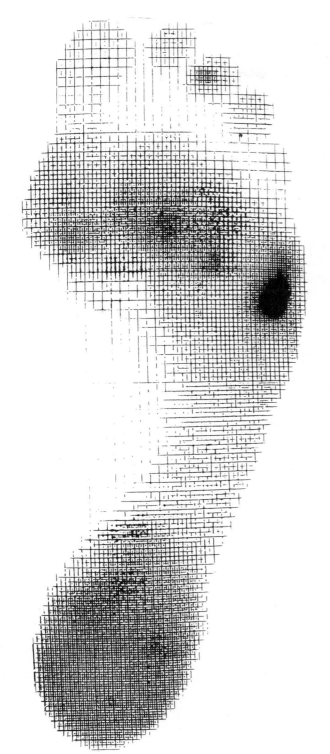

FIGURE 19-36 Floor reaction imprint (Harris mat) serves as pattern for plantar off-loading. (Courtesy of Theradynamics, Milwaukee, Wisconsin.)

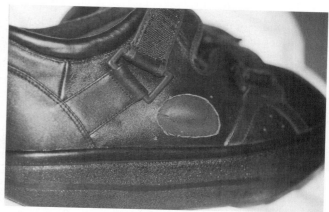

B

FIGURE 19-37 A. Lateral foot ulceration; not a weight-bearing surface; **B.** Upper construction allows relief of pressure for nonplantar ulcerations without window edema consequence.

not always sufficient to treat aggressive, virulent foot infections.[99] Surgical intervention may be in the best interest of the patient if conservative therapy is not an option or has proven ineffective. Options should be discussed with the patient and the family, and they should be involved in the final outcome, when possible. Surgical debridement of all osteomyelitis and nonviable tissue must be completed.[100] The surgeon will preserve as much length and width as possible to balance the motor function.[9] The goal of amputation is ambulation and reconstruction.

Metatarsal osteotomies can eliminate the intrinsic stresses caused by elongated or plantarflexed metatarsal joints in neuropathic limbs and decrease number of amputations.[101] Toe resections are the most distal amputation choices available. Expected outcomes of each toe resection are as follows:

- First toe—Interphalangeal disarticulation for an infected distal phalanx gives good balance. When possible, a wafer of the proximal phalanx should be left to maintain the position of the sesamoids beneath the first metatarsal head.
- Second toe—Disarticulation results in loss of lateral support of the first toe. A second ray resection is usually better to avoid secondary hallux valgus.
- Third or fourth toes—The remaining toes will tend to shift to close the gap.
- All five toes—A long forefoot lever is left with good weight-bearing properties.[9]

The advantages of the partial foot amputation are the following:

- It preserves end weight-bearing function.
- It preserves proprioception.
- It provides for limited disruption of body image.
- It requires shoe modification/orthosis or limited prosthesis.

Limitations of the partial foot amputation are the loss of normal foot function related to loss of forefoot lever length and associated muscles, and the challenges presented in selecting appropriate adaptive equipment.

The Chopart's amputation is selected when a patient retains sensation in the heel pad. Metatarsals and tarsals are removed, leaving a very short limb. It is difficult to suspend a shoe without the aid of an AFO or prosthesis.

The transmetatarsal/Lisfranc amputation is preferred for the resultant length of foot; amputation is through the metatarsals. The longest partial foot amputation is the distal metatarsal amputation, in which the toes are amputated. This level will require a short shoe or forefoot block to prevent forward motion.

In all partial feet, it is important to watch for an equinus deformity. The toes are no longer present, and visual inspection is more difficult without their reference.

Whether from trauma or chronic infection, the partial removal of the calcaneus is a follow-up challenge for the orthotist. Removing weight bearing from the heel is difficult, and the patient who has had a calcanectomy must be followed carefully.

The most successful methods of controlling future breakdown have involved the patellar tendon-bearing (axial resist) orthosis or the neuropathic walker. A soft RTV foam has been used to fill a void between the orthosis and the heel area. The same orthotic treatment is useful for chronic heel ulcers and plantar skin grafts that require reduction in weight-bearing and shear forces.

Documentation

Documentation continuity is essential for all patients and requires a standard form to be used for assessment and future follow-up (see Exhibit 19-4). Tracing the ulceration on transparent film will allow for accuracy of detailed healing progression. Providing the patient with a duplicate tracing can improve compliance because the patient can follow his or her own progress. Photographs of ulceration sites are important for noting improvement in depth and granulation of ulceration. Methods for making tracings and taking photos are described in Chapter 5.

Care of the Skin and Nails of the Neuropathic Foot

The Skin

Routine noninvasive skin and nail care is an important asset to any clinical team. The basic foot care can also be taught to the patient and family as promotion of foot health, along with daily examination for early detection of complications. This section includes the procedures, implements, and techniques for optimal results. The professional treatment of skin and nails is vital to the patient with neuropathy. The medical community has recognized the need for this skilled area of clinical expertise. Routine foot conditioning should not include any sharp debridement, which is addressed in other chapters.

Healthy skin is soft, flexible, moist, and acidic. It is the largest organ of the body, covering 3,000 square inches on the average adult. The skin weighs approximately 6 pounds (twice the weight of the brain and liver). The skin receives about one-third of all circulating blood of the body. Its two main parts, the epidermis and the corneum (the dermis), serve as a protective barrier against microorganisms. The skin insulates against heat and cold and helps to eliminate body wastes in the form of perspiration. Its sense receptors enable the body to feel pain, cold, heat, touch, and pressure. The epidermis is thickest on the palms and soles of the feet and becomes thinner over the surface of the trunk. It is important to promote conditions as close as possible to normal skin for neuropathic patients because they already have compromised utility of the skin's attributes. With routine care, the performance of the skin as protection of the body can be improved (see Chapter 4).[102]

The Nails

Nails are composed of hard keratin, a modification of the horny epidermal cells of the skin. The white crescent shape of the lunula at the proximal end of each nail is caused by air mixed in the keratin matrix. The nail plate originates from the proximal nail fold and attaches to the nail bed (Figure 19-38A, B). It grows about 1 mm per week unless inhibited by disease. Regeneration of a lost toenail occurs in 6–8 months.[102]

Noninvasive Skin and Nail Care

Before beginning skin and nail care, thoroughly inspect feet and ankles for breaks in the skin. Look for ulcers, heel fissures, maceration between the toes, or imbedded objects. When nails are neglected and overgrown, they can break the skin of the neighboring toe. Abnormal nails that are not given routine care can accumulate excess keratin and debris under

Facts about Nails

- Nails grow approximately 0.1 mm per day, or 3 mm per month.
- Nails grow faster in daytime and summer.
- Fever and serious illness slow growth rates.
- Pregnancy enhances growth.
- Nails grow more rapidly in men and young people than in women and the elderly.
- Toenails grow one-half to one-third the rate of fingernails.[103]

the nails and in the nail folds, creating an ideal environment for bacteria to grow.[104] Poor hygiene necessitates routine foot care. The poorly managed foot will require professional treatment twice a month until the skin and nails are conditioned; routine care can be managed monthly. All tools should be cleaned and sterilized, or disposed of, to reduce cross-contamination. The procedure for basic skin and nail care for neuropathic feet (Figure 19-39A through H) is as follows:

1. Wash hands and prepare sterilized tools. (Figure 19-39A1–A5)

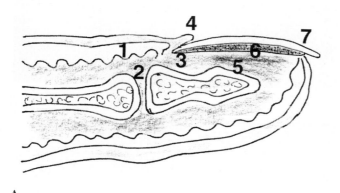

A

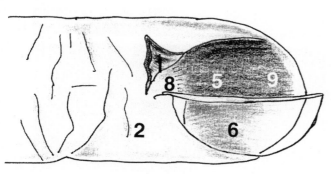

B

FIGURE 19-38 Anatomy of the nail. **A.** Cross-section. **B.** Nail diagram. 1. nail matrix, 2. nail root, 3. nail fold, 4. eponychium, 5. nail bed, 6. nail body, 7. free edge, 8. lunula, 9. hyponychium.

2. Submerge feet into warm water (not to exceed 95° F, use thermometer). You can also use water that is three parts water to one part vinegar in cleaning the feet. Vinegar softens the skin and nails.[105]
3. While wearing gloves, make a paste of baby shampoo (or any mild soap) and baking soda in the palm of your hand and gently massage over the entire foot.
4. Rinse and wrap feet individually in towels.
5. Expose toes and apply Blue Cross cuticle remover.
6. Using the curette, gently remove dead skin and loose cuticle from the toes (Figure 19-39B).
7. Rinse.
8. Using the nail clippers, cut the nail straight across. Don't cut what you can't see. Always have good lighting (Figure 19-39C).
9. Thinner, more fragile nails can be cut using the smaller cuticle nippers (Figure 19-39D).
10. Ingrown toenails are a puncture wound. To prevent them, use the ingrown nail file to smooth sharp corners that can dig into the skin (Figure 19-39E).
11. Smooth rough edges of nails with an emery board. The patient may take the emery board home for self-care (Figure 19-39F).
12. Massage emollient into feet but not between toes. Avoid lotions with fragrance, because they contain alcohol that will dry the skin. Vaseline, lanolin, or even Crisco may be used as a moisture barrier to contain the moisture within the skin. Remind the patient to use caution when using emollient to prevent slipping and falling. Removing excess and covering with socks will help to minimize the hazard.
13. Educate the patient regarding appropriate footwear.

There are nails that are difficult to trim. The safest way to trim the pincer nail is to file it straight across, rather than to risk cutting the skin (Figure 19-39G). Some nails have grown into a "tent" shape. This tenting is usually caused by years of wearing pointed shoes. When trimming this type of nail, be aware of the skin under the nail at the dorsal apex. A condition called *onycholysis*, separation of the nail plate from the nail bed, can be caused by nail traumas and disorders. If onycholysis has been present for an extended period (6 months or more), the structure of the nail bed can change, and the nail plate will no longer attach to the nail bed. At this point, the condition becomes permanent. Keep the patient's nails short to prevent them from catching on surroundings and tearing off.[106] Some patients will have nails that are atrophied, due to their illness. Figure 19-39H reveals an atrophied nail with a hematoma.

Heel Fissures

Patients with autonomic neuropathy can have very dry, nonelastic skin, due to the lack of sweat and oil production. Deep heel fissures develop from the dry skin and may compromise the integrity of the skin. When the fissures occur, there is an opportunity for bacteria and debris to invade the skin, causing ulcerations and infection (Figure 19-40A).

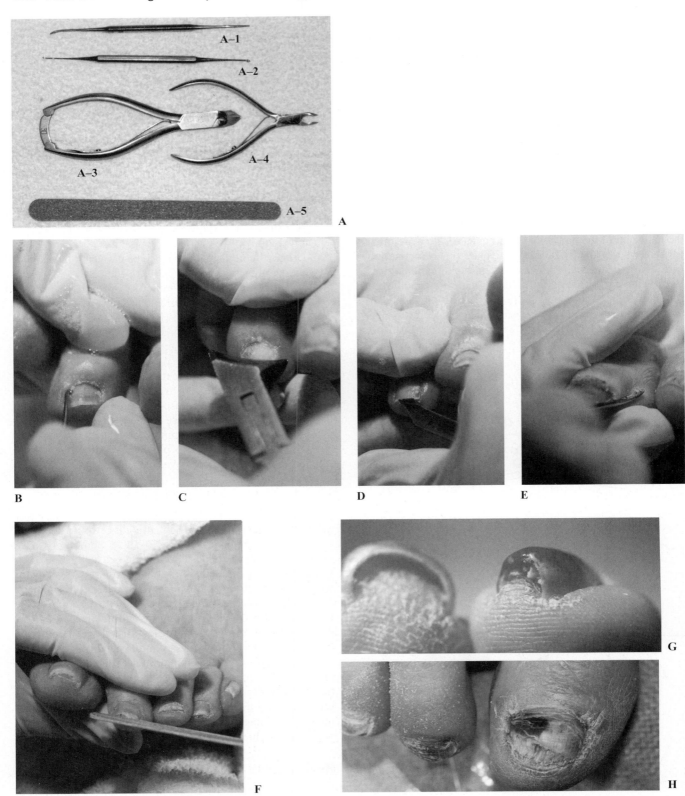

FIGURE 19-39 A. Tools for nail care: 1. ingrown nail file, 2. curette, 3. clippers, 4. cuticle nippers, 5. emery board. **B.** Use curette to loosen and remove debris. **C.** Clippers to cut nails. **D.** Cuticle nipper for fragile nails and small spaces. **E.** Ingrown nail file to round sharp corners. **F.** Emery board to smooth edges. **G.** Pincer nail. **H.** Nail with hematoma.

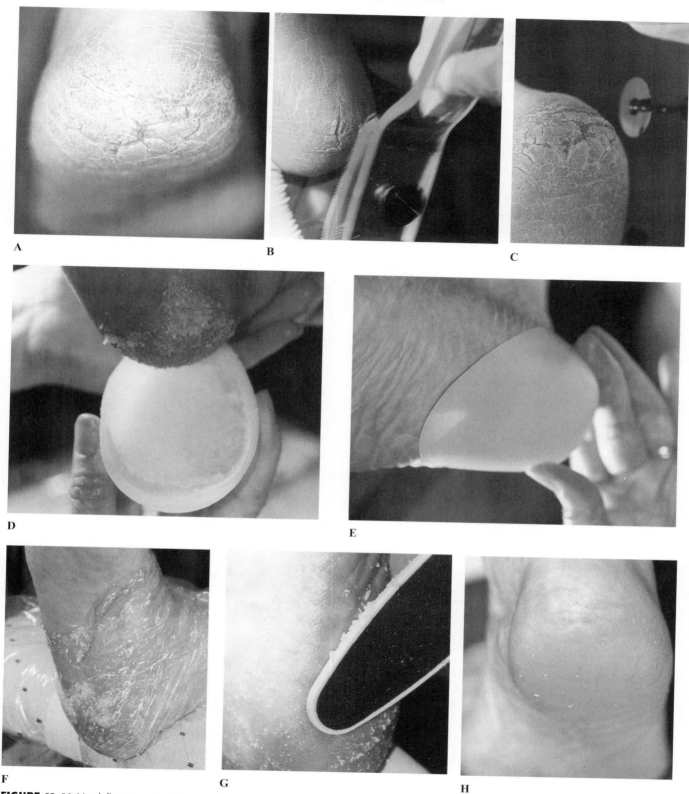

FIGURE 19-40 Heel fissures: **A.** Dry, cracking hyperkeratotic heel. **B.** Callus reducer; used dry on dry skin. **C.** Dremel tool to reduce callus. **D.** Heel cup to concentrate basic callus paste. **E.** Heel cup on foot. **F.** Plastic wrap to apply and contain basic callus paste on large areas. **G.** Foot file to exfoliate heel callus. **H.** Heel fissures after first treatment.

Care of heel fissures begins with the basic callus care procedure. Use a dry callus reducer on dry skin with one-directional strokes. When skills for using the Dremel (Moore Medical, New Britain, CT) are developed, the tool can be used in the same fashion for very thick hyperkeratotic skin. Do not attempt to finish a difficult case in one session; several appointments will be required to reduce the buildup.

Heel Fissure Care

1. Wash hands and don gloves.
2. Use the callus reducer (Figure 19-40B) or Dremel tool (Figure 19-40C) to decrease the hyperkeratotic thickness.
3. Wrap the foot in a warm, moist towel for 5 minutes.
4. Remove towel, apply Vick's VapoRub to heel, followed by Back to Basics Callus Paste (Figure 19-40D, Exhibit 19-5). The paste can be held in place with a plastic heel cup or plastic wrap, followed by a towel wrap, for 10 minutes (Figures 19-40E, F).
5. Unwrap foot and remove paste from the heel with a wet foot file (Figure 19-40G).
6. Rinse the foot and apply a moisture barrier emollient (Figure 19-40H).
7. Wipe excess emollient off and don socks and shoes.

Once the patient's feet are conditioned, routine foot care can be maintained with 4- to 6-week follow-up appointments.

Hypertrophic Nail (Onychauxis) Care

The hypertrophic nail may be caused by damage to the matrix, fungal infection, age and/or vascular complications. Hypertrophic nails that have been neglected need to be thinned to make shoe fit possible and to prevent secondary infections due to traumatization of the prominent nail.

The most effective and expedient method for thinning the nail is to use the cordless rotary Dremel tool with a disposable abrasive disc. These discs (emery medium 1/8 inch) are easily interchangeable and are discarded after each patient. It is important for the practitioner and the patient to don masks, and coverings for eyes and hair to protect from airborne dust. Use of a HEPA air filter device would give added protection.

Procedure for reducing hypertrophic nails:

1. Wash hands, don gloves, have practitioner and patient don masks and coverings for hair and eyes.
2. Examine the skin around the nail for damage (Figure 19-41A).

EXHIBIT 19-5   Back to Basics Paste

1 cup kosher salt
1/2 cup Epsom salts
8 tbsp baking soda
8 tbsp mineral oil[107]

3. If there are no signs of broken skin or infection, secure toe with thumb and index fingers and move other toes away from the working area.
4. Turn Dremel on and move sanding disc in a proximal to distal direction, with slow, even strokes until nail is thinned (Figure 19-41B). Caution must be exercised when thinning the nail, due to unanticipated raised nail beds (Figure 19-41C).
5. Wash and dry the thinned nail and apply a conditioning agent, i.e., Tineacide. Use of this or comparable product will allow future nail care to be more effective by keeping the nail and surrounding skin conditioned (Figure 19-41D).

■ CASE STUDY

The neuropathic patient may neglect foot care. Figure 19-42A–D is a pictorial case study of a neuropathic patient who neglected regular foot and nail care. In spite of the overgrown, hypertrophic nails and callus formation, he continued to don his shocks and shoes. Once foot and nail care were initiated, the skin and nails improved in appearance and there was reduced risk of injury to adjacent skin.

Callus (Hyperkeratosis) Care

A callus is located in an area of high pressures and shear forces. It is the body's protective mechanism for an area of chronic irritation. To the neuropathic patient, the callus is indicative of chronic trauma (repetitive stress injury) that may lead to skin breakdown and serious complications.[108] Lack of sensation prevents the neuropathic patient from reacting to high pressures that can produce an ulceration. Reduction of callus is required on an ongoing basis to prevent the callus and eventual ulceration. The majority of plantar ulcerations in neuropathic patients are located in the forefoot, especially at the great toe and first, second, and fifth metatarsal heads.[104]

CLINICAL WISDOM

Callus Care

Avoid corn medications that can produce chemical burns; they contain salicylic acid. Vick's VapoRub will act quickly to soften the hardened skin. Vaseline is the daily treatment to provide a moisture barrier after bathing.

Procedure of callus reduction:

1. Wash hands.
2. Don gloves and hold foot securely with one hand. In the other hand, use the dry callus reducer in one direction over the dry callused area. When the screen fills with debris, tap on a hard surface, clear the screen, and continue the process. After the callus is reduced, give the screen to the patient with instructions on home use.
3. When the callus is reduced, ulceration may be revealed under the callus. Reduce the callus but do not open the

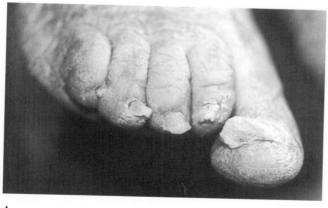

A

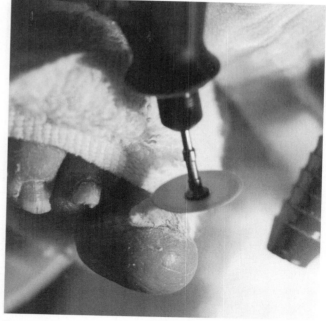

B

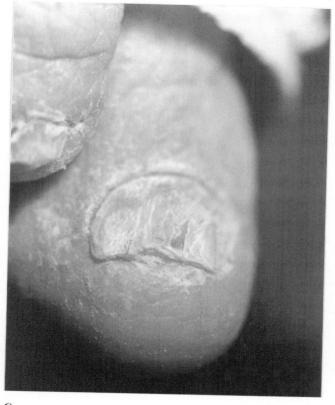

C

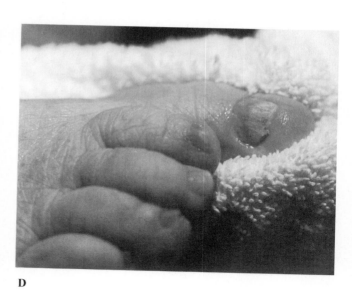

D

FIGURE 19-41 Reducing hypertrophic nails: **A.** Hypertrophic nails. **B.** Dremel tool to reduce nail thickness. **C.** Reduced nail with raised nail bed. **D.** Completed nail procedure after conditioning.

skin. An off-loading insole will be necessary to reduce the pressure and shear to the area (Figure 19-43).

4. Once the callus is reduced, wrap the foot in a warm, moist towel for 5 minutes.

5. Remove the towel and apply Vick's VapoRub, followed with Back to Basics Paste (see Exhibit 19-5). Cover with plastic wrap and towel for 10 minutes.

6. Gently remove paste with foot file, rinse, and pat dry.

7. The patient may need to be seen weekly to reduce the callus in stages.

8. Assess footwear to determine what is causing callus formation. Therapeutic depth shoes with accommodative inserts should be worn by all patients with neuropathic feet (unable to feel the 5.07 monofilament).[104]

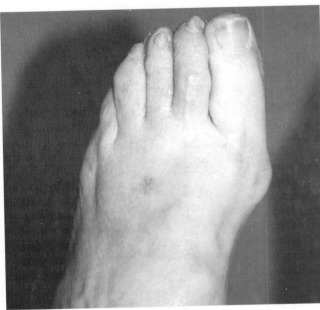

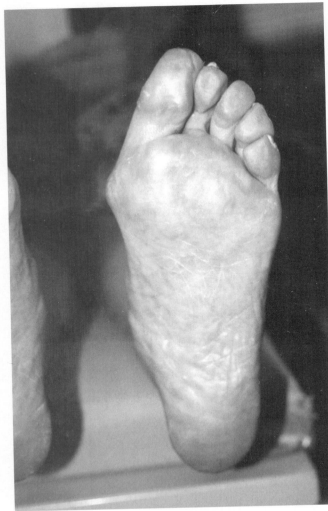

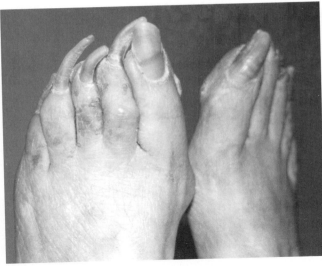

A

B

C

D

FIGURE 19-42 The neuropathic patient may neglect foot care. **A, B.** Patient continues to don shoes over excessive nail growth. **C, D.** Condition of feet after an extensive foot care procedure.

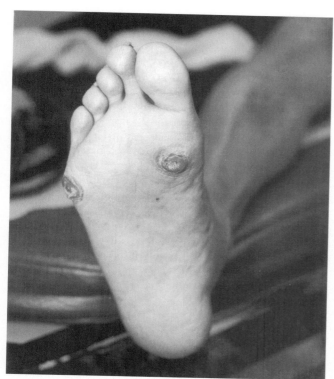

FIGURE 19-43 Foot requiring callus reduction and redistribution of weight-bearing forces at first and fifth metatarsal head.

CLINICAL WISDOM

Bathroom Surgery

Remind patients to never perform "bathroom surgery." Self-inflicted wounds due to razor blades and other sharp objects are common with patients who lack protective sensation.

Using a cordless Dremel rotary tool to reduce callus:

1. When learning to use the Dremel, begin with the less powerful Mini-Mite cordless model until skills are developed. Practicing on hoof trimmings purchased from a pet supply company will give similar experience to working on callus and hypertrophic nails. When proficient, the more powerful Multi-Pro model can be used.
2. When using a Dremel, thin the callus thickness by sanding in one direction (proximal to distal). Do not work in an area for a long period because the prolonged friction can cause overheating at the skin surface.
3. Continue with steps 2 through 7 in the procedure for callus reduction above.

Conclusion

As the post-World War II generation ages, the medical community will be faced with the increasing demand for basic, noninvasive foot care with minimal risk of transmitted infections and skin conditions. Attention to foot care has become a recognized requirement for aging and, especially, neuropathic patients. Health-care professionals are seeking information and specialized training relating to foot care in the clinical setting. Their efforts are being rewarded with fewer amputations, and patients are being educated in self-care. Self-care has allowed early detection and medical attention to conditions that would otherwise result in catastrophic events. Routine foot care is an integral part of comprehensive care for the neuropathic patient, and its presence will greatly improve the quality of life to those in the greatest need. See Chapter 20 for more information about foot and nail care in the nondiabetic foot.

Self-Care Teaching Guidelines

Foot Inspection

The patient is the most important member of a clinical team approach to the treatment of a neuropathic limb. There is no complication too small to be addressed, and the patient must bring abnormalities to the team's attention. Self-care begins with daily inspections of the feet, with the help of mirrors, magnifying glasses, and family members, when necessary. Examination includes footwear and orthotics for wear and foreign objects. The diabetic patient must understand that this examination may be complicated by other disease processes, including retinopathy, autonomic neuropathy (loss of smell and sensory signals), and decreased mobility of joints. These patients are handicapped by the lack of pain as a warning signal and require systematic instruction to educate them in the proper skills required for daily inspection and detection of impending trauma.

Precautions and Risk Reduction Methods

There are several precautions for the patient with a neuropathic limb. The skin is very susceptible to damage and infection, and it must be treated carefully. It is advised that the patient not soak the feet in water because the chance of burns is always present, and the soaking will leave the skin moist and susceptible to fungal infection. Prolonged soaking can remove the natural protective barrier from the skin and lead to other infections. Feet should be washed with a nondrying soap and towel dried. After the foot wash, petroleum jelly can be applied to retain natural moisture and the feet covered with socks. Care should be taken not to use creams with perfumes (alcohol) because they will further dehydrate the skin.

Dehydrated skin is especially susceptible to trauma. Adhesives of any form should never be applied directly to the skin of a neuropathic limb. On removal of the adhesive, there is a risk of loss of the outer layer of skin, leaving an area open to infection. The adhesives could be in the form of tape, a Band-Aid, or over-the-counter self-adhesive pads.

When the patient selects footwear, he or she should choose not only the correct size and width, but also shoes with no stitching over the forefoot. The stitched areas will never mold to the foot; instead, they will cause breakdown of the skin, especially over bony areas.

Socks for the neuropathic foot should be seamless and without holes or repairs (Figure 19-44). Tube socks do not contour to the foot without folds that can cause irritation. The socks should be a blend to wick perspiration and should be nonconstricting at the calf. The use of white or light colors will enable the patient to detect drainage due to trauma easily. With a new shoe, the break-in period should be completed with two thin socks on each foot. The double socks will allow shear to occur between them and will decrease the probability of blistering from new leather.

The partial foot sock is designed of highly elastic fibers. The sock shape will conform to partial foot length and shape. The single size fits a Chopart's amputation, as well as a long transmetatarsal amputation. There are no folds or seams to cause friction.

Toe socks decrease maceration between toes. The moist environment between the toes encourages fungal growth and may lead to ulceration and bacterial infection. The seamless construction helps to reduce overlapping of lesser toes but must be compensated for in shoe size if they are to be worn with shoes.

Keep current on recalled products. For example, one hair removal system published a product alert on its device because of problems occurring with diabetic patients. Small

areas were bleeding after hair was removed, leaving an entrance for bacteria and possible infection! Over 50% of the over-the-counter foot care products should never be used by a patient with a neuropathic limb or diabetes. There are occasionally warnings, but they are in very fine print.

Care must be taken with exercise programs. When we walk, each step carries one and one-half times our body weight; jogging increases the force to three times the body weight.[109] The patient with a neuropathic limb would be advised to choose an exercise program that includes aerobics, swimming, cycling, dance, or chair exercises. Even walking should include slow, short steps only—no jogging.[110]

The patient with a neuropathic limb should never walk barefoot. Even in the pool or on the beach, water shoes should be worn. Hot sand can cause burns, and undetected objects in the sand can cause injury. Burns can be caused by the floorboard of an automobile, as well as by any warmth-producing equipment. The interior of the shoe must be examined before every donning. Small objects can easily drop into a shoe.

Compliance Issues

The practitioner must understand compliance problems of patients with neuropathic limbs, especially diabetic patients. They do not willfully neglect self-care activities but simply are not aware of the possible dangers and are not taught adequately or motivated sufficiently.[2] Diabetic patients may have other complications that the practitioner does not consider in the compliance of their activities. Many cannot see (retinopathy), feel (sensory neuropathy), or smell (autonomic neuropathy) that there is an infection or a potential problem. Those with vision impairments will need help from a family member or caregiver to perform self-care guidelines.

Patients with neuropathic and dysvascular limbs require knowledge and skills to administer self-examination and self-care. The medical community must educate the patients, as well as the medical team, to treat conservatively and accommodate the chronic complications that exist in a growing portion of the population. Exhibit 19-6 is a checklist of instructional items with documentation to verify learning and understanding for the patient with neuropathic foot.

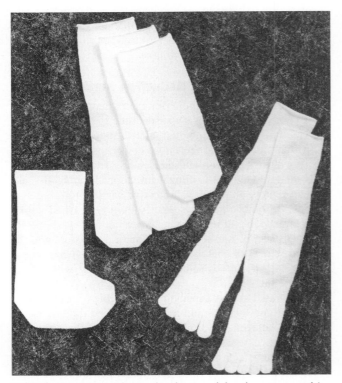

FIGURE 19-44 Specialty socks designed for the neuropathic, partial, and macerated foot. (Courtesy of Knit Rite, Inc., Kansas City, Kansas.)

REVIEW

1. Loss of sensation in the upper and lower extremity that is equidistant from the spine is classified as peripheral neuropathy.
2. A rigid hallux deformity requires a rigid rocker sole on the shoes.
3. An increase in local surface temperatures indicates that an area has healed and the patient may resume previous activity level.
4. The acute Charcot foot is cool and blue, and pulses are absent.

Exhibit 19-6   Self-Care Guidelines for the Patient with Neuropathic Foot

Self-Care Guidelines for Patient with Neuropathic Foot	Instructions Given (Date/Initials)	Demonstration or Review of Material (Date/Initials)	Return Demonstration *or* States Understanding (Date/Initials)
1. Foot Inspection Methods a. Use mirror to check feet b. Use magnifying glass to check feet c. If blind, family member performs foot inspection			
2. Foot Inspection Item a. Toe nails: check for broken, cracked, or sharp nails b. Broken skin: check between toes, along sides of feet, tops and ends of toes, sole of foot c. Soft toe corns: check between toes d. Callus: check for cracks e. Drainage: check for any drainage from a sore f. Odor: check for odor from any source on the foot			
3. Patient Understands a. Significance of findings of foot inspection: break in nails, skin, or callus b. When to notify health-care provider if there is break in nails, skin, or callus c. To notify health-care provider immediately if there is any injury to the feet			
4. Foot Care Routine a. Wash feet with nondrying soap and towel dry b. Apply coating of petroleum jelly to all skin surfaces of feet c. Cover coated feet with clean white socks			
5. Foot Care Precautions a. Never walk barefoot b. Never use adhesive tape products on the skin c. Never put feet in hot water or apply a heating pad or hot pack d. Never soak feet e. Never apply over-the-counter foot care products to remove corns or callus, or to treat nails			
6. Shoe Wear Orthotic Inspection a. Choose shoes that are correct size and width b. Make sure there is no stitching over the forefoot of shoe c. Check for wear: heels, soles, tops, inside, bottom, edges, counter d. Always check shoes, socks, and orthotics for foreign objects; remove objects before donning			
7. Exercise Precautions a. Never jog b. Walk with short, slow steps			
8. Preferred Exercises a. Aerobic: low impact b. Swimming (wear soft bathing shoes in water to protect feet, dry feet thoroughly following) c. Cycling: protect feet and ankles from trauma d. Dancing e. Chair and mat exercises			
9. Importance of Follow-Up with Health-Care Provider			

RESOURCES

Acor Orthopedic
18530 South Miles Pkwy
Cleveland, OH 44128
(800) 237-2267 fax (216) 662-4547
Materials/fabrication tools
Prefab orthoses
Custom and diabetic shoes

Alimed, Inc.
297 High Street
Dedham, MA 02026
(800) 225-2610 fax (800) 437-2966
Materials/wound supplies
Wheel chairs/positioning
Specialty diabetic products

Apex Foot Health
170 Wesley St.
South Hackensack, NJ 07606
(800) 526-2739 fax (800) 526-0073
Materials/tools
Prefab orthoses
Modifiable footwear

Boston Brace International
20 Ledin Dr.
Avon, MA 02322
(800) 262-2235 fax (800) 634-5048
Soft ankle foot orthosis (AFO)

Brown Medical Industries
481 South 8th Ave. East
Hartley, IA 51346
(800) 843-4395 fax (712) 336-2874
Cast and bandage protector

Comfort Products, Inc.
705 Linton Ave.
Croydon, PA 19021
(800) 822-7500 fax (215) 785-5737
Diabetic socks

Darco International, Inc.
810 Memorial Blvd.
Huntington, WV 25701
(800) 999-8866 fax (304) 522-0037
Wound healing shoe system
P/O med/surg shoe/cast boot
Neuropathic shoes/walker

Deltatrak, Inc.
5653 Stoneridge Dr.
Pleasanton, CA 94588
(800) 962-6776 fax (925) 467-5949
Infrared thermometer

Hands on Foot, Inc.
2076 Bonita Ave.
La Verne, CA 91750
(909) 596-7674 fax (909) 596-5211

Neuropathic limb courses
Wound off-load courses
Callous reducers

Ipos, North America, Inc.
2045 Niagara Falls Blvd. #8
Niagara Falls, NY 14304
(800) 626-2612 fax (716) 297-0153
Heel and forefoot relief shoes

Juzo-Julius Zorn, Inc.
P.O. Box 1088
Cuyahoga Falls, OH 44223
(800) 222-4999 fax (800) 645-2519
Neuropathic/compression stockings
Sleeves/gloves/gauntlets
Prosthetic shrinker/suspension

Knit-Rite, Inc.
120 Osage Ave.
Kansas City, KA 66105
(800) 821-3094 fax (800) 462-4707
Diabetic/partial foot socks
Prosthetic socks/shrinkers
Prosthetic suspension

Measurements, Inc.
2946 Ponce de Leon
New Orleans, LA 70119
(504) 949-1192 fax (504) 943-3489
Infrared thermometer

Moore Medical, Inc.
389 John Downey Dr.
New Britain, CT 06050
(800) 234-1464 fax (800) 944-6667
Wound care supplies/material
Tools/tube foam/crest pad support
Medical supplies

North Coast Medical, Inc.
187 Stouffer Blvd.
San Jose, CA 95125–1042
(800) 821-9319 fax (408) 277-6824
Monofilaments

Theradynamics
7283 W. Appleton Ave.
(800) 803-7813 fax (414) 438-1051
Milwaukee, WI 53216
Floor reaction imprint (Harris)
Material/fabrication equipment
Prefabricated orthoses

UCO International, Inc.
16 E. Piper Ln. # 130
Prospect Heights, IL 60070
(800) 541-4030 fax (847) 541-4144
Material/specialty pads (MTH)
Tools and equipment
Prefabricated orthoses

Care of the Skin and Nail of the Neuropathic Foot Resources

Antoine de Paris
P.O. Box 1310
Solvang, CA 93464
(805) 688-0666 fax (805) 686-00330
(800) 222–3243
Pedicure tools
Nail clipper #30
Cuticle nipper #14
Ingrown nail file #86

Hands on Foot, Inc.
P.O. Box 7674
2076 Bonita Ave.
La Verne, CA 91750
(909) 596-7674 fax (909) 596-5211
Callus reducers
Socks
Shoes (Gentle Step)

Moore Medical Products
389 John Downey Dr.
P.O. Box 2740
New Britain, CT 06060–2740
(800) 234-1464 http://www.mooremedical.com
Tube foam
Lamb's wool
Curette
Dremel tool

Sally's Beauty Supply (nationwide franchise)
Blue Cross cuticle remover
Foot files
Emery boards

Sussman, C. *Diabetic Foot Care and Ulcer Prevention, Wound Care Patient Education and Resource Manual*, Gaithersburg, MD: Aspen Publishers; 1999.

Tineacide
(800) 307-8818

REFERENCES

1. Brenner M. *Management of the Diabetic Foot*. Baltimore: Williams & Wilkins, 1987.
2. Shipley D. Clinical evaluation and care of the insensitive foot. *Phys Ther* 1979;59:13–22.
3. Veves A, Boulton A. Commentary. *Diabetes Spectrum* 1992;5:336–337.
4. Bowker J. Commentary. *Diabetes Spectrum* 1992;5:335.
5. Brenner M. Management of the diabetic foot. *Podiatr Products* May 1988;54–58.
6. Ellenberg M. Diabetic neuropathic ulcer. *J Mt Sinai Hosp* 1968;35:585–594.
7. Green D, Waldhausl W. A forum on neuropathy. *Diabetes* 1988;10.
8. Bowker J. Neurological aspects of prosthetic/orthotic practice. *J Prosthet Orthot* 1993;5(2):52–54.
9. Bowker J. Partial foot and Syme amputations: An overview. *Clin Prosthet Orthot* 1987;12:10–13.
10. Letts M. The orthotics of myelomeningocele. In: *Atlas of Orthotics*. St. Louis, MO: CV Mosby, 1985, pp. 300–306.
11. Weingarten M. Commentary. *Diabetes Spectrum* 1992;5:342–343.
12. Pecoraro R, Reiber G, Burgess E. Pathways to diabetic limb amputation: Basis for prevention. *Diabetes Care* 1990;13:513–521.
13. Fylling C. Conclusions. *Diabetes Spectrum* 1992;5:358–359.
14. Bamberger D, Stark K. Severe diabetic foot problems: Avoiding amputation. *Emerg Decis* 1987;3(8):21–34.
15. Olin J. Peripheral arterial disease. *Diabetes Forecast* October 1992;78–81.
16. Newman B. A diabetes camp for Native American adults. *Diabetes Spectrum* 1993;6:166–202.
17. Harkness L, Lavery L. Diabetes foot care: A team approach. *Diabetes Spectrum* 1992;5:136–137.
18. Jerrell M. Management of the diabetic foot. *O & P Business News*. Aug 15, 2005, 28–33.
19. Robbins D. Office guide to diagnosis and classification of diabetes mellitus and other categories of glucose tolerance. *Diabetes Care* 1991;14(suppl 2):3–4.
20. Brand P. Neuropathic ulceration. *The Star* May/June 1983:1–4.
21. Ashbury A. Foot care in patients with diabetes mellitus. *Diabetes Care* 1991;14(suppl 2):18–19.
22. Brand P. In: *Insensitive Feet—A Practical Handout on Foot Problems in Leprosy*. London: The Leprosy Mission, 1977.
23. Brand P. Management of sensory loss in the extremities: management of peripheral nerve problems. *J Rehab* 1980;862–872.
24. Myerson M, Papa J, Eaton K. The total contact cast for management of neuropathic plantar ulceration of the foot. *Diabetes Spectrum* 1992;5:352–353.
25. Edelstein J. Foot care for the aging. *Phys Ther* 1988;68:1882–1886.
26. Utley R. Nutritional factors associated with wound healing in the elderly: The role of specific nutrients in the healing process. *Diabetes Spectrum* 1992;5:354–355.
27. Knighton D, Fiegel V, Doucette M. Treating diabetic foot ulcers. *Diabetes Spectrum* 1990;3:51–56.
28. Ellenberg M. Don't be fooled by peripheral neuropathy. *Diabetes Forecast* 1983;January/February.
29. Yale J. *Yale's Podiatric Medicine*. 3rd ed. Baltimore: Williams & Wilkins, 1980.
30. Cailliet R. *Foot and Ankle Pain*. Philadelphia: F.A. Davis; 1983, 181–189.
31. Jahss M. Shoes and shoe modifications. In: *Atlas of Orthotics*. St. Louis, MO: CV Mosby, 1985, pp. 267–279.
32. Tsairis P. Differential diagnosis of peripheral neuropathies. In: *Management of Peripheral Nerve Problems*. Rancho los Amigos:, 1980, pp. 712–725.
33. Thomas P. Clinical features and differential diagnosis. In: *Peripheral Neuropathy*. Philadelphia: WB Saunders, 1984, pp. 2:1169–1185.
34. Wakelee-Lynch J. Relieving pain with peppers. *Diabetes Forecast* June 1992;35–37.
35. Dailey G. Effect of treatment with capsaicin on daily activities of patients with painful diabetic neuropathy. *Diabetes Care* 1992;15:159–165.
36. *Diabetes Mellitus: Management and Complications*. New York: Churchill Livingstone, 1985, pp. 234–235, 277–293, 360–361.
37. Apelqvist J, Castenfors J, Larsson J. Prognostic value of systolic ankle and toe blood pressure levels in outcome of diabetic foot ulcer. *Diabetes Care* 1989;12:373–378.
38. Cherry G, Ryan T, Cameron J. Blueprint for the treatment of leg ulcers and the prevention of recurrence. *Wounds* 1992;3:1–15.
39. Field M. The use of garments to create compression. *Biomech Desk Ref;*6:139–140.
40. Perry J. Normal and pathological gait. In: *Atlas of Orthotics*. St. Louis, MO: CV Mosby, 1985, pp. 83–96.
41. Mann R. Biomechanics of the foot. In: *Atlas of Orthotics*. St. Louis, MO: CV Mosby, 1985, pp. 112–125.
42. Barber E. Strength and range-of-motion examination skills for the clinical orthotist. *J Prosthet Orthot* 1993;5(2):49–51.
43. Thomas P, Eliasson S. Diabetic neuropathy. In: *Peripheral Neuropathy*. Philadelphia: WB Saunders, 1984, pp. 2:1773–1801.
44. Boughton B. Experts debate long and short of limb length discrepancy. *Biomechanics* 2000;7:139–140.
45. Oakley W, Catterall R, Martin M. Aetiology and management of lesions of the feet in diabetes. *Br Med J* 1956;56:4999–5003.
46. Sinacore OR, Elsner R, Rubenow C. *Healing Rates of Diabetic Foot Ulcers in Subjects with Fixed Charcot Deformity*. Platform Presentation, Physical Therapy 1997 APTA Scientific Meeting and Exposition; San Diego, CA: APTA, May 30–June 4, 1997.
47. Sussman C, Strauss M, Barry D, Ayyappa E. Consideration of the motor neuropathy for managing the neuropathic foot. *J O & P Suppl* April 2005;17:(2)s28–s31.

48. Tiberio D. Pathomechanics of structural foot deformities. *Phys Ther* 1988;68:1840–1849.

49. Yale J. *Yale's Podiatric Medicine.* 3rd ed. Baltimore: Williams & Wilkins, 1980, pp. 135–136.

50. Wilson J, Foster D. *Textbook of Endocrinology.* Philadelphia: WB Saunders, 1992, pp. 1294–1297.

51. Olefsky J, Sherman R. Diabetes. In: *Insensitive Feet—A Practical Handout on Foot Problems in Leprosy.* London: The Leprosy Mission, 1977.

52. Yale J. *Yale's Podiatric Medicine.* 3rd ed. Baltimore: Williams & Wilkins, 1980, pp. 159–160.

53. Wagner FEW. The dysvascular foot: A system for diagnosis and treatment. *Foot Ankle* 1981;2:64–122.

54. Glugla M, Mulder G. The diabetic foot. In: Krasner D, ed. *Medical Management of Foot Ulcers in Chronic Wound Care: A Clinical Source Book for Healthcare Professionals.* St. Louis, MO: Mosby/Health Management Publications, 1990, pp. 223–239.

55. Wagner F. A classification and treatment program for diabetic, neuropathic and dysvascular foot problems. *Foot Ankle* 1983;1–47.

56. Sosenko J, Kato M, Soto R. Comparison of quantitative sensory threshold measures for their association with foot ulceration in diabetic patients. *Diabetes Care* 1990;13:1057–1062.

57. Omer G. Sensibility testing. In: *Management of Peripheral Nerve Problems.* Philadelphia: W. B. Saunders, 1980, pp. 3–14.

58. Birke J, Sims D. Plantar sensory threshold in the ulcerative foot. *Br Lepr Relief Assoc* 1986;57:261–267.

59. Birke J. Management of the diabetic foot. *Wound Care Manage* 1995.

60. Ashbury A. Diabetic neuropathy. *Diabetes Care* 1991;14(suppl 2):63–68.

61. Thivolet C, Farkh J, Petiot A. Measuring vibration sensations with graduated tuning fork. *Diabetes Care* 1990;13:1077–1080.

62. National Aeronautics and Space Administration. Mission accomplished (thermography aids in the detection of neuromuscular problems). *NASA Tech Brief.* January 1993, p. 92.

63. Apelqvist J, Larsson J, Agardh C. The influence of external precipitating factors and peripheral neuropathy on the development and outcome of diabetic foot ulcers. *J Diabetic Complications* 1990;4:21–25.

64. Huntley A. Taking care of your hands. *Diabetes Forecast* August 1991;11–12.

65. Bergtholdt H. Temperature assessment of the insensate. *Phys Ther* 1979;59:18–22.

66. Horzic M, Bunoza D, Maric K. Contact thermography in a study of primary healing of surgical wounds. *Ostomy Wound/Manage* 1996;42(1):36–43.

67. Lavery L, Higgins K, Lanctot D, et al. Home monitoring of skin temperatures to prevent ulceration. *Diabetes Care* 2004;27:2642–2647.

68. Chan A, MacFarlane I, Bowsher D. Contact thermography of painful neuropathic foot. *Diabetes Care* 1991;14:918–922.

69. Zhu H, Maalej N, Webster J. An umbilical data acquisition system for measuring pressures between foot and shoe. *IEEE Trans Biomed Eng* 1990;37:908–911.

70. Wertsch J, Webster J, Tompkins W. A portable insole plantar measurement system. *J Rehabil Res Dev* 1992;29:13–18.

71. Lord M. Clinical trial of a computer-aided system for orthopaedic shoe upper design. *Prosthet Orthot Int* 1991;15:11–17.

72. McAllister D, Carver D, Devarajan R. An interactive computer graphics system for the design of molded and orthopedic shoe lasts. *J Rehabil Res Dev* 1991;28:39–46.

73. Sims D, Cavanagh P, Ulbrecht J. Risk factors in the diabetic foot: Recognition and management. *Phys Ther* 1988;68:1887–1916.

74. DeJong R. *The Neurologic Examination.* New York: Harper & Row, 1969, pp. 742–743.

75. Newman L, Palestro C, Schwartz M. Unsuspected osteomyelitis in diabetic foot ulcers: Diagnosis and monitoring by leukocyte scanning with indium in oxyquinoline. *Diabetes Spectrum* 1992;5:346–347.

76. Kuncir E, Wirta R, Golbranson F. Load-bearing characteristics of polyethylene foam: An examination of structural and compression properties. *J Rehabil Res Dev* 1990;27:229–238.

77. Levin M, O'Neal L. *The Diabetic Foot.* St. Louis, MO: CV Mosby, 1988.

78. Pratt D. Medium term comparison of shock attenuating insoles using a spectral analysis technique. *J Biomed Eng* 1988;10:426–428.

79. Pratt D. Long term comparison of shock attenuating insoles. *Prosthet Orthot Int* 1990;14:59–62.

80. Lockard M. Foot orthosis. *Phys Ther* 1988;68:1866–1873.

81. Hack M. Fitting shoes. *Diabetes Forecast* 1989;January.

82. McPoil T. Footwear. *Phys Ther* 1988;68:1857–1865.

83. McPoil T, Adrian M, Pidcoe P. Effects of foot orthoses on center-of-pressure patterns in women. *Phys Ther* 1989;69:66–71.

84. Coleman W, Brasseau D. Methods of treating plantar ulcers. *Phys Ther* 1991;71:116–122.

85. Dwyer G, Rust M. Shoe business. *Diabetes Forecast* June 1988;60–63.

86. Mueller M, Diamond J, Sinacore D. Total contact casting in treatment of diabetic plantar ulcers. *Diabetes Care* 1989;12:384–388.

87. Sinacore D, Mueller M, Diamond J. Diabetic plantar ulcers treated by total contact casting. *Phys Ther* 1987;67:1543–1549.

88. Birke J, Novick A, Graham S, et al. Methods of treating plantar ulcers. *Phys Ther* 1991;71:41–47.

89. Diamond J, Sinacore D, Mueller M. Molded double-rocker plaster shoe for healing a diabetic plantar ulcer. *Phys Ther* 1987;67:1550–1552.

90. Armstrong DG, Lavery LA. Healing the diabetic wound with pressure offloading. *Biomechanics* 1997;4:67.

91. Fleischli JG, Laughlin TJ. TCC remains the gold standard for off-loading plantar ulcers. *Biomechanics* 1998;5:51–52.

92. Giacolone VF. Diabetic footwear: Pressure relief modalities. *Podiatr Today* 1998;10:16–20.

93. Birke J, Nawoczenski D. Orthopedic walkers: Effect on plantar pressures. *Clin Prosthet Orthot* 1988;12:74–80.

94. Lauridsen K, Sorensen C, Christiansen P. Measurements of pressure on the sole of the foot in plaster of paris casts on the lower leg. *J Int Soc Prosthet Orthot* 1989;13:42–45.

95. Nawoczenski DA, Birke JA. Management of the neuropathic foot in the elderly. *Top Geriatr Rehab* 1992;7:36–48.

96. Ovington LG. Wound healing forecast looks wet. *Biomechanics* 1998;5:39–70.

97. Pieper B, Templin T, et al. Wound prevalence, types and treatments in home care. *Adv Wound Care* April 1999;117–126.

98. Armstrong DG, Lavery LA, et al. Infrared dermal thermometry for the high-risk diabetic foot. *Phys Ther* 1997;77:169–171.

99. McIntyre K. Control of infection in the diabetic foot: The role of microbiology, immunopathology, antibiotics, and guillotine amputation. *J Vasc Surg* 1987;5:787–802.

100. Lai C, Lin S, Yang C. Limb salvage of infected diabetic foot ulcers with microsurgical free-muscle transfer. *Diabetes Spectrum* 1992;5:356–357.

101. Tillow T, Habrshaw G, Chrzan J. Review of metatarsal osteotomies for the treatment of neuropathic ulcerations. *Diabetes Spectrum* 1992;5:357–358.

102. Stanley J. *Structure and Function in Man.* 3rd ed. Philadelphia: WB Saunders, 1974, pp. 65–68.

103. Kechiijian P. How do nails grow? *Nails* May 1993;78–79.

104. O'Neal LW. Surgical pathway of the foot and clinicopathologic conditions. In: Bowker JH, Pfeifer MA, eds. *The Diabetic Foot.* 6th ed. St. Louis, MO: CV Mosby, 2000, pp. 501–506.

105. Ruscin C, Cunningham G, Blaylock A. Foot care protocol for the older client. *Geriatr Nurs* July/Aug 1993;210–212.

106. Sher RK. The nail doctor. *Nails* December 1977;94–95.

107. Levin SM, Jacoby S. *Your Feet Don't Have To Hurt.* New York: St. Martin's Press; 2000. pp. 65–68.

108. Harkless LB, Satterfield VK, Dennis KJ. Role of the podiatrist. In: Bowker JH, Pfeifer MA, eds. *The Diabetic Foot.* 6th ed. St Louis, MO: CV Mosby, 2000, p. 690.

109. Furman A. Give your feet a sporting chance. *Diabetes Forecast* April 1989;17–22.

110. Graham C. Neuropathy made you stop. *Diabetes Forecast* December 1992;47–49.

Management of Common Foot Problems

Teresa J. Kelechi

CHAPTER OBJECTIVES

At the completion of this chapter, the reader will be able to:

1. Describe the clinical presentation of three foot problems: tinea pedis, onychomycosis, and plantar fasciitis.
2. List two interventions each for the treatment of tinea pedis, onychomycosis, and plantar fasciitis.
3. Describe four patient education points related to the prevention of foot disorders.
4. List three referral criteria for foot complications.

Foot problems plague approximately 70% of individuals 65 years of age and older.[1] Many problems are related to the nails and skin. Nail deformities are among those conditions that require intervention, particularly onychomycosis, which is a fungal infection that causes the nails to discolor and thicken. Loss of nail integrity from a deformed toenail can lead to more serious complications, such as infections, osteomyelitis, wounds, and, in some cases, amputation. Patients with diabetes and impaired circulation can be at greater risk for such complications. Skin problems, such as xerosis, tinea pedis, and fissures, can also place patients at risk for more serious complications. Plantar fasciitis, which presents as a painful heel, can plague both the young and older populations. Skin and nail problems, as well as plantar fasciitis, can reduce functional ability and thus impair quality of life. Therefore, it becomes critical that health-care providers address the feet by inspecting the skin and nails, investigating complaints of heel and plantar foot pain, and providing interventions to ameliorate or prevent more serious foot problems.

Foot care interventions, such as debriding toenails, paring hyperkeratotic lesions (corns and calluses), and prevention/management of diabetic foot complications, are beyond the scope of this chapter (see Chapter 19 for care of the skin and nails of diabetic patients). The literature is replete with references and texts related to the assessment, identification of risk factors, interventions, and patient education specific to diabetic patients.[2,3] This chapter focuses instead on common foot problems.

Tinea Pedis

Tinea pedis, most commonly known as "athlete's foot," is a mycotic disorder. It is the most common form of dermatophytosis, or fungal infection of the feet. Dermatophytes are aerobic fungi and the most commonly isolated fungal organisms.[4] They invade, infect, and persist in the stratum corneum and, rarely, penetrate below the surface of the epidermis and its appendages. The skin responds to the superficial infection by increased proliferation, which leads to scaling and epidermal thickening.[5]

The causes of tinea pedis are classified into three anamorphic genera: *Trichophyton, Microsporum,* and *Epidermophyton,* depending on their conidial structures. Trichophyton rubrum is the most prevalent fungal pathogen in the feet.[4] Dermatophytes can be acquired from the soil, animals, and other humans. The most common source in the United States is infected individuals. A higher incidence in modern times can be attributed to the increased use of broad-spectrum antibiotics, the expanding number of immunocompromised patients, such as those with HIV or AIDS, and lifestyle changes. Those individuals with hepatic, renal, and endocrine diseases (e.g., diabetes mellitus) are at higher risk.

The prevalence of fungal foot infections in people with diabetes is often underestimated. Marked mycoses on the soles of the feet is often considered to be dry skin by patients and health-care providers; therefore, people with diabetes require more diagnostic, therapeutic, and preventive care in terms of mycotic diseases than previously thought.[6]

There is also an increased incidence of fungal infections among gardeners and farmers; individuals who regularly wear boots or sports shoes; and individuals who frequent sports facilities, pools, and communal leisure facilities. Ten percent of the population is estimated to be infected by a dermatophyte; of these, tinea pedis is the most common, occurring in up to 70% of adults.[1] Contributing factors include warmth and high humidity, with constant occlusion.

Signs and Symptoms

Exhibit 20-1 presents the clinical findings of tinea pedis. Symptoms include pruritus, scaling, redness, painful or uncomfortable breaks in the skin, weeping, odor, and disability.[1,4]

Diagnosis

Laboratory studies are generally indicated, because greater diagnostic accuracy occurs when the clinical diagnosis is verified by laboratory tests. This verification is especially important when the use of systemic therapy is anticipated. Aqueous potassium hydroxide preparation (KOH) and fungal cultures can be performed.

KOH specimens should be obtained from the active border or edge of a lesion or scale by scraping a skin sample from the site of infection. If a vesicle or bulla is present, the roof is an appropriate specimen. In pustular lesions, the purulent debris is acceptable. Place the material on a glass slide, add 10%–20% KOH, with or without dimethyl sulfoxide (DMSO). If DMSO is added, heating is not necessary. A fungal stain, such as chlorazol black E or Parker's blue black ink, can be added to highlight the hyphae. A positive KOH specimen will show multiple septate hyphae.[5] A negative result does not necessarily exclude the possibility of dermatophyte infection; therefore, a culture of the sample helps identify the causative fungal organism.[4]

Fungal cultures are recommended for persistent and difficult conditions that require specific identification. Various methods of obtaining cultures have been described in the literature, such as using a sterile toothbrush or rubbing moistened sterile swabs or gauze pads over the affected area, and then pressing into the surface of the dermatophyte test medium to be cultured. The laboratory should be contacted for the acceptable method of obtaining the culture and which medium is to be used.

Differential diagnosis is indicated to rule out psoriasis, parapsoriasis, eczema, candidiasis, bacterial infection, and other dermatoses.

The diagnosis of tinea pedis is generally classified into three categories: interdigital toe web infections, plantar moccasin-type infection, and vesiculobullous tinea pedis.

Interdigital toe web infections usually start as dermatophyte infections (*Trichophyton rubrum* and *Trichophyton mentagrophytes*), with an interplay between various bacterial species and, although rare, *Candida* species. Scaling is the initial feature, and, when the bacteria proliferate, maceration occurs (Figure 20-1). The terms *dermatophytosis simplex* and *dermatophytosis complex* have been proposed to address two forms of interdigital infection. *Simplex* refers to the features of scaling and, at times, fissures, whereas *complex* includes a highly macerated, leukokeratotic symptomatic process in which dermatophytes can be recovered in only one-third of patients. This variety of interdigital infection is mainly caused by an overgrowth of a myriad of bacterial species.[7]

Plantar moccasin-type infection results in diffuse, hyperkeratotic scaling of the plantar surface and is often associated with toenail involvement. The skin can become red, with severe itching in some cases. The main feature is small scales that often appear as small, round areas of peeling skin (Figure 20-2).

Vesiculobullous tinea pedis presents as acute, highly inflammatory eruptions, particularly on the arch and side of the foot. *T. mentagrophytes* is primarily responsible. People with recurrent episodes tend to have low-grade scaling between exacerbations of acute inflammation. Differing environmental factors, such as seasonal temperature, sweating from physical activities, and types of shoe wear, influence

---

EXHIBIT 20-1 Clinical Presentation of Tinea Pedis

1. Whitish, macerated interdigital spaces, most often the fourth and fifth digits
2. Erythematous skin with vesicles, scales, or fissures
3. Malodor from bacterial superinfection, which can mask the underlying fungal infection
4. Thickened, scaly, dry patches on the soles and sides of feet
5. Lesions that are noninflammatory scaly, acute or subacute eczematous-like, chronically lichenified, nodular and granulomatous, bullous and pustular, or resembling pyoderma
6. Associated infections involving the hair follicle and nail, persistent hyperpigmentation and/or hypopigmentation, and secondary bacterial infection

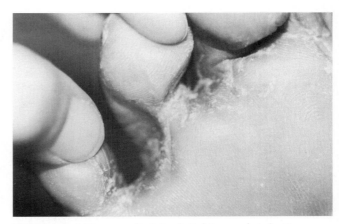

FIGURE 20–1 Tinea pedis interdigital toe web infection.

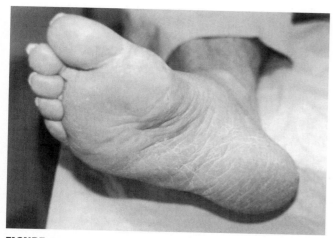

FIGURE 20–2 Moccasin-type tinea pedis.

the growth of the fungus. When sufficient proliferation and penetration of the stratum corneum occur, the epidermis comes into contact with fungal antigens, and a T cell-mediated immune contact allergic response occurs.[7]

Management

Treatment modalities for tinea pedis include general and specific interventions, which are often varied and include both topical and oral medications. General interventions involve the use of topical antifungal agents, which are indicated for simple interdigital and noninflammatory moccasin-type dermatophytoses. However, topical antifungal agents may not penetrate far enough into the keratinous tissue to eliminate the fungal organisms, resulting in relapses and chronic tinea pedis.[4] Exhibit 20-2 presents common topical products.

CLINICAL WISDOM

Terbinafine hydrochloride cream (Lamisil Cream 1%, available over the counter) should be applied twice daily until clinical signs and symptoms of tinea pedis significantly improve, usually by day 7. Drug therapy should be provided for a minimum of 1 week, not to exceed 4 weeks. Interdigital tinea pedis caused by *T. rubrum, T. mentagrophytes,* and *E. floccosum* in which the toe web space is moist has been responsive to ciclopirox 0.77% gel, applied twice daily for 4 weeks.[8]

Specific interventions for tinea pedis depend on the type of infection. For dermatophytosis complex, the use of a topical fungicidal agent, such as an allylamine (terbinafine), alternated with a double antibiotic ointment, such as Polysporin, or with broad-spectrum antibacterial agents, such as Castellani paint, aluminum chloride, and various tinctures of dye (gentian violet), can be used. If the toenails are infected, this reservoir of fungi must also be treated. Topical therapy is often recommended for several weeks to eradicate residual fungus and prevent relapse, but this should be

closely monitored. The use of 40% urea cream as an adjunct to topical antifungals such as ciclopirox cream has been found to be beneficial in the treatment of the erythema, scaling, and pruritus. Patients are instructed to apply the 40% urea cream once daily and the ciclopirox cream twice daily for 2 to 3 weeks.[9]

RESEARCH WISDOM

For most dermatophytic infections of the foot, topical agents are usually effective and less expensive than oral agents.[10]

Severe moccasin-type or dermatophytosis complex infections that are resistant to topical therapy alone require systemic therapy, such as itraconazole (Sporanox) 200 mg daily for 1 week (increase to 12 weeks if toenails are involved, and refer to package insert for more detailed prescribing information) or terbinafine hydrochloride 250 mg daily for 1 week (protocol will change if the patient has onychomycosis; see prescribing information in package insert). Although not well studied, oral therapy for tinea pedis is limited to patients with more extensive infections, such as vesicobullous and moccasin-type resistant infections and chronic infections.[10]

CLINICAL WISDOM

Tinea pedis can mimic dry skin. Dry skin tends to be flaky, whereas infected skin tends to produce small, round scales that give the appearance of the skin peeling.

Vesiculobullous tinea pedis with acute, highly inflammatory eruptions requires topical or systemic corticosteroids in conjunction with antifungal agents for acute attacks. The choice of topical or systemic therapy depends on the extent and severity of the process. Caution must be exercised in the use of combination topical corticosteroid-antifungal mixtures, which contain potent fluorinated corticosteroids. Combination products containing a low-potency nonfluorinated corticosteroid can initially be used for symptomatic inflamed lesions of tinea. Steroid therapy should be withdrawn once the cell-mediated immune response is curtailed or there is evidence that symptoms are relieved, and it should never exceed 4 weeks. Contraindications for the use of these combinations include application on occluded areas and use in children less than 12 years of age and immunosuppressed patients.[11]

Surgical intervention is usually not indicated. However, some clients elect to have the infected toenail plate permanently removed, due to continuing nail deformity. The complications of both topical and systemic therapy should be discussed with each client. The most common side effects of topical therapy include irritation, burning, itching, and dryness. Systemic therapy side effects can occur with terbinafine (Exhibit 20-3) and itraconazole (Exhibit 20-4). Clients who have known hypersensitivities to topical and systemic antifungal therapy should not take these drugs.

Outcome measures for successful treatment of tinea pedis include skin that is free of scaling, flakiness, and peeling, and relief of symptoms, such as itching or discomfort. Treatment failure should be suspected if the skin has not improved after 1 month of treatment. Skin cultures can be obtained if the infection is suspected to be recalcitrant to therapy. It is important to treat both tinea pedis and onychomycosis, as mycologically proven foot dermatomycosis is a significant risk factor for the development of acute bacterial cellulitis.[12]

CLINICAL WISDOM

Liver function studies are indicated prior to treatment with oral itraconazole and terbinafine, per package insert.

Prevention

Prevention of tinea pedis is a lifelong goal. Many individuals experience several acute exacerbations during their lifetimes. Prevention goals are to minimize damp, moist skin caused by footwear and avoid environments that promote fungal growth, such as contaminated showers. The following self-care tips can help to prevent recurrences:

1. Dry feet well after bathing and showering, making sure to dry between the toes.
2. Use antifungal powders or sprays twice daily to minimize moisture on the feet and between the toes.
3. Use skin sealant/antiseptic products such as Liquid Band-aid, which act as moisture barriers between the toes.
4. Use lamb's wool or another absorptive product between the toes when maceration, the whitish overhydrated epidermis, first appears.

5. Change socks frequently, especially when damp.
6. Wear fabrics that are most conducive to wicking moisture away, including synthetics such as nylon; cotton tends to absorb moisture and "hold" it next to the skin.
7. Change shoes frequently and apply antifungal powders and sprays to the inside of the shoes, which helps to reduce fungus in the shoes.

Members of households may choose to use separate tubs and showers from those who are affected to prevent the transmission from one person to another; the surface should be cleaned after each use with a solution that kills fungus.

Plantar Fasciitis

Plantar fasciitis is the most common form of heel pain. It is caused by inflammation, microruptures, hemorrhages, and collagen degeneration of the plantar fascia. The sequelae are fibrosis and possible ossification between the origin of the flexor digitorum brevis and the fascia.

The cause of plantar fasciitis is variable and multifactorial.[13] The major underlying factor is overuse injury to soft tissue, involving repetitive, excessive loading impact on heel strike over time. Anatomic, biomechanical, and environmental factors contribute to damage. Anatomic risk factors include pes planus, subtalar joint pronation, cavus foot, unequal leg length, tarsal coalition, and low or high foot arch. Biomechanical forces include tight Achilles tendon with inflexibility, weak plantar flexors, weak ankle flexors, weak intrinsic muscles, obesity, sudden weight gain, pregnancy, and sudden trauma. Changes in activity level; a rapid increase in training activities related to speed, intensity, and duration; running on steep hills, poor/hard surfaces, or barefoot on sand; wornout running shoes; poor shoe supports; inadequate stretching; excessive walking on the job; and excessive standing on hard, unyielding surfaces are examples of environmental risk factors. Athletic activities that have been linked to plantar fasciitis are running, distance running, tennis, gymnastics, and basketball.

EXHIBIT 20-3   Side Effects of Terbinafine (Lamisil)

- Gastrointestinal disorders, including diarrhea and dyspepsia
- Dermatologic disorders, including rash, pruritus, and urticaria
- Liver enzyme abnormalities
- Taste disturbance
- Visual disturbance

EXHIBIT 20-4   Side Effects of Itraconazole (Sporanox)

- Gastrointestinal disorders
- Edema
- Fatigue
- Fever
- Malaise
- Skin disorders, including rash and pruritus
- Central and peripheral nervous system problems, including headache
- Psychiatric disorders, including decreased libido
- Hypertension
- Hypokalemia
- Albuminuria
- Abnormal hepatic function
- Impotence

Signs and Symptoms

The clinical features of plantar fasciitis include subjective symptoms of pain or discomfort. The pain can be described as a slow, dull ache; intense achiness; or burning sensation. The pain can be sharp, pinpoint, or knifelike. Patients often complain of pain in the heel when standing after periods of rest, especially during the first step in the morning.[14] This pain diminishes with each successive step, but can return late in the afternoon after prolonged weight bearing. It is usually described as nonradiating and well localized to the medial aspect of the heel pad. The symptoms are predominantly unilateral, but bilateral involvement occurs in 10% of cases.[13]

CLINICAL WISDOM

One of the most common complaints of heel pain associated with plantar fasciitis is the report that the pain is excruciating upon first rising in the morning, when the foot touches the floor. This is a hallmark symptom of fasciitis.

Diagnosis

Objectively, pain can be evaluated as localized point tenderness with palpation over the medial calcaneal tuberosity. The pain can be reproduced during passive dorsiflexion of the ankle or toes and when standing on the toes to tighten the plantar fascia. If the condition is chronic, thickening, nodularity, and tautness can be palpated along the fascia. Diagnostic tests such as radiographs, bone scans, and blood studies are generally reserved for ambiguous presentation. A radiograph can be normal or reveal a horizontal bone spur projecting from the calcaneal tuberosity. The spur is not necessary in making the diagnosis, but its presence indicates chronic inflammation.[15]

Other related problems that can mimic plantar fasciitis include, but are not limited to:[16]

- Heel pad atrophy
- Tarsal tunnel syndrome
- Achilles tendinitis
- Calcaneal fracture
- Stress fracture
- Compartment syndrome
- Complete or partial plantar fascia rupture
- Systemic disorders, such as lupus erythematous, rheumatoid arthritis, ankylosing spondylitis, Reiter syndrome, gout, and vascular insufficiency

Client assessment and diagnosis include a thorough history (e.g., reports of heel pain) and physical examination. The procedure for examining the client is as follows:

1. Ask client to stand. Assess for a rigid cavus foot (high arch) or pes planus (flat foot).
2. Ask client to walk. The gait should be observed for any excessive pronation (ankles turning inward) on heel strike. Observe for a limp that might occur with weight bearing when the foot touches down on its lateral aspect.
3. Ask client to dorsiflex (move foot upward toward leg) and plantar flex (push toes downward toward floor). Assess range of motion of the ankle and to identify a tight heelcord. Ask the client to repeat these movements, using only the toes, to identify a tight heel cord or limitation in flexing and extending the great toe.
4. Inspect the shoes for any abnormal wear and the quality of arch support within them. Shoes that do not fit properly or are in poor condition should be replaced. Athletic-type walking shoes with proper arch supports are indicated.

Management

Interventions include treating pain, restoring flexibility to the ankle and arch, strengthening the muscles in and around the foot, and gradually resuming activities. Conservative measures are described.[17]

General measures include rest, ice application, stretching, and muscle strengthening. A conservative rest program involves a decrease in activity for 6 weeks. Local ice application several times per day (conservative) includes ice massage for 6–7 minutes or application of an ice pack for 20–40 minutes 4-6 times a day. Ice should be applied long enough to achieve a numbing affect, while avoiding frostbite injury.

CLINICAL WISDOM

A bag of frozen vegetables, such as peas, can be placed in a plastic zipper bag and labeled *ice bag*. A paper towel should be placed around this ice bag and applied to the heel several times a day. Or, the client can place a foam cup filled with water in the freezer. When frozen, place the cup in a plastic zipper bag and massage the foot with the ice. Another method is to fill a 20 oz soda bottle with water and freeze. The frozen bottle can be placed on the floor, and the affected foot can be "rolled" over the bottle to ice the foot.

Conservative stretching is considered by some to be the most important aspect of the treatment regimen. Demonstrate gastrocnemius and soleus stretches to the patient and have him or her repeat the demonstration. Gastrocnemius stretch is performed by having the client lean forward into a wall and place the affected foot 12–18 inches from the wall, with the foot flat against the floor and the knee straight. The soleus stretch is performed in the same manner, but with the back knee slightly bent. The stretch can be obtained in the seated position by placing a towel under the ball of the foot and gently pulling it upward. Proper stretching involves a gentle pulling pressure in the muscle with the tendon being stretched, without causing an increase in pain. Ice or medication (nonsteroidal antiinflammatory drugs [NSAIDs] or other antiinflammatory agents) can be used prior to stretching. It is recommended that a 10- to 20-second stretch be performed on rising in the morning, with 15 repetitions performed at least two to five times per day.

Conservative muscle strengthening exercises can also be taught to the patient. Instruct the patient to pick articles off the floor, using only the toes. Patients should observe the clinician demonstrating exercises and then perform these exercises several minutes each day for at least 6 weeks.

Specific interventions include the use of medications, support devices, strapping, shoe wear, and orthotics.[13] NSAIDs can be prescribed for pain management. In acute cases, NSAIDs are prescribed for a 7- to 10-day course up to 1 month, depending on the drug and degree of symptom management required. Patients should be encouraged to check with their health-care provider before starting a regimen of NSAIDs, because of the side effects.

Conservative support devices include use of heel cups, pads, lifts, and arch support inserts placed in both shoes. These devices relieve tension on the plantar fascia by reestablishing the arched shape of the foot. Cups and pads are especially beneficial to the elderly when there is atrophy of the plantar heel pad. If tenderness is localized, a cutout can be made into any of these three types of shoe inserts to relieve pressure over the tender area. Pedorthists, physical therapists, chiropractors, and podiatrists can recommend the proper inserts and orthotics when needed.

Conservative strapping, splinting, and other methods of immobilizing the foot help to reestablish or maintain the arch of the foot, stabilize the first metatarsal head, decrease forefoot pronation, control heel valgus (turning outward), and change the foot strike position. Strapping is considered to be beneficial in the acute phase of plantar fasciitis. Night splints can be obtained from specialty shoe stores and pharmacies and worn at night to keep the foot in proper alignment (dorsiflexed), thus preventing relaxation of the fascia, which, when supported, is less painful. Sports medicine or physical therapy professionals can perform the strapping procedure and recommend splints. The splints can also be obtained from specialty footwear and online stores.

Shoes—good walking shoes and athletic-type footwear—are part of the treatment plan. Shoes with a firm heel, proper heel cushioning, and adequate longitudinal arch support are recommended. Orthotics are devices that relieve symptoms by providing adequate resistance to the mechanical forces applied to the foot. Clients can be referred to an orthotist, pedorthist, podiatrist, or other foot care-related specialist for orthotic devices.

If no improvement is noted within 6 weeks, the client can be referred to physical therapy, although there are conflicting data regarding the benefit of physical therapy modalities, such as pulsed ultrasound, phonophoresis, monochromatic near infrared light, and high-energy shock wave therapy.[18,19] Additionally, contrast soaks can be recommended. Contrast soaks involve using hot and cold soaks for 15 minutes twice a day, beginning with a warm soak for the first half and followed by cold soaks for the remainder.

If improvement is only minimal after another 6–8 weeks, a steroid injection may be necessary. A corticosteroid injection into the calcaneal attachment can help control the inflammation of plantar fasciitis. The major risks are fascia rupture, associated with degeneration of the fascia, and fat-pad atrophy. Steroid injections tend to be very painful. Measures to reduce the pain include use of a local anesthetic and corticosteroid cryospray before the injection, and use of medial injection parallel to the fascia. Three injections may be given 2–4 weeks apart.[20] If pain is recalcitrant to treatment, surgery may be an option. Candidates for surgery are limited to those with significant pain and disability in activities of daily living after conservative therapy has been exhausted.[21,22] Exhibit 20-5 presents complications related to plantar fasciitis treatment.

CLINICAL WISDOM

When historical or physical findings of plantar heel pain are unusual or routine treatment proves ineffective, consider an atypical cause of heel pain, such as stress fracture of the calcaneus or heel spur syndrome.[16]

Outcomes measures of successful treatment of plantar fasciitis include a reduction in pain after 4–6 weeks of conservative treatment and cessation of symptoms after 8 months to a year. Referral criteria include clients whose symptoms last longer than 6 months or who present with chronic symptoms of many months to years duration. Consultation with a foot-care specialist in sports medicine, orthopedics, podiatry, pedorthy, or physical therapy depends on the client's responsiveness to conservative treatment. Follow-up is generally appropriate within 6 weeks from onset of treatment.

Prevention

Self-care strategies for prevention of exacerbations include wearing proper footwear with adequate arch supports and avoiding extreme dorsiflexion of the feet, such as bending down on the forefoot, which puts excessive pressure on the toes and metatarsal heads of the feet. This position causes extreme tension on the fascia and can induce microtears. Avoiding excessive trauma from sports-related "pounding" of the feet during activities on hard surfaces, such as concrete, is also recommended.

EXHIBIT 20-5 Complications of Plantar Fasciitis Treatment

A. Orthotics—Toe jamming, heel irritation, and slippage from an improper fit

B. Nonsteroidal anti-inflammatory drugs—Gastrointestinal upset most common (see package insert for comprehensive list of adverse reactions)

C. Strapping—Allergy to tape or prep adhesive, blistering, and irritation

D. Shoes—Ill-fitting footwear, leading to blisters, corns, calluses, and pain

E. Steroid injections—Fat-pad atrophy, pain and degeneration of the fascia, and plantar fascia rupture

F. Surgery—Decrease in strength and function

Onychomycosis

Onychomycosis (tinea unguium) is an infection of the toenails in which fungal organisms invade the nail unit via the nail bed or nail plate, causing insidious, progressive destruction of the nail plate if left untreated (Figures 20-3 and 20-4). It is precipitated by environmental factors, repeated microtrauma to the nail and its structures, moisture, and skin fungal infection. It is also related to aging, extensive use of chemotherapeutic, systemic antibiotic and immunosuppressive therapies, and human immunodeficiency virus (HIV). Fungal infections appear more commonly in males between 40 and 80 years of age and in the elderly rather than the younger population. A history of cancer, psoriasis, tinea pedis interdigitalis, the moccasin form of tinea pedis, and regular swimming activity can double the risk of developing onychomycosis.[23]

There are three main classes of fungi that cause onychomycosis. Dermatophyte fungi account for 90% of fungal infections and include *T. rubrum, Epidermaophyton floccosum,* and *T. mentagrophytes.* Yeasts, including *Candida albicans,* account for 8%, and nondermatophyte molds, including *Aspergillus* species, *Scopulariopsis brevicollis, Scytalidium dimidiatum, Scytalidium hyalinum, Fusarium* species, and *Acremonium* species, account for 2% of onychomycosis. Mixed infections involving two or more fungi can occur.

The initial pathophysiology involves a mild inflammatory response to the fungi once they have invaded the nail bed, causing hypertrophy of the bed. Hyperkeratosis and hypertrophy of the nail plate results in a discolored, deformed, thick, crumbly nail that can become loosened from the nail bed.[24]

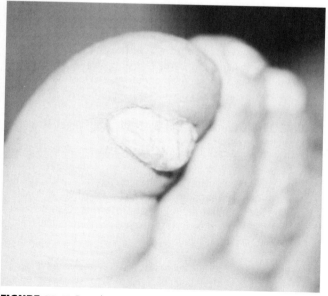

FIGURE 20-3 Onychomycosis demonstrating hyperkeratosis and hypertrophy of the nail plate with a deformed, thick, crumbly nail. The plate is thickened, deformed, brittle, and crumbly.

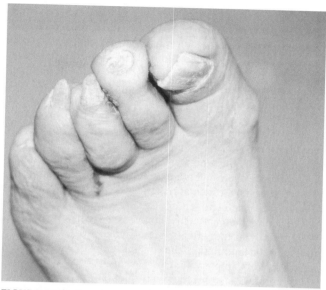

FIGURE 20-4 Onychomycosis involving multiple nail plates.

Signs and Symptoms

There are four patterns of onychomycosis nail infection: distal subungual, proximal subungual, white superficial, and Candida. Each pattern is associated with a different entry point of the fungi into the nail unit and a different appearance of the infected nail.

Distal subungual onychomycosis is the most common type, and *T. rubrum* is the most common cause. The distal nail plate turns yellow or whitish brown, with hyperkeratotic debris accumulation under the nail. The plate often becomes thickened, deformed, brittle, and crumbly, and can make wearing shoes uncomfortable or painful.[25]

Proximal subungual onychomycosis, which is caused by dermatophytes, appears more frequently in immunocompromised patients. Fungi invade the proximal nail fold and cuticle, and then infect the deeper portion of the plate. The proximal nail plate develops a white color in patchy areas. The surface remains smooth and intact. Hyperkeratotic debris can accumulate under the plate.

White superficial onychomycosis (WSO) is most often caused by the dermatophyte *T. mentagrophytes* and a variety of molds. There are three types of WSO: classical; dual invasion of the nail plate, superficial and ventral; and pseudo-WSO with deep fungal invasion of the nail plate.[26,27] Fungi directly invade the surface of the plate, producing a white, soft, dry, powdery, crumbly appearance. The plate does not thicken and continues to adhere to the nail bed. It can occur in patients with HIV disease.

Candida onychomycosis is mainly caused by *C. albicans.* It is a rare syndrome, limited to patients with chronic mucocutaneous candidiasis. The nail plate thickens and turns yellow-brown.[25]

The predisposing factors to nail infections include chronic tinea pedis and other foot infections, male gender, poor hygiene, chronic exposure of nails to water, advanced age with slower growth of the nail and decreased circulation, and athletics in which trauma to the nail weakens the seal between the nail plate and nail bed, allowing fungal organisms to penetrate the nail unit.[25] Athletes are at high risk because of profuse sweating, with runners particularly prone to onychomycosis. Exogenous heat and moisture, which worsen the condition, as well as hyperhidrosis (excessive sweating), as seen in people who wears shoes or boots every day for 12 or more hours at a time, also increase risk. Data suggest that people who wear sandals are less vulnerable to fungi because their feet are exposed to the air. Immunosuppressed patients are also at risk. Postmenopausal women are affected because estrogen appears to exert a protective effect in younger women. Onychomycosis appears to manifest itself initially in individuals in their 40s and 50s. It is common in older populations and in individuals with diabetes and circulatory impairment.[28-30]

Onychomycosis presents with three common signs. The nail plate becomes discolored, with white, brown, or yellow patches or streaks. Resulting subungual hyperkeratosis and debris as the plate loses its structural integrity and onycholysis (loosening or separation of all or part of the nail plate from the bed) are common. Symptoms include pain; trauma to adjacent soft skin folds from the thickened nails; and embarrassment from disfigured, discolored, and deformed nails. Pain can result from the thick nail plate because it causes pressure on the nail bed from ill-fitting footwear.

Diagnosis

As a rule, laboratory studies are conducted when onychomycosis cannot be managed by standard mechanical or pharmacologic treatments. Histologic analysis via nail culture should be conducted in resistant clinical situations in which fungal infection is suspected. It can take up to 30 days to obtain results. Because specimen processing can require special techniques, contact a local laboratory for requirements. If a diagnosis is still not possible using microscopic exam or histologic analysis, biopsy of the nail bed is indicated. Several diagnostic approaches are described in detail in the literature.[31-33]

CLINICAL WISDOM

Many nail conditions can mimic onychomycosis, such as trauma-induced dystrophic nail (abnormal in appearance, shape, and texture), psoriasis, eczema, lichen planus, ischemic conditions, congenital nail disorders, yellow nail syndrome, and pseudomonas.

Management

Treatment of onychomycosis includes general measures of mechanical manual debridement with nippers and more specific measures, such as topical nail reduction using urea compound (20%–40%) in petrolatum under thin film dressing, topical and oral antifungal agents, and surgical nail removal. Monotherapy is often ineffective in the treatment of onychomycosis. The overall cure rates of topical therapy are relatively low, and relapse rates are relatively high. Nail lacquers and creams can be used in conjunction with manual debridement and can include (but are not limited to) ciclopirox (8% Penlac Nail Lacquer applied to affected nails before bedtime or more than 8 hours before washing nails), oxiconazole nitrate (Oxistat 1% cream), sulconazole nitrate (Exelderm 1% cream), terbinafine hydrochloride (Lamisil AT 1% cream or spray), and others (sodium pyrithione, amorolfine, allylamines, bifonazole/urea, propylene glycol-urea-lactic acid, imidazoles, organic acids).[34] Systemic antifungal agents, such as itraconazole (Sporanox) or terbinafine (Lamisil), are useful (Exhibit 20-6). Data from a plethora of studies of drug therapies yield inconsistent findings about the efficacy, best treatment regimens, and cost-effectiveness.[35-42] Fluconazole (Diflucan) is a newer oral agent that is undergoing study for treatment of onychomycosis.[43]

Baseline liver function studies are obtained prior to initiation of oral therapy and during its course. Refer to package insert for prescribing information.[44] Most recent data suggest the combination of topical and oral therapies is most effective when nail fungus is resistant to topical treatments of greater than 2 months duration.[44] Combination therapy can reduce the duration and cumulative dosage of oral therapy.[25] In the future, combined therapies with new oral antimycotics and antifungal lacquers, and treatments combined with surgical, laser, or chemical removal of the affected nail regions, may improve results. It is important to review the literature pertaining to the best practices for prescribing oral antifungal therapy, as open studies and randomized controlled trials are proliferative, and newer findings could change prescribing practices.

The optimal clinical effect for systemic therapy is seen some months after cessation of treatment and is related to the period required for outgrowth of healthy nail. It can take up to 12 months for nail cure. The duration of treatment is based on prescribing recommendations, mycological cure,

---

EXHIBIT 20-6 Guidelines for Systemic Antifungal Therapy for Onychomycosis[32]

- Itraconazole, 200 mg twice a day for 7 days per month for 3 months. Advise clients to take with a full meal. Adverse reactions include elevated liver enzymes (> 2 times normal range), gastrointestinal disorders, rash, hypertension, orthostatic hypotension, headache, malaise, myalgia, hypokalemia, albuminuria, and vertigo.
- Terbinafine, 250 mg every day for 12 weeks. Adverse reactions include headache; gastrointestinal symptoms, such as diarrhea, dyspepsia, abdominal pain, nausea, diarrhea, and flatulence; dermatologic symptoms, such as rash, pruritus, and urticaria; liver enzyme abnormalities; taste disturbance; and visual disturbance.

and outcome measures, including a nail free of discoloration, thickness, and crumbly texture.[34] It is important to remind clients that a "perfect" nail may not be an attainable goal. However, a nail plate that is much less thick is cosmetically more appealing and does reduce the risk of injury to the underlying nail bed.

Prevention

Measures to prevent fungal infection or reinfection are critical.[45] Novel treatment approaches are evolving, such as the use of low-voltage direct current, which exerts an antifungal effect.[46] Clients should be instructed on the following key points:

1. Wear properly fitting shoes. Alternate between two pairs so you do not wear the same pair every day. Shoes with a high toe box of extra depth can accommodate thickened nails.
2. Wear thin acrylic or acrylic-blend socks, such as those worn by runners. These wick the moisture away from the skin, rather than absorbing it, keeping the skin drier. The socks should be changed frequently if they do become moist.
3. Wash the feet daily and pay close attention to drying well between the toes.
4. Trim toenails straight across, smoothing any rough or jagged edges and following the contour or shape of the toe.
5. Alert health-care professionals of any changes in the nail or skin.

Anecdotal data suggest that patients who use various herbal preparations and over-the-counter products have experienced a reduction in symptoms associated with onychomycosis. Vick's VapoRub, tea tree oil, and vinegar have been reported to lessen the severity of symptoms.[47]

Referral criteria include treatment failure with systemic agents (after 9–12 months of nail growth, even after systemic therapy has been completed) and client dissatisfaction with mechanical debridement. Patients who are unable to take systemic therapy should be referred to foot-care specialists for evaluation of more aggressive treatment, such as removal of the nail plate by surgical or chemical methods, particularly when severe toenail deformities exist. Clients who elect conservative measures, such as mechanical debridement, should see foot-care professionals every 2 to 3 months.[2] Quality of life is important to consider during all aspects of treatment and should be included as part of the history.[48]

Miscellaneous Conditions

This section presents information on miscellaneous foot conditions, including xerosis and anhidrosis, hyperhidrosis, cellulitis, maceration, hyperkeratotic lesions, fissures, and onychauxis. For each, the definition, pathophysiology, key points, and general guidelines for management are provided.

Xerosis and Anhidrosis

Xerosis and anhidrosis describe excessively dry, flaky skin that can be particularly severe on the heels and bottoms of the feet. Anhidrosis is often related to autonomic dysfunction caused by endocrine or neurologic disorders, which results in loss of moisture production in the skin and severe flaking (Figures 20-5 and 20-6).

Management of xerosis and anhidrosis includes:

1. Teach client to avoid prolonged soaking of feet in hot water because it can cause excessive drying by depleting moisture from the skin. Soaking should be limited to 10 minutes.
2. Apply topical hydrating products and seal them with petrolatum-based products several times each day and at bedtime. The condition can require a prescription-strength product if symptoms do not resolve after 4 weeks. Products containing humectants attract and retain moisture on the skin.
3. Wear proper footwear and socks, which are barriers between the skin and shoe, to reduce friction.

Hyperhidrosis

Hyperhidrosis is excessive moisture production related to endocrine/neurologic or sweat gland disorders. Management includes:

1. Teach client to change acrylic or acrylic-blend socks several times each day.
2. Consider using spray antiperspirants on skin and absorptive powders daily or more frequently as needed. Prescription-strength antiperspirant (e.g., Drysol) may be needed to treat recalcitrant sweating.
3. Footwear should be of leather or canvas/cloth material that is breathable.

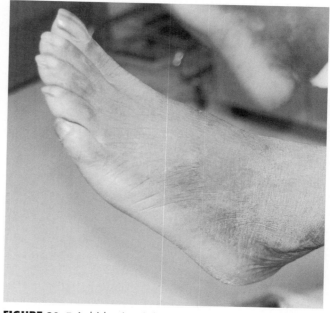

FIGURE 20–5 Anhidrosis of the foot.

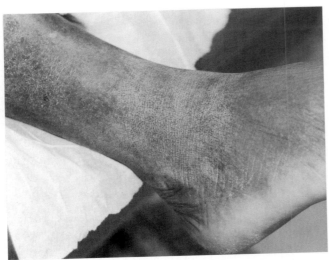

FIGURE 20–6 Close-up photo of the skin in Figure 20-5. Note the cracking in the skin.

Cellulitis

Cellulitis is inflammation and subsequent infection of the connective tissue between adjacent tissues and organs, and commonly results from bacterial infection. It gives the overlying skin a reddish appearance. Infection can be located in the toes, dorsum and plantar surface of the feet, and lower leg skin. This can result from trauma, wounds, and immunodeficiency syndromes.

Management of cellulitis includes:

1. Order diagnostic testing, such as radiographs or magnetic resonance imaging, to rule out osteomyelitis.
2. Initiate proper antibiotic therapy.
3. Initiate wound care, if wound is present.
4. Teach patient to dress the wound and prevent mechanical, thermal, and chemical injury to the area.
5. Instruct patient to report worsening of symptoms, such as increased size, drainage, redness, pain, and fever.
6. Instruct patient to take pain relievers.

Maceration

Maceration describes macerated toe web spaces that result from rigid or fixed toe deformities or functional impairments, such as stiffness, which prevent the client from bending over to dry the feet and areas between the toes. Excessive moisture gets trapped and can lead to fungal and bacterial infections.

Management of maceration includes:

1. Implement moisture control practices, such as drying well between toes after bathing or showering and wiping toe web spaces with drying agents (e.g., alcohol) for up to 1 week. Spray antiseptics can be used, which also offer a drying effect.
2. Use lamb's wool, cotton, or other absorptive material between toes to reduce moisture. This should be changed daily.
3. Skin sealants applied to the toe web spaces act as a moisture barrier. Liquid antiseptic products such a Liquid Band-Aid and New-Skin are available from drug stores and major discount chains and can be sprayed or "painted" between the toes.
4. Apply absorptive powder between toes and in shoes to reduce moisture.
5. Instruct client to wear thin acrylic or acrylic-blend socks when wearing shoes.
6. Advise client to change shoes frequently.
7. Once maceration is treated, skin moisture barrier/protectant wipes can be used between the toes as a moisture barrier.

If maceration persists for longer than 10 to 14 days, consider the presence of an interdigital tinea pedis and/or superimposed bacterial infection. Topical antifungal and antibacterial agents should be used for up to 1 month. Oral antifungal agents may be warranted if the fungal infection is recalcitrant to topical therapies.

Hyperkeratotic Lesions

Hyperkeratotic lesions include corns and calluses. Corns (helomas; Figure 20-7) and calluses (tylomas; Figure 20-8) are circumscribed masses of a hornlike collection of epidermal cells that are thicker in the center and gradually taper, becoming thinner at the periphery. Hard corns arise on top of or on the sides of the toes; soft corns arise between the toes. Calluses are found on the plantar surface of the feet under prominent weight-bearing areas and on the medial and lateral aspects of the sides of the feet and great toes. Corns and calluses form as a result of abnormal intermittent or chronic weight-bearing pressure and/or shear sliding stresses.

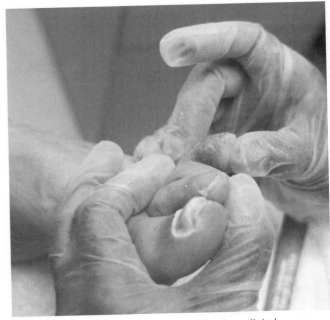

FIGURE 20–7 Example of a corn in the interdigital space.

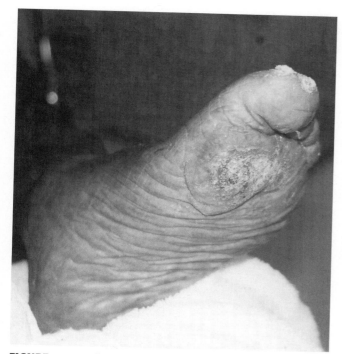

FIGURE 20–8 Callus formation.

Management of hyperkeratotic lesions includes:

1. Reduce amount of thickened keratoses by either mechanical debridement (buffing) or paring with sharp debridement. Topical keratolytic agents containing urea for example Carmol lotion, cream or gel can also be used to "thin" the thickened epidermis and reduce hyperkeratoses, especially on the heels.
2. Pad with sheet hydrogel and silicon-based products that are nonmedicated. Foam pads can also be used.
3. Recommend pressure relief shoes, such as those with a high toe box and padded cushion inserts. There are numerous commercially available inserts and orthotics that can further reduce the build-up of calluses by redistributing weight from highly prominent bony prominences.
4. Instruct client to gently buff areas two to three times per week with a pumice stone and file board before taking a shower or bath and to pad with proper over-the-counter pads, as directed. There is an abundance of silicon-based products, for example Silipos, for the feet and toes, such as sleeves that fit over the toes that are nonadhesive and reusable.

Fissures

Fissures are cracks in the dermis that cause a partial-thickness wound. Management includes:

1. Reduce keratotic tissue around fissure, if present, by mechanical or chemical debridement.
2. Cleanse area and apply dressing, such as thin film, thin hydrocolloid, sheet hydrogel, and dressing cloth tapes, to close the wound. A skin sealant or adhesive such as Dermabond can be used to fill and seal the fissure.
3. Change dressing weekly to allow for closure of wound. If the fissure is draining, red, inflamed, or extremely painful, consider an infection and treat accordingly.
4. Instruct client on moisturizing protocol to prevent further fissures.
5. Instruct client to wear shoes at all times and to avoid slippers or sandals that "flop" against the heel, causing excessive friction.

Onychauxis

Onychauxis describes hypertrophic toenails or excessively thick toenails that result from trauma, aging, genetic predisposition, etc., and is not related to onychomycosis. Management includes:

1. Mechanical debridement is required.
2. Teach client to reduce toenails at home if functionally able, using proper equipment such as nail files.
3. Instruct client to obtain extra-depth shoes or shoes with a high toe box to accommodate thickened toenails.

Self-Care Teaching Guidelines

Specific self-care teaching guidelines have been presented under each specific foot problem. The following include general guidelines for self-care for all foot problems. It is important to instruct clients to purchase shoes that accommodate structural deformities and swelling, offer support and cushion, and are easy to put on and take off. Proper shoes are important for preventing a variety of complications. Those that are too narrow can cause blisters and corns, and shoes that are too short can cause toenail injury and hammertoes. Shoes that offer little support can lead to foot pain. Finally, shoes should be considered functional aids, rather than stylish accompaniments to clothing. Unfortunately, culture often dictates dress codes. The health-care professional can be very influential in helping clients to understand the need for proper footwear, which can prevent serious foot complications, provide relief from excessive pressure and mechanical stress, and add to quality of life by reducing foot pain.

Teaching guidelines for general foot care should address the following:

1. Proper self-care practices to include general information on bathing, drying well between toes, and avoiding excessive soaking. No bathroom surgery!
2. The importance of daily self-inspection of feet and the areas between the toes. A mirror can be placed on the floor so the client can inspect the plantar surface of the foot for any cracks, discolorations, drainage, redness, and swelling. For individuals with limited vision, help from family members and caregivers can be required to inspect the feet.
3. The need to wear shoes at all times, even when getting up at night to go to the bathroom.

4. Information on purchasing proper shoes to accommodate structural deformities, diabetes, and other individuals needs.

5. When to report problems to the health-care provider, such as abnormal sensations and pain in the legs at night or when ambulating.

6. Reminding the health-care provider to inspect the feet routinely during each visit.

Conclusion

Foot problems continue to plague a disproportionately high percentage of older adults, affecting functional abilities and quality of life. In particular, problems affecting the toenails, skin and plantar structures of the foot can have profound consequences such as severe infections or foot deformities. Health-care providers play a key role in the overall care and management of foot health by routinely including questions about the feet in the history, inspecting the skin and nails during the physical examination, and vigorously investigating complaints of heel and plantar foot pain. There are a plethora of evidence-based interventions to guide practice for the purpose of ameliorating and/or preventing more serious foot problems and improving quality of life.

REVIEW QUESTIONS

1. How does the clinical presentation of tinea pedis differ from dry skin (xerosis)?
2. What is the hallmark symptom of plantar fasciitis?
3. Why is wearing shoes one of the most important prevention activities for a variety of foot problems?
4. Why is it important to refer patients for recalcitrant heel pain?

REFERENCES

1. Gupta AK, Chow M, Daniel CR, Aly R. Treatments of tinea pedis. *Dermatology Clin.* 2003;21:431-462.
2. American Diabetes Association Clinical Practice Recommendations. *Diabetes Care.* 2005;28:S20-S21.
3. Armstrong G, Lavery L. Clinical Care of the Diabetic Foot. Alexandria, VA: American Diabetes Association, 2005.
4. Foster KW, Ghannoum MA, Elewski BE. Epidemiologic surveillance of cutaneous fungal infection in the United States from 1999 to 2002. *J Am Acad Dermatol.* 2004;50:748-752.
5. Daniel CR, Daniel MP, Daniel J, et al. Managing simple chronic paronychia and onycholysis with ciclopirox 0.77% and an irritant-avoidance regimen. *Cutis.* 2004;73:81-85.
6. Mayser P, Hensel J, Thoma W, et al. Prevalence of fungal foot infections in patients with diabetes mellitus type I – underestimation of moccasin-type tinea. *Exp Clin Endocrinol Diabetes.* 2004;112:264-268.
7. Gupta AK, Skinner AR, Cooper AE. Interdigital tinea pedis (dermatophytosis simplex and complex) and treatment with ciclopirox 0.77% gel. *Int J Dermatol.* 2003;42(Suppl 1):23-27.
8. Aly R, Fisher G, Katz J, et al. Ciclopirox gel in the treatment of patients with interdigital tinea pedis. *Int J Dermatol.* 2003;42(Suppl 1):29-35.
9. Elewski BE, Haley HR, Robbins CM. The use of 40% urea cream in the treatment of moccasin tinea pedis. *Cutis.* 2004;73:355-357.
10. Tan JS, Joseph WS. Common fungal infections of the feet in patients with diabetes mellitus. *Drugs Aging.* 2004;21:101-112.
11. Erbagci Z. Topical therapy for dermatophytoses: Should corticosteroids be included? *Am J Clin Dermatol.* 2004;5:375-384.
12. Roujeau JC, Sigurgeirsson B, Korting HC, et al. Chronic dermatomycoses of the foot as risk factors for acute bacterial cellulites of the leg: A case-control study. *Dermatology.* 2004;209:301-307.
13. Landorf KB, Keenan AM, Herbert RD. Effectiveness of different types of foot orthoses for the treatment of plantar fasciitis. *J Am Pod Assoc.* 2004;94:542-549.
14. Cole C, Seto C, Gazewood J. Plantar fasciitis: Evidence-based review of diagnosis and therapy. *Am Fam Phys.* 2005;72:2237-2242.
15. Lane GD, London B. Heel spur syndrome: A retrospective report on the percutaneous plantar transverse incisional approach. *J Foot Ankle Surg.* 2004;43:389-394.
16. Weber JM, Vidt LG, Gehl RS, Montgomery T. Calcaneal stress fractures. *Clin Podiatr Med Surg.* 2005;22:45-54.
17. Young B, Walker MJ, Strence J, Boyles R. A combined treatment approach emphasizing impairment-based manual physical therapy for plantar heel pain: A case series. *J Orthop Sports Phys Ther.* 2004;34:725-733.
18. Zhu F, Johnson JE, Hirose CB, Bae KT. Chronic plantar fasciitis: Acute changes in the heel after extracorporeal high-energy shock wave therapy—observations at MR imaging. *Radiology.* 2005;234:206-210.
19. Rompe JD. Shock-wave therapy for plantar fasciitis. *J Bone Joint Surg Am.* 2004;86:2216-2228.
20. Genc H, Saracoglu M, Nacir B, et al. Long-term ultrasonographic follow-up of plantar fasciitis patients treated with steroid injection. *Joint Bone Spine.* 2005;72:61-65.
21. Hogan KA, Webb D, Shereff M. Endoscopic plantar fascia release. *Foot Ankle Int.* 2004;25:875-881.
22. Filippou DK, Kalliakmanis A, Triga A, et al. Sport related plantar fasciitis. Current diagnostic and therapeutic advances. *Folia Med.* 2004;46:56-60.
23. Sigurgeirsson B, Steingrimsson O. Risk factors associated with onychomycosis. *J Eur Acad Dermatol Venereol.* 2004;18:48-51.
24. Huang DB, Ostrosky-Zeichner L, Wu JJ, et al. Therapy of common superficial fungal infections. *Dermatol Ther.* 2004;17:517-522.
25. Campbell AW, Anyanwu EC, Morad M. Evaluation of the drug treatment and persistence of onychomycosis. *Scientific World.* 2004;4:760-777.
26. Baran R, Hay R, Perrin C. Superficial white onychomycosis revisited. *J Eur Acad Dermatol Venereol.* 2004;18:569-571.
27. Piraccini MB, Tosti A. White superficial onychomycosis: Epidemiological, clinical, and pathological study of 79 patients. *Arch Dermatol.* 2004;140:696-701.
28. Theodosat A. Skin diseases of the lower extremities in the elderly. *Dermatol Clin.* 2004;22:13-21.
29. Weinberg JM, Vafaie J, Scheinfeld NS. Skin infections in the elderly. *Dermatol Clin.* 2004;22:51-61.
30. Pattillo MM. Therapeutic and healing foot care: A health feet clinic for older adults. *J Gerontol Nur.* 2004;31:26-32,50-51.
31. Fletcher CL, Hay RJ, Smeeton NC. Onychomycosis: The development of a clinical diagnostic aid for toenail disease. Part I. Establishing discriminating historical and clinical features. *Br J Dermatol.* 2004;150:701-705.
32. Qureshi HS, Ormsby HA, Kapadia N. Effects of modified sample collection technique on fungal culture yield: Nail clipping/scraping versus microdrill. *J Pak Med Assoc.* 2004;54:301-305.
33. Summerbell RC, Cooper E, Bunn U, et al. Onychomycosis: A critical study of techniques and criteria for confirming the etiologic significance of nondermatophytes. *Med Mycol.* 2005;43:39-59.
34. Sidou F, Soto P. A randomized comparison of nail surface remanence of three nail lacquers, containing amorolfine 5%, ciclopirox 8% or tioconazole 28% in healthy volunteers. *Int J Tissue React.* 2004;26:17-24.
35. Gupta AK, Ryder JE. How to improve cure rates for the management of onychomycosis. *Dermatol Clin.* 2003;21:499-505.
36. Gupta AK, Ryder JE, Skinner AR. Treatment of onychomycosis: Pros and cons of antifungal agents. *J Cutan Med Surg.* 2004;8:25-30.
37. Gupta AK, Ryder JE, Johnson AM. Cumulative meta-analysis of systemic antifungal agents for the treatment of onychomycosis. *Br J Dermatol.* 2004;150:537-544.
38. Frankum LE, Nightengale B, Russo CL, Sarnes M. Pharmacoeconomic analysis of sequential treatment pathways in the treatment of onychomycosis. *Manag Care Interface.* 2005;18:55-63.
39. Sanmano B, Hiruma M, Mizoguchi M, Ogawa H. Combination therapy consisting of week pulses of oral terbinafine plus topical application of terbinafine cream in the treatment of onychomycosis. *J Dermatolog Treat.* 2004;15:245-251.

40. Krob AH, Fleischer AB, D'Agostino R, Feldman SR. Terbinafine is more effective than itraconazole in treating toenail onychomycosis: Results from a meta-analysis of randomized controlled trials. *J Cutan Med Surg.* 2003;7:306-311.

41. Pavlotsky F, Armoni G, Shemer A, Trau H. Pulsed versus continuous terbinafine dosing in the treatment of dermatophyte onychomycosis. *J Dermatolog Treat.* 2004;15:315-320.

42. Wenig JA. The systemic treatment of onychomycosis. *Clin Podiatr Med Surg.* 2004;21:579-589.

43. Chen X, Hiruma M, Shiraki Y, Ogawa H. Combination therapy of once-weekly fluconazole (100, 150, or 300 mg) with topical application of ketoconazole cream in the treatment of onychomycosis. *Jpn J Infect Dis.* 2004;57:260-263.

44. Gupta AK, Carney PS, Jegasothy SM, et al. Onychomycosis: Management and treatment. Proceedings of a clinical roundtable. *Cutis.* 2004;74(1 Suppl):16-25.

45. Treating Nail Fungus: Take the Right Steps. Patient Tips from Industry. *Diab Educ.* 2004;30:389-391.

46. Kalinowski DP, Edsberg LE, Hewson RA, et al. Low-voltage direct current as a fungicidal agent for treating onychomycosis. *J Am Podiatr Med Assoc.* 2004;94:565-572.

47. Kelechi TJ, Stroud S. The four V's for foot care: Vaseline, vegetable shortening, vinegar and Vicks VapoRub. *Adv for Nur Pract.* 2004;12:67-70,84.

48. Firooz A, Khamesipour A, Dowlati Y. Itraconazole pulse therapy improves the quality of life of patients with toenail mycosis. *J Dermatolog Treat.* 2003;14:95-98.

Management of Malignant Cutaneous Wounds and Fistulas

Barbara M. Bates-Jensen and Susie Seaman

CHAPTER OBJECTIVES

At the completion of this chapter, the reader will be able to:

1. Explain the significance of symptom assessment in malignant cutaneous wounds.
2. Describe methods of managing bleeding, exudate, and odor in malignant cutaneous wounds.
3. Describe interventions for management of pain related to malignant cutaneous wounds.
4. List and explain factors to be considered when assessing the client with a draining wound or fistula.
5. Examine management methods for the client with a fistula.
6. Design a pouching procedure for a draining wound or fistula.

Significance of Malignant Cutaneous Wounds

Malignant cutaneous wounds, also known in the literature as *fungating tumors/wounds, ulcerating malignant wounds*, or *tumor necrosis*, present both a physical and emotional challenge for patients and even experienced clinicians. Fungating or ulcerating wounds are often unsightly, malodorous, and painful (see *Color Plates 61–65*). These wounds are a blow to self-esteem and may cause social isolation at the very time when the patient needs more time with family and friends. In treating patients with malignant cutaneous wounds, the goal of care is to improve quality of life through symptom palliation. Treatment is directed at alleviation of the distressing symptoms associated with these lesions, with attention focused on minimizing pain and infection, managing exudate and odor, and controlling bleeding. The wound care clinician plays a pivotal role in the development of a treatment plan aimed at decreasing the effect that these lesions have on the patient's quality of life.

Malignant cutaneous lesions may occur in up to 5% of patients with cancer and 10% of patients with metastatic disease. Lookingbill and colleagues[1] retrospectively reviewed data accumulated over a 10-year period from the tumor registry at Hershey Medical Center in Pennsylvania. Of 7,316 patients, 367 (5.0%) had cutaneous malignancies. Of these, 38 patients had lesions as a result of direct local invasion, 337 had metastatic lesions, and 8 had both. A secondary analysis from the same registry found that 420 patients (10.4%) out of 4,020 with metastatic disease had cutaneous involvement.[2] In women, the most common origins of metastasis were breast carcinoma (70.7%) and melanoma (12.0%). In men, melanoma (32.3%), lung carcinoma (11.8%), and colorectal cancer (11.0%) accounted for the most common primary tumors. Although these types of cancer account for the majority of skin involvement, it is important to note that metastatic cutaneous lesions may arise from any type of malignant tumor.[3,4]

Cutaneous metastasis of internal cancer may predict survival time. In a retrospective study of 200 patients who developed cutaneous metastasis over a 46-year period, the median survival time after cutaneous involvement was 6.5 months (mean 22.8 ± 43.8 months).[5] Survival time varied by primary diagnosis. Median survival after cutaneous metastasis of the three most commonly observed cancers were: 2.9 months for bronchopulmonary cancer, 13.8 months for breast cancer, and 15.5 months for melanoma.

Pathophysiology of Malignant Cutaneous Wounds

Malignant cutaneous lesions may be secondary to local invasion of a primary tumor or metastasis from a distant site.[6] Local invasion may initially manifest as inflammation with induration, redness, heat, and/or tenderness. The skin may have a *peau d'orange* appearance, and the area may be fixed to underlying tissue. As the tumor infiltrates the skin, ulcerating and/or fungating wounds develop. In metastatic disease, tumor cells detach from the primary site and travel via blood and/or lymphatic vessels or tissue planes to distant organs, including the skin.[3,4] Infiltration of the skin involves spread of cancerous cells along tissue planes, blood and lymph capillaries, and via perineural spaces because these areas offer little resistance.[7] These lesions may initially present as well-demarcated nodules, ranging in size from a few millimeters to several centimeters. Their consistency may vary from firm to rubbery. There may be pigmentation changes noted over the lesions, from deep red to brown-black. In general, these nodules are painless. Over time, these nodules may ulcerate, drain, and become very painful.

Tumor cells secrete growth factors that promote angiogenesis and extracellular matrix deposition and, thus, tumor growth. Abnormalities in capillary development and lymphatic flow cause changes in local tissue perfusion that lead to increased tumor growth with simultaneous tissue death and alterations in local edema and exudate.[8,9] As the tumor grows larger, it is unable to sustain sufficient vascular growth to support the entire mass. This results in fragile capillaries, poor perfusion, altered collagen synthesis, and resultant tissue ischemia and necrosis.[8] Additional tissue destruction occurs secondary to proteolytic enzymes secreted by tumor cells.[10] The resulting lesion may be fungating, in which the tumor mass extends above the skin surface with a fungus or cauliflower-like appearance, or it may be erosive and ulcerative.[10] The wound bed may be pale pink to red with very friable tissue, completely necrotic, or a combination of both. The fragile capillary bed may result in bleeding, which is frequently a challenge to control. The presence of necrotic tissue results in increased bacterial colonization and offensive odor. Typical organisms that infiltrate metastatic wounds include *Escherichia coli, Pseudomonas aeruginosa,* and strains of *Staphylococcus, Proteus*, and *Klebsiella.*[8,10] Necrotic tissue provides an excellent medium for growth of anaerobes such as *Bacteroides.*[8] The surrounding skin may be erythematous, edematous, fragile, and exceedingly tender to touch. Maceration may occur in the presence of excessive wound exudate.

Malignant Cutaneous Wound Assessment

Assessment of malignant cutaneous wounds includes all parameters of wound assessment, with particular attention to evaluation for potential complications and evaluation of treatment appropriateness. Wound assessment of malignant cutaneous wounds is intended for use not only to document wound improvement or deterioration but also as a precursor to determining treatment needs and evaluating of treatment effectiveness. In particular, attention to size and shape of the lesion, exudate characteristics, wound appearance, including necrotic tissue characteristics and bleeding or ulcerations, odor, presence of infection, and surrounding skin condition are important wound characteristics to consider in planning for topical dressing application.[11,12] Haisfield-Wolfe and Baxendale-Cox[10] have proposed a staging classification system for assessment of malignant cutaneous wounds. Use of wound classification increases communication effectiveness among health-care practitioners and makes treatment evaluation consistent. The proposed classification system was tested in a pilot study with 13 wounds. The wounds were evaluated using wound depth as described with clinical descriptors, predominate color of the wound, hydration status of the wound, drainage, pain, odor, and presence of tunneling or undermining. Use of the Haisfield-Wolfe and Baxendale-Cox classification system provides a basis for a standard set of descriptors that clinicians can use both to understand and to assess malignant cutaneous wounds.

Malignant cutaneous wounds are expected to increase in size over time and to change in appearance. They may occur singly or in groups, and nodules may enlarge and remit, depending on response to treatment.[13] Although chemotherapy and/or radiation therapy may bring about regression of fungating lesions from breast cancer,[14] usual treatment is only palliative to ease suffering, as it can be expected that lesions will eventually recur.[15] Reduction in the size of the lesion may result in decreased exudate and pain, in addition to decreasing bleeding from lesions.[13]

Assessment is composed of the following categories: location, surface appearance, infection, surrounding skin, symptoms, and potential for serious complications. Location of the wound may impair mobility and functional level of the patient. Occupational therapy can help in facilitating activities of daily living and functional ability. Wound location will impact the dressing selection and dressing fixation because malignant cutaneous wounds may be located in wrinkled skin or highly uneven anatomic sites. The location of the wound also has significant psychological impact. If the wound is located in an area where it is easily covered from public view, the patient will respond differently than if the wound is located such that hiding the wound is not possible.

Assessment of wound appearance is not so different from assessment of any other wound type. However, there are some special considerations for malignant cutaneous wounds.[11,12] Wound appearance should be evaluated for size, specifically looking for undermining and deep structure exposure. The wound should be assessed as fungating or ulcerative, with objective assessment of the percentage of viable versus necrotic tissue. Tissue should be assessed for friability and bleeding. Odor and exudate amount should be monitored and the presence of a fistula documented. Evaluation of the wound appearance also includes assessment of wound colonization versus infection. Identification of heavy bacterial colonization provides information on the deterioration or response of the wound to palliative care and can impact dressing selection. Malignant cutaneous wounds that are heavily colonized require special attention to cleansing, odor-reducing dressing selection, and exudate management. Clinically infected malignant cutaneous wounds with associated cellulitis and fever require systemic antibiotic therapy.

The skin surrounding the wound should be evaluated for color, integrity, and presence of nodules or other signs of progression of malignancy. Typically, the skin surrounding malignant cutaneous wounds is erythematous. The skin may be fragile, macerated, or denuded as a result of excess exudate. Many times, extension of the wound can be predicted by the presence of nodules or eruptions in the skin surrounding the wound site. Surrounding skin may also exhibit signs of radiation skin damage, with erythema and other evidence of poor tissue perfusion. Tumor extension or metastasis will impact dressing type selection and fixation methods, such as using nonadherent dressings or methods other than tape for affixing the dressing. Significant deterioration in the surrounding skin becomes problematic in determining appropriate dressing selection because of the need for larger and larger dressings and the problems associated with securing the dressing on the site.

Symptom assessment is also important in malignant cutaneous wounds. The degree of symptoms experienced by the patient will depend on wound location, depth of tissue invasion and damage, nerve involvement, and the patient's previous experience with pain and use of analgesia.[16] The symptoms of pain and pruritus are characteristically associated with these wounds. Pain may include deep pain that is characterized by continuous aching or stabbing and superficial pain such as burning and stinging that may be associated only with dressing changes. If pain symptoms are the result of dressing changes, use of a short-acting topical analgesic with a rapid onset will be beneficial for total management of the wound. These fast-acting pain medications make dressing changes more bearable for the patient. If the pruritic symptoms are related to dressings, the remedy may be as simple as trying a different dressing. More typically, pruritus may be a side effect of systemic analgesia and, if significant to the patient, may warrant change in pain medication or new systemic medications.

Assessment of the malignant cutaneous wound must include assessment of the potential for serious complications. Evaluation should include potential for hemorrhage, especially for patients in which the lesion is located close to major blood vessels. Lesions in these areas may also lead to blood vessel compression and obstruction. Lesions in the neck and chest area pose the threat of airway obstruction. Assessment includes attention to potential complications of bleeding and hemorrhage, swelling, pain, tissue necrosis, and airway obstruction.

Assessment of potential complications also involves evaluation of the patient's risk for infection and local bleeding secondary to capillary fragility. The presence of bacterial colonization results in increased odor and exudate. This may be a common observation in patients with cutaneous tumors, and its presence indicates a need for a change in local care. If accompanied by signs of infection such as increased erythema, exudate, pain, and/or fever, there is an invasive infection that necessitates systemic care. Observation of local bleeding necessitates use of extreme care in dressing removal and the need for preparation to control it. Assessment of treatment effectiveness must occur at each dressing change. If the wound is noted to be degenerating, the treatment may need to be changed more frequently than in other wound types. Pain assessment is critical, because these wounds are often very painful, and adequate analgesia can control the pain and improve quality of life.

Malignant Cutaneous Wound Management

Control of bacterial colonization, exudate, odor, bleeding, and pain are the cornerstones of management for malignant cutaneous wounds.[6,11,17–22] In determining the appropriate treatment regimen, the abilities of the caregiver must also be considered. The limited information on treatment effectiveness reflects the absence of evidenced-based care in this area and the extreme need for further research and dissemination of findings.[18]

Infection Control: Wound Cleansing and Debridement

Infection control is facilitated by focusing on wound cleansing and wound debridement. Because malignant cutaneous lesions are frequently associated with necrotic tissue and odor, wound cleansing is essential to remove necrotic debris, decreasing bacterial counts and, thus, reducing odor.

CLINICAL WISDOM

If the lesion is not very friable, the patient may be able to get in the shower. This not only provides for local cleansing but also gives the added psychological benefit of helping the patient to feel clean. The patient should be instructed to allow the shower water to hit the skin above the wound, then allow the water to run over the wound.

If there is friable tissue (tissue that bleeds easily with minimal trauma) or the patient is not able to shower, the nurse/caregiver should gently irrigate the wound with normal saline or a commercial wound cleanser. For wounds without tissue friability that have increased necrosis and/or odor requiring more aggressive cleansing, low-pressure irrigation with normal saline can be performed using a 35-cc syringe and a 19-gauge needle held a few inches away from the wound. Saline has the advantage of not disturbing any tissue that might be healthy, but a disadvantage is the lack of odor-reducing ingredients. Skin cleansers are highly efficacious at controlling odor in cutaneous tumors that have significant tissue necrosis and a high bacterial burden because they contain antiseptics. In many cases, the use of skin cleansers alone will be sufficient to control odor without the need for further products. They are also useful to gently cleanse the surrounding skin. However, the patient may experience burning from skin cleansers, especially if the wound has a large amount of viable tissue, and in that case, they should be avoided in favor of saline or wound cleansers.

RESEARCH WISDOM

For wound cleansing in malignant cutaneous wounds, Collinson[23] suggests using warmed saline, and Cormier and colleagues[24] have suggested use of a handheld shower head and tepid water with liquid soap.

Use of antimicrobial solutions, such as povidone-iodine, sodium hypochlorite solution, chlorhexidine, or hydrogen peroxide are not recommended by some;[6,15] however, sodium hypochlorite solution and chlorhexidine are recommended by others.[8] If these products are utilized, no more than two weeks of treatment should be considered because of significant burning, wound desiccation, and skin irritation that can be associated with their use. The rationale for antimicrobial solution use is the decrease of bacterial burden on the surface of the wound, with resultant decrease in odor. However, the antimicrobial solutions do not inhibit further bacterial proliferation because they are inactivated by body fluids, blood, pus, and slough (all of which are found in abundance in malignant cutaneous wounds).[25,26] In addition, these chemicals can have their own offensive odor that may be troublesome for the patient. For these reasons, skin cleansers may be worth a try before using the stronger antimicrobial solutions. Wound cleansing is followed by necrotic tissue debridement, if necessary.

Necrotic tissue in malignant cutaneous wounds is typically dry, encrusted material, slough, or black eschar. Necrotic tissue in malignant cutaneous wounds may be extremely malodorous. Conservative debridement strategies are the basis for odor control. Use of autolysis, enzymatic, and/or conservative sharp debridement are the preferred options. Debridement of dry, encrusted material and black eschar may be best accomplished with a protocol described by Collinson,[23] involving warm normal saline cleansing, application of an amorphous hydrogel primary dressing, and covering with a thin film dressing as secondary dressing. The dressing is changed daily at first and less frequently as debridement occurs. It should be noted that use of the thin film dressing will significantly increase wound odor (which may not be tolerable for patients and caregivers), and the adhesive backing may damage the fragile surrounding skin. Collinson[23] describes initiation of liquefaction of necrotic tissue within 24 hours of starting the dressing. The hydrogel dressing allows for rehydration of the necrotic tissue and manages drainage associated with autolytic debridement. Use of hydrogel dressings is a gentle debridement technique with the additional advantage of decreasing pain.[20]

Procedures for sloughy, wet, necrotic tissue differ. Collinson[23] advocates using calcium alginate dressings as a primary dressing and covering with either a thin film dress-

ing or a foam dressing. The use of the calcium alginate dressing has the additional advantage of controlling bleeding in the wound site. Secondary foam dressings will result in less odor than will use of secondary transparent film dressings; foam dressings will not damage fragile surrounding tissues. Use of this procedure adequately debrides soft, sloughy, necrotic tissue while protecting surrounding skin from maceration by controlling exudate.

CLINICAL WISDOM

Debridement is best done by enzymatic, autolytic, or conservative sharp methods and gentle mechanical methods (such as low-pressure irrigation), as opposed to wet-to-dry dressings, which are traumatic, painful, and can cause significant bleeding upon removal.

If eschar on the tumor is extensive and thickly adherent to the tissues, sharp debridement may be indicated to allow for infection prevention, odor control, and exudate management. Clinical wound infection, as evidenced by clinical signs of infection (increased exudate, erythema, induration, pain, and/or fever) may be effectively treated with topical antibiotic preparations or topical antimicrobial dressings (such as silver impregnated products), in conjunction with systemic antibiotics. The topical preparation may work better in malignant cutaneous wounds, because of the decreased perfusion and vasculature throughout the tumor that impedes systemic antibiotic dissemination, making the combination approach most successful.

Management of Exudate and Odor Control

The goal in management of exudate is to provide a moist wound environment to prevent trauma from drying and fissuring, or dressing adherence.[27] The wound should be kept moist, but not wet. Dressings should be chosen both to conceal and to collect exudate *and* odor.[12] It is crucial to use dressings that absorb and contain exudate because a patient who experiences unexpected drainage on clothing or bedding may experience significant feelings of distress and loss of control. Specialty dressings, such as foams, alginates, or starch copolymers, are notably more expensive than gauze pads or cotton-based absorbent pads. However, if the use of these dressings reduces cost by reducing the need for frequent dressing changes (improving quality of life for the patient), they are cost-effective, both in terms of dollars spent and quality of care. In wounds with low exudate, the goal is to maintain a moist environment and to prevent dressing adherence and bleeding. Dressing choices for wounds in this category include nonadherent contact layers, such as Adaptic (Johnson & Johnson), Dermanet (DeRoyal), Mepitel (Mölnlycke), petrolatum gauze (numerous manufacturers), and Tegapore (3M Health Care). Amorphous hydrogels, sheet hydrogels, and hydrocolloids may also be helpful for low exudate wounds. Hydrocolloids are contraindicated with fragile surrounding skin and may increase odor. Semipermeable film dressings are also contraindicated with fragile surrounding skin. Nonadherent dressings are best for the primary contact layer because they minimize the trauma to the wound associated with dressing changes.

Wounds with high exudate require attention to absorbing and containing exudate. Dressings such as alginates, foams, starch copolymers, gauze, and soft cotton pads are all possible selections. Seaman[28] suggests nonadherent contact layers (such as petrolatum gauze) for the primary dressing on the wound bed, covered with soft, absorbent dressings (such as gauze and abdominal binder dressings) for secondary dressings to contain drainage. The dressing should be changed one to two times daily. When drainage increases, the use of calcium alginate dressings to decrease the frequency of dressing changes may be considered. Grocott[29] also recommends use of calcium alginate dressings and discusses use of hydrocolloids for less exudative wounds. Hydrocolloids may be difficult to apply to the uneven surface of malignant cutaneous wounds, and gel dressings may be easier for caregivers to manage. Protection of the surrounding skin and tissues is another goal with exudate management.

CLINICAL WISDOM

Use of menstrual pads as wound dressing selection may be helpful for wounds with heavy exudate. These pads have the added benefit of clothing protection because of the outer plastic lining.

Using skin barriers on the skin surrounding the wound, then taping dressings to the skin barriers (changing the barriers every 5–7 days), is one method of protecting surrounding skin from both excess drainage and tape, and the resultant skin stripping with dressing changes. Another method of protecting the surrounding skin is use of a barrier ointment to the skin surrounding the ulcer. The barrier protects fragile tissue from maceration and the caustic effects of the drainage on the skin. Dressings can then be held in place with Montgomery straps or tape affixed to a skin barrier placed on healthy skin, flexible netting, tube dressings, sports bras, panties, and the like.[12]

Odor control is by far the most challenging management aspect of malignant cutaneous wounds. Literature supports use of metronidazole (Flagyl, Helidac, MetroCream, MetroGel, Noritate Cream) topically in controlling wound odor.[30–37] Application of MetroGel (Galderma Laboratories), a 0.75% topical antibiotic, to the wound results in a decrease in wound odor in 2–3 days, even in the presence of resistant odor.[14,30–33] Typically, dressings are changed once to twice daily, and the topical gel may be supplemented with irrigant solution. Topical therapy is available by crushing metronidazole tablets in sterile water and creating either a 0.5% solution (5 mg/cc) or a 1% solution (10 mg/cc).[13,35] Additionally, as an irrigant solution, 500 mg metronidazole in 100 mL normal saline IV solution can be used to irrigate the wound and may be used as a wet-to-moist gauze dressing (this may be very effective for packing undermined or tunneled areas of the wound).[36,37] Cau-

tion must be used with this method to prevent adherence of the gauze to the wound and subsequent bleeding and pain. Others have reported odor reduction with use of 0.8% metronidazole gel, with or without systemic therapy. Systemic metronidazole 500 mg three to four times a day may also be administered when clinical infection is suspected or for severe wound odor management, but caution should be used because of the adverse gastrointestinal effects that may occur.[38,39]

Another topical antimicrobial agent is Iodosorb gel, an iodine complexed in a starch copolymer (cadexomer iodine). This product contains slow-release iodine and has been shown to decrease bacterial counts in wounds without cytotoxicity.[40,41] Seaman has had clinical experience with this product in reducing odor associated with venous ulcers. Cadexomer iodine is available in a 40-g tube and is applied to the wound in a 1/8-inch layer. An advantage of this product is exudate absorption, in that each gram absorbs 6 mL of fluid. Disadvantages include cost (comparable with metronidazole 0.75% gel) and possible burning on application.

CLINICAL WISDOM

Use of peppermint oil or other aromatherapy products in the environment around the patient may help in eliminating wound odor. Charcoal also acts to absorb the odor from the wound. A basket of charcoal under the bed or table may also help in ridding the environment of wound odor for the home care patient.[24] Kitty litter under the bed may also decrease odor in the patient's room. Use of charcoal dressings may also be helpful in odor management. Many charcoal dressings are expensive and less flexible, so their use must be individualized as appropriate. Charcoal dressings typically are applied after the primary and secondary dressings have been applied and may be reused with each dressing change unless strike-through of wound drainage has occurred.

Less conventional methods of odor management are also available. The topical use of yogurt or buttermilk has been reported to be successful in eliminating some malignant cutaneous wound odors.[38,42,43] The yogurt or buttermilk is applied topically to the wound after cleansing. The use of yogurt or buttermilk may work by decreasing the wound pH, thus stunting bacterial proliferation and the resultant odor. It is theorized that the low pH of the lactobacilli present in the yogurt and buttermilk is responsible for the alteration in wound pH. There are limited studies supporting the use of yogurt or buttermilk, and none have addressed specific limitations or contraindications for use of the treatment.

The following case illustrates the positive effect that the wound care clinician can have on patients with malignant cutaneous wounds. Not all wounds will heal, and palliative management of these wounds is just as important as taking other types of wounds to complete closure.

CASE STUDY

An anxious 82-year-old woman with breast cancer with cutaneous metastasis to the left chest wall was referred to the Wound Healing Center. She was accompanied by her daughter, who was also very anxious and worried. The patient had undergone a mastectomy and radiation therapy 4 years prior and had developed chest wall metastasis 8 months before referral. Current wound care included no cleansing, and she kept the wound covered with dry gauze, which would adhere to the wound. Her main complaint was of severe pain, which she rated an "8" on a scale of 0–10 and described as a constant ache with intermittent sharp pains in the area of the tumor metastasis. Current pain management consisted of oral hydrocodone with acetaminophen, one tablet four times a day. She felt that pain was something that could not be controlled and that she would have to live with it. Her second complaint was of severe malodor associated with the wound, and she stated that her main goal in coming to the Wound Healing Center was to learn how to care for the wound and decrease the odor. Assessment revealed a 5 × 5 cm moderately dry necrotic wound on the left chest wall (see *Color Plate 61*) with severe malodor, scant tan exudate from the lower edge, and very thin, fragile surrounding skin.

The necrotic tissue was sharp debrided, taking care not to damage viable tissue or cause pain or bleeding. The wound was then thoroughly cleaned and rinsed with a skin cleanser, resulting in almost total elimination of odor. It was noted that the superior edge of the wound was fungating and mildly friable and there was rib exposure at the base of the wound (see *Color Plate 62*). The daughter was instructed on the following daily wound care:

1. Cleanse the wound and skin with skin cleanser and pat dry.
2. Apply a thin coat of metronidazole gel 0.75% across the wound.
3. Cover with one to three layers of petrolatum gauze (one layer to start and add more layers if the wound dries out and the dressing adheres to the tissue).
4. Cover the wound and surrounding skin with an absorbent ABD pad and secure with chest stockinette.

A long discussion was undertaken with the patient and daughter regarding pain management. The oncologist was contacted, who started the patient on Duragesic patch 25 mcg to be changed every 72 hours, and the patient was continued on the hydrocodone for breakthrough pain.

The patient returned to the clinic two weeks later. She was in much better spirits and reported complete control of the odor. She was now on Duragesic patch 50 mcg, with use of two to four hydrocodone per day and reported pain at a 2–3 on a scale of 0–10, which was acceptable to her. She felt very encouraged by her progress, and her daughter reported that she was much more interactive with the family. The patient and daughter were extremely appreciative of the simple interventions that had been undertaken to improve the patient's quality of life.

The patient continued with monthly reassessments in the Wound Healing Center, and 3 months later, reported problems with bleeding from the tumor. She had been hospitalized for one significant episode of bleeding and had undergone angiography and catheter embolization of the artery feeding the tumor. This had stopped any major bleeding but she reported continued seepage from the friable areas of the tumor and was quite scared by this. Assessment revealed an area of friable tissue with no large vessels visible. Bleeding was easily controlled in the clinic with pressure and silver nitrate application. She was reassured that bleeding was normal and that she and her daughter could handle all but the most severe of bleeding episodes with the following steps, advancing to each subsequent step if bleeding was not controlled:

1. Rest in reclined position with chest and head elevated.
2. Apply local pressure with water-moistened gauze for 15 minutes.
3. Apply oxidized regenerated cellulose and collagen (Promogran) to any bleeding areas and continue pressure for 15 minutes.
4. Apply ice packs to the area for 15–20 minutes.
5. Gently apply silver nitrate with the use of silver nitrate sticks (the daughter was instructed in this and the patient was given a prescription for same).
6. Contact physician or Wound Healing Center if bleeding continues. As the patient was not on hospice care, she was instructed to go to the Emergency Room for any significant, high-volume bleeding.

When the patient was assessed the next month, she reported mild episodes of bleeding that were controlled with pressure alone. She stated that once she had been taught that bleeding was normal from these types of wounds, she had not worried about it and it had not been a problem. Pain and odor remained under good control, despite the fact that the wound was obviously larger, with increased rib exposure.

Controlling Bleeding

Wound bleeding is common in malignant cutaneous wounds. Prevention is the best therapy for controlling bleeding. Prevention involves use of a gentle hand in dressing removal and thoughtful attention to use of nonadherent dressings or moist wound dressings. Dressings should be soaked off with normal saline for easy, nontraumatic removal.[14] On wounds with low exudate, the use of hydrogel sheets, or amorphous hydrogels under a nonadherent contact layer, may keep the wound moist and prevent dressing adherence. Even highly exudating wounds may require a nonadherent contact layer to allow for nontraumatic dressing removal. When dressings stick to the wound on removal, they should be soaked away with normal saline or water to lessen the trauma to the wound bed. Even with use of nonadherent or moist wound dressings, bleeding may occur in malignant cutaneous wounds. Applying direct pressure to visible bleeding vessels for 10–15 minutes is the first intervention. The addition of ice packs may be helpful and also contribute to local comfort. If pressure alone is ineffective, several other options exist.

One suggestion is use of calcium alginate or collagen dressings because both have hemostatic properties.[13] Others advise use of gauze soaked in 1:1000 epinephrine over the bleeding point or application of sucralfate (Carafate) paste (crush a 1-g sucralfate tablet in 2–3 mL of water-soluble gel) over widespread oozing.[14,22] As an alternative, use of a topical absorbable hemostatic products, such as purified gelatin (Gelfoam, Pfizer) or oxidized regenerated cellulose (Surgicel, Johnson & Johnson), may be appropriate. Oxidized regenerated cellulose/bovine collagen (Promogran, Johnson & Johnson) has not been studied for control of bleeding, but may be of use in controlling mild bleeding. Small bleeding points can be handled with silver nitrate sticks. If bleeding continues, more aggressive palliation may be necessary. Radiation therapy may be useful in achieving hemostasis.[14] Additionally, super-selective angiography with transcatheter embolization of the arteries supplying the tumor may control bleeding and shrink the lesion.[44] Uncontrolled bleeding, as well as continuous capillary oozing, can result in acute and chronic anemia.

Minimizing Pain

There are several types of pain associated with malignant cutaneous wounds, deep aching and/or sharp pain, burning/stinging sensations, and superficial pain related to procedures. Deep pain should be managed by regularly scheduled oral, subcutaneous, or parenteral analgesics, with extra premedication prior to dressing changes. Opioids for pre-procedural medication may be needed, and rapid-onset, short-acting analgesics may be especially useful for those already receiving other opioid medication. Use of non-steroidal anti-inflammatory drugs may be beneficial.[14]

For management of superficial pain related to procedures, Seaman[28] recommends use of Hurricaine Topical Anesthetic Aerosol Spray, which is a reasonably priced, over-the-counter aerosol of benzocaine 20%. The onset of action is 15–30 seconds, and the spray is applied after removing the dressing prior to wound cleansing and again after wound cleansing, for residual action. If the spray is applied to the chest wall or head/neck wounds, the patient's face should be covered to prevent mouth and throat numbness if inhaled. Topical lidocaine cream in a liposomal matrix for enhanced tissue penetration (L.M.X.™ 4%, Ferndale Laboratories) is an over-the-counter product that provides good superficial anesthesia to cuts and abrasions.[45] It may be more effective that benzocaine or lidocaine gel or spray in managing superficial tumor pain. Use of ice packs over tender areas may be beneficial to some patients for pain relief.[28]

Another emerging option for topical analgesia is the use of topical opioids, which bind to peripheral opioid receptors.[46–50] Back and Finlay[47] reported the use of diamorphine 10 mg added to an amorphous hydrogel and applied to the wounds of three patients on a daily basis. Two of the patients had painful pressure ulcers, and the third had a painful malignant ulceration. All three patients were on systemic opioids. The patients noted improved pain control on the first day of treatment. Krajnik and Zbigniew[48] reported the case of a 76-year-old woman with metastatic lesions on her scalp that caused severe tension pain. Ibuprofen 400 mg three times a day was ineffective, and because the pain was in a limited area, the authors applied morphine 0.08% gel (3.2 mg morphine in 4 g of amorphous hydrogel). The patient's pain decreased from 7 on a 10-point visual analogue scale (VAS) to 1 within 2 hours of gel application. Pain increased back to 6 on the VAS at 25.5 hours postapplication. Therefore, the gel was reapplied daily and maintained pain control with no side effects. Similar results have been obtained by other authors in the care of patients with painful ulcers.[49,50] In addition, Ballas[51] noted success in treating two patients with painful sickle cell ulcers using topical crushed oxycodone on one patient and topical crushed meperidine on another one. Wound care clinicians should consider this option for topical pain relief in the care of patients with localized pain from a cutaneous tumor. Because wound care is performed frequently in these patients, the addition of topical opioids may be an excellent adjunct to the pain management plan.

Other Management Options

Many patients in the early stages of cutaneous metastasis or local invasion may be candidates for more aggressive care aimed at tumor shrinkage and the resulting decrease in pain, exudate, bleeding, and odor. These treatments may include transcatheter embolization,[44] local radiation therapy,[14] and/or intra-arterial chemotherapy.[52] Bufill, Grace, and Neff reported the case of a 59-year-old woman with an extensive fungating chest wall tumor secondary to breast cancer whose tumor completely resolved following local intra-arterial chemotherapy.[52] She died 10 months later with only a palpable breast mass but no open wound.

Despite the fact that patients may eventually succumb to the underlying cancer and that there may no longer be a curative treatment available, individual patients may benefit from temporary improvement in the lesion through more aggressive palliative treatments. The wound care clinician should speak with the patient's primary provider about the feasibility of these treatments for individual patients.

Malignant Cutaneous Wound Outcome Measures

The expected outcome for most malignant cutaneous wounds is that the wound will deteriorate and increase in size. Outcome measures are, therefore, related to palliation of symptoms, not wound healing. The major goals of therapy are to reduce odor, manage exudate, minimize pain, and control bleeding. Outcomes of therapy relate to the ability and success of the treatment in meeting these goals. Patient or caregiver reports of wound odor or even of the amount of time family members spend with the patient on a daily basis are good measures of outcomes related to achieving effective odor control. Outcomes related to effective management of exudate include the amount and type of exudate and possibly the number of dressing changes per day to manage exudate. Other options for outcome measures related to exudate are the number of accidental leaks of exudate through to clothing or maceration of surrounding skin because of moisture.

Pain outcome measures must include patient self-report with an evidence-based tool for assessment of pain. Additional outcomes related to pain and discomfort may be related to the patient's perception of the wound dressing itself. The dressing should be perceived as comfortable, accessible, user-friendly, and as staying in place for the desired time period.[13] The amount of analgesia required by the patient is not a good outcome measure for pain because the implication is that as the analgesia amount decreases the outcome improves, and this is generally not the case with palliative care. In fact, in many instances, the amount of analgesia will increase over the course of therapy.

Outcome measures for controlling bleeding may include monitoring of hemoglobin and hematocrit status and prevention of excessive trauma to the wound by the wound dressing, as well as frequency of bleeding events. Outcome measures typically will reflect the goals of therapy; therefore, with malignant cutaneous wounds, outcomes are focused on alleviation of suffering related to the wound. Achievement of comfort, general psychological well-being, and a satisfactory level of physical functioning can all be measures of patient outcomes.[13]

Patient and Caregiver Education Related to Malignant Cutaneous Wounds

The same education provided to the patient and caregiver about basic wound care should be provided to those with malignant cutaneous wounds. Frequency and procedures for dressing changes, including time of premedication for pain management and alternatives for odor control, should be presented and reinforced. Education regarding reportable conditions is important. Patient and caregivers should be taught to report the following conditions to their health-care provider:

- Excessive or malodorous exudate
- Pruritus or cellulitis
- Severe emotional distress
- Increased or change in pain
- Bleeding
- Fever
- Unusual or major change in the wound appearance
- Inability of the caregiver to manage wound care
- Inability to obtain needed wound care supplies[13]

Patient and caregiver education must also focus on the psychosocial aspects of malignant cutaneous wounds. Patients are often unable to separate themselves from the wound and may feel as though their body is rotting away. Indeed, patients are often unable to view the wound, may become nauseous or retch when dressing changes are performed, or provide other signs of low self-esteem related to the wound. The clinician can facilitate a trusting relationship with the patient by reviewing the goals of care and by openly discussing issues that the patient may not have talked about with other providers. For example, it is helpful to acknowledge odor openly, then to discuss how the odor will be managed. Attention to cosmetic appearance of the wound with the dressing in place can assist the patient in dealing with body image disturbances. Use of flexible dressings (such as foam dressings and thin film dressings) and use of dressings that can fill a defect (such as pastes or calcium alginates) may be appropriate in restoring symmetry and providing adequate cosmesis for the patient.[13]

Isolation may result from embarrassment, shame, or guilt. Family caregivers may be overcome by the appearance of the wound or the other associated characteristics, such as the odor. Assisting the patient and the caregiver to deal with the distressing symptoms of the malignant cutaneous wounds such that odor is managed, pain is alleviated, and exudate is contained will allow for time to deal with the psychosocial issues related to body image disturbance. Improving cosmetic appearance of the wound, eliminating odor, and containing exudate will help to achieve the goal of satisfactory psychological well-being.

Education must include realistic goals for the wound. Both the patient and the caregiver must understand the realistic goals of care. In malignant cutaneous wounds, the goal of complete wound healing is seldom achievable, but through attention to exudate, odor, and pain, the patient's quality of life can be maintained, even as the malignant cutaneous wound degenerates. Determination of priority goals in palliation may be the first step in patient and caregiver education. For example, if the patient is most disturbed by odor, measures to address wound odor should be foremost in the treatment plan. Continual education and evaluation of the effectiveness of the treatment plan are essential to maintaining quality of life for those suffering with malignant cutaneous wounds.

Significance of Fistulas

A fistula is an abnormal passage or opening between two or more body organs or spaces. The most frequently involved organs are the skin and digestive tract, although fistulas can occur between many other body organs/spaces. Often, the organs involved and the location of the fistula influence management methods and may complicate care, although the goal of care is fistula closure. For example, fistulas involving the small bowel and the vaginal vault and those involving the esophagus and skin both create extreme challenges in care related to both the location and the organs involved in the fistula. The enterocutaneous fistula (ECF) and fistulas involving the pancreas are also typically problematic. This chapter predominantly addresses ECFs.

Spontaneous closure of ECFs with adequate medical management can occur in 60%–85% of all enteric or small bowel fistulas.[53–56] Adequate medical management includes nutrition supplementation and support e.g., enteral or parenteral with or without Somatostatin infusion. The time required to achieve closure ranges from 5 to 26 days, thus requiring long-term treatment plans for all patients with fistulas. Of the ECFs that will close spontaneously, 90% will do so within a 4- to 7-week time frame.[55,57–59] Therefore, if the fistula has not spontaneously closed with adequate medical treatment (e.g., management of sepsis and parenteral or enteral nutrition with or without Somatostatin infusion) within 7 weeks, the goal of care may change from fistula closure to management of the fistula for quality of life. Palliative care is particularly needed when the chances of fistula closure are limited by other nonmodifiable factors. Factors that inhibit fistula closure include complete disruption of bowel continuity, distal obstruction, presence of a foreign body in the fistula tract, an epithelium-lined tract contiguous with the skin, presence of cancer, previous radiation, and Crohn's disease.[59] The goal for fistula care is closure of the fistula (either spontaneous or surgical) through attention to fluid and electrolyte balance, prevention of sepsis and infection control, maintenance of adequate nutrition, and protection of surrounding tissues.[59] Goals of care for palliative fistula management involve containment of effluent, management of odor, increased comfort, and protection of the surrounding skin and tissues. Patients with a fistula demonstrate 5%–21% mortality despite advancements in care practices, including fluid and electrolyte stabilization, nutritional support, surgical management, and diagnosis and treatment of infection.[53–55,59]

Surgical management may be indicated for fistula closure and for palliative care. However, fistula recurrence has been reported in 20% of persons within 3 months following surgery.[60] Optimizing the patient prior to surgical procedures is desired, and the exact timing of the intervention is highly individualized. Management involves surgical resection, bypass, diversion, or endoscopic use of fibrin tissue glue. Surgical resection involves removal of the diseased area of the intestine, including the fistula site, with end-to-end anastomosis and temporary diversion to protect the healing site. Surgical bypass involves using end-to-end anastomosis of the intestinal tract, bypassing or going around the fistula site. The intestinal tract just before and just after the fistula opening are anastomosed together, effectively isolating and separating the area of the intestine containing the fistula opening. Surgical diversion involves creation of an ostomy located proximal to the fistula site, thus diverting the fecal stream before it reaches the fistula site. Use of endoscopic procedures and fibrin tissue glue has also been used to seal low-output fistulas and anal fistulas, with no adverse effects and early healing reported.[61–63] Fistulas involving the bladder (e.g., enterovesical fistulas) require surgical intervention for closure.

Pathophysiology of Fistula Development

In cancer care, those with gastrointestinal cancers and/or those who have received irradiation to pelvic organs are at highest risk of fistula development. Fistula development occurs in 1% of patients with advanced malignancy.[64] In most cases of advanced malignancy, the fistula develops in relation to either obstruction from the malignancy or from irradiation side effects. Radiation therapy damages vasculature and causes damage to underlying structures. In cancer-related fistula development, management is almost always palliative. However, fistula development is not limited to those with cancer.

In addition to cancer patients or those who have received radiation therapy, postsurgical adhesions, inflammatory bowel disease (e.g., Crohn's disease), and small bowel obstruction all place an individual at high risk for fistula development. One major cause of fistula development is postsurgical adhesions. Adhesions are scar tissues that promote fistula development by providing an obstructive process within the normal intestinal passageway. Many clinicians have reported the majority of fistula cases as arising from anastomotic breakdown immediately following surgical procedures.[57,65] Inadequate blood supply and aggressiveness of surgical procedure can create vulnerability to fistula formation in surgical patients.

Those with inflammatory bowel disease, Crohn's disease in particular, are prone to fistula development by virtue of effects of the disease process on the bowel itself. Crohn's disease often involves the perianal area, with fissures and fistulas common findings. Because Crohn's disease is a transmural disease, involving all layers of the bowel wall, patients with Crohn's are prone to fistula development. Crohn's disease can occur anywhere along the entire gastrointestinal tract, and there is no known cure. Initially, the disease is managed medically with steroids, immunotherapy, and metronidazole for perianal disease. If medical management fails, the patient may be treated with surgical creation of an ostomy in an attempt to remove the bowel affected with the disease. In later stages of disease, if medical and surgical management has failed, multiple fistulas may present clinically, and the goal for care becomes palliative, with symptom control the primary objective.

Other factors contributing to fistula development include the presence of a foreign body next to a suture line, tension on a suture line, improper suturing technique, distal obstruction, hematoma/abscess formation, tumor or additional disease in the bowel anastomotic site, and inadequate blood supply.[66] Each of these can contribute to fistula formation by promoting an abnormal passage between two body organs. Typically, the contributing factor provides a path of least resistance for evacuation of stool or urine along the tract, rather than through the normal route. Such is the case with a foreign body next to the suture line and hematoma or abscess formation. In some cases, the normal passageway is blocked, as with tumor growth or obstructive processes.

Finally, in many cases, the pathology relates to inadequate tissue perfusion, as with tension on the suture line, improper suturing, and inadequate blood supply.

Fistula Assessment

Assessment of the fistula involves assessment of the fistula source, surrounding skin and fistula output, and fluid and electrolyte status. Evaluation of the fistula source may involve use of diagnostic tests, such as radiographs, to determine exact structures involved in the fistula tract. Additional tests with computed tomography and magnetic resonance imaging may be required to rule out abscess or complicated fistula tracts.[59] Assessment of the fistula source involves evaluation of fistula output for odor, color, consistency, pH, and amount.[67] These all provide clues to the fistula origin.

Fistulas with highly odorous output likely originate in the colon or may be related to cancerous lesions. Fistula output with minimal odor may be from small bowel origins. Color of fistula output also provides clues to the source of the fistula. Clear or white output is typical of esophageal fistulas. Green output is usual of fistulas originating from the gastric area. Light brown or tan output may indicate fistula output from small bowel sources. Small bowel output is typically thin and watery to thick and pasty in consistency, whereas colonic fistulas have output with a pasty to a soft consistency.

The volume of output is often an indication of the source of the fistula. For small bowel fistulas, output is typically high with volumes from 500 mL over 24 hours for low-output fistulas, to 3,000 mL over 24 hours for high-output fistulas. Esophageal fistula output may be as high as 1,000 mL over 24 hours. Fistulas can be classified according to output, with less than 500 mL over 24 hours classified as low-output fistulas and those with greater than 500 mL over 24 hours classified as high-output fistulas.[59, 66]

Assessment of the anatomic orifice location, the proximity of the orifice to bony prominences, regularity and stability of the surrounding skin, number of fistula openings, and the level the fistula orifice exits onto the skin all influence treatment options. Fistulas may be classified according to the organs involved in the defect and according to the location of the opening of the fistula orifice. Fistulas with openings from one internal body organ to another (such as from small bowel to bladder or from bladder to vagina) are *internal* fistulas, whereas those with cutaneous involvement (such as small bowel to skin) are termed *external* fistulas. Exhibit 21-1 presents common fistula terminology related to internal and external fistula types.

CLINICAL WISDOM

The location of the fistula often impedes containment of fistula output. Skin integrity should be assessed for erythema, ulceration, maceration, or denudement from fistula output. Typically, the more caustic the fistula output, the more impaired the surrounding skin integrity. Multiple fistula tracts may also hamper containment efforts.

EXHIBIT 21-1   Fistula Terminology

Fistula Name	Organs Involved/Fistula Type
Pancreatico-colonic	Pancreas to colon/internal
Enterocutaneous	Small bowel to skin/external
Enterovesical	Small bowel to bladder/internal
Enterovaginal	Small bowel to vagina/internal
Colocutaneous	Colon to skin/external
Colovesical	Colon to bladder/internal
Rectovaginal	Rectum to vagina/internal
Vesicocutaneous	Bladder to skin/external

Assessment of fluid and electrolyte balance is essential in fistula assessment. Patients with ECFs are at high risk for fluid volume deficit or dehydration and metabolic acidosis, because of the loss of large volumes of alkaline small bowel contents. Significant losses of sodium and potassium are common with small bowel fistulas. Laboratory values should be monitored frequently. Evaluation for signs of fluid volume deficit is also recommended. Fistulas of gastrointestinal origins are more prone to electrolyte and fluid disruptions. Exhibit 21-2 presents typical composition of output from gastrointestinal organs involved in fistulas.

Fistula Management

Nutrition management and fluid and electrolyte maintenance are both essential in adequate fistula care. One of the cornerstones of fistula management is attention to nutrition. Most fistula patients are malnourished and become more so as the duration of time with the fistula increases. Fluid and nutritional requirements may be greatly increased with fistulas, and there are difficulties using the gastrointestinal system with ECFs. Lack of adequate intake of protein and calories, inadequate digestion and absorption of nutrients, extreme losses of nutrient-rich output, and increased metabolic demands from infection also contribute to the nutritional deficits present in patients with fistulas. Consultation with a nutritionist or dietician is highly encouraged early in the management of the fistula patient.

Protein and calorie needs vary, based on the type of fistula, amount of output, status of the patient prior to fistula development, and infection status. The route for nutritional supplementation depends on the anatomic location of the fistula and on the patient's ability to take in adequate nutrition orally. As a general guideline, the intestinal system should be used whenever possible for nutritional support. Using the gastrointestinal tract allows the intestines to continue performing usual functions, thus maintaining normal physiology of the tract. When the intestinal tract is not used, there is always the possibility of damage to it from atrophy of the villi, with subsequent loss of absorption capabilities. If nutrition can bypass the fistula site, absorption and tolerance are better with use of the intestinal tract. Enteral nutrition is preferred when the fistula is located in the *most* proximal or distal portions of the gastrointestinal tract.

EXHIBIT 21-2 **Fistula Output Characteristics**

Organs Involved	Approximate Amount of Secretions/ Output (24 hr)	Characteristics
Esophagus	1,000 mL	Alkaline pH, clear-colored liquid
Stomach	2,000 mL	Acidic pH, green, clear liquid, major losses of Cl and some Na
Duodenum, Jejunum, and Ileum	3,000 mL	Alkaline pH, light brown liquid, major losses of Na, K, & Cl
Pancreas	1,200 mL	Alkaline pH, clear liquid, major losses of Na, Cl, and HCO3
Gall Bladder	600 mL	Alkaline pH, bile—yellow brown liquid—major losses of Na and Cl
Colon	150 mL	Alkaline pH, brown color, may be soft, pasty consistency

For ECFs, bypassing the fistula orifice is not always feasible. If the small bowel fistula is located distally, there may be enough of the intestinal tract available to absorb nutrients adequately prior to the fistula orifice. If the fistula is located more proximally, there may not be enough intestinal tract available for nutrient absorption prior to the fistula orifice. Specific solutions or feeding regimens should be ordered in consultation with the dietician because he or she can recommend the most appropriate supplement. Many of these patients must be managed with intravenous hyperalimentation (TPN) during the early stages of fistula management. The specific goals of fluid and electrolyte and nutritional support for fistula management must be discussed with the patient and family, particularly with the patient receiving palliative care. Typically, patients with ECFs should see a reduction in fistula output within 7 days of TPN therapy. If after 7 days there is no change in fistula output, adding Somatostatin infusion has demonstrated improvements and spontaneous closure in some patients [54,55,59]

Wherever anatomically possible, the fistula should be managed with an ostomy pouching technique. The surrounding skin should be cleansed with warm water, without soap or antiseptics; skin barrier paste should be used to fill uneven skin surfaces to create a flat surface to apply the pouch, and pouch types should be chosen based on fistula output. Pediatric pouches are often smaller and may be useful for hard-to-pouch areas where flexibility is needed, such as the neck for esophageal fistulas. For example, if the fistula output is watery and thin, choose a pouch with a narrow spigot or tube for closure, and, in contrast, a fistula with a thick, pasty output would be better managed with a pouch with an open end and closure clamp for closure. Pouches must be emptied frequently, at least when one-third to one-half full. There are several wound drainage pouching systems that will allow for visualization and direct access to the fistula through a valve or door that allows opening and reclosing of the pouch. These wound management pouches are available in large sizes and often work well for abdominal fistulas.[68–70] Pouching the fistula allows for odor control (many fistulas are quite malodorous), containment of output, and protection of the surrounding skin from damage. Gauze dressings with or without charcoal filters may be used when the output from the fistula is less than 250 mL over 24 hours and is not severely offensive in odor.

Colostomy caps (small, closed-end pouches) may be very useful for low-output fistulas that continue to be odorous.

There are specific pouching techniques that are useful in complex fistula management, including troughing, saddle-bagging, and bridging.[66] These techniques are particularly helpful when dealing with fistulas that occur in wounds, most commonly the small bowel fistula that develops in the open abdominal wound. Troughing is useful for fistulas that occur in the posterior aspect of large abdominal wounds.[71] Line the skin surrounding the wound and fistula with a skin barrier wafer and seal edge the nearest wound with skin barrier paste. Then apply thin film dressings over the top or anterior aspect of the wound, down to the fistula orifice and the posterior aspect of the wound. Last, use a cut-to-fit ostomy pouch to pouch the opening in the thin film dressing at the fistula orifice. Wound exudate drains from the anterior portion of the wound (under the thin film dressing) to the posterior portion of the wound and out into the ostomy pouch, along with fistula output. The trough technique does not prevent fistula output from contaminating the wound site. Figure 21-1 shows the trough technique.

A similar method of managing fistulas is by a closed suction wound drainage system. Jeter and colleagues[72] describe the use of a Jackson-Pratt drain and continuous, low suction in fistula management. After cleansing the wound with normal saline, the fenestrated drain of the Jackson-Pratt is placed in the wound on top of a moistened gauze opened up to line the wound bed (primary contact layer); a second fluffed wet gauze is placed over the drain, and the surrounding skin is prepared with a skin sealant. Next, the entire site is covered with a thin film dressing, crimping the dressing around the tube of the drain where it exits the wound. The tube exit site is filled with skin barrier paste, and the Jackson-Pratt is connected to low, continuous wall suction. The connection site may have to be adjusted or may require use of a small "Christmas tree" connector or device and secured with tape. Jeter and colleagues advise changing the system every 3 to 5 days.[72]

Others have used a similar setup for pharyngocutaneous fistulas.[73] Some have reported success with high-output fistulas and suction catheters attached to low, intermittent suction, using the approach described by Jeter and colleagues.[72,74,75] Topical dressings and skin protection around the suction catheter are still required with this approach be-

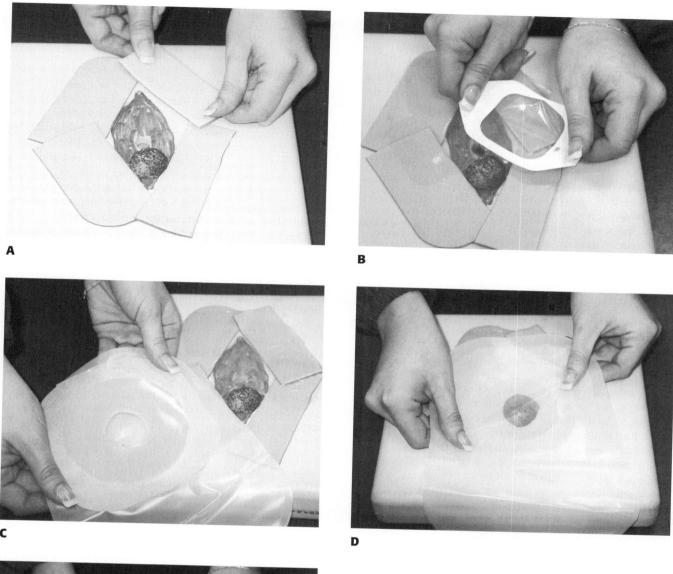

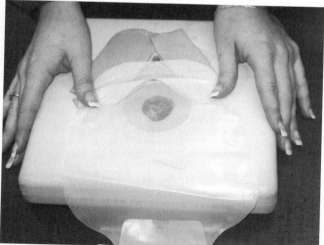

FIGURE 21-1 Photo series depicting the trough procedure. **A.** Skin barrier wafers or hydrocolloid wound dressings are used to protect the skin surrounding the wound. **B.** Thin film dressings or transparent dressings are applied to the anterior portion of the wound on top of the hydrocolloid dressing or skin barrier wafers. The thin film dressings can be overlapped to obtain continuity and provide adequate coverage. The fistula area is left open and not covered by the thin film dressings. **C.** An ostomy pouch is sized for the fistula opening and prepared appropriately. **D.** The ostomy pouch is applied over the open fistula site. **E.** The ostomy pouch is applied over and on top of the thin film dressing covering the anterior portion of the wound. (Courtesy of Barbara Bates-Jensen.)

cause the suction catheter will not provide for complete containment of drainage.[74,75] The suction catheter technique is most effective when fistula output is liquid and watery. Fistula output that is pasty, thick, or chunky will clog the suction catheter, making the system ineffective. Insertion of the suction catheter into the fistula opening will prevent fistula closure because the body responds to the catheter as a foreign object. However, laying the catheter in the wound around the fistula opening will not prevent fistula closure. A soft catheter should be used to prevent undue trauma to the wound bed.

Vacuum-assisted closure with the V.A.C.™ (Kinetic Concepts, Inc, San Antonio, Texas) is similar therapy and may assist in promoting healing of ECFs. Vacuum-assisted closure is suggested for two goals: obtaining complete pressure-related closure of acute fistulas as an aid to ECF closure and segregating the fistula from the abdominal wound to obtain sufficient healing and stabilization of the patient to allow for surgical repair of a chronic fistula. In both cases, the device is not intended as a method of containing or managing ECF output. Patients must be on TPN therapy with nothing by mouth and the fistula must be assessed prior to initiation of therapy. Pressure is usually continuous at 150 to 175 mm Hg for acute ECFs and slightly lower for chronic ECFs.[76]

The bridging technique prevents fistula output from contaminating the wound site and allows for a unique wound dressing to be applied to the wound site. Bridging is appropriate for fistulas that occur in the posterior aspect of large abdominal wounds, where it is important to contain fistula output away from the wound site. Using small pieces of skin barrier wafers, a bridge is built by consecutively layering the skin barriers together until the skin barrier has the appearance of a wedge or bridge and it is the same height as the depth of the wound.[66] Using skin barrier paste, the skin barrier wedge is adhered to the wound bed (it will not harm the healthy tissues of the wound bed) next to the fistula opening. An ostomy pouch is then cut to fit the fistula opening, using the wedge or bridge as a portion of intact surrounding skin to adhere the pouch.[66] The anterior aspect of the wound may then be dressed with the dressing of choice. Figure 21-2 presents the bridging technique.

Saddlebagging is used for multiple fistulas, where the fistula orifices are close together and it is important to keep the output from each fistula separated. Using two (or more for multiple fistulas) cut-to-fit ostomy pouches, the fistula openings are cut on the back of the pouch, off-center or as far to the side as possible; the second pouch is cut to fit the next fistula and is cut off-center as far to the other side as possible. The skin is cleansed with warm water, and skin barrier paste is applied around the fistulas orifices. The ostomy pouches are applied, and, where they contact each other (down the middle), they are affixed/adhered to each other in a "saddlebag" fashion. Figure 21-3 presents the saddlebag procedure, and Figure 21-4 shows the procedure in use. Multiple fistulas can also be managed with one ostomy pouching system accommodating the multiple open-

ings. This method is appropriate when fistula openings are close together and there is no need to separate drainage.[77] Figure 21-5 demonstrates multiple fistulas managed with one large pouching system.

Vaginal fistulas present complex management problems. Whether the fistula involves the bladder or intestine, manifestations are continual leakage of stool or urine (depending on fistula origins) through the vaginal vault, with erosion and denudation of the sensitive vaginal epithelium, as well as the perineal skin. Containment of the fistula output is extremely difficult because of the anatomic constraints of the perineal area. Female urinary containment pouches can be tried, as can soft, cuplike devices inserted into the vaginal vault to direct output flow into a tube and drainage bag system. Use of skin protector ointments, attention to odor control, and some form of fistula output containment are essential for these patients. Consultation with the enterostomal therapy (ET) nurse or ostomy nurse is extremely advantageous in any of these cases because clinical experience plays a major role in successful management of the complex fistula.

Pouching to contain the fistula output will usually contain odor as well. If odor continues to be problematic with an intact pouching system, internal body deodorants may be helpful, such as bismuth subgallate, charcoal compositions, or peppermint oil.[78] Taking care to change the pouch in a well-ventilated room will also help with odor. If odor is caused by anaerobic bacteria, some clinicians suggest use of 400 mg metronidazole orally three times a day.[64]

Management of high-output fistulas may be improved with administration of octreotide acetate 300 μg subcutaneously over 24 hours.[64,79] Octreotide is an analog of Somatostatin and as such has fewer side effects and a longer half life. Somatostatin has a half life of less than 3 minutes and therefore must be administered as a continuous intravenous infusion for the duration of the therapy. Octreotide and lanreotide are two synthetic analogues of somatostatin and may be administered subcutaneously over a period of hours or days. Octreotide may be given for the prevention of ECF with pancreatic involvement following pancreatic surgery in high risk patients.[79] Typically, octreotide is given subcutaneously as 100 μg every 8 hours for a period of at least 7 days. Evidence supporting use of octreotide or somatostatin for treatment of existing ECFs is mixed.[59,79] The current suggested approach is to treat the ECF initially with nutrition support (e.g., enteral or TPN) and if no response in fistula output with a week to add therapy with somatostatin or octreotide.[59]

Outcome Measures for Fistulas

Outcome measures for fistula care relate to the potential for fistula closure, maintenance of fluid and electrolyte balance, and management of the fistula output. Of course, for a newly developed fistula, the goals of care are fistula closure, and the major outcome measure is slowing of fistula output, with eventual closure of the fistula site. In some cases, when fis-

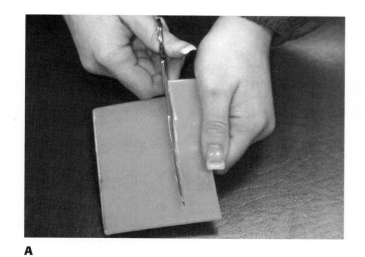

A

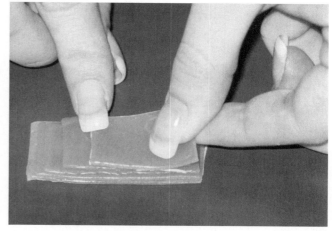

B

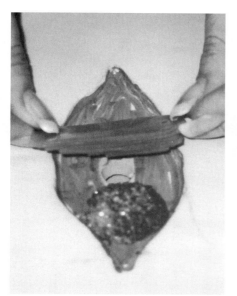

C

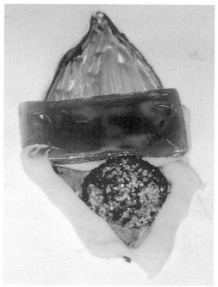

D

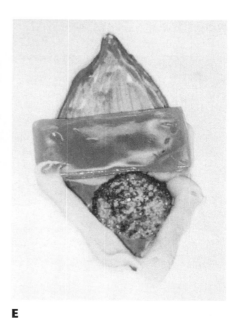

E

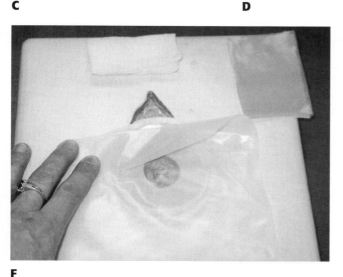

F

FIGURE 21-2 Photo series depicting the bridging procedure. **A.** A skin barrier wafer is cut into strips. **B.** The strips of skin barrier wafer are applied on top of each other to create a "bridge." **C.** The skin barrier "bridge" is applied to the wound. **D.** The skin barrier "bridge" is secured in the wound bed using skin barrier paste. The paste is also used around the fistula site as necessary to create an even surface. **E.** The skin barrier "bridge" is in place and the anterior portion of the wound can be seen to be clear of the fistula area. **F.** An ostomy pouch is sized and cut to fit the fistula area. The ostomy pouch is applied over the fistula, using the skin barrier "bridge" as part of the adhesive surface area for pouch application. **G.** A wound dressing can be applied to the anterior portion of the wound that is now protected from fistula output by the ostomy pouch. **H.** The wound dressing can be changed more frequently than the fistula pouch system if necessary. This system allows the wound to be treated with a different approach than the fistula area. (Courtesy of Barbara Bates-Jensen.)

(Continued)

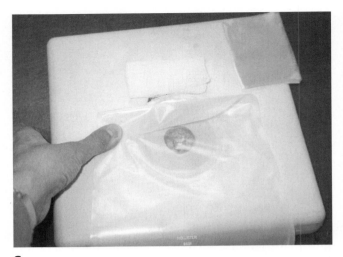

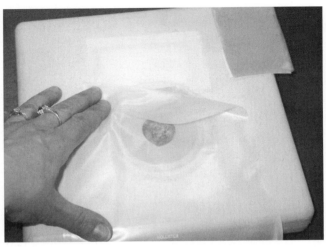

G

H

FIGURE 21-2 *(Continued)*

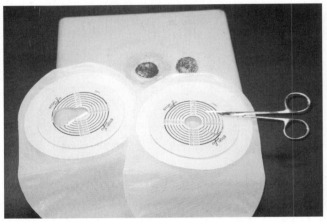

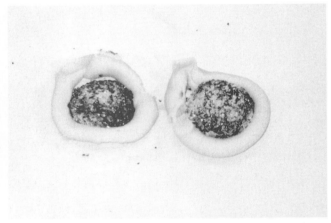

A

B

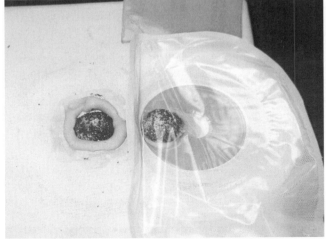

C

FIGURE 21-3 Photo series depicting the saddlebagging procedure. **A.** Two ostomy pouches are used to pouch each of the fistulas present separately. This will allow for unique containment of fistula output for each site. Ostomy pouches are sized and cut to fit the fistula openings. The fistula openings are cut off-center, as far to one edge of the pouch skin barrier backing as possible. **B.** Skin barrier paste is used around the fistula openings to provide for a smooth adhesive area and fill in any dips or crevices around the fistula openings. **C.** Each ostomy pouch is applied to the fistula site. The adhesive area of the pouch closest to the second fistula site is not firmly adhered to the skin; rather, it is left (or bent up) in a nonadhered manner.

(Continued)

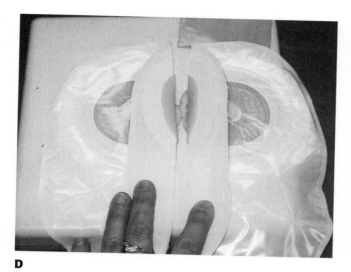

D

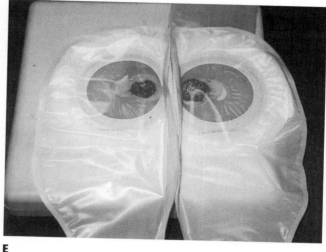

E

FIGURE 21-3 (Continued) **D.** The second ostomy pouch is applied over the second fistula and, as with the first pouch, the adhesive area closest to the other fistula is left in a nonadhered fashion. **E.** The nonadhered middle sections of the two pouches are adhered to each other to create the "saddle." Both pouches will require simultaneous changing as it is nearly impossible to change one without changing the other because of the adherence of one pouch to the other in the middle section. (Courtesy of Barbara Bates-Jensen.)

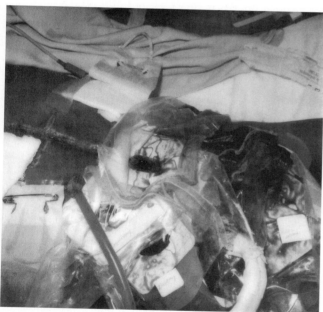

FIGURE 21-4 Saddlebagging procedure in use. Photo demonstrates an abdomen with multiple fistula sites and draining wound sites. Each site was pouched separately with the saddlebagging technique used for most because of the close proximity of many of the sites. The midline abdominal wound shows a posterior fistula that was pouched using the bridging technique. (Courtesy of Copyright © Barbara Bates-Jensen.)

tula closure is not likely to occur spontaneously and the patient is not a surgical candidate, outcomes of care become targeted to quality of life with the fistula. The outcome measures may include decrease in fistula output; management of fistula odor, as measured by patient/caregiver self-report;

and maintenance of fluid and electrolyte balance, as monitored by frequent laboratory values.

Patient and Caregiver Education for Fistulas

Patient and caregiver teaching first involves adequate assessment of the patient's self-care ability and the caregiver's ability. The patient and caregiver must be taught the management method for the fistula, including pouching techniques, how to empty the pouch, odor control methods, and strategies for increasing fluid and nutritional intake. Many of the pouching techniques used to manage fistulas are complicated and may require continual surveillance by an expert, such as an ET nurse or ostomy nurse.

Conclusion

Fistulas and malignant cutaneous wounds require attention to basic care issues, creativity in management strategies, and thoughtful attention to psychosocial implications of cutaneous manifestations. Both malignant cutaneous wounds and fistulas are often palliative care conditions. Palliative care intervention strategies for both skin disorders reflect a similar approach to curative care, with the goals of treatment to reduce discomfort, manage odor and drainage, and provide for optimal functional capacity. In each area, involvement of the caregiver and family in the plan of care is important. To meet the needs of the patient and family, access to the multidisciplinary care team is crucial, and consultation by an ET or certified wound, ostomy, or continence nurse is highly desirable. Goals of care, although not always to cure the condition, are at all times to alleviate the distressing symptomatology and improve quality of life.

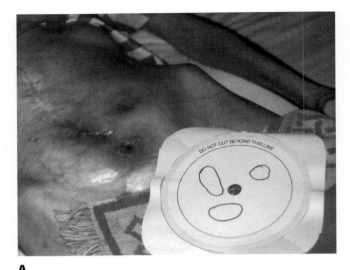

A

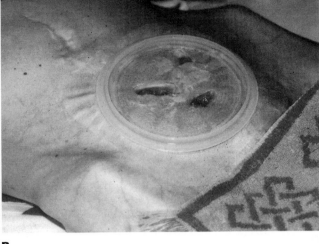

B

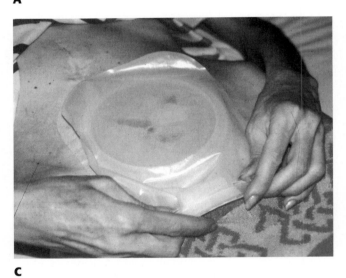

C

FIGURE 21-5 Photo series depicting the use of one pouch for multiple fistulas. **A.** Three major fistula sites evident on abdomen (from long-standing Crohn's disease). A two-piece pouch is used and the skin barrier wafer portion is cut to fit the fistula openings. Pouch with large opening has been cut to fit the three fistula sites. Caution must be used to cut the pouch barrier so that the fistula openings are cut with attention to how the skin barrier will be applied on the skin (it is common to accidentally reverse the images if not aware). **B.** Skin barrier portion of two-piece pouch applied. Skin barrier paste has been used around the fistula openings to help apply the pouch. **C.** Pouch attached to skin barrier and closure clamp applied. (Courtesy of Barbara Bates-Jensen.)

REVIEW QUESTIONS

1. Malignant cutaneous lesions may occur:
   a. In up to 5% of patients with cancer and 10% of patients with metastatic disease
   b. In up to 25% of all cancer patients
   c. Very rarely, no studies have documented the occurrence
   d. In up to 10% of all cancer patients and 50% of patients with metastatic disease
2. Malignant cutaneous wounds occur secondary to:
   a. Local invasion of a tumor
   b. Spread via lymphatics and blood vessels
   c. Surgical removal of primary tumor
   d. a. and b.
3. Enterocutaneous fistulas are usually managed initially by:
   a. Surgically "oversewing" the fistula (intestinal bypass)
   b. Medical management consisting of bowel rest and nutritional support
   c. High-dose antibiotics and steroids to reduce infection and inflammation
   d. Surgical resection and end-to-end anastomosis
4. Which of the following best exemplifies conditions and treatments that predispose to fistula development?
   a. Intra-abdominal sepsis, surgery, chronic diverticulitis
   b. Surgery, anal malformation, chronic diverticulitis
   c. Chronic diverticulitis, intra-abdominal sepsis, surgery, Crohn's disease
   d. Radiation therapy, intra-abdominal sepsis, surgery, Crohn's disease

REFERENCES

1. Lookingbill DP, Spangler N, Sexton FM. Skin involvement as the presenting sign of internal carcinoma. *J Am Acad Dermatol* 1990;22:19–26.
2. Lookingbill DP, Spangler N, Helm KF. Cutaneous metastases in patients with metastatic carcinoma: A retrospective study of 4020 patients. *J Am Acad Dermatol* 1993;29:228–236.
3. Rosen T. Cutaneous metastasis. *Med Clin North Am* 1980;64:885–900.
4. Brodland DG, Zitelli JA. Mechanisms of metastasis. *J Am Acad Dermatol* 1992;27:1–8.

5. Schoenlaub P, Sarraux A, Grosshans E, Heid E, Cribier B. Survival after the occurrence of cutaneous metastasis: A study of 200 cases. *Ann Dermatol Venereol* 2001;128:1310–1315.

6. Ivetic O, Lyne PA. Fungating and ulcerating malignant lesions: A review of the literature. *J Adv Nurs* 1990;15:83–88.

7. Collier M. The assessment of patients with malignant fungating wounds—A holistic approach: Part 1. *Nurs Times* 1997;93(suppl):1–4.

8. Goodman M, Hilderley LJ, Purl S. Integumentary and mucous membrane alterations. In: Groenwald SL, Hansen-Frogge M, Goodman M, Yarbro CH, eds. *Cancer Nursing, Principles and Practice*. Boston: Jones & Bartlett Publishers, 1997, pp. 768–821.

9. Grocott P, Cowley S. The palliative management of fungating malignant wounds—generalizing from multiple-case study data using a system of reasoning. *Int J Nurs Stud* 2001;38:533-545.

10. Haisfield-Wolfe ME, Baxendale-Cox LM. Staging of malignant cutaneous wounds: A pilot study. *Oncol Nurs Forum* 1999;26(6):1055–1064.

11. Moody M, Grocott P. Let us extend our knowledge base: Assessment and management of fungating malignant wounds. *Prof Nurs* 1993;8:586–590.

12. Bates-Jensen BM, Early L, Seaman S. Skin disorders. In: Ferrell B, Coyle N, eds. *Textbook of Palliative Care in Nursing*. New York: Oxford University Press, 2001.

13. Haisfield-Wolfe ME, Rund C. Malignant cutaneous wounds: A management protocol. *Ostomy/Wound Manage* 1997;43(1):56–66.

14. Waller A, Caroline NL. Smelly tumors. In: Waller A, Caroline NL, eds. *Handbook of Palliative Care in Cancer*. Boston: Butterworth-Heinemann, 1996, pp. 69–73.

15. van Leeuwen BL, Houwerzijl, Hoekstra HJ. Educational tips in the treatment of malignant ulcerating tumours of the skin. *Eur J Surg Oncol* 2000;26:506–508.

16. Naylor W. Assessment and management of pain in fungating wounds. *Br J Nurs* 2001;10(22 Suppl):S33–36,S38,S40.

17. Hallet A. Fungating wounds. *Nurs Times* 1995;91(39):78–85.

18. Fairburn K. A challenge that requires further research: Management of fungating breast lesions. *Prof Nurse* 1994;9:272–277.

19. Clark L. Caring for fungating tumours. *Nurs Times.* 1992;88(12):66–70.

20. Young T. The challenge of managing fungating wounds. *Community Nurse* 1997;3(9):41–44.

21. Whedon MA. Practice corner: What methods do you use to manage tumor-associated wounds? *Oncol Nurs Forum* 1995;22:987–990.

22. Grocott P. The management of fungating wounds. *J Wound Care* 1999;8:232–234.

23. Collinson G. Improving quality of life in patients with malignant fungating wounds In: Harding KG, Cherry G, Deale C, Turner TD, eds. *Proceedings of the 2nd European Conference on Advances in Wound Management*. London: MacMillan Magazines, October 20–23, 1992, pp. 59–63.

24. Cormier AC, McCann E, McKeithan L. Reducing odor caused by metastatic breast cancer skin lesions. *Oncol Nurs Forum* 1995;22(6):988–999.

25 Butler GA. Desloughing agents at work. *Nurs Mirror* 1985;160(13):29.

26. Leaper D. Antiseptics and their effect on healing tissue. *Nurs Mirror* 1985;82(22):45–47.

27. Seaman S. Dressing selection in chronic wound management. *J Am Podiatr Med Assoc* 2002;92:24–33.

28. Seaman S. Home care for pain, odor, and drainage in tumor-associated wounds. *Oncol Nurs Forum* 1995;22(6):987.

29. Grocott P. Application of the principles of modern wound management for complex wounds in palliative care. In: Harding KG, Leaper DL, Turner TD, eds. *Proceedings of the 1st European Conference on Advances in Wound Management*. London: MacMillan Magazines, 1991, pp. 88–91.

30. Newman V, Allwood M, Oakes RA. The use of metronidazole gel to control the smell of malodorous lesions. *Palliative Med* 1989;3:303–305.

31. Bower M, Stein R, Evans TRJ, Hedley A, Pert P, Coombs RC. A double-blind study of the efficacy of metronidazole gel in the treatment of malodorous fungating tumours. *Eur J Cancer* 1992;28A:888–889.

32. Poteete V. Case Study: Eliminating odors from wounds. *Decubitus* 1993;6(4):43–46.

33. Finlay IG, Bowszyc J, Ramlau C, et al. The effect of topical 0.75% metronidazole gel on malodorous cutaneous ulcers. *J Pain Symptom Manage* 1996;11:158–162.

34. Clark J. Metronidazole gel in managing malodorous fungating wounds. *Br J Nurs* 2002;11(6 Suppl):S54–S60.

35. Rice TT. Metronidazole use in malodorous skin lesions. *Rehabil Nurs* 1992;17:244, 245, 255.

36. Ashford RFU, Plant GT, Maher J, Teares L. Double-blind trial of metronidazole in malodorous ulcerating tumours. *Lancet* 1984;1(8388):1232–1233.

37. McMullen D. Topical metronidazole. Part II. *Ostomy/Wound Manage* 1992;38(3):42–46.

38. Forman WB, Sheehan DC. Symptom management. In: Sheehan DC, Forman WB, eds. *Hospice and Palliative Care*. Sudbury, MA: Jones & Bartlett Publishers, 1996, pp. 83–97.

39. Jacob M, Markstein C, Liesse M, Deckers C. What about odor in terminal care? *J Palliative Care* 1991;7(4):31.

40. Holloway GA, Johansen KH, Barnes RW, et al. Multicenter trial of cadexomer iodine to treat venous stasis ulcer. *West J Med* 1989;151:35–38.

41. Danielsen L, Cherry GW, Harding K, et al. Cadexomer iodine in ulcers colonised by *Pseudomonas aeruginosa. J Wound Care* 1997;6:169–172.

42. Welch LB. Simple new remedy for the odour of open lesions. *RN* 1981;44(2):42–43.

43. Schulte MJ. Yogurt helps to control wound odor. *Oncol Nurs Forum* 1993;20(8):1262.

44. Rankin EM, Rubens RD, Reidy JF. Transcatheter embolisation to control severe bleeding in fungating breast cancer. *Eur J Surg Oncol* 1988;14:27–32.

45. Kundu S, Achar S. Principles of office anesthesia: Part II. Topical anesthesia. *Am Fam Physician* 2002;66:99–102.

46. Stein C. The control of pain in peripheral tissue by opioids. *N Engl J Med* 1995;332:1685–1690.

47. Back IN, Finlay I. Analgesic effect of topical opioids on painful skin ulcers. *J Pain Symptom Manage* 1995;10:493.

48. Krajnik M, Zbigniew Z. Topical morphine for cutaneous cancer pain. *Palliative Med* 1997;11:325.

49. Zeppetella G, Paul J, Ribeiro M. Analgesic efficacy of morphine applied topically to painful ulcers. *J Pain Symptom Manage* 2003;25:555–558.

50. Flock P. Pilot study to determine the effectiveness of diamorphine gel to control pressure ulcer pain. *J Pain Symptom Manage* 2003;25:547–554.

51. Ballas SK. Treatment of painful sickle cell leg ulcers with topical opioids. *Blood* 2002;99:1096.

52. Bufill JA, Grace WR, Neff R. Intra-arterial chemotherapy for palliation of fungating breast cancer. *Am J Clin Oncol* 1994;17(2):118–124.

53. Berry SM, Fischer JE. Classification and pathophysiology of enterocutaneous fistulas. *Surg Clin North Am* 1996;76(5):1009.

54. Ryan JA, Adye BA, Weinstein AJ. Enteric fistulas. In: Rombeau, JL, Caldwell, MD, eds. *Clinical Nutrition, Volume II. Parenteral Nutrition*. Philadelphia: WB Saunders, 1986, pp. 419–36.

55. Rose D, et al. One hundred and fourteen fistulas of the gastrointestinal tract treated with total parenteral nutrition. *Surg Gynecol Obstet* 1986;163(4):345.

56. Rombeau J, Rolandelli R. Enteral and parenteral nutrition in patients with enteric fistulas and short bowel syndrome. *Surg Clin North Am* 1987;67(3):551.

57. Fischer JE. Enterocutaneous fistulas. In: Najarian JS, Delaney JP, eds. *Progress in Gastrointestinal Surgery*. St. Louis, MO: CV Mosby, 1989.

58. Kurtz R, Heimann T, Aufses A. The management of intestinal fistulas. *Am J Gastroenterol* 1981;76:377.

59. Makhdoom, ZA, Komar, MJ. Nutrition and enterocutaneous fistulas. *J Clin Gastroenterol* 2000;31(3):195–204.

60. Lynch AC, Delaney CP, Senagore AJ, Connor JT, Remzi FH, Fazio VW. Clinical outcome and factors predictive of recurrence after enterocutaneous fistula surgery. *Ann Surg* 2004;240(5):825–31.

61. Hwang TL, Chen MF. Short note: Randomized trial of fibrin tissue glue for low-output enterocutaneous fistula. *Br J Surg* 1996;83(1):112.

62. Hammond TM, Grahn MF, Lunniss PJ. Fibrin glue in the management of anal fistula. *Colorectal Disease* 2004;6:308–319.

63. Singer M, Cintron J, Nelson R, Orsay C, Bastawrous A, Pearl R, Sone D, Abcarian H. Treatment of fistulas-in-ano with fibrin sealant in combination with intra-adhesive antibiotics and/or surgical closure of the internal fistula. *Dis Colon Rectum* 2005; 48(4): 799–808.

64. Waller A, Caroline NL. Stomas and fistulas. In: Waller A, Caroline NL, eds. *Handbook of Palliative Care in Cancer*. Boston: Butterworth- Heinemann, 1996, pp. 81–86.

65. Chamberlain RS, Kaufman HL, Danforth DN. Enterocutaneous fistula in cancer patients: Etiology, management, outcome and impact on further treatment. *Am Surg* 1998;64(12):1204.

66. Rolstad BS, Bryant RA. Management of drain sites and fistulas. In: Bryant RA, ed. *Acute and Chronic Wounds: Nursing Management* 2nd ed. St. Louis, MO: CV Mosby, 2000, pp. 317–341.

67. Hess CT. Assessing a fistula, part 1. *Nurs* 2002;32(8):22.
68. Schaffner A, Hocevar BJ, Erwin-Toth P. Small bowel fistulas complicating midline surgical wounds. *J Wound/Ostomy Continence Nurs* 1994;21(4):161–165.
69. O'Brien B, Landis-Erdman J, Erwin-Toth P. Nursing management of multiple enterocutaneous fistulae located in the center of a large open abdominal wound: A case study. *Ostomy/Wound Manage* 1998;44(1):20.
70. Benbow M. The use of wound drainage bags for complex wounds. *Br J Nurs* 2001;10(19):1298–301.
71. Wiltshire BL. Challenging enterocutaneous fistula: A case presentation. *J Wound/Ostomy Continence Nurs* 1996;23(6):297–301.
72. Jeter KF, Tintle TE, Chariker M. Managing draining wounds and fistula: New and established methods. In: Krasner D, ed. *Chronic Wound Care*. King of Prussia, PA: Health Management Publications, 1990, pp. 240–246.
73. Harris A, Komray RR. Cost-effective management of pharyngocutaneous fistulas following laryngectomy. *Ostomy/Wound Manage* 1993;39(8):36–44.
74. Beitz JM, Caldwell D. Abdominal wound with enterocutaneous fistula: A case study. *J Wound/Ostomy Continence Nurs* 1998;25(2):102.
75. Lange MP, et al. Management of multiple enterocutaneous fistulas. *Heart Lung* 1989;18:386.
76. V.A.C.(r) *Therapy Clinical Guidelines. A Reference Source for Clinicians*. San Antonio, TX: KCI, January, 2005.
77. Wessel LC. Application of a wound pouch over an enterocutaneous fistula: A step-by-step approach. *Ostomy Wound Manage* 2002;48(9):26–8,30.
78. McKenzie J, Gallacher M. A sweet smelling success. *Nurs Times* 1989;85(27):48–49.
79. Gray M, Jacobson T. Are somatostatin analogues (octreotide and lanreotide) effective in promoting healing of enterocutaneous fistulas? *J WOCN* 2002; 29(5): 228–233.

Management of Wound Healing with Biophysical Agent Technologies

Carrie Sussman

The management of wound healing with biophysical agent technologies is presented in Part IV. Biophysical agents presented include: electrical stimulation, pulsed radio frequency stimulation (a variant of electrical stimulation), phototherapy (ultraviolet, infrared and laser light) ultrasound (different delivery methods), whirlpool, pulsed lavage with suction, and negative pressure therapy. Chapters 22 to 28 describe the physical science associated with each technology, what is currently known about the science and clinical efficacy, the safety and rationale for its use, devices, procedures for application, and case studies. Each device mentioned in Part IV has the ability to affect one or more of the barriers (e.g. ischemia, infection or moisture balance) to healing. How to choose between them remains the key question. This introduction will provide some guidelines about why, when, for who, and how to chose a biophysical agent. The individual chapters will discuss the what and how to use them.

Relationships Between Biophysical Interventions and Components of the Electromagnetic Spectrum

Chapters 22–24 deal with technologies that exploit the properties of the Electromagnetic Spectrum (EMS). Perhaps looking at the physical relationship between the different biophysical agents to the EMS will shed some insight into why there is so much interest in them and why they are useful for wound healing and why many of the effects appear to be so similar. Although effects described in each chapter appear to be similar, no optimal EMS frequency or wavelength signal from these devices or optimal outcomes has as yet been identified. Patient characteristics, clinician intervention expertise and device availability in addition to evidence are often the deciding point

Exposure to electromagnetic radiation is on-going for all living systems. Sources of exposure are both natural (e.g., sunlight and earth's electromagnetic field) and man-made (e.g., cell phones, power lines, computers, and sunlamps). Man recognized long ago that the sun had healing properties and has tried to take advantage of those properties by harnessing the energy of the sun in different way to exploit those properties. As science has progressed, scientists have been able to analyze the components of the electromagnetic radiation and develop a

scale to describe the relationship between them, called the electromagnetic spectrum (EMS). EMS is the whole range of wavelengths or frequencies of electromagnetic radiation, extending from very short gamma rays to visible light and the longest radio waves (see Figure IV-1). Further scientific advances have led to the development of technologies that use segments of the EMS for biologic purposes. As mentioned before, several biophysical agents discussed in Part IV are designed to take advantage of the properties of the EMS family. Electric and magnetic fields are two component properties of electromagnetic radiation that are perpendicular to each other. The EMS is categorized according to frequency and wavelength. As the frequency increases, the wavelength decreases. All EMS wavelengths share the property of passing through space (e.g body tissue or wound dressings) without requiring a medium for transmission. The different wavelengths are like family members that differ from each other only in their wavelength or frequency, and there is often overlap between the neighbors. At low frequencies, 30–300 kHz, there are the long radiowaves that are used in the radiofrequency stimulators and electric stimulators. In the middle are the mid-frequency wavelengths, shorter than radio or microwaves but longer than visibile light, infrared radiation (IR) (75-10-6 cm). These wavelengths overlap the radiowaves of the long end and have the same properties as visible light on the short end. Laser and monochromatic light are components of this segment of the EMS.

One of the properties of IR is thermal radiation. This feature is used in thermography and also to heat superficial tissues such as with IR stimulators. The rainbow is the visible light part of the EMS, and this part of the spectrum stimulates many body cellular systems including the system that produces vitamin D. Beyond the visible light segment is the still shorter wavelengths of ultraviolet light (UV) (UV A,B,C), which is a component of sunlight and has the ability to heal as well as burn the skin. The frequency of UV is 10^{13} to 10^{17} Hz or wavelengths of 400 to 4 nanometers. Low frequencies through UV range are considered to be nonionizing radiation and cannot break molecular bonds or produce ions, which makes them safe for therapeutic applications. [1]

Shorter wavelength relatives of the EMS family are the X-rays and Gamma rays, which are ionizing and have the potential to inhibit cell growth or have the ability to damage cells. They are used therapeutically to exploit those

FIGURE IV-1 The electromagnetic spectrum.

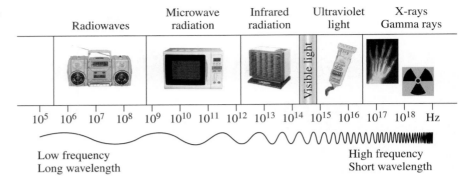

properties in treatment of cancer, for example but are avoided for purposes of wound healing. Ultrasound (US) is also nonionizing but it is not a part of the EMS; it is high-frequency sound waves that require a medium for transmission of the energy into tissues [2] (see Chapter 24).

It has been firmly established that each of these EMS members, as well as ultrasound, presented here have abilities to affect complex cellular process and influence tissue growth. This should not be a surprise since the body is continuously bombarded with wavelengths from the EMS in the environment. Cells over time have learned to respond to signals from the environmental bombardment. Now as a result of extensive research efforts, the effects of the EMS component on cellular systems are being applied clinically through the use of complex delivery systems to trigger responses needed for wound healing. Details about the physical properties of each segment of the EMS used in the different technologies are described in the individual chapters in Part IV, along with the results of research efforts.

Medial applications

The devices described in Part IV are all FDA approved for medical application but most are not specifically approved for wound healing applications. Individual chapters have information about FDA premarket approval for specific application of that technology. While having little apparent risk, all have best-practice methods that will provide optimal outcomes, and some do have significant health risks if used improperly. Any adverse medical events that result from using any of these products should be reported to the FDA. Prior reports can be viewed at the FDA web site; this is the link to MAUDE, the database on devices and adverse events: http://www.access-data.fda.gov/scripts/cdrh/cfdocs/ cfMAUDE/search.CFM.

Therapeutic use of Biophysical Agents

Although biophysical agents are efficacious for healing, the dosing regimens remain largely empirical because the science of the interactions at the cellular level is only just being discovered. Innovative scientists, engineers, designers, and manufacturers are working continuously to discover the underlying science and clinical effects, and to develop products that will deliver these biophysical signals to target tissues and exploit them for therapeutic benefit. Biophysical stimulation is an alternative to pharmacologic interventions with benefits theoretically of sustained increases in cellular processes at the local and, in some cases, systemic levels, without risk of local or systemic toxicity.

Biophysical agents are categorized by the American Physical Therapy Association (APTA) as electrotherapeutic modalities and physical agents with long histories of clinical application, clinical effectiveness, and use by physical therapists (PTs). The two categories of electrotherapeutic modalities are defined as follows:

"Electrotherapeutic modalities include physical agents that use electricity to modulate or decrease pain, reduce or eliminate soft tissue inflammation caused by musculoskeletal, peripheral vascular, or integumentary injury, disease, or surgery; or increase the rate of healing in open wounds."[3] These modalities include alternating, direct, and pulsed current (e.g., high-voltage pulsed current, low-voltage pulsed current, and transcutaneous electrical nerve stimulation [TENS]).

"Physical agents use heat, sound, or light energy to increase the connective tissue extensibility, modulate pain, reduce or eliminate soft tissue inflammation and swelling caused by musculoskeletal injury or circulatory dysfunction, increase the healing rate of open wounds and soft tissue, remodel scar tissue, or treat skin conditions."[3] These modalities include deep thermal modalities (e.g., thermal ultrasound, pulsed short-wave diathermy), nonthermal modalities, (e.g., pulsed ultrasound, pulsed radio frequency energy, ultraviolet light), and hydrotherapy (e.g., whirlpool, pulsatile irrigation with suction).

Practice Patterns

Are the uses of these devices limited to supervision of a PT? In current clinical practice, other licensed health-care practitioners are including biophysical agents in their care plans and providing many of these interventions for their patients. Does that indicate that they have the knowledge base for making these clinical decisions? Each health-care professional group has certain backgrounds that make them especially qualified to provide safe and effective clinical care. Practice areas are typically based on three pillars:

1. Basic academic education
2. History of use in clinical practice
3. Licensing and legal statutes.

Physical therapists meet all three requirements and provides a high level of knowledge about using most biophysical agents. The Center for Medicare and Medicaid Services (CMS) recognizes, for example, the knowledge base of the PT for appropriate use of electrical stimulation by providing reimbursement under the Part B program for this service when provided by a PT. That knowledge base may not be valued the same way under capitated systems of reimbursement.

The physical therapy education curriculum includes instruction in the selection, protocols, and application of electrotherapeutic modalities and physical agents (biophysical agents). Licensing examination includes testing of knowledge in appropriate, safe use; protocols; and interpretation of the results. Liability issues also suggest that PTs should be the health-care professional responsible for treatment or instruction in the use of these interventions because the PT is the legally licensed and most qualified practitioner to refer to for these interventions. Wound management is no longer a standard part of general PT practice as it once was, and additional training and certification in current wound management would be highly recommended. Wound ostomy continence nurses (WOCN) have specialized skills in wound management and have special expertise in use of physical agents like negative pressure therapy.

Procedures and protocols to achieve optimal outcomes are not well understood by less knowledgeable practitioners. Many of the devices presented in this section are easy to apply and have a perceived low level of skill requirement (e.g., electrical stimulation, ES), yet a sound knowledge base needed for best outcomes is high.

Nurses are usually the initial wound treatment provider and often initiate referral to the PT, as well as serving as case managers and medical reviewers. Physicians and podiatrists are required in most cases to approve the referral and certify medical necessity. Therefore, it is very important that these health-care professionals understand the candidacy, referral criteria, and clinical outcomes expected from the therapy. The chapters in Part IV contain technical information that may be beyond the interest of many health-care professionals, but there are also clinical decision-making sections that will guide them through the rationale for referral and the treatment selection by the PT. Collaborative practice requires mutual understanding of the treatment recommended and the expected results. In addition, nurses, patients, or caregivers may be the individuals who deliver the direct treatment established by the PT's plan of care. Those modalities suited to self-care or care by a provider other than a PT are explained in each chapter's section on self-care treatment guidelines (Exhibit IV-1).

Candidacy for Intervention

The interventions discussed in Part IV chapters are often classified as adjunctive or advanced therapies. Eaglstein suggested adding new, alternative, or adjunctive therapies at four "points" in the course of care:[4]

1. Initially when predictors such as ulcer size and duration indicate a likely failure of standard care
2. When the rate of healing with standard care predicts failure

3. After failure to heal in the "magic" time (2–4 weeks)
4. Under special circumstances such as unusual diagnosis or patient demand

The mode of intervention best suited to the patient, the treatment setting, and the wound will be determined by the PT and recommended to the wound management team.

As a guide, patients should be referred to a PT for intervention with a biophysical agent when the additional following candidacy criteria are met:

- Medical comorbidities exist that predict that a wound needs extra help to heal (e.g., arterial occlusive disease, spinal cord injury, diabetes, venous insufficiency, hematoma or deep tissue injury).
- Healing will be speeded by the therapy.
- The wound has a large size or is of long duration.
- The wound has been recalcitrant to other methods of healing.
- There is an acute wound in a patient with a comorbidity such as chronic obstructive pulmonary disease or atherosclerosis, or diabetic neuropathy, indicating a high probability of delayed healing.
- The acute traumatic wound(s) is associated with neuromuscular or musculoskeletal problems that may require immobilization.
- The wounds extend into subcutaneous tissue and deeper underlying structures and interfere with functional activities (e.g., the patient is unable to sit up in a wheelchair because of the wounds over the ischial tuberosities or coccyx).
- The patient's functional status is impaired by slow wound healing (e.g., gait will be helped if the wound is healed more rapidly, or the patient may be able to return to work).
- Patient or family preference.

Reasons for Referral

The patient referred for biophysical interventions is usually an individual who has not shown signs of normal wound repair. Often other treatment interventions are or have been tried with limited or no success. Based on research, presented in the individual chapters, optimal time for intervening with biophysical agents is during the first 72 hours immediately after injury, when cellular events are most likely to be positively influenced to produce a successful healing cascade. However, in reality, more chronic wounds than acute wounds are referred to a PT for these advanced therapies, in spite of evidence from several studies showing that intervention by a PT soon after onset of the problem (e.g., stroke,[5,6] acute musculoskeletal pain[7,8]) reduces cost and the consequences of costly

EXHIBIT IV-1   Definition of Standard Wound Care

- Cleansing
- Debridement
- Bacterial balance
- Moisture balance
- Compression for venous ulcers
- Off-loading for diabetic neuropathic ulcers
- Pressure relief for pressure ulcers
- Good nutrition

health problems. As a reflection of clinical reality, most of the clinical research has focused on healing chronic wounds. Results provide evidence of these technologies for healing of chronic wounds or to alter factors related to chronic wound healing such as circulation, tissue oxygenation, cellular processes, pain, and edema. Expected outcomes would be based on the identified target problems.

Functional Diagnosis for Wound Healing

Like a medical diagnosis, multiple functional diagnoses may be determined that would benefit from one or multiple interventions with biophysical agents. For example, *absence of an inflammation phase and an inability to progress to proliferation* is a functional diagnosis about functional impairment of the healing cascade at the cellular or tissue level. The application of biophysical agents such as negative pressure therapy and pulsed radiofrequency that would increase circulation and stimulate cellular responses could speed healing and progression through the phases of healing.

Although traditionally patients with nonhealing wounds are referred for physical therapy, patients with musculoskeletal injuries and soft tissue trauma should also be considered patients with closed wound. Hunt and Hussain found that open- and closed-wound healing physiology are similar.[9] Therefore, it is reasonable to assume that they would respond similarly to the same treatment interventions. Patients with the following types of wounds should be viewed as candidates for intervention with biophysical agents:

- Skin tears
- Hematomas; deep tissue injury
- Stage I pressure ulcers
- Stage 0 neuropathic ulcers
- Superficial and partial-thickness burn wounds
- Donor sites
- Surgical wounds that do not heal in an orderly manner
- Abrasions that interfere with one's ability to walk, work, or compete in a sport

In patients with metabolic diseases (e.g., lupus or diabetes) who suffer superficial or closed wounding, acute wounds can, and often do, become chronic. In these patients, the impairment is a closed tissue wound.

In summary, a patient who has a functional diagnosis of impairment of a body system at the cellular, tissue, or organ level (or a combination) related to tissue repair should be considered a candidate for a biophysical intervention for closed or open wound healing. Unfortunately, practice is often based not on best practice or evidence but on reimbursement.

Prognosis

Can clinical research studies help guide prognosis? Clinical research studies are useful guides for predicting outcomes of wound care. However, they should not be relied upon with complete confidence because these studies are usually carried out in ideal settings under optimal conditions. Candidates are carefully chosen to meet specific admission criteria, which does not necessarily coincide with the clinical presentation of patients. Studies also set their own outcome measures that they report, which again may not be a match for the clinical practice. For example, most clinical studies of chronic wound healing interventions do not continue until closure; other ways of reporting the effectiveness of therapeutic agents have been chosen. One of these ways is to graph the percentage of healing over time to see the path or trajectory of wound healing or nonhealing[10]. (see Chapter5)

Normal wound healing takes three to four weeks. [11] The definition of a chronic wound is a wound healing that has not occurred in an orderly manner in the expected time without help [12]The concept of using biophysical agents is to provide help to initiate or accelerate the rate of repair of acute or chronic wounds. For example, Dyson and Young[13] found that application of low-intensity ultrasound during the early inflammatory phase of acute wounds accelerated the inflammatory phase of repair, leading to an earlier proliferative phase.

The prognosis is initiation of the inflammatory phase followed by progression of the wound through the proliferative phase of healing with reduction of 30% in surface area size in two to three weeks.

Multiple clinical randomized controlled studies report that a healing rate of 30% to 47% in two to three weeks from start of care is predictive of wound healing, whether the etiology is pressure ulcers, venous ulcers, or diabetic ulcers[14-18] (see Chapter 5). Therefore, patients with wounds that do not meet this target healing rate with standard care should be referred for adjunctive therapy intervention. It is the responsibility of the clinician to track and report the results of that care.

Primary or Adjunctive Therapy

Are all the treatment interventions in this section considered adjunctive rather than primary treatment modalities? Negative pressure therapy and pulsed lavage with suction usually are used as primary treatment interventions. Photo stimulation and ultrasound are used on a case-by-case basis determined by the health-care professionals treating the patient. Electrical stimulation is now considered a primary treatment modality rather than adjunctive therapy by some experts. [19,20] However, Medicare still considers it adjunctive for purposes of reimbursement. The Center for Medicare and Medicaid Services (CMS) coverage policy, for example, does not reimburse for ES or PRFS for wound healing until the wound shows chronicity of at least 30 days and is a full-thickness or deeper ulcer (stage III or IV). Patients need to be informed that they have this treatment option early but that reimbursement by the Medicare program will probably not be paid. See the CMS website for details www.hhs.cms and search for electricals stimulation coverage policy.

Choosing Between Interventions

A frequently asked question is, How do I know which intervention to choose? The purpose of presenting information about many different biophysical interventions in this section is to provide the clinician with choices and enough information about each intervention to determine if the presenting patient is a candidate for one or more of them. Figure IV-1 is an algorithm showing the phases of wound heal-

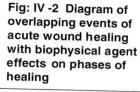

Fig: IV -2 Diagram of overlapping events of acute wound healing with biophysical agent effects on phases of healing

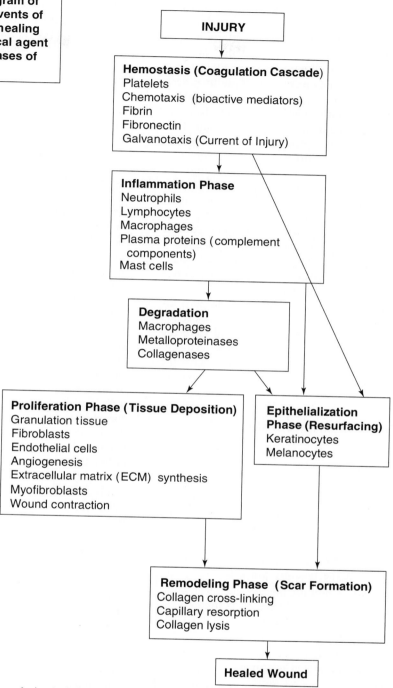

FIGURE IV-1 Putative treatment effects of physical therapy technologies on phases of wound healing. (Adapted with permission from Sussman CA. The role of physical therapy in wound care. In: Krasner D, ed. *Chronic Wound Care: A Clinical Source Book for Health Professionals. Health* Management Publications, Inc. 1990:327–367. Wayne, PA.)

ing with a key that highlights which are the putative effects on the phase or factor of healing of the ten biophysical technologies described in this part.

The rules for selection of treatment interventions include consideration of the patient's medical status, the status of the wound healing phase, and all treatments used to achieve the expected outcome. Wounds receive multiple treatment interventions, (e.g. topical agents, dressings and a biophysical agent) requiring that all treatment interventions be compatible with the patient, one another, and the wound. This will require collaboration of the team members—nurse, physician, pharmacist, and PT—to select interventions that are compatible with and efficacious for wound healing. Exhibit IV-2 lists three rules of treatment selection, an example of how each is used, and a formula for selection of treatments to achieve a desire outcome in a prescribed period. The letters "A," "B," and "C" in the formula represent three treatment interventions. The number of treatments usually given is often three but is not limited to three. Each chapter in Part IV will address the issue of treatment interactions and compatibility with other interventions.

If more than one of the technologies affects the same aspect of the phase, other criteria would be used to choose the modality. For instance, most devices described have the ability to increase tissue perfusion. What differs is the mechanism by which it acts. The thermal modalities have the ability to heat and increase circulation to produce a mild in-flammatory reaction by vasodilation of the blood vessels of the skin or deeper tissues. Care must be exercised in applying them to ischemic tissues that cannot dissipate the heat. The nonthermal devices use different mechanisms that have proven efficacy in increasing tissue perfusion.

The mechanisms of action on the biologic system are different, but the expected treatment outcomes of progression through the phases of healing are similar for each of the devices. Chronic wounds often develop because of underlying problems of inadequate perfusion, ischemia, or infection. Therefore, reperfusion of the tissues may be the stimulus needed to reinitiate the inflammatory phase and to control infection.

In evidence-based practice, research is highly valued as the basis for selecting an intervention, and consequently the intervention with the highest level of research and or the most supporting research may be given higher value and acceptance over less-tested devices; however, clinical experience and patient preference are important components of evidence-based medicine. For example, pulsatile lavage with suction (PLS) has no controlled clinical trials for efficacy of wound healing but has been used in the operating room for many years to cleanse and débride wounds, and studies and clinical experience show that it is effective in removing debris and bacteria. Since wound cleansing and debridement are standards of care, selection of PLS would be use of good clinical judgment to meet this standard. The patient may have a very painful wound, so minimal handling of the wound and surrounding tissues using a treatment like pulsed radio frequency stimulation is indicated for comfort and compliance by the patient and by the facility. Hospitals, nursing homes, and outpatient clinics accredited by the Joint Commission on Accreditation of Healthcare Organizations (Joint Commission) must meet standards requiring that every patient's pain be assessed regularly, managed aggressively and effectively, and documented.[21] Pain relief has been studied using the biophysical agents presented here that could be considered for incorporation into a nonpharmacologic plan of care for pain management of a wound along with the benefit of wound healing as a means of achieving compliance with this standard.

Practical considerations in choosing an intervention include the treatment setting, the treatment provider, the treatment payer, the treatment availability, medical contraindications, and adjunctive treatments (e.g., dressings and multiple biophysical agents). If the treatment provider is to be other than a PT or physical therapist assistant (PTA), the treatment must be safely and correctly applied by a person not trained in physical therapy. This would involve evaluation of the person and his or her ability to provide the care. Policies, procedures, and job descriptions could be used in facilities to establish who will have this responsibility. For the most predictable outcomes and for patient safety, a PT with wound management skills may be the best qualified to act as the supervising clinician when using most of these agents.

The treatment payer often must be agreeable to paying for the biophysical intervention selected. For example, Medicare has an exclusion policy for payment of UV light

EXHIBIT IV-2   Rules of Treatment Selection

1. **Medical assessment and tissue assessment determine the selection of treatment.**

   Example: Client has a venous stasis ulcer in inflammatory phase and has a cardiac pacemaker implant. Whirlpool, HVPC, PRFS, and PSWD are contraindicated. Ultrasound would be a good choice for local application.

2. **Treatment changes during the progression of healing so as to affect the recovery process.**

   Example: Client has a necrotic hip pressure ulcer with eschar. Treatment starts with whirlpool, scoring eschar, enzymes, and occlusive dressing. Necrotic tissue is removed. Treatment changes.

3. **Each selected treatment is goal specific based on how it affects the predicted outcome.**

   Example: Client has a clean full-thickness wound in the acute proliferative phase. Prognosis is wound closure. Treatment selected: clean with normal saline, use hydrogel-impregnated gauze dressing, apply HVPC through dressing, and cover with secondary dressing.

Formula To Select Treatment

Wound Healing Phase of Tissue + Treatment A + Treatment B + Treatment C = Wound Healing Phase of Tissue in X Period of Time

to treat wounds. However, there is now evidence that UV light is a useful treatment to control infection and reinitiate an inflammatory response. At this time, the cost of the UV treatment could not be billed separately. Other rationale would be needed to justify its selection, such as the short treatment time (e.g., 30 seconds) and rapid wound disinfection that would speed healing and reduce long-term costs. Electrical stimulation and pulsed radiofrequency stimulation as described in Chapters 22 and 23 are other examples of Medicare coverage policy restrictions. However, these restrictions should not preclude their availability as a choice for patients who would benefit from their use.

Treatment availability is a practical reality. If the preferred intervention is not available and cannot be obtained, another choice must be made. Medical contraindications exist for all of the different technologies, but the medical contraindication that rules out the use of one will not necessarily rule out the use of others. For example, a semicomatose patient should not be seen in the whirlpool, but wound cleansing with pulsatile lavage with suction at bedside would be an appropriate alternative. Sometimes treatment availability leads to overuse of a particular intervention and restricts choice of other possibilities. Examples of overuse may be negative pressure or whirlpool.

The following case study illustrates how thoughtful evaluation of the history and systems review narrowed down the choice of treatment intervention to one appropriate technology after considering all the factors.

■ CASE STUDY

Choosing the Appropriate Treatment Intervention

A case example in which multiple factors had to be considered when making a choice of intervention was required for E.F. An elderly lady, E.F. lived in a nursing home because of incompetence related to Alzheimer disease. She had venous disease and a history of recurrent venous ulcers of the lower leg. A new episode of ulceration occurred, and the patient was referred to the PT. The patient had a pacemaker, would not stay in bed or in a wheelchair for 5 minutes, and would not tolerate dressings or compression devices. The venous disease diagnosis ruled out whirlpool. The pacemaker ruled out any form of diathermy. The low tolerance for compression ruled out compression devices. The inability to tolerate staying in one place more than 5 minutes and intolerance for dressings ruled out electrical stimulation. Pulsatile lavage with suction was not available and would not have been tolerated by the patient. The only choice remaining was ultrasound because she could be kept still and amused for the 5 minutes required for a periwound ultrasound treatment. This was also an appropriate choice because ultrasound is particularly effective during the acute inflammatory phase and effects absorption of hemorrhagic materials. This patient is included as one of the case histories in Chapter 24. The results are viewed in *Color Plates 74 to 76*.

Functional Wound Cost Outcomes Management

How do costs for treatment with biophysical agents for wound healing compare? Does this group of interventions provide good value for the money spent? Based on data from Swanson,[22] Maver,[23] and Birke,[24] biophysical technologies used by PTs are competitive for certain wounds. Swanson compared the costs of a course of wound care with hydrotherapy (whirlpool) with a high-voltage pulsed-current (HVPC) type of electrical stimulation. She found that the course of 3 months (90 days) of care with hydrotherapy treatment (whirlpool) for necrotic wounds with an unknown outcome was $4,500, compared with $2,100 for a 7.5-week (52 days average) course of care with outcome of wound closure following treatment with HVPC electrical stimulation. Maver[23] compared the cost of conventional treatment for stage III pressure ulcers that did not heal during a course of care with a mean time of 34.62 weeks at a cost of $7,946.33, with 8.5 weeks course of care to healed status with Diapulse, pulsed radiofrequency stimulation,[24] combined with conventional care cost of $2,929.62. The reported savings per ulcer in this study was $4,484.

Birke[24] reported on numerous studies using total-contact casting (TCC) to heal plantar ulcers in patients with neuropathy. The average time to closure was 42 days. The average cost for a closed wound was $1,250. These cost savings do not include savings derived from reduced mortality, morbidity, and reduction in amputations. Comparative lengths of care and expected outcome for hydrotherapy, HVPC, and TCC are illustrated in Figure IV-2.

Cost comparison allows for a profile of wound cost outcomes and comparative analysis of the results of a course of care. Physical therapy is cost competitive for certain wounds (Figure IV-3). Health-care professionals including the entire team and program directors need to understand the information required to predict and manage cost for proper utilization of services. The necessary information to predict cost and outcome are available from several sources: clinical trials, program evaluation reports, the facility's clinical database, evidence-based clinical practice guidelines, and payer databased reports.

Does your clinic know your cost outcomes? Cost outcomes are differentiated from the technical outcome for the wound (e.g., closure). Cost outcomes are what it costs to provide a course of care compared with the billed charges. This determines the cost to the provider as differentiated from the charges to the payer. The cost outcome is based on all the related costs for providing the service: labor cost, supply cost, and equipment cost. To determine the cost of treating a wound the clinical manager needs to predict the number of expected visits to achieve a predicted outcome. For example, if an outcome of closure is expected in 49 visits, a cost analysis can be done as follows:

Labor cost at \$30/visit × 49 = \$1,470
Supply cost at \$6.25/visit × 49 = \$306.25

FIGURE IV-3 Length of stay dependent on wound type and procedure.

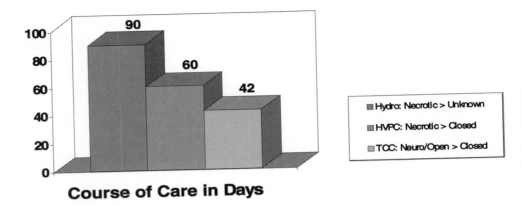

Equipment cost at $0.50 × 49 = $24.50
Total cost = $1,800.75
Billed charges at $60/visit × 49 = $2,940
Net profit = $1,139.25

The cost for a different outcome to convert the wound to clean and stable may take half the time to closure. Cost to the payer would be reduced by half, to $1,470. The case manager for the payer may be more willing to authorize an interim step for a known cost than an unknown outcome at unmanaged cost.

Reducing variability in healing rates and being able to predict outcomes helps the management of wound care costs. Recent research is there to help with clinic management. For example, Kantor and Margolis[25] found that with good wound care, 56% of venous ulcers healed in 16 weeks, but only 28% of diabetic neuropathic ulcers healed in the same time period. Further results suggest that there was a steady rate of healing for venous ulcers during the first 12 weeks, but the linear rate begins to diminish rapidly after that point. For the diabetic neuropathic ulcer group there was little improvement in proportion healed after 16 weeks. Based on these data, an average healing rate for two-thirds of the chronic leg ulcers of 49 days (7 weeks) with standard care plus biophysical agents was significantly less than the healing rates reported and was cost effective. This is an example of how to compare the results of one clinic's outcomes with reports in the literature.

Utilization Review and Cost Outcomes Management

Utilization review and cost outcomes management mean that continued on-going evaluation of patient candidacy for the advanced therapy intervention be reviewed. Candidacy determined at the initial evaluation may change as the patient experiences a course of care (Figure IV-4). The Sussman wound healing tool, described in Chapter 5, was developed as a diagnostic tool to evaluate progression through the phases of healing when wounds were treated with biophysical technologies. For example, reduction in wound depth is a finding that the wound has progressed to the

acute proliferative phase. Reduction in wound size is a measure of wound contraction, also part of the proliferative phase and of the epithelialization phase. The Bates-Jensen Wound Assessment Tool (BWAT) and the pressure ulcer scale for healing (PUSH) tool, also described in Chapter 5, meet the criteria for documentation of wound progress over time represented by a numeric change. If these benchmarks of healing are not occurring in an orderly and timely manner, it may be due to a poor response to treatment, perhaps because of changes in medical status, and should trigger a change in the treatment approach. The following are some examples of situations that trigger a change:

- *Failure to progress:* If the wound is not progressing through the biologic sequence of repair and reducing in size significantly after 2 to 4 weeks of treatment with HVPC, the entire wound management plan needs to be reviewed to determine whether it is the HVPC treatment or other factors that are responsible for failure to progress. Since all wounds have multiple associated interventions, including wound cleansing, topical treatments, dressings, and debridement, along with the HVPC, each intervention should be reviewed to determine whether continuation is appropriate or if there needs to be a change in these interventions or with the HVPC protocol.
- *Wound regression:* If the wound has gotten larger or deeper or has developed undermining or tunneling from the separation of the fascial planes, or is invading named structures or areas or has become infected, this is referred to as wound *regression*. It may be the result of debridement or ischemia or infection. The PT, PTA, or nurse should be able to recognize the signs and symptoms of regression and take responsibility to report the change in condition to the physician.
- *Medical instability:* If the patient has become medically unstable (e.g., pneumonia, sepsis, renal failure), the body's ability to heal is impaired, and the situation requires a change in medical management before continuing with physical therapy. The PT may determine that the physical therapy intervention should be put on hold until the medical condition is stabilized.
- *Other management required:* If the wound has progressed to a clean and stable wound in the proliferative phase, it

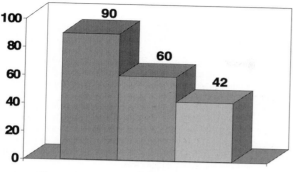

Course of Care in Days

FIGURE IV-4 Cost comparison for different wound interventions and outcomes. Physical therapy is competitive for certain wounds.

■ Hydro: Necrotic > Unknown

■ HVPC: Necrotic > Closed

■ TCC: Neuro/Open > Closed

may indicate that the wound is ready for grafting or artificial skin to cover the wound more quickly and perhaps reduce scarring. It may be the best prognosis for the wound and/or for the patient and may have been the reason for referral, the objective of the patient, the family, the therapist, and the physician.

- *Wound needs less skilled care:* The wound is now at a phase of repair on the trajectory of healing that demonstrates that the healing response is sustained. Now the patient/caregiver or nurse may be able to continue to provide standard wound care procedures until healed, and the PT would bow out.
- *Goals met:* Sometimes, the patient and family have reached their goals and do not wish to continue or become noncompliant with treatment. In other cases, the wound has healed.
- *Closure and beyond:* Wound closure may be the intent of the treatment, but closure does not include remodeling. Wounds that are minimally closed are at very high risk for recurrence, especially when located over areas of friction, shear, and pressure, such as on the seating surface or plantar surface of the foot. Wounds in those areas of high risk would benefit from further stimulation of collagen synthesis by treatment like electrical stimulation until the minimally healed scar is acceptably healed.[12] Acceptable healing is achieved when there is a thickening of the scar formation and the color of the scar blanches from bright red or pink to light pink or white (see Chapter 14 for more information about scar).

Plan of Care/Treatment

Part IV focuses primarily on the use of externally applied treatments for wound repair and does not address specific dressings. It must be reinforced, however, that all of the described technologies are supplemental to standard wound management which is covered in other chapters throughout the book. It is noted where specific requirements of the technology are compatible with the dressing regimen or vise versa.

Chapter Organization

Each chapter in Part IV covers the following information about each modality:

- Related definitions and terminology
- Associated physical science
- The theory and science of the therapy
- Clinical trials, when available, that relate to efficacy
- Indications, contraindications, and precautions
- Expected outcomes and outcomes measures
- Equipment use and safety
- Procedures, including protocols and patient set-ups
- Clinical and research-related wisdom
- Self-care treatment guidelines, if appropriate
- Case study, using the functional outcome report

REFERENCES

1. Cameron MH, Perez D, Otano-Lata S. Electromagnetic Radiation.In: Cameron M, ed. Physical Agents in Rehabilitation: from Research to Practice. Philadelphia: Saunders; 1999:304–306.
2. Kloth L, Ziskin MC. Diathermy and pulsed radio frequency radiation. In: Michlovitz SL, ed. *Thermal Agents in Rehabilitation,* 3rd ed. Philadelphia: FA Davis; 1996:213–220.
3. American Physical Therapy Association. A guide to physical therapist practice, Vol. 1: a description of patient management. *Phys Ther.* 1995;75:707–764.
4. Eaglstein W. What is standard care and where should we leave it? In: *Evidence Based Outcomes in Wound Management.* Dallas, TX: ConvaTec;2000.
5. General Accounting Office, US Congress, reported in PT Bulletin. *American Physical Therapy Association,* Vol. 12, No. 10, March 7, 1997.
6. Hayes S, Carroll S. Early intervention care in the acute stroke patient. *Arch Phys Med Rehabil.* 1986;67:319–321.
7. Linton S, Hellsing A, Andersson D. A controlled study of the effects of early intervention on acute musculoskeletal pain problems. *Pain.* 1993;54(3):353–359.
8. American Physical Therapy Association. *Outcome Effectiveness of Physical Therapy: An Annotated Bibliography.* Alexandria, VA: APTA; 1993.
9. Hunt T, Hussain MZ. Can wound healing be a paradigm for tissue repair? *Med Sci Sports Exerc.* 1994;26:755–758.
10. Robson MC, Hill DP, Woodske ME, Steed DL. Wound healing trajectories as predictors of effectiveness of therapeutic agents. *Arch Surg.* 2000;135(7):773–777.
11. Harding K. Wound care: putting theory into clinical practice. In: Krasner D, ed. *Chronic Wound Care: A Clinical Source for Health Care Professionals.* King of Prussia, PA: Health Management Publications Inc; 1990:19–30.

12. Lazarus GS, Cooper DM, Knighton DR, et al. Definitions and guidelines for assessment of wounds and evaluation of healing. *Arch Dermatol.* 1994;130:489–493.

13. Dyson M, Young S. Acceleration of tissue repair by low intensity ultrasound applied during the inflammatory phase, APTA/CPTA Joint Congress, Abstract No. R-186, presented in Las Vegas, Nevada, June 1998.

14. Skene AI, Smith JM, Dore CJ, Charlett A, Lewis JD. Venous leg ulcers: a prognostic index to predict time to healing. *Br Med J.* 1992;305(6862):1119–1121.

15. Tallman, P, Muscare E, Carson P, Eaglstein WH, Falanga V. Initial rate of healing predicts complete healing of venous ulcers. *Arch Dermatol.* 1997;133(10):1231–1234.

16. Phillips T. Machado F, Trout R, Porter J, Olin J, Falanga V. Prognostic indicators in venous ulcers. *J Am Acad Dermatol.* 2000;43(4):627–630.

17 vanRijswijk L. Full-thickness pressure ulcers: patient and wound healing characteristics. *Decubitus.* 1993;6(1):16–21.

18. Marston W, Carlin RE, Passman MA, Farber MA, Keagy BA. Healing rates and cost efficacy of outpatient compression treatment for leg ulcers associated with venous insufficiency. *J Vasc Surg.* 1999;30(3):491–498.

19. Garber, SL, Biddle AK, Click CN. *Pressure Ulcer Prevention and Treatment Following Spinal Cord Injury: A Clinical Practice Guideline for Health-Care Professionals.* Jackson Heights, NY: Paralyzed Veterans of America; 2000:12–14.

20. Dolynchuk K, Keast D, Campbell K. Best practices for the prevention and treatment of pressure ulcers. *Ostomy Wound Management.* 2000;46(11):38–52.

21. Joint Commission on Accreditation of Healthcare Organizations (Joint Commission). Pain Management Standards (Standard RI 2.8 and PE 1.4). In: Joint Commission, ed. *Comprehensive Accreditation Manual for Hospitals.* Oakbrook Terrace, IL: Joint Commission; 2001.

22. Swanson G. Use of cost data, provider experience, and clinical guidelines in the transition to managed care. *J Ins Med.* 1991;23(1):70–74.

23. Maver RW. An actuarial report on the cost-effectiveness of a new medical technology. *J Ins Med.* 1991;23(2):120–123.

24. Birke J. Management of the diabetic foot instructional course. Wound Care Management Conference. November 1995.

25. Itoh M, et al. Accelerated wound healing of pressure ulcers by pulsed high peak power electromagnetic energy (Diapulse). *Decubitus.* 1991;4(1):24–34.

26. Kantor J, Margolis DJ. Expected healing rates for chronic wounds. *Wounds: A Compendium of Clinical Research and Practice.* 2000;12(6):155–158.

Electrical Stimulation for Wound Healing

Carrie Sussman

CHAPTER OBJECTIVES

At the completion of this chapter, the reader will be able to:

1. Explain the physical properties of electrical stimulation used for wound healing treatment, including their significance.
2. Describe evidence of the physiologic effects of electrical stimulation on body systems: cellular, circulatory, and neuronal.
3. Describe the results of animal and clinical studies using different types of electrical stimulation waveforms.
4. Select the appropriate candidates for wound healing with electrical stimulation.
5. List the contraindications and precautions of electrical stimulation for wound healing.
6. Apply electrical stimulation for different wound healing situations, including home self-care, and evaluate outcomes of care.

Use of exogenous electrical current for wound healing of chronic indolent ulcers of many etiologies has been reported in the literature since the 1960s. There are many descriptive reports, quality assurance documents, case reports, and experimental research, including randomized controlled trials (RCTs), evaluating efficacy and safety. For a long time there was skepticism about use of this intervention. Recently the skepticism has been replaced by recognition of its value as an evidenced-based tool for tissue healing. That recognition is demonstrated by inclusion of electrical stimulation (ES) as a recommended treatment choice in clinical practice guidelines, in a meta-analysis, in a national coverage policy by the Center for Medicare and Medicaid Services (CMS) for reimbursement, and through frequent mention in the wound literature.

Some reasons for the skepticism include the variation in modes of stimulation delivery, different protocols, and limited data available for each specific ES device as well as small sample sizes and lack of homogeneity of subjects in the studies. Not all ES procedures are alike, creating confusion about which one to use for wound healing. Chapter 22 presents the evidence available currently about ES and wound healing needed for clinical decision making. The CMS national coverage policy is found at the CMS website (www.cms.hhs.gov). Search for electrical stimulation coverage policy.

Evaluating the Evidence

In 1993, the Agency for Health Care Policy and Research (AHCPR), now the Agency for Health Care Research and Quality (AHRQ), convened a panel of experts to review the literature related to adjunctive treatments for pressure ulcers. In 1994, this panel published guidelines[1] for pressure ulcer treatment. The literature review by the AHCPR panel (1993) focused on several adjunctive therapies used to facilitate healing of pressure ulcers. Usually, an adjunctive therapy is selected to restart or accelerate wound healing. The adjunctive therapies considered by the panel were ES, hyperbaric oxygen, infrared, ultraviolet and low-energy laser irradiation, ultrasound, miscellaneous topical agents, and systemic drugs (not antibiotics). At the time of the review, only ES had sufficient supporting evidence to warrant better than a "C" recommendation by the panel. ES was given an evidence rating of "B" based on five clinical trials[2,3] in which ES was used to treat pressure ulcers in 147 patients. The recommendation read: "Consider a course of treatment with electrotherapy for stage II and IV pressure ulcers that have proved unresponsive to conventional therapy. Electrical stimulation may also be useful for recalcitrant Stage II ulcers.[1]" In 1996, the American Medical Directors Association published clinical practice guidelines for pressure ulcers and supported the recommendation of the AHRQ panel to consider a course of electrotherapy.[4]

In an update of the AHCPR *Guidelines for Pressure Ulcers*, Ovington[5] revisited the issue by reviewing the literature through May 1998 to determine the status of adjunctive therapy evidence in the 5 years since the AHCPR review. The goal was to determine whether any new data existed that would change or strengthen the evidence of the AHCPR recommendations. In her review, Ovington[5] changed the designation of "*controlled clinical trials (CCTs)*" for the five studies used by AHCPR to "*randomized controlled trials (RCTs)*" and added one additional RCT study for treatment of pressure ulcers in 74 patients. [6] Based on an additional RCT not included in the 1993 AHCPR evidence review, she recommended that ES be upgraded to an "A" from a "B" for the treatment of pressure ulcers. In August 2000, the Consortium for Spinal Cord Medicine published *Pressure Ulcer Prevention and Treatment Following Spinal Cord Injury* clinical practice guidelines.[7] In these guidelines, ES treatment was recommended (grade level A) as primary treatment for use to promote closure of stages III or IV pressure ulcers, along with standard wound care interventions.

Review of the literature (through December 2005) found several RCTs studying ES efficacy for treating chronic wounds of different etiologies, including individuals with spinal cord injury (SCI) who had a total of 185 pressure ulcers[8] and had a positive treatment effect with a protocol using ES. Patients with 42 leg ulcers—venous, arterial, and diabetic—benefited from 4 weeks of ES treatment but those benefits were negated 4 weeks after treatment stopped.[9] Two studies of 81 and 42 subjects with chronic venous ulcers[10,11] were conducted in Poland. Two RCTs were published that evaluated ES treatment for patients with diabetic foot ulcers[12] and ischemic ulcers.[5,13,14] In an unpublished RCT study of 37 human subjects with pressure ulcers, the ES group showed significant decrease in volume measurements.[15] This information is mentioned here to demonstrate the on-going accumulation of a body of evidence about ES efficacy for wounds of different etiologies. All of the cited studies are reviewed more completely in other parts of this chapter.

Meta-Analysis

A meta-analysis is a mathematical synthesis used in statistics to average the findings across multiple studies quantitatively. It is used to estimate better the magnitude of a treatment effect. Gardner and Frantz[16] recognized the problem of analyzing the efficacy of ES for wound healing when the methods are variable. They undertook to examine the entire body of evidence available at that time, irrespective of device and parameters, and performed a meta-analysis to acquire information about the merits of using ES as an adjunctive wound healing therapy. Another goal of the Gardner/Frantz meta-analysis was to provide clinicians and researchers with valuable information about the utility of pursuing further research in this area. This goal has been met given the number of additional studies now available. (A new meta-analysis looking at the additional body of published work would be useful.) The methods and findings of the meta-analysis are discussed below.

Efficacy and Reimbursement

Part of the skepticism that has surrounded this treatment stems from events pertaining to reimbursement. For close to 20 years, care providers of Medicare recipients with chronic wounds who had medical necessity, decided on a case-by-case basis, were reimbursed for ES wound treatment. In 1997, that changed. The Health Care Financing Administration (HCFA) reported findings in a review of ES by an independent group, ECRI, a health-care technology assessment consulting firm, that ES in all forms is no *more or less* effective than standard care. Based on this report, HCFA announced that it would exclude reimbursement for all forms of ES therapy for wound healing for Medicare recipients. Its findings contradicted the findings of the AHCPR panel. The meta-analysis of ES had not been prepared at that time. Opposition to this decision came from providers, patients, health-care professionals, and the American Physical Therapy Association (APTA), which observed the benefits of treatment of chronic wounds with ES. In November 1997, the federal court enjoined HCFA from implementing this policy. [17]

In July 1998, HCFA notified program carriers and intermediaries that the court order remained in effect until further notice and to disregard Section 35–98 of the Medicare Coverage Issues Manual issued in 1997 that excluded ES reimbursement for the treatment of wounds and to pay for claims based on supporting documentation.[18] The tide turned in favor of ES wound treatment coverage when an HCFA medical and surgical procedures panel unanimously voted that there was sufficient evidence that ES has obvious public benefits and that they could classify this therapy as *more* effective than standard care alone for the treatment of nonhealing chronic wounds.[2] Still, doubts remain among some in the healthcare community about the use of ES for chronic wound healing. Doubt seems to have changed to broader acceptance following the issuance of a national coverage policy for ES treatment of chronic wounds issued by HCFA, now the Center for Medicare and Medicaid Services (CMS), in 2002.

The goal of this chapter is to present the evidence based on a review of the current literature (through December 2005) about what is known regarding the efficacy and utility of using ES as adjunctive therapy for wound healing. The chapter begins with definitions and terminology used to discuss and distinguish ES parameters. The second section details the science and theory of the therapy and relates back to the parameters. Clinical decision making applies the science and theory by considering the indications for the therapy, reasons for referral, medical history, and systems reviews that are part of the diagnostic process. This section is followed by a description of the equipment and accessories used, the rationale for selection of protocols, the expected outcomes, and the patient set-up. Because ES is a treatment intervention that can be taught to patients or other caregivers, self-care teaching guidelines are included. Case studies applying the functional outcome report (FOR) to document the rationale for selection of ES as the intervention, followed by a discussion revealing the clinical decision-making process and the actual outcomes, conclude the chapter.[19] Chapter 2 describes the FOR.

Definitions and Terminology

Electrical stimulation for wound healing is defined as the use of a capacitive coupled electrical current to transfer energy to a wound. The type of electricity that is transferred to the target tissue is controlled by the electrical source.[1] Clinicians need to be familiar with the terminology and characteristics associated with ES to better understand the interrelationships between the various stimulation characteristics and the clinical effects desired. This is not meant to be a comprehensive description of all ES characteristics but instead emphasize those that have an evidence-based role in wound healing in clinical practice. For more information, see the suggested readings listed at the end of this chapter.

Capacitive Coupling

Capacitively coupled ES involves the transfer of electric current through an applied surface electrode pad that is in wet (electrolytic) contact (capacitively coupled) with the external skin surface and/or wound bed. When capacitively coupled ES is used, at least two electrodes are required to complete the electric circuit. Electrodes are usually placed over wet conductive medium: (1) in the wound bed or on the skin a distance away from the wound—monopolar technique, or (2) straddling the wound—bipolar technique. Bipolar technique along the wound edge has advantages of not having to disrupt the wound bed or dressing, thus chilling the wound, as well as not introducing contaminants into the wound or spreading disease when the electrode is removed. It is the method reported in most of the biphasic studies that will be discussed later in this chapter.

Polarity

Polarity refers to the property of having two poles that are oppositely charged. The positive pole is called the *anode* and the negative pole the *cathode*. The positive pole lacks electrons and attracts electrons from the negative pole. If the wound is placed between the poles as in the bipolar technique described above, and the electrodes are relatively close together, no one polarity predominates, and this is referred to as tangential polarity.[20] Polarity can be chosen or emphasized for biologic effects that are described throughout this chapter by taking into account the placement of the electrodes (see the section on active and dispersive electrodes). In a review of the literature,[20] it was concluded that alternating polarity (negative initially) was more effective for potential wound healing results than maintaining either positive or negative polarity throughout the course treatment.

Amplitude and Voltage

Amplitude refers to the measure of the magnitude of the voltage and should not be referred to as the intensity.[21] Voltage is a measure of the force of the flow of electrons, and amperage is the measure of the rate of flow of the current. When voltage is turned up, the current will also go up, and vice versa. Some stimulators provide a readout of voltage and some a readout of current. The relationship between voltage and current is expressed as Ohm's law. The formula for this is current times resistance equals voltage [$V = RI$, where V is voltage, I is current, and R is resistance]. In general, low-voltage devices produce voltages of different ranges from 60 to 100 V. High-voltage devices range from 100 to 500 V. These are peak ranges. Peak amplitude is the highest amplitude of the current or voltage. Amplitude for wound healing is adjusted until the patient with sensation can feel a tingling sensation (paresthesia) at the edge of the wound. Insensate individuals, of course, cannot respond to this sensation. The voltage is usually turned up until there is a mild muscle contraction or fasciculation, and then backed down until that muscle contraction is no longer visible. For wound healing treatment with high-voltage pulsed current (HVPC), the amplitude is usually set between 75 and 150 V to achieve this response.[22]

Amperage

The unit of current is the ampere (A), which is defined as the rate at which electrons move past a certain point. A milliampere (mA) is one-thousandth of an ampere, and a microampere (µA) is one-millionth of an ampere. Microamperage current is usually between 5 and 20 µA of current (less than 1.0 mA).

Waveforms

Waveforms are classified by the direction of current flow. Current flow is either unidirectional or bidirectional. Direct current is unidirectional and continuous. Two basic waveforms are used for rehabilitation purposes. They are direct current (DC) and pulsatile current (PC).[23] A unidirectional current that is of one second or longer duration is defined as direct current. Pulsatile currents differ from direct currents because they are introduced into the tissues in the form of a pulse with a duration of a few milliseconds or less. The waveforms that are classified as pulsatile currents include monophasic, biphasic, and polyphasic. Waveforms are the graphic representations of a current on a current/time or voltage/time plot.[24] Figure 22-1 shows examples of different current waveforms including: monophasic square wave pulsed current and twin-peaked pulsed current, symmetrical biphasic and asymmetric biphasic and polyphasic alternating waveforms. In the following sections, electrical characteristics that are relevant to reports in the literature about bioelectricity are described with the intent of helping the reader interpret the findings.

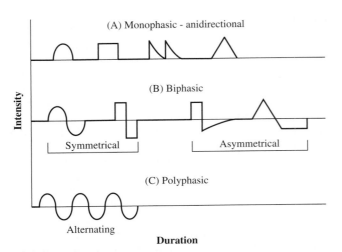

FIGURE 22-1 Classification of waveforms in clinical electrical stimulation. (Adapted with permission from Alon G, De Dominico G. *High Voltage Stimulation: An Integrated Approach to Clinical Electrotherapy*, 1st ed. Hixton, TN: The Chattanooga Group; 1987:34.)

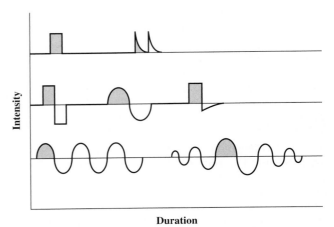

FIGURE 22-2 Single phases for different wave forms (*gray area*). (Reprinted with permission from Alon G, De Dominico G. *High Voltage Stimulation: An Integrated Approach to Clinical Electrotherapy*, 1st ed. Hixton, TN: The Chattanooga Group; 1987:37.)

Reporting of ES Parameters

To use the evidence produced from clinical studies, several parameters have been identified that are needed to help define the effective treatment dose, to make studies reproducible, and to compare studies.[22,25,26] They include:

- Type of current delivered
- Current amplitude (often termed intensity)
- Pulse frequency (rate) and width
* Pulse duration
- Electrode size or average current density/area of the electrode (i.e., mA/cm^2)
- Duty cycle for pulsed currents
- Phase charge and current density, including calculation of the phase charge delivered to the tissues
- Treatment time

Direct Current

Unidirectional current is also called *galvanic* or *direct current*. Direct current is continuous, uninterrupted, unidirectional current. Direction of the flow is determined by the polarity selected. Direct current waveforms may be modulated into pulsatile currents with specific phases.

Phase, Phase Duration, and Interpulse Interval

A phase is the time that elapses from the start of a pulse until it ends. The phase duration is the length of time that the pulse is on. Figure 22-2 illustrates the concept of phase for different wave forms.) The time between pulses is termed the *interpulse interval* (see Figure 22-3). For monophasic waveforms, the phase duration and pulse duration are synonymous. For biphasic waveforms there are two phases and the pulse duration is the same for both phases.[23] Phase mod-

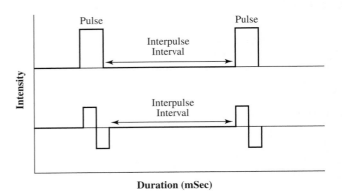

FIGURE 22-3 Interpulse interval. (Reprinted with permission from Alon G, De Dominico G. *High Voltage Stimulation: An Integrated Approach to Clinical Electrotherapy*, 1st ed. Hixton, TN: The Chattanooga Group; 1987:35.)

ulations are possible and useful for rehabilitation purposes. The possibilities include change of phase duration, change of phase and pulse intensity, and change in pulse frequency or rate.

On some stimulators the pulse duration is labeled incorrectly as "pulse width." Pulse duration affects biologic responses. For example, direct current has a continuous duration that can raise tissue temperature and change the pH under the electrode, which can produce blisters under the electrode. However, a short pulse duration (5–100 µsec), typical of HVCP, produces insignificant changes in both tissue pH and tissue temperature.[23,27,28] Such a current is therefore very safe but raises questions about the effect of polarity when the pulse duration is so short. For purposes of muscle stimulation, the stimulation must be provided at an amplitude and a duration that will stimulate a muscle contraction, which is a minimum of 1 msec.[28]

If the goal is to keep the stimulation tolerable, the amplitude must be kept as low as possible, forcing the duration of the stimulus to be longer. Because high-voltage pulsed monophasic current has a pulse duration shorter than 1 msec, it cannot be used to stimulate denervated muscle. Even at maximum pulse rates, the phase duration for HVPC represents less than 1% of the on time, and the interpulse interval 99% percent of the total time.[23] Despite this, HVPC stimulators can cause excitation of sensory, motor, and pain-conducting fibers. The laws of excitation state that "at a shorter phase duration, less charge is needed to cause threshold excitation."[29] For pain management and wound healing, the pulse duration and the amplitude of the current are variable. Some clinicians and researchers suggest that this current must be on for at least 1 second to produce strong polarity effects of the tissue under the electrodes. Yet, even at these very short pulse durations of HVPC, different effects related to polarity are reported. Many of these effects will be presented in this chapter.

Frequency or Pulse Rate

Pulsed current is defined as an electrical current that is conducted as a signal(s) of short duration. Each pulse lasts for a few milliseconds (msec) or microseconds (μsec), followed by an interpulse interval, then repeated.[30]

Pulse rate or frequency is the number of pulses delivered per unit of time. The *rate* of the off and on cycle is defined as pulses per second (pps). Alternating current frequency is usually expressed in Hertz (Hz) and pulsed monophasic current in pps. Thus, Hz and pps represent the same property, that is, the number of pulses delivered each second.[30]

The range of pps is usually from 0.1 to 999 Hz. A pulse of 0.1 Hz is on for 10 seconds, and a pulse of 999 Hz is on for 1 msec. The time between pulses when no electrical activity occurs is the interpulse interval (Figure 22-3). Pulsed ES (PES) has a train of pulses that are repeated at regular intervals and are termed the *pulse rate* or *pulse frequency*. Pulsed current can be either unidirectional or bidirectional.

Duty Cycle

The on/off ratio is the ratio of the time the current is on to the time the current is off. A duty cycle is the ratio of *on time* to the *total cycle time*, including both the on and off time. A ratio is used to express the relative proportion of the on and off time and can be expressed as a percentage. For instance, if the total cycle is 60 μsec, the on time is 20 μsec, and the off time is 40 μsec, there is a 1:2 on/off ratio and the duty cycle is a 1:3 ratio, or a 33% duty cycle. The calculation for duty cycle is pulse duration in seconds × frequency (Hz) = fraction of time during which current is actually applied.

Pulsatile Currents
Monophasic Pulsed Current

Pulsed current is phasic. Monophasic pulsed current is defined as pulsed current that deviates from baseline and returns to baseline after a designated time period. The monophasic pulsed current waveform may be either a square wave or the traditional twin-peaked pulsed wave of the HVPC. Monophasic pulses and phases are identical (see Figure 22-2). Monophasic waves are such that, at one electrode, the polarity is positive and the other is negative. This stays constant throughout the treatment unless changed by the clinician. Polarity appears to have specific effects on biologic responses.

High-Voltage Pulsed Current

HVPC typically has a twin-peaked monophasic waveform (see Figure 22-4). HVPC is a misnomer if *galvanic* is used with it. This current was named incorrectly by the manufacturers. The acronym HVPC does not have *galvanic* in the acronym. The pulse rate most frequently used for wound healing is 50–120 pps (0.83–1.25 msec). Each peak or spike has an effective 5- to 20-μsec phase duration. Voltage can be selected with intensity between 100 and 500 V. The amplitude selected for wound healing is usually between 80 and 200 V, and the polarity and pulse rate are varied. There is a long interpulse interval between pulses that makes a low average current. The high-voltage stimulation has a high peak current that means greater penetration into tissue, allowing for stimulation of deep motor points. [23] On the skin surface, alkaline/acidity changes under the electrodes have not been measured.[27,28] Because HVPC is not galvanic, this explains why there are no alkaline/acidity effects.

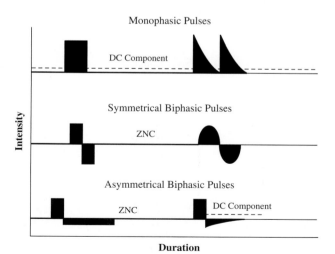

FIGURE 22-4 Typical pulse characteristics of a high-voltage stimulator. (Reprinted with permission from Alon G, De Dominico G. *High Voltage Stimulation: An Integrated Approach to Clinical Electrotherapy*, 1st ed. Hixton, TN: The Chattanooga Group; 1987:62.)

Absence of chemical changes under the electrodes has led to questions about how polarity effects can be the factor that stimulates cellular responses when the duration of the HVPC pulse is so short. However, multiple studies demonstrate different effects on blood flow, edema, and bacteria under the anode and cathode when using HVPC (Table 22-1). One study showed that fibroblasts were attracted to the cathode of an HVPC stimulator, suggesting that there may be some cellular polarity effects under the electrode.[31] Although multiple studies show cellular effects and responses to HVPC, each study shows something different; therefore, corroborating research would be useful to support the findings of these single studies (see the section on galvanotaxis).

Microcurrent Electrical Stimulation

A pulsed monophasic stimulus is referred to as *monophasic low-voltage microcurrent electrical nerve stimulation* (MENS). This refers to a pulsed current at an intensity less than 1 mA (1–999 µA), and the voltage is less than 100 V. MENS is delivered at amplitudes that have minimal detectable sensation and are incapable of motor nerve stimulation. MENS typically has a single modified monophasic square waveform. The pulse duration of these devices ranges from 0.1 to 999 Hz, equivalent to an on time of 10 seconds to 1 µsec. The pulse duration is inversely related to the frequency. Microcurrent stimulation has a prolonged pulse duration at the lower frequencies, which will have a different tissue polarity effect than a shorter-duration pulse, most typically used in high-voltage stimulation. For example, a low-voltage pulsed stimulus at 0.1 Hz is on for 10 seconds, whereas the high-voltage monophasic simulators are used at 80–120 pps and are on for only 0.83–1.25 msec. Thus, pulsed low-voltage current of at least 1 pps can maintain the polarity effect delivered to the tissues under the electrode. The peak amplitude is usually 600 µA/60 V. The average amplitude commonly used is 200–300 µA for soft tissue[32] and 20 µA for bone healing in rabbits.[33] MENS current has been used in bone healing; however, in this clinical application, the amplitude recommended is 20–50 µA.[34,35,36,12,37,38,39,40]

When pulsed slowly, there are reported cellular and tissue polarity effects under the electrodes.[41] This type of current may be used to restore the normal bioelectrical resting current or reverse the injury current.[41] There is some concern that the voltage may be too low to push the current through the resistance of the skin and the subcutaneous tissues, but no specific studies could be found to confirm this.

Alternating/Biphasic Current

Bidirectional waveforms are referred to as *faradic* or *alternating*, as well as *biphasic* or *bipolar*. British literature uses the term *"faradic"* for all alternating current (AC), probably in reference to the scientist Faraday. In the United States, faradic is no longer designed in ES units because it is very

TABLE 22-1 Polarity Effects of Electrical Stimulation

Effect	Pole	Researcher	Type of Current
↑ Blood flow	Negative	Mohr et al[69]	HVPC
		Politis et al[71]	PES
		Pollack[72]	PES
		Gentzkow et al[3]	PES
		Goldman et al[14,93]	HVPC
↓ Edema	Negative	Mendel and Fish[101]	HVPC
		Reed[100]	HVPC
		Ross and Segal[99]	HVPC
Debridement	Negative	Sawyer and Deutch[109,110,111]	DC
Thrombolysis	Negative	Sawyer and Deutch[109,110,111]	DC
Thrombosis	Positive	Williams and Carey[164]	DC
Oxygen (tc P0₂)	Anode	Byl et al[117]	MENS, 100 µA low volt
Oxygen (tc P0₂)	Negative bias	Baker et al[165]	Asymmetric biphasic
Wound contraction	Alternating (±) every 3 days	Stromberg[62]	PES
Tendon repair	Positive	Owoeye et al[166]	HVPC
Bacteriostatic effects	Both	Barranco et al[112]	DC
		Rowley et al[113]	DC
		Kincaid and Lavoie[115]	HVPC
		Szuminsky et al[116]	HVPC

uncomfortable. Alternating current is uninterrupted bidirectional current flow. The waveforms may be symmetric, in which the shape of the waveform is always balanced. Both the shape and size are the same. An asymmetric waveform can be balanced or unbalanced (see Figure 22-1). One of the most common outputs from an electrical stimulator is balanced asymmetric. A balanced asymmetric waveform is typical of transcutaneous electrical nerve stimulation (TENS) used for pain modulation.

Biphasic waves are such that the polarity is constantly changing. They are opposite at any moment in time. However, the waveform can be biased so that one polarity is emphasized. Several studies using this type of current for wound healing have been reported in the literature, which are described in this chapter. The best wound healing effects seem to be achieved when a biphasic waveform is asymmetric and biased, so that the polarity at one pole predominates, which is usually the negative pole. Pain modulation and edema reduction in patients with diabetic neuropathy have been reported with a biphasic waveform.[42,43] The effects of stimulation with a biphasic waveform on wound healing are discussed further in following sections.

Phase Charge and Charge Density

Phase charge and charge density, also known as current density, have not been considered closely in the past. How important are phase charge and current density to tissue healing? Phase and pulse charge refer to the total charge or "dose of electric current" within each phase of each pulse[29] (see Figure 22-5). Phase charge is a time- and amplitude-dependent characteristic.[21] It is possible to calculate the pulse charge for any type of electrical waveform if waveform, frequency (rate) and duration (width) of the pulse, and amplitude (voltage) are known. The unit of measure for charge is the coulomb. One coulomb is the quantity of electricity transferred by a current of one ampere in one second. Figure 22-4 shows the effect of waveforms on charge accumulation.

Brighton et al[44] studied the relationship between charge, current density, and the amount of new bone formed in rabbits. They reported that a classical dose–response relationship exists between current amplitude, charge delivered, and biologic effect. At a low, constant DC current regime there is minimal or no effect. A regime of optimal or maximal effect occurs at 20 µA (36.29 C) and a gradual occurrence of cellular necrosis as currents increase significantly higher, 80 µA (145.15 C). The findings indicated that the amount of bone formed by the cathode is related to both the current density and charge. The amount of bone formation by pulsed DC approached that of constant DC, *only* as the total charge delivered by the pulsed current approached that delivered by the constant current (27.20 coulombs, pulsed vs 36.3 coulombs constant current). To achieve this pulse charge with pulsed current at 20 µA, a frequency of 750 Hz[44] is needed. The relationship between charge delivered and biologic effect has thus been established for bone healing, and it appears that a significant relationship has been estab-

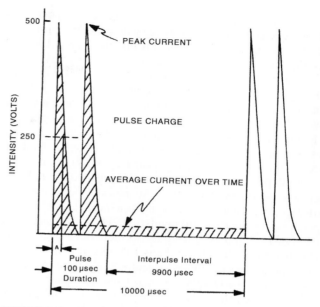

FIGURE 22-5 The effect of waveform on charge accumulation (*darkened area*). (Adapted with permission from Alon G, De Dominico G. *High Voltage Stimulation: An Integrated Approach to Clinical Electrotherapy*, 1st ed. Hixton, TN: The Chattanooga Group; 1987:41.)

lished between charge delivered and biologic effect for soft tissue healing.

Waveforms are either symmetric or asymmetric Symmetric waveforms have equal phase characteristics with respect to the baseline for each phase and thus the phase charges of each are equal. An asymmetric waveform phase characteristics are unequal with respect to the baseline. (Figure 22-1) These waveforms may be either charge balanced or unbalanced with the phase charge being the same or different.[21] (Figure 22-5). For instance, when considering a monophasic square wave pulse (LVPC), the phase charge (q) is represented by the area under the curve and is expressed as the product of the phase duration (t) and the peak current amplitude (I).[29]

In biologic systems, the charges are small and are usually expressed in microcoulombs (µC).[42] One µC is equivalent to 10^{-6} coulombs. To calculate the amount of phase charge per second, the number of µC is multiplied by the frequency of the pulse. See example of this calculation in Exhibit 22.1. A typical high-voltage stimulator with very short duration (5–20 µsec), twin-peaked (triangular-shaped) pulses, for example, has a maximum pulse charge of only 10 to 15 µC, which is very low and within safety limits.[43] One of the deficits of the high-voltage stimulator is that at a tolerable voltage level it has insufficient phase charge to excite skeletal muscle of large muscle groups to produce a vigorous muscle contraction. However, it can cause threshold excitation of sensory, motor, and pain-conducting fibers because at very short phase duration, less charge is needed to cause threshold excitation.[29]

The pulse charge of a sine wave can be compared with the pulse charge of a square wave by doubling the charge delivered by one phase. The result is that the charge delivered by the square wave is significantly greater than that of the sine wave. Thus, more pulse amplitude is required to provide the same charge with a sine wave than a square wave, making it less efficient for excitation.[29] It makes no difference what type of current is used (high or low voltage, monophasic, biphasic, or AC time, or amplitude modulated); as long as there is sufficient phase charge for a given phase duration, excitation of the nerve and cellular effects will occur.[29]

Kloth presented evidence to the HCFA Medical and Surgical Procedures Panel that the phase charge quantity (dosage) needed to enhance soft tissue healing can be computed for monophasic (triangular) HVPC and square wave (PES or LVPC) pulses using the formula described here to quantify the dose (phase charge) delivered to the tissues across a number of studies, regardless of device used.[22] In his review of the literature, Kloth found that four studies[45,46,47,3] reported the pulse charge. Two of the studies used HVPC[45,47] and two[46,3] used PES or LVPC. He then went on to calculate the charge quantity per unit for other studies using the data in those reports. Based on the calculations derived from his review of these studies, Kloth found that the charge quantity varied somewhat, but that the effective "window of charge" dosage is between 200 and 600 μC.[22]

EXHIBIT 22-1 Calculation of Pulse Charge for Monophasic Square Wave Pulse

Amplitude of current (I) × pulse duration (t) × pulse frequency = pulse charge/time

Example: 30 mA × 140 μsec = 4.2 μC × 128 pps = 537.6 μC/second[30]

Calculation of Pulse Charge for Monophasic Triangular Wave Pulse

Area of one phase = phase charge = (1/2) × phase duration × amplitude = (1/2) × 20 μsec × .325 amp = 3.25 μC

Total charge per second = phase charge × frequency = 3.3.25 microcoulombs × 105 pps = 342 μC/sec[47]

The second measurement of dosage is the current density. Current density is an indicator of the electrochemical effects of stimulation.[27,25] The charge or current density is the electrical charge per cross-sectional area of the electrodes. The larger the size of the electrode, the smaller the charge current density and conversely the smaller the electrode the greater the current density. Reich et al reviewed 17 studies of pulsed stimulation and computed the absolute spatial current density for each of them.[20] The findings indicated the parameter obtained by multiplying the average spatial current density by the effective duty cycle (duty cycle = 1 for DC) by the total duration of treatment is essential in measuring dosage delivered to the tissues. To perform this calculation, it is essential to know the size of the elec-

trode or to have a report of current density (A/cm²) as part of the study methods. A follow-up calculation of importance is to multiply the absolute current density by the time of the treatment. This gives the total amount of charge delivered per unit area (coulombs/centimeter squared).[25]

Unfortunately, most researchers fail to provide all of the data needed for these calculations. Most notably the electrode size is omitted.[25,26] These authors went the extra mile and contacted some of the researchers or manufacturers to obtain the information needed to perform the calculations. Based on their review, they found a trend that an absolute charge density transfer (dose) on the order of 0.1–2.0 C/cm² may be effective and that further research is indicated to verify this range.

An adequate but not excessive charge amount must be delivered to stimulate the desired response in the tissues.

EXHIBIT 22-2 Example of Calculating Current Density

Current amplitude ÷ area of the electrode

Example: Current amplitude is 10 A and the electrode is 10 cm². Current density equals 1 A/cm².[25]

Different tissues or cells receive a different pulse charge per unit area depending on their physical structure. For instance, sensory nerve fibers of the skin may receive up to 100 times more stimulation (pulse charge per unit area) than epidermal cells and fibroblasts due to their physical properties.[48] The sensitivity of the nerve fiber to sensory stimulation may be responsible for the vascular changes associated with ES. On the other hand, the weak stimulation of the epidermal and fibroblast cells may be what enhances the metabolism of these cells to speed up wound healing.[48]

Transcutaneous Electrical Nerve Stimulation

Except for true DC and subliminal stimulators, most clinical stimulators are TENS. In TENS, the electrodes are applied transcutaneously, with the physiologic objective of exciting peripheral nerves. As long as surface electrodes are used and peripheral nerves are excited, the stimulator is a TENS unit, regardless of the names used by commercial companies or the waveforms.[30] However, for clarification, the studies that report use of TENS stimulators are usually using biphasic or modified AC currents. Some stimulators are identified as DC, HVPC, LIDC, PES (also LVPC), or microamperage current.

Theory and Science of Electrical Stimulation

Bioelectrical Systems

The body has its own bioelectrical system. This system influences wound healing by attracting the cells of repair, changing cell membrane permeability, enhancing cellular secretion through cell membranes, and orientating cell structures.

Sodium Current of Injury

The intact skin surface maintains an average constant electronegative charge of approximately −23 mV with respect to the deeper epidermal layers. The negative charge on the surface is created by negatively charged chloride ions (Cl−), which stay on the surface after positively charged sodium ions (Na+) are pumped into the inner layers of the epidermis by the sodium ion pump. Thus, the skin has electrical potentials across it, and it acts as a battery. When there is a break in the skin surface, current can flow between the parts of the skin transmitted through the ionic fluids of the tissues between the outer and inner layers of the skin (Figure 22-6).[49] Regenerating tissues show a distinct pattern of unidirectional current flow and polarity switching. As healing is completed, or *arrested*, these currents disappear. When ulcers become dry, the voltage gradient is eliminated, and the current disappears.[41] This has been suggested as an explanation of why moist wounds heal better than dry wounds.

CLINICAL WISDOM

Moist Wounds Promote the "Current of Injury"

Keeping a wound moist with normal (0.9%) saline (sodium chloride) maintains the optimal bioelectric charge because it simulates the electrolytic concentration of wound fluid. Dressings such as amorphous hydrogels and occlusive dressings help to promote the body's "current of injury" by keeping the wound environment moist.

To test the hypothesis that ulcers kept moist maintain a higher electrical potential than do dry wounds, Cheng[50] measured the electrical potentials of partial-thickness wounds treated with occlusive dressings. He devised a system of electrodes connected to a voltmeter that could be used for measuring the electrical potential during the 4 days that it took for the wound to epithelialize. The device was placed with one electrode in the center of the wound and a second electrode placed on the adjacent normal skin sur-

face. He compared the changes in electrical potential between wounds that were occluded to retain moisture and those that were air exposed and allowed to dry out. On day zero, day of wounding, both groups had the identical electrical potential (35–38 mV). The occluded wounds maintained a high electrical potential of 29.6 mV for the 4-day period. The air-exposed wounds' electrical potential dropped to 5.2 mV. After epithelialization was completed in the occlusion group, the electrical potential returned to a similar potential to that of the air-exposed group. This work seems to support the hypothesis that occlusive dressings can help to promote the electrical current of injury.

One rationale for applying ES is that it mimics the natural current of injury and will jump-start or accelerate the wound healing process.[3] Sumano and Mateos[51] applied a protocol of modified biphasic stimulation to recalcitrant wounds and burns. Part of the protocol called for the wounds and burn injuries never to be closely covered with heavy dressings or gauzes, and the patients were instructed to allow air contact to the wounds in the home and minimal coverage outdoors. Of the 44 wounds treated, 41 (93%) had > 90% healing, and 3 (7%) had > 60–90% healing. None of the wounds healed less than 60%. Perhaps the ES that was delivered for 20 minutes on a daily or every-other-day basis imitated the current of injury sufficiently that, even with the dry wound environment, the wounds progressed toward healing. Further investigation is needed to clarify the role of ES in imitating the current of injury and the benefit of maintaining a wound environment that is moist versus dry.

CLINICAL WISDOM

Use ES in conjunction with moist wound healing methods to enhance the effect of the current of injury.

Galvanotaxis and Polarity

Unidirectional electrical current flow in the tissues attracts the cells of repair and is called *galvanotaxis*. There is a significant body of research that demonstrates that polarity influences healing in different ways at different phases. Table 22-1 summarizes the polarity effects on other aspects of biologic systems related to wound healing. Table 22-2 summarizes the cellular effects by phases of wound healing.

Neutrophils, lymphocytes, platelets, macrophages, keratinocytes, and epidermal cells are early responders following injury and play significant roles in development of the inflammatory response. The neutrophils are attracted to the negative pole if the wound is infected, to the positive pole if not infected.[52] Lymphocytes and platelets are attracted to the negative pole[31] as are epidermal cells[53] and keratinocytes.[54] These cells fight infection and produce chemotactic and growth-stimulating cytokines needed to repair or regenerate the tissue. The addition of an electric field and fibronectin also have been associated with the upregulation of epidermal growth factor receptors (EGFRs), which is significant for early response to injured tissue. However, for

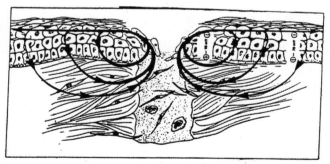

FIGURE 22-6 Current path in wounded section of the skin. Disruption in the epidermis has provided a return path for current driven by transepithelial potential. (Reprinted with permission from *Clinics in Dermatology*, Vol. 2, L.F. Jaffe and J.W. Vanable, Electric Fields and Wound Healing, 1984, with permission from Elsevier Science.)

TABLE 22-2 Galvanotaxic Effects on Cells by Phases of Healing

Effect	Cells and Charge	Attraction Pole	Type of Current	Researcher
Inflammatory: autolysis and phagocytosis	Macrophages (+)	Anode	DC Sinusoidal	Orida and Feldman[57,58]
	Neutrophils (±)	Anode/cathode	DC	Fukushima et al[52]; Kloth[132]
	Mast cells (decreased) (-)	Anode	PES, 35 mA, 128 pps	Weiss et al[63]; Gentzkow and Miller[49]
Proliferative: fibroplasia (collagen formation)	Fibroblasts (+)	Cathode	HVPC, 50 V, 100 pps	Bourguignon and Bourguignon[167]
			DC, 10–100 mV/cm	Canaday and Lee,[69] Erickson and Nuccitelli[60]
			DC, 1,500 mV/cm	Yang et al[168]
Wound contraction	Myofibroblasts (+)	Alternating	HVPC	Stromberg[62]
Epithelialization	Epidermal cells (-) Keratinocytes (-)	Cathode Cathode	DC, 50 mV/mm DC 100-200 mV	Cooper and Schliwa[169,53]

this to occur there needs to be an aqueous serum available for the cellular migration and the presence of substrates, fibronectin, and laminen.[54] Animal studies demonstrate that, in the early acute inflammatory phase of healing, the rate of epidermal cell migration in dermal wounds is enhanced by 3 days of stimulation with a negative pole, followed by stimulation with the positive pole for 4 days. Closure was achieved in 100% of the treatment group and in only 87% of the control group. Comparison of tensile strength and mitotic activity between the treated and control groups was comparable.[55,56] This corresponds to a 0- to 3-day inflammatory phase and a 4- to 7-day repair phase of healing.[55,56]

Orida and Feldman found that macrophages are attracted to the positive pole.[57] Cho et al have now shown that macrophage motility occurs in a 1-Hz low-amplitude (2 V/cm) sinusoidal electric field.[58] Again, laminin- or fibronectin-coated substrates need to be present for the macrophage migration to proceed. In the presence of an electric field, the organization of the macrophages is improved and random movement is suppressed. Ferrier recognized that different cell types, when subjected to the same electrical signal, can react differently,[59] and that has implications for the concept of galvanotaxis that remains to be developed.

Fibroblasts are key cells in contraction and connective tissue formation. Fibroblasts are attracted by the negative pole to proliferate and synthesize collagen and to contract the wound rapidly.[31,60] Protein and DNA synthesis are enhanced by negative stimulation. Perhaps this helps to explain the effect of the negative pole on wound healing, as reported in several studies reviewed in this chapter. Under similar parameters, calcium ion (Ca^{2+}) or uptake by fibroblast cells is increased, which immediately produces an increased exposure of insulin receptors on the fibroblast cell surface. If insulin is available to bind, the additional receptors on the fibroblasts will significantly increase protein

and DNA synthesis. If insulin is added after exposure to HVPC stimulation, further increase in Ca^{2+} uptake and a twofold increase in protein and DNA synthesis occur. Therefore, timing of insulin delivery and HVPC treatment to diabetic patients with wounds may have a different outcome. Conversely, these same receptors are inhibited by Ca^{2+} channel blocker medications.[31] Slower healing can be expected in wounds if the patient is taking Ca^{2+} channel blocker medication.

Studies with guinea pigs showed that pulsed low-voltage microamperage direct current (LIDC) caused a rapid calcium flux in the epidermis. The researchers concluded that the growth of fibroblasts and keratinocytes may be enhanced by pulsed LIDC, due to changes in calcium homeostasis.[6] LIDC clinical study results are presented in Table 22-3.

CLINICAL WISDOM

During the review of the medical history, the pharmaceutical history should be reviewed with these factors in mind. Drug effects could change the prognosis for healing with ES.[3]

Very low-current density electric fields can be used to enhance the efficacy of biocides and antibiotics against biofilm bacteria. Costerton called this the "bioelectric" effect. Biofilms are colonies of sessile bacteria that adhere to surfaces, like the wound bed, and are not readily affected by antibiotics or electrical stimulation individually, but when combined there is effective electrical enhancement of the antibiotic efficacy against biofilm bacteria within the electric field.[61] Wound bed biofilm bacterial colonization is an identified healing problem. The potential for clinical application of this dual approach to treat chronic wounds that are colonized with bacteria biofilms needs to be researched clinically. Chapter 4 describes biofilms and their significance for chronic wounds.

TABLE 22-3 LIDC Clinical Study Protocols and Results

Investigator	Type of Study	Polarity	Amplitude/Rate	Frequency and Duration	Disease State	Mean Healing Times
Wolcott et al[84]	Uncontrolled clinical trial	3 days cathode followed by anode; reversed daily or every 3 days if wound plateaus	200–800 μA	2 hr twice or three times daily	Ischemic dermal ulcers	9.6 weeks 10.4%/week
Gault and Gatens[130]	Uncontrolled clinical trial	3 days cathode followed by anode; reversed daily or every 3 days if wound plateaus	200–800 μA	2 hr twice or three times daily	Ischemic skin ulcers	5.0 weeks 20%/week
Carley and Wainapel[2]	Randomized controlled clinical trial	3 days cathode followed by anode; reversed daily or every 3 days if wound plateaus	200–800 μA pulsed	2 hr twice daily	Pressure ulcers	8 weeks for 58% of group treatment 12.5%/week
Katelaris et al[131]	Comparative clinical study	Negative throughout	20 μA	Not stated	Venous leg ulcers	No significant difference between groups except much longer mean healing rate for ES/povidone-iodine group (12.2 weeks) 8.2%/week
Wood et al[6]	Randomized clinical trial	Starting negative	300–600 μA; .8 Hz	3 times/week, duration not stated	Pressure ulcers	6.5–7 weeks 14.3%/week

Note: Calculations of mean healing times based on study data.
Data from references listed in the table.

Research on rapid wound contraction can also provide clinical guidance for treatment selection. Stromberg[62] found that alternating polarity using monophasic current, every 3 days at 128 pps and amplitude at 35 mA accelerated wound contraction during the first 4 weeks after injury. Conversely, he found that constant polarity, either negative or positive, was less effective. Thoughtful application should be considered in areas where rapid wound contraction would not be desirable, such as in the hand or neck.

The goal of wound healing is a scar whose characteristics are most like the original skin. Mast cells regulate this process throughout the healing cycle. A large number of mast cells in the healing wound are associated with diseases of abnormal fibrotic healing, such as keloid and hypertrophic scar formation (see Chapter 14). After exposure to positive polarity current (PES 150 μsec, 128 pps, peak current 35 mA), a decrease in mast cells, decreased scar thickness, softer scar, and better cosmetic results were observed in donor sites used for partial-thickness skin grafts. Control scars on the same patients showed evidence of hypertrophy. Differences were clinically apparent at 1 month postoperatively, and subtle differences persisted after 6 months. A side benefit of the ES treatment was the reduction in pruritus in the treated wounds, compared with intense pruritus in the control scar on the same patient.[63]

Since a principle rational for applying ES to a wound is to initiate or recreate the galvanotaxic environment needed for cells to migrate to the wound site and the cells affected by the negative pole are the first responders essential to initiate the healing cascade, the basic science supports use of the negative pole over the wound site at the start of treatment. Most researchers using monophasic ES report that they used the negative pole as the active treatment electrode over the wound site at the beginning of the treatment period until the wound was granulating, or they used only the negative pole during the entire study period. See the section of clinical studies with high-voltage pulsed current for more details.

In an uncontrolled study, Alon et al[64] used positive polarity with HVPC throughout the course of care. Refining the choice of polarity for specific effects has been the subject of many research studies (see Tables 22-1 and 22-2). There remains a need for additional research to explain and validate the efficacy of procedures and protocols. Meanwhile, reading and interpreting the current literature builds understanding of the rationale for this treatment intervention and professional judgment about its use.

In practice, the issues of polarity and wound healing are appropriate when referring to continuous or monophasic pulsed current. Even though the electrodes are marked as positive and negative for units that deliver AC and biphasic current, the imbalance of the charge of the electrodes is very small and not enough to affect the movement of the ions under the electrodes. When using continuous current, a change in polarity is a change in the direction of the current and a change in the flow of the ions under the electrode.

The studies demonstrating these polarity effects have been done with continuous and pulsed currents, usually with the current on for more than 1 second. One of the concerns in wound healing research is whether the polarity effects of monophasic pulsed current predictably occur under the electrodes when the duration of the current is on for such a very short period of time. For example, with high-voltage stimulation, the monophasic waveform pulduration is less than 1 second (100 sec) (Fig 22-5), and no measurable changes occur relative to alkalinity (H^+) or acidity (OH).[27] The question is whether some cell migration is still facilitated by the polarity of the electrodes at the wound site or whether some other factors explain the physiologic effectiveness of externally applied HVPC for healing wounds. More research is needed to show that high-voltage stimulation creates measurable polarity effects or that other physiologic processes of healing are facilitated.

Although the effects of polarity and wound healing have focused primarily on the movement of ions under the electrodes, there are other issues about current flow that could facilitate healing. For example, Wolf's law[65,66] states that, under conditions of repetitive stress, collagen is remodeled. One type of stress on a tissue is a mechanical force, such as weight bearing. This weight bearing facilitates the deposition of collagen in soft tissue and bone along the lines of the force on the tissue. Mechanical forces on the tissue can also be created when other types of energy are delivered to the tissue, such as ultrasound or electricity. When a sound wave pulsates or an electrical current pulsates, a force is created on the cell, and it expands and contracts, creating a piezoelectric effect. It has been suggested that this piezoelectric effect accounts for the increased collagen deposition.[67,68] Thus, in pulsed current, it is possible that wound healing repair (collagen deposition) measurement is facilitated by this mechanism, independent of the polarity effects of the electrode. If this is true, biphasic current should have a piezoelectric effect. However, at this time, biphasic current is rarely used for wound healing. In the future, this may change, given that recent results of several studies document significant healing effects with biphasic current.

Blood Flow, Oxygen, and Edema

Blood Flow Studies

Numerous studies in the literature that have looked at the effects of ES on blood flow in animals and humans, both healthy and with disease, are described in this section. The results reported are inconsistent. Reasons for the inconsistencies are related to the dissimilarity of study populations, electrical current characteristics (polarity, frequency, waveform), and methods of recording measurements. Standardization from one study to another is lacking. Human studies are summarized in Table 22-4.

Animal Studies. Treatment with HVPC with negative polarity induced greater blood flow in rats than did positive polarity. The blood flow volume was increased nearly instantaneously at the pulse rates tested: 2, 20, 80, and 120

TABLE 22-4 Effects of Electrical Stimulation on Blood Flow in Human Subjects

Researcher	Hecker et al[75]	Cramp et al[76]	Dodgen et al[87]	Forst et al[88]	Gilchreast et al[90]	Peters et al[88]	Kaada[79]	Cosmo et al[80]	Mawson et al[82]	Goldman et al[14]
Type stimulator	PES	TENS	TENS HVPC	TENS	HVPC	DC	TENS	TENS	HVPC	HVPC
Frequency Low	2 Hz, 8 Hz	4 Hz	Not stated	Not stated	100 pps	N/A	2 Hz	2 Hz	10 pps	100 Hz
Frequency High	32 Hz, 64 Hz, 128 Hz	110 Hz		Not stated				Not tested		
Polarity	Negative/positive	Biphasic	Biphasic positive/negative	Biphasic	Negative		Biphasic	Biphasic	Negative	Negative
Amplitude	Mean 22.56 mA	Not stated	Not stated	Not stated	100 V	Not stated	15–30 mA	10–45 mA	75 V	Sensory or max 360V
Duration of stimulation	60 min at each FQ	15 min	30 min	Not stated	30 and 60 min	4, 60-min periods	30 min 3 times daily	60 min	30 min	1 hour daily x 14 weeks
Effect during Rx	High ↑ BF trend at 32, 64, 128 Hz, negative polarity; no temperature variations from baseline	Low ↑ BF High, no change; no change in skin temp	Both stimulators produced ↑ tcPO₂ levels Response not polarity dependent	↓ BF axon reflex vasodilation in neuropathic group; induced hyperemia associated with suppressed sweat response in all groups	Bimodal response ↓ BF (73%) (N = 97) ↑BF 2770 N=35	No significant increase unless PVD present; transient rise in PVD group	Widespread vasodilation; release of vasoactive polypeptide	35% ↑ BF in ulcer 15% ↑ BF periwound skin	35% ↑ sacral TcPO₂ supine	↑ tcPO₂ from 10 mm Hg to 30 mm Hg and laser Doppler flow threefold increase in dermal peri wound perfusion compared with controls
Effect post Rx (15–30 min)	Not stated	Not stated	Rose further for 30 min	Not stated	Not tested	No increase in BF	30–45 min post stimulation increase in skin temperature (5.2°C)	29% ↑ BF in ulcer 9% ↑ BF periwound skin	Fell slightly after 15 min	Gradual rise over 14-week study period
Method of measurement	Photoplethysmography and cutaneous thermistors	Laser Doppler flowmetry and thermistor	TcPO₂	Laser Doppler flowmetry	TcPO₂	TcPO₂	Skin temperature	Laser Doppler imaging	TcPO₂	TcPO₂, Laser Doppler imaging
Population tested and N	Healthy adults (N = 10)	Healthy adults (N = 30)	Diabetes (N not stated)	Controls; (N = 21) Diabetics: (1) without complications (N = 14), (2) with neuropathy and without retinopathy (N = 14), (3) with retinopathy and without neuropathy (N = 8), (4) with neuropathy and retinopathy	Diabetics (N = 132)	Diabetics (N = 19)	Diabetes; Raynaud disease; mixed etiologies Note: Stimulation given at HoKu point between first and second metacarpals	Chronic leg ulcers (N = 15)	Spinal cord injured (N = 29)	Ischemic (N = 8)

Data from references listed in the table.

pps. In addition, blood flow was enhanced by increasing the amplitude of the current (up to stimulating muscle contraction). In a small number of cases, however, blood flow volume increased without visible muscle contraction. Blood flow velocity remained elevated from 4 to 20 minutes after treatment. [69]

Mehri et al[70] showed that there is an age-related decline in skin vascular reactivity by the sensory nerves that correlates with a decline in wound repair efficacy. They used low-frequency TENS (20 V, 5 Hz for 1 minute) and compared the effect on blood flow, using laser Doppler flowmetry (LDF), with high frequency (20 V, 15 Hz for 1 minute). At the high frequency, the vascular response in old rats was significantly reduced (46%) compared with young controls. At low frequency, however, older rats produced similar vascular responses to the young. Results suggest that sensory nerves respond preferentially to low-frequency ES.

Necrosis of skin flaps and free full-thickness skin grafts are a major problem following plastic surgery. Two skin flap studies in rats and pigs showed greater blood flow increases and improved survival of anode-treated flaps than did controls or those treated with the cathode.[71,72,73] Another study[74] with pigs used PES (128 pps, 35 mA, 30 minutes twice daily) and a protocol of alternating polarity every 3 days. Treated flaps that were given PES twice on the first day postoperatively had a 92% survival rate, compared with those treated only once on that day (19% survival). None of the control flaps survived.

Human Studies. LDF, laser Doppler imaging (LDI), intravital video microscopy, and computerized image analysis technologies have made it possible to evaluate and quantify circulatory changes induced by ES at the microcirculatory levels. Earlier researchers used a variety of methods to report results of blood flow following ES, including photoplethysmography, cutaneous thermistors, transcutaneous oxygen partial pressure (tcPO$_2$) measurement, and laboratory tests for vasodilator substances.

Hecker et al[75] chose to look at the effects of pulsed galvanic stimulation on peripheral blood flow in 10 healthy adult volunteers. They systematically varied both current polarity and frequency to maximize the likelihood of observing blood flow and/or temperature effects. The electrodes were placed over the left brachial artery in the axilla, negative polarity, and over the left radial artery at the wrist, positive polarity. Stimulation was given for 1 hour at each of five frequencies: 2, 8, 32, 64, and 128 Hz. A 30-minute period between changes in frequency was allowed to return to baseline. Current amplitude was adjusted to the highest level attainable, not exceeding the subjects' perceived discomfort. Testing was repeated on two separate occasions. On the second test, polarity was reversed. Measurements were made with thermistors attached to fingers and photoplethysmography. Results showed that current frequency, polarity, and varying combinations of the two had no significant effect on blood flow. A trend toward greater blood flow corresponded to the highest frequencies (32, 64, 128

Hz) with negative polarity. No significant temperature variations, compared with baseline, were found. The authors postulated that healthy individuals may have transient blood flow increases but that they rapidly return to baseline.

Cramp et al[76] compared the sensitivity to change in blood perfusion during treatment with TENS, using LDF and a skin thermistor. Low- and high-frequency (4 and 110 Hz) TENS was applied to the forearm skin of 30 healthy human volunteers. Double-blind conditions were implemented. Blood flow and skin temperature readings were recorded before, during, and for 15 minutes after TENS application. Analysis of the results showed significant increases in blood perfusion during the treatment period in the low-frequency group, when compared with the other two groups, and no significant changes in skin temperature.

Wikstrom et al[77] quantified blood flow changes at two different frequencies (2 Hz, 100 Hz, and sham) when TENS was applied to nine healthy adults. Changes in blood flow were measured, using LDI every 5 minutes. Results showed mean blood flow increases of 40% during low-frequency TENS, compared with a 12% increase at high frequency and no change during sham stimulation. In the second part of this study, Wikstrom and associates looked at circulatory changes in blister wounds of the leg induced in the same nine healthy adults before and during a 45-minute application of TENS (2 and 100 Hz). The blister wound is a new standard wound used for clinical studies. Microcirculatory blood flow was measured, using intravital video microscopy and computerized image analysis, as red blood cell velocity (RBC-V) in 5–14 individual capillaries in each wound. Mean RBC-V increased by 23% during low-frequency TENS (n = 6) and by 17% during high-frequency TENS (n = 8).

Kaada[78,79] reported a causal relationship between TENS and mechanisms involved in widespread microvascular cutaneous vasodilatation. Results showed that a 15- to 30-minute period of TENS-induced vasodilatation produced a prolonged vascular response with a duration of several hours or longer, potentially indicating the release of a long-lasting neurohumoral substance or metabolite. Kaada attributed the effects to three possible modes of action: inhibition of the sympathetic fibers supplied to skin vessels; release of an active vasodilator substance, vasoactive intestinal polypeptide; or a segmental axon reflex responsible for affecting local circulation. The Kaada studies included reports of clinical results, wherein patients served as their own controls of stimulation-promoted healing in cases of chronic ulceration of various etiologies.[79]

LDI was used to study the effects of TENS in and around chronic lower leg ulcers. Cosmo et al[80] enrolled 15 older adult patients with chronic leg ulcers of various causes in the study. Duration of the ulcers ranged from 3 months to 16 years. Low-frequency TENS (2 Hz, 10–45 mA) was applied for a 60-minute period. The changes in blood flow were measured every 5 minutes by LDI. After the treatment period, mean blood flow had increased in the ulcer by 35% and in the intact skin surrounding the ulcer by 15%. Mean blood flow increases of 29% in the ulcer and 9% in the skin were measured 15 minutes after the cessation of TENS treatment.

Oxygen Studies

Blood flow is the mechanism of oxygen transport to the tissues. Treatment interventions that increase blood flow consequently will enhance oxygen delivery to the tissues, improve healing, and possibly prevent tissue damage from tissue loads.

Constant delivery of oxygen is required to meet high metabolic demands of the tissues, oxidative killing of infectious organisms, protein and collagen synthesis, and hydroxylation of proline to make useful collagen. Measurement of partial pressure of oxygen ($tcPO_2$) in millimeters of mercury (mm Hg) taken at the skin level is a reflection of the oxygen available to the tissues and is the measurement frequently reported in studies. Chapter 7 has more information about partial pressure of oxygen measurements.

Mawson et al[81] wanted to determine whether tissue oxygenation at the sacrum is reduced in individuals with spinal cord injury (SCI), due to the interactive effects of prolonged immobilization and injury related to autonomic nervous system dysfunction. This group of investigators compared the $tcPO_2$ levels in 21 subjects with SCI and 11 able-bodied subjects lying prone and supine on egg-crate mattresses. $TcPO_2$ levels of SCI individuals were lower than those of controls in prone position (65.3 ± 16 mm Hg versus 76.4 ± 13 mm Hg; $p = .053$) and markedly lower in supine position (49.1 ± 26 mm Hg versus 74.2 ± 13 mm Hg; $p = .004$). $TcPO_2$ levels were monitored following supination, and the results showed that the levels of oxygen in controls fell slightly after supination but returned to previous levels within 15 minutes. In contrast, the oxygen levels of the SCI group fell rapidly by 18 mm Hg and stabilized after 15 minutes at a level 27 mm Hg below that of controls. Next, SCI subjects above and below the median supine $tcPO_2$ value were compared in terms of presence or absence of pressure ulcers. Five of the 10 (50%) of SCI subjects with $tcPO_2$ levels below the median supine $tcPO_2$ level had a pressure ulcer, compared with one among the 11 (9%) SCI subjects with $tcPO_2$ levels above the median ($p = .055$ by Fisher's exact test). These findings suggest the need for further studies on the role of reduced oxygen in the etiology of pressure ulcers.

Mawson et al[82] next looked at the possibility of developing a new way of preventing pressure ulcers in SCI individuals. They chose to study whether HVPC could increase sacral $tcPO_2$ levels in SCI persons lying prone and supine. They conducted four experiments, with the following results:

1. When HVPC was applied to the back at the spinal level T6, dose-related increases in sacral $tcPO_2$ were measured in three subjects lying prone.
2. In the second experiment, carried out on 29 subjects lying supine on egg-crate mattresses, HVPC (75 V, 10 Hz) produced a 35% increase in sacral $tcPO_2$ from baseline level (mean $\pm$ SD) or 49 ± 21 mm Hg to 66 ± 18 mm Hg after 30 minutes of stimulation ($p = 0001$).
3. Simulated HVPC was found to have no effect on sacral $tcPO_2$ in five subjects lying supine.
4. HVPC was repeated on 10 subjects, and its effects were found to be highly reproducible. The mode of action attributed by the researchers to these effects is that the HVPC restores the sympathetic tone and vascular resistance below the level of the spinal cord lesion, thereby increasing the perfusion pressure gradient in the capillary beds.

Another approach for preventing pressure ulcers in SCI individuals with ES may be an implanted neuromuscular stimulation (NEMS) system with percutaneous leads. Spinal cord injury produces many health problems, including decreased muscle bulk and reduced capillary network associated with the bulk loss over the sitting surfaces reducing blood volume that could be supplied to the tissues, as well as loss of blood pumping function, decreased sympathetic nervous system activity resulting in decreased blood pressure and vascular patency that makes the blood vessels in the area less capable of withstanding normal tissues load and maintaining blood flow.[83] The result is decreased tissue health below the level of the injury, resulting in increased risk for pressure ulcer development. Although the intent of developing a NEMS system was to provide muscle stimulation that will be useful to provide the SCI patient with standing time and facilitate transfers, secondary health benefits appear possible. A study of eight SCI individuals with NEMS implants found that there are additional health benefits, including increased $tcPO_2$ levels in the ischial region, in the unloaded state, after 8 weeks. The ischial pressure distribution changed, probably due to the increase in gluteal muscle thickness, which increased by 50% but not the total pressure unloading of interface pressures on the seating surfaces.[83]

Lack of adequate oxygen could be a partial explanation for difficulty in healing diabetic ulcers.[84] Baker et al[85,86] measured oxygen enrichment to the cells of wound repair in a study of age-matched older normal adults and diabetic subjects. Oximetry readings of $tcPO_2$ were taken 30 minutes prior to stimulation, during 30 minutes of stimulation, and 30 minutes after stimulation. The ES waveforms used were monophasic-paired spikes with negative polarity and a compensated monophasic waveform. Both waveforms were introduced with the cathode over the wound. The older normal adults showed higher $tcPO_2$ levels at the end of 30 minutes of stimulation, regardless of waveform used. However, there were differences in response time for the diabetics. The normal adults showed increased oxygen levels earlier in the treatment period than did the diabetics. Diabetic subjects showed measurable but not significant increases in $tcPO_2$ at the end of the 30 minutes of stimulation but did show significant increases 30 minutes after cessation of the stimulation with the monophasic and submotor compensated monophasic waveforms. The authors' analysis of the study was that diabetic subjects demonstrate a compromised ability to increase transcutaneous oxygen during submotor stimulation, *regardless* of the waveform used. When trace level muscle contraction was elicited with the compensated monophasic waveform, there was no change in the $tcPO_2$ levels in the diabetics. For some reason, the trace muscle contraction blunted the $tcPO_2$ response in the diabetics. The same effects were found for both waveforms and with stimulation by either the positive or the negative pole.

In another study of diabetics, Dodgen et al[87] compared the effects of a monophasic paired spike waveform, using both negative and positive polarity, with a symmetric biphasic waveform. Measurements of $tcPO_2$ from baseline 30 minutes prior to stimulation, during 30 minutes of stimulation, and 30 minutes after treatment were compared. The findings showed that the $tcPO_2$ levels were significantly increased, regardless of waveform or polarity. Increases were present at the end of the stimulation period and continued to rise during the next 30 minutes after stimulation. Therefore, researchers concluded that the mechanism of action of ES on increasing transcutaneous oxygen was unrelated to polarity and did not require any net ion flow. Both the Baker and Dodgen studies cited here were reported as abstracts. Details about the variables of frequency and amplitude are missing from these reports.

Comparison of the microvascular response to TENS and postocclusive ischemia in the diabetic foot was reported by Forst et al.[88] LDF was used to measure the "flare" response (hyperemia) following TENS and to compare this axon reflex vasodilatation with postischemic hyperemia in the skin of the foot of diabetic and nondiabetic subjects. Twenty-one control subjects and 57 diabetic subjects were enrolled. The diabetics were stratified into four groups:

1. 24 without complications
2. 14 with neuropathy and without retinopathy
3. 8 with retinopathy and without neuropathy
4. 21 with both neuropathy and retinopathy

Following TENS, there was increased skin blood flow across all groups. However, compared with the control group, axon reflex vasodilatation was significantly reduced in groups 2 and 4. All groups had equivalent increased blood flow after arterial occlusion. There was a good association observed between postocclusive and TENS-induced hyperemia at the dorsum of the foot, but poor association at the base of the big toe. An observation reported was that the TENS-induced hyperemia was associated with a diminished sweat response but not with pathologic cardiovascular function tests. The conclusion reached was that electrical axon reflex vasodilatation is diminished in diabetic patients suffering from peripheral autonomic C-fiber injury, especially in skin rich in thermoregulatory blood flow. The diminished neurovascular response is independent of vascular alteration due to diabetes mellitus.

Peters et al[89] evaluated the effects of galvanic ES on vascular perfusion in 19 diabetic subjects. Eleven of these were diagnosed with impaired peripheral perfusion, based on their initial $tcPO_2$ values (<40 mm Hg). Stimulation was given at the lateral side of one leg, and measurements were taken at the dorsum of the foot and at the base of the great toe of *both* feet. On the first day, one foot was treated with ES for four 60-minute periods and vascular perfusion assessed before and after the stimulation session. Measurements were taken for 1 hour on day 1 of the experiment. Methods of measurement were transcutaneous oximetry and LDF. Findings were that, during the first 5 minutes of stimulation, there was a significant rise in tissue oxygenation as compared with the control measurements in the group of diabetics with impaired vascular perfusion. However, for those without vascular disease ($tcPO_2$ levels >40 mm Hg), there was no significant increase, compared with baseline. Also, after the stimulation periods, the stimulated feet did not show any significant increase in blood flow over the control feet. The data suggest to the researchers that external subsensory ES induces a transient rise in skin perfusion in persons with diabetes and impaired peripheral perfusion.

Gilcreast et al[90] tested the effect of HVPC (100 pps, 100 V, negative polarity) on foot skin perfusion in diabetics at risk for foot ulceration. A sample of 132 subjects was tested. Baseline $tcPO_2$ levels were obtained, stimulation applied, and the repeat $tcPO_2$ measurements recorded at 30- and 60-minute intervals. Initial $tcPO_2$ levels were significantly higher than subsequent readings. However, the oxygen response was distributed bimodally: 35 (27%) subjects showed increased $tcPO_2$, and 97 (73%) experienced a *decreased* $tcPO_2$ reading. This treatment appears to increase blood flow in a subset of diabetics.

Byl et al[91] found that, when supplemental oxygen was given by mask prior to and during microamperage stimulation (100 μA for 45 minutes), there were significant increases in subcutaneous oxygen measured. Maximal oxygen saturation may be necessary prior to and during ES to facilitate the dissociation of oxygen from the hemoglobin.[91]

Ischemia, $tcPO_2$ levels below 20 mm Hg, is a predictor of poor healing outcomes of lower extremity wounds. Ischemic wounds not only do not heal but also often increase in size unless reperfused with bypass surgery. Many patients do not meet the criteria for reperfusion surgery, including patients with diabetes and end-stage renal disease. For these individuals, amputation may be required. Goldman et al reported a six-subject case series that showed HVPC induced a slow persistent increase in $tcPO_2$, levels in the periwound skin of patients with diabetes. After $tcPO_2$, levels exceeded 20 mm Hg, four of the six wounds eventually healed.[92] This case series prompted them to do a chart review of retrospective data to determine patients with critical ischemia ($tcPO_2 < 10$ mm Hg) with arteriosclerosis and who were high-risk nonsurgical candidates with ischemic wounds.[93] They located 22 patients (the six cases mentioned were among this group) that met the inclusion criteria of critical ischemia. Half had only standard wound care and the others had taken a course of HVPC. Those in the HVPC group tended to rise out of the critical ischemic range (5 +/- 8 mm Hg initial values elevated to 26+/- 20 mm Hg). The control group also had increased tcPO$_2$, but not as great. The wounds in the HVPC group closed by 32 weeks after the start of treatment. By contrast, the control group wound area increased more than three times the initial area by 16 weeks.

The nature of the case studies and retrospective analysis have potential for bias. The parties realized this and based on the preliminary trends observed, undertook a pilot investigation, a small prospective RCT (N = 8) lasting 14 weeks. In this study, by week 14 the HVPC treated wounds averaged 30 mm Hg in the periwound tissues, well above the ischemic range, and the control group had an increase in tcPO$_2$ averaging 15 mm Hg. Laser Doppler evaluation of these two groups showed a threefold significant increase in dermal periwound perfusion in the HVPC group by week eight, compared with controls. The plan is to expand this into a larger controlled trial. For details about treatment parameters for blood flow and oxygen studies cited cases, see Table 22-4.

In transferring technology from the lab bench to the bed, the clinician could take the information from these research studies and formulate a protocol for wound healing for patients with ischemia such as diabetics. For example, nasal supplementation of oxygen could be provided during ES treatment for patients with diabetes to accelerate the oxygen uptake. A trial to evaluate the difference in wound healing outcomes for diabetics treated with ES while breathing room air or supplemental oxygen could yield useful clinical data. The result would be development of a new clinical protocol for treating diabetic wounds.

Although a number of the studies reviewed here looked at changes in tcPO$_2$ levels before and up to 15–30 minutes after treatment, they did not look at the long-term effects of regular electrical stimulation over a period of weeks. The increased tcPO$_2$ levels in ischemic tissues over time (8–14 weeks), as reported by Goldman et al and Bogie and Reger in these small studies using HVPC, suggests that it takes more than a few minutes of ES treatment time to have a carryover effect on oxygen transport in ischemic tissues. So far, this application has had limited prospective study with small sample size. Further study with larger sample sizes could be useful in determining if this approach would be beneficial as primary care for prevention as well as healing.

Venous System Response. Alon and De Domenico[23] reviewed the literature on the effects of ES on venous circulation. As yet, ES is not used extensively for management of venous circulation problems but merits inclusion in this section for thoughtful application. There is no support for intervention in the acute phase of varicose hemorrhage or deep vein thrombosis, but ES can effectively treat chronic conditions, including deep vein thrombosis and venous stasis. When muscle groups in the calf and posterior thigh are stimulated to produce intermittent tetanic muscle contraction, there is very effective enhancement of venous return in cases of venous insufficiency or deep vein thrombosis. The required stimulation parameters are those needed to provide motor excitation leading to evoked intermittent

tetanic muscle contraction. Augmentation of the venous return initiates a response of vasodilatation of the arterioles to bring blood flow to the muscles.

In SCI individuals, there is a loss of normal vasomotor tone in the abdomen and lower extremities. Peripheral edema and a high incidence of deep vein thrombosis have been associated with the circulatory stasis that occurs. One case study of a patient with edema, cyanosis of the feet, and toe ulcers demonstrated the benefits of using computer-controlled neuromuscular ES to stimulate numerous muscle groups, resulting in reduced edema, improved skin color, and healed ulcers by the fifth week of the treatment regimen.[94] The use of the ES-induced leg muscle contractions in individuals with paraplegia to augment cardiovascular responses, probably via reactivation of the skeletal muscle pump and resulting increased venous return, has been reported in several studies.[95,96,97] Benefits include ameliorating blood pooling in the lower extremities and prevention of edema in the extremities by promoting lymph flow. Use of ES as a preventive treatment is being investigated, and results indicate that it may be useful in situations in which the motor pump function is lost, due to paralysis or other lifestyle situations.[98]

Enhanced blood flow to tissues will support tissue demands for increased oxygen and nutrients required for healing. In the case of the patient with venous insufficiency, stimulation of enhanced blood flow will need to be evaluated and may require aftercare of compression to avoid pooling of blood at the ankles, due to the incompetent valves (see Chapter 10). If the arterioles are severely occluded, the vasodilatation response may not occur, and electrically evoked muscle contraction may not be desired. In fact, the muscle contraction may cause severe pain by curtailing limited blood flow to the area, leading to ischemia. There are very limited clinical data to support specific protocols for this effect. Therefore, it is up to the PT to evaluate the vascular impairments, based on the diagnostic process, and to select a protocol to support the desired effect. The section on protocols and procedures provides an example for guidance.

Summary. To summarize, transcutaneous application of ES has been shown in several studies to increase blood flow, microcirculation of the skin, and tissue oxygen levels (see Table 22–4) in animals, healthy individuals, diabetics, patients with SCI, and around chronic ulcers of the lower extremity. Blood flow increases in most studies were greatest when low-frequency stimulation was applied. There are conflicting reports about the effects of ES on circulation in healthy adults, in those with spinal cord injuries, vascular disease, and in diabetics that merit further investigation. The bimodal effects reported by Gilcreast et al[90] may be explained by use of high-frequency stimulation (100 pps) and/or the impairment of the electrical axon reflex vasodilatation in diabetics with neuropathy and not in others without neurologic complications, as described by Forst et al.[88]

Increasing oxygenation of tissues for healing and prevention of tissue damage are important reasons to consider treatment intervention with ES. In light of the accumulating body of evidence that low-frequency ES is a potent enhancer of blood flow, randomized clinical trials are needed to verify the benefits of using ES for preventing pressure ulcers, as has been suggested by Mawson et al,[82] and to determine the best treatment protocols to take advantage of the information now available about enhancement of microcirculation with low-frequency stimulation.

Edema and Pain Studies

Edema is a consequence of disruption in circulation and blood flow to the tissues. Following traumatic injury, there is hemostasis and margination to halt bleeding. The biologic events that follow (see Chapter 2) result in edema formation as a component of the acute inflammatory phase of repair. In systemic breakdown, such as loss of valvular competency in venous disease or loss of autonomic nervous system function in SCI, edema results. Use of ES as a modality to reduce edema has many anecdotal reports. However, evidence of the efficacy of ES to reduce or prevent edema is limited to a few animal studies, some human studies, and limited clinical trials.

Edema reduction under the negative pole is attributed to a phenomenon called *cataphoresis*.[99] Cataphoresis is the movement of nondissociated colloid molecules, such as droplets of fat, albumin, particles of starch, blood cells, bacteria, and other single cells, all of which have an electrical charge, due to the absorption of ions, under the influence of a direct current toward the cathode.

Animal Studies. Several attempts have been made to learn whether edema reduction occurs with application of HVPC.[100] Reed[100] reported reduction of post-traumatic edema in hamsters following HVPC and attributed the effect to reduced microvessel leakage. Post-traumatic edema was curbed in frogs treated with HVPC when the cathode was used. There was no effect if the anode was applied. Treatment effect was significant from the end of the first treatment session until the end of data recording 17 hours later.[101] A similar study using HVPC on rat hind paws found significant treatment effects after the second 20-minute treatment with the cathode.[69]

The above studies showed efficacy in curbing post-traumatic edema in one species of rat and one species of frog. Thornton and colleagues[102] found that edema formation was curbed in Zucker-Lean and Brown Norway rats but not in Sprague-Dawley rats when cathodal HVPC (120 pps) at 10% less than needed to induce visible muscle contraction was applied. The fact that not all species of rat react the same suggests a caveat in extrapolating data to human subjects.

Matylevich et al[103] observed the effect of 40 mA DC on plasma albumin extravasation after partial-thickness burn injury in Sprague-Dawley rats. Silver nylon wound dressings were used as the anodes. Burn rats with no treatment or treated with silver-nylon dressing without current were used as controls. Quantitative analysis of fluorescein isothiocyanate (FITC)-albumin leakage and accumulation in the wound tissue was performed using confocal fluorescence microscopy. When DC was applied, leakage was reduced by 30%–45% and approached normal rates by 8 hours postburn. FITC-albumin concentration peaked at 4 hours postburn, was 18%–48% less than in burned control, and approached the level observed in unburned control by 18 hours postburn. The conclusion of the study was that direct current has a beneficial effect in reducing plasma protein extravasation after burn injury. Chu et al,[104,104] who worked with the Matylevich group on the study reported above, then considered the effect of direct current on wound edema after full-thickness burn injury in the same rat species. Using the same study design as described, the main results were that continuous direct current reduced burn edema by 17% to 48% at different times up to 48 hours postburn. Neither reversal of electrode polarity nor change in current density had any significant effect on the results of treatment. Starting treatment during the first 8 hours postburn produced the least edema accumulation, but the reduction was significant even when direct current was applied 36 hours after burn. If started immediately after injury, treatment had to be continued for a minimum of 8 hours to be most effective.

Human Studies. There is a paucity of human studies on the effects of ES on edema and pain. The few studies located are described in this section. Albumin is a colloidal protein found in blood, is negatively charged, and is repelled by negative polarity, causing a fluid shift and, thereby, a reduction of edema. Ross and Segal[99] claimed benefit in treating postoperative edema, healing, and pain with HVPC in 25 postoperative patients. Effects of direct current on edema were attributed to cataphoresis. They formulated a protocol based on the use of the cathode to reduce edema. The treatment parameters were negative polarity, four paired pulses per second for 15 minutes. After 15 minutes, the polarity was switched to positive and pulse rate increased to 80 paired pulses per second for another 15 minutes. Treatment was over the surgical site.

Griffin et al[105] compared the efficacy of intermittent pneumatic compression (IPC) and HVPC in reducing chronic post-traumatic hand edema in an RCT. Thirty patients were assigned to one of three groups (10 to each) to receive a single treatment for 30 minutes of IPC, HVPC, or sham HVPC. Chronic edema was defined as edema following traumatic injury persisting for 14 to 21 days. The HVPC stimulator was set at 8 pps, with a reciprocal mode of stimulation alternating between the ulnar and median nerves at the elbow. Intensity was adjusted to produce minimal muscle contraction of thumb flexion and finger abduction, and polarity was set at negative for the active sites. The results reported were that there was no significant difference between HVPC and IPC ($p = .446$), and the difference between the HVPC and placebo HVPC groups did not quite reach statistical significance. The single 30-minute IPC session produced significant reductions in edema. There was also wide variability reported between the HVPC and IPC groups.

Kumar et al,[42] in a randomized controlled, single-blinded trial with biphasic TENS and amitriptyline (Elavil, Etrafon, Limbitrol) (N = 23), found that there was a beneficial effect from TENS for relief of painful diabetic peripheral neuropathy beyond the effect of the amitriptyline. The treatment unit used was a proprietary device called *H-wave* (Electronic Waveform Laboratory, Huntington Beach, CA), with characteristics of biphasic exponentially decaying waveform with pulse widths of 4 msec, <35 mA, <35 V, and 2–70 Hz. Treatment was applied at the knee region but treatment effect was in the foot. Results of a survey of patients using H-Wave TENS showed the following: 41 patients reported a 44% ± 4% subjective reduction in pain; 13 patients had no improvement.[43] Those who had no improvement also reported a significantly higher incidence of foot ulcers than did the responder group. Nineteen patients reported swelling over the ankles. Twelve reported some decrease in the swelling with the TENS treatment, six claimed no change, and one had an increase. Only one of the 12 responders was using compression stockings. However, four of six of those who reported no change were wearing compression stockings. Data from this survey suggest that the beneficial effects of electrotherapy for neuropathic pain continue with prolonged usage. Why the nonresponders had more foot ulcers than the responders deserves further investigation. Pruritus is also classified as pain treatment with PES, effectively reducing pruritus associated with healing of donor sites.[63]

Dobbins et al[106] reported no statistically significant decreases in acute knee edema pain or function after use of HVPC on postoperative days 1–4 following total knee arthroplasty in an RCT with 32 patients. All participated in an exercise protocol daily. The methodology for determining the difference in volume was the truncated cone equation but, because the knee is not really a cone, the results may have been flawed. Using this methodology, the study reported a clinical significance—65 cm³ less volume in the treatment group than in controls. The treatment may be effective in decreasing postsurgical knee edema and pain and in increasing function. Treatment parameters, supplied by personal communication with the researcher, were 120 pps and amplitude to patient tolerance but below muscle contraction. In some cases, the amplitude was almost 200 V. The negative pole was used for 20 minutes daily.[107] Based on the studies of effect of ES frequency on blood flow already discussed, perhaps a lower frequency would have improved the outcomes. Further work is needed to determine the most effective parameters.

Fakhri and Amin[108] reported that, if edema was present around a burn wound, there was an immediate discharge of pus and tissue fluids during application of the low-voltage DC that ceased when the current was terminated. Sumano and Mateos[51] included a case study as part of their clinical trial report. Using modified biphasic stimulation on a pa-

tient with a second-degree burn wound, there was significant reduction of the signs of inflammation, including edema and pain, after three treatments. Investigation on a larger scale on the efficacy of ES in reducing edema in humans is needed to verify this phenomenon and to determine the effective treatment parameters.

Debridement, Thrombolysis, and Thrombosis

Review of the research is a guide for the clinician and provides evidence to support a protocol for wound healing initiated with the negative pole at the wound site. Debridement is facilitated if the tissue is solubilized or liquefied, such as occurs with enzymatic debriding agents or autolysis. For example, necrotic tissues are made up of coalesced blood elements. ES using negative current can solubilize this clotted blood.[109,110,111] The term for this is thrombolysis.

Reperfusion of tissues is rapidly followed by autolytic debridement. Increased blood flow, stimulated by ES at the negative pole, has been attributed to having this effect. For example, two studies reported that on average there was nearly complete debridement of pus and necrotic tissue with cathode stimulation during the first 2 weeks of treatment.[10,11]

The positive electrode has been found to induce clumping of leukocytes and forming of thromboses in the small vessels. Another example of thrombolysis with the negative electrode is reversal of clumping and thrombotic effects.[3] This may explain a clinical observation by this author, in which hematoma and hemorrhaging at the wound margin or on granulation tissue are lysed and reabsorbed following application of HVPC with the negative pole. This is of clinical importance because hemorrhagic material goes on to necrosis if not lysed and reabsorbed quickly. Perhaps continuous use of positive polarity produces the clumping of leukocytes, as well as explaining why a protocol of intermittently changing polarity restarts the healing process. These are critical issues that need to be researched.

> **RESEARCH WISDOM**
>
> Deep tissue injury involves hemorrhage of capillaries and initiation of the clotting cascade. If tissues are not reperfused early, ischemia reperfusion injury may occur, along with cell death. More on deep tissue injury and ischemia reperfusion injury is presented in Chapter 2. Early treatment with ES has the potential to reverse the downward course of these injuries and deserves clinical research to evaluate the benefits.

Antibacterial Effects

Because infection is a contributing factor in chronic wound healing, methods to control infection are of clinical importance. Bactericidal effects have been attributed to ES. Research suggests that there is evidence to support this theory. In vitro and in vivo studies applying direct current have both been shown to inhibit bacterial growth rates for organisms commonly found in chronic wounds at the cathode.[112,113] Passage of positive current (anode) through silver wire electrodes was found to be bactericidal to Gram-negative bacteria in wounds and inhibitory to Gram-positive wound bacteria.[114] At low levels of amplitude, 0.4–4 µA, there were negligible bactericidal effects.[112] Kincaid and Lavoie[115] tested in vitro stimulation, using HVPC at the cathode and anode, and Szuminsky et al[116] tested HVPC in vitro at the cathode. Both studies found inhibition of *Staphylococcus aureus, Escherichia coli,* and *Pseudomonas aeruginosa.* However, the amplitude of the stimulation reported by Kincaid and Lavoie was 250 V, and Szuminsky et al reported 500 V. Patients would likely find this voltage amplitude intolerable.

Because there is inconsistency in these findings and because there are no chemical changes (acidity or alkalinity) measured under the electrodes of HVPC, it is not clear whether the antibacterial effects are due to polarity or to another mechanism. For example, increased subcutaneous oxygen was found under the anode when a microamperage current (at 0.3 Hz) was passed through the electrode.[117] It is possible that the oxygen, rather than the polarity, is the variable that is responsible for the bactericidal effects on pathogens.

Chu et al[118] used microamperage current (0.4–40 µA) conducted through a silver nylon dressing placed in the wound of male Sprague-Dawley rats. Chu induced burn wounds in rats, then inoculated them with a lethal dose of *P. aeruginosa* bacteria. Treatment with the silver nylon dressing as the anode was effective as a barrier to infection. Even the silver nylon dressing alone, without the current applied, had a significant protective barrier effect. However, when the silver nylon dressing was used with the cathode or just the nylon cloth without a metal coating, an effective protective barrier did *not* occur.

Thurman and Christian,[119] Gault and Gatens,[120] Webster et al,[121] Fitzgerald and Newsome,[122] and Sumano and Mateos[51] published case studies of patients with infected wounds who had positive outcomes following treatment with ES.[11] Polak reported cleaning of ulcers with "pus" and necrotic tissues during the first two weeks of care using HVPC at the negative pole. No organisms were mentioned.[11] Organisms mentioned in the prior listed studies included *S. aureus and P. aeruginosa.* Infectious conditions reported included septic abscess, chronic osteomyelitis, infected burn, and thoracic spinal infection. Stimulation types used were low-intensity pulsed direct current, constant current, HVPC, and modified biphasic. Wound asepsis was normally accomplished within 3–7 days, using negative polarity.[120] Concurrent use of antibiotics and alternating the polarity during the treatment session with HVPC (negative 20 minutes, followed by 40 minutes of positive polarity) was mentioned by Fitzgerald and Newsome.[122] Webster used electrically activated silver dressings with the dressing as the anode to treat chronic osteomyelitis wounds. Sixteen (64%) of the cases resulted in closed, stable, pain-free wounds, and nine of twelve cases, complicated by nonunion, achieved union. The authors suggest that the silver anode dressing is an effective treatment for chronic bone infection, when combined with surgical debridement, and reduces the need for prolonged systemic antibiotics.

Sumano and Mateos[51] reported that use of antiseptics and antibiotics was precluded in all cases enrolled in their study and attributed the reduction in observable signs of infection to the ES treatment. One case included was a patient who had recurrent osteomyelitis. The patient response to the ES protocol was fair (> 60–90% healing) but complete recovery was not achieved. These authors suggest that, under these circumstances, ES may be regarded as beneficial and harmless, and may even have a preparatory role for further medical care. Presence of osteomyelitis has long been considered a contraindication for ES therapy. After review of the cases reported, further investigation of the use of ES for bactericidal effects in human subjects should be undertaken. Table 22-5 summarizes the beneficial results of ES on infected wounds.

Biofilms are implicated in chronic wound infections. Biofilm bacteria are sessile and attached to a surface such as the wound bed. Chapter 4 has additional information about biofilm infections as they relate to chronic wounds. Antibiotics are unable to effectively destroy bacteria in biofilm communities except when administered at intolerably high doses. However, low-intensity DC electric fields (1.5 to 20 V/cm and current density 15µ A/cm^2) have been shown to completely override the inherent resistance of biofilm bacteria to biocides and antibiotics.[61] Costerton has called this the "bioelectric effect." Under laboratory conditions, all biofilm bacteria within the electric fields were readily killed by an antibiotic on all areas of the active electrodes. The benefit of the bioelectric effect is the reduction in the concentration of antibacterial agents needed to kill biofilm bacteria to levels very close to those needed to kill planktonic, floating bacteria of the same species. However, this killing effect has not been seen in the electric field alone but during dual treatment.[61]

Pain

A large body of literature supports the use of TENS for both acute and chronic pain management. Techniques for pain modulation can be used, along with the wound healing protocols. For example, one electrode may be placed on the painful area, which includes the wound and adjacent tissues, and the indifferent electrode over the related spinal nerve. The electrodes can also be bracketed proximal and distal to the areas of pain around the wound, such as with a bipolar technique described later in this chapter.[123] Pain management would be a good reason to use electrodes of equal size so that there would be sufficient current density at the both electrodes.

Sensory Nerve Activation

Khalil and Merhi[124] as a second part of their study, induced thermal wounding of aged rats. One group received TENS stimulation twice daily for 5 days, and the second group received sham TENS stimulation. Using healing, full wound

TABLE 22-5 Case Study Reports of Beneficial Results of ES on Infected Wounds

Source	Infection Type	Stimulation Type Used	Results
Thurman and Christian[119]	Abscess in diabetic	HVPC	Healed
Fitzgerald and Newsome[122]	Spinal wound with *Staphylococcus aureus*	HVPC	Healed
Webster et al[121]	Chronic osteomyelitis	DC	Healed
Sumano and Mateos[51]	Osteomyelitis	Modified biphasic	Improved
	Infected burn		Healed

Data from references listed in the table.

contraction as the outcome measure, they found a statistically significant improved rate of healing for the TENS group (14.7 ± 0.2 days versus 21.8 ± 0.3 days). Their contention is that TENS can accelerate peripheral activation of sensory nerves at low-frequency ES parameters. Khalil and Merhi[124] and Mawson et al[82] may be talking about the same or similar mode of activation of the sensory nerves.

Scar Formation

In animal and human studies, flaps and grafts treated with monophasic pulsed current ES heal without ischemia and result in flatter, thinner, and more resilient scars than in controls.[2, 62,55] Pulsed ES was used to stimulate healing of burned rat skin.[125] The repaired skin of the electrostimulated group had an appearance similar to that of the control skin, and the overall appearance of the repaired skin was compatible with a well-organized healing process.

Adamian et al[126] reported that 12 patients with slow healing postburn wounds received local ES treatment. Morphologic and biochemical studies confirmed marked stimulating effects of local ES-associated acceptance of dermal autografts and healing. Fakhri and Amin[108] reported a descriptive study in which they treated 20 indolent burn wounds with DC stimulation twice a week for 10 minutes per session until healed or ready for regrafting. All patients had failed one or two surgical skin grafts and served as their own controls. The wounds were deep dermal wounds or full-thickness or mixed. Epithelialization began by day three after start of the ES treatment. The largest wounds took the longest to heal (up to 3 months). Autologous skin grafts were successful after 2–4 weeks of ES treatment. The paper particularly cites the appearance of islands of epithelial cells in full-thickness skin burns that would have been expected to be destroyed. Benefits to scar formation from the treatment were better elasticity, more durability to stress, better cosmesis, and better regeneration of the skin pigments.

From case studies and clinical trials, evidence is being compiled to look at the outcomes of the treatments with ES on all phases of wound healing. Currently, there is a positive trend to treatment with ES, with an expected outcome of a functional, improved quality scar. More studies with human subjects are needed to compare different current waveforms and treatment parameters and their effects on collagen formation and scar.

Comparison of Monophasic and Biphasic Stimulation Effects

Animal Studies

A comparison of biphasic with monophasic stimulation of acute incisional wounds in rats by Bach et al[127] showed that both types of current caused a significant increase of collagen content around the incision line, compared with controls, but did not affect the tensile strength or the energy absorption of the collagen formation in the early postoperative period. Reger et al[128] also compared biphasic and monophasic stimulation of wounds induced in new monoplegic pigs with wounds in normal pigs and denervated controls. When compared with controls, both biphasic- and monophasic-stimulated wounds showed reduced healing time and increased perfusion in the early phases of healing. Monophasic stimulation reduced the wound area more rapidly than did biphasic, but biphasic stimulation reduced the wound volume more rapidly than did monophasic. Their impression was that the applied current appears to orient new collagen formation, even in the absence of neural influences. Collagen organization is considered an important factor in improved tensile strength of the scar. This study found that the ES did not reduce the strength of the healing wounds below those of the nonstimulated controls.

Human Studies

Stefanovska et al[129] compared the efficiency of monophasic (600 µA, 2 hours daily) and biphasic (40 Hz, 15–25 mA to produce minimal muscle contraction, 2 hours daily) in healing pressure ulcers in 150 patients with spinal cord injuries. Treatment was applied across the wounds using a bipolar technique. As in the Reger study,[128] monophasic was less effective for reducing the depth of deep wounds than was biphasic, and biphasic was less effective for reducing the wound area of large wounds. Frantz[15] reported that full-thickness pressure ulcers had a statistically significant reduction in depth but not in surface area when treated with biphasic.[49] Table 22-6 summarizes the treatment effects attributed to biphasic and monophasic.

Clinical Studies

Since the 1960s, a series of clinical trials has been undertaken to evaluate the effect of ES on wound healing. The early studies are classics in this field.

TABLE 22-6 Summary of Treatment Effects Attributed to Direct Current and Alternating Current

Investigator	Subjects and Disease States	Direct Current	Alternating Current (Biphasic)
Stromberg[62]	Healthy pigs	Faster wound contraction if polarity alternated	
Reger et al[128] Stefanovska et al[129]	Spinal cord injury, pigs Spinal cord injury, humans	Faster wound contraction Less effective for deep wounds	Faster volume reduction Less effective for large wounds
Frantz[15]	Pressure ulcers, humans		Fast volume reduction; slow wound contraction

Data from references listed in the table

Low-Voltage Microamperage Direct Current Studies

LIDC was used in six clinical studies. Wolcott et al,[84] Gault and Gatens,[130] Carley and Wainapel,[2] Katelaris et al,[131] and Wood et al[6] studied treatment of ischemic and indolent ulcers. In the first three studies, a positive (anode) polarity was used after a period of three or more days at the cathode. The polarity was reversed every day or every 3 days if wound healing did not progress. Rationale for initial cathode application was the solubilization of necrotic tissue[132] and bactericidal effects.[112,113] All studies except the Katelaris study used an amplitude of 200 to 800 µA. Duration of treatment was very long: 2 hours, two or three times per day, or 42 hours per week for the first two studies, and 20 hours per week for the third study. Treatment in the Wood study was administered three times per week, but length of treatment was not stated. Katelaris et al incorporated ES treatment with dressings, did not state how long current was applied, and used negative polarity throughout. A combined total of 225 patients were treated, and 75 served as controls. In most cases, the patient served as his or her own control. Mean healing times reported were 9.6 weeks, 4.7 weeks, 5.0 weeks, 8 weeks, and 6.5–7 weeks, respectively, for the five studies (see Table 22-3).

The difference in healing time between these studies is not clear. Perhaps in the Wolcott et al study the wounds were more extensive. Carley and Wainapel[2] noted that the pulsed LIDC treatment group healed 1.5–2.0 times faster than did the control subjects, who were treated with wet to dry dressings and whirlpool. Katelaris et al[131] found no statistical difference in healing times between normal saline, normal saline with electrode, and povidone-iodine treated wounds. However, results when povidone-iodine was used with the negative electrode showed that the mean healing rate was statistically longer, 85.3 days (12.2 weeks). The researcher theorized that the retardation effect may be due to the negative pole ionization of the iodine and forcing iodine ions down an electrochemical gradient into the cell, where they act as intracellular toxins.

Microcurrent stimulation has been studied in animal models in which current was applied only one or two times

---

RESEARCH WISDOM

Make certain that any form of iodine, if used to treat a wound, is thoroughly removed before application of electrotherapy.[131]

---

per day for 30 minutes for 1–2weeks; no significant clinical effects were demonstrated on wound healing.[117,133] In another study, there were significant increases in subcutaneous oxygen measurements when supplemental oxygen was given by mask during the MENS stimulation[91] There was no acceleration in healing.

Modified Biphasic Stimulation Studies

Barron et al[134] reported a study of six patients with pressure ulcers who were treated three times a week for 3 weeks, for a total of nine treatments with microcurrent stimulation. The waveform was a modified biphasic square wave. The treatment characteristics were 600 µA, 50 V, and 0.5 Hz. The electrode probes were placed 2 cm away from the edge of the ulcer, then moved circumferentially around the ulcer. Each successive placement of the probes was 2 cm from the prior placement. In this small study, two ulcers healed 100%, three healed 99%, and one decreased in size 55%.

Sumano and Mateos[51] reported the use of acupuncture-like ES for the treatment of unresponsive wounds of mixed etiologies and burns. In this clinical trial, in which patients served as their own controls, the device used had the parameters of 300 mV, 67 Hz, 0.04 mA, and a calculated absolute charge density of 0.4–0.8 C/cm². The method of delivery for most wounds was via electrodes clipped to stainless steel acupuncture filiform needles that were inserted subcutaneously along the edges of the lesion and placed to form an almost complete, closed peripheral circuit. In very large burn wounds, the current was applied by means of covering the wound with saline-soaked gauze, and then randomly attaching alligator clips from the stimulator to the gauze, maximally separating the positive and negative electrodes. Delivery of current through the gauze in this manner without a conductor is problematic. Treatments were administered either daily or every other day, based on the severity of the lesion and compliance of the patient.

Throughout the course of the treatment protocol, no local antiseptics or antibacterials (either systemic or local) were administered. Dry wound healing methods, as described in an earlier section, were used. Only normal saline was used to cleanse wounds. Forty-four wounds (34 wounds/10 burns) were treated. Patients and wounds were assessed using a stratified classification method of lesion and medical condition severity. When wounds were classified according to their severity, as well as the overall condition of the patient, a closer statistical correlation between the lesion grade and number of treatments to total cure was observed (r = 0.98). Number of treatments were less (8.4 ± 2.3) for grade I severity lesions (N = 10) than for those of grade III severity (N = 17)(41.38 ± 6.58). The authors reported a positive correlation between the severity grade and the time of the first visit for alternative treatment. Mean time from lesion identification to first presentation was 11.8 ± 4.49 days for grade I, 15.44 ± 8.58 for grade II, and 24.5 ± 5.21 days for grade III.

This study was conducted in Mexico, where patients are familiar with acupuncture. All patients in the study requested this alternative type of medical treatment when their wounds/burns did not heal quickly (2–4 weeks) with conventional wound healing procedures and drugs. Although this procedure uses acupuncture needles, it is not an orthodox acupuncture procedure. Authors reported that the patients were compliant with the treatment and attributed the compliance to high patient satisfaction, with the evident improvement seen from the first treatment session. Early intervention with the ES procedures seems to have accelerated the healing process, reduced risk for increased wound severity, and required less treatment interventions to achieve an excellent outcome. In all patients, healing proceeded in a thoroughly organized manner, almost regardless of the severity of the type of wound or burn treated.[51]

High-Voltage Pulsed Current Studies

Nine randomized controlled and controlled clinical prospective studies were found in a literature review reporting the use of HVPC for wound healing. Reporting investigators included Kloth and Feedar,[47] Griffin et al,[45] Unger et al,[135] Gogia et al,[136], Houghton et al,[9] Peters et al,[13] Polak et al,[11] Franek et al,[10] and Goldman et al[14] using HVPC. A brief summary of each study follows; Table 22-7 summarizes the data.

Kloth and Feedar[47] studied wounds of mixed etiologies and found a mean healing time of 7.3 weeks, and 100% of the treatment group healed. Positive polarity was used initially, then switched to negative if the wound plateaued. Unger et al[135] reported on a controlled study of nine subjects in the treatment group and eight controls. The average wound size in the treatment group was 460 mm², compared with the control group, whose average wound size was 118.5 mm². Mean healing time was 7.3 weeks for the treatment group, with 88.9% completely healed. The protocol started with negative polarity for 3 days or until the wound was clean, then switched to positive. Gogia et al[136] treated for 20 minutes following a 20-minute whirlpool session 5 times a week, beginning with 4 days of negative polarity, then switched to positive polarity. The rate of healing in the experimental group was particularly high during the first 2 weeks of treatment (31.45%), then slowed considerably and was not statistically different from the control group after 5 weeks.

The above study populations were heterogeneous, but subsequent studies have been homogenous or stratified by etiology of the population and separate results reported. Griffin et al[3] demonstrated an 80% reduction in size of pressure ulcers in SCI-injured patients in 4 weeks, when treated with negative polarity, but ulcers were not treated until healed. Houghton et al's[9] RCT focused on treatment of vascular leg ulcers (N = 27 subjects, 42 ulcers). The study time was not intended to take the wounds to closure but to evaluate the effect of HVPC on size and tissue appearance over a 4-week period. The vascular leg ulcers were stratified into three groups: diabetic, arterial, or venous. Then the ulcers were randomly assigned to one of two treatment groups. One group received HVPC treatment and the other placebo treatment. All HVPC treatment was given at negative polarity, three times weekly treatment of 45 minutes per session. Outcome measures reported included percentage reduction in surface area and wound tissue appearance as evaluated with the photographic wound assessment tool (PWAT). (Chapter 5 describes this assessment tool.) Surface area for the total experimental group decreased 44.3 % ± 8.8%, or 11% per week during the four weeks of the study, and the ulcers in the control group did not decrease. Seven patients had bilateral venous ulcers and they were used as their own controls. Data was stated in two ways: combined healing for the combined group of vascular ulcers (above) and separately for the seven. In patients who were their own controls, the treated ulcer had a surface area reduction that was significantly greater (57% +/- 15) than the control ulcer (20% +/- 18.16%) and PWAT scores reduction over the time of the study.

Polak et al[11] also reported an RCT using HVPC for venous leg ulcers. English translation of the Polish published study was provided by the first author as a personal communication. In this study, 22 patients were enrolled for treatment and 20 as controls. The study lasted 7 weeks. Treatment was six times weekly for 50 minutes per session. Outcomes were reported two ways: percentage of healing and weekly healing rate of both volume and surface area. Findings were that the treated ulcer had a 73.4% reduction of area compared with 47% reduction for control. Volume reduction for the experimental group was 91.3% versus 68%. Weekly healing rate was a volume reduction of 1 cm³ for treated ulcers and 0.6 cm³ for controls. The number of healed or percentage of healed ulcers was not reported.[11] Likewise, the rate of area reduction was faster for the experimental group (1.4 cm² per week versus 1.0 cm² per week). A second RCT from Poland by Frane, Polak and Kucharzewski also investigated the effect of HVPC on venous ulcers.[10,11] Three groups were used: group A (N = 33)

TABLE 22-7 **HVPC Clinical Studies**

Researchers	Number of Patients	Percentage Healed	Mean Time To Heal
Alon et al[64]	15 treated, 0 controls (diabetic)	80%	10.4 weeks (9.6%/week)
Kloth and Feedar[47]	9 treated, 7 controls, 3 cross-overs (mixed wound etiology)	100%	7.3 weeks (13.7%/week)
Griffin et al[45]	8 treated, 9 controls (pressure ulcers)	80% reduction in size	4-week treatment period (20%/week)
Unger[137]	223 treated, 0 controls	89.7%	10.85 weeks (9.27%/week)
Unger et al[135]	9 treated, 8 controls (pressure ulcers)	88.9%	7.3 weeks (13.7%/week)
Gogia et al[136]	6 controls treated with sterile whirlpool	35% (ES with whirlpool) vs 28% (whirlpool) area reduction	20 days (20%/week)
	6 treated with sterile whirlpool and HVPC	30% (ES with whirlpool) vs 58% (whirlpool) depth reduction	
Polak et al[11]	22 treated, 20 controls treated with medications Venous leg ulcers	Treated group reduction: area 73%; volume 91% Controls reduction area: 47% volume 68%	7-week treatment 6.5-week controls Number healed not reported
Houghton et al[9]	42 ulcers, 27 patients Leg ulcers: diabetic, venous, arterial	44.% mean reduction in size	4-week study (healing rate 11%/week)
Goldman et al[14]	4 treatment 4 control Infrapopliteal Ischemic Ulcers	3 healed; (one patient expired) 3 healed; one amputation	Decreased in size during first 4 weeks then went on to heal Increased in size 50% during first 4 weeks then turned around but healing rate slower than treatment group

Source: Data from references listed in the table

received HVPC treatment and compression bandaging, group B (N = 32) received topically applied medicine and compression therapy, and group C (N = 14) received Unna boot compression. Outcome measures analyzed were rate of healing, rate of "pus" debridement/cleansing, and degree of granulation formation after 2 weeks. Findings were that the rates of wound healing and pus cleansing were highest in group A. An inclusion criterion was ankle brachial index ABI greater than 0.8. Negative polarity was used until wound was clean of pus, typically 1–3 weeks, then changed to anode for the rest of the study. (Note: From an accompanying photograph, pus appeared to include necrotic tissue.)

Peters et al reported a 12-week RCT study of ES efficacy on healing of diabetic foot ulcers (N = 40) using an unusual protocol.[13] All patients received off-loading, debridement as needed, and moist wound healing dressings that were changed twice daily. Treatments and dressing changes were performed by the patient or a family member. The object was to test outcome as related to compliance using a unique treatment schedule. The treatment took place in the patient's home during night sleep, the purpose being to improve compliance because the patient's regular schedule of activities would be minimally impacted. The device used was a small microcomputer strapped to the leg and the electric current was delivered through a Dacron mesh silver nylon stocking. The device used compliance metering. Current was delivered as twin peak pulses at 50 V amplitude in 3 phases: high pulse rate (80 pps) for 10 minutes followed by low pulse rate (10pps) for 10 minutes, then a 400-minute rest period. Polarity was not reported. Programming of the computer allowed for this sequence to be repeated throughout the night, presumably for seven to eight cycles per night. Conductivity was assured with a slowly evaporating electrolyte fluid applied to the skin.

Compliance was evaluated and the findings were that: 1) compliance from both groups was essentially the same; 2) compliant patients only used the device correctly 50% of the time; and 3) compliant patients in both groups had better outcomes than both noncompliant groups. Two dropouts occurred in each group. Healing outcomes were as follows: 75% of treatment group healed and 35% in placebo group healed. Among the healers in both group, the average healing times were essentially the same: 6.8 +/- 3.4 weeks and 6.9 +/- 2.8 weeks. Conclusion: Patients who used the ES protocol for 20 hours or more per week were more likely to heal than those who used placebo or less than 20 hours of stimulation per week.

Goldman reported a small RCT pilot study (N = 8 ; 4 in each group) of patients with ischemic ulcers. Ischemic ulcers have a predisposition to be unstable and rapidly expand into gangrenous eschar.[14] Patient inclusion criteria for this study was critically ischemic wounds occurring below the knee diagnosed by vascular study that had not healed in at least 4 weeks. The groups were appropriately matched. Risk was evaluated by the clinical team; expectation that the wound would not increase in size over the 14-week study period was another inclusion criteria. A significant finding from this small study was that both $tcPO_2$ levels and laser Doppler flow measurements were increased out of the ischemic range in the treatment group and not in the controls.

At the 1-year follow-up there were was one unrelated death but no amputations in the HVPC group. There was one amputation in the control group even though the controls elected to transfer to HVPC after the 14-week trial period. Impetuous for this RCT prospective pilot study was a 5-year retrospective RCT observational study previously reported by the same principal author. In that study, they identified criteria met by 22 patients with ischemic wounds below the ankle who were poor candidates for revascularization. Eleven subjects had received HVPC plus standard care and the other eleven subjects received only standard care. At the end of one year from start of treatment, 90% of wounds (9/10) were healed in the HVPC group, compared with 29% (2/7) who only received standard care. In addition, there were observations of a marked increase in $tcPO_2$ levels in the HVPC-treated group of patients over the study period and that ulcer healing tended to improve after the start of ES (see the section on ES and oxygen earlier in this chapter). The study authors recognized correctly that a small number of subjects have the ability to skew the results and calculated an N of 24, 12 each group, to test their hypothesis about increasing microcirculation with an ES phase 2 study.

Unger[137] reported an uncontrolled study using HVPC treatment and the same protocol as above for 223 pressure ulcers. The mean healing time for the 223 wounds in the uncontrolled study was 10.85 weeks (see Table 22-7). Two additional published uncontrolled studies included 30 patients. Alon et al[64] used positive polarity and stimulated wounds three times a week for 1 hour; 12 of the 15 (80%) of the ulcers treated healed. One patient died, one did not respond, and the ulcer in one decreased significantly in size but did not heal in 21.6 weeks. Akers and Gabrielson[138] published a study that compared (1) HVPC direct application to the wound; (2) application of HVPC using the whirlpool as a large electrode; and (3) whirlpool alone. The direct application of the active electrode to the wound site had the best outcome, followed by HVPC using the whirlpool as an electrode. Whirlpool alone was the least effective.

In all the studies except the Gogia, Houghton, and Peters studies, the treatment frequency was five to seven times per week for 45–60 minutes. At this time, it is hard to state what is the optimal amount of stimulation needed to effect healing, However, it does seem apparent that HVPC is an effective adjunct to standard wound care for the populations studied.

Low-Voltage Pulsed Electrical Current Studies

Two CCTs with low-voltage pulsed current, labeled PES, were located in the literature. Gentzkow et al[3] reported a study of 40 ulcers in 37 patients. Nineteen pressure ulcers were stimulated, and 21 were sham stimulated. The trial lasted for 4 weeks. The treated ulcers healed more than twice as much as the sham-stimulated ulcers (49.8% versus 23.4%), healing at a rate of 12.5% per week, compared with 5.8% for the sham-stimulated group. Cross-over results for 15 of the 19 sham-treated ulcers showed a fourfold greater healing during the 4 weeks of stimulation, compared with 4 weeks of sham treatment. This difference was statistically significant.[3]

Feedar et al[46] published a study on pressure ulcers. The 61 patients served as their own controls. The treatment phase of the study was preceded by a 4-week control phase of optimal nonelectrically stimulated wound care. Only the stage III or IV ulcers with need of surgical debridement, necrotic/purulent drainage, or exudate seropurulent drainage that did not improve during the control phase went on to the treatment phase. After 4 weeks of treatment, 58.8% of the wounds had improved. After an average of 8.4 weeks, 23% completely healed and 82% improved significantly.

CLINICAL WISDOM

Best Method for Effective HVPC Treatment

Apply HVPC directly to the wound for best expected outcome. Conducting current to the tissues during whirlpool is not recommended because it is less effective, and some clinicians report that stimulator leads have become entangled in the agitator. There have even been stories of stimulators falling into the water.

Biphasic Stimulation Studies

Controlled Animal Study

Khalil and Merhi[124] decided to test the effect of frequency on wound healing in aged rats. Aged rats were wounded and then divided into an active treatment group and a sham treatment group. Low-frequency TENS (20 V, 5 Hz for 1 minute) was applied twice daily to the treatment group, and sham treatment was applied to the controls. The active group required 14.7 ± 0.2 days for complete healing, which was a significant improvement over the sham group (21.8 ± 0.3 days). The conclusion reached was that wound healing in aged rats can be accelerated by peripheral activation of sensory nerves, using low-frequency parameters.

Human Studies

There are reports in the literature by Kaada,[79] Lundeberg et al,[139] Stefanovska et al,[129] and Baker et al[8,140] of clinical trials of wound healing with biphasic waveforms. Frantz's[15]

RCT has been submitted for publication. Kaada,[79] Lundeberg et al,[139] and Frantz[15] each used biphasic symmetric waveforms with significant improvement in both ulcer area and healed ulcers. Kaada[79] reported results of TENS on 10 subjects, who served as their own controls, with recalcitrant ulcers of different etiologies. Stimulation was provided indirectly over the web of the thumb daily (HoKu point) during three 30-minute sessions with rests of 45 minutes between, for a total of 11/2 hours of stimulation. Stimulation was below visible muscle contraction. Lundeberg et al[139] conducted an RCT on 64 patients with chronic diabetic ulcers due to venous stasis. All patients received standard treatment with paste bandage, in addition to the sham or TENS treatment. Asymmetric biphasic stimulation was determined to produce significant wound healing effects, whereas the other waveforms did not increase the healing rate.

The RCT study by Stefanovska et al[129] compared direct current and asymmetric biphasic current. In two RCTs, Baker et al[8,140] compared asymmetric biphasic, symmetric biphasic, and microcurrent (DC). The asymmetric biphasic waveform has a potential for some polar effect that should not be discounted. The polar effect may explain why it was more effective than the symmetric biphasic waveform. However, another likely explanation of the effects is stimulation of neural mechanisms that effect healing.[8] In all of the studies except Kaada, stimulation was delivered to the skin at the wound perimeter, rather than into the wound bed. An advantage of the perimeter stimulation was less disruption of the wound bed, less cross-contamination of the wound, and less interference with the dressing.

Benefits were found in patients with spinal cord injury who had pressure ulcers[8,129] and in patients with diabetic ulcers, including those with peripheral neuropathy[140] and venous stasis.[139] Franz[15] combined the indirect stimulation over the web of the thumb daily (HoKu point) protocol of Kaada with a protocol of bipolar biphasic stimulation on either side of the wound at the wound perimeter. The patients were elderly nursing home patients with pressure ulcers. The number of days to achieve a 50% or greater reduction in wound size was chosen as the outcome measure using two measurements of the size of wound surface area and wound volume. The 50% closure was selected as the study outcome, rather than 100% healing, due to the relatively short study period of 8 weeks and the chronicity of the wounds entered in the study. Based on surface area measurements, the median time to 50% healing was 42 days for the TENS group and 54 days for the control group. The rate failed to reach significance based on surface area. However, according to volume measurements with stereographic photography, there were significant differences in the time to 50% closure, with a median time of 28 days for the TENS group and 53 days for the control group. Volume data were applicable only to full-thickness ulcers (N = 31). Complete healing was reported for 8 of 20 (40%) of the TENS group and 5 of 17 (29.4%) in the control group. Six

of the 17 full-thickness ulcers in the TENS groups healed, compared with 2 of 14 in the control group. Another research finding has been made in this study that more rapid reduction in wound depth occurs when alternating current (AC) is used. One animal RCT[128] and two human RCTs[15,129] have noted this observation. Table 22-8 summarizes the protocols used and results for all of the biphasic studies.

Meta-Analysis of Effect of ES on Chronic Wound Healing

Gardner and Frantz[16] used meta-analysis to average quantitatively the findings across multiple ES studies. The meta-analysis for ES for wound healing was undertaken by the authors for three purposes:

1. To quantify the effect of ES as an adjunctive therapy for chronic wound healing
2. To explore the influence that the type of ES may have on efficacy of the ES treatment
3. To explore the influence that the wound etiology may have on ES effectiveness for healing

To achieve these goals, the meta-analysis estimated the rate of healing of chronic wounds treated with ES. To be included in the meta-analysis, the following criteria had to be met:

1. The study was on the use of ES for ulcer or periulcer stimulation
2. The subjects were humans
3. Reports would include all types of chronic wounds (arterial, diabetic, pressure, and venous)

The outcome measure chosen for evaluation was the percentage of healing per week because it was the most common measurement either reported or that could be calculated from study data. Fifteen studies, which included 24 ES and 15 samples, were analyzed and the average rate of healing per week calculated for each sample. The 15 studies included have been described in the preceding text. Ninety-five percent confidence intervals were also calculated. The 95% confidence intervals of the ES (18–26%) and control samples (3.8–14%) did not overlap. Then the samples were grouped by type of ES device and chronic wound, and reanalyzed. The rate of healing per week was 22% for ES samples and 9% for control samples. The net effect of ES was 13% per week. Net increase in rate of healing was 10.9%. DC healing rate was 12.6% per week vs. pulsed current healing rate net increase of 15.5%. ES treatment was most effective for treatment of pressure ulcers (net effect = 13% per week). Findings regarding the relative effectiveness of different ES devices were inconclusive. The authors felt that the problem was extensive overlap in the confidence intervals.

The conclusion reached by these authors was that ES produces a substantial improvement in the healing of chronic wounds, and further research is needed to identify which ES

TABLE 22-8 Biphasic Treatment Protocols and Results

Parameters	Kaada[79]	Lundeberg et al[139]	Stefanovska et al[129]	Baker et al[8,140]	Frantz[15]	Barron et al[134]	Sumano and Mateos[51]
Phase duration	Not reported	1 msec	0.25 msec	100 µsec	150 µsec	Not stated	Not stated
Pulse rate	100 Hz	80 Hz	40 Hz	50 Hz	85 Hz	0.5 Hz	65 Hz
Waveform	Symmetric	Symmetric	Asymmetric, charge balanced	Asymmetric	Symmetric square	Modified square	Symmetric square
Amplitude	15–30 mA muscle contraction	15–25 mA evoking paresthesias	15–25 mA below contraction	24–25 mA below contraction	10 mA	600 µA/50 V	0.04 mA current charge density: 0.4–0.8 C
Frequency and duration	Daily; three 30-min sessions (off 45 min between sessions)	Twice daily for 20 min	Daily for 2 hours	Daily; three 30-min sessions (short break between sessions)	Three times daily 30 min	Three times per week	Daily or every other day 20 min
Location	Negative electrode Web between 1st and 2nd metacarpal bones	Wound edge	Wound edge	Less than 1 cm from edge; proximal and distal to ulcer	(1) web space both hands (2) + proximal to wound edge (3) – distal to wound edge	.2 cm from ulcer edge, moved around wound edge	Along wound edges
Patient population and study type	Multiple diagnoses (N = 10) CCT	Diabetics with venous stasis ulcers (N = 64) RCT 7%/week decrease in size	SCI with pressure ulcers (N = 150) RCT	Study 1 SCI with pressure ulcers (N = 185) RCT Study 2 Diabetic ulcers (N = 80) RCT	Pressure ulcers (N = 37) RCT	Pressure ulcers (N = 6) Case Series	Mixed wounds and burns (N = 44) CCT
Results of treatment	Healing of chronic ulcers	42% healed in treatment group control group 15% healed 4.25%/week decrease in size	Monophasic less effective for reducing depth than biphasic Monophasic more effective for reducing area than biphasic Experimental 25.2%/week decrease in size Control 15.4%/week decrease in size	Asymmetric biphasic significantly improved healing rates by 60% over controls	Median time to closure using volume measurements for TENS group: 28 days; controls 53 days. No statistical difference in surface area change.	Healing and decreased size	Healing in organized manner

Data from references listed in the table.

devices are most effective and which wound types respond best to this treatment. Evaluation of the meta-analysis showed that the studies chosen for the meta-analysis were both published and unpublished, randomized and nonrandomized clinical trials, and descriptive studies. Only three were reports of TENS, alternating was classified separately, and the rest were either direct current or pulsed direct current. Many of the studies chosen for this analysis had very small subject samples (3–7). Controls received a variety of treatments, including moist dressings (13), antiseptics (4), and whirlpool (4). However, the evidence of effectiveness of this adjunctive therapy compares favorably or surpasses treatment with other interventions used for wound healing.

Summary

Electrical stimulation studies have varied from continuous waveform application with direct current to pulsed short-duration monophasic pulses to biphasic pulses. What is known and acknowledged is that ES seems to have positive effects on wound healing or on the components necessary for wound healing (e.g., blood flow and oxygen uptake, DNA and protein synthesis), but there is still ambiguity about the type of ES characteristics that are most important or critical. For instance, polarity has played an important role in protocols used, even though the likelihood of polarity effects of currents with pulses of very short duration is questionable. One possible reason for the wound healing effects of ES with any type of current may result from the effect of low-level sensory stimulation on the peripheral nerves, which is not wholly dependent on the polar nature of electrical current. Kaada[78] describes effects that include inhibition of sympathetic input to superficial vessels, release of an active vasodilator, and axon-reflex stimulation. Study results are beginning to show evidence that stimulation with direct current, alternating current, and pulsed current have somewhat different physiologic effects. As identification of the specific effects of different currents is more thoroughly tested, the clinician will be able to choose the type of stimulation and a protocol to derive a specific outcome for prevention or healing.

Choosing an Intervention: Clinical Reasoning

Applying Theory and Science to Clinical Decision Making

The previous section evaluated the efficacy of ES on many components of healing, as well as clinical trials of human wound healing. The studies basically looked at six components:

1. Galvanotaxis and effect at the cellular level
2. Circulatory effects
3. Effects on edema
4. Antibacterial effects
5. Effects on pain

6. Effects on repair, regeneration, and completeness of healing

The clinician should consider these variables when selecting ES intervention and choosing a protocol.

The specific medical diagnosis may not be a significant factor in selecting ES for wound healing. The medical diagnoses of patients in the studies included burns, pressure ulcers, diabetic ulcers (vascular and neuropathic), vascular ulcers (venous and arterial), and vasculitic ulcers. The surgical wounds included in the studies were acute incisions, skin flaps, donor sites, and dehiscence. Acute and chronic wounds were included. Electrical stimulation had demonstrated efficacy for wound healing across diagnoses and pathogeneses. Reported effects were related to the stimulation of the mechanisms of healing at the cellular, tissue, and/or systems levels. Healing follows a predictable pattern, regardless of etiology; what affects the outcome are the intrinsic, extrinsic, and iatrogenic factors that alter healing, described in Chapter 2. The PT intervenes in wound management specifically to facilitate the functional mechanisms of healing. Electrical stimulation is just one of the interventions that can be used.

Wound attributes that have positively responded to electrical stimulation were necrotic tissue and pus, inflammation, wound contraction, infection, and wound resurfacing. Wounds of all depths, from partial-thickness to full-thickness and deeper, have been successfully treated with electrical stimulation (e.g., stage II to stage IV pressure ulcers). Wounds have traditionally been classified by medical diagnosis, by depth of tissue disruption, and/or by phase of wound healing. Depth of tissue disruption is a description of the tissue loss and function that is broader and more generic than that in the medical diagnosis system. The depth of tissue disruption system can be used for wounds, regardless of the wound etiology, and is referred to as wound severity diagnosis. Classification by phase of wound healing is also independent of the medical diagnosis. This is the wound healing phase diagnosis. Change in wound phase is an outcome of the process of wound healing (see Chapter 4 and Table 22-9).

The typical subjects selected for clinical trials with ES had nonconforming wound healing with long chronicity. The chronic wounds were the reason for referral for ES. There is significant scientific evidence to support that early intervention with externally applied electrical currents will also accelerate healing for the acute healthy wound. Early intervention with ES could be a useful method to prevent chronicity and return the individual earlier to a functional status. This is consistent with other areas of physical therapy practice, such as stroke and low back rehabilitation, where early intervention can reduce the development of costly chronic health problems.

Summary

In summary, selection of ES for wound healing is not dependent on the wound etiology or patient medical diagno-

TABLE 22-9 Appropriate Wound Classifications for Electrical Stimulation

Level of tissue disruption (wound severity)	Superficial, partial thickness, full thickness, subcutaneous, and deep tissues
Etiologies/diagnostic groups	Burns, neuropathic ulcers, pressure ulcers, surgical wounds, vascular ulcers (venous and arterial)
Wound healing phase	Inflammatory phase: acute, chronic, absent Proliferative phase: acute, chronic, absent Epithelialization phase: acute, chronic, absent Remodeling phase: acute, chronic, absent
Age	Older than 3 years

sis. ES intervention and treatment characteristics are appropriate when there are impairments to the systems that interfere with healing at one or more levels: cellular, tissue, or organ. Functional loss at any of these levels suggests that the wound will not or has not healed with the current level of intervention. The reason for referral to the PT is for the development of another strategy to facilitate healing. The use of externally applied currents is one such strategy.

Precautions

Signs of adverse effects using ES for wound healing were evaluated in the various clinical trials. The only two adverse signs were some skin irritation or tingling under the electrodes in a few cases and pain in some other cases. Patients with severe peripheral vascular occlusive disease, particularly in the lower extremity, may experience some increased pain with ES, usually described as throbbing. An alternative acupuncture protocol has been suggested in these cases— placing the active electrode on the web space of the hand between the thumb and first finger instead of over the ulcer located on the leg.[78,79] Children less than 3 years of age should not be considered candidates for intervention with ES. Healing mechanisms for this group are not well understood and, although there are no known adverse effects, the benefits are not defined. However, older children may benefit from use of an ES intervention to stimulate sensory nerves and accelerate the rate of healing.[141]

Contraindications

Contraindications for the use of ES as described are from various sources and fall into the following categories:

1. When stimulation of cell proliferation is contraindicated (e.g., malignancy)
2. Where there is evidence of osteomyelitis

3. Where there are metal ions
4. Where the placement of electrodes for treatment with ES could adversely affect a reflex center
5. Where electrical current could affect the function of an electronic implant[132,123]

Carefully evaluate the medical history and review body systems when considering candidates for use of this intervention.

Presence of Malignancy

When there is a malignancy in the area to be treated, ES should not be used (e.g., malignant melanoma, basal cell carcinoma). Electrical stimulation stimulates cell proliferation and could lead to uncontrolled cell growth. If the malignancy is distant from the wound (e.g., breast cancer in a patient with a pressure ulcer on an ankle), however, local use of ES should be considered, weighing the risks and the perceived benefit of the treatment, mindful that ES has demonstrated systemic effects.[78,142] In such a case, it would be a precaution but not a contraindication, although this is not consistent with required manufacturer labeling.

Active Osteomyelitis

There has been concern that stimulation of tissue growth with ES may cause superficial covering of an area of osteomyelitis. This could blind the site from observation. A medical record that documents a history of a bone infection should trigger an investigation of the current status of the infection. If the osteomyelitis is being treated actively with antibiotic therapy, some clinicians are recommending that treatment with ES be started. It is not unusual for the osteomyelitis to be resolved but not to be noted in the medical record. The contraindications listed here have been included in physical agent texts and manufacturer literature for many years. Based on the publication of the case studies reported earlier, in which patients with osteomyelitis were treated successfully with ES, it is time to re-evaluate the contraindication to use of ES in an area of osteomyelitis. Controlled clinical trials are indicated to test the benefits of ES for treating wounds in which there is evidence of osteomyelitis.

CLINICAL WISDOM

Identification of Osteomyelitis

If a wound penetrates to the bone, as determined by inserting a probe, it must be assumed that osteomyelitis is present and the patient should not be treated with ES. An immediate referral to a surgeon for evaluation[143] must be initiated.

Topical Substances Containing Metal Ions

Topical substances containing metal ions (e.g., povidone-iodine, zinc, Mercurochrome, and silver sulfadiazine [Silvadene, SSD] that might be used as part of the wound treatment regimen) should be removed before the application of ES. Direct-current ES has the ability to transfer ions into the tissues by iontophoresis. Heavy metal ions may have toxic properties when introduced into the body. If removal of the topical substance is not appropriate, however, ES could be used on other areas of the skin where the topical agent has not been applied.

Electronic Implants

Demand-type cardiac pacemakers and other electrical implants raise concerns regarding the use of electrical current. ES is contraindicated *over* electrical implants because the current and electromagnetic fields could disrupt function of the implant. Use of ES with a demand-type cardiac pacemaker is one of its contraindications. Studies to evaluate safe utilization of TENS in the presence of a cardiac pacemaker report mixed results. Application of TENS in 51 patients with 20 different cardiac pacemakers at four sites (lumbar area, cervical spine, left leg, and lower arm area ipsilateral to the pacemaker) without episodes of interference, inhibition, or reprogramming of the pacemakers was reported by Rasmussen et al.[144] Shade[145] reported successful use of a TENS unit in conjunction with a temporary cardiac pacemaker. No interference was seen on the EKG readout.

Sliwa and Marinko[146] reported an EKG artifact with routine EKG produced by surface TENS electrodes applied to the thoracic and lumbar regions. Chen et al[142] reported two cases in which cardiac pacemaker dysfunction occurred and was undetected by electrocardiograms. It showed up with extended cardiac monitoring with the Holter monitor. The pacemaker sensitivity was then reprogrammed, and the abnormalities did not recur. The recommendation was extended cardiac monitoring for patients with cardiac pacemakers during prolonged use of TENS to ensure safety and to determine any need for reprogramming of the pacemakers.

Patients with cardiac pacemakers should not be excluded from the use of TENS but require careful evaluation and extended cardiac monitoring. The risks and benefits of using ES for wound healing need to be carefully weighed.

Natural Reflexes

There are areas of the body that are particularly sensitive to any stimulation (e.g., carotid sinus, heart, parasympathetic nerves, ganglion, laryngeal muscles, phrenic nerve). Sensory levels of ES might create a vasospasm or some type of vasoconstriction that could lead to a vasovagal response and other neural responses that could interfere with the function of vital centers and be harmful to the patient. Thus, ES is contraindicated to run current through the upper chest and anterior neck.

Equipment

Regulatory Approval

Under what is called *premarket approval* (PMA), manufacturing companies are allowed to make claims of effectiveness and safety about medical devices. PMA requires ex-

tensive clinical trials, typically 2,000–3,000 cases for approval. "Off label" means treatment not approved by the FDA. No electrical stimulators have received PMA by the FDA for wound healing. Externally applied currents for wound healing are considered as off-label use at this time. Off-label use for medical devices is an accepted and common practice in medicine as innovative therapy, as long as the participants are not closely associated with the manufacturer.[147] For example, the on-label uses for neuromuscular stimulators, such as HVPC, include application for increased circulation, relaxation of muscle spasms, and muscle re-education. The on-label use for TENS is pain management.

Expect to find an FDA-mandated instruction manual accompanying each electrical stimulator. Listed in the manual are labeled indications, contraindications, warnings, and precautions (Exhibit 22-3). The FDA indications and contraindications do not exactly match what is described in the previous text. The PT must be aware of these limitations when selecting a protocol with ES and use thoughtful clinical judgment.

Devices

Electrical stimulators have three basic components: a source of power, an oscillator circuit, and an output amplifier. There are two size ranges: clinical models and portable models. The latter can be as small as a beeper. Two basic power sources are used: batteries and house line current. Batteries are used in portable stimulators; house line current is usually used in the clinic setting. Batteries need to be fully charged to deliver the output expected. A spare battery

---

EXHIBIT 22-3 FDA Indications and Contraindications for Electrical Stimulation

- Relaxation of muscle spasms
- Prevention or retardation of disuse atrophy
- Increasing local blood circulation
- Muscle re-education
- Immediate postsurgical stimulation of calf muscles to prevent venous thrombosis
- Maintaining or increasing range of motion
- Pain
- Edema

FDA Contraindications for Electrical Stimulation

- Should not be used on patients with demand-type cardiac pacemakers
- Should not be used on persons known to have cancerous lesions
- Should not be used for symptomatic pain relief unless etiology is established or unless a pain syndrome has been diagnosed
- Should not be used over pregnant uterus
- Electrode placements must be avoided that apply current to the carotid sinus region (anterior neck) or transcerebrally (through the head)

should be kept on hand. Rechargeable batteries may be more cost-effective than single-use types. House line current is usually available.

Many electrical stimulators now use microprocessors with a choice of several waveforms and pulse rates, and even include preset protocols for wound treatment. The clinician should not assume that this is the "correct" protocol for the wound. It is the clinician's responsibility to know the rationale for protocol characteristics and what the settings are on the chosen stimulator. Most programs allow clinicians to override the preset programs.

Select a stimulator based on the available waveform, pulse characteristic, and ability to adjust intensity and polarity. A desirable stimulator should allow for flexibility to set up and deliver a variety of protocols, based on changes dictated by clinical trials and current concepts of physiologic rationale. Manufacturers are an important source of helpful information about the characteristics of their devices.

Testing Equipment

Meters are useful to the clinician to check on the current flow between two electrodes. Use the device meter if available; if no meter is available on the stimulator, pursue other options. Patient sensation is always a good indicator, if the patient can give a report. The use of ES for wound healing is usually done at a sensory level, but many of the patients are insensate or unable to communicate, or the wounds are deep and below the level of sensation and the patient will not be able to indicate if the current is not felt. Another test method is to position the dispersive/indifferent electrode over a muscle motor point to determine whether there is a muscle twitch or tingling under the electrode. The electrode pads can be checked by the PT by placing a wet contact on both positive and negative electrodes, and then resting the forearms on each electrode pad. Ask a colleague to turn up the device until a sensation of prickling is felt.

Electrical stimulation equipment should have regular calibration checks. In between checks, a multimeter can be used for periodic spot checking to see that the equipment is functioning properly. Multimeters, which are a combination of volt-ohm-milliammeter, have the ability to determine current flow. They are inexpensive, easy to use, and readily available. A broken lead wire, weak battery, or resistant electrode may not be apparent because the stimulation in the wound bed is below the level of sensation or the patient is insensate or cognitively impaired and cannot report changes in sensation. Checking for good electrical conduction is the responsibility of the clinician.

Electrodes

Electrode Materials

The electrode is the contact point between the electrical circuit and the body. The electrode must be a good conductor, provide very little resistance to the current, and conform well to the surface. All metals are good conductors of electricity. Aluminum foil is an excellent conductor to use for electrodes (Figures 22-7A and 22-7B). It is nontoxic, inexpensive, disposable, conformable, and can be sized as needed. Carbon-impregnated electrodes are sold to go with most electrotherapeutic devices. They are designed for multiple uses and are relatively inexpensive, but they need to be disinfected between uses, even if restricted to a single patient. They are less conformable than aluminum foil and will become resistive over time as they lose carbon and accumulate body oils and cleaning products. Self-adhesive electrodes can be used for bipolar techniques but not for direct wound applications. A novel approach to electrodes is a Dacron mesh conductive silver nylon garment (stocking and glove, etc.) (Prizm Medical, Inc.; Duluth GA 30096). A slowly evaporating electrolyte fluid is applied to the skin under the garment to reduce skin resistance and allow conduction of the current to the tissues.[13] This application allows delivery of the stimulation over a large surface area without concern about size, shape, or electrode placement around the wound. The company makes an HV stimulator that interfaces with the garment electrodes.

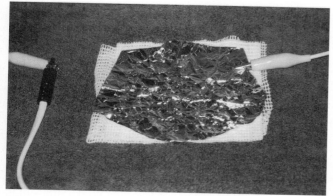

A

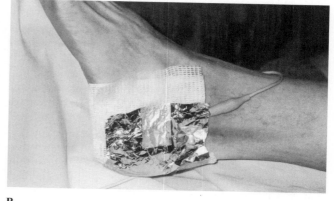

B

FIGURE 22-7 Electrode materials. **A.** Aluminum foil electrode. **B.** Electrode with alligator clip.

Electrode Arrangements

Size and Shape of Electrodes. Size, shape, and arrangement of electrodes affect the current density and depth. Current density as described is the amount of current flow per unit area. Current density is a measure of the quantity of charged ions moving through a specific cross-sectional area of body tissue. The unit of measurement is mA or mA/cm^2. This measure will affect the reaction of the tissues being stimulated. In general, the greater the current density, the greater the effect on tissue biology. Two determinants of current density are *size* of the electrode and the *amplitude* of the current applied,[148] and for pulsed currents, it is also important to know the duty cycle. Small electrodes concentrate the current for local effects more than do larger electrodes, which tend to disperse the charge. Also, the farther apart the electrodes, the deeper the current penetrates.

Active and Dispersive Electrodes. For monophasic stimulation, the small electrode is commonly referred to as the *active or treatment electrode*, and the large electrode is called the *dispersive electrode*. If the two are of nearly equal size or have equal current, the current will be divided between the two, with the current density at the two treatment sites the same. If the two are not of equal size, the larger electrode will have less current density than the smaller electrode. A rule of thumb is that the combined area of the active electrodes should not exceed the overall area of the dispersive electrode. Usually, a larger size dispersive electrode is used because it's more comfortable due to the lesser charge density and perception under it. The effects of the tangential electric field extends and affects events from 2 to 3 cm up to 11+ cm beyond the edge of the stimulating electrodes.[149] Maximum tangential electric field occurs on the body surface in the edge regions where the two electrodes of opposite polarity faced each other, and maximum tangential fields are stronger than the perpendicular fields directly under the stimulating electrodes.[149] Therefore, to achieve polarity effects, avoid placement of the active and dispersive electrodes so that they touch each other or are too close to avoid the possibility that the wound is receiving stimulation from both poles. Wounds treated with tangential fields and those treated with perpendicular fields have nearly the same rate of healing.[150] Studies that report patients having two wounds, one of which is used as the control and the second treated with ES, may report results that are better than studies when external controls are used.[130]

At times in clinical practice, it is necessary to treat multiple wound sites with a single electrical circuit, using one or two bifurcated lead wires (Figure 22-8). The advantage of bifurcation is that more sites can be treated simultaneously. A disadvantage is that, although the same amount of current and charge per phase passes through all the bifurcated leads, the physiologic responses can vary significantly because of the different skin impedances. Physiologic reactions can be very different when subliminal stimulation is perceived under one electrode and the sensory stimulation under the other. Also, significant levels of stimulation may

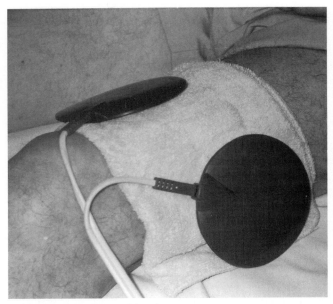

FIGURE 22-8 Bifurcated leads.

affect the healing results of wounds that are distant from each other but on the same body.[20]

Another disadvantage is that, if there is a difference in the total surface area of the electrode(s) connected to one lead compared with the other, the stimulation will be stronger under the electrode with the smaller total surface area because there will be greater current density under that electrode. Often, the wound sites are different sizes. It is important to recognize that the depth and undermining can make the effective electrode size of a small wound significantly larger than the surface area appears. The PT must consider these physical properties of electric current when planning treatment and correct them to provide the "window of charge" (200–600 μC) dose identified by Kloth[24] and the current density recommended by Reich.[20] It may be prudent to use a stimulator with two channels or to have two treatment sessions if there are multiple wounds with a large discrepancy in wound sizes or if there are different phases of healing. In these situations, it would be important to optimize the phase charge and current density.

Dispersive Pad Placement. Attempts have been made to apply scientific findings to electrode placement. Most studies use the active electrode for direct application (Figure 22-9A) to the site,[47, 135,137,9] but some use the bipolar technique (Figure 22-9B) at the wound edges.[8,129,139,140] The dispersive electrode placement has more variation. For example, in two similar studies, the dispersive electrode was placed differently. In one study,[47] it was placed cephalad on the neural axis, whereas in the second study it was placed 30.5 cm from the wound.[4] One study on SCI patients with pressure ulcers in the pelvic region used a protocol in which the dispersive was always placed on the thigh. Another method is to place the dispersive proximal to the

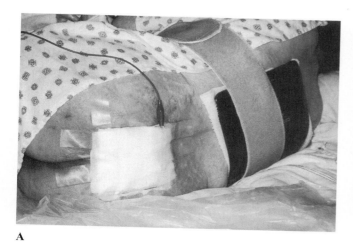

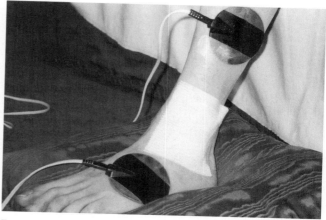

FIGURE 22-9 Dispersive Pad Placement. **A.** Monopolar technique. **B.** Bipolar technique.

wound.[135,137] Current thinking suggests that the dispersive should be moved around the wound to induce the current to enter the wound from different sides. At this time, there is not an established, proven method that has been shown to change the effect of the treatment. All reported treatment methods had statistically significant treatment results. The amount of separation of the poles may have been contributory to these effects.

Monopolar Technique. Monopolar technique is used with monophasic continuous or pulsed waveforms. With the monopolar technique, an electrode is placed to control the polarity at the wound site. Usually, one active electrode is placed on a wet, conductive medium in the wound bed, and the dispersive electrode, in a wet conductive medium at a distance from the wound site, is placed on the intact skin (see Figure 22-9A). Polarity for the two electrodes will be opposite. Current will flow through the intervening tissues between the two electrode poles. The current under the active electrode will reflect the polarity selected on the stimulator provided that there is adequate separation of the poles. There is a uniform electrical potential with strong electrical field at the edges of the electrodes and perpendicular to them. However, the amplitude of the electrical field has been found to decrease as the distance between the electrodes increases. The electrical field has maximum value at the edges of the electrodes where the positive and negative stimulating electrodes face each other.[149] As stated before, the farther apart the two electrode poles are, the deeper the current will flow into the intervening tissues. Current will flow through the tissues by following the path with the lowest resistance, which is usually through the muscles and nerves and deeper tissues. More research needs to be done that examines current amplitude in the tangential fields at different depths. Increasing the distance between the electrodes is a good position choice if wounds are deep and extend into underlying tissues, such as stage III and stage IV pressure ulcers, and/or having tunneling and undermined spaces.

The electrodes can be arranged to target the stimulation to specific tissue sites. Remember to visualize the path of the current flow when placing the dispersive pad. The poles are usually set up in parallel fashion, enabling current to flow between the positive and negative electrodes, no matter how many electrodes are used at either pole. When the surface area of the electrodes is unequal, the current density will not be the same under the two sites. Current density will also vary, according to the impedance of the intervening tissues and the size of the electrodes. Impedance is the opposition to current flow within the circuit. Different body tissues have different impedances to current flow. Skin, bone, and fat have high impedance and are poor electrical conductors. When there is a break in the skin, however, there is a significant lowering of the skin impedance to current. Techniques to reduce skin impedance include abrasion of the skin surface to remove the hard layers of keratin on the surface, tissue warming, and hydration. High-voltage currents of approximately 100 V have the demonstrated ability to cause sudden, spontaneous breakdown in skin impedance.[148] Because of the fluid in muscles and blood vessels, these tissues are good electrical conductors, and it can be expected that current will flow directly through them, with little impedance.

It is important to understand these principles of tissue impedance and current flow and then to apply them correctly to derive the optimal benefits from treatment with ES. For example, if the dispersive electrode is to be placed on the back, place it *below* the scapula to avoid impedance by the bone to current flow. Patients with thick layers of callus on the feet will have high impedance to current. Paring the callus should precede ES treatment, or another placement must be found where the electrode does not lie on callus. The muscular tissue of the thigh is a good placement for the dispersive electrode when treating wounds of the lower leg or foot. One suggestion is to switch the dispersive electrode for each treatment so that the current flows into the wound from each side of the wound through different surrounding tissues and through a different wound edge.[149,151] It is not only the active electrodes that can be bifurcated; the dispersive electrode can also be bifurcated. This allows use of a pair of smaller electrode pads that can be made to conform to smaller body parts, such as an arm or a lower leg (see Figure 21-8).

CLINICAL WISDOM

Enlarging the Dispersive Electrode

If the dispersive electrode area size needs to be increased, this can be accomplished by using a wet washcloth wrapped around a limb or extending a wet washcloth out from the edges of the dispersive electrode to cover a larger skin area. If the wound area size is nearly as large as or larger than the skin area under the dispersive electrode, it will be more comfortable for the patient, but the amplitude of the current or the treatment time may need to be increased to deliver the same total amount of current.

Bipolar Technique. The definition of bipolar technique is the placement of the two leads with their respective electrodes on either side of the target area. This brackets the stimulation to the area associated with the clinical problem.[30] For instance, the two electrodes with opposite polarity may both be placed on the intact skin adjacent to the wound site so that the current passes between the electrodes through the wound tissue. The closer they are together, the more superficial will be the effect; the greater will be the effects of the electric fields of positive and polarity negative at electrode facing edges, and the more the two fields will overlap. This is a reasonable choice for superficial or partial-thickness wound disruptions.

The bipolar technique is used with either monophasic or biphasic waveforms. An application of the bipolar technique is to place the electrodes on either side of the wound or to place the treatment electrode in the wound and use four bifurcated dispersive leads connected to electrodes placed around the wound so that current will flow through the wound from all sides at once. Finally, one active electrode could be placed in the middle of the wound and a dispersive electrode fashioned like a donut, made from aluminum foil, slipped over the treatment electrode with an intervening space between so that stimulation would flow into the wound bed from all sides of the wound edges simultaneously. The foil electrode would connect to the dispersive lead with an alligator clip, just like the active leads (see Figure 22-9B).

CLINICAL WISDOM

Aluminum foil may be used as the dispersive as well as active electrode material. It can be cut to size and conforms easily to all body contours.

Wound Healing Protocol Selection for Electrical Stimulation

Aspects

There are many different ES protocols for wound healing. This section first describes some of the aspects of the protocols described, including electrode polarity, rationale, frequency, and amplitude, as described by the researchers.

Polarity

Polarity must be considered when using galvanic and monophasic pulsed current. Electrode polarity varies, depending on the protocol selected. Most researchers studying ES for wound healing start their protocols with the negative pole as the active electrode, then change the polarity after a period of treatment.[2,62,55,99] Griffin et al,[45] Houghton et al,[9] and Goldman et al[14] maintained negative polarity to the wound site throughout the assessment period of 4 weeks or longer. The other researchers recommend using negative polarity for 3–7 days, then changing polarity. Another recommendation is to use negative polarity until the wound is cleansed of necrotic tissue and drainage is serosanguineous, and then to continue with the negative polarity for three additional days or change to the positive pole.[135,137,10, 11] If the wound is not infected, positive polarity can be used to start the treatment.[47] Some researchers suggest that the polarity should be changed back to negative for 3 days when the wound plateaus. Another method is to change the polarity every 3 days until the wound is healed to a partial-thickness depth. Once that outcome is achieved, change the polarity by alternating daily until the wound is closed. Several animal studies demonstrate better healing when polarity is initiated at the negative pole, then switched to positive.[55,56,152] See earlier sections on theory and science for additional rationale for selecting polarity.

Rationale

Usually, the negative electrode is used as the active electrode when infection is suspected. The polarity is often switched back and forth during the course of healing. Electrode polarity switching accommodates the variability in the skin battery potentials that occurs during the course of healing. Thus, electrode polarity may need to be alternated during treatment to achieve an optimal rate of healing. Additional research is needed to ascertain whether wound healing with ES is dependent on matching treatment electrode polarity with fluctuations in wound injury potential polarity.[47] So far, studies have not reported on this important issue. Still, the idea of polarity switching has some demonstrated merit.

Biphasic Protocols

Protocols demonstrating significant benefit for wound healing with biphasic current are now appearing regularly in the literature.[8,48,129,130,134,139,140] The eight studies reported in this chapter have similar protocols, except that the two studies by the Baker et al[8,140] research group found that the best outcome was achieved when the biphasic waveform was asymmetric and biased toward the negative pole. Sumano and Mateos[51] used filiform needles to conduct the current and not carbon electrodes. Biphasic treatment protocols and the results are shown in Table 22-8.

Frequency Pulse Rate

Frequency, or pulse rate, is another variable that varies from study to study without much explanation. Several studies used a pulse rate of 100–128 pps for treatment with HVPC.[45, 47] One investigator starts treatment at 50 pps.[135,137] The author uses 30 pps based on the effect of lower frequency on blood flow. In several ES research studies, lower-frequency pulse rates produced higher mean blood flow velocity than did higher pulse rates and had a longer mean recovery time following cessation of ES, compared with control levels.[69] Frequency rate switching during the healing process is also not well understood but becomes more relevant as more information about pulse charge is discovered. For example, in one study, the rationale given for reducing the pulse rate for the final phase of healing from 128 to 64 pps was "because we believed the higher pulse frequency might be harmful to the newly healed tissue."[46] This concern is probably due to the higher pulse charge delivered to the tissue at the higher pulse rate.

Amplitude

Wound healing protocols for amplitude are usually constant, repeated in either milliamperes or voltage. The HVPC protocols all report amplitudes of 100–200 V, the low-voltage DC protocols call for a 35-mA amplitude, and the low-voltage microamperage stimulation units have an amplitude less than 1 mA. The ability of the patient to tolerate high-intensity current will depend on the sensory perception of the individual. For example, in superficial or partial-thickness tissue disruption, if there is intact sensation, an amplitude above 100 V may be very uncomfortable. In deeper wounds or in cases of impaired sensation, these higher amplitudes are well tolerated. Adjust the amplitude to patient comfort. It has been suggested to test the amplitude by stimulating until there is a visible muscle contraction under the electrode. This is not practical if the active electrode is located in a wound within a muscle because the sensory nerves will not be stimulated. If the dispersive electrode is secure over a large body area, the intensity of the stimulation required to cause a muscle contraction will be very high and probably uncomfortable, and may not be visible to the PT.

Conclusion

Clearly, more investigation is needed to achieve an optimal treatment protocol with ES. In the meantime, the protocols and dosage presented in this chapter are for use with low- and high-voltage monophasic and biphasic waveforms, which represent these authors' interpretation of the literature and the application to clinical treatment. The author has used these protocols for several years, with good clinical re-

sults. Protocols are listed for wound healing for the three phases of repair and for the treatment of an edematous limb in which the edema extends beyond the wound area. Protocols change for each phase of repair and have expected outcomes for each. Expected outcomes are based on the literature and clinical experience.

Selecting the Device and Treatment Protocol

In today's health-care system and use of interdisciplinary wound teams, different clinicians from different disciplines are using ES for wound treatment. Yet it is the physical therapist who is the best-educated and trained practitioner in the physical properties of different ES devices, the bioelectric and physiologic effect of each, and the best able to understand and interpret the research and clinical application pertaining to electrotherapeutic modalities. As such, the PT has the unique qualifications to select equipment and protocols, to be responsible for accurately predicting outcomes and instructing others in the proper use of the ES equipment.

Depending on the stimulator selected, the protocol for treatment will vary. In some cases, the characteristics of ES for different current type may not always be based on the wound healing phases. For example, asymmetric biphasic stimulation parameters are not varied during the progression through the phases of healing.[8, 140]

The most common stimulator used for wound healing today is probably the HVPC neuromuscular stimulator. However, now there are more RCTs and CCTs showing efficacy using biphasic and LVPC (TENS) than using HVPC. Protocols and results for using biphasic (TENS) are found in Table 22-8. Depending on the wound status (full versus partial thickness), different stimulator current effects should be considered. The protocols presented below are based on use of the HVPC stimulator. Because the protocol and dosage are similar to the studies reported with low-voltage pulsed electrical current,[3, 46] the protocol would also be appropriate to use with those stimulators. The protocols are based initially on the wound healing phase diagnosis, and there are changes in polarity and pulse rate as the wounds progress through the phases of healing.

Sussman Wound Healing Protocol

Sussman uses a wound healing protocol for HVPC, based on the completed diagnostic process (see Chapter 1). Table 22-10 lists the Sussman Wound Healing Protocols for HVPC for all four phases of wound healing and edema control. In using this method, the clinician initiates an HVPC treatment protocol based on the assessed wound healing phase diagnosis and predicts an expected outcome for that protocol. Because the polarity of the healing wound changes during the phases of healing, different treatment characteristics are used as wound healing progresses. In the protocol given below, the stimulation selected for treatment is a monophasic current and monopolar technique used with HVPC. For wounds in the acute inflammatory phase, with an absence of inflammation phase, or in a chronic inflammatory phase,

TABLE 22-10 Protocols for HVPC Treatment

Parameters	Edema	Inflammation	Proliferation	Epithelialization	Remodeling	Venous Return[46]
Polarity	Negative	Negative	Alternate negative/ positive every 3 days	Alternate daily	Alternate daily	Not critical; adjust for patient comfort
Pulse rate (frequency)	30–50 pps	30 pps	100–128 pps	60–64 pps	60–64 pps	40–60 pps
Intensity	150 V or less depending on patient tolerance	100–150 V	100–150 V	100–150 V	100–150 V	Surge mode, on time, 3–15 sec; off time, 9–40 sec (1:3 on/off ratio) to motor excitation
Duration	60 min	60 min	60 min	60 min	60 min	5–10 min, progress to 20–30 min
Treatment frequency	5–7 times/week for first week, then 3 times/ week for 1 week	5–7 times/week, once daily	5–7 times/week, once daily	3–5 times/week, once daily	3 times/week, once daily	Daily; modify to biweekly

the PT would start treatment with parameters to stimulate circulation and cellular responses for healing that induce an inflammatory phase. The protocol calls for a change of parameters as the wound healing phases progress. Likewise, for a wound healing phase, diagnosis of the repair (proliferative) phase, and a wound in the remodeling phase, the PT would start treatment using a different set of parameters, as outlined.

Predictable Outcomes with Sussman Wound Healing Protocol

Predictable outcomes are expected for each protocol, which are equivalent to a change in the wound phase characteristics. For example, if the wound healing phase diagnosis is *acute inflammatory phase*, the *expected outcomes* are hemorrhage free, necrosis free, erythema free, edema free, exudate free, red granulation, and progression to the next phase—the proliferative phase. If there is absence of inflammation or chronic inflammation, an acute inflammatory phase needs to be initiated, to restart the healing process. Expected outcomes would indicate change to an acute inflammatory phase, described as increased erythema (change in skin color), edema, and warmth. The phase change outcome predicted is *initiation of acute inflammatory phase*. Each wound healing phase has its own diagnosis and expected outcomes that are independent of wound etiology.

When the wound healing phase diagnosis is *acute proliferative phase*, the *expected outcomes* are reduction in size (e.g., open area, depth, undermining/tunneling), red granu-

lation tissue-filled wound bed, minimal serous or serosanguineous wound exudate, odor free, adherence of wound edges, and, at the end of the phase, a change in wound healing phase to the epithelialization phase. When the wound healing phase diagnosis is absence of or chronic proliferative phase, the predicted outcome must be acute proliferative phase: reduction in depth, reduction in open area size, and closing of tunnels or undermining. Chronic proliferation may be due to infection of the granulation tissue. There would be clinical signs of infection, including purulent exudate, malodor, and change in appearance of the granulation tissue from beefy red to dull pink. The additional expected outcome for a chronic proliferative phase would then enable the wound to become infection-free and to restart the proliferative phase.

A wound healing phase diagnosis of *acute epithelialization phase* has the *expected outcome* of resurfacing and a change in wound healing phase to *remodeling*. A wound in the remodeling phase has an immature scar formation that lacks optimal healing and could benefit from continued stimulation with ES to enhance the migration of the epidermal cells and the maturation of the vascular system of the scar tissue. Absence of an epithelialization phase may result from a drying out of the wound tissues, due to either a poor dressing choice or an absence of dressing. Epidermal cells require a moist environment to migrate across the wound surface. Correction of the inadequate wound treatment would be a necessary part of the plan of care. Chronic epithelialization is associated with rolled wound edges that have become fibrotic and stuck without resurfacing the wound. Other adjunctive measures may be required to reinitiate an inflammatory response in the wound edges that, in turn, will reinitiate the epithelialization process.

Once closure is achieved, the patient is usually discharged from a treatment protocol, including ES. However, the remodeling phase is often overlooked as a point at which treatment with ES can be beneficial in reducing the risk of immature scar breakdown. The remodeling phase is the longest of all the phases of healing, lasting from 6 months to 2 years. A scar that is thicker, better vascularized, softer, and flatter is more resistant to stress from shearing, friction, and pressure, all of which account for a high incidence of recurrence of ulceration on the seating surface or plantar surface of the foot. Electrical stimulation enhances the remodeling of the scar.[63] Of course, other methods also need to be considered to protect the new scar tissue, including pressure-relief devices and dressings. The PT also would include a program of stretching, exercise, and soft tissue mobilization techniques to enhance the elasticity of the mature scar. *Color Plates 1–6* illustrate a case taken through the four phases of healing with ES.

Procedures for High-Voltage Pulsed Current

The procedure section of this chapter is outlined in a stepwise fashion to help the PT and PTA deliver the treatment intervention with ES in a systematic and time-efficient way for both the patient and the clinician. Unfortunately, treatment with ES requires a number of supply items and steps. First of all, consider having a PTA set up the treatment station where the equipment and supplies are available (see list of equipment and supplies needed). The same set of instructions would be useful to give to a patient or caregiver for home treatment. The PTA can also be responsible to see that the supplies are ordered and available in the department. Always have enough supplies on hand so that treatment is not delayed while someone is running around chasing down the needed equipment.

CLINICAL WISDOM

Ultraviolet Light Stimulation to Restart the Epithelialization Phase

One method suggested to restart the epithelialization phase is to use ultraviolet C light stimulation to create an erythema of the wound edges.[153] By using a dosage that produces a second-degree burn, there is a burning back of the leading edge of the cells that have stopped migration. The erythema response to ultraviolet light may lead to shedding of the outer layer of the skin, followed by a mild inflammatory response that includes vasodilatation and capillary permeability and reinitiates the epithelialization process. Ultraviolet light also has the benefit of being bactericidal (see Chapter 23). Another approach is use of topical or oral vitamin A to stimulate an erythema in the tissues. Treatment with electrical stimulation should cease if a method to restart the epithelialization process is not also attempted.

Protocol for Wound Healing

Equipment Needed:

- Normal saline (0.9%)
- Clean gloves
- Irrigation syringe, 35 mL with 19-gauge needle or angiocatheter
- Clean gauze pads
- Aluminum foil electrode or carbon electrode
- Alligator clips or electrode lead
- Bandage tape
- Nylon stretch strap
- Wet washcloth
- Dispersive pad
- HVPC machine leads
- Infectious waste bag

Instructions for Patient and Caregiver:

1. Explain the procedure, the reason for treatment, and how long it will last. Explain that a mild tingling will be felt and where it will be felt.
2. Advise the patient not to handle, replace, or remove electrodes during the treatment. Patients who cannot understand these directions or will not cooperate need to be monitored closely.
3. Give patient a call light to use.

Procedure for Setting Up the Patient for HVPC Wound Treatment:

1. Have supplies ready before undressing the wound.
2. Position the patient for ease of access by staff and for the comfort of both.
3. Remove the dressing and place in infectious waste bag (usually a red bag).
4. Cleanse wound thoroughly to remove slough, exudate, and any petrolatum products.
5. Sharply débride necrotic tissue, if required, before HVPC treatment.
6. Open gauze pads and fluff, then soak to moisten in normal saline solution; squeeze out excess liquid before applying.
7. Fill the wound cavity with gauze, including any undermined/tunneled spaces. Gauze pad can be opened to full size, then pulled diagonally to form a thin "spaghetti" strip. Insert into undermined/tunneled spaces like roller gauze. Pack gently.
8. Place electrode over the gauze packing; cover with a dry gauze pad and hold in place with bandage tape.
9. Connect an alligator clip to the foil.
10. Connect to the stimulator lead to output device.
11. Place the dispersive electrode.
    a. The dispersive electrode is usually placed proximal to the wound (see section on electrode placement for alternative locations).
    b. Place over soft tissues; avoid bony prominences.
    c. Place a moist washcloth over the dispersive electrode.
    d. Place a washcloth against the skin and hold it in good contact at all edges with a nylon elasticized strap.

(Covering the wet dispersive setup with a plastic sheet to separate it from the bed and the patient's clothing to keep them dry will be appreciated by the patient and the nursing staff.)

e. If placed on the back, the weight of the body plus the strap can be used to achieve good contact at the edges.

f. Dispersive pad should be larger than the sum of the areas of the active electrodes and wound packing. If the size of a self-adhesive electrode is large enough to disperse the current, it can be used instead of a carbon dispersive pad.

g. The greater the separation between the active and dispersive electrode, the deeper the current path. Use greater separation for deep and undermined wounds.

h. Dispersive and active electrodes should be at least 20–30 cm apart for monopolar effects. Current flow will be more shallow when they are closer together.

Additional Treatment Methods:

• Up to four wounds can be set up with a single-channel stimulator, using double bifurcated leads from the stimulator to the electrodes. However, this will not provide maximum current density at the treatment sites. For a patient with multiple wounds, it is not practical to run several series of treatments. An alternative is to use two HVPC stimulators, if available. Electrode placement will require careful planning so that the current flows through target tissues. For example, if there is a wound on the right hip, coccyx, left foot, and right heel, the dispersive electrode should be placed on either the right or left thigh. The thigh has a good blood supply and good conductivity. This setup will send the current flowing through the deep tissues to the feet, the hip, and the coccyx.

• Alternating placement of the dispersive electrode for each treatment, if possible, to direct current flow to opposite sides of the wound has been suggested.[131] This will be more difficult when wounds are located in the feet.

• If a limb is involved, the circumference may be too small to wrap with the large dispersive electrode and maintain good contact. An alternative is to use bifurcated leads, which are available to use with the dispersive cable for some stimulators, or a self-adhesive pad. When using this setup, attach two round, carbon-impregnated electrodes or a foil electrode to make the surface area of the dispersive electrode larger than the active electrode. Place the electrodes on either side of the limb. It is easier to conform the two pads to a small limb segment than the large rectangular dispersive electrode, standard with most stimulators. Use wet gauze under the electrodes; if a greater conductive surface is required, extend the wet gauze out from the edges of the electrode over the surrounding skin. Hold the dispersive electrode in place with nylon elasticized straps. If the patient complains of excessive tingling under the dispersive setup, check for good contact and see whether the size can be increased further (see Figure 22-8, which shows bifurcated leads spread out on a washcloth for a dispersive electrode).

Alternative Methods of Conducting Current to the Wound.
Alternative methods of conducting current to the wound using dressing products have been of interest for many years. A recent study of conductivity of different wound dressings reported that: (1) transparent films are poor conductors, (2) fully hydrated hydrocolloids and alignates[154] will conduct current very well, (3) hydrogel amorphous gels and sheet forms are good conductors because of their high water content,[155] and (4) silver dressings have demonstrated benefits when used in animal and human studies for bactericidal effects and reduction of edema that has been enhanced with the addition of anodal DC electrical current.[103,104] Silver dressings should be discontinued when infection is controlled; they are not an appropriate dressing choice for wounds with eschar. The eschar must be débrided first (see Chapter 11 for indications and contraindications and evidence about the application of silver dressings). Although silver dressings are in clinical use for wound treatment, use with ES has not been clinically adapted.

There is a definite need to advance this technology for the treatment of infected and edematous wounds. An animal study using pigs with burn wounds demonstrated that use of a hydrogel dressing with PES delivered through the dressing increased the levels of collagenase during the critical period of epithelialization initiation. Collagenase enhancement may be one mechanism by which the ES accelerated the wound healing of these burns.[156] See Chapter 11 and Table 11-1 for a description of amorphous and sheet hydrogel characteristics.

CLINICAL WISDOM

Suggestions for Setup to Maximize Treatment Effectiveness and Efficiency

• Assemble the setup supplies into kits before the start of the treatment day to make the delivery of service more time efficient.

• Pre-cut and shape the aluminum foil electrodes. Size and shape should be close to the size of the wounds. Round is preferable to rectangular.

• To make an electrode, cut a strip of household aluminum foil the width of the electrode. Fold the strip in half and turn in the edges to make a smooth pad.

• To make a packing strip from gauze, open a gauze pad, pull on the bias or diagonal, and twist to make a spaghetti strip or use stretch gauze strips.

• Warm saline or a package of amorphous hydrogel by placing bottle between a folded hot pack before use to avoid chilling the wound tissue and slowing mitotic activity. Check the temperature with a digital thermometer. The temperature should not be greater than 98°F to avoid burns. Myer[157] reported keeping the wound care products, including a 16-oz bottle of saline, warm for 3–4 hours. She observed that warming of the wound care products before electrical stimulation treatment resulted in brighter redness of granulation tissue and contributed to reduction of pain.

Irrigation Devices

Spray bottles and bulb syringes may not deliver enough pressure (2.0 psi or less) to cleanse wounds adequately. The Water Pik at middle to high settings may cause trauma to the wound tissue and drive bacteria into wounds; it is not recommended for cleansing soft tissue wounds. Use a cleanser delivery device such as syringe with a 19-gauge catheter to deliver water at 4–8 psi.[158] Warm the solution before application.

Perform Sharp Debridement before HVPC Treatment

Complete sharp debridement of necrotic tissue before setting up the patient for HVPC treatment so that the wound packing will act as a pressure dressing to control any bleeding and so that the wound environment will not have to be disturbed again after HVPC treatment.

Hydrogels. Use an amorphous hydrogel-impregnated gauze to conduct current. This type of dressing is used for partial-thickness, full-thickness, and subcutaneous lesions extending into deep tissue wounds. Hydrogels can be left in the wound for up to 3 days. This product class can benefit the wound management by:

- Conducting electrical current when covered with an electrode
- Promoting the "sodium current of injury"
- Absorbing light to moderate wound exudate
- Maintaining a moist wound environment
- Gradually absorbing wound moisture (is also a moisture donor to the wound)
- Retaining the cell growth factors in the wound bed
- Reducing trauma and cooling of the wound, through less handling
- Reducing product and labor costs by serving a dual purpose

Hydrogel sheets also have high water content and can also be used to conduct current when placed under the electrode.[155] They have benefits similar to the amorphous hydrogels, except that they should not be left on an infected wound. They are used for lightly exudating wounds and are best used for superficial partial-thickness wounds, such as donor sites after skin grafting.

Amorphous hydrogel-impregnated gauze or a hydrogel sheet can be used as the wet contact coupler under an electrode. Although manufacturers say that all that is required is to clip the alligator clips to the dressing to conduct current, Alon[159] explained that this will focus the current at one small area of the dressing and not disperse it throughout the wound area unless the entire dressing surface is covered with a conductive electrode. Follow the setup steps described above, but substitute the saline-soaked gauze with the amorphous hydrogel-impregnated gauze or hydrogel sheet. Dressings may be left in place for up to 3 days. The

amorphous hydrogel should be warmed before application, but be careful not to overheat the product and cause burns. Check temperature with a digital thermometer. Temperature should not be greater than 97°F. If wound conditions permit, cover with a moisture/vapor-permeable transparent film or another dressing to retain moisture without maceration and to maintain body warmth. For amorphous hydrogel-impregnated gauze, on the second day, lift the secondary dressing and slip an aluminum foil electrode underneath; connect an alligator clip lead to the dressing and the stimulator. Replace secondary dressing. Repeat on the third day. The same approach would apply to the hydrogel sheet.

Remove Petrolatum Before Stimulation

All petrolatum products, including enzymatic debriding agents such as collagenase (Santyl) and Papain urea (Accuzyme), which are petrolatum-based products, must be removed before treatment or current will not be conducted into the wound tissues.

Protocol for Treatment of Edema

Soft tissue trauma and a closed or minimally open wound would benefit from ES to control, eliminate, or reduce edema formation. Edema stimulates pain receptors because of the tension in the tissues, blocks off circulation inflow to the tissues, and impairs mobility. Edema eliminated, controlled, or reduced would be the expected outcome from this intervention. Table 22-10 shows a protocol for treatment for edema reduction using HVPC stimulation. There are limited reports and no clinical trials to support this treatment.[99,100,101,109,110,111]

Procedure for Setting Up the Patient for Treatment of Edema:

1. Use the method for setting up the wound described under the protocol for wound healing.
2. Elevate the limb and support it on a pillow or foam wedge, above the heart if possible.
3. Use three or four electrodes.
4. Place one electrode over the wound and arrange the other electrodes over the vascular areas of the limb.
   a. If the wound is in the lower leg, place the second electrode over the medial aspect of the foot and the third over the popliteal area.
   b. If the edema is in the foot distal to the wound, a "foot sandwich" can be made by surrounding the foot with a foil electrode that wraps around the top and bottom of the foot.

Note: Apply the same clinical reasoning for the upper extremity.

Protocol for Circulatory Stimulation in Spinal Cord Injured Patients

The procedure for sacral and lower extremity circulatory stimulation of spinal nerves in spinal cord injured persons is listed below:

Preliminary testing found that use of HVPC for increasing circulation and oxygenation of tissues of the sacrum may have a preventive effect on pressure ulcer formation in spinal cord injured patients.[82] Motor stimulation of an SCI patient with acrocyanosis (cyanosis of the extremity) also reversed some circulatory problems of the lower extremity.[94] Rationale for this application is that ES restores the sympathetic tone and vascular resistance below the level of SCI. Vasodilator polypeptides have also been identified in the blood following ES.[78,79] The following procedure is based on the Mawson et al[82] methods. Further testing and reporting are recommended.

1. Clean the skin surface where the electrodes will be placed to remove oils and sweat. Alcohol can be used.
2. Use the bipolar technique.
3. Use a sponge or gauze pad moistened with water under the electrodes to conduct the current.
4. Place one electrode or bifurcated electrodes over the pad on the soft tissue adjacent to the T10 spinal level. Bifurcated electrodes could be used on either side of the spinal column.
5. Place the second single or bifurcated electrodes on the soft tissue of the buttocks, adjacent to the sacrum.
6. Frequency: 10 pps
7. Amplitude: 75 V (below muscle contraction)
8. Duration: 30–60 minutes daily or 5 times per week

Protocol for Infection Control and Disinfection

A clean technique is recommended for treatment of chronic wounds. The use of aluminum foil electrodes is a good method of controlling infection and eliminates the need for disinfection of the electrode pads. If carbon electrodes or electrodes with sponges are used over the wound, they need to be disinfected between each use, even if used for a single patient. A cold disinfection solution, such as Cydex+, will disinfect for all organisms within 10 minutes, according to the material data sheet. Cydex+ comes with an activating solution that is added to the main solution when the bottle is opened. The activated solution can be reusable for up to 28 days. The product is available in quart and gallon sizes. Unless large quantities of electrodes are going to be disinfected at one time, the quart solution has been found to be most cost effective.[160]

Another cold disinfectant, Milkro-Quat, at a dilution of 18.6 g (2/3 oz) in 3.8 L (1 gal) of water, has been tested for disinfection of electrodes and electrode sponges after treatment of colonized wounds. The electrodes and sponges were soaked in the disinfecting solution for 20 minutes and then tested for bacterial counts. Both the efficacy of the disinfectant and the protocol for disinfection were evaluated. Samples taken from 92% of the posttreatment electrode sponges after they were disinfected contained no bacterial growth. The remaining 8% contained two or fewer colonies. The results were the same for samples cultured anaerobically.[160] The dispersive pad, which is placed on intact skin, should be cleaned between uses with soap and water or wiped with an alcohol-soaked pad. Alligator clips that come in contact with wound contaminants should be disinfected between uses. One company furnishes alligator clips with packs of hydrogel-impregnated gauze that can be kept for single patient use. Over time, the carbon electrodes will absorb oil and detergent products and will become resistant to current flow. A periodic check (e.g., every 30 days) of the conductivity of the electrodes is highly recommended.

■ CASE STUDY 1

RR, a 50-year-old male, 15 years post-SCI quadriplegic, has had two flap procedures for ischial tuberosity pressure-related ulcers. Wound healed slowly. Cyanosis over the ischial tuberosity occurred when sitting on his pressure relief cushion in his wheelchair for 1 hour and took about 2 hours to resolve. He had been confined to very short trips out of the house to the doctor.

Reason for the referral: (1) concern that he would have a reoccurrence of skin breakdown, and (2) bed-bound status was interfering with his social interaction with family and friends and ability to go out into the community.

A program of preventive ES was initiated to resolve the cyanosis and increase tissue perfusion and oxygen. After 5 days of 60-minute per day ES with HVPC using the procedure described here, up time in his wheelchair increased to 3 hours, and cyanosis was 50–75% less intense and resolved in about 30 minutes. By day 10, he was able to be up in the wheelchair for 6 hours with pressure relief of 5 minutes per hour, and resolution of the cyanosis occurred consistently within 30 minutes. Further testing is indicated to determine efficacy of ES as a preventive procedure for pressure ulcers.

CLINICAL WISDOM

Benefits of Aluminum Foil Electrodes

Aluminum foil electrodes are very cost effective and time efficient for treatment of open wounds. They are easily made, are good conductors, can be molded to fit the body part, can be sized for maximum current density to the wound, and are disposable. Saline-soaked gauze packed in the wound and covered with an electrode is also cost efficient and is particularly good on deep lesions.

Aftercare. After the ES treatment is complete, slip the electrode out from between the wet and dry gauze. The wound can be left undisturbed. If saline-soaked gauze is the conductive medium, it should be changed before it dries or be covered with an occlusive dressing. If additional topical treatments are required, such as enzymatic debriding agents or antibiotics, the packing will need to be removed. Frequent dressing change is being discouraged because it disturbs the wound healing environment by removing important substances in wound exudate and cooling the wound. It takes 3 hours for a chilled wound to rewarm and slows leukocytic and mitotic activity.[161,162,163]

Protocol for Treatment of Chronic Venous Insufficiency or Chronic Deep Vein Thrombosis

This protocol from Alon and De Domenico[23] is based on using HVPC to elicit the pumping action of skeletal muscles (see Table 22-10, showing HVPC protocols). The best muscle-pumping action is achieved from active exercise, but for some patients, this is not an option or is inadequate to facilitate the venous pump mechanisms. Therefore, ES can be used as an intermittent method for stimulation of muscle pump action. Patients with chronic lymphedema may also benefit.

Setting Up the Patient:

1. A bipolar technique is usually used.
2. Place both electrodes over the plantar flexors, one proximal and one over the muscle bellies.
3. Use a surge or interrupted mode, with an on time of 3–15 seconds and an off time of 9–40 seconds. This 1:3 on/off ratio is essential to avoid muscle fatigue.
4. Begin with shorter on/off time, then increase the stimulation time as patient accommodates.
5. Polarity is not critical and can be adjusted for patient comfort.
6. Pulse rate is between 40 and 60 pps and can be adjusted for patient comfort.
7. Intensity that will produce intermittent, moderate *tetanic* muscle contraction is required. Increase intensity gradually for patient comfort and compliance.
8. Expect that a few treatment sessions will be required to reach the desired level of muscle contraction.
9. Treatment time is pathology dependent.
   a. Chronic thrombophlebitis: 30–60 minutes biweekly
   b. Venous stasis: commence 5–10 minutes daily; progress to 20–30 minutes biweekly
10. Precaution: Plantar flexors have a tendency to cramp; proceed slowly to avoid cramping. Such cramping must be avoided. To avoid cramping, place the feet against a footboard that limits full range of plantar flexion.
11. Expected outcome: enhanced venous return, measured by reduced edema. May facilitate healing of venous ulceration.

Self-Care Teaching Guidelines

Selecting the Candidate for Self Care

HVPC stimulation and TENS are very safe and easy-to-apply treatments that a patient or caregiver can be taught for self treatment at home. Several investigators used a home treatment protocol for their studies, as reported above. HVPC stimulators, as described, are available as portable, battery pack units. Some units come with compliance meters. TENS are also portable. This is a simple treatment, but it requires several steps and clear instructions. Review the procedures with the person who will deliver the care to ensure that adequate care will be given to achieve the predicted outcomes. If the PT does not believe that the person

is able to be taught safe, appropriate procedures, this should be documented and might be a rationale for skilled services or another intervention.

To achieve success in a self-care program, psychosocial concerns need to be addressed before establishing the program. Select the patient and/or caregiver who is alert, motivated, and able to learn the directions for application. It will require clinician support and encouragement to convince the patient/caregiver to accept the responsibility for self-care. Patients and caregivers are accustomed to receiving medical care at the clinic or by a home care practitioner, rather than doing self-care. The concept of sharing the problem between patient and clinician is new to many people. It takes a step-by-step process to gain patient cooperation.

Begin in the clinic or at the home visit by encouraging and teaching the patient and/or the caregiver to participate in the setup process. Many people are repulsed by the sight of a dirty, smelly, ugly wound. That is often the first hurdle. Take it slowly, with patience and understanding of these feelings. Explain in simple language why the wound is dirty, smelly, and ugly, and how the treatment will improve the problem. Wound measurements and photographs can be used as motivation to encourage continued participation. "Before and after" photographs of other clients treated in this way are particularly effective ways of showing the patient/caregiver how other wounds improved. Move the patient or caregiver increasingly into the role of treatment provider as soon as possible. Observe, instruct, and offer words of support and praise.

Instructions

Independence in the treatment routine must be established before dispensing electrical stimulator for self-care at home. Although it may seem overwhelming to give five steps of instructions for a single treatment protocol, understanding the five steps of instructions listed here will ensure that the patient or caregiver is able to achieve the goal of independence in the treatment routine. Keep instructions as simple as possible so that the responsible party will not be overwhelmed. Because of the number of steps required, prepared instruction sheets listing the five steps would be helpful. Simple drawings can be helpful in teaching the proper placement of the electrodes. Don't assume that the patient will know where to place the electrodes or how to put on the dressing when he or she arrives home. Two or three visits with the PT may be necessary to complete the instruction. Schedule regular follow-up assessments, usually weekly, to evaluate outcomes and change protocols.

Five Steps of Instruction:

1. The list of needed supplies: Make sure that the patient can acquire all the necessary items or help make arrangements to acquire those that are needed (e.g., a portable HVPC stimulator and electrodes).
2. Setup of the patient and the wound for treatment, including all the steps listed: Review what is on paper, then

do a demonstration and return demonstration to confirm understanding.

3. The treatment protocol: Review the treatment protocol by dialing in the characteristics for the selected protocols on the stimulator to be used. The dials can be left at the correct setting to help the patient, but they may be moved and should be rechecked at each treatment session. Give *only* the treatment protocol for the current wound healing phase. Tell the patient or caregiver what outcomes to expect and what findings should be reported promptly. Change instructions as the wound heals.

4. The aftercare procedures: Aftercare procedure instructions should include how to apply the prescribed dressing product and disposal of the disposable waste products from the treatment in the home setting (see Chapter 11). It is important to make sure that the patient or caregiver understands the proper use of the prescribed aftercare dressing products. Damage to the wound and failure to achieve predicted outcomes can be avoided by instruction in use of products. Again, practice and a return demonstration are proven methods of teaching new techniques.

5. A list of expected signs and symptoms: The patient and the caregiver need to be aware of the importance of any expected changes in signs and symptoms related to the treatment and must know when to report any undesirable results.

CASE STUDY 2

Pressure Ulcer Treated with ES

Patient ID: S.A. Age: 85 Onset: December (color photo 32)

INITIAL ASSESSMENT: BRIEF MEDICAL HISTORY AND SYSTEMS REVIEW

Reason for Referral

The patient has developed pressure ulceration along the lateral border of her left foot. She is not a candidate for surgical intervention because of multiple comorbidities.

Medical History

The patient is an 85-year-old woman who is unresponsive, with fetal posture and fixed contractures of all four extremities. She has a history of multiple cerebrovascular accidents. She does not reposition herself in bed and cannot sit up in a wheelchair. She is on nasogastric tube feeding for nutrition; a Foley catheter is in place to control incontinence of urine. The wound onset was 2 weeks prior to referral to physical therapy. The wound has deteriorated and become necrotized. The nursing staff has been using enzymatic and autolytic debridement methods.

Systems Review

Circulatory System. The patient has systemically impaired circulation due to arteriosclerotic vascular disease. The circulation to the lower extremity is further impaired as a result of contractures of the hips and knees.

Respiratory System. The patient has shallow, impaired respiration due to inactivity and her bed-bound status.

Musculoskeletal System. The patient has impaired joint mobility due to contractures, resulting in severe disability of the musculoskeletal system.

Neuromuscular System. The patient lacks the ability to respond to the need for self-repositioning and is cognitively unaware.

EXAMINATIONS INDICATED AND DERIVED DATA

Vascular Examination

Palpation of pulses indicates a weak dorsal pedal pulse. Determination of the ankle-brachial index is not possible due to contractures at the elbow. Pulse oximetry of the great toe shows an oxygen saturation of 96%.

Musculoskeletal Examination

There is limited passive range of motion (less than 90° at either the hips, knees, or elbows). There is no active motor movement.

Integumentary Examination

The surrounding skin is erythematous, seen as a red glow under darkly pigmented skin. The tissue is edematous. The temperature of the wound is elevated compared with surrounding tissues. There are hemorrhagic areas along the wound margin indicating deep tissue injury, and necrotic tissue covers the wound surface.

Evaluation of the Examination Findings and Relationship to Function

The specific dysfunction that generated a referral for the services of a PT is loss of wound healing capacity. The patient's loss of function is due to generalized impairments (circulatory, cardiopulmonary, musculoskeletal, and neuromuscular). Limited bed mobility and limited cognitive ability further complicate the ability to heal without physical therapy intervention for integumentary management.

DIAGNOSIS

Musculoskeletal Disability

Impaired flexibility and strength lead to increased susceptibility to pressure ulceration of the feet.

Neuromuscular Disability

The patient has neuromuscular disability associated with insensitivity and inability to reposition and make needs known.

Wound Healing Impairment

The signs and symptoms identified by the wound assessment, including edema, erythema, heat, and the presence of necrotic tissue, indicate that the wound healing phase diagnosis is a chronic inflammatory phase of healing and impaired wound healing associated with a chronically inflamed wound.

Functional Diagnosis

- Undue susceptibility to pressure ulceration on the feet
- Impaired wound healing
- Chronic inflammatory phase
- Insensitivity to need for position change

Need for Skilled Services: The Therapy Problem

The patient has failed to respond to interventions with dressing changes for the last 2 weeks. She now requires the following four interventions:

1. Debridement of the necrotic tissue from the wound bed to determine level of tissue impairment and to initiate the healing process
2. HVPC to enhance circulation to the foot, facilitate debridement, and restart the process of repair
3. Therapeutic positioning to remove pressure trauma on the foot
4. Range-of-motion exercises to all four extremities to maintain tissue extensibility and increase circulation

PROGNOSIS

Healing is not expected without intervention; however, the prognosis is good for a clean, stable wound. Initiation of the acute inflammatory phase with electrical stimulation is expected in 2 weeks with progression to a proliferative phase in 4 weeks, and a clean, stable wound in 6 weeks.

(Continued)

■ **CASE STUDY 2** *(Continued)*

TREATMENT PLAN

- Instruction will be given to nurses' aides in range-of-motion needs of the patient; it will include initial instruction and follow-up for two different shifts (four visits).
- Instruction will be given to the nursing staff in therapeutic positioning; it will include initial instruction and follow-up for two different shifts (three visits).
- HVPC parameters:
  1. The active electrode will be placed on the wound site.
  2. The dispersive electrode will be placed on the thigh.
  3. Polarity initially will be negative, then alternated between positive and negative, as described under the Sussman Wound Healing Protocol, as the wound changes phases.
  4. The pulse rate will be changed from 30 pps to 120 pps to 64 pps as phases change.
  5. The current intensity will be set at 150 V throughout.
  6. HVPC will be of a 60-minute duration, seven times a week.

Debridement will be achieved by HVPC, enzymes, and sharp instruments daily as needed to remove necrotic tissue.

INTERVENTIONS

Passive Range-of-Motion Exercises

Passive range-of-motion exercises will be performed to all four extremities, ranged twice daily by the restorative nurse's aide as instructed by the PT.

Targeted Outcome. The nurse's aide will be able to provide the optimal amount of range of motion for all four extremities; increase tissue extensibility at elbows, hips, and knees; and increase perfusion to the lower extremities; due date: 2 weeks.

Healing Pressure Relief

Therapeutic positioning with adaptive equipment will be used to keep feet off the bed, and a pressure-relief mattress replacement will be provided.

Targeted Outcome. The nursing staff will be able to use therapeutic positions to reduce the risk of pressure ulcer formation on the feet, including elimination of pressure on the lateral border of the foot with pressure ulcer; due date: 1 week.

Electrical Stimulation with HVPC 7 Days per Week

Targeted Outcome. The intervention will stimulate perfusion and cellular responses of the inflammatory phase, and wound debridement will progress to the acute inflammatory phase followed by progression to the proliferative phase; due date: 6 weeks.

Debridement

Sharp debridement will be used for nonviable tissue; enzymatic debridement will be used to solubilize the necrotic tissue between sharp debridement sessions.

Targeted Outcome.
The wound will be necrosis free; due date: 4 weeks.

DISCHARGE OUTCOME

Within 4 weeks the wound was clean, granulating wound edges were contracting, and epithelialization was starting. Because it was now evident that there was potential for wound closure, the prognosis was changed to healed wound from clean and stable; HVPC treatment was continued, and at 12 weeks the wound was fully epithelialized and closed.

CASE STUDY 3

Vascular Ulcer Treated with ES

Patient: C.Z. Age: 80
(Color photos of the case are *Color Plates 55* and *56*.)

INITIAL ASSESSMENT

Reason for Referral

The patient came to the PT because a vascular ulcer on the posterior right calf would not heal. The patient and his wife reported that they had been caring for the ulcer for more than 6 months, and they wanted it to heal so they could resume their usual activities in the community.

Medical History

The patient has a history of severe arterial vascular occlusive disease of the lower extremities. Old World War II burn scarring covered the surrounding area of the calf, with hyperkeratotic scarring that kept breaking down. The recurrent skin breakdown on his leg resulted in protracted periods of healing (e.g., more than 1 year). One ulcer had healed in 6 months after a course of care using electrical stimulation (HVPC). The previous ulcer took more than a year and did not heal. The patient was ambulatory and alert, with mild confusion. His wife reported that any moisture left on the surrounding skin caused maceration and skin breakdown. A femoral angioplasty had been done the week before the patient was seen in the outpatient clinic.

FUNCTIONAL DIAGNOSIS AND TARGETED OUTCOMES

Integumentary Examination

Adjacent Skin.
Hyperketosis; scar tissue; flaky, friable, dry skin; and pallor are present.

Functional Diagnosis. The patient has loss of functional mobility due to integumentary impairment.

Targeted Outcome. The patient will have improved skin texture and integrity; due date: 6 weeks.

Wound Tissue Examination

The wound edges are poorly defined. There is necrotic tissue along the margins. There is a small island of skin in the middle of the wound bed. The wound has partial-thickness skin loss with moderate exudate. The wound is about 200 cm^2.

Functional Diagnosis. There is absence of an inflammatory phase.

Targeted Outcome: Acute inflammation will be achieved; due date: 2 weeks.

Associated Impairment. Necrotic tissue is present.

Targeted Outcome: A clean wound bed will be achieved; due date: 4 weeks.

Functional Diagnosis. There is absence of a proliferative phase.

Targeted Outcome: The wound will exhibit granulation tissue and be ready for grafting; due date: 6 weeks.

Vascular Examination

Medical Diagnosis. The patient has severe arterial vascular occlusive disease, status postangioplasty.

Functional Diagnosis. The patient has vascular impairment contributing to impaired healing.

Targeted Outcome: Perfusion will be enhanced; due date: 2 weeks.

The patient's loss of function in these systems is responsible for the undue susceptibility to skin breakdown on the legs and inability to heal without integumentary intervention. The patient has improvement potential. The wound will heal partially, and the wound bed will be prepared for grafting following intervention.

NEED FOR SKILLED SERVICES

The patient has failed to respond to treatment with wound dressings and conservative management of the leg ulcer. It requires debridement of necrotic tissue to initiate the healing process and HVPC to initiate the healing phases and to enhance perfusion so that the wound bed is prepared for grafting.

TREATMENT PLAN

- The patient and wife will be instructed to perform HVPC as a daily home treatment program with a portable HVPC rental unit.
- Wound debridement will be performed to remove necrotic tissues; methods will include autolysis, sharp debridement, and enhanced perfusion with the use of HVPC.
- The wife will be instructed in wound dressing changes with alginate to absorb moderate exudate, including how to cut the dressing to fit the wound to avoid maceration.

DISCHARGE OUTCOMES

- The patient started care in mid-December.
- The wound was necrosis-free.
- The wound phase changed to both proliferative and epithelialization. The wound size was reduced to less than half the original area.
- The wound was grafted at the end of February.
- The wound graft was successful. A smaller graft was needed than originally expected because of the epithelialization. Surrounding integumentary integrity was improved: the skin was softer and smoother, and no new hyperkeratosis developed in the scar tissue area.

GENERAL COMMENTS

The patient and his wife were compliant with the home treatment regimen. The femoral angioplasty apparently opened the vessels enough to permit the enhanced perfusion from the HVPC to reach the tissues or possibly the two months of regular HVPC treatment effected the microcirculation as described in the clinical studies by Goldman et al.[14,93,92] Grafting was the best option for this couple because it provided faster closure and allowed them to live more functional lives without having wound care duties. It also provided a better covering with healthier skin from the opposite thigh to cover the open area. New scar tissue was better-quality tissue than that surrounding older scars, possibly due to the improved collagen organization and vascularization associated with the HVPC.

REVIEW QUESTIONS

1. What are three ways that ES can aid wound healing?
2. What is the most frequently used type of electrical current for wound healing studies?
3. Based on the evidence presented, what different effects are attributed to biphasic and monophasic currents?
4. Name three contraindications or precautions that apply to ES.

REFERENCES

1. Bergstrom N, Allman RM, Alvarez OM, Bennet MA, Carlson CE, Frantz R. *Clinical Practice Guideline: Treatment of Pressure Ulcers (AHRQ Publication No. 95-06-0652*. Rockville MD: US Department of Health and Human Services Public Health Service Agency for Health Care Policy and Research (AHCPR) now Agency for Health Care Research and Quality (AHRQ); 1994. 15.
2. Carley PJ, Wainapel SF, . Electrotherapy for acceleration of wound healing: low intensity direct current. *Arch Phys Med Rehabil.* 1995;66(7):443-446.
3. Gentzkow G, Pollack S, Kloth L, Stubbs H. Improved healing of pressure ulcers using dermapulse, a new electrical stimulation device. *Wounds.* 1991;3(5):158-170.
4. Taler G, Bauman T, Breeding C, Cali TJ, al e. *Pressure ulcers: clinical practice guideline.* Columbia, MD: American Medical Directors Association; 1996.
5. Ovington LG. Dressings and Ajunctive Therapies: AHCPR Guidelines Revisited. *Ostomy wound Management.* January 1999;45(Suppl 1A):94s-106s.
6. Wood JM, Evans PE 3d, Schallreuter KU, et al. A multicenter study on the use of pulsed low intensity direct current for healing chronic Stage II and Stage III ulcers. *Arch Dermatol.* Aug 1993;130(5):660-661.
7. Garber SL, Biddle AK, Click CN, et al. *Pressure ulcer prevention and treatment following spinal cord injury: A clinical practice guideline for health-care professionals.* Jackson Heights, NY: Paralyzed Veterans of America; August 2000.
8. Baker LL, Rubayi S, Villar F, Demuth SR. Effect of electrical stimulation waveform on healing of ulcers in human beings with spinal cord injury. *Wound Rep Reg.* 1996;4:21-28.
9. Houghton PE, Kincaid CB, Lovell M, et al. Effect of Electrical Stimulation on Chronic Leg Ulcer Size and Appearance. *Physical Therapy.* January 2003;83(1):17-28.
10. Franek Andrzej, Polak Anna, Kucharzewski Marek. Modern application of high voltage stimulation for enhanced healing of venous crural ulceratio. *Medical Engineering and Physics.* 2000;22:647-655.
11. Polak Anna, Franek Andrzej, Hunika-Zurawinska Wieslawa, Bendkowski Witold, Kucharzewski Marek, Swist Daria. High Voltage Electrostimulation in Treatment of Venous Crural Ulceration. *Wiadomosci Lekarskie.* 2000;LIII:7-8.
12. Bassett CAL, Pawluk RJ, Becker RO. Effects of electric currents on bone in vivo. *Nature.* 1964;204:652-654.
13. Peters EJ, Lavery LA, Armstrong DG, Fleischli JG. Electric Stimulation as an adjunct to Heal Diabetic Foot Ulcers: A randomized Clinical Trial. *Arch Phys Med Rehabil.* June 2001;82(June):721-725.
14. Goldman Robert, Rosen Mark, Brewley Barbara, Golden Michael. Electrotherapy Promotes Healing and Microcirculation of Infrapopliteal Ischemic Wounds: aprospective pilot study. *Adv in Skin and Wound Care.* 2004;17:284-290.
15. Frantz RA. Nursing intervention: healing pressure ulcers with TENS, submitted.
16. Gardner SE, Frantz RA, Schmidt FL. Effect of electrical stimulation on chronic wound healing: a meta-analysis. *Wound Repair and Regeneration.* 1999;7(6):495-503.
17. Anonymous. Aitkin, Noecker, Heyen, Langill, Sharp, Turner and American Physical Therapy Association vs Shalala. United States District Court, District of Massachusetts, Civil Action No. 97-11726-GAO, November 18, 1997.
18. Administration HCF. *Suspension of national coverage policy on electrostimulation for wound healing.* Baltimore, MD: Dept of Health and Human Services; July 1999. Transmittal No. AB-99-52.
19. Swanson G. Functional outcomes report: the next generation in physical therapy reporting. In:. Stewart DL, Abeln SH, eds. *Documenting Functional Outcomes in Physical Therapy.* St Louis, MO: Mosby-Year Book. 1993:101-134.
20. Reich J, Cazzaniga A, Tarjan P, Mertz P. The reporting and characterization of exogenous electric fields. In: Brighton C, Pollack SR, eds. *Electromagnetics in Biology and Medicine.* San Francisco, CA: San Francisco Press, Inc.; 1991:355-360.
21. Alon G, Robinson AJ, Spielholz N, et al. *Electrotherapeutic Terminology in Physical Therapy.* 2 ed. Alexandria, VA: American Physical Therapy Association; 2000.
22. Medical and Surgical Procedures Panel. *Medicare Coverage Policy-MCAC: Electrical Stimulation for the Treatment of Wounds.* Baltimore, MD: Health Care Financing Administration. 2000:1-73.
23. Alon G, De Domenico G. High Voltage Stimulation: An Integrated Approach to Clinical Electrotherapy. *Hixton,* TN: The Chattanooga Group. 1987.
24. Kloth L, Alon G, Baker L, et al. Electrotherapeutic Terminology in. *Physical Therapy.* Alexandria, VA: Section on Clinical Electrophysiology, American Physical Therapy Association;. 1990.
25. Reich J, Tarjan P. Electrical Stimulation of Skin. *International Journal of Dermatology.* July/August 1990;29(6):395-400.
26. Mertz PM. Electrical Stimulation and Wound Healing: Commentary. *Wounds: a compendium of clinical research and practice.* November/December 2000;12(6):172-173.
27. Newton RA, Karselis TC. Skin pH following high voltage pulsed galvanic stimulation. *Physcial Therapy.* October 1983;63(10):1593-1596.
28. Newton RA. High-voltage pulsed current: theoretical bases and clinical applications. In:. Nelson R, Currier D, eds. *Clinical Electrotherapy.* Norwalk, CT: Appleton & Lange. 1991:201-220.
29. Alon G. Principles of electrical stimulation. In: Nelson R, Hayes KW, Currier DP, eds. *Clinical Electrotherapy.* third ed. Stamford, CT: Appleton & Lange; 1999:55-124.
30. Alon G. Principles of electrical stimulation. In: Nelson R, Currier D, eds. *Clinical Electrotherapy* Norwalk, CT: Appleton & Lange; *1991:35-114.* 1991:35-114.
31. Bourguignon GJ, Jy W, Bourguignon LYW. Electric stimulation of human fibroblasts causes an increase in Ca2+ influx and the exposure of additional insulin receptors. *J Cell Physiol.* 1989;140:379-385.
32. Gersh M. Microcurrent electrical stimulation: putting it in perspective. *Clin Manage.* 1989;9(4):51-54.
33. Friedenberg ZB, Andrews ET, Smolenski BI, et al. Bone reaction to varying amounts of direct current. 1970;131:894-899.
34. Bassett CAL, Becker RO. Generation of electric potentials by bone in response to mechanical stress. *Science.* 1962;137:1063.
35. Friedenberg B, Roberts PG, Didizian NH, Brighton CT. Stimulation of fracture healing by direct current in the rabbit fibula. *J Bone Joint Surg.* 1971;53A:1400-1408.
36. Bassett CAL. Electromechanical factors regulating bone architecture. In: Fleish. R, Backwood HJJ, Owen M, eds. *Third European Symposium on Calcified Tissues.* New York: Berlin, Springer-Verlag; 1966:78.
37. Friedenberg ZB, Kohanim M. The effect of direct current on bone. *Surg Gynecol Obstet.* 1968;127:97-102.
38. Friedenberg ZB, Harlow MC, Brighton CT. Healing of nonunion of the medial malleolus by means of direct current: a case report. 1971;11:883-885.
39. Brighton CT. Current concepts review: the treatment of nonunions with electricity. *J Bone Joint Surg.* 1981;63-A:847-851.
40. Goh JCH, Bose K, Kang YK. Nugroho B. Effects of electrical stimulation on the biomechanical properties of fracture healing in rabbits. *Clin Orthop.* 1998;223:268-273.
41. Jaffe LS, Vanable JW. Electric fields and wound healing. *Clin Dermatol.* 1984;3:34.
42. Kumar D, Alvaro MS, Julka IS, Marshall HJ. Diabetic Peripheral Neuropathy Effectiveness of electrotherapy and amitriptyline for sympotomatic relief. *Diabetes Care.* August 1998;21(8):1322-1325.
43. Julka IS, Alvaro MS, Kumar D. Beneficial effects of electrical stimulation on neuropathic symptoms in diabetes patients. *The Journal of Foot and Ankle Surgery.* May/June 1998;37(3):191-194.

44. Brighton CT, Friedenberg ZB, Black J, Esterhai JL, Mitchell JEI, Montique F. Electrically Induced Osteogenesis: Relationship between Charge, current density and the amount of bone formed. *Clinical Orthopedics and Related Research.* Nov/ Dec 1981;161(Nov/ Dec 1981):122-131.

45. Griffin JW, Tooms RE, Mendius SK, Clifft R, Vander Zwaag R, El-Zeky F. Efficacy of high voltage pulsed current for healing of pressure ulcers in patients with spinal cord injury. *Phys Ther.* 1991;71:433-444.

46. Feedar JA, Kloth LC, Gentzkow GD. Chronic dermal ulcer healing enhanced with monophasic pulsed electrical stimulation. *Phys Ther.* 1991;7(19):639-649.

47. Kloth Luther, Feedar Jeffery. Acceleration of wound healing with high voltage, monophasic, pulsed current. *Phys Ther.* 1988;68:503-508.

48. Cheng K, Mertz PM, Tarjan P. Theoretical study of rectangular pulse electrical stimulation (RPES) on skin cells (in vivo) under conforming electrodes. Paper presented at: Biomedical Sciences Instrumentation; April 2-3, 1993.

49. Gentzkow G, Miller K. Electrical stimulation for dermal wound healing. *Clin Podiatr Med Surg.* 1991;8:827-841.

50. Mertz P, Davis SC, Oliveira-Gandia M, Eaglstein WH. The wound environment: implications from research studies for healing and infection. In:. Krasner D, Kane D, eds. *Chronic Wound Care.* 2nd ed. Wayne, PA: Health Management Publications. 1997;58.

51. Sumano H, Mateos G. The use of acupuncture-like electrical stimulation for wound healing of lesions unresponsive to conventional treatment. *Am J of Acupuncture.* 1999;27(1/2):5:14.

52. Fukishima K SN, Inui H, Miura, H, Tamai Y, Murakami Y. Study of galvanotaxis of leukocytes. *Med J Osaka University.* 1953;4:195-208.

53. Nishimura KY IR, Nuccitelli R. Human Keratinocytes migrate to the negtive pole in direct current electric fields comparable to those measure in mammalian wounds. *Journal of Cell Science.* 1996;109:199-207.

54. Zhao Min, Pu Jin, Forrester John V, McCaig Colin D. Membrane lipids, EGF receptors, and intracellular signals colocalize and are polarized in epithelial cells moving directionally in a physiological electric field. *FASEB J.* June 1, 2002;16(8):857-859.

55. Brown M, McDonnell M, Menton DN. Polarity effects on wound healing using electrical stimulation in rabbits. *Arch Phys Med Rehabil.* 1989;70:624-627.

56. Alvarez O. The healing of superficial skin wounds is stimulated by external electrical current. *J Invest Dermato.* 1983;8(12):144-148.

57. Orinda N FJ. Directional protrusive pseudopodial activity and motility in macrophages induced by extracellular electric fields. *Cell Motil.* 1982;2:243-255.

58. Cho MR, Thatte HS, Lee RC, Golan DE. Integrin-dependent human macrophage migration induced by oscillatory electrical stimulation. *Ann Biomedical Engineering.* March 2000;28(3):234-243.

59. Ferrier J, Ross SM, Kanehisa J, Aubin JE. Osteoclasts and osteoblasts migrate in opposite directions in response to a constant electrical field. *J Cell Physiol.* Dec 1986;129:283-288.

60. Erickson CA, Nuccitelli R. Embryonic fibroblast motility and orientation can be influenced by physiological electrical fields. *J Cell Biol.* 1984;98:296-307.

61. Costerton J William, Ellis B, Lam K, Johnson Frank, Khoury Antoine E. Mechanisms of Electrical Enhancement of Efficacy of Antibiotics in Killing Biofilm Bacteria. *Antimicrobial Agents and chemotherapy.* 1994;38(12):2803-2809.

62. Stromberg BV. Effects of electrical currents on wound contraction. *Ann Plast Surg.* 1988;21(2):121-123.

63. Weiss D, Eaglestein W, Falanga V. Exogenous electric current can reduce the formation of hypertrophic scars. *J Dermatol Surg Oncol.* 1989;15:1272-1275.

64. Alon G, Azaria M, Stein H. Diabetic ulcer healing using high voltage TENS. *Phys Ther.* 1986;66:77. Abstract.

65. Wolf J. Das *Gesetz der Transformatin der Knochen.* Berlin, Germany: Hirschwald; 1897.

66. Forrester JC, et al. Wolf's law in relation to the healing of skin wound. *J Trauma.* 1970;10:770-778.

67. Byl NN, McKenzie A, Wong T, West J, Hunt TK. Incisional wound healing: a controlled study of low- and high-dose ultrasound. *JOSPT.* 1993;18(5):619-627.

68. Byl NN, McKenzie A, West JM, Whitney JD, Hunt TK, Scheuenstuhl HA. Low-dose ultrasound effects on ultrasound healing: a controlled study with Yucatan pigs. *Arch Phys Med Rehabil.* 1992;73:656-664.

69. Mohr T, Akers T, Wessman HC. Effect of high voltage stimulation on blood flow in the rat hind limb. *Phys Ther.* 1987;67:528-533.

70. Mehri M, Helme R, Khalil A. Age related changes in sympathetic modulation of sensory nerve activity in rat skin. *Infamm Res.* 1998;47(6):239-244.

71. Politis MJ, Zankis MF, Miller JE. Enhanced survival of full-thickness skin grafts following the application of DC electrical fields. *Plast Reconstr Surg.* 1989;84(2):67-72.

72. Pollack S. The effects of pulsed electrical stimulation on failing skin flaps in Yorkshire pigs. Paper presented at the Meeting of the Bioelectrical Repair and Growth Society; 1989; Cleveland, OH. 1989.

73. Lundeberg T, Kjartansson J, Samuelsson U. Effect of electrical nerve stimulation on healing of ischemic skin flaps. *Lancet.* 1988;2:712-714.

74. Im MJ, Lee WPA, Hoopes JE. Effect of electrical stimulation on survival of skin flaps in pigs. *Phys Ther.* 1990;70:37-40.

75. Hecker B CH, Schwartz DP. Pulsed Galvanic Stimulation: Effects of Current Frequence and Polarity on Blood Flow in Health Subjects. *Arch Phys Med Rehabil.* June 1985 1985;66:369-371.

76. Cramp A, Gilsensan C, Lowe A, Walsh D. The effect of high and low frequency transcutaneous electrical nerve stimulation upon cutaneous blood flow and skin temperature in healthy subjects. *Clin Physiol.* 2000;20(2):150-157.

77. Wikstrom S, Svedman P, Svensson H, Tanweer H. Effect of transcutaneous nerve stimulation on microcirculation in intact skin and blister wounds in healthy volunteers. *Scand J Plastic Reconstr Surg Hand Surg.* 1999;33(2):195-201.

78. Kaada B. Vasodilation induced by transcutaneous nerve stimulation in peripheral ischemia (Reynaud's phenomena and diabetic polyneuropathy). *Eur Heart J.* 1982;3(4):303-314.

79. Kaada B. Promoted healing of chronic ulceration by transcutaneous nerve stimulation (TNS). *Vasa.* 1983;12:262-269.

80. Cosmo P, Svensson H, Bornmyr S, Wikstrom SO. Effect of transcutaneous nerve stimulation on the microcirculation in chronic leg ulcers. *Scan J Plast Reconstr Surg Hand Surg.* 2000;34(Mar):61-64.

81. Mawson AR, Siddiqui FH, Connolly B, Sharp CJ, Sammer WR, Bjundo JJ. Sacral transcutaneous oxygen tension levels in the spinal cord injured: risk factors for pressure ulcers. *Arch Phys Med Rehabil.* 1993;74(7):745-751.

82. Mawson A, Siddiqui F, Connolly G, et al. Effect of high voltage pulsed galvanic stimulatioon on sacral transcutaneous oxygen tension levels in the spinal cord injured. *Paraplegia.* May 1993;31(5):311-319.

83. Bogie KM, Reger SI, Levine SP, Sahgal V. Electrical Stimulation for Pressure Sore Prevention and Wound Healing. *Asst Technol.* Jan 2000;12(1):50-66.

84. Wolcott L, Wheeler P, Hardwicke H, et al. Accelerated healing of skin ulcers by electrotherapy: preliminary clinical results. *South Med J.* 1969;62:795-801.

85. Baker LL. The effect of electrical stimulation on cutaneous oxygen supply. *Rehabil Res Dev Prog Rep.* 1988:176.

86. Baker LL, Chamber R, Merchant L, Park D, Sokolski D, Yoneyama C. The effects of electrical stimulation on cutaneous oxygen supply in normal older adults and diabetic patients. *Phys Ther.* 1986;66:749.

87. Dodgen PW, Johnson BW, Baker LL, Chambers RB, PT. The effects of electrical stimulation on cutaneous oxygen supply in diabetic older adults. *Phys Ther. 67.* 1987;(5):S4.

88. Forst T, Pfutzner A, Bauersachs R, al e. Comparison of the microvascular response to transcutaneious electrical nerve stimulation and post occlusive ischemia in the diabetic foot. *Journal of Diabetes Complications.* 1997;11(5):291-297.

89. Peters EJ, Armstrong DG, Wunderlich RP, Bosma J, Stacpoole-Shea S, LA L. The benefit of electrical stimulation to enhance perfusion in persons with diabetes mellitus. *Journal of Foot and Ankle Surgery.* 1998;37(5):396-400.

90. Gilcreast D, Stotts N, Baker L. Effect of electrical stimulation on foot skin perfusion in persons with or at risk for diabetic foot ulcers. *Wound Repair and Regeneration.* 1998;6(5):434:441.

91. Byl N, McKenzie A, West J, Whitney J, Hunt T, Scheuenstuhn H. Microamperage stimulation: effects on subcutaneous oxygen (II). Presented at the Annual Conference of the California Chapter of the American Physical Therapy Association; 1990; San Diego, CA. 1990.

92. Goldman Robert J, Brewley Barbara I, Golden Michael A. Electrotherapy reoxygentes inframalleolar ischemic wounds on diabetic patients: a case series. *Adv in Skin and Wound Care.* May-Jun 2002;15:112-120.

93. Goldman R., Brewley B., Zhou L., G. Michael Electrotherapy Reverses Inframalleolar Ischemia: a retrospective observationl study. *Adv in Skin and Wound Care.* March/April 2003 2003;16:79-89.

94. Twist D. Acrocyanosis iln a spinal cord injured patient- effect of computer-controlled neuromuscular electrical stimulation: a case report. *Physical Therapy.* 1990;70:45:49.

95. Thomas AJ, Davis GM, Sutton JR. Cardiovascular and metabolic responses to electrical stimulation-induced leg exercise in spinal cord injury. *Methods In Med.* 1997;36(4-5):372-375.

96. Raymond J, Davis GM, Bryant G, Clarke JE. Cardiovascular responses to an orthostatic challenge and electrical-stimulation-induced leg muscle contractions in individuals with paraplegia. *Eur J Appl Physiol Occup Physiol.* 1999;80(3):201-212.

97. Phillips W, Burkett LN, Munroi R, Davis M, Pomeroy K. Relative changes in blood flow with functional electrical stimulation during exercise of the paralyzed lower limbs. *Paraplegia.* 1995;33:90-93.

98. Faghri PD, Votto JJ, Hovorka CF. Venous hemodynamics of the lower extremity in response to electrical stimulation. *Arch Phys Med Rehabil.* 1998;79:842-848.

99. Ross C, Segal D. HVPC as an aid to post-operative healing. *Curr Podiatry.* 1981(May):19-25.

100. Reed BV. Effect of high voltage pulsed electrical stimulation on microvascular permeability to plasma proteins: a possible mechanism in minimizing edema. *Phys Ther.* 1998;68:491-495.

101. Mendel F, Fish D. New perspectives in edema control via electrical stimulation. *J Athlet Train.* 1993;28:63-74.

102. Thornton RM, Mendel FC, Fish DR. Effects of electrical stimulation on edema formation in different strains of rats. *Phys Ther.* 1998;78:386-394.

103. Matylevich NP, Chu CS, McManus AT, Mason AD Jr, Pruitt BA Jr. Direct current reduces plasma protein extravasation after partial thickness burn injury in rats. *J Trauma.* 1996;4(3):424-429.

104. Chu CS, Matylevich NP, McManus AT, Mason AD Jr., Jr PB, et al. Direct current reduces wound edema after full-thickness burn injury in rats.*J Trauma.* 1996;40(5):738-742.

105. Griffin JW, Newsome LS, et al. Reduction of chronic posttraumatic hand edema: A comparison of high voltage pulsed current, intermittent pneumatic compression and placebo treatments. *Phys Ther.* 1990;70:279-286.

106. Dobbins GM, Henderson RJ, Schuit D. Effects of high voltage pulsed current on acute edema following total knee arthroplasty. *Abstract. Section on Clinical Electrophysiology Newsletter.* 1999;January 1999.

107. Dobbins GM. Personal communication August 30, 2000.

108. Fakhri O, Amin MA. The effect of low-voltage electric therapy on the healing of resistant skin burns. *J Burn Care Rehabil.* 1987;8(1):15-18.

109. Sawyer PN. Bioelectric phenomena and intravascular thrombosis: the first 12 years. *Surgery.* 1964;56:1020-1026.

110. Sawyer PN, Deutch B. The experimental use of oriented electrical fields to delay and prevent intravascular thrombosis. *Surg Forum.* 1995;5:163-168.

111. Sawyer PN, Deutch B. Use of electrical currents to delay intravascular thrombosis in experimental animals. *Am J Physiol.* 1956;187(473-478).

112. Barranco S, Spadaro J, Berger TJ, Becker RO. In vitro effect of weak direct current on staphylococcus aureus. *Clin Orthop.* 1974;100:250-255.

113. Rowley BA MJ, Chase G. 1974;238:543-551. The influence of electrical current on an infecting microorganism in wounds. *Ann NY Acad Sci.* 1974;238:543-551.

114. Kloth LC. *Bactericidal effect of passing an electrical current through a silver wire* [poster presentation]. Presented at the Symposium on Advanced Wound Care; April 1996; Atlanta, GA. 1996.

115. Kincaid CB, Lavoie K. Inhibition of bacterial growth in vitro following stimultion with high voltage, monophasic, pulsed current. *Phys Ther.* 1989;69:29-33.

116. Szuminsky NJ, Albers AC, Unger P, Eddy JG. Effect of narrow, pulsed high voltages on bacterial viability. *Phys Ther.* 1994;74:660-667.

117. Byl N, McKenzie A, West J, et al. Pulsed micro amperage stimulation: A controlled study of healing of surgically induced wounds in Yucatan pigs. *Phys Ther.* 1994;74:201-218.

118. Chu CS, McManus AT, Pruitt BA Jr, Mason AD Jr. Therapeutic effects of silver nylon dressings with weak direct current on Pseudomonas aeruginosa-infected burn wounds. *J Trauma.* 1998;28(10):1488-1492.

119. Thurman BF, Christian E. Response of a serious circulatory lesion to electrical stimulation. *Phys Ther.* 1971;51(10):137-140.

120. Gault W, Gatens, PF. Use of Low Intensity Direct Current in Management of Ischemic Skin Ulcers. *Phys Ther.* 1976;56(3):141:145.

121. Webster DA, Spadaro JA, Becker RO, Kramer S. Silver anode treatment of chronic osteomyelitis. *Clin Orthop Relat Res.* 1981;161:106-114.

122. Fitzgerald GK ND. Treatment of a large infected thoracic spine wound using high voltge pulsed monophasic current. *Phys Ther.* June 1993;73(6):355-360.

123. Barr JO. Transcutaneous electric nerve stimulation for pain management. In: Nelson R, Currier D, eds. *Clinical Electrotherapy.* Norwalk, CT: Appleton & Lange. 1991:280.

124. Khalil Z, Merhi M. Effects of aging on neurogenic vasodilator responses evoked by transcutaneous electrical nerve stimulation: relevance to wound healing. *J Gerontology biol Sci Med Sci.* 2000;55(6):B257-263.

125. Castillo E, Sumano H, Fortoul TI, Zepeda A. The influence of pulsed electrical stimulation on the wound healing of burned rat skin. *Arch Med Res.* 1995;26(2):185-189.

126. Adamian AA, Shloznikov BM, Muzykant LI, Zaidenberg MA. Clinico-morphological changes in a burn wound after electric stimulation with pulsatile current. *Khururgiia(Mosk).* 1990;1990(6):77-81.

127. Bach S, Bilgrave K, Gottrup F, Jorgensen TE. The effect of electrical current on healing skin incision. An experimental study. *Eur J Surg.* 1991;157(3):171-174.

128. Reger SI, Hyodo A, Negami S, Kambic HE, Sahgal V. Experimental wound healing with electrical stimulation. *Artif Organs.* 1999;23(5):460-462.

129. Stefanovska A, Vodovnik L, Benko H, Turk R. Treatment of chronic wounds by means of electrical and electromagnetic fields, 2: value of FES parameters for pressure sore treatment. *Med Biol Eng Comput.* 1993;31:213-220.

130. Gault W, Gatens P Jr. Use of low intensity direct current in management of ischemic skin ulcers. *Phys Ther.* 1976;56:265-269.

131. Katelaris PM, Fletcher JP, Little JM, McEntyre RJ, Jeffcoate KW. Electrical stimulation in the treatment of chronic venous ulceration. *Aust NZ J Surg.* 1987;57(9):605-607.

132. Kloth LC. Electrical stimulation in tissue repair. In: McCulloch J, Kloth L, Feedar J, eds. *Wound Healing Alternatives in Management.* 2nd ed. Philadelphia: FA Davis. 1995:275-310.

133. Leffmann DJ, Arnall DA, Holmgren PR. Effect of microamperage stimulation on the rate of wound healing in rats: a histological study. *Phys Ther.* 1994;74(195-200).

134. Barron JJ, Jacobson WE, Tidd T. Treatment of decubitus ulcers. *Minn Med.* 1985;68(2):103-106.

135. Unger P, Eddy J, Raimastry S. A controlled study of the effect of high voltage pulsed current (HVPC) on wound healing. *Phys Ther.* 1991;71 (suppl):S119.

136. Gogia P, Marquez R, Minerbo G. Effects of High Voltage Galvanic Stimulation on Wound Healing. *Ostomy/ Wound Management.* Jan/Feb 1992;38(1):29-35.

137. Unger PC. A randomized clinical trial of the effect of HVPC on wound healing. *Phys Ther.* 1991;71 (suppl):S1118.

138. Akers T GA. The effect of high voltage galvanic stimulation on the rate of healing of decubitus ulcers. *Biomed Sci Instrum J.* 1984;20:99-100.

139. Lundeberg TCM, Eriksson SV, Mats M. Electrical nerve stimulation improves healing of diabetic ulcers. *Ann Plast Surg.* 1992;29(4):328-330.

140. Baker LL, Chambers R, Demuth S, Villar F. Effects of electrical stimulation on wound healing in patients with diabetic ulcers. *Diabetes Care.* 1997;20(3):1-8.

141. Alon G, Smith GV. Kid Care: Helping heal with E-Stim. *Adv Directors Rehabil.* 1999(March):47-50.

142. Chen D, Philip M, Phillip PA, Monga TN. Cardiac pacemaker inhibition by transcutaneous electrical nerve stimulation. *Arch Phys Med Rehabil.* 1990;71(1):27-30.

143. Donayre C. Diagnosis and management of vascular ulcers: arterial, venous and diabetic. Presented at Wound Care Management 96; Torrance, CA; October 1996.

144. Rasmussen MJ, Hayes DL, Vlieststra RE, Thorsteinson G. . Can transcutaneous electrical nerve stimulation be safely used in patients with permanent cardiac pacemakers? *Mayo Clin Proc.* 1998;63:443-445.

145. Shade SK. ,Use of transcutaneous electrical nerve stimulation for a patient with a cardiac pacemaker. A case report. *Phys Ther.* 1985;65(2):206-208.

146. Sliwa JA, Marinko MS. Transcutaneous electrical nerve stimulatorinduced electrocardiogram artifact. A brief report. *Am J Phys Med Rehabil.* 1996;75(4):307-309.

147. Eaglestein W. Off-label uses in wound care. Paper presented at the Symposium on Advanced Wound Care; Atlanta, GA; April 1996.
148. Cook T, Barr JO. Instrumentation. In: Nelson R, Currier D, eds. *Clinical Electrotherapy.* Norwalk, CT: Appleton & Lange. 1991:11-33.
149. Brown M. *Electrical stimulation for wound management.* In Gogia PP, ed. *Clinical Wound Management.* Thorofare, NJ: Slack, Inc; 1995:176-183.
150. Cheng K, Tarjan P, Thio Y, Mertz P. In vivo 3-D distributions of electric fields in pig skin with rectangular pulse electrical stimulation (RPECS). *Bioelectromagnetics.* 1996;17:`.
151. Kloth LC. *Electrical stimulation for wound healing.* Exhibitor presentation at American Physical Therapy Association Conference; Minneapolis, MN; June 1996.
152. Davis S. The effect of pulsed electrical stimulation on epidermal wound healing. *J Invest Dermatol.* 90:555.
153. Cummings J, Kloth LC. Role of light, heat and electromagnetic energy in wound healing. In McCulloch J, Kloth L, Feedar J, eds. *Wound Healing Alternatives in Management.* 2nd ed. Philadelphia: F.A Davis. 1995:275-314.
154. Selkowitz DM. Electrical currents. In: Cameron MH, ed. *Physical Agents in Rehabilitation.* Philadelphia: WB Saunders. 1999;402.
155. Bourguignon GL, et al. Occlusive wound dressings suitable for use with electrical stimulation. *Wounds.* 1991;3(3):127.
156. Agren MS, Mertz MA. Collagenase during burn wound healing: influence of a hydrogel dressing and pulsed electrical stimulation. *Plast Reconstr Surg.* 1993;94:518-524.
157. Myer A. Observable effects on granulation tissue using warmed wound care products. Presented at Symposia, "Future Directions in Wound Healing"; American Physical Therapy Association Scientific Meeting; June 1997; San Diego, CA.
158. Beltran K, Thacker JG, et al. Impact pressures generated by commercial wound irrigation devices. Unpublished research report. Charlottesville, VA: University of Virginia Health Science Center. 1994.
159. Alon G. Antibiotics enhancement by transcutaneous electrical stimulation. *Presented at Symposia, "Future Directions in Wound Healing";* American Physical Therapy Association Scientific Meeting; June 1997; San Diego, CA. 1997.
160. Kalinowski DP, Brogan MS, Sleeper MD. A practical technique for disinfecting electrical stimulation apparatuses used in wound treatment. *Phys Ther.* 1996;12:1340-1347.
161. Lock P. The effect of temperature on mitosis at the edge of experimental wounds. In: Lundgren A, Sover A, eds. *Symposia on Wound Healing: Plastic, surgical and Dermatologic Aspects.* Molndal, Sweden; 1980.
162. Myers JA. Wound Healing and use of modern surgical dressing. *Pharm J.* 1982;229:103-104.
163. Thomas ST. *Wound Management and Dressings.* London: The Pharmaceutical Press; 1990.
164. Williams RD, Carey LC. Studies in the production of "standard" venous thrombosis. *Ann Surg.* 1959;149::381-387.
165. Baker L, Dogen P, Johnson B, Chambers R. The effects of electrical stimulation on cutaneous oxygen supply in diabetic older adults. *Phys Ther.* 1987;67:773.
166. Owoeye I, Spielholtz NI, Fetto J, et al. Low intensity pulsed galvanic current and the healing of tenotomized rat Achilles tendons: preliminary report using lead to break measurements. *Arch Phys Med Rehabil.* 1987:415-418.
167. Bourguignon GJ, Bourguignon LYW. Electric stimulation of protein and DNA synthesis in human fibroblasts. *FASEB J.* 1987;1:398-402.
168. Yang W, et al. Response of C3H/10T1/2 fibroblasts to an external steady electric field stimulation. *Exp Cell Res.* 1984;155:92-104.
169. Cooper MS, Schliwa M. Electrical and ionic controls of tissue cell locomotion in DC electrical fields. *J Cell Physiol.* 1995;103:363-370.

Induced Electrical Stimulation: Pulsed Radio Frequency and Pulsed Electromagnetic Fields

Carrie Sussman

CHAPTER OBJECTIVES

At the completion of this chapter, the reader will be able to:

1. Describe the physical properties of thermal and nonthermal pulsed electromagnetic fields.
2. Identify and differentiate between the physiologic effects of three different pulsed electromagnetic fields used for wound healing.
3. Evaluate radiofrequency devices based on their potential uses.
4. Analyze animal and clinical studies to evaluate the efficacy of different pulsed electromagnetic field therapies for wound healing.
5. Evaluate a patient's candidacy for pulsed short-wave diathermy and pulsed radiofrequency stimulation based on indications, precautions, and contraindications.
6. Prepare a patient for treatment and evaluate outcomes of care.

Short-wave diathermy was introduced in Germany in 1907 and spread throughout Europe and the United States. The word *diathermy* was introduced by Nagelschmidt to describe the relatively uniform heating produced in tissue by the conversion of high-frequency currents into heat.[1] In the following decades, diathermy was used to treat all types of illnesses and injuries. The stimulator used electromagnetic short waves from the short-wave radio portion of the spectrum, and was called *continuous short-wave diathermy* (CSWD). CSWD was an application of electromagnetic energy to medicine that became widely popular because it made possible subcutaneous tissue heating and the targeting of deep tissue structures. This was in contrast to the superficial heating available by means of hot packs and infrared, in which heat is rapidly dissipated by the superficial vasculature.

During the 1960s and 1970s, many clinical studies used animals and biologic systems to determine the possible biologic mechanisms of the action of electromagnetism on tissue. Unfortunately, many of these studies were not blinded, controlled, or randomized. In the 1980s, 1990s, and within the past decade, there have been case studies, clinical trials, and some randomized clinical trials with both animal and human subjects designed to determine the effects of nonthermal pulsed radiofrequency stimulation (PRFS) and pulsed electromagnetic fields (PEMF). During this time,

manufacturers have supported research using their own products, and have applied their proprietary names to therapies such as Diapulse (Diapulse Corporation of America, Great Neck, NY), or more recently the Provant Wound Closure System with Cell Proliferation Induction (CPI) technology (Regenesis Biomedical, Inc., Scottsdale, AZ).

All class III diathermy nonthermal medical devices licensed by the Federal Drug Administration (FDA) induce electrical current in the tissues. Research efforts supported by manufacturers deserve recognition for their contribution to our understanding of the efficacy and utility of their technological products. Unfortunately, the use of proprietary terminology to report these findings adds another level of confusion for the clinician trying to search the literature, identify treatment parameters, and compare, evaluate, and apply these technologies appropriately. Although they have improved over time, study designs and reporting methods are other issues that have made comparison and evaluation of these interventions problematic.

The goal of this chapter is to encapsulate the available evidence based on a review of the literature concerning what is known about the benefits and disadvantages of using pulsed short-wave diathermy (PSWD), PRFS, and PEMF as adjunctive therapy for patients with acute and chronic wounds. The chapter begins with definitions and terminology related to the properties of the devices involved. The next section details the science and theory of the therapy and the studies that support its use. Following is an outline of the clinical reasoning relating to the selection of both a candidate for treatment and the appropriate device for use, including the reasons for referral, medical history, and systems reviews that are components of the diagnostic process. Procedures and protocols for application of specific devices are provided, as are precautions, contraindications, and expected outcomes.

Definitions and Terminology

Electromagnetic Fields

The equipment we are concerned with here operates in one small portion of the electromagnetic spectrum (sometimes referred to as the *radio, radiation,* or *frequency spectrum*). In its entirety, the spectrum ranges in energy from below power transmission waves (very-low frequency) to above cosmic rays (very-high frequency), and includes radiowaves, microwaves, visible light, infrared, ultraviolet light, and X-rays. All frequencies within the spectrum have certain characteristics in common. For example, they all travel at the speed of light, which is 300,000 km (186,000 mi) per second. They all travel unimpeded through a vacuum. They all consist of two parts, a magnetic field, and an electrostatic field, traveling at right angles to each other.

One of many important differences between waves from different portions of the spectrum is what happens when they encounter an object. Are they absorbed (like heat waves)? Do they have some other effect on the object? Are they reflected (like light waves striking a mirror)? Or do they fail to affect the object at all (like cosmic rays passing through Earth)?

It should be noted that the electromagnetic waves discussed here do not include sound or ultrasonic waves, which require a physical medium through which to travel. They are "pure energy" and do not have any mass. Also, the techniques for using the equipment discussed in this chapter are not the same as those appropriate for use of either high- or low-voltage electrical stimulation equipment, which operates on pulsed direct current, not the 27.12 MHz of the typical CSWD or PRFS equipment discussed in this chapter. At the 27.12 MHz used by short-wave diathermy and pulsed radiofrequency medical equipment, some of the energy will pass through a patient's body, some will be reflected from a patient's skin, some will be absorbed by the tissue and converted to heat, and some will cause the tissue cells within the patient's body to react in a certain way. The effect that will be produced on the tissues depends on the extent of absorption and energy release in the tissues, which depends on the wavelength. It is also important to note that, when an electrical field reacts with body tissues, a magnetic field is created, and, similarly, a magnetic field produces an electrical field. Exhibit 23-1 is a reference list of the devices discussed in this chapter and their acronyms. Table 23-1 compares the four types of stimulators and their effects. Exhibit

23-2 lists identified factors that affect the effectiveness of electrotherapeutic devices that are explained in the following sections.

Units of Measurement

There are several units of measurement associated with electromagnetic fields (EMFs) of which the reader should be aware. The frequency of a wave may be expressed in two ways, as a frequency, meaning the number of cycles occurring within a 1 second period (e.g., 27.12 million cycles for a 27.12 MHz wave), or as a wave length, which measures how far a wave has traveled during one cycle. For our 27.12 MHz example, this would be 11 m. Signal (or wave) strength is measured in volts per meter (V/m). This unit represents how much voltage would be induced by the magnetic flux portion of the wave while traveling through free space and going through a wire 1 m long.

Carrier Frequency and Waveforms

When studying diathermy equipment, there are two frequencies to be aware of, the carrier frequency and the waveform or modulation frequency. The carrier frequency is the basic operating frequency of the equipment. For example, the carrier of a radio station is the frequency at which the station broadcasts. For PSWD equipment, the carrier (or broadcast) frequency is 27.12 MHz. The waveform or modulation frequency is the frequency at which the carrier frequency is modulated (i.e., the music from the radio station). For PSWD and PRFS equipment, modulation frequency is the rate at which the carrier frequency is turned on and off (i.e., 600 pulses per second [pps]). For the pulsed high-voltage equipment discussed in Chapter 22, the waveform is monophasic pulsed current. The waveform frequency may be the same as that used for PRFS equipment.

When radiofrequency energy is transmitted as a continuous wave or signal, enough energy can be absorbed by an object to cause noticeable heating, for example in a microwave oven. To control these heating effects and still maintain the benefits to tissue of the EMF stimulation, several manufacturers have developed generators that deliver bursts or trains of short-wave radiofrequency pulses. These bursts are another example of modulating frequency.

Diathermy equipment, including CSWD, PSWD, and PRFS, operates at a frequency specified by the Federal Communications Commission, which allows use of radio frequencies of 13.56, 27.12, and 40.68 MHz for these medical devices. Typically, PSWD and PRFS equipment use 27.12 MHz.

TABLE 23-1 **Comparison of Characteristics of Electromagnetic Field Devices**

Device	Signal	Typical Pulse Duration	Induced Voltage	Effects
Continuous Shortwave Diathermy (CSWD)	13.57, 27.12, 40.68 MHz sinusoidal	Continuous	V/cm	Tissue heating, no off time for heat dissipation. Unable to depolarize nerve
Pulsed Shortwave Diathermy (PSWD)	27.12 MHz sinusoidal; Duty cycle 3.9%	95 μsec	V/cm	Tissue heating allows for heat dissipation. Unable to depolarize nerve
Pulsed Radio-frequency (PRF)	27.12 MHz 80–600 pps sinusoidal	65 μsec	V/cm	Nonthermal, cellular and circulatory effects. Unable to depolarize nerve
Pulsed Electromagnetic Field (PEMF)	1–100 pps sinusoidal low energy	1–100 msec	mV/cm	Nonthermal, cellular effects

Signals at these frequencies can travel through the body relatively unhindered, without requiring contact between the applicator and the body. This is an important attribute for treatment. Radiofrequency waves transport electromagnetic energy through the air or a vacuum without the need for a conductive medium such as water or air. The energy delivered to the tissues is reduced, however, as the gap between the tissues and the applicator head increases, because a portion of the energy is dispersed away from the target. One clinical application of this effect is reduce the heating created by a PSWD device by increasing the gap between the applicator head and the tissue for patients with heat sensitivity, or where only mild heating is required. On the other hand, when using PRFS equipment, any gap should be very small, 0.5 cm, in order to avoid reducing the energy too much.

CLINICAL WISDOM

Modifying Heating Effects

Increase the gap between applicator and tissue when using PSWD for patients with heat sensitivity or where mild heating effects are desired (Exhibit 23-3).

EXHIBIT 23-2 **Factors That Affect the Effectiveness of Electrotherapeutic Devices**

- Waveform Shape
- Amplitude
- Pulse shape and duration
- Pulse frequency and repetition rate
- Exposure time in each 24-hour period
- All of the above must be adequate and matched to the biologic needs of the tissues.

Source: Adapted with permission from M.S. Markov and A. Pilla, *Electromagnetic Field Stimulation of Soft Tissues: Pulsed Radiofrequency Treatment of Postoperative Pain and Edema, Wounds,* Vol. 7, No. 4, pp. 143–151, © 1995, Health Management Publications.

Pulse Rate and Pulse Duration

Both PSWD and PRFS use radio waves that are pulsed (that is, interrupted) at regular intervals. The pulse rates for PSWD vary from 1 to 7,000 pps. The pulse duration (or width) varies from 65 to 400 microseconds (μsec)(1 μsec = 10^{-6} seconds). While the pulse is on, the signal is generated. For example, during a 65-μsec pulse period, some 1,763 waves of 27.12 MHz energy are generated. During the intervals between pulses, no energy is generated.

Longer pulse duration, coupled with greater pulse frequency, delivers more energy to the tissues and has a greater thermal effect. With high pulse rates (which result in short interpulse intervals), heat builds up in the tissues because the short interpulse interval does not allow heat to dissipate. Conversely, a low-frequency pulse rate, along with a short pulse duration (which means a long interpulse interval), produces insignificant tissue heating because the interpulse interval is long enough to allow heat dissipation.

Nonthermal PRFS medical devices generally have a fixed pulse duration of 65 μsec (of the basic 27.12-MHz wave), with pulse rates that can vary from 80 to 600 pps. They are classified as low frequency. This type of signal does not have adequate intensity to heat tissues.

It is very important for the physical therapist (PT) to be familiar with the device he or she intends to use. Some devices offer a large range of variability of pulse rates and pulse durations from which to choose. Treatment effects will be different, depending on the parameters selected. Read and understand the instruction manual that comes with the device and choose parameters that provide the physiologic response required.

EXHIBIT 23-3

Greater Pulse Frequency and Width ⟶ More Energy ⟶ More Heat

Testing Thermal and Nonthermal Effects at Different Settings

Try combinations of different on/off times and pulse rates on normal subjects over superficial tissues. Evaluate their effects before and after treatment and over various time intervals by measuring changes to the surface temperature of the skin with a liquid crystal skin thermometer, or to deeper tissue with an infrared scanner.

Duty Cycle

The duty cycle is the ratio of on time to total cycle time, which includes both the on and off times. As an example, at a pulse duration having an on time of 65 μsec and a pulse rate of 600 pps, each complete period lasts 1/600 seconds or 1,667 μsec. The interpulse interval, or off time, is then $1.667 - 65 = 1,602$ μsec. At 600 pps, the duty cycle is 65 μsec/1, 667 μsec = 3.9%.[2] This means that, in a 30-minute treatment (30 × 60 seconds × 3.9%), a total of only 70 seconds of energy is delivered.[2] This information is important because most clinical studies use a 30 minute treatment time period. Therefore, adjustment of treatment time would need to be carefully considered in order to make sure that there was an adequate but not excessive amount of energy delivered to the tissue.

Amplitude

Historically, power was the way in which the amplitude of a generated field was measured, but this has nothing to do with the energy is delivered to the tissues. For example, 1,000 watts (W) of generated power is transferred to the drum applicator, where it undergoes significant transformation into the EMF that is then delivered to the patient. Until the transformation into an EMF, it is appropriate to speak of power, but at the last step, it is more correct to speak of the amplitude of the EMF delivered to the tissues. The power driving the applicator coil can be measured either as peak pulse power (which for the Diapulse ranges from 185 to 275 W) or as mean power, which (for both Diapulse and Provant devices) ranges from 7.5 to 38 W. These values are determined by settings of peak power and pulse frequency. The benchmark for measurement of heating effects is 38 W or more mean. Less than 38 W is, therefore, used as an indicator of minimal heating or nonthermal therapy.[3] The heating effect of a PSWD device is related to the magnitude of the mean power output and can be adjusted to achieve appropriate treatment effects by either direct or indirect application. Treatment outcome can be measured by measuring the skin temperature where heating is desired or by measuring skin blood flow with a laser Doppler.

Commonly, the amplitude of the EMF is described in terms of flux density with the units in gauss (G) or tesla (T), where 10,000 G = 1 T. For example, the magnetic resonance imaging device operates on the order of 1–2 T.[4] Manufacturers include tables in their instruction manuals, listing the approximate values of average output power in watts at different pulse rates and widths. This information should be used only as a guide, not as a definite amount of power delivered to the tissues. The electric or magnetic field itself can be measured, but it is not yet possible to measure the intensity *received* by the tissues.

Comparison of Electromagnetic Field Devices

The devices have been labeled in the literature as PEMF, pulsed electromagnetic induction, pulsed electromagnetic energy, and pulsed radiofrequency (PRF). However, these terms are not synonymous, nor should they be considered interchangeable, because they have significantly different characteristics. Electromagnetic field modalities used for medical purposes can be categorized into four groups:

1. Static magnetic fields
2. Low-frequency sine waves
3. PEMF
4. PRF

Low-frequency sine waves have a very low signal (smaller than 1 G) and induce 1–10 mV/cm electric field at frequencies below 100 Hz. The PEMF waveform is considered relatively low frequency, pulse duration 1–100 μsec and a repetition rate of 1–100 pps, and the PRF signal may be a rectangular envelope of sinusoidal waves with a duration of 65 μsec. The PRF repetition rate varies between 80 and 600 pps, and the duty cycle is less than 4%. The signals of PEMF are in the mV/cm range and those of PRF in the V/cm range.[2] The PEMF signal has been used primarily for osteogenesis, although soft tissue repair studies with this signal have been published recently.[5–10] By contrast, PRF is used mainly for the treatment of pain, edema, and soft tissue injuries as well as cellular stimulation.

Several differences in the signal characteristics exist, the main difference being the signal shape. A PEMF waveform is typically an asymmetric train of pulses, whereas the PRF signal represents a burst of pulses within a rectangular envelope (Figure 23-1). Asymmetry of the stimulus pulse was at one point thought to be necessary to achieve a therapeutic effect. Asymmetric pulses require significant electrical energy, however, constraining clinical delivery systems to suboptimal designs. The results of a study on rabbit fibula osteotomy suggest that asymmetry is not in fact necessary for clinical therapeutic effect.[11] Other differences include the repetition rate of the PRF pulsed signal, which is 80–600 pps and classified as high frequency.[2] The PEMF signal is longer than that of the PRFS.[2]

Thus, it is important to recognize that the acronym *PEMF* is not generic for all EMF devices, and that there are important differences between the therapeutic modalities. These distinctions are relevant to the PT when reviewing studies reporting on the use of these different EMFs and when selecting therapeutic devices.

The Health Care Financing Administration, now the Center for Medicare and Medicaid Services (CMS) in 1997 in-

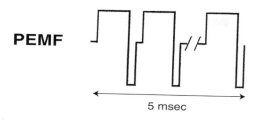

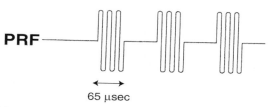

FIGURE 23-1 Pulse electromagnetic field (PEMF) signal was designed for bone growth stimulation, whereas pulse radiofrequency (PRF) waveform is mainly used in treatment of soft tissues. Note: PEMF signal is asymmetric, whereas PRF represents rectangular envelope of pulse burst of 65 μsec. (Reprinted with permission from *Wounds: A Compendium of Clinical Research and Practice*, Vol. 7, No. 4, © 1995, Health Management Publications.)

cluded PEMF in an exclusion policy for reimbursement of wound treatment along with capacitative electrical stimulation for wound healing of Medicare beneficiaries.[12] (See Chapter 22) Because that policy was stalled by a court injunction,[13] reimbursement for Medicare beneficiaries was made on a case-by-case basis until a national coverage policy for use of induced electrical stimulation (PRFS) for treatment of nonhealing wounds of different etiologies was issued. That occurred in 2004. The policy explanation states that it is essentially equivalent therapy to electrical stimulation, but by a different application method.[14] The coverage policy can be accessed at www.hhs.cms.gov by searching for electrical stimulation coverage policy. Published treatment guidelines for pressure ulcers have not distinguished PRFS-induced current from capacitative electrotherapy as an adjunctive treatment.[15-17] Electrical stimulation is included as a recommended modality for best practice in recommendation no. 9 of the *Canadian Association of Wound Care Guidelines: Pressure Ulcer Prevention* and the Paralyzed Veterans of America pressure ulcer prevention and treatment guidelines following spinal cord injury.[17,18]

PEMF studies have primarily been conducted or reported in the literature outside of the United States, and only since communication has improved across borders, as a result of the internet and clinical databases, has this information become available to other clinicians. PEMF devices have been used in the United States primarily for osteogenesis, but several studies on soft tissue repair for venous ulcers have been reported (these are reviewed in the clinical section). Equipment to provide this type of treatment is not readily

available in U.S. therapy clinics at this time. The Magnatherp electromagnetic (PEMF) unit (Meditea Electromedica, Buenos Aires), operating at 3–50 Hz and an amplitude of up to 200 Gauss, was the type of equipment used by researchers in some of the animal studies discussed earlier in this chapter (see Figure 23-2).

Comparison of PSWD and PRFS Equipment

Both PSWD and PRFS apply radio waves from the short-wave range of the spectrum at 27.12 MHz. Both modulate the 27.12-MHz carrier frequency with square or pulse bidirectional waveforms (see earlier discussion regarding carrier frequency and waveforms). Like all radio wave signals, the 27.12-MHz signal travels through air and is not impeded by nonmetallic structures (otherwise, your radio would not play indoors). Heating effects are adjusted by changing the pulse rate and intensity. Higher pulse rates have greater thermal impact. Low pulse rates, in the 90- to 200-pps range, produce mild heating and are nonthermal at lower rates. Both transmit radiation from a coil contained in the drum head to the target tissues. This method of energy transfer to the tissues is called *induction*. An electrical current is induced in the tissues, as described above.

Both PSWD and PRFS penetrate deeply into the tissues and most affect those tissues with good conductivity. Because they are so similar, it is easy to equate them; however, they are not synonymous—their effects are based on two different physiologic phenomena. PSWD has the ability to heat the tissues, whereas PRFS affects the tissues at the cellular level. Because PSWD energy penetrates deeply, it heats from the inside out, just as, when cooking food in the microwave the center is heated first. Heating effects may continue even after the stimulation is removed. Delayed response to stimulation is an important concept to remember; the patient may not report heating right away because the skin is not heated first, such as when a hot pack is applied. Follow the guidelines listed in the protocols for treatment parameters.

Because both PSWD and PRFS deliver a signal to the tissues at 27.12 MHz, they have an equal ability to penetrate

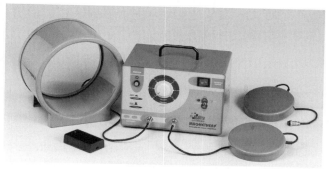

FIGURE 23-2 Magnatherm electromagnetic (PEMF) unit (3–50 Hz) and amplified up to 200 Gauss. (Courtesy of Meditea Electromedica, Buenos Aires, Argentina.)

tissues. The depth of penetration of the magnetic field decreases by approximately the square of the distance as it moves away from the surface of the applicator. Guy et al[1] measured thermal changes in the tissues at a depth of 5–6 cm up to 15 cm from the applicator. Markov and Pilla[2] found that the magnetic field of 27.12 MHz radio waves is 30% of the initial value at 5 cm distance from the applicator, 10% at 10 cm, and 3–5% at 15 cm. As already described, treatment effects would be expected to be altered by the distance of the applicator from the target tissues.

PRFS and High-Voltage Pulsed Current Fields

PRFS induces electrical currents in the body through the action of an electromagnetic or a radio field. As such, it has no positive or negative poles, and the current goes in concentric circles (see Figure 23-3).[4] This induced alternating current is not related to intervening tissue, but is related to the distance from the coil, with the current intensity being greatest just beneath the coil edges.

For treatment purposes, high-voltage pulsed current (HVPC) has, in general, the same amplitude as do PSWD/PRFS. HVPC, however, has a unidirectional flow, with a specific polarity,[19] whereas the electromagnetically generated current is a circular flow of current without polarity, as shown in Figure 23-3. The mechanism of action for PSWD/PRFS is a direct effect of the magnetic field and induced electric current in the cells. HVPC, on the other hand, has a negligible magnetic field, and the method of cellular stimulation is by electric current. The direct effect of magnetic and electrical fields in the tissues cannot be distinguished because they come together with high-frequency fields. The methods of delivery are different for PSWD/PRFS and HVPC. PSWD/PRFS is delivered without skin contact, and the signal is "broadcast" through the air (Exhibit 23-4). HVPC by contrast is delivered by capacitive coupling from an electrode, through a wet contact medium applied to the skin. HVPC has a negligible magnetic field (Figure 23-4), and its stimulation is mainly by electric current. PRFS delivers a more uniform and predictable signal to the tissues than do capacitative coupled electrodes.[2]

The effects of both PSWD and PRFS stimulation are detailed in Exhibit 23-5, and the attributes that make them useful for the treatment of wounds are as follows:

1. The penetration of the magnetic field into the tissues is not restricted by impedance from intervening structures, such as skin, bone, or plaster. However, metal (e.g., rings) will alter penetration and/or localized heating (see safety issues, below).
2. Stimulation at the skin level is not sufficient to depolarize the pain nerve endings in the skin and is therefore painless.
3. Treatment is nondisruptive and compatible with other interventions. For instance, treatment may be delivered over a bandaged wound or over a splint or cast.
4. There is relative uniformity of the induced magnetic field in the entire volume of the wound.[2]
5. Relatively good dosimetry can be achieved because the magnetic field lines are essentially parallel and remain in this alignment throughout the healing process.[2]

Theory and Science

Both PSWD and PRFS send EMF signals to the tissues, but they are not considered synonymous therapies. Both are classified as diathermy by the Food and Drug Administration (FDA) but in two separate classes: thermal and nonthermal. The cellular effects of PSWD have not been reported in the literature, but ongoing research is being

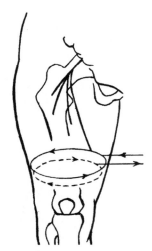

FIGURE 23-3 A PSWD or PRFS coil placed over the anterior thigh, showing the exciting current (solid line) and the resultant induced current (broken line). (Reprinted with permission from R. Kellogg, Magnetotherapy: Potential Clinical and Therapeutic Applications, in *Clinical Electrotherapy*, D.P. Currier and R.M. Nelson, eds., pp. 390–391, © 1991, Appleton & Lange.)

EXHIBIT 23-4 PSWD/PRFS Characteristics

- 27.12-MHz radio waves
- Modulation waveform square or pulse bidirectional
- Signal travels through air
- Not impeded by nonmetallic structures
- Pulse rates: 1–7,000 pps maximum;
  PR = maximum average intensity
- 200 pps → moderate to vigorous heating
- 90–200 pps → mild heat
- <90 pps → nonthermal
- Applicator: wire coil covered by housing
- Uniform magnetic field
- Induce electric current in tissues
- Deep penetration 5–6 cm up to 15 cm (MF value decreased by approximately the square of the distance)

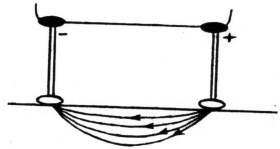

FIGURE 23-4 A pair of direct-contact electrodes used for HVPC and placed over the skin, showing the resultant current flow through the skin. (Reprinted with permission from R. Kellogg, *Magnetotherapy: Potential Clinical and Therapeutic Applications*, in *Clinical Electrotherapy*, D.P. Currier and R.M. Nelson, eds., pp. 390–391, © 1991, Appleton & Lange.)

conducted using radiofrequency in the thermal range for treatment of tumors; there are, however, numerous reports concerning the cellular effects of PRFS and PEMF. This is not to say that PSWD does not have similar effects on cells that are as yet unknown. CSWD and PSWD are considered thermotherapy but PRFS and PEMF are classified as non-thermal induced electrotherapy.

Thermotherapy

The practice of warming wounds to promote healing has been performed since ancient times, and warm soaks and warm compresses are still used for healing. Only recently have scientists begun to understand and explain why wounds respond to warmth. Under normal conditions, the skin is always colder than the core. The average periwound and wound temperature has been measured to be 4.5–5.6° F lower, respectively, than core temperature, so core temperature may not actually reflect the temperature of the wound bed.[20] Core hypothermia has been recognized as a factor in inhibition of platelet activation, decreased resistance to wound infection, and slowed wound healing. The inhibitory effects of hypothermia on platelet activation are completely reversed by warming the blood to 37° C.[21] Heat is also thought to counter the inhibitory effects of chronic wound fluid on fibroblasts. Raising the temperature of the wound by a degree or more could reduce the wound fluid inhibitory activity and assist in the healing of chronic wounds.[22]

Continuous Short-Wave Diathermy

The primary benefits of CSWD are attributed to the deep heating effects on muscle and joint tissues, which have a subsequent effect on tissue physiology. Early experimental and clinical research was focused on the effects associated with tissue heating that can occur when tissue temperatures are raised to 41–45° C in the deep tissue structures. CSWD and PSWD can be used to raise deep tissue temperature 5° C for therapeutic effects.[23] This was determined to be a safe

EXHIBIT 23-5   Wound Healing-Related Effects with PSWD/PRFS

- Perfusion of tissues is increased, either directly or indirectly.
- Deep tissue heating with PSWD allows heating within deep wounds and tunnels, including areas with abscess or infection.
- PSWD raises tissue temperatures.
- Painful wounds and associated soft tissue can be treated without direct contact.
- PSWD and PRFS provide analgesia of pain endings.
- PSWD and PRFS produce edema reduction.
- PRFS stimulates cellular activity and cell membrane signal transduction mechanisms.
- PRFS stimulation can take place over clothing, wound dressings, elastic wraps, splints and casting materials.
- No disruption of the wound healing environment is needed with PRFS.
- Stimulation of deep structures with PSWD, including nerves and blood vessels, can effect physiologic changes.
- PSWD and PRFS provide relative uniformity of the induced magnetic field in the entire volume of the wound.
- PSWD and PRFS provide relatively good dosimetry.

tissue temperature range when the body could respond to pain stimuli, and when there was a sufficient reservoir of blood with adequate cooling capacity to dissipate the heating through blood flow. Where circulatory occlusion is present, however, heating is contraindicated because, in limited circulatory systems, there is poor heat dissipation and consequently a higher risk for burns.[24]

Researchers in the 1930s, 1940s, and 1960s were interested in testing indirect diathermy applications (to the abdomen and sacrum) to effect peripheral blood flow dynamics in the feet and hands, resulting in several published studies. One study of blood-flow changes in normal adult women was published by Wessman and Kottke.[25] The parameters of the treatment were not stipulated, unfortunately. They did find statistically significant heating at the hands and toes, but less marked effects in the calf, from 13 to 37 minutes after CSWD, with effects lasting up to approximately 80 minutes after application of the diathermy. Heating was noted in the calf later than in the foot and in a two-step pattern. Researchers attributed the results to the ways that circulatory control of the two areas functions. In the foot, there are many arterioanastomoses, allowing greatly increased blood flow to occur in the foot. This shunting with indirect heating occurs to a lesser extent in the calf. It was apparent that changes of blood flow in the hand and foot do not represent changes of cutaneous flow throughout the body, nor do changes of blood flow to the calf or forearm indicate changes of muscular flow only.[25]

Clinical application of these findings suggests the use of indirect heating when direct application of heat to patients with peripheral vascular disease (PVD) may be dangerous. Conversely, heating of the torso may be dangerous for patients with cardiac disease. The fact that indirect heating effects lasted an average of 80 minutes after application of diathermy demonstrates that there is a long-lasting effect on the metabolism of the limbs.[25]

Early CSWD did not have a pulsed option and was, therefore, contraindicated for impaired circulatory conditions. In response, there was an effort to reduce the effects of continuous heating by developing pulsed short-wave equipment. The equipment that was developed allowed adjustment of the pulse rate, the interpulse interval, and the energy output, so that the heat created in the tissues during the on time would dissipate during the off time. Because the signal was pulsed, it was called *pulsed short-wave diathermy* and was described in early literature as "athermal." *Diathermy*, which means "heat through," is an inappropriate descriptor for a phenomenon without heat. Despite use of the term *athermal* that appears in the literature, this is not scientifically accurate. Biophysicists suggest that a better descriptor is the term *nonthermal* because the movement of atoms and molecules in all bodies produces some heat.

Tumors are more sensitive to heat than normal tissue because they are hypoxic, acidic, and poorly nourished. Hypoxic cells, as well as cells in the late S phase of the mitotic cycle (DNA synthesis), are normally more resistant to ionizing radiation, but are vulnerable to hyperthermia. There are reports of complete regression or partial regression of cancerous tumors when direct thermotherapy with radiofrequency, 8 or 13.6 MHz for 30–60 minutes, is used to raise local tissue temperatures to 41–44°C following radiation therapy. Tissues can be targeted and treatment methods adjusted, depending on the depth and size of the tumor. Currently, hyperthermia is being used only as an experimental treatment in late-stage cancers.[26] Irradiated tissues often develop fibrosis and are subject to skin breakdown, even many years after radiation therapy. Irradiated tissues treated with low frequency (8 MHz) high intensity (1.5 kW) CSWD for 30–60 minutes show an increase in blood flow and cell membrane permeability, resulting in increased ability to revascularize, repair, and prevent ischemia and fibrosis.[27]

Pulsed Short-Wave Diathermy

As described earlier, PSWD is a thermal agent that can heat both deep and superficial tissues. Silverman and Pendleton,[27] and Santoro et al[28] wanted to know whether indirect tissue heating in the abdomen and lumbosacral areas would raise the distal tissue temperature in the foot and the calf. In both studies PSWD, CSWD, and a placebo were used to treat young adults by placing the treatment head over the lower abdomen. Silverman and Pendleton's treatment protocol lasted 20 minutes at a high average power setting of 65 W and low average power of 15 W for both treatment machines. To achieve the high power, the pulse rate was set at 2,400 pps, and the low power pulse rate was 600 pps. Peripheral circulation was then measured in the calf and in the foot. The result was that the change in circulation was most prominent in the foot, and occurred only with high average power. The mean increase was 165% with pulsed high power and 195% with continuous high power. No circulatory effects were found in the foot with low power using either type of device. Temperatures were recorded under the treatment head. The mean increase in skin temperature was 5.3°C with continuous treatment and 5.8°C with pulsed treatment. The foot temperature increased 1.9°C and 2.2°C, respectively. Local heating occurred on the abdomen of the subjects who received low power, with mean changes of 3.1°C and 3.4°C respectively for CSWD and PSWD. Subjects reported a comfortable sensation under the treatment heads. These are statistically significant changes in temperature and blood flow overall, but not significantly different between the pulsed and continuous generators, confirming the ability of a PSWD generator to heat tissue.

In Santoro's study,[28] 10 patients with moderate to severe arterial PVD were treated with PSWD 5 days a week for 20 days, spread over a period of 1 month. The treatment consisted of a 30-minute, two-part protocol. During the first 20 minutes, the treatment was at maximum amplitude for the unit, which was a high-dose heating level, 95 μsec at a rate of 7,000 pps. During the last 10 minutes, the intensity was reduced to a low heating level, 95 μsec at a rate of 700 pps, in what was called a *cooling phase*. Two applicator heads were used, with one placed over the plantar surface of the foot and the second over the area of the anterior thigh. In cases in which both limbs were affected, both applicators were placed over the plantar surfaces of the feet. Variables measured included surface temperature, transcutaneous partial pressure of oxygen ($tcPO_2$), segmental Doppler blood pressure, superficial blood flow (measured with a laser Doppler flowmeter), and patient perceptions.

Findings were that temperature peaked at the end of the 20 minutes of high heat, and then gradually reduced. The $tcPO_2$ readings increased in the treated and the untreated limbs. They were insignificant in the treated limbs but significant in the untreated limbs, possibly because of reflex vasodilation from the warm circulating blood and sympathetic nervous system activity. Sixty percent of the patients reported subjectively that they felt that the treatment had improved their quality of life. No adverse effects were reported.[22] Exhibit 23-6 lists the effects of PSWD, and Table 23-2 summarizes clinical study reports on the effects of PSWD and PRFS on circulation.

EXHIBIT 23-6   Summary of Effects of PSWD

↑ Perfusion
↑ Local tissue $tcPO_2$
↑ Tissue metabolism
↑ Antibiotic delivery to tissue
↑ O_2 antimicrobial effect
↑ Cellular processes

TABLE 23-2 Clinical Studies of the Effects of PSWD and PRFS on Circulation

Researcher	Silverman and Pendleton[27]	Santoro et al[28]	Erdman[54]	Mayrovitz and Larsen[55]	Mayrovitz and Larsen[56]
Type of study Type of stimulator Frequency	Case series PSWD 80–2600 pps	Uncontrolled PSWD 7000 pps 90 μsec; 700 pps 95 μsec	Case series PRFS (Diapulse) 400 pps; 500 pps; 600 pps 65 μsec	Controlled PRFS (MRT Sofpulse) 600 pps 65 μsec	Controlled PRFS (MRT Sofpulse) 600 pps, 65 μsec
Amplitude	Average high power 65 W Average low power 15 W	Maximum power	Moderate power level (4) to peak (6) Av power 16 W at (4) Max of 40 W at (6)	Peak power 35 W Peak power	1 Gauss at skin surface
Duration of stimulation	20 min indirect heating at abdomen	20 min max amp indirect heating 10 min mod amp direct heating	Indirect stimulation at epigastrum	45 min 1x direct stimulation at the arm	45 min 1x direct stimulation of lower limb
Effect of Rx	Average increases tissue temp with pulsed high power at abdomen 5.8° C At foot 2.2° C Increase of 165% at foot Average increases tissue temp at low power at abdomen 3.1–3.4° C at foot no significant change	Insignificant temp increase in tx limb; Significant temp increase contralateral limb Increased tcPO₂ both limbs (Note: Temp peaked at 20 min)	↑ Av temp at foot 2.0° C ↑ Volume increase of 1.75 at max power	Blood flow: Mean group increase: 29% in treated limb Untreated: no change Skin Temp: Mean group 1.8° C ↑ skin temp treated limb Untreated limb: 0.5° C ↑ skin temp	↑ Blood flow volume at tx site; No increase at contralateral control site (Note: at baseline the ulcerated limb had higher BFV than contralateral) No increase in skin temp
Effect post Rx (15–30 min)	Not reported	Not reported	↑ Volumetric change Returned to baseline within 30 min post	Not reported	Not reported
Method of Measurement	Temperature	Temperature tcPO₂	Volumetric plethysmography Skin temperature readings	Skin temperature (thermistor) Laser Doppler Flowmeter	Skin temperature (thermistor) Laser Doppler Flowmetry
Health Status Tested and N	Healthy adults N not stated	Arterial PVD N = 10	Healthy young adults N = 20	Healthy adults N = 9	Diabetics N = 15 with foot ulceration, 9 with PVD

(Data from references listed in the table)

Further study is needed to determine the efficacy of thermotherapy (CSWD and/or PSWD) in prevention of tissue fibrosis and enhancement of healing of irradiated tissues. Like tumors, the chronic wound environment is often hypoxic, acidotic, and poorly nourished. Application of thermotherapy should be investigated clinically for its effects on chronic wound healing. At this time, the reports of successful outcomes for wound healing remain anecdotal.

Nonthermal PRFS and PEFS

Pulsing the radio waves did not solve all the problems of creating a truly nonthermal device. The next modification was to change the signal so that the signal was pulsed at lower rates and longer intervals. PRFS was introduced in the late 1950s, just as use of diathermy was waning. The first device that was approved by the FDA for medical use and appeared on the market was the Diapulse. The FDA allows the Diapulse Corporation to market the device as a short-wave diathermy class III device. Diathermy class III devices that are currently being marketed are described in the equipment section later in the chapter. It should be made clear that, although there are similarities between PSWD (thermal) and PRFS (nonthermal), they are not synonymous (Table 23-3). Several studies report the effects of nonthermal PRFS using commercially available PRFS devices.

The way in which manufacturers handle the technical specifications for their devices is the way in which the outputs are reported. Diapulse is constructed with vacuum tubes. Provant and MRT SofPulse were both solid-state analogues of Diapulse. Diapulse, MRT SofPulse, and Provant devices use fixed pulse duration, 65μsec for the former two and 42μsec for the latter. MRT Sofpulse used 3 milliseconds with pulse rate adjustable from 80 to 600 pps at the maximum generated power. When pulsed at the maximum rate, power was applied only 3.9% of the time. Equipment in this classification was designed to allow for dissipation of heat, and to reduce its accumulation. The FDA has designated all three of these devices as equivalent. Based on recent research and a change in product ownership, the MRT SofPulse is no longer on the market, having been replaced by a new SofPulse, sold by Ivivi Technologies (Northvale, NJ) with pulse durations from 2–5 μsec and repetition rates from 1–5 pps. This new device requires less than 20 watts input power and induces a magnetic field one-tenth the strength of the other three PRFS units.

Basic Science of Nonthermal PRFS and PEMF

Evidence has accumulated over the years that the body is positively affected by electrical currents, both capacitive and induced. However, the underlying processes that take place in the microenvironment are still not well understood. With the intent of improving the understanding of the mechanisms of action induced by applying PRFS to tissues, researchers have been focusing on its effects on different cellular systems. This section presents a synopsis of the effect of PRFS and PEMF on some cellular systems. Care must be taken when attempting to extrapolate findings in the laboratory to the human body.

The electromagnetic field (EMF) has been identified as the signal to the tissues that is the therapeutic factor, with the ability to modulate biologic phenomena.[2,29] EMF modulation of biologic processes depends first on the physiologic state of the injured tissues and whether or not a physiologically relevant response can be achieved and, second, on the use of an effective dose of EMF to the injury (target) site.[2,29] Effective dosimetry is achieved by configuring the waveform to satisfy the target response time and minimum amplitude required for nonthermal effects.[2,29] Cellular activity can be modified by induced changes in the electrical status of the cell, the cell membrane, and the cell-to-cell communications. Cell-to-cell communications via electrically conducting gap junctions increase EMF sensitivity by several orders of magnitude versus a single cell exposed to the same EMF source.[2,29] The PEMF signal modulates Ca^{2+} binding kinetics, stimulates all types of cell proliferation, affects the cell membrane diffusion and/or permeability, and moves negatively charged plasma proteins toward lymph capillaries. Cellular changes following treatment with PRFS have been observed to alter processes that are essential to tissue repair, including proliferation of parenchymal and connective tissue cells, synthesis of extracellular matrix proteins, collagenization, and acquisition of wound strength.[2,29]

The processes involved in cellular membrane signal transduction that research has shown are affected by an applied electric field of specific strength and form are receiving considerable attention. Normally cell membranes are impermeable to all compounds carrying a charge. Ions can move through specific protein membrane channels, and the application of an electric field of appropriate strength can open these channels. For example, the opening of the cal-

---

TABLE 23-3 Comparison of CSWD, PSWD, and PRFS Characteristics

Device	Signal	Pulse Rate	Effect
Continuous short-wave diathermy	27.12 MHz	Continuous	Heating, No heat dissipation
Pulsed short-wave diathermy	27.12 MHz	High repetition rate, moderate repetition rate	Limited heat dissipation, moderate heat dissipation
Pulsed radiofrequency stimulation	27.12 MHz	Low repetition rate	Heat dissipation, cellular effects

cium ion (Ca^{2+}) channels causes an increase of Ca^{2+} influx of Ca^{2+} that is released from intracellular stores.[30] Inflow of Ca^{2+} into the cells will activate cellular processes through the binding to calmodulin, which will then activate calmodulin-dependent kinases whose function is to phosphorylate proteins using ATP. What ensues is a biochemical cascade that has the potential to have far-reaching effects on cells, including cell orientation and migration, immune-cell functions, cell proliferation, cell shape changes, and ultimately on the optimal function of the body.[31,32] One application used by clinical researchers to test these effects involved the use of low-frequency EMF applied at a distance from the surface of venous ulcers to promote healing based on the concept that the EMF will interact with peripheral blood mononuclear cells (PBMC) via Ca^{2+} channels activating signal transduction cascades, promoting cytokine synthesis, and changing cell proliferation patterns.[33] More information about the methods and results of this study are provided below.

There is supporting research that EMF of appropriate strength also opens Na^+ and Na^+/K^+ channels. Enhanced Na^+ inflow causes an action potential resulting in the depolarization of the cell.[31] Another cellular study looked at the effect of EMFs on transduction pathways that regulate lymphocyte proliferation, and found that 0.1mT, 60 Hz EMFs can induce a 20% mean increase in the anti-CD3 binding to T-cell receptors of Jurkat cells. There was a relationship between cell proliferation and the amount of energy given. T-cells are key modulators of inflammation, and potentially EMF technology can be used to treat inflammatory diseases.[34]

Both electric and electromagnetic fields have demonstrated ability to produce a sustained upregulation of growth factors. A mechanism ascribed to stimulating cells with EMF is the induction of growth factors that in turn stimulate cell replication through a Ca^{2+} pathway is one mechanism ascribed to the effects of EMF cell stiumulation.[32] ES and EMF stimulate and regulate the expression of genes and the synthesis of growth factors in connective tissues for structural extracellular matrix (ECM) constituents, and dosimetric relationships have been described.[35] PEMF exposure stimulates mRNA expression of several bone morphogenic proteins (BMPs) and upregulates TGF beta mRNA. It has been suggested that the increase in TGF Beta-1 mRNA protein synthesis in osteoblast cultures is a direct result of the effect of the EMF on calcium/calmodulin-dependent pathways.[36] TGF Beta-1 is instrumental in the cascade of regulatory events involved in ECM formation, cell growth, and accelerated chondrogenesis. TGFBeta-1 actions and hypertrophic scarring are explained in Chapter 2. This process has been identified as one mechanism involved in the stimulation of osteogenesis. Originally, the exogenous application of PEMF was designed to mimic the asymmetric waveform that is detected when bone is dynamically deformed.[37] Now that the mechanism of PEMF effects is better understood, it is clear that waveform configuration plays an important role in dosimetry.[30] PEMF thresholds appear to encompass more

factors than dose response alone. Frequency, amplitude, and timing, singly or in combination, appear to be involved in the results of many of the experimental studies.[30,32,37]

PEMF safety appears to be well established. No toxicologic or teratologic effects have been demonstrated by in vitro or in vivo safety testing.[35,37] When adult human fibroblasts and chondrocyte cells were exposed to PSWD, there was a relationship between cell proliferation and the dose in terms of amplitude and time duration of energy given.[38] Mean input power to the applicator of 13.8 W (< 1 W in situ) and exposure for 10 minutes increased fibroblast proliferation significantly compared with control groups. Lower power to the applicator (6W) for 10 minutes increased proliferation of chondrocytes cells and response is dose and, most important, time dependent.[38] The purpose of the study was to determine the influences of different dosages applied to different cell types. This clearly demonstrates that a single treatment protocol may not have optimal benefits, and that more work is needed to understand and to develop protocols to meet the desired outcomes of treatment, depending on the phase of healing that is to be influenced.

Fibroblast proliferation varies significantly with treatment dose and duration. Twenty-four hours after treatment, fibroblasts that were exposed to 10 minutes of treatment at a dose of 32 mw/cm^2 showed half-maximally enhanced proliferation, but those subjected to longer durations of 15–60 minutes showed maximal cell proliferation.[32] Under the same treatment dose parameters, epithelial cells also showed maximal mitogenesis with treatment durations of 30 minutes. These treatment durations correspond with what is recommended in treatment protocols.

Knowledge is accumulating that support the potential of EMF to promote healthy responses at key points in the healing process, but specifics as to time and duration of application, and the necessary amplitude of the EMF signal for optimal outcomes is not yet available. That does not mean that their use should be postponed until more conclusive studies are completed. There is wide recognition of the value of these tools, and they have a proven safety and efficacy record (e.g. the hundreds of thousands of bone osteogenesis studies and patients treated) that suggests that they are appropriate interventions for the treatment of complex soft tissue wounds, as well as bone.

In fact, the current state of knowledge of the mechanism of PRFS bioeffects has recently allowed the peak input power to the applicator to be reduced from 300 W to < 10 W in the Ivivi SofPulse. This leads to more efficacious and faster therapeutic outcomes.[39] In addition, there is negligible radiofrequency interference on monitoring and life-sustaining electronic equipment. The reduced power requirement of modern PRFS devices has allowed the development of portable, battery-operated units which can be sent home with the patient. To achieve all of this, the PRFS signal now typically has a burst duration of 3 msec, vs 65 μsec, which repeats at 5 bursts per second, versus 600/sec, at a peak amplitude of 0.05G, versus 2G.

Hematoma and Thrombolysis

Rupture of small or large vessels accompanies both surgical and traumatic wounding, and produces thrombosis and hematoma in the tissues. Hematomas produced by pressure are often referred to as "purple ulcers" or more recently as a "deep tissue injury."[40–42] More information about hematoma and deep tissue injury is found in Chapter 4.

Basic Science and Animal Studies

Fenn[43] found that hematoma absorption in rabbit ears was accelerated compared with the control group, and that the acceleration became statistically significant on the sixth day after initiation of treatment with a Diapulse PRFS. One nonthermal phenomenon observed after application of PRFS with Diapulse was called a *pearl chain phenomenon*. When fat globules in milk were exposed to PRFS, the fat globules aligned into an order array of pearl chains and remained in that formation until the energy was removed. A second test using thermal energy caused agglomeration of the fat particles that was irreversible. This pearl chain phenomenon is also reproducible with blood and lymph cells.[44] Cameron[45] looked at wound healing in 20 dogs, comparing a control group of untreated animals with a Diapulse PRFS-treated group. He took specimens from 24 hours to 10 days after wounding and studied the tissues under the microscope. At 48 hours, the hematoma had been absorbed and replaced by fat that was arranged in strands migrating toward the ends of the wounds. By comparison, the control animals had minimal fat activity by the fourth day after wounding.

Human Clinical Trial

Sambasivan[46] treated four cases of extradural hematomas with a Diapulse PRFS. Treatment was applied twice daily for 10 days at a maximum pulse rate of 600 pps and a 65-μsec duration for 30 minutes per session, alternating right and left sides of the head. The treated cases showed clearance of their hematoma. If the results are reproducible, this could have tremendous potential for shortening healing times.

A high level of concern about the issue of deep-tissue injury and hematoma exists, but there is limited information about tested methods for thrombolysis of clotted blood associated with hematoma. Information presented here is a starting place for more study, both to validate the current findings and to develop clinical procedures. Clinicians can begin gathering data about wounds or soft tissue areas that are treated in the clinic that have hemorrhagic areas and report results. Based on what has been done before, there is little risk associated with this. The FDA allows PSWD manufacturers to list hematoma as an indication for application of PSWD, although no further evidence to support the efficacy was found in the literature review. Clinically, neither CSWD nor PSWD are widely used in the United States. However, a survey of 41 hospital-based physical therapy departments in Ireland found that PSWD was the preferred mode of treatment, often used more than once daily. Treatment efficacy was reported anecdotally for soft tissue injury and hematomas as well as other inflammatory conditions.[47]

Effects on Attributes of the Inflammatory Phase

The following clinical studies investigated the role of an intervention with PRFS and PSWD on attributes of the inflammatory phase: edema, pain, circulation, and tissue oxygen.

Edema and Pain

Ionescu et al[48] observed that, when burn wounds were treated with PRFS, there was prevention of edema formation, pain, and reduction in local symptoms. These observations led to further investigation to understand the mechanisms involved and to demonstrate objective proof. Local skin enzymatic activity was chosen as an indicator of the viability of the tissue. Samples of proteins and some principal enzymes in normal and burned tissue were compared before and after PRFS therapy. The enzymatic activities of the skin decrease when traumatized or burned. The data showed that, compared with normal skin, the enzymatic activity was significantly modified after the treatment. The earlier the application of treatment, the sooner the normal enzymatic activities were restored.

Reduction of soft-tissue edema resulting from trauma has been reported following treatment with PRFS for 20–30 minutes, and has persisted for several hours after treatment. The mechanism by which this occurs is postulated to be the effect of PRFS on sympathetic nervous system outflows, inducing vasoconstriction and restriction of blood flow from blood vessels to the interstitial areas around the wound site.[2]

Some PSWD devices can be set at a protocol that is mildly thermal. The Magnatherm and the Curapulse are such devices. (International Medical Electronics, Kansas City, MO), the Curapulse (Enraf Nonius, Delft, The Netherlands and Henley International, Sugarland, TX), A study of 25 podiatric surgical patients was conducted by Santiesteban and Grant[49] at a dosage of 700 pps and a power setting of 12, or approximately 120 W. This intensity is now called *mildly thermal*, but was reported in the study as *athermal*. A control group of 25 did not receive this treatment. Two electrodes were used, one over the plantar aspect of the postoperative foot and the other on the inguinal region. If both feet were operated on, the electrodes were placed over the plantar aspects of both feet. Two treatment sessions were given. One was given as soon after surgery as possible and the other 4 hours later. Nurses noted the number and types of pain medications used and the length of the hospital stay, measured in hours. There were significant differences between the treatment group and the control group. The former had a length of stay that was on average 8 hours shorter, and used weaker analgesic medication.[49]

Early intervention with PRFS (Diapulse) in the treatment of hand injuries was studied by Barclay et al[50] to compare the effects on edema, pain, and improvement of function.

Sixty matched pairs of patients who had hand injuries were evaluated within 36 hours of admission. In the treated group, with the exception of two cases, there was a complete resolution of edema by the third day, compared with the control subjects, whose swelling greatly increased. The 17 patients in the treated group were symptom free by the third day, and by day 7, only one in the treated group had slight loss of function; the 29 other patients had been discharged. By contrast, in the control group of 30 patients, 3 had been discharged, and the remaining 27 were still symptomatic with edema, pain, and loss of function.[50]

Acute ankle sprains have a rapid onset of edema and pain and are common injuries in athletes and in the military. Pennington et al[51] studied the effect of PRFS (Diapulse) on 50 patients with grade I and II ankle sprains at 1–24 hours, 25–48 hours, and 49–72 hours after injury and found a statistically significant decrease in the edema (0.95% versus 4.7%) and pain in the treatment group. Reduced pain was reported for 64% of the treated patients, compared with 33% for the control group. Because of the small sample size in the three different time-elapsed groups, no analysis was performed on this component but, overall, those patients who were treated within the 72-hour time frame had a statistically significant effect, including a significant decrease in the time lost from military training.[51]

In another study, two hundred acute head trauma patients with a Glasgow Coma Scale of 8 or less were alternately assigned to treatment with PRFS or to serve as controls.[46] The patients in this category had diffuse brain damage, multiple contusions, and brain edema, and were in poor states of consciousness. Except for the addition of the PRFS stimulation, the same management protocol was followed in the intensive care unit (ICU). PRFS stimulation at 600 pps for 30 minutes was given every 12 hours, with the drum alternating on the right and left sides of the head. Treatment began at the time of admission into the ICU. Serial computed tomography scans were done to evaluate the outcomes and for comparison with controls. In all cases, on the first day of admission to ICU, there was clear evidence of edema, and the ventricles appeared slitlike. By the tenth day, for those in the PRFS treatment group, the edema had disappeared, and the ventricles were seen well. However, in the control cases, it took 12–15 days to see the ventricles. Another measure reported for 20 cases was intracranial pressure (ICP). In the 10 cases receiving PRFS, the ICP diminished by the fifth day after injury and by day 7 came to near normal levels. Controls' ICP began to diminish by day 7. Mortality at the end of one month for the PRFS group was 24% in the PRFS group and 29% among controls.[46]

Early intervention during the inflammatory phase of healing was given credit for the successful outcomes in terms of reduced swelling and pain and early return to functional activities in the studies by Barclay et al,[50] Pennington et al,[51] and Ionescu et al.[48] Research information such as this can be used as a clinical guide for referral to the PT for evaluation of the appropriateness of this treatment following acute trauma. Then it is up to the PT to evaluate the treatment outcomes and to compare them with the research studies.

CASE STUDY

R.J., a 74 year old male, had hand surgery to remove a synovial mass located between the first and second metacarpal bones of his left (dominant) hand. There were incisions on both the dorsum of the hand and the palm because of the extent of the mass. Surgery was carried out with a regional anaesthetic block. Numbness prevailed for several hours after the surgery. Approximately 3 hours after surgery, a PRFS coil (Sofpulse) was used over the wound pressure dressing for a 30 minutes treatment. The treatment was repeated about 4 hours later. At bedtime, R.J. reported that the anaesthetic had worn off, he took two plain acetaminophen 500 mg tablets as a prophylactic for possible pain during the night and went to bed. Those were the only pain medications that he took. He continued to use the PRFS device several times daily for 30 to 60-minute sessions. When the pressure dressing was removed 5 days later, the incision was tender to pressure but otherwise the hand was free from pain. Edema was present in all the fingers and did not seem to be affected by the PRFS. He was able to use the hand functionally for self-care (dental hygiene, eating, dressing) from the first postoperative day. He continued to use the PRFS device for 3 weeks to facilitate the healing process and potentially improve the quality of the scar. There were no complications.

Circulatory Effects

Increased blood flow benefits wound healing by autolytic debridement of necrotic tissue, delivering critically needed oxygen and nutrients and removing metabolites. Local application of heat causes vasodilation of the vasculature and allows for increased blood flow. Infection rates are inversely proportional to blood flow and oxygen levels because, in this situation, oxygen functions equivalent to an antibiotic by oxygenation of the leukocytes, which are critical to fighting infection.[52] All of the processes of wound healing are oxygen dependent, including collagen deposition. Heat is a simple and effective method to enhance blood flow.[19, 53] For example, if blood flow can increase to the lower extremities without elevating body heat and if it can be maintained, it can then be applied as a helpful treatment of vasospastic PVD and could be beneficial in controlling infection. Treatment interventions that can increase perfusion to the tissues are important tools. The following studies report the effects of CSWD, PSWD, and nonthermal PRFS on blood flow to the extremities. Table 23-2 summarizes studies on circulatory effects.

Erdman[54] studied the effect of the Diapulse PRFS device, with the inductive head placed over the epigastrium, in a study measuring changes in blood flow to the feet of 20 normal young adults. The findings included a mean increase in foot temperature of 2.0° C and an average volume increase of 1.75-fold at the maximum generated power. Rectal temperatures did not change, nor did pulse rates. Furthermore, in all 20 cases, increased blood flow was directly proportional to the energy applied at the three highest settings. A short period of effect followed cessation of the treatment.

Mayrovitz and Larsen[55] reported that treatment with PRFS increased skin blood perfusion in the treated region. PRFS stimulation with the MRT SofPulse at 65 μsec at a pulse rate of 600 pps and peak power, applied for 40 minutes on the forearm skin of nine healthy men and women, produced enhanced microvascular perfusion, averaging 30% compared with pretest levels. Skin temperature was increased by an average of 1.8° C, but the rise occurred ahead of the measured increased perfusion. This is similar to the study by Erdman.[54] The mechanisms of action are not understood.

Mayrovitz and Larsen[56] conducted another study using the MRT SofPulse, also to study effects on perfusion. Laser Doppler red blood cell (RBC) perfusion, volume, velocity, and skin temperatures were evaluated for 15 subjects, each of whom had had diabetes for at least 5 years and each of whom had an ulcer on the foot or toe of one limb. Ulcer duration was a minimum of 8 weeks. The contralateral limb was intact and served as the control. Nine subjects had PVD, as confirmed by noninvasive vascular testing. Baseline data were collected for the multiple variables. The ulcerated limb had pretreatment perfusion and volume much greater than the control limb. A single treatment was administered at the periulcer site. The result was an increase in perfusion, measured by a laser Doppler, and increased skin temperature related to PRFS treatment. These preliminary findings suggest that, if the resting perfusion is marginally inadequate for healing, giving this small boost in perfusion may be sufficient to aid the healing of the ulcer. The parameters of the stimulation were 65 μsec, 600 pps, at peak power, with the head 1.5 cm above the surface of the ulcer.[56] Table 23-4 summarizes changes in tissue temperature after application of PSWD/PRFS.

Wound Healing Clinical Studies

The only studies on the efficacy of PSWD have been described under changes in tissue temperature and blood flow. There are no controlled clinical trials specifically investigating the efficacy of PSWD for wound healing. Several randomized, double-blind, controlled, and case study reports on PRFS efficacy for wound healing in animals and humans will be reviewed. A significant problem with the studies that was identified while reviewing the literature on electromagnetic radiation therapy for wound healing and related systemic factors was the inability to compare or combine the results of these studies because, in most cases, the study results reported are subjective, observational, qualitative data, rather than quantitative, statistically analyzed data. For example, most of the studies reviewed did not have data about the percentage of change in wound size per unit of time reported or data from which that information can be calculated. Systematic reviews of the literature are usually quantitative. No such reviews of the literature on the use of PSWD, PRFS, or PEMF have been made. The data from clinical studies are presented by disease state and intervention used. Using the levels of evidence and grades of recommended quality ratings, PRFS would have level II, III, IV, and V evidence and a recommendation grade of "B."

Researchers have branched out from investigating the effect of PEMF on osteogenesis to also look at its effects on soft tissue healing in animals and human subjects. However, stimulation periods using very low-frequency devices that demonstrate efficacy have been much longer than other treatments, up to 3 or 4 hours per day. Treatment at higher frequency and shorter duration had similar effects. The need for longer treatment periods or higher frequency and shorter duration is probably due to the need to accumulate sufficient pulse charge in the tissues to have a biologic effect on the target tissues (see chapter 22). There is a positive trend to the results for healing of venous ulcers. Although PEMF is not yet a typical application for wound healing, the results of the studies will be presented.

Additional quantitative studies are needed to support the limited evidence presented here. Several of the studies located were performed in countries outside of the United States, some were reported in peer-reviewed U.S. journals,

TABLE 23-4 PSWD/PRFS Change in Tissue Temperature

Device	Area Stimulated	Pulse Rate	Intensity	Tissue Temperature
PSWD	Abdomen	2,400 pps	High dose	↑ 1.5°C at abdomen[48] ↑ 2.2°C at foot[50]
PRFS	Abdomen	600 pps	Peak power	↑ 2.0°C at foot[22]
PRFS	Arm (normal subjects)	600 pps	Peak power	↑ 1.8°C[23]
PRFS	Foot (diabetics)	600 pps	Peak power	↑ 0.5°C[22]

and others were published in the journals of other countries. They are presented here for thoughtful consideration.

Animal Studies

Studies on nerve regeneration in rats treated with Diapulse (30 minutes daily for 3 weeks) showed that surgical incisions healed in 4 days in the treated rats and in 7 days in the controls. Early recovery of mobility (weight bearing) occurred in the treated group (10 days), compared to controls (21 days). Nerve conduction as evidence of tissue regeneration of peripheral nerves in the active treatment group was accelerated, and there was less scar tissue and fibrosis.[57]

Randomized controlled studies of the effects of PEMF on healing of cutaneous surgical wounds in animals (rats,[58,60] dogs,[61] rabbits[62]) demonstrate that PEMF significantly enhances wound epithelialization and provides significant short-term changes in other variables indicative of healing. In one study, PEMF was able to significantly reverse the impaired healing effect of corticosteroids.[58] In another study comparing PEMF and pulsed magnetic field (PMF) therapy (17 Hz), there was better collagen alignment in repaired tendons in the PMF (17 Hz) group than in a group treated with PEMF, and the PMF group suppressed extravascular edema better during early inflammation.[63] PEMF at different intensity was tested on ligament wound healing. Tissue stimulated by PEMF showed earlier increases in capillaries and fibroblasts, with better organization of collagen than controls. Amongst three intensities tested, the group treated with 50 G consistently had the best results during the study period.[63]

Human Clinical Studies

Human clinical studies reported in this section have been sorted by etiology of the wounding and include pressure ulcers, postsurgical wounds, and venous ulcers. Studies within each subsection are described in chronologic order, from oldest to most recent. Venous leg ulcer studies all have the use of PEMF in common. However, the parameters for treatment vary. Tables 23-5 (pressure ulcer clinical studies), 23-6 (postsurgical clinical studies), and 23-7 (venous ulcer clinical studies with PEMF) summarize the studies for each section.

Pressure Ulcers. Pressure as the wound etiology was the criteria for participation in the following clinical studies. Itoh et al[64] studied the effect of PRFS on stage II partial-thickness and stage III full-thickness ulcers. Comorbidities included cerebrovascular accidents, multiple sclerosis, organic brain syndrome, spinal cord tumor, diabetes, spinal cord injury, and spinal stenosis. Conventional treatments, dressings and topical agents, were continued. In all, 22 patients were included during the 9-month study. All ulcers healed. Stage II ulcers healed in 1–6 weeks (mean 2.33 weeks), and all stage III ulcers healed in 1–22 weeks (mean 8.85 weeks). Treatment was provided using the Diapulse PRFS device at a setting of 600-pps pulse frequency and a

setting of 6 (peak power) for 30 minutes twice daily. Treatment sessions were scheduled at approximately 8-hour intervals.[64]

Wilson[65] reported on results of recalcitrant pressure ulcers treated with PRFS (Diapulse). Twenty-five stage II, 11 stage III, and 14 stage IV pressure ulcers affecting 32 patients were enrolled in the uncontrolled study. Duration of ulcers was reported to be up to 2 years. Ages ranged from 77 to 88 years. All received conventional treatment for several weeks up to 2 years prior to inclusion in the PRFS study. Significant wound healing was observed on the most difficult ulcers in 3–7 days. Initially, wound exudate increased for 1–2 days, then ceased by the third day. All but one patient completely healed, and that individual's wound showed marked improvement before the patient died from other causes.[59]

Salzberg et al[66] studied 20 patients with spinal cord injuries, 10 of whom had stage II pressure ulcers and 10 who had stage III pressure ulcers. The group was randomized to 10 treated and 10 sham-treated groups. Again, the device tested was the Diapulse. Although the study did not list the treatment parameters, an inquiry to the principal author and the Diapulse Corporation provided the information that the settings were 600-pps pulse frequency and 6, peak power. The treatment lasted for 30 minutes twice daily for 12 weeks or until the ulcers healed. Results were that the active treatment group with stage II ulcers had a shorter mean time to complete healing than did the control group (13.0 days versus 31.5 days). The stage III ulcers also healed faster than the controls, but the size of the group was very limited. The study authors' conclusion was that the treatment significantly improved healing.[66]

Seaborne et al[67] randomized 20 nonambulatory individuals with pressure ulcers of the trochanter and sacrum into four groups of five subjects each for a study with PSWD. Allocations were concealed and assessors blinded. Each group was treated with one of four different protocols. Protocols were electrostatic field (electrical stimulation) at 20 and 110 pps, and PEMF nonthermal at 20 and 110 pps. An ABAB repeated measures experimental design was used, with each treatment regimen lasting one calendar week. Multifactorial analysis showed highly significant reduction in the pressure ulcer surface area in all treatment groups, without significant difference between the groups.[67]

Postsurgical Wounds. Cameron[68] undertook three studies on the effect of PRFS (Diapulse) on postsurgical wound healing. Study 1 was a 100-patient, double-blind study of postsurgical patients, study 2 was an observational uncontrolled study of 81 postsurgical and orthopaedic patients, and study 3 was a 465-patient observational uncontrolled study of nonsurgical orthopedic patients. In studies 1 and 2, each patient was treated twice daily for 20 minutes over the liver and 20 minutes over the wound (400 pps, 4-inch penetration) for 4 days after their operation. Patients in the third study were outpatients and were given the regimen twice daily 3 days a week for 2 weeks, then twice a day on Mon-

TABLE 23-5   Pressure Ulcer Clinical Studies

Researcher	Itoh et al[64]	Wilson[65]	Salzberg et al[66]	Seaborne et al[67]
Type of study	Uncontrolled Unblinded Observational	Uncontrolled Observational	Double Blind-RCT	Blinded-RCT
Type of stimulator	PRFS (Diapulse)	PRFS (Diapulse)	PRFS (Diapulse)	ES Vs PEMF
Frequency	600 pps 65 μsec	Not stated	600 pps 65 μsec	20 pps ES 110 pps ES 20 pps PEMF 110 pps PEMF
Amplitude	Peak power	Not stated	Peak power	
Duration of stimulation	30 minutes BID	Not stated	30 minutes BID for 12 weeks	
Effect during Rx	All patients healed Stage II healed mean 2.33 weeks Stage III healed mean 8.85 weeks Mean size: 5.56 cm² ± 4.18 Mean size: 8.78 cm² ± 11.96 *Mean healing/week: Stage II 57% Stage III 8.87%	Initial increase in wound exudate (1–2 days) All wounds healed except 1	Stage II Active group: 84% healed at 1 week Median no. days to complete healing: 13.0 Placebo: 40% healed at 1 week Median no. days to complete healing: 31.5 Stage III Ulcer area Active group: decreased average of 70.6% (*5.9%/week) Placebo: 20.7% (*1.7%/week)	All groups showed highly significant reduction in surface area size. No statistical difference between groups
Method of Measurement	Size measurement Photographs	Observational	Prospective Size measurement	Reduction in surface area size
Disease state tested and N	Pressure ulcers N = 9 stage II 13 stage III	Pressure ulcers N = 25 stage III 11 stage III 14 stage IV	Pressure ulcers/SCI N = 10 stage II 10 stage III	Pressure ulcers N = 20 (4 groups of 5)

* Percentage size change per week calculated from the study data.

TABLE 23-6 Postsurgical Clinical Studies

Researcher	Goldin et al[69]	Cameron[68]	Santiesteban and Grant[49]	Kaplan and Weinstock[70]	Aronofsky[71]	Comorosan et al[73]
Type of study	DB-RCT	Study I DB Controlled Study 2 Uncontrolled	RCT	DB-RCT	CT (nonrandomized, unblinded)	CT
Type of stimulator	PRFS (Diapulse)	PRFS (Diapulse)	PSWD	PRFS (Diapulse)	PRFS (Diapulse)	PRFS (Diapulse)
Frequency	400 pps/600 pps 65 μsec	400 s 65 μsec	700 pps 95 μsec	400 pps/600 pps 65 μsec	600 pps 65 μsec	400 pps/600 pps 65 μsec
Amplitude	25.3 W/38 W	Med power (4)	120 W (max power setting)	Peak power (6) Med power (4)	Peak power	Peak power (6) Med power (4)
Duration of stimulation	10 min (hepatic) 20 min (wound) every 6 hours × 7 days	Study 1 20 min (hepatic) 20 min over wound BID × 4 days Study 2 Same as in study 1	30 min after surgery and 4 hrs later	Before surgery 10 min BID post 15 min to wound and 15 min epigastrium (hepatic)	Gr 1: 15 min 24 hr preop and 10 min just preop Postop: 24 hr, 48 hr, 72 hr Gr 2: 10 min postop Postop: 24 hr, 48 hr, 72 hr Gr 3: no PRFS	10 min (hepatic) 15 min (wound)
Rx Effect	90% or greater healing for 59% of tx group 29% healing for sham group Evaluated but not reported statistically significant results for healing	Study 1 Tx group little improvement for abdominal incision with regard to suture removal; all other had sutures removed on day 5 postop Study 2 Shorter hospital stay for tx group	Active group had 8 hr shorter length of hospital stay than controls and significantly less pain medication	Postop day 3: Severe/moderate edema Placebo 80% PRFS 58%	Inflammation and pain 72 hr post: Gr 1: None 75% Mod 20% High 3.% Gr 3: None 2% Mod 57% High 37% Pain: Gr 1: None 63% Mod 30% High 6.7% Gr 3: None 7% Mod 57% High 37%	Plasma; fibronectin concentrations ↑ on postop day 7 in tx group; lower than baseline in control group

(Continued)

TABLE 23-6 *(Continued)*

Researcher	Goldin et al[69]	Cameron[68]	Santiesteban and Grant[49]	Kaplan and Weinstock[70]	Aronofsky[71]	Comorosan et al[73]
Method of Measurement	Degree of pain	Retrospective review of medical records Subjective measurements	Retrospective review of medication and length of stay records	Likert-like scale grading for edema, erythema, and pain	Healing in group 1: 3–5 days postop Group 2: 5–7 days postop Group 3: 10–12 postop	Observation of inflammatory and infectious process and scar formation Lab measurements
Etiology tested and N	Split-thickness skin graft donor sites N = 29 active 38 sham	Heterogenous surgical patients Study 1 N = 100 Study 2 N = 81	Post podiatric foot surgery N = 25 active 25 control	Postsurgical podiatric patients	Oral surgery N = 90 (30/group)	Heterogenous surgical wounds N = 15 active 10 control

(Data from references listed in the table.)

TABLE 23-7 Venous Ulcer Clinical Studies with PEMF

Researcher	Ieran and Zaffuto[74]	Todd et al[76]	Duran et al[75]	Stiller et al[77]	Kenkre et al[78]
Type of study	DB CT	DB-RCT	Observational	DB-RCT	DB-RCT
Type of stimulator	PEMF	PEMF	PEMF	PEMF	PEMF
Frequency	75 Hz	5 Hz	Not available	25% duty cycle	600 Hz 800 Hz
Amplitude	28 mT	Field strength 60	Not available	0.06 mV/cm 22 Gauss	25 μT
Duration of stimulation	4 hr daily × 90 consecutive days	15 min twice weekly	15 min × 10 treatments	3 hr daily × 8 weeks	30 min 5x/week × 30 days
Effect during Rx	Healing of exp group Av 71 days 30% decrease in size of ulcers in controls	• Mean reduction of ulcer size: 7% was the same for treatment and control groups • Girth of affected leg: Active: decrease 2.77% Control: increase 1.16%	33% reduction in mean surface area	• Wound surface area: 47.1% decrease for active 48.7% increase for placebo • Wound depth decrease: 46% for active; 3.8% for placebo • Granulation tissue: quantity and quality 14.1% decrease in unhealthy granulation in active 0% decrease for placebo • Clinical Assessment based on 8-pt scale: 50% of active group healed or markedly improved 54% of placebo group rated worse 0% of active group rated worse	Wound surface area: Gr A Placebo ↓ 14.2% (20 days) ↓ 21.8% (30 days) Gr B1 600 Hz ↑ 28.15% (20 days) ↑ 76% (30 days) Gr B2 800 Hz ↓ 24.7% (20 days) ↓ 38% (30 days)
Effect post Rx	Healing continued post-tx period for the tx group 25% reoccurrence in tx group vs 50% in controls				4 week observation period. Day 50 B2 800 Hz group had significantly greater healing (63% vs 34% Gr A) + improved mobility
Method of Measurement	Healing	Reduction in surface area size	Reduction in surface area of ulcer	Wound characteristics	Reduction in surface area size Pain reduction; QOL
Etiology tested and N	Venous ulcers N = 44	Venous leg ulcers N = 19	Venous ulcers N = 18	Venous ulcers N = 31	Venous leg ulcers N = 19

(Data from references listed in the table.)

TABLE 23-7   continued with additional study

Researcher	Canedo-Dorantes[33]
Type of study	CCT (patient own control)
Type of stimulator	PEMF
Frequency	60 Hz
Amplitude	120 V (36.36 Gauss Field Strength)
Duration of stimulation	2-3 hours 3 × weekly for 4 months
Effect during Rx	Responders:
	Arterial ulcers 15/ 17 healed or decreased >50%
	Venous ulcers 14/25 healed or decreased > 50% in size
	* healing rates were same both groups
	Nonresponders:
	Arterial ulcers: 2/ 17 healed poorly or increased in size
	Venous ulcers: 11/ 25 healed poorly or increased in size
Effect post Rx	Responders remained healed 6 months to 2 years post Rx
Method of Measurement	Digitized photography measured size and tissue appearance
Etiology state tested and N	Predominently Arterial : N :17 ulcers ; 8 patients
	Venous: 25 ulcers ; 18 patients
	Median ulcer duration all patients 639 days.

day and Friday, then once weekly (twice a day). The PRFS was used as an adjunctive treatment to other standard methods of care.

Outcomes were evaluated by the surgeon, who was asked to complete a questionnaire rating whether the patient's condition was the same, better, or worse, as compared with other patients in their experience. The groups analyzed by same, better, or worse showed no statistically significant difference in the treatment and control groups. There was a moderate reduction in length of hospital stay in the treatment group except in those with back surgery. The 81-patient study results demonstrated short hospital stays, despite the fact that some of the patients had osteomyelitis. The outpatient study of 465 patient results showed that acute trauma and inflammatory processes responded the best, but less than 20% were well within 3–4 weeks, which is what would have been expected normally. There also appeared to be no significant benefit from the PRFS treatment of chronic cases.

There were some methodologic problems with the Cameron studies. Too much emphasis was placed on subjective clinical findings. Use of other treatment modalities along with the PRFS did not allow for an accurate evaluation of the PRFS stimulation, and absence of inferential statistics further compounds the methodologic problems associated with this study.

A double-blind, controlled clinical trial by Goldin et al[69] used Diapulse PRFS to study the effects on healing an pain in medium-thickness split-skin grafts. The patients were randomized into two groups, 29 in the active treatment group and 38 in the sham treatment group. The parameter for the treatment group was peak output frequency, 400 pps. The average pulse was fixed at 65 μsec. Mean energy output was nonthermal, 25.3 W. Treatment was given preoperatively and postoperatively every 6 hours for 7 days. Two variables were evaluated: the stage of healing and the degree of pain during the healing phase. Healing rates on day 7 were 90% or greater healing for 59% of the treatment group and 29% of the sham-treated group. Mechanisms of healing are not clear. Theories to explain the results include increased blood flow and reduced incidence of edema. The stimulation of the cells of repair and repolarization of the depolarized cell membranes of damaged cells that reversed the "injury potential" and the electrical field were thought to be the mechanisms of action.[69]

A double-blind randomized clinical evaluation of PRFS (Diapulse) following foot surgery in 100 patients was reported by Kaplan and Weinstock.[70] The average number of surgical procedures performed was slightly less than five. As in other studies with Diapulse, the protocol called for 400 pps over the epigastrium and 600 pps over the surgical site. Power level was at 4 for 15 minutes and 6 for 15 minutes to the respective areas. Treatment began before surgery with a 10-minute treatment. A Likert-type scale was used to grade the tissue for symptoms of edema, erythema, and pain. Results reported were statistically significant reduction in severe to moderate edema in the treatment group at the third post operative day (80%) versus controls (58%); however, the data were reported descriptively.

Dental surgery procedures are often the cause of pain, edema, ecchymosis pressure, and disfigurement. In a nonrandomized controlled clinical trial, 90 dental surgery patients were divided into three groups of 30 each.[71] They were treated with Diapulse at 600 pps peak power 72 hours preoperatively and postoperatively, only postoperatively 72 hours, or with placebo. Results reported were statistically significant absence of inflammation and pain at 72 hours postoperatively for the pre/post operative treatment group.

Children undergoing orchidopexy were treated in a double-blind clinical trial. A total of 50 paired boys were involved in the trial. Circumferential measurements of the scrotum were made before and after surgery and treatment of the scrotum, and photographs were taken. Repeat measurements and photographs were taken, with the objective of reducing subjective observation reports of edema and bruising. Treatment was with Diapulse at 500 pps and level 5 intensity for 20 minutes over the scrotum and at 500 pps level 4 intensity over the epigastrium for 10 minutes. The treatment regimen was repeated three times daily for the first 4 postoperative days. Matched pairs of boys were used, with one as the control. Investigators chose this operation as a model because of its classic edema and bruise formation. Results suggest that there was a trend toward improvement in edema formation, and resolution of posttraumatic bruising was found to be significantly accelerated.[72]

Another study of postsurgical wounds treated with Diapulse over the wound site and over the hepatic area was reported by Comorosan et al.[73] Fifteen patients were selected for treatment, and 10 served as the control group. The local application was at 600 pps at maximum power output for 20 minutes and the hepatic application at 400 pps at a power setting of 4 for 10 minutes. Treatment started on the second postoperative day and continued for 5 days. Comorosan et al[73] reported that the results of this protocol were evaluated by looking at the clinical criteria for wound healing, including the disappearance of edema, hematoma, and parietal seroma; the lack of inflammatory and infectious processes; the suppleness and presence or absence of keloids in the scar; and the degree of postoperative sensitivity. All clinical wound attributes evaluated showed clear-cut improvement. An additional analysis of the effects of the hepatic stimulation showed increased fibronectin levels in the treated patients and lower fibronectin levels in the controls. This is another measure of healing.

Venous Leg Ulcers. No clinical studies reporting results of PRFS or PSWD on treatment of venous ulcers were located, but the results of PEMF stimulation of venous ulcers have been reported in several studies. The nature of PEMF stimulation is that it is undetectable by the patient or the clinician.

Ieran and Zaffuto[74] carried out a double-blind study of 44 patients with skin ulcers of venous origin using a coil electrode to generate a PEMF with 75 Hz and 2.8 mT intensity for 4 hours daily for 90 consecutive days. Healing was within 71 days, on average. Success was significantly higher in the experimental group, both on day 90 and in the follow-up period. Twenty-five percent of the patients in the experimental group and 50% in the control group experienced recurrence of the ulcer.[74]

Duran et al[75] reviewed 18 cases with venous ulcers who were treated 10 times with PEMF, each session lasting 15 minutes. They found a significant reduction in the mean surface area of 33% by reepithelialization following treatment with PEMF. A double-blind randomized controlled clinical trial of 19 patients with venous ulcers used a protocol applying PEMF two times weekly over a 5-week pe-

riod.[76] Treatment parameters were field strength of 60, 5 Hz intensity, and duration of 15 minutes. Treatment was carried out by placing coils on either side of the ulcer over the wound dressings. Parameters measured were ulcer size, lower leg girth, degree of pain, and presence of infections. The findings were that there was no statistically relevant difference noted between the active and inactive treatment groups. However, there was a trend in favor of a decrease in ulcer size and lower leg girth in the active treatment group and no proliferation of bacterial populations. No effect was noted on report of pain. One patient in the study in the active treatment group had an initial ulcer size that was so large that it skewed the mean ulcer pre- and posttreatment areas. Removing this patient's ulcer from the study group reflected truer results that showed a trend toward improved healing but was not statistically significant (17.5% in active treatment versus 7.1% in sham treatment). Another study defect was the mean initial duration of the venous ulcer, which ranged from a mean 3.5 years for the active treatment group to a mean of 18.3 years for the sham group.[76] The results of this pilot study are inconclusive, due to the small sample size and lack of rigor in selecting the patients. Also, the duration and frequency of the treatment were perhaps too minimal to have a more statistically significant treatment effect.

Thirty-one patients were enrolled in a prospective, randomized, double-blind, placebo-controlled multicenter study by Stiller et al[77] of venous ulcer healing to determine the efficacy of PEMF treatment.[77] Recalcitrant venous ulcers showed after 8 weeks that the active treatment group of 18 had a 47.7% decrease in wound surface area versus 42.3% for the placebo group of 13 ($p < .0002$). A global evaluation of the wounds indicated that 50% of the ulcers in the active group healed or markedly improved versus 0% in the placebo group. None of the active group of ulcers worsened versus worsening in 54% of the placebo group ($p < .001$). Likewise, there were statistically significant decreases in wound depth and pain intensity in the active group. Results were achieved using a portable home device that the patient or caregiver applied for 3 hours daily for 8 weeks or until the ulcer healed, if prior to 8 weeks. Treatment parameters were 3.5-msec pulse width, bidirectional delta B of approximately 22 G. The protocol was derived from the study of PEMF used effectively to treat nonunion fractures. Researchers concluded that PEMF is a safe and effective nonsurgical therapy for recalcitrant venous leg ulcers. The subjects in this trial may have done better than the earlier group because the duration of the stimulation, given on a daily basis, allowed for enough pulse charge accumulation to reach the target tissues and produce a biologic effect.

Kenkre[78] reported the results of a study with 19 patients with venous leg ulcers enrolled in a prospective, randomized, double-blind controlled clinical trial. Outcome measures were rate and scale of ulcer healing, changes in pain levels, quality of life, degree of mobility, side effect profile, and acceptability to patients and staff. The device used was the Elmedistraal electromagnetic device (available in the

United Kingdom) that delivered perpendicular electric and magnetic fields through a pulse generator, creating frequencies of 100, 600, and 800 Hz. The magnetic field produced was 25 μT. These parameters appear to be similar to PRFS, although the study is called "electromagnetic therapy." Sixty-eight percent of the active treatment group achieved improvement in ulcer size, and 21% of those experienced complete healing. Reduction of pain levels was also statistically significant, despite the chronicity of the ulcers. Those treated at 800 Hz were found to have statistically greater healing and pain relief than either those in the 600-Hz group or the control group at day 50. However, the treatment phase ended at day 30, and, at that time, the trend for healing was better in the control group and the 800-Hz group, compared with the 600-Hz group but reduction of pain scores was greatest in the 600-Hz group. In all three groups, some ulcers with a long history of chronicity healed. It appears that, as in the Ieran study,[74] the effects of the treatment continued after cessation of the treatment. Adverse effects reported were sensations of heat, tingling, pins and needles in the lower half of the limb, and headaches (unusual for two patients), but patients who experienced these sensations continued with the study. Psychosocial benefits of improved mobility and community activity were reported.

Canedo-Dorantes et al [33] evaluated healing of patients with chronic arterial and venous leg ulcers that were resistant to medical and surgical treatment. The subjects were grouped as follows: group I, 8 patients with 17 ulcers of predominantly arterial origin, and group 2, 18 patients with 25 chronic leg ulcers of predominantly venous origin. Systemic treatments for pain, rheumatoid arthritis, arterial hypertension and diabetes were continued but other systemic medications and preventive treatments were discontinued. Local wound care was limited to wound cleansing with soap and water and covering with an unspecified dressing. The team of researchers used a novel approach, applying the EMF to either *arm* not the ulcer directly. The purpose of this alternative application was to determine whether the EMF could alter systemic effects by interaction with EMF action potentials at a peripheral location. The hypothesis was that peripheral blood mononuclear cells could be induced in the body of the patients with chronic leg ulcers by using EMF frequencies that were previously tested on normal human blood samples. The treatment method described was to place an arm into an exposure chamber so as to achieve a homogeneous magnetic field. Average exposure time was 2-3 hours per day three times a week for a 4 month period. EMF strength of 36.36 G was generated inside the chamber. Wound surface area size and appearance were documented at baseline and during follow ups photographically and the information digitized and processed electronically. Results were reported by groups, with "responders" fully healed or experiencing a greater than 50% reduction, while "nonresponders" had at least one ulcer that experienced a less than 50% reduction or increased in size. Healing or deleterious effects were observed in all patients within the first two weeks after initiation of the treatment. No negative secondary effects were reported either during treatment or the follow up period. Responders with 29 previously unresponsive ulcers began to heal by week 2 and by the end of the study period 15 arterial and 14 venous ulcers were in the responder groups; 2 arterial and 11 venous ulcers were in the nonresponder groups. Group demographics showed the following associations: Responders healed at the same rates, the arterial ulcer group showed the development of visible vascular networks and increased periwound temperatures after 4–8 weeks of treatment. Nonresponders in the venous group had higher body mass index, had nonpitting edema and severe lipodermatosclerosis. The arterial group had severe arterial occlusion and or uncontrolled arterial hypertension. Pain among nonresponders only partially reduced in 4–6 weeks of treatment. In the responders with venous ulcers, pain, edema, and weeping reduced significantly or were eliminated 3–6 weeks after start of care.

All of these studies represent a small sample of patients with leg ulcers but there seems to be a trend that shows treatment efficacy with PEMF for patients with this wound etiology. More work is needed to establish treatment parameters and the utility of this treatment for venous ulcers.

Summary

The prior section reviewed and evaluated the scientific studies of the mechanisms and efficacy of PSWD, PRFS, and PEMF on components related to tissue repair and clinical trials of wound healing. PSWD studies described the thermotherapy effects on the body. PSWD effects are attributed to changes to the circulatory system and the autonomic nervous system, whereas the effects of PRFS and PEMF are attributed to changes in the cellular activity of the tissues and mechanisms that control blood flow and edema that are not heat related. PRFS and PEMF studies reported effects on the cells' and the body's bioelectric systems. Both PSWD and PRFS devices showed that they can increase blood flow, which increases oxygen transport essential to support the metabolic demands of the tissues and to control infection. All three modes of electromagnetic stimulation affect pain and edema during the inflammatory phase. Because the treatment outcomes desired are edema-free and pain-free, and these are benefited by enhanced circulation, it is logical to choose a treatment approach with demonstrated outcomes for these aspects of the inflammatory phase. If the circulatory effects desired require deep heating such as to raise core body temperature, then PSWD would be the first choice. A protocol for PSWD is given that is based on the circulatory effect on acute, subacute, and chronic inflammation. How PSWD or PRFS could affect ischemia reperfusion injury (see Chapter 2) would be a useful study. The effects on the inflammatory phase of healing are well established, but information about the affect on phases of healing following inflammation until closure is very limited. Enhanced circulation and oxygen are requirements of all the phases of healing, so continuation during all phases is appropriate. PRFS is the preferred choice if the objective is to stimulate the body's bioelectric system at the cellular level, over a dressing, cast, or bandage; to increase peripheral micro-circulation; to prevent or minimize edema; to avoid and relieve pain; or if the patient has a medical history that rules out heat (see "Selection of Candidates" section, below). Treatment effects should be seen within hours for acute wounds and in 3–7 days from the start of the protocol for chronic wounds.[65-67] Reported effects include increased wound exudate for the first 1–3 days. Progress through the phases of healing should continue throughout the episode of care.

PSWD and PRFS are similar but not identical. They both are radio wave signals from the short-wave spectrum. PSWD has the ability to heat tissue; PRFS does not. Both have reported increased perfusion and blood flow in normal adults. Only two studies by Santoro et al[28] and Mayrovitz and Larsen[42] looked at the effect of PSWD and PRFS on blood flow changes in individuals with PVD. Cellular changes are reported for stimulation with PRFS but not for PSWD, although that does not rule them out, and they should be investigated. Exhibits 23-4 and 23-7 list the characteristics and rationale for selecting PSWD and PRFS.

PEMF stimulators have distinctly different parameters than the radiofrequency stimulators and are not found in PT clinics or wound clinics because they are typically used by orthopedic surgeons for nonunion fracture healing. Initially used for osteogenesis of nonunion fractures, PEMF has now been tested for soft tissue wound healing in venous ulcers with good outcomes in pilot studies. More research with PEMF is needed to standardize the methodology of treatment, to produce objective data about healing, and to verify results. A limited number of studies have been reviewed, and the most recent are animal and PEMF studies. Although the results presented look promising, more new studies are needed to answer questions about the effects of PSWD, PRFS, and PEMF on wound healing. There remain many unknowns about mechanisms of action, and there is a need for improved study designs and reporting of the data with objective quantitative results. For example, the rate of healing has been identified as a predictor of healing outcome and the trigger for referral for adjunctive therapy.[79-83] The study data for most of the research projects testing these interventions did not provide quantitative information about the rate of healing of the control or the treatment groups, making it impossible to compare rate of healing between study intervention and controls and between other adjunctive therapy interventions. Except for two studies where the percentage of change could be derived from the data reported, the best available data are the percentage of patients that healed in a study and those that did not. One factor is evident from compiling the matrices of studies for different applications of PRFS, namely that the Diapulse protocol, 400 pps, power level 4 over the epigastrium, and 600 pps peak power over the target tissue, has been followed consistently, with treatment efficacy reported for each application. Although many of the studies are reported as double-blind randomized controlled trials, it is also evident that many of the data reported are observational descriptive data, rather than quantitative.

To review, the studies looked at seven components that the PT should consider when selecting this intervention.

1. PRFS and PEMF stimulate cellular activity and cell permeability.
2. PRFS and PEMF affect the body's bioelectric system.
3. PSWD and PRFS affect edema formation but possibly through different processes.
4. PSWD, PRFS, and PEMF prevent or modulate pain.
5. PSWD and PRFS affect circulation, as measured by increased blood flow and $tcPO_2$, but through different processes.
6. PRFS promotes absorption of hematoma.
7. PSWD heats tissue; PRFS does not.

Patients who were treated in the clinical studies had acute postsurgical wounds, including split-thickness skin grafts, or posttrauma, and chronic pressure ulcers, venous or arterial leg ulcers. The wounds were either partial- or full-thickness tissue disruption, extending into deeper tissues (e.g., stages II through IV pressure ulcers). None of the effects of treatment described are dependent on the medical diagnosis, the wound etiology, or the depth of the wound. However, wounds that are deep, large, or of long duration have been identified as slower to heal. Those wounds will probably heal faster with one of these adjunctive therapy interventions.

EXHIBIT 23-7 Wound Classification and Characteristics

Wound Classification	PSWD/PRFS
Level of tissue disruption	Superficial, partial thickness, full thickness, subcutaneous and deep tissues
Etiologies/diagnostic groups	Burns, neuropathic ulcers, pressure ulcers, surgical wounds, vascular ulcers
Wound phases	*Inflammatory phase:* necrosis, exudate, edema, pain
	Proliferative phase: Granulation, contraction, collagen synthesis, angiogenesis
	Epithelialization phase: epidermal migration
	Remodeling: collagen organization

Applying Theory and Science to Clinical Decision Making

Selection of Candidates

A comprehensive patient history, systems review, and examination are very important in making a clinical decision to choose either PSWD or PRFS. Review the history and systems for information about sensation, circulation, edema, metal and electronic implants, acute osteomyelitis, cancer, and pregnancy. According to the manufacturer's labeling requirements, PSWD is contraindicated for all conditions for which heat is contraindicated. PSWD should not be used over areas of insensitivity that prevent the patient from reporting a sensation of heating. One way to mitigate the heating effect of PSWD is to leave a greater air gap or more toweling between the applicator and the tissues. Check pulses and perform other visual examinations to detect circulatory deficits. If findings show diminished circulation, noninvasive vascular testing may be required. Do not use PSWD over ischemic tissue (e.g., an ankle-brachial index of less than 0.8) because the body requires adequate perfusion to regulate tissue temperature. If circulatory perfusion is obstructed, it may not allow for the heat to dissipate and result in burning. However, consider indirect heating with PSWD or PRFS over the lumbar area or the abdomen that will produce reflex vasodilation in areas remote from the site of heating, e.g., the foot.[54,56] This is also suggested for patients with vasospasm.

Do not use PSWD over metal, including surgical metal hardware; foreign bodies, such as shrapnel, bullets, or metallic sutures; or intrauterine devices. The metal may become heated and reflect high levels of energy that will cause burns. Do not use PSWD if the patient has electronic implants or is connected to electrical or electronic equipment because the EMF of the PSWD may cause interference with these electronic devices. PSWD is contraindicated over any area where there is primary or metastatic malignant tissue growth or over organs or tissues containing high fluid volumes (e.g., the heart, edematous extremity, and over the abdomen and lumbar areas during pregnancy). Treatment is contraindicated over areas with acute osteomyelitis without adequate drainage or before drainage has been established. A diagnosis of active tuberculosis would be a contraindication for PSWD. Review the patient's vital signs. Patients who are febrile should not be treated with additional heat; however, nonthermal PRFS could be used. Check the pharmacy history for blood-thinning medications and tendency for hemorrhage. Patients in the first 24–48 hours after traumatic injury should not be selected for treatment with PSWD because the treatment can increase bleeding and edema. Hemorrhaging tendency, including heavy menstruation, is a precaution for use of PSWD. Changing the parameters of the treatment would be indicated to modify the amount of heating. If wound examination findings are acute inflammation, direct heating should be avoided, but indirect heating could be useful (e.g., inflammation in the foot can be treated with PSWD or PRFS applied over the abdomen or sacrum).

Examination for wound drainage is important. If PSWD is used, wounds that have a heavy amount of wound exudate would require special handling to absorb all of the moisture before treatment, to avoid burns.[2,84] Because treatment with PRFS is reported to increase wound exudate significantly for the first 1–3 days, management of the wound exudate should be planned by either changing the dressing more frequently or using more absorbent dressing materials. The surrounding skin may also require protection from maceration by application of a skin barrier.

Age should be considered when selecting candidates for PRFS or PSWD. Application of PRFS or PSWD over growth plates is probably not harmful because of the short duration of the wound healing treatment application, compared with the lengthy period of stimulation required to alter bone formation in bone healing studies using pulsed EMFs. Children have growth plates until about 16 years of age, depending on race, sex, and the bone involved (use over immature bone is a listed contraindication). Children usually do not have the underlying comorbidities that lead to chronic wounding, but forced immobility due to pain would be detrimental to a child. Some of the most common wounds in children are burns. A child with burn wounds would benefit from PRFS early intervention to normalize skin enzymes and to eliminate edema and pain, resulting in less scarring and quicker return to play and school activities.

Sometimes, the risk is insignificant, compared with the benefit. For example, children were treated for subdural hematoma with PRFS without complications and had more rapid resolution of edema and hematoma than did controls who were not treated.[46] If the benefit of accelerated wound healing outweighs the small risk of interference with a bone plate, prudent judgment should be used. Heat applications must always be applied carefully to the elderly because of impairments of circulatory system functions and changes in sensory perceptions. Exhibit 23-8 shows a list of contraindications, warnings, and cautions to be taken when using PSWD and PRFS equipment.

PRFS has fewer precautions and contraindications because it does not heat tissues. Key information to check in the medical history is the presence of electronic or metal implants (including intrauterine devices), osteomyelitis, cancer, or pregnancy. Avoid using this intervention in the presence of any of these conditions.[2,85] Metals reflect radiofrequency energy common to both PSWD and PRFS, so application over metal implants will reflect the energy back into the tissues, creating more intense energy levels in the tissues over the implant than usual, or the energy may be blocked from reaching the target tissues. Location of the metal should guide the PT to consider an alternative method of application, such as moving the applicator head above or below the area of metal (whichever is closest to the wound) to treat the surrounding wound tissues. Contrary to the recommendation to wait until acute hemorrhaging or acute inflammation have passed to treat with PSWD, PRFS should

EXHIBIT 23-8   FDA Contraindications, Warnings, and Cautions for PSWD and PRFS

PSWD

- Do not treat over ischemic tissue with inadequate blood flow
- Do not treat over or near metallic implants
- Do not use with patients with cardiac pacemakers
- Do not treat in any region where presence of primary or metastatic malignant growth is known or suspected
- Do not treat over immature bone
- Do not treat over acute osteomyelitis without adequate drainage or before adequate drainage has been established
- Do not treat patients who have a tendency to hemorrhage (including menses)
- Do not treat over pelvic or abdominal region or lower back during pregnancy
- Do not treat transcerebrally
- Do not use over anesthetized areas
- Avoid situations that could concentrate the field, including moist dressings, perspiration, adhesives
- Use caution when treating patients with heat sensitivity
- Use caution when treating patients with inflammatory processes

PRFS

- Do not use as a substitute for treatment of internal organs
- Do not use over metal implants
- Do not use with patients with cardiac pacemakers
- Do not use with patients who are pregnant
- Do not treat over immature bone

(Data from International Medical Electronics, *Magnatherm*® *Model 1000 Instruction Manual* and Electropharmacology, *MRT*® *sofPulse*™ *User's Manual*.)

be applied early after wounding. As described, studies have shown that application of PRFS during the first 72 hours reduces pain, posttraumatic edema, and, in burn patients, the enzymes associated with trauma.

Safety Issues

PSWD

Contact with any metal (e.g., jewelry, zippers, brassiere fasteners, and brassiere underwires) should be avoided when using PSWD because of the risk of burns and distortion of the EMF is possible from metal objects placed near the cables. Also avoid contact with metal furniture or parts (e.g., mattress springs). PSWD should not be used over synthetic materials that may melt and cause burns.[1] Electronic devices (e.g., hearing aids, watches) should not be worn during treatment with these devices because the EMF may cause disruption of the device. Hearing aids may produce annoying noise feedback.

PRFS

Electronic devices (e.g., hearing aids, watches) should not be worn during treatment with PRFS devices for the same reasons cited above. Do not administer PRFS directly over metal (e.g., jewelry, zippers) because the energy will be reflected and not reach the target tissues.

Therapist Safety

Many sources of EMFs are present in the environment, and most do not affect the human body. By the nature of the PSWD and PRFS devices described in this chapter, the EMFs do not pass 100% of the energy into the tissues being treated. Some energy is dissipated into the area close to the equipment. Operators and persons close to the equipment will absorb a small amount of an EMF. EMFs from PSWD at distances of 0.5 m from the cables and 0.2 m from inductive applicators are low at low and medium pulse settings. A study of PT work habits found that most remain at least 1 m from the applicator and 0.5 m from the cables during the operation of PSWD equipment. At those distances, there is little danger of excess absorption.[86] However, some older model PSWDs may not have shielded cables. The device should be checked for leakage of EMF energy. For personnel working with this equipment who have electronic implants, however, it would be prudent not to be exposed to the EMF because the stray radiation can affect the operation of those devices. The same holds true for other patients or family members occupying the same treatment areas. A timer is usually part of the equipment, and it will turn the equipment off automatically, but if the patient needs to be assisted during the treatment, the staff member can approach the console without standing close to the cables. Several studies have attempted to measure the effects of EMFs on personnel working in areas where frequent exposure to SWD occurs. An epidemiologic study looked at the risk of birth defects, perinatal deaths, and late spontaneous abortions affecting fetuses of female therapists working with SWD. The result of this retrospective study showed that the risk of a miscarriage was not associated with reported use of SWD.[87] Patients, except as mentioned, have no measurable risk from the EMF associated with this equipment, and the benefits probably outweigh any negative effects.

Equipment

Regulatory Approval

The PSWD generators are classified as Class II short-wave diathermy devices, used for therapeutic deep heating for purposes of treatment of pain, muscle spasms, and joint contractures. PRFS generators are classified as Class III short-wave diathermy for all other uses (except treatment of malignancy), intended to treat medical conditions by means other than deep heating as nonthermal units, and are sold to control pain and edema.[88] State licensing agencies regulate what is physical therapy. Medicare guidelines state that the use of diathermy should always be by or under the supervision of a licensed PT. Exhibit 23-8 lists FDA contraindications, and Exhibit 23-9 lists FDA indications.

Devices

Pulsed Short-wave Diathermy

A PSWD generator uses a coil mounted within a case (called a *head*) as the radiating element. This coil is driven by a crystal-controlled amplifier contained within the main chassis of the unit. The output of this head is an EMF with a radiofrequency of 27.12 MHz. The head is mounted on a movable, adjustable arm. Depending on the unit design, the head may be rectangular or round. Some devices allow the frequency to be delivered continuously or pulsed. The range of heating and nonthermal effects will depend on the pulse rate and duration. A PSWD device that can be operated at a broad range of pulse rates and pulse durations will have the most potential clinical applications. Heating effects are the principal action of the device at high pulse rates of long duration, and nonthermal effects are achieved at low pulse rates and over short durations. At the nonthermal settings, the PSWD may have effects equivalent to those of the PRFS devices, which are limited to this range. PSWD devices are on the market, including the Magnatherm (International Medical Electronics, Kansas City, MO), the Curapulse (Enraf Nonius, Delft, The Netherlands and Henley International, Sugarland, TX), and Megapulse (Electro-Medical Supplies, Ltd, UK and PTI Corporation, Topeka, KS). They are considered equivalent; however, there are differences in available pulse rates, pulse duration, and average outputs.

The Curapulse method of creating the electric and magnetic fields uses a different technology than do the other devices described. Each field is delivered in isolation by means of the condenser electrodes and a monode head, and transformation to an EMF occurs within the body tissue. Curapulse is available with either one or two electrodes that can be operated with different protocols. For example, the pulse rate and the duration of treatment must remain constant for both heads, but the other parameters can be set separately for each. Two models are available: (1) Model 670 allows for variation of pulse duration from 65 to 400 µsec, adjustable in seven steps, and an adjustment of frequency from 26 to 400 Hz, adjustable in 10 steps, that can be used for both thermal and nonthermal effects; (2) Model 970 has a fixed pulse duration of 400 µsec and a frequency of 15–200 pps, and is considered a thermal device. Maximum outputs are also different. Table 23-8 shows the available parameters for these different models

The Megapulse pulse-width settings range from 25 to 400 µsec. Three pulse modes are offered with the device on/off cycles consisting of one-third on time and two-thirds off time; two-thirds on time and one-third off time; and continuous. The pulse duration and frequency can be changed during those three modes. When longer on time and shorter off time are selected, there will be more thermal effects. Shorter on and longer off time will be less thermal, and the effects will be stimulation of the cells, rather than heating. It can be used like a PSWD or PRFS device. The wide range of settings may be confusing to new users, but they enhance the choice and variety of applications and conditions that can be treated.

The Magnatherm SSP unit is designed so that each of the two round inductive treatment heads can be set at the same or different settings to deliver controlled dosages for individualized treatment effects. Each is controlled and monitored from its own panel. There is a full range of pulse rates to choose from (see Figure 23-5). The unit is designed to be used on a cart for mobility, or to be lifted off the cart and packed in its own carrying case for portability. However, the 25-pound weight would be a real workout for a therapist carrying it from car to house several times a day. A wheeled attachment would facilitate this application.

RESEARCH WISDOM

Pattern of Treatment Effect

The pattern of treatment effect for PSWD and PRFS stimulators is in the form of the shape and size of the applicator head.

Pulsed Radiofrequency Stimulators

PRFS generators, like PSWD generators, consist of a radiating treatment head or applicator coil and an electronic console with the power generator. The output of this head is an EMF with a radiofrequency of 27.12 MHz that is the same for all three devices described here. Other parameters vary.

EXHIBIT 23-9   FDA Indications

PSWD	PRFS
Improved blood flow	Relief of pain and edema
Improved oxygenation	Increased blood flow
Increased metabolic rate	
Inflammatory conditions	
Relief of pain and edema	

TABLE 23-8   Typical Equipment Parameters

Device	Operating Frequency (MHz)	Pulse Rates (pps)	Pulse Widths (μsec)	Generated Power (W)
Magnatherm	27.12	700–7,000	95 Fixed	
Megapulse	27.12	50–800	20–400	0.2–100% (1,000 peak)
Nonthermal mode		< 200	< 200	150 Peak, 5–40 average
Thermal mode		> 200	> 100	
Curapulse				
Model 970	27.12	15–200	400 Fixed	1,000 Peak, 80 average
Model 670	27.12	26–400	65–400	200 Peak, 32 average
Diapulse	27.12	80–600	65 Fixed	293–975 Peak, 1.5–38 average
SofPulse,	27.12			
Model Roma		1-5	2-5 msec	1-10 W
Model Torino		2	3msec	2 W

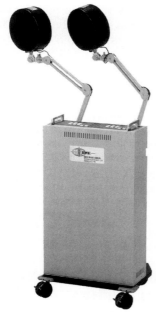

FIGURE 23-5 Shortwave diathermy unit (Magnatherm SSP). (Courtesy of International Medical Electronics Ltd., Kansas City, MO.)

Diapulse

The Diapulse has a pulse length of 65 μsec and an interpulse interval that can be varied from 12.4 to 1.6 msec by altering the pulse frequency. This allows ample time for heat to be dissipated.[89] Electromagnetic effects at the cellular level are the actions to expect from these devices, not heating.[2] The Diapulse has a stronger magnetic field and a weaker electrical field, and both are emitted simultaneously.[90] The frequency can be set in six steps (80, 120, 200, 300, 400, 500 pps) in conjunction with six intensity settings. Peak power output is 38 W delivered to the tissues.

Provant Wound Closure System

The Provant Wound Closure System product is designed with a treatment coil enclosed in a pad and a lead attaching it to the power generator. The signal is a pulsed square wave with a pulse duration of 42 μsec and frequency of 1 KHz. Output strength delivered to the tissues is 187V/m at 5.0 cm.

Ivivi Technologies Roma and Torino Models

The Ivivi Technolgies Roma model is a clinical model with three outputs for application to three wound areas. The treatment coil comes in different size diameters for treatment of different size wound or multiple wounds in a given area, The EMF field is projected equally in all directions around the coil and has the ability to reach and treat a large volume of tissue. For example, an 8" coil loop will treat the whole head. Since there is no sensation when using PRFS it is difficult to know that the active coil is transmitting the energy. To compensate for this the manufacturer has designed two failsafe alarm systems that are built into the unit. One alarm sends a flashing light error message letting the operator know that the output is not intact. The second alarm is a beeping sound to call attention to a problem. Based on the basic science research reported elsewhere in this chapter, the manufacturer has adjusted the energy delivery to provide longer duration signal (1 msec) and reduced output from 300 W to 10 W. The Torino model is a disposable single patient design that consists of a coil loop and a small generator (see Fig 23-6).

The current state of knowledge of the mechanism of PRFS' bioeffects has recently allowed the peak input power to the applicator to be reduced from 300 W to <10 W. This leads to more efficacious and speedier therapeutic outcomes.[39] Like all PRFS units in this class, the radiofrequency used remains at 27.12 Hz, but with this low power output there is negligible radiofrequency interference on monitoring and life-sustaining electronic equipment. The low power requirement of modern PRFS devices has allowed the development of portable, battery-operated units which can be sent home with the patient. To achieve all of this the PRFS signal now typically has a burst duration of 3 msec, versus 65 μsec, which repeats at 5 bursts/sec, as opposed to 600/sec, and a peak amplitude of 0.05G, versus 2G. So far the only company to use this new technology is Ivivi, in their two Sofpulse models, the Roma clinical model and Torino portable and single-subject use model. Another innovation of this product line is the use of a radiating coil loop instead of a drum housing the radiating coil. Loops come in varying sizes to assure adequate dosimetry for wounds of different sizes. Manufacturers are marketing these devices for home use by patients and caregivers under a medical prescription and the supervision of a licensed health care practitioner. All are FDA approved devices for pain, edema, and circulation but NOT for wound healing.

Procedures

Protocols

Protocols are established to achieve a predictable outcome. PSWD is a thermal agent and, as such, has predictable effects on tissue temperature and blood flow. Normal resting body temperature is between 36.3° C and 37.5° C. PSWD at thermal levels has the ability to raise deep tissue temperature to 45° C. Vigorous heating is defined as raising tissue temperature to between 40° C and 45° C.[23] This is estimated to be the maximum safe upper limit to raise tissue temperature and corresponds to the pain threshold of the skin. Maintaining a tissue temperature of 45° C for a sufficiently long period will result in irreversible tissue damage. Three factors influence the maximum tissue temperature reached: the square of the intensity, the tissue impedance, and the length of time the tissue is heated. Also, tissue perfusion determines how quickly the blood flow will dissipate the heat.[2] The observable effect of heating is hyperemia due to increased blood flow. This is a mild inflammatory response, initiating the biologic cascade associated with the process of inflammation (see Chapter 2). Vasodilation occurs, along with increased capillary hydrostatic pressure and vessel permeability. This promotes movement of fluid from the vessels into the interstitial spaces. Symptoms associated with this process are *edema, pain,* and *warmth.* Raising the tissue temperature within a 5- to 15-minute period will raise the tissue temperature to the maximum range. The resulting vasodilation will produce a marked increase in blood flow that will then dissipate the heat and decrease the temperature by several degrees. A total exposure period of 20–30 minutes is described in the literature as the required time for the optimal therapeutic benefits of heating to occur. Studies show that this can be achieved with inductive coupling using PSWD while avoiding excessive heating of the superficial tissues and subcutaneous fat.[1] Tissue heating below 40°C temperature is considered mild.[19]

PRFS protocols used in the reported studies have a single set of parameters, regardless of whether perfusion, reduction of edema or pain, or tissue healing was the outcome. It is not currently known, however, what may be the optimal parameters of dosage that affect different levels of tissues at different stages of repair. This determination requires further research. In the current situation, the experimental protocols

have validity and reliability, and can be used safely. These are listed below, in the "Setup for Treatment" sections.

Expected Outcomes

Change in temperature measures the change in tissue perfusion after the treatment. How the tissue responds functionally to the enhanced perfusion is the functional outcome (e.g., progression to the proliferative phase—red, neovascularized granulation tissue). The sequence of predictable biologic events occurs during the process of healing as the wound progresses from an initial phase of healing (inflammatory) to a later phase of healing (epithelialization or contraction). The steps of the progression are outcome measures for measuring and predicting wound healing. See Chapter 1 for possible wound outcomes and prognoses. The expected outcome for a chronic wound treated with a physical agent such as PSWD or PRFS should be progress from one phase to the next phase in a 2- to 4-week period. Research evidence can be used as a guide for the mean time for healing. For example, in two pressure ulcer studies using PRFS (Diapulse),[64,66] closure was reported at a rate of 8.7% and 5.9% per week for stage III pressure ulcers. The healing time will be at the end of the range for patients with the factors that affect healing, such as older age, immobility, comorbidities, long duration of wound, large wound size, and the depth of tissue involvement. If reassessment does not confirm the expected outcomes, treatment must change. Change here can mean a change in protocol (e.g., mild heating changed to vigorous heating), an increase in the length of treatment time, a change in frequency from three times per week to daily, or a change in dressing or topical agent. Any or all of the above are ways to consider changing the treatment to affect the wound status and reach a predictable outcome. Below are expected outcomes for the protocols for both PSWD and PRFS.

Wound Healing Phase Diagnosis: Acute or Chronic Inflammation

Expected Outcome Protocol

- Hyperemia: change in skin color to red, blue, or purplish, depending on color of surrounding skin
- Temperature: increased tissue temperature, due to increased tissue perfusion
- Edema: resolution or prevention and restoration of tissue turgor
- Wound progression to the proliferative phase

Wound Healing Phase Diagnosis: Subacute Inflammation

Expected Outcome Protocol

- Skin color: change to that of surrounding skin
- Temperature: change to that of adjacent tissues or same area on corresponding opposite side of the body
- Edema-free
- Necrosis-free
- Wound progression to the proliferative phase

TABLE 23-9   Magnatherm Protocol Used by Sussman for Case Study

Magnatherm Settings	Duration	Effect
PR 5,000 pps power level 12 (thermal)	5 min	Vigorous heating—warm up
PR 700 pps power level 12 (nonthermal)	25 min	No perceived sensation of heat

Magnatherm PSWD Protocol

The protocol used by Sussman and reported in Case Study 1 at the end of this chapter was for treatment of a patient with a pressure ulcer, and parameters were proposed by the manufacturer (International Medical Electronics) of the Magnatherm. This protocol called for a short initial phase (5 minutes) of heating at a high pulse rate and peak power output, followed by a reduction in the pulse rate to the lowest level, which also reduced the heating effect (see Table 23-9). The lower pulse rate was maintained for 25 minutes. The total treatment time was 30 minutes. The rationale was that the effects of the high-dose heating treatment would rapidly raise the tissue temperature and cause vasodilation. The lower pulse rate produced mild heating, and the longer interpulse interval would allow for heat dissipation. Additional rationale for this setting was that this would sustain the vasodilation effects of the high heating phase throughout the duration of the treatment.

Protocols for PSWD

Kloth and Ziskin[2] devised a protocol for using PSWD, based on the definitions of Lehman and deLateur[23] of vigorous and mild heating, to write a protocol for the acute, subacute, and chronic inflammatory phases of healing. The power level of the PSWD unit is divided into four levels. The four levels range from quarter power, which has a sensory effect below sensation of heat, to full power, which is vigorous heating. Table 23-10 shows the PSWD dosages and effects, and the aspect of the inflammation phase of healing to be treated at that level. Table 23-11 shows the dosage, level, duration, frequency, and expected temperature changes in the tissues.

Change Moist Dressing during PSWD Treatment

According to the PSWD instruction manual, it is necessary to remove wound dressings before PSWD.[84] To avoid burns of wound tissue during treatment with PSWD, replace any moist wound dressing with a dry sterile gauze pad. Check the gauze pad during the treatment when there is much wound exudate observed during the setup. If the dressing is moist, remove and replace it with another dry gauze dressing.

There are anecdotal clinical reports that the use of PSWD over wound dressings does not have harmful effects. Also, clinical practice for wound management has changed since the PSWD instruction cautions were first issued in 1981. Further evaluation of the effects of PSWD on wound fluids and dressing adhesives is needed to update this position.

TABLE 23-10   PSWD Power, Effects, and Application

Dose	Level	Effect	Phase of Healing
I (1/4 power)	Lowest	Below sensation of heat	Acute inflammation
II (1/2 power)	Low	Mild heat sensation	Subacute, resolving inflammation
III (3/4 power)	Medium	Moderate, comfortable heat sensation	Subacute, resolving inflammation
IV (full power)	Heavy	Vigorous heating, well tolerated; reduce to just below maximum tolerance	Chronic conditions

(Reprinted with permission from L. Kloth and M. Ziskin, Diathermy and Pulsed Radio Frequency Radiation, in *Thermal Agents in Rehabilitation*, 3rd ed, S. Michlovitz, ed., © 1996, F.A. Davis Company Publishers.)

TABLE 23-11   PSWD Dosage, Duration, and Outcomes

Dose	Duration*	Outcome
I	15 min one or two times daily for 1–2 weeks	Temperature ↑ 37.5–38.5°C
II	15 min daily for 1–2 weeks	Temperature ↑ 38.5–40.0°C
III	15–30 min daily for 1–2 weeks	Temperature ↑ 40.0–42.0°C
IV	15–30 min daily or two times per week for 1 week to 1 month	Temperature ↑ 42.0–44.0°C

* Continue for 2 weeks. If outcomes are achieved through the phases of healing, continue.

(Reprinted with permission from L. Kloth and M. Ziskin, Diathermy and Pulsed Radiofrequency Radiation, in *Thermal Agents in Rehabilitation*, 3rd ed, S. Michlovitz, ed., © 1996, F.A. Davis Company Publishers.)

Setup for Treatment with Pulsed Short-wave Diathermy

1. Explain the procedure to the patient and caregiver.
2. Inspect and remove all metal items, including jewelry, wristwatches, brassieres with metal fasteners, and clothing with zippers.
3. Remove hearing aids and external electronic devices.
4. Place the patient on a nonmetal surface.
5. Avoid contact with synthetic materials, including pillows.
6. Remove clothing from body area.
7. Position the patient for comfort in a position that can be maintained for 30 minutes.
8. Remove the wound dressing and absorb excess exudate; cover with dry gauze.
9. Cleanse the wound of debris and metallic and petrolatum-based products; blot dry.
10. Cover the wound and surrounding skin with a 1/2-inch thickness of toweling.
11. Cover the drum with a disposable surgical head cap or terry cloth towel for hygiene.
12. Place the drum 0.5–1 cm above the terry cloth.
13. Set the protocol and treatment duration. Start.

Patient Monitoring

- Never leave a patient who is confused or disoriented alone and unsupervised while receiving treatment.
- When using PSWD, remember that pain is a warning that excessive heating is occurring. Give the patient a call light and pay immediate attention to a call. Reduce power level. Increase air space, either by positioning the drum farther from the target tissue or by layering towels between the drum and the body area.
- Check skin before application for unguents that may have been applied (e.g., oil of wintergreen, Ben-Gay); clean thoroughly, and dry.

Aftercare for Pulsed Short-wave Diathermy

Because the dressing is always removed before this treatment, it is important that the wound be dressed with the appropriate dressing as soon as possible after conclusion of the treatment. A dressing should be selected that will match the frequency of the PSWD treatment and other components of the wound healing. Rapid redressing of the wound safeguards against wound contamination and desiccation of the wound tissues, sustains the warmth of the wound that has occurred from the increased profusion, and promotes optimal cell mitosis.

CLINICAL WISDOM

Tissue Perfusion

When tissue perfusion is the treatment effect, the wound will be warmed, and the cells will divide and proliferate faster in the warm environment. Therefore, dress the wound *immediately after* PSWD and *before* PRFS.

CLINICAL WISDOM

PSWD (Magnatherm) for Venous Disease

Patients with venous disease do not tolerate high heating and subsequent effects of vasodilation. Two phases are used. For the first phase of treatment, energy is adjusted to deliver a pulse rate of 1,600 pps for 15 minutes. This is followed by a second phase at 700 pps for a 15-minute period. Power levels are kept at power level 12.[91]

Pulsed Radiofrequency Stimulation Protocol

The protocol suggested for PRFS is based on the parameters used in the several controlled clinical trials with the Diapulse described earlier. These are nonthermal parameters but have a demonstrated ability to enhance microvascular tissue perfusion. Mechanisms of action may be different. Consider this therapy intervention if microvascular perfusion is desired and/or heating is contraindicated, if wound dressing is to be left intact during the treatment, or if the wound is inside a cast and is painful.

Setup Treatment with Pulsed Radiofrequency Stimulation

Diapulse

1. Explain the procedure to the patient and caregiver.
2. Position the patient for comfort, with the treatment site accessible, so that it can be maintained for 30 minutes.
3. Cover the drum with a disposable surgical head cap or terry cloth towel for hygiene.
4. Place the drum 0.5–1 cm above the terry cloth over the wound site.
5. Leave clothes, dressings, casts, bandages, splints in place unless there is strikethrough or it is time to change dressing.
6. Drum can lay on top of bandages, casts, splints, Unna boot
7. Set the protocol and treatment duration. Start.

Sofpulse

Roma Model This is a clinical model with 3 output leads for treatment to three areas during the same 30 minute treatment period. Dose of treatment will be equal to all areas regardless of coil loop size. Coil loops of different diameters are available to best meet the wound size. Large coils could be laid over near wounds e.g. hip and coccyx for more efficient treatment.

Precautions:

1. Do not bend the loop into a different shape. If it is configured into a "U" the signal polarity will cancel itself out. If twisted into a pretzel or squeezed like a sausage the area of treatment will be restricted and the depth of penetration reduced.
2. Place the generator unit on a stable surface.
3. The coil loop is designed for single patient use and can be cleaned and disinfected between uses and discarded at end of care.

Set Up:

1. Explain the procedure to the patient and caregiver.
2. Position the patient for comfort, with the treatment site accessible, so that it can be maintained for 30 minutes.
3. Leave clothes, dressings, casts, bandages, splints in place unless there is strikethrough or it is time to change dressing.
4. Match loop coil size to the wound area to be treated.
5. Position the loop so it stays in the position and is not likely to be dislodged by gravity or patient movement.
6. Lay the loop coil **flat** over the wound area and tape in place as shown in Figure 23-6.
7. Coil loop can lay on top of clothing, bandages, casts, splints.
8. DO NOT bend or twist the loop as this will interfere with delivery of the signal from the coil (see precaution 1 above).
9. Error alarm messages are built into this unit and include a flashing light that will indicate the output is not intact and also there is a beeping signal to alert patient and caregiver of operational problems.
10. A home care model (Torino) is also available that is totally disposable after use.
11. Preset protocols and 30 minute timer. Roma 1-5 pps, 2-5msec, 1-10 W; Torino2pps, 3msec, 2 W; Torino is designed for unattended home use.

Frequency for all the PRFS devices described is once or twice daily or every 4 hours for pain management, 30 minutes per session.

Adjunctive Treatments

It has already been mentioned that PSWD and PRFS can be used in conjunction with adjunctive treatments, such as compression bandages, casts, splints. It can also be used following whirlpool or pulsatile lavage with suction (PLS) for cleans-

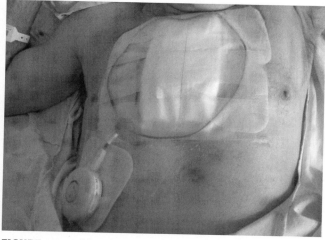

FIGURE 23-6 Ivivi Soft Pulse device. (Courtesy of Ivivi Technologies, Inc, Northvale, NJ.)

ing or debridement. If dressings are to be removed, it may be preferable to treat with PSWD or PRFS immediately after the other interventions to keep the wound temperature from declining. Another choice could be to treat the wound with ultraviolet light for bactericidal effects or to initiate a mild inflammatory process, then follow with either PSWD or PRFS to enhance the circulation and cellular activation. It also can be used along with negative pressure therapy as shown in the pictorial case study Figures 23-7A–E. More information about negative pressure therapy is found in Chapter 28. The combination of therapies could enhance results, since the mechanisms of action are different. Benefits of multiple treatments with different or multiple biophysical agents are anecdotal and have not been proven. The clinician should assess whether the addition of these interventions has potential benefit and support it with a rationale and documentation. This is an area that merits further research for best utilization management of services and best efficacy for the patient.

Another adjunctive treatment with well-established effects on circulation is exercise. Exercise following PSWD or PRFS would use the muscle pump for exchange of nutrients and oxygen brought to the tissue by the PSWD or PRFS treatment and removal of waste products, as well as to help dissipate the effects of heating and avoid burning. Exercise encourages movement of fluids from the venous system into the lymphatics and is a way to avoid stasis in the area of heating. For those patients who are unable to exercise actively, assisted or passive range of motion would encourage change in fluid dynamics in the affected area. Therapeutic positioning should also be considered as an adjunctive treatment because improper positioning may have blood flowing away from the target tissues or applying pressure to the area that is to be perfused.

Self-Care Teaching Guidelines

Both PSWD and PRFS labels state that "federal law restricts the sale and use of this equipment to a licensed health practitioner."[45,85] However, the manufacturers and distributors of the PRFS nonthermal devices report that patients are using them as home therapy units under physician prescription and unattended supervision. SofPulse and Provant come in a portable home care model. PSWD should not be used unsupervised and unattended in the home.

Documentation

The functional outcome report (FOR) described in Chapter 1 is an accepted method to meet Medicare and third-party payer guidelines for documentation of the need for physical therapy intervention for wound healing. The two cases presented as examples of the use of PSWD and PRFS are documented by using the FOR method. A sample form and case are found in Chapter 1. Also, try to apply the method to wound cases in the clinic.[92] Data collected about treatment outcomes in a systematic manner can be of great value to report the success of the therapy and to predict outcomes.

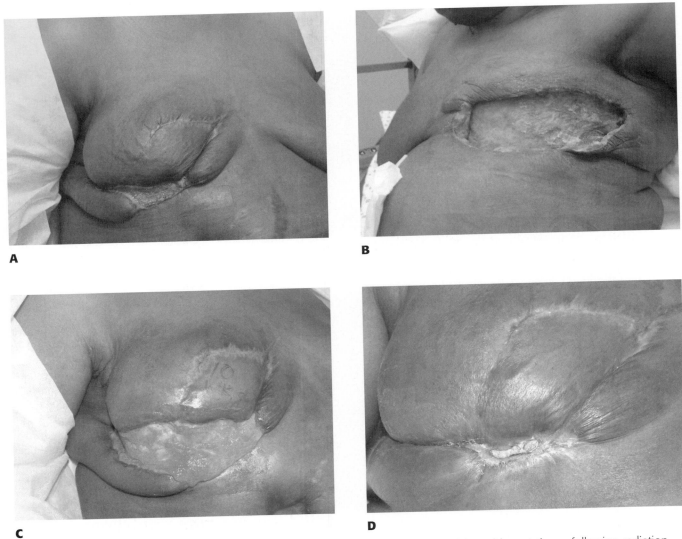

FIGURE 23-7 Pictorial case study. **A.** Post surgical view of woman with surgical excision of breast tissue following radiation skin necrosis. Two prior flaps had been lost trying to close the defect. **B.** PRF with Ivivi Romeo (Ivivi Technologies, Northvale, NJ) and V.A.C. (KCI, San Antonio, TX) negative pressure devices in place. This combined treatment was provided for one week post op, and then the negative pressure was discontinued. **C.** View of tissue 11 days post op. Treatment now only with PRF and dressings. **D.** View of epithelializing and contracting wound at 2 months post op. (Pictorial case study provided courtesy of Berish Strauch, MD, Department of Plastic and Reconstructive Surgery, Montefiore Medical Center, Albert Einstein College of Medicine of Yeshiva University. Bronx, NY.)

■ **CASE STUDY**

Pressure Ulcer Treated with Pulsed Short-wave Diathermy

Patient ID: S.D. Age: 86

FUNCTIONAL OUTCOME REPORT: INITIAL ASSESSMENT

Reason for Referral

The patient is minimally mobile and has developed a pressure ulcer on the left heel and fifth metatarsal head. She is alert but lacks the ability to reposition. Autolytic debridement with occlusive dressing has not been successful.

Medical History and Systems Review

The patient experienced a left fractured hip with open reduction and internal fixation 3 years ago. She never regained the ability to ambulate after the hip fracture. She also has a history of multiple cerebrovascular accidents that suggests that her circulatory system is impaired. She is placed in a wheelchair for a few hours a day. She takes food orally and eats most of the diet offered. There has been no recent loss of weight. She is incontinent of bowel and bladder and has a Foley catheter in place.

Evaluation

The patient has an impaired healing response that is due to impairment of the circulation and loss of the muscle pump function due to immobility of the lower extremities. These functional losses contribute to the inability of the wounded tissue to progress through the phases of repair without intervention. The patient has improvement potential for the wounds, but will remain at risk for future pressure ulceration. The following examinations are indicated:

- Mobility: muscle function and joint integrity
- Circulatory status function
- Integumentary system: surrounding skin and wound

Examination Data

Muscle Function and Joint Integrity. The patient has a fixed varus deformity of the leg, and no active mobility of the left hip joint exists. There is minimal mobility of the left knee, and a knee flexion contracture at 75° limits function of the left leg. The hip and knee deformities have created a positioning problem, with the left ankle crossing over the right leg and the lateral aspect of the foot, from toes to heel, in a position that is subject to pressure. Ankle joint range and mobility is also severely impaired.

Mobility. The patient is immobile. She does not attempt to self-reposition in either bed or wheelchair.

Circulation. There is edema of the left foot, extending to the ankle. The foot is warm (98.6° F), with 1+ palpable pulses. No dependent rubor is noted when the patient is seated in a wheelchair.

Integumentary System.
There is an ulcer on the left lateral heel; it has eschar necrosis, inflammatory signs of changes in skin color (red), warmth (98.6° F), and local edema. The whole foot to the ankle is edematous. There is an ulcer on the left fifth metatarsal head with eschar necrosis, signs of mild inflammation, no pain, changes in skin color (red), and warmth (98.6° F) and

edema. It is 6.9 cm². (See *Color Plates 68* and *69* for pictures of the wounds at evaluation and during treatment)

Functional Diagnosis

- Undue susceptibility to pressure ulceration on the feet
- Both wounds chronic inflammatory phase
- Tissue impairment due to presence of eschar

Need for Skilled Services: The Therapy Problem

The patient has failed to respond to interventions with dressing changes for the last 2 weeks. She now requires debridement of the eschar from both wounds to determine the extent of tissue involvement and to initiate the healing process; PSWD would be of benefit to enhance circulation to the foot, facilitate debridement, and restart the process of repair; and therapeutic positioning to avoid trauma from pressure to the foot.

Targeted Outcomes

- The wound bed will be clean.
- There will be an enhanced inflammatory response: erythema, edema, and warmth.
- The patient will progress through the phases of healing from inflammation to epithelialization.
- The patient will be properly positioned to remove pressure from the left foot.

TREATMENT PLAN

Debridement Strategy

Score eschar and use an enzymatic debriding agent and occlusion for autolysis. Sharply débride when eschar is softened. Apply PSWD for perfusion and cellular stimulation

Prognosis. Clean wound bed; *due date:* 21 days

PSWD

Apply PSWD for increased circulation to the foot, using the protocol of one applicator over the abdomen and the second applicator over the plantar surface of the foot. Use the device at the vigorous heating setting for 5 minutes, followed by mild heating (nonthermal) for 25 minutes.

Prognosis

- Acute inflammation; *due date:* 14 days
- Progression through phases to closure; *due date:* 8 weeks

Frequency. Apply PSWD daily seven times per week, twice daily for 30 minutes.

Therapeutic Positioning

Use therapeutic positioning with pillows to eliminate pressure on the left foot; instruct nurses' aides in proper positioning.

Discharge Outcome

The wound on the fifth metatarsal head was healed by day 15. The wound on left heel had full-thickness skin loss after removal of eschar and necrotic tissue. The wound had a clean wound bed by week 4. Closure was achieved by week 7. (See *Color Plate 70.*)

RESOURCES

Diapulse
Diapulse Corporation of America
3321 E Shore Rd.
Great Neck, NY 11023
Phone: 516-829-8069
www.Diapulse.com

Magnatherm
International Medical Electronics, LTD.
PO Box 45030
Kansas City, MO 64171
Phone: 1-800-432-8003
www.magnatherm.com

Provant Wound Closure System
Regenesis Biomedical Inc.
1435 N Hayden Road
Scottsdale, AZ 85257-3773
Phone: 1-877-970-4970
www.regenesismedical.com

SofPulse
Ivivi Technologies
224-S Pegasus Ave,
Northvale, NJ 07647
201-784-8168
www.ivivitechnologies.com

REVIEW QUESTIONS

1. Discuss how PRFS differs from other types of electrical stimulation. Should PRFS and electrical stimulation be considered equivalent modalities? Provide rationale.
2. Describe the three benefits of using PRFS.
3. Explain how PRFS and PSWD differ and when you would choose each.
4. Describe the putative effects of PRFS. Is this supported by evidence?
5. What treatment outcomes would you expect from PSWD? From PRFS?

REFERENCES

1. Guy A, Lehmann J, Stonebridge J. Therapeutic applications of electromagnetic power. *Proc IEEE.* January 1974:55–75.
2. Markov MS, Pilla A. Electromagnetic field stimulation of soft tissues: pulsed radio frequency treatment of postoperative pain and edema. *Wounds.* 1995;7(4):143–151.
3. Kloth L, Ziskin M. Diathermy and pulsed radiofrequency radiation. In: Michlovitz SL, ed. *Thermal Agents in Rehabilitation.* Philadelphia: FA Davis; 1996:213–254.
4. Kellogg R. Magnetotherapy: potential clinical and therapeutic applications. In: Nelson R, Currier D, eds. *Clinical Electrotherapy.* Norwalk, CT: Appleton & Lange; 1991:390–391.
5. Skerry TM, Pead MJ, Lanyon LE. Modulation of bone loss during disuse by pulsed electromagnetic fields. *J Ortho Res.* 1991;7:600–608.
6. Blumlein H, McDaniel J. Effect of the magnetic field component of the Kraus-Lechner method on the healing of experimental nonunion in dogs. In: Burny F, Herbst E, Hinsenkamp M, eds. *Electric Stimulation of Bone Growth and Repair.* New York: Springer-Verlag; 1978:35–46.
7. Herber H. Cordey J, Perren SM. Influence of magnetic fields on growth and regeneration in organ culture. In: Burny F, Herbst E, Hinsenkamp M, eds. *Electric Stimulation of Bone Growth and Repair.* New York: Springer-Verlag; 1978:35–40.
8. Mooney V. A randomized double-blind prospective study of efficacy of pulsed electromagnetic fields for interbody lumbar fusion. *Spine.* 1990;15:708–712.
9. Sharrard WJ. Double blind trials of pulsed electromagnetic fields of delayed union of tibial fractures. *J Bone Joint Surg.* 1990;72-B:347–355.
10. Skerry TM, Pead MJ, Lanyon LE. Modulation of bone loss during disuse by pulsed electromagnetic fields. *J Ortho Res.* 1991;9:600–608.
11. Pienkowski D, Pollack SR, Brighton CT, Griffith NJ. Comparison of asymmetrical and symmetrical pulse waveforms in electromagnetic stimulation. *J Orthop Res.* 1992;10(2):247–255.
12. Medicare Coverage Issues Manual (MCIM)—Medical Procedures, Section 35–98, 5 Medicare and Medicaid Guide (CCH). In: *Health Care Financing Administration (HCFA).* Baltimore: Department of Health and Human Services; 1997:35–98.
13. *Anonymous, Aitken, Noecker, Heyden, Langill, Sharp, Turner and American Physical Therapy Association vs Shalala.* Civil Action No. 979–1127. United States District Court, District of Massachusetts: 1997.
14. National Coverage Decision for Electrical Stimulation (ES) and Electromagnetic Therapy for the Treatment of Wounds. Vol 270.1; 2004. Department of Health and Human Services, Center for Medicare and Medicaid Services.
15. Bergstrom N, Allman RM, Alvarez OM. *Treatment of Pressure Ulcers.* Clinical Practice Guideline. Rockville, MD: Agency for Health Care Research and Quality (AHRQ), formerly known as the Agency for Health Care Policy and Research (AHCPR), U.S. Department of Health and Human Services, Public Health Service; 1994.
16. Ovington LG. Dressings and adjunctive therapies: AHCPR guidelines revisited. *Ostomy/Wound Manage.* 1999;45(Suppl 1A):94s–106s.
17. Dolynchuk K, Keast D, Campbell K. Best practices for the prevention and treatment of pressure ulcers. *Ostomy/Wound Manage.* 2000;46(11):38–52
18. Garber SL, Biddle AK, Click CN, et al. *Pressure ulcer prevention and treatment following spinal cord injury: A clinical practice guideline for health-care professionals.* Jackson Heights, NY: Paralyzed Veterans of America; August 2000.
19. Rabkin J, Hunt TK. Local heat increases blood flow and oxygen tension in wounds. *Arch Surg.* 1987;122:221–225.
20. Bello YM, Lopez AP, Philips TJ. *Wound Temperature is Lower than Core Temperature.* Abstract. In: Symposium for Advanced Wound Care and 8th Annual Medical Research Forum on Wound Repair. Miami, FL: Health Management Publications; 1998.
21. Michaelson AD, MacGregor H, Barnard MR. Reversible inhibition of human platelet activation by hypothermia in vivo and in vitro. *Thromb Haemost.* 1994;71(5):633–640.
22. Park H-Y, Shon K, Phillips T. The effect of heat on inhibitory effects of chronic wound fluid on fibroblasts in vitro. *Wounds.* 1998;10(6):189–192.
23. Lehman JF, deLateur BJ. Therapeutic heat. In: Lehmann JF, ed. *Therapeutic Heat and Cold.* 4th ed. Baltimore: Williams & Wilkins; 1990.
24. Brown G. Diathermy: a renewed interest in a proven therapy. *Phys Ther Today.* Spring 1993:78–80.
25. Wessman HC, Kottke FJ. The effect of indirect heating on peripheral blood flow, pulse rate, blood pressure and temperature. *Arch Phys Med Rehabil.* 1967;48:567–576.
26. Tortorici L, Purdy S. Laser and electromagnetic fields in the treatment of cancer. *Rehabil Oncol.* 2000;18(3):18–22.
27. Silverman D, Pendleton L. A comparison of the effects of continuous and pulsed short-wave diathermy on peripheral circulation. *Arch Phys Med Rehabil* 1968;49:429–436.
28. Santoro D, Ostranderl, Lee B, Cagir B. *Inductive 27.12 MHz: Diathermy in Arterial Peripheral Vascular Disease.* 16th International IEEE/EMBS Conference; October 1994; Montreal, Canada.
29. Pilla AA. Mechanisms and therapeutic applications of time-varying and static magnetic fields. In: Barnes F GB, ed. *Handbook of Biological Effects of Electromagnetic Fields.* 3rd ed: CRC Press; 2006. In press.
30. Brighton CT, Wang W, Seldes R, et al. Signal transduction in electrically stimulated bone cells. *J Bone Joint Surg.* 2001; October 83A (10): 1514–1523.
31. Seegers JC, Engelbrecht A, van Papendorp DH. Activation of signal-transduction mechanisms may underlie the therapeutic effects of an applied electric field. *Medical Hypotheses.* 2001;57(2):224–230

32. George FR, Lukas RJ, Moffett J, et al. In-vitro mechanisms of cell proliferation induction: a novel bioactive treatment for accelerating wound healing. *Wounds* 2002;14(3):107–115

33. Canedo-Dorantes L, Garcia-Canto R, Barrera R, et al.. Healing of chronic arterial and venous leg ulcers with systemic electromagnetic fields. *Arch Med Res.* 2002;33:281–289.

34. Nindl G, Balcavage WX, Vesper DN, et al. Experiments showing that electromagnetic fields can be used to treat inflammatory diseases. *Bimed Sci Instrum.* 2000;36:7–13.

35. Aaron RK, Boyan BD, McKCiombor D, et al. Stimulation of growth factor synthesis by electric and electromagnetic fields. *Clin Orthop.* 2004;419:30–37.

36. Pilla A. A Synopsis of Published Peer Reviewed Studies, not dated, Ivivi Technologies

37. Bassett C. Low energy pulsing electromagnetic fields modify biomedical processes. *BioEssays.*1987;6(1):36–40

38. Hill J, Lewis M, Mills P, et al. Pulsed short-wave diathermy effects on human fibroblast proliferation. *Arch Physical Med Rehab.* 2002;83(6):832–836.

39. Strauch B, Patel M, Navarro JA, et al. Pulsed magnetic fields accelerate cutaneous wound healing in rats. *Plast Reconstr Surg* 2006, In press.

40. Ankrom MA BR, Sprigle S, Langemo D, et al. National Pressure Ulcer Advisory Panel. Pressure-related deep tissue injury under intact skin and the current pressure ulcer staging systems. *Adv Skin Wound Care.* 2005;18(1):35–42.

41. National Pressure Ulcer Advisory Panel. *Deep tissue injury - White paper.* Washington, DC 2005.

42. Witkowski JA. Purple ulcers. *J ET Nurs.* 1993; 20:132.

43. Fenn JE. Effect of pulsed electromagnetic energy (Diapulse) on experimental hematomas. *Can Med Assoc J.* 1969;100:251.

44. Ginsberg AJ. Pearl Chain Phenomenon. Abstract. Presented at the 35th Annual Meeting of the American Congress of Physical Medicine and Rehabilitation; 1958;36:112–115.

45. Cameron BM. Experimental acceleration of wound healing. *Am J Orthop.* 1961;336–343.

46. Sambasivan M. Pulsed electromagnetic field in management of head injuries. *Neurol India.* 1993;41(Suppl):56–59.

47. Shields N, Gormley J, O'Hare N. Short-wave diathermy: current clinical and safety practices. *Physiother Res Int.* 2002;7(4):191–202.

48. Ionescu A, Ionescu D, et al. *Study of Efficiency of Diapulse Therapy on the Dynamics of Enzymes in Burned Wound.* Presented at the Sixth International Congress on Burns; August 31, 1982; San Francisco.

49. Santiesteban J, Grant C. Post-surgical effect of pulsed shortwave therapy. *J Am Podiatr Med Assoc.* 1979;75:306–309.

50. Barclay V, Collier R, Jones A. Treatment of various hand injuries by pulsed electromagnetic energy (Diapulse). *Physiotherapy.* 1983;69(6):186–188.

51. Pennington G, Daily D, Sumko M. Pulsed, non-thermal, high-frequency electromagnetic energy (Diapulse) in the treatment of grade I and grade II ankle sprains. *Mil Med.* 1993;158:101–104.

52. Knighton D, Halliday B, Hunt TK. Oxygen as antibiotic: a comparison of inspired oxygen concentration and antibiotic administration on in vivo bacterial clearance. *Arch Surg.* 1986;121:191–195.

53. Jonsson K, Jensen J, Goodson WH III. Tissue oxygenation, anemia, and perfusion in relation to wound healing in surgical patients. *Ann Surg.* 1991;214(5):605–613.

54. Erdman W. Peripheral blood flow measurements during application of pulsed high frequency currents. *Orthopedics.* 1960;2:196–197.

55. Mayrovitz H, Larsen P. Effects of pulsed electromagnetic fields on skin microvascular blood perfusion. *Wounds.* 1992;4(5):197–202.

56. Mayrovitz H, Larsen P. A preliminary study to evaluate the effect of pulsed radio frequency field treatment on lower extremity peri-ulcer skin microcirculation of diabetic patients. *Wounds.* 1995;7(3):90–93.

57. Wilson D, Jagadesh P, Newman P, et al. The effects of pulsed electromagnetic energy on peripheral nerve regeneration. *Ann NY Acad Sci.* 1974;230:575–585.

58. Dindar H, Renda N, Barlas M. The effects of electromagnetic field stimulation on corticosteroids-inhibited intestinal wound healing. *Tokai J Exp Clin Med.* 1993;18(1–2):49–55.

59. Patino O, Grana D, Bolgiani A. Effect of magnetic fields on skin wound healing. Experimental study. *Medicina (B Aires).* 1996;56(1):41–44.

60. Patino O, Grana D, Bolgiani A. Pulsed electromagnetic fields in experimental cutaneous wound healing in rats. *J Burn Care Rehabil.* 1996;17(6 Pt 1):528–531.

61. Scardino M, Swaim SF, Sartin, EA. Evaluation of treatment with a pulsed electromagnetic field on wound healing, clinicopathologic variables, and central nervous system activity of dogs. *Am J Vet Res.* 1998;59(9):1177–1181.

62. Lin Y, Nishimura R, Nozaki K. Effects of pulsing electromagnetic fields on the ligament healing in rabbits. *J Vet Med Sci.* 1992;54(5):1017–1022.

63. Lee E, Maffuli N, Li CK, et al. Pulsed magnetic and electromagnetic fields in experimental Achilles tendonitis in the rat: a prospective randomized study. *Arch Phys Med Rehabil.* 1997;78(4):399–404.

64. Itoh M, Montemayor J, Matsumoto E, et al. Accelerated wound healing of pressure ulcers by pulsed high peak power electromagnetic energy (Diapulse). *Decubitus.* 1991;4(1):24–34.

65. Wilson CM. Clinical Effects of Diapulse Technology in Treatment of Recalcitrant Pressure Ulcers. In *Clinical Symposium on Pressure Ulcer and Wound Management.* Orlando, FL: Silver Cross Hospital and *Decubitus*; 1992.

66. Salzberg A, Cooper-Vastola S, Perez F, et al. The effects of non-thermal pulsed electromagnetic energy (Diapulse) on wound healing of pressure ulcers in spinal cord-injured patients: a randomized, double-blind study. *Wounds.* 1995;7(1):11–16.

67. Seaborne D, Quirion-DeGirardi C, Rovsseau M, et al. The treatment of pressure sores using pulsed electromagnetic energy (PEME). *Physiother Can.* 1996;48(2):131–137.

68. Cameron BM. A three phase evaluation of pulsed high frequency radio short waves (Diapulse), 646 patients. *Am J Orthop.* 1964:72–78.

69. Goldin JH, Broadbent JD, et al. The effects of Diapulse on the healing of wounds: a double-blind randomised controlled trial in man. *Br J Plastic Surg.* 1981;34:267–270.

70. Kaplan EG, Weinstock R. Clinical evaluation of Diapulse as adjunctive therapy following foot surgery. *J Am Podiatr Assoc.* 1968;58(5):218.

71. Aronofsky DH. Reduction of dental postsurgical symptoms using nonthermal pulsed high peak power electromagnetic energy. *Oral Surg Oral Med Oral Pathol.* 1971;32(5):688–696.

72. Bentall R, Eckstein H. A trial involving the use of pulsed electro-magnetic therapy on children undergoing orchidoplexy. *Hippokrates Verlag Stuttgart.* 1975;17(4):380–388.

73. Comorosan S, Paslaru L, Popovici Z. The stimulation of wound healing processes by pulsed electromagnetic energy. *Wounds.* 1992;4(1):31–32.

74. Ieran M, Zaffuto S. Effect of low frequency pulsing electromagnetic fields on skin ulcers of venous origin in humans: a double blind study. *J Orthop Rev.*1990;8:276–282.

75. Duran V, Zamurovic A, Stojanovk S, et al. Therapy of venous ulcers using pulsating electromagnetic fields—personal results. *Med Pregl.* 1991;44(11–12):485–488.

76. Todd D, Heylings D, Allen G, et al. Treatment of chronic varicose ulcers with pulsed electromagnetic fields: a controlled pilot study. *Ir Med J.* 1991;84(2):54–55.

77. Stiller M, Pak G, Shupack J, et al. A portable pulsed electromagnetic field (PEMF) device to enhance healing of recalcitrant venous ulcers: a double-blind, placebo-controlled clinical trial. *Br J Dermatol.* 1992;127(2):147–154.

78. Kenkre J, Hobbs F, Carter Y, et al. A randomized controlled trial of electromagnetic therapy in the primary care management of venous leg ulceration. *Fam Pract.* 1996;13(3):236–240.

79. Bates-Jensen B. *A Quantitative Analysis of Wound Characteristics as Early Predictors of Healing in Pressure Sores.* Dissertation Abstracts International, Vol. 59, No. 11. Los Angeles: University of California; 1999.

80. Margolis DJ, Gross EA, Wood CR, et al. Planimetric rate of healing in venous ulcers of the leg treated with pressure bandage and hydrocolloid dressing. *J Am Acad Dermatol.* 1993;28(3):418–421.

81. Robson MC, Hill DP, Woodske ME, et al. Wound healing trajectories as predictors of effectiveness of therapeutic agents. *Arch Surg.* 2000;135(7):773–777.

82. Van Rijswijk L. Full-thickness leg ulcers: Patient demographics and predictors of time to healing. Multi-center leg ulcer study group. *J Fam Pract.* 1993;36(6):625–632.

83. International Medical Electronics. *Megatherm (Model 1000) Short-wave Therapy Unit Instruction Manual.* Kansas City, MO: International Medical Electronics LTD; 1981.

84. Van Rijswijk L, Polansky M. Predictors of time to healing deep pressure ulcers. *Ostomy/Wound Manage.* 1994;40(8):40–42, 44, 46–48.

85. Electropharmacology. *MRT SofPulse User's Manual.* Pompano Beach, FL: Electropharmacology, Inc.; 1994.

86. Martin CJ, McCallum HM, Strelley S, et al. Electromagnetic fields from therapeutic diathermy equipment: A review of hazards and precautions. *Physiotherapy.* 1991;77:3–7.

87. Ourllet-Hellstrom SR. Miscarriages among female physical therapists who report using radio- and microwave-frequency electromagnetic radiation. *Am J Epidemiol.* 1993;138:775–786.

88. CFR Ch. 1 (4–1–93 Edition). Device described in paragraph (BX1); see section 890.3, 48 FR 53047, Nov. 23, 1983, as amended in 52 FR 17742, May 11, 1987, Document No. A779269 (PSWD Instruction Manual).

89. Low JL. The nature and effects of pulsed electromagnetic radiations. *NZ J Physiother.* 1978;:18–22.

90. Hayne CR. Pulsed high frequency energy—its place in physiotherapy. *Physiotherapy.* 1984;70:459.

91. Frankenberger L, *personal communication.* 1997.

92. Swanson G. Functional outcomes report: The next generation in physical therapy reporting. In: Stewart DL, Abeln SH, eds. *Documenting Functional Outcomes in Physical Therapy.* St. Louis, MO: Mosby-Year Book; 1993.

Phototherapy in Wound Management

Teresa Conner-Kerr, Karen W. Albaugh, Lynda D. Woodruff,
Michelle Cameron, and Autumn Bill

CHAPTER OBJECTIVES

At the completion of this chapter, the reader will be able to:

1. Define phototherapy and list the portions of the electromagnetic spectrum commonly used in the application of this therapeutic modality.
2. List the biologic effects of ultraviolet, visible, and infrared radiation.
3. Describe the preclinical and clinical science studies supporting the use of phototherapy in wound management.
4. List indications and contraindications to treatment of open wounds with phototherapy.
5. Describe the procedures for applying phototherapy to open wounds.

Phototherapy, also known as light therapy, is a form of radiant energy that has been utilized for healing purposes by humans since the time of primitive man. Radiant energy from the sun was used by both the early Greco-Romans and ancient Egyptians for its curative powers; including its effects on wounds and skin disorders. Herodotus, known as the "father of history,"[1,2] was one of the first individuals to surmise a relationship between sun exposure and a heightened biologic response. He was credited with having observed the difference in degree of calcification between the skull bones of vanquished Egyptian and Persian soldiers. He ascribed the increased thickness of Egyptians soldiers' skull bones to greater sun exposure because of the cultural practice of shaving the scalp from an early age. As a result of these observations, Herodotus and others became advocates of sun therapy, and sunlight was prescribed for numerous ailments including epilepsy, paralysis, asthma, malnutrition, and obesity.

Historical Perspective

The sun and the light that it provides was recognized as having potential healing properties by many early cultures, among them the Egyptians, Romans, Greeks, Sumerians, Chinese, Indians, and Japanese.[3] Because of the sun's s integral role in ancient societies, many of the ancient gods were named for the sun. One such god was Helios, Greek god of physical light and sun.[1,2] Evidence of the role that the Greeks believed that the sun god played in healing can be seen in ancient stone inscriptions.

However, with the advent of Christianity, little was written about heliotherapy or sun therapy until the 18th century.[1,2] It was not until 1796 that significant attention was refocused on the question of whether sunlight was beneficial to humans. At this time, a prize was offered by the University of Gottingen for the best essay on the effects of light on the human body. The winning essay by Ebernaier was the first to propose a relationship between the lack of sun exposure and the development of rickets. Some years later, Niels Finsen prepared a paper on the influence of light on skin. Using his own forearm, he demonstrated the ability of sunlight to induce a delayed erythema on unprotected skin exposed to sunlight.

It was also around this time that the germicidal properties of sunlight were discovered. The bactericidal properties of light were first demonstrated in 1877.[1,2] Using an unboiled Pasteur's solution, Downes and Blunt showed that sunlight could prevent the growth of bacteria. In later experiments, Downes and Blunt were able to demonstrate that light near the violet end of the electromagnetic spectrum had the greatest bactericidal potency. However, it was not until Duclaux in 1885 and Ward in 1892 demonstrated the bactericidal effects of sunlight in the absence of heat generation that the bactericidal properties of sunlight became generally accepted.

Some years later, Bernhard and Morgan were the first to show that ultraviolet (UV) radiation below 329 nm was bactericidal.[1,2] Between 1890 and 1909, UV energy was shown to be bactericidal to many bacteria, including *Mycobacterium tuberculosis, Staphylococcus, Streptococcus, Bacillus,* and *Shigella dysenteriae.* It was during this time that UV radiation became a common treatment for tuberculosis of the skin. In fact, the Nobel Prize for Medicine and Science was awarded to Finsen in 1903 for his work on the treatment of tuberculosis-induced skin lesions.

In the following decades, much of the UV research focused on the use of UV radiation to control or prevent surgical wound infection.[1,2,4] This interest continues today with several groups investigating the utility of using UV radiation to prevent or control infection of orthopedic surgical wounds.[5,6,7,8] Additionally, with the emergence of antibiotic-resistant wound pathogens, the role of ultraviolet light in the C band (shorter wavelength ultraviolet) for the treatment of infected acute and chronic wounds is being re-examined along with its putative ability to stimulate wound healing processes.[9,10,11,12]

Similarly, interest in the potential health benefits of other wavelengths of light and novel delivery systems has also evolved over the past 50 years. Focused monochromatic beams of light energy (lasers) have been studied for their potential health benefits since the 1960s.[3,13] Work in this area began with the discovery by Charles Townes and coworkers at Columbia University in New York and Drs. Basov and Prochorov at the Lebedev Institute in Moscow of the maser (**m**icrowave **a**mplification by **s**timulation **e**mission of **r**adiation).[14,15,16] The maser is the longer wavelength predecessor of the laser (**l**ight **a**mplification by **s**timulation **e**mission of **r**adiation). Both the maser and laser use electromagnetic energy (microwave-masers; light-lasers) to excite or add energy to atoms or molecules.

Shortly after the discovery of the maser in 1954, Dr. Thomas Maiman published his work on the ruby laser.[17] Interest in this novel technology quickly grew with the establishment of the first medical laser laboratory at the University of Cincinnati in 1961. By 1971, Mester published his first study in an English-based journal demonstrating a positive effect of the ruby laser on wound healing.[18] Since that time, more than 100 positive, double-blind clinical studies have been published demonstrating positive health benefits of laser on tissue healing and pain control or reduction.[19]

Radiant Energy Definitions

Radiant energy is defined as energy in the form of electromagnetic waves.[20] Different forms of radiant energy are represented by the electromagnetic spectrum (EMS), and these energy forms are arranged in order of their wavelength, frequency, or both. Wavelengths represent the interval between respective peaks in an energy wave. Wavelengths of radiant energy extend from millions of meters (electrical power) to as short as a million-millionth (10^{-12}) of a meter (gamma and cosmic rays).[3] The wavelength of radiant energy determines its depth of penetration. Longer wavelengths penetrate deeper into tissue than do their shorter counterparts. For example, a wavelength of 850 nm penetrates to 40 mm, an 800-nm wavelength penetrates to 30 mm, while a 660-nm wavelength penetrates to approximately 10 mm.[21] It is also important to distinguish between depth of penetration and depth of effect, as the biologic cascade of events set in motion by radiant energy treatment can extend beyond the treatment depth.

It is also important to consider factors that affect absorption of radiant energy other than wavelength. These include angle of application and intensity, as well as tissue factors such as density and skin color. Less heavily pigmented tissues are more sensitive to the detrimental effects of radiant energy due to decreased amounts of melanin present in the epidermis to protect the nucleus of keratinocytes. Denser tissues or tissues with greater melanin content may prevent or limit radiant energy from reaching deeper levels due to absorption. As a result of this absorption, less energy is available for transmission to deeper tissues. The effect of the angle of application and the intensity or power will be considered in the following section, Physical Science of Phototherapy Radiant Energy Forms.

Other radiant energy definitions that are important to understand when studying or considering phototherapy include power, power density, energy, and energy density (see Exhibit 24-1 for definitions).[3] Power is the amount of work performed and is measured in watts. Power is used to determine treatment time. An inverse relationship exists between these two parameters, power and time. As a result, when power increases, treatment times generally decrease.

Power density describes the relationship of the power of the light source to the area irradiated or treated.[3] Thus, power density equals average power divided by area irradi-

EXHIBIT 24-1   Definition of Radiant Energy Terms[3]

Term	Definition	Système International (SI unit)
Power	Rate at which work is performed	Watts
Power density (irradiance)	Power per unit area	Watts/cm^2
Energy (work)	Power (watts) $\times$ time (seconds)	Joules
Energy density (fluence)	Power density $\times$ time	Joules/cm^2
Dose	Reported as energy density	Joules/cm^2

ated. At a given power, if the area irradiated increases, then the power density decreases.

Energy is power multiplied by time. Energy density or dose is the amount of energy per unit area and can be calculated by multiplying power density by time.[3]

Therapeutic Radiant Energy Forms

Radiant energy is used by a number of health-care professionals for a variety of purposes. For example, therapeutic radiation involves the use of very short wavelength, high-energy radiant energy (x-rays and gamma rays) by medical physicists, oncologists, and surgeons in the management of tumors. We will not be addressing these forms of radiant energy in this chapter, as the focus will be on the radiant energy used in the management of open wounds. Radiant energy from the mid-portion of the EMS (UV, visible, and infrared radiation [IR]) is used for this application. Longer wavelength radiant energy from the upper portion of the EMS (microwave and short-wave diathermy) is also used in the management of open wounds and their periwound areas but is covered in Chapter 23. The first part of this chapter focuses on ultraviolet radiation and the latter half on lasers, light-emitting diodes, and super luminescent (luminous) diodes .

Ultraviolet energy: As mentioned above, the three energy forms that have been used historically to provide phototherapy include UV, visible, and IR. UV light is a form of radiant energy that falls between X-rays and visible light on the EMS (Figure 24-1). However, UV light is a misnomer, as this portion of the EMS is largely invisible to the human eye. UV light is more appropriately described as UV energy or radiation. UV energy encompasses the wavelengths between 180 nm and 400 nm and has been commonly separated into three distinct bands, UVA, UVB, and UVC,[22,23,24] based on their wavelength and associated biologic activities.

According to the International Commission on Illumination (CIE), UV wavelengths can be subdivided as follows: 400–315 nm (UVA), 315–280 nm (UVB), and 280–100 nm (UVC).[23] The World Health Organization (WHO) definition of the three UV bands differs somewhat as compared with the CIE. The WHO defines UVA as wavelengths 400–320 nm, UVB as wavelengths 320–280 nm, and UVC as wavelengths 280–200 nm. Recently, UVA has been subdivided into UVA1 and UVA2, since UVA2 rays are thought to have actions more similar to those of UVB. UVA1 encompasses wavelengths from 340 to 400 nm while UVA2 encompasses wavelengths from 320 to 340 nm.[22]

Long-wave UV radiation, or UVA, is referred to as black light or near UV radiation and is closest to the visible light portion of the EMS. The middle band of UV radiation, or UVB, is known as sunburn radiation and is thought to mediate most of the harmful effects of sunlight on human skin, including photo-aging and carcinogenesis.[25,26,27,28,29] UVA and UVB account for approximately 6.3% and 0.5% of sunlight during the summer, respectively.[22,24] On the other hand, UVC, or shortwave UV, radiation is known for its germicidal effects, and almost all of these rays are prevented from reaching the earth by the ozone layer.

Visible energy: The visible wavelengths of light fall between 400 and 800 nm in length and are detectable by the human eye.

Infrared energy: Similar to UV, IR can be divided into two separate bands, a short or near band and a long or far band. Short or near IR wavelengths of light fall between 800 and 1500 nm, whereas long or far infrared wavelengths fall between 1500 and 15000 nm.

Physical Science of Phototherapy Radiant Energy Forms

Radiant energy forms are characterized by specific wavelengths and frequencies. As the wavelengths of energy increase across the EMS, from cosmic rays to electric power, the frequency decreases.[20] For example, gamma rays have short wavelengths but are high frequency compared with broadcast or electric power waves that are long wave and

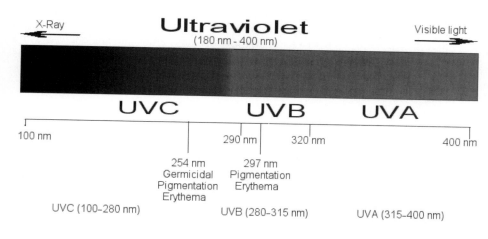

FIGURE 24-1. UV spectrum. (Courtesy of Teresa Conner-Kerr and John Kerr)

low frequency. In biologic tissues, longer wavelengths typically penetrate more deeply than do short ones. Therefore, longer wavelengths allow treatment of deeper structures.

Time to delivery of radiant energy is affected by the density of the medium in which it travels.[3,20] Radiant energy travels in a straight line at high speed while in a vacuum. However, as the density of the medium increases (skin, muscle, bone), the speed of the radiant energy wave decreases. Delivery of radiant energy to a biologic medium is also affected by its interaction with the medium in the following ways:

1. Reflection (decrease in energy to the medium as some waves are reflected away from the medium)
2. Absorption (energy captured by the medium with a decrease in waves traveling completely through the medium)
3. Refraction (bending and dividing wavelengths into component parts)
4. Penetration or transmission through the medium (decreased absorption by the medium with loss of energy from the medium)

Three physical laws govern the use of radiant energy in the treatment of biologic tissues.[20] The first, Grotthus-Draper law, states that the effect of a wavelength on a tissue is determined by the amount of energy that the tissue absorbs. Different wavelengths are known to produce different effects. The second law, the inverse square law, states that the intensity of the energy wave is inversely related to the square of the distance from the radiant source. The third law, the cosine law, states that energy absorption is at its greatest when energy waves strike a medium at right angles. All of these laws must be taken into consideration for the proper and optimal application of radiant energy.

Phototherapy Delivery Systems

Modern approaches to phototherapy began with the use of ultraviolet light boxes and infrared lamps in the early part of the 20th century.[1] By the late 1950s, a new technology emerged that produced a uniform and coherent, monochromatic beam of light, the laser.[17,30,31] Early use of the laser focused on high-power units that operated at an intensity high enough to produce coagulation of body proteins due to thermal effects; hence the term hot laser. In comparison, low level or cold lasers, which do not produce significant elevation of tissue temperatures, were adopted for applications in wound/tissue healing and pain control due to their photobiomodulation effects. Low-level lasers were first used in Europe, China, and Canada and have only recently gained acceptance in the United States for use in wound healing.

Recent developments in phototherapy involve the use of clusters of light-emitting diodes (LEDs), laser diodes (LDs), super luminescent (luminous) diodes (SLDs), or a mixture of these light sources (cluster probes).[3,17,21,30,31] Energy emitted from a laser differs from that emitted by an LED or SLD because it is a stimulated emission and not a spontaneous one. Laser diodes (LDs), on the other hand, are true lasers.

With laser, a photon of the absorption wavelength, is fired at an atom already in its high energy state from prior absorption. The atom absorbs this photon, and then quickly emits two photons to get back to its lower energy state. Both of these newly emitted photons are of the same wavelength. This produces light that is coherent (beam stays together), collimated (directional) and monochromatic (one wavelength/color). In contrast, light produced by LEDs and SLDs is polychromatic, although it may have a narrow range of wavelengths, and is not collimated or coherent.[21,30] Since LEDs and SLDs are not collimated or coherent, they produce a wider beam of energy. However, the importance of this lack of coherence or collimation by LEDs and SLDs is not known since. As light enters tissue, it is refraction or bent and this changes the direction that the light travels. As a result, the light beam is widened and the coherent quality of the laser light is lost. It has been proposed that the effects of LEDs and SLDs may be comparable to those of lasers because of the changes that laser light undergoes once it enters tissue. Large randomized, controlled trials have yet to answer this question definitively.

Light-Emitting Diodes

LEDs emit a form of radiant or light energy in the visible or invisible range of the electromagnetic spectrum. They are made from semiconductors and when a charge is applied to the material, electrons move from a conduction band to a lower energy orbital releasing photons of light. LEDs spontaneously release a narrow range of wavelengths with similar shades of light colors that are minimally divergent.

Laser Diodes

LDs derive light from an LED and produce positive feedback in a chamber/resonator that leads to a stimulated emission of photons. LDs are true lasers and produce a collimated and monochromatic beam of light.

Super Luminescent (Luminous) Diodes

SLDs are high-intensity, narrow-frequency, light-emitting diodes. SLDs produce an amplified spontaneous emission with a narrow frequency range and beam angle that is wider than a LD but between that of an LED and LD. The SLD is not a laser because there is no stimulated emission of light energy.

Cluster Probes

The above technologies may also be combined to produce cluster probes that take advantage of their unique properties. The advantage of combining these different technologies is that treatment times are reduced, larger tissue areas can be treated, and the biologic effects of different wavelengths may be accessed.

Ultraviolet Energy

Biologic Effects of Ultraviolet Energy

The three bands of UV radiation differ in their ability to penetrate human skin (Figure 24-2) and to produce certain biologic effects.[20,22,24] The UVA band constitutes the longest wavelengths of the UV energy spectrum, and these rays are known to penetrate human skin to the level of the upper dermis. In contrast, UVB rays penetrate only to the stratum basale, the lowermost level of the epidermis. UVC rays (which have the least ability to penetrate human skin) reach only the upper layers of the epidermis.

Specific UV wavelengths have been associated with particular biologic responses (see Figure 24-1). For example, the germicidal effects of UV radiation are associated with UV wavelengths from 250 to 270 nm,[20,22,24] while UV wavelengths of 254 nm and 297 nm have the greatest ability to induce an erythematous or reddening reaction in the skin. The tanning response, on the other hand, is predominantly associated with wavelengths of 254 and 299 nm.

UV energy has been used to treat a variety of skin conditions, including open wounds, because of its biologic effects.[6,7,8,11,32,33,34,35,36] UV radiation is known to promote exfoliation of the outer skin layers, enhance healing through the induction of an erythematous response in the skin, and inactivate a variety of microorganisms. The biologic effects of UV have been classified as immediate or long term (Exhibit 24-2).[23,27,37] Stenbak[27] lists the induction of erythema and its accompanying inflammatory changes along with increased pigmentation as examples of acute skin reactions to UV exposure. In comparison, late cutaneous effects are

EXHIBIT 24-2   Immediate and Long-Term Effects of High-Level Exposure to UVB Radiation

Immediate
  Early (0–60 hours)
    Immediate hyperpigmentation
    Epidermal hyperplasia
    Inflammatory reactions
  Late (60–336 hours)
    Secondary hyperpigmentation
    Hyperplasia
    Fibrosis
  Long standing (CHRONIC exposure)
    Elastosis
    Carcinoma

identified as elastosis, or the loss of skin elasticity, and carcinogenesis.

Early Cutaneous Effects

Skin reddening or erythema is a well-known effect of UV at certain exposure levels. UV radiation produces this reddening of the skin via stimulation of an inflammatory response that leads to increased vascularity of the dermis.[23,27,37] Erythema is most effectively produced by the 297 nm and 254 nm UV wavelengths.[22,24] These wavelengths encompass both the B and C bands of UV. Erythema that results from the longer wavelengths has a greater latency and lasts for a longer period of time than that produced by shorter wavelengths. However, the shorter wavelengths have a greater potency.

UV-induced erythema is associated with a latent period of 2 to 3 hours.[23] The exact mechanism that underlies this latent appearance of erythema is unknown, but several theories have been offered. The latent development of the erythemal response has been ascribed to the production of some diffusable biologic mediator from damaged epidermal cells.[23,37] It is thought that this mediator then diffuses to the dermis, where it enhances blood vessel permeability. The identity of this diffusable mediator is unknown. Several substances including histamine, bradykinin, and prostaglandins have been implicated in this role. In the past, prostaglandins were thought to be the most likely candidate for this role as a diffusable mediator. However, work by Hensby[38] utilizing prostaglandin antagonists has been inconclusive, and the role that prostaglandins play in mediating erythema is unclear.

Recent studies by Brauchle[39] have demonstrated a significant increase in vascular endothelial growth factor (VEGF) expression in cultured keratinocytes after irradiation with both sublethal and physiologic levels of UVB. Irradiation of quiescent keratinocytes lead to both an increase in mRNA levels as well as increased levels of VEGF. Since VEGF is known to enhance vascular permeability, it is thought that VEGF may be a potential target for the above-described diffusable mediator. However, the identity of this

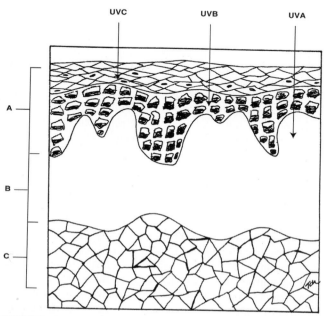

UVC   UVB   UVA

FIGURE 24-2. Depth of penetration into the integument by UVA, UVB, and UVC rays. (Courtesy of Teresa Conner-Kerr)

diffusable mediator(s) remains unknown. Congruent with the findings of Brauchle,[39] Holtz[40] has shown that UV-induced erythema is accompanied by an intercellular edema in the prickle or spiny cell layer of the skin and an accumulation of white cells in local blood vessels. The development of intercellular edema is also consistent with the separation of the upper and lower epidermal layers that occurs upon exposure to high-intensity UV radiation. These effects on the skin most likely underlie the ability of UV radiation to stimulate debridement. Debridement would result from this sloughing of the upper layers of the epidermis as well as recruitment of phagocytic white blood cells. Increased lysosomal activity and leakage of lysosomal enzymes that has been detected with UV exposure may also contribute to this debridement effect.

Another immediate effect of UV exposure includes skin thickening, or hyperplasia.[26,27] UV rays induce a hyperplasia or cellular proliferation in the stratum corneum, or outermost layer of the skin. This process is thought to be protective against subsequent sunlight-induced skin damage. Research indicates that DNA changes are seen within 4 to 7 hours after irradiation of the epidermis. Epidermal cells in stratum basale have been shown to accumulate glycogen at 12 hours, and increased RNA levels are seen at 24 hours in both the basal and lower prickle cell layer. These increased levels of RNA are thought to reflect an increased rate of transcription, indicating on-going repair. These increased levels of RNA are consistent with the finding that UV radiation stimulates the production of IL-1α by keratinocytes.[41] IL-1α is known to play a role in enhancing wound epithelialization.[42]

Work by Kaiser et al.[41] demonstrated that UVB stimulated epithelialization, thus providing further evidence of a role for UVB in stimulating epidermal migration by enhancing IL-1α production. This work supports the current treatment approach of utilizing UV to enhance epithelialization, especially with indolent wounds that exhibit fibrotic edges. In these wounds, UV may stimulate or restart the epithelialization process.

When low-level UV radiation exposure occurs, it is thought that the above-described effects are confined to the upper third or one half of the epidermis.[28] As a result, no long-lasting effects are thought to occur as the cells in these layers are differentiating in transit to becoming part of the outer dead layer of the skin. Therefore, these data among others lend support to the supposition that UV radiation stimulates repair processes and that these effects may be harnessed at a low enough level to prevent long-term damage. The wound clinician may find the induction of epidermal hyperplasia by UV radiation to be beneficial in promoting rapid epithelialization in acute and chronic wounds.

High levels of UVB exposure have also been shown to affect Langerhans cells.[23,43,44] These cells inhabit the middle region of the epidermis and appear to have an immune function. They are part of the macrophage lineage and are derived from the bone marrow. High-level UVB exposure is known to produce Langerhans cell necrosis within 24 hours. This pattern of cellular necrosis is seen in both experimental rodent models and humans. The destruction of these cells is thought to account for the immunosuppressive ability of high levels of UVB. Interestingly, this immunosuppressive effect of high-level UVB exposure has been harnessed by researchers to enhance graft take in individuals with burn wounds.[45] However, since the Langerhans cells are derived from the bone marrow, no long-term effects are expected as a result of this local immunosuppression of the treated skin. Furthermore, the effects of short treatment times at low intensities with UVB or UVC are unknown. It is possible that the effects may be different from those seen with high-level UV radiation.

Late Cutaneous Effects

Late cutaneous effects include elastosis,[28] or loss of skin elasticity, and carcinogenesis.[25,28,37] Elastosis has been observed traditionally in the skin of individuals who labor in the sun for most of their lives. It is characterized by the degeneration of collagen and elastin fibers in the dermis. Histologic analysis of skin, which exhibits elastosis, includes basophilic degeneration and enlarged, blunted elastic fibers. These changes are not found in adjacent skin areas that have been protected from prolonged exposure to the sun.

Prolonged or lifetime exposure to UV radiation, particularly rays in the B band, is well accepted as a causative factor in certain types of skin cancers. According to Moseley,[23] supporting evidence for UVB-related carcinogenesis includes:

1. Increased number of skin cancers on sites exposed to the sun chronically
2. Decreased numbers of certain types of skin cancers with increased natural pigmentation
3. Increased incidence of skin cancer in light-skinned people, especially those who spend significant time outdoors
4. Increased incidence of skin cancer in light-colored people who live near the equator
5. UVB readily produces skin cancer in experimental animal models with prolonged continuous exposure (hours)
6. Individuals with deficient DNA repair mechanisms in the skin are more prone to skin cancers

However, these effects are associated with prolonged exposure to sunlight, particularly high-intensity UVB over a period of years. Therefore, the relevance of these concerns when deciding whether to employ short duration, low-intensity UV radiation for stimulation of wound healing or treatment of wound infection especially with UVC rays should be questioned. Additionally, these carcinogenic effects are linked to cellular changes in the epidermis, and the greatest number of wounds that are candidates for UV treatment are of at least partial thickness. If warranted with this low level of UV energy exposure, the periwound could be protected with draping or a UV blocking ointment such as petrolatum.

Bactericidal Effects

Research has shown that UV radiation from all three bands, A, B and C, has the ability to kill numerous microorganisms. As a result of its effectiveness in killing microorganisms, UV light has been used in a variety of ways, including water purification, serum sterilization, pharmaceutical clean room, and surgical theatre decontamination.[26] It has also been used to treat a variety of skin infections and heavily contaminated wounds.

Because of continuing issues with surgical infections, there has been renewed interest in the potential role of UV light in preventing surgical wound infections. Taylor et al[6,46] in the United Kingdom examined the effectiveness of UVC radiation on reducing bacterial numbers in individuals undergoing total joint arthroplasty. UVC energy was delivered by tubing placed overhead in a conventional plenum-ventilated surgical theatre. The UVC tubes were activated 10 minutes after the surgical procedure was initiated. Results of the study showed that the UVC application was effective in significantly reducing bacterial levels in both the theatre air and surgical wounds. Bacterial levels in the surgical wounds fell 87% with UVC delivered at 100 microW/cm^2 (N = 18) and 92% with UVC delivered at 300 microW/cm^2 (N = 13).

In a similar study, Moggio et al[7] also found that UV irradiation significantly lowered the average number of airborne bacteria detected over the surgical site. The rate of infection for 1,322 individuals that underwent hip arthroplasties was found to be only 0.15% with application of UVC. Similar findings were obtained by Berg et al[8] when UVC application in operating rooms was compared with a sham blue light application. These authors concluded that the air quality was similar to that produced by ultraclean air ventilation systems. It is also interesting to note that both Berg et al[8] and Taylor et al[46] recorded no adverse effects of UVC exposure on operating room personnel.

A growing interest in the use of UV energy for treatment of established wound infections has also been seen in the past two decades. This renewed interest in UV light comes at a time when antimicrobial resistance is rampant among common wound pathogens and when the health-care community is increasingly under pressure to find the most cost-effective and time-efficient method of treatment for various health-care problems.

The effectiveness of UV radiation in killing microbes has been demonstrated by many researchers using in vitro testing. High and High[47] demonstrated that broad-spectrum UV radiation delivered by the Kromayer lamp (model 10), which produces wavelengths from all three UV bands, was effective in eliminating a wide range of wound pathogens in vitro. Exposure times tested in this study are consistent with treatment times that have been recommended in the past for skin and wound infections. The times were based on the previously described classification of erythemal responses with E2, E3, and E4 doses (see section on UV treatment times for a description) being effective in killing common wound pathogens. Complete eradication of all wound pathogens tested was only obtained at an E4 dose. In contrast, Nordback et al[48] did not find a difference in colonization levels in rats with acute surgical wounds that were exposed to broad-spectrum UV radiation. Since the UV radiation source emitted a broad spectrum of UV A, B, and C wavelengths and the proportion of each type of wavelength is not described, it is difficult to determine if the wavelengths that are known to have the greatest germicidal activity (UVC at 250–270 nm) were present at adequate doses.

Using a halogen lamp that emits predominantly UVC, we have shown that a broad range of wound pathogens including those expressing antibiotic resistance can be effectively eliminated with short treatment times (Exhibit 24-3).[49,50] Using the V-254 lamp, which selectively emits UVC energy, we have been able to obtain a 99.99% kill rate for all tested common wound pathogens. Using an in vitro model with optimal growth characteristics for the microorganisms tested, we have shown that UVC irradiation is effective in eradicating both procaryotic organisms such as bacteria and eucaryotic organisms such as yeast or multicellular fungi at short exposure times. In fact, we have found that UVC is effective in killing multicellular eucaryotic wound pathogens at treatment times shorter than those currently advocated for procaryotic (bacterial) organisms. However, our data does indicate that multicellular eucaryotic organisms require 10 times the exposure time (30 seconds) for a 99.9% kill rate as compared with the most susceptible eucaryotic organism (3 seconds).

Work conducted in our laboratory has also demonstrated that short UVC exposure times can produce a 99.99% kill rate for common antibiotic resistant bacterial pathogens in vitro and in vivo.[9,10] Using an optimal growth model in vitro, we have found that 99.99% of methicillin-resistant

EXHIBIT 24-3 Exposure Times for 99.99% Inactivation of Common Procaryotic and Eucaryotic Wound Pathogens by UVC Radiation

	UVC Treatment Times (seconds)				
	in vitro				*in vivo*
	3	5	15	30	30
Procaryotes *(bacteria)*					
MRSA		*			*
VRE		*			
Group A streptococcus		*			
Pseudomonas aeruginosa		*			
Mycobacterium abscesses		*			
Unicellular eucaryote *(yeast)*					
Candida albicans		*			
Multicellular procaryote *(fungi)*					
Aspergillus fumigatus		*			
Mixed cultures	*				
Pseudomonas aeruginosa					
Candida albicans					
Aspergillus fumigatus					

Staphylococcus aureus (MRSA) and vancomycin-resistant *Enterococcus* (VRE) are eliminated with only 5 seconds of exposure to UVC. Additionally, data from our laboratory indicates that once-daily exposure to UVC for 5 days is adequate to produce 100% eradication of MRSA from acute rat surgical wounds.

Studies by Taylor et al[51] using an in vitro model also found UVC to be effective in killing bacteria. In this study, the effects of UVC on bacteria alone and in combination with pulsed jet lavage was compared with commonly used antiseptics. All of the tested topical agents including 3% hydrogen peroxide, 1% and 10% povidone-iodine, and 0.05% chlorhexidine were found to reduce bacterial numbers on agar. However, the bactericidal effects of only hydrogen peroxide and povidone-iodine were effectively eliminated when tested on muscle tissue treated with whole blood or plasma. The effects of UVC application and pulsed jet lavage were found to be additive, suggesting a clinical role for co-application of these modalities in treating wound infection.

UV Preclinical Studies

The effects of UVA and UVB radiation on wound healing has been examined using a number of different animal models, including the rat, hairless guinea pig, rabbit, and pig.[52,53,54,55,56] Positive effects of UVB on wound healing were observed in both the rat[48] and rabbit[52] animal models but not in the hairless guinea pig[53,54,55] model. Irradiation of the acute surgical wound bed of rats with a UVA and UVB energy source resulted in a significantly increased rate of wound closure between the fourth and fifteenth days of treatment compared with untreated controls on the contralateral side of the animal.[48] Additionally, no decrement in wound tensile strength was found at either day 7 or 15 compared with the untreated controls. The results from this study also suggest that the effects of UVA and UVB are localized and not systemic, as healing of the contralateral wounds was not enhanced.

Similarly, El Batouty et al[52] found a modestly higher rate of tissue regeneration in acute full-thickness wounds to the pinna of rabbit ears using a hot quartz lamp (UVA and UVB). UV-treated wounds healed more rapidly than their untreated controls. Additionally, histopathologic analysis demonstrated significant increases in epithelization rates and collagen deposition as compared with untreated controls.

In contrast, acute surgical wounds induced in hairless guinea pigs that had been pretreated with UVA or UVB radiation every other day for 16 weeks did not exhibit enhanced wound closure rates.[54,55] Additionally, wound tensile strength was found to be significantly less in both the UVA- and UVB-treated animals. Histopathologic analysis also demonstrated marked endothelial swelling and eosinophilic infiltration in the irradiated group. Similar findings for decreased wound tensile strength were found using hairless guinea pigs pretreated with pure UVA radiation prior to wounding. Due to the extraordinarily long duration of treatment (16 weeks in the first study and 21 weeks in the second study) and the use of a pretreatment UV paradigm rather than UV treatment postwounding, the relevance of these findings are not clear. Furthermore, additional work by the same investigators found that there were no significant differences in tensile strength of wounds made to UV-treated versus untreated skin by recovery day 90.[56]

At this point in time, examination of the effects of UVC on wound healing rates in both the pig and rodent model have shown no grossly detectable facilitation of wound closure. In the porcine model, no significant effect of UVC radiation on wound tensile strength was detected.[56] However, recent studies in our laboratory demonstrated that a 30-second UVC treatment once daily for 5 days in a rodent model resulted in a cleaner and smoother transition area between the periwound and the wound bed with no tissue curling.[12] This treatment paradigm also produced a change in wound morphology due to altered wound contraction. The induction of a change in wound contraction by UVC is consistent with the findings of Morykaw et al.[57] Using cultured fibroblasts, Morykaw et al[57] demonstrated increased secretion of fibronectin into the culture medium after UVC irradiation. Fibronectin is an extracellular matrix protein that appears to play a role in wound contraction.

UV Clinical Studies

Although there is significant experimental data to suggest a positive role for UV radiation in enhancing wound healing, relatively few clinical studies have been conducted. However, the majority of studies that have been conducted have found positive effects. Documented positive effects of UVA and UVB on wound healing can be found in the literature as far back as 1945.[32] Stein and Shorey[32] published an article detailing the increased rate of wound healing and reduction of wound infection in two soldiers, one with a traumatic wound and the other with a pressure wound. Both wounds had been resistant to healing prior to the institution of UV radiation. The traumatic wound healed within 10 days of the initiation of UV therapy, and the pressure wound healed in less than 2 months.

A randomized controlled trial examining the effects of both UVA and UVB energy on superficial pressure sores in the elderly has also demonstrated enhanced healing rates.[33] In this study, UV-treated ulcers closed in an average time of 6.25 weeks compared with an average of 10 weeks for control wounds. Additionally, a clinical study by Crous and Malherbe[34] also examined the effects of UVA and UVB on wound healing in individuals with venous insufficiency. Treatment parameters were based on the commonly accepted method of determining UV dosage by determining the degree of erythemal response by the skin upon exposure to successively longer treatment times (Exhibit 24-4). An E_1 dose was used for periwound skin and granulation tissue and an E_4 dose for necrotic tissue. At these doses, UV radiation appeared to facilitate wound healing, but wound closure was not achieved with any of the wounds.

EXHIBIT 24-4 Erythemal Dosages Used with UV Radiation Exposure

Dose	Skin Reaction	Time to Develop	Time to Resolution
SED	None noted		
E_1 (MED)	Subtle reddening	4–6 hrs	24 hrs
E_2	Similar to mild sunburn Skin exfoliation and pigmentation	4–6 hrs	3–4 days
E_3	Similar to severe sunburn Intense erythema Marked increase in exfoliation and pigmentation	2 hrs	Several days
E_4	Same as E_3 with significant tissue swelling and exudate	2 hrs	Several days

SED = suberythemal dose
E_1 (MED) = minimal erythemal dose
E_2 = second-degree erythemal dose
E_3 = third-degree erythemal dose
E_4 = fourth-degree erythemal dose

The effects of UVC on chronic wound healing have also been examined. A study by Nussbaum et al[35] examined the effects of UVC combined with ultrasound on pressure ulcer healing. Their treatment parameters were similar to those used with the Crous and Malherbe[34] study. The treatments parameters included E_1 for clean/granulating wounds, E_3 for purulent/slow healing wounds, E_4 for heavily infected wounds, and $2E_4$ for necrotic wounds. Combination of the UVC and ultrasound treatment was found to enhance healing over that of cold laser or moist wound healing. However, it is difficult to ascribe the enhanced healing effects observed in this study to a UVC-mediated effect, as the UVC treatment employed was delivered in combination with ultrasound. Therefore, it is not clear as to what effect either of the modalities had separately.

Taylor[36] also examined the effectiveness of UVC in treating 56 individuals with infections of the skin including the following lesions: tinea pedis, tinea capitis, sporotrichosis, and tinea corporis. The treatment times were between 2 and 5 minutes, with individuals receiving an average of 3.2 treatments over a period of 5 to 7 days. Fifty patients showed a good response to therapy, with most showing significant clearing of the infection within 1 week.

Recently, Thai et al[11] found that UVC was effective in decreasing bacterial numbers in chronic wounds. *Pseudomonas aeruginosa, Staphylococcus aureus,* and methicillin-resistant *Staphylococcus aureus* numbers among other bacterial species were reduced with a single application of UVC for 180 seconds. Consistent with in vitro testing, UVC was shown to be most effective in reducing the level of *Pseudomonas aeruginosa* in chronic wounds. However, the effects of UVC on MRSA was not as robust as the effects on other bacteria in the wounds with only a one-level reduction in numbers after the standard 180-second treatment time. The present data indicates that multiple treatments of 180 seconds may be required to completely eradicate common bacterial pathogens from chronic wounds.

UVC: Current Recommended Treatment Approaches
UVC Treatment Algorithm

Based on recent work[9,10,49,50] performed in the Collaborative Laboratory for Wound Healing, we propose the use of the algorithm found in Figure 24-3 to determine treatment times for infected wounds when using UVC radiation. This algorithm is based on a review of the available research. This approach would be in place of the older system that utilized degree of skin erythema to determine treatment times. Our algorithm is based on the theoretical principle of choosing UVC treatment times according to minimal lethal dose for the infecting organism. The author advocates this approach as it specifically addresses the susceptibility pattern of the infecting organism to UVC and not the response of the host to UVC. As a result, an adequate dose for killing or inactivation of a particular pathogen can be selected while preventing or minimizing any damage to host cells. As outlined in the previous sections, longer treatment times, especially those used with UVB, are known to produce deleterious effects.

Procedure for Administration

Equipment Selection. The primary decision to be made concerning equipment selection is whether a UVA/UVB or UVC energy source is to be utilized for treatments. Presently, research appears to indicate that either source is germicidal, although the peak germicidal wavelengths are in the UVC band from 250 to 270 nm. In vitro testing has shown that 99.99% killing or inactivation of common procaryotic wound pathogens occurs at 5 seconds with a UVC energy source[9,49,50] compared with greater than 180 seconds (an E_4 dose) with a UVA/UVB source.[47] Additionally, once-daily treatments for 30 seconds by UVC has been shown to produce greater than 99.99% eradication of MRSA in living tissue.[10] Furthermore, the role of UVC in

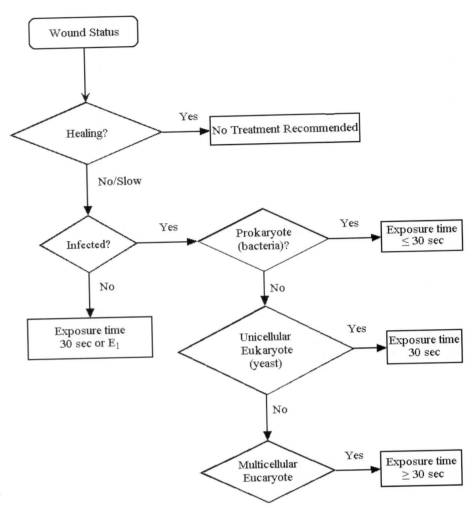

FIGURE 24-3. UVC treatment algorithm. (Courtesy of Teresa Conner-Kerr)

preventing surgical wound infections during operative procedures has been demonstrated.[46] A recent study by Thai et al[11] found that a one-time UVC treatment of chronic wounds for 180 seconds produced reduction in bacterial numbers. The authors of this study suggest the need for multiple treatment sessions to obtain complete wound bed clearance of bacterial pathogens. At this time, it is not clear whether multiple replications with shorter treatment times or longer treatment times with fewer replications would be more beneficial. Therefore, it is recommended at this time that UVC be applied to clinically infected wounds for either a single 180-second treatment or for 30 seconds daily for 5 days.

The greatest number of wound healing studies (many of which are sited in this text) have been conducted using UVA and UVB radiation. Results from both preclinical and clinical studies indicate that UVB in particular stimulates wound healing through the promotion of increased epithelialization rates and increased dermal vascularity. Recent molecular studies suggest a role for UVB radiation in facilitating wound healing. As outlined previously, a putative mechanism for the effects of UVB on wound healing may be through the stimulation of cytokines such as IL-1(or VEGF.[58,59]

Data from several studies also support a role for the use of UVC radiation in stimulating healing. Nussbaum et al[35] demonstrated increased rates of pressure ulcer healing in individuals treated with UVC and ultrasound combined. Healing rates obtained by Nussbaum et al in this study were greater than those seen in a randomized controlled clinical trial using UVB radiation.[33] However, it is difficult to compare these two studies because of the age difference between the two subject groups.

Positive effects of UVC treatment on wound healing have also been seen in our laboratory using an acute surgical wound model.[12] Once-daily treatments of UVC radiation for 30 seconds were found to produce a more organized transitional area between the periwound and wound tissue with no apparent rolling over of the wound margins. Changes in the pattern of wound contraction were also noted with UVC treatment of these acute wounds. This finding is consistent with results from an in vitro study that showed increased fibronectin secretion by cultured fibroblasts and enhanced lattice contraction post-UVC irradiation.[57]

Therefore, the decision to use one particular UV energy source for wound healing is less clear than that for germicidal effects. Since most of the literature has linked chronic exposure to high-dose UVB to carcinoma formation,[28,37] the author recommends that low-dose or MED (E_1) UVB be utilized for treatment and that treatment sessions be limited in number. Individual response to therapy should dictate length and number of treatments with the minimum number of treatment sessions conducted to stimulate angiogenesis or re-epithelialization. Observation of increased rates of granulation tissue formation and/or re-epithelialization support cessation of therapy.

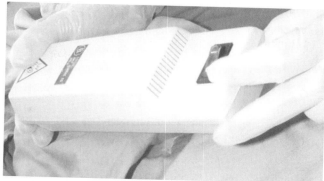

FIGURE 24-5. UVC treatment of infected sacral pressure ulcer. (Courtesy of Teresa Conner-Kerr)

RESEARCH WISDOM:

Select a UVC Lamp for Clinical Infections

The peak germicidal effects of UV radiation are seen with wavelengths of 250 to 270 nm. These wavelengths are found in the UVC band. Therefore, when treating fungal or bacterial skin or wound infections, use low-dose UVC radiation.

Several different lamp types are available that selectively emit UVC radiation; examples of these can be seen in Figure 24-4. One of the early UVC generators that was commonly used by PTs and physical medicine physicians was the Birtcher cold quartz lamp. The cold quartz lamps emit better than 90% UVC at approximately 254 nm.[22] This emission falls within the peak germicidal range for UV radiation. The V-254" lamp also has a similar emission range. Either of these lamps will provide a good germicidal effect. However, the halogen lamp is lighter and has a larger face plate that allows for more rapid treatment of larger wounds.

Preparation of Wound and Periwound Area for UV Treatment. A variety of approaches have been used in the past to prepare the wound bed for treatment with UV radiation. Most authorities recommend protecting the periwound and any nontreatment area with draping materials (Figure 24-5). UV-resistant ointments such as petrolatum jelly may also be

used to protect the periwound area that is immediately adjacent to the wound bed. On the other hand, it has been argued that protecting the adjacent periwound eliminates a potential source of epithelial cells and wound healing factors that would also be stimulated with the treatment. The author recommends protecting the periwound area if high-level (greater than E_2) UV radiation is to be used. It is not clear as to whether periwound protection is warranted with very low UV exposure times in the clinical situation, as most of the information available on carcinogenic potential of UV radiation addresses chronic or high-level exposure times. Furthermore, most of the research has examined the carcinogenic potential of UVB and not UVC. Presently, low-dose UVC appears to be a relatively safe treatment alternative, especially in the treatment of antibiotic-resistant pathogens.

Other considerations for preparation of the wound bed are removal of all dressing materials and cleansing of particulate matter in the wound bed. This can be accomplished by a variety of mechanisms, including pulsatile lavage or normal saline flush. At this point in time, there is one study that found added benefit to decreasing microorganism numbers in an in vitro wound model when co-administering jet lavage and UV radiation.[51] Cleansing of the wound bed is also important, as the depth of penetration for all UV wavelengths is only at best less than 100–200 um.[23] Therefore, cleansing of particulate increases wound bed exposure.

CLINICAL WISDOM

Cleanse Wound and Remove Necrotic Tissue Prior to UV Treatment

To maximize exposure of the wound bed to the UV rays, the wound should be cleansed with a gentle cleanser such as normal saline and debridement to remove as much necrotic tissue as possible.

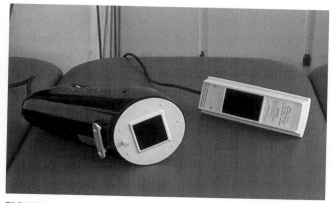

FIGURE 24-4. Germicidal UVC lamps. The black lamp on the left is a Birtcher cold quartz lamp and the lamp on the right is the V-254" halogen lamp. (Courtesy of Med Faxx, Inc., Wake Forest, North Carolina)

It is also recommended that all dressings be removed for treatment. Mackinnon and Cleek[60] had previously suggested that UV radiation could be used with transparent dressings. However, we were unable to detect any bacterial inactivation or killing when bacterial cultures covered with either Tegaderm or Bioclusive were irradiated with UVC for treatment times as long as 120 seconds.[50]

Treatment Times.   In the past, UV dose has been calculated according to the MED response (Exhibit 24-4) of each individual client.[22,23,24] However, the author questions the appropriateness of this system for determining UVC treatment times as the recommended treatment times for necrotic and/or infected wounds are at levels high enough to produce significant cellular necrosis. Findings in our laboratory using both in vitro and in vivo modeling indicate that many wound pathogens, especially MRSA, can be eradicated at very low treatment times (see Exhibit 24-3).[9,10,49,50]

Therefore, we advocate the use of the shortest exposure time that have been shown to be effective in eradicating the offending wound pathogen (see Exhibit 24-3). We also encourage the use of the shortest treatment times (MED; ~30 seconds) or UV dosages that have been found to stimulate the synthesis or secretion of biologic factors[57,58,59] involved in wound healing or that have been found to induce positive wound healing effects[12] (see Exhibit 24-4).

At this time, it is also recommended that treatment times be considered in relation to the existence of UV recovery mechanisms. Recovery and repair post-UV radiation exposure has been documented in many different types of organisms, including viruses, bacteria, fungi, protozoa, and vertebrates, among others.[37] Recovery or photoreactivation of an organism that has been damaged by exposure to UV radiation is defined as the ability of an organism to regain its propagative potential. One of the primary mechanisms by which photoreactivation appears to work is the induction of a repair enzyme upon exposure to near UV or short wavelength visible light. This enzyme effectively reconnects two components of DNA that had been cleaved during exposure to UV radiation. The effectiveness of photoenzymatic repair is expressed by a single numeric index called the fluence reduction or fluence modification factor. The fluence reduction factor indicates the degree to which UV radiation-induced damage is reversed as a result of photoenzymatic repair.

It is important that the clinician who is considering using UVC for wound infections or to stimulate healing recognize the presence of this UV recovery mechanism. Treatment times should be designed to exceed the ability for pathogens to reactivate but not for mammalian cells to recover from any detrimental effects of UV exposure. Since research has shown that increasingly complex organisms[49] are less susceptible to the detrimental effects of UVC radiation at a given dose, theoretically it should be possible to design a treatment paradigm for wound infections that would prevent or minimize host cell damage. In a recent study, we found that multicellular eucaryotic organisms required 6–10 times the UVC exposure time for 99.99% eradication as compared with common bacterial wound pathogens when tested in vitro. In another study[10], we showed that UVC decreased the bacterial load in living tissue by 99.99% with once-daily treatment for 30 seconds over a 5-day period.

It is also thought that many of the positive biologic responses elicited by UV radiation can be effected by lower doses than currently recommended. Therefore, it is recommended that an initial low dosage (MED, 30 seconds of UVC or UVA/UVB) be used in the treatment of wounds.

Treatment Distance.   Recommended treatment distances for the UVC lamps are 1 inch or 2.54 cm from the UVC source to the wound bed.[22,24] UVC lamps are available with built-in spacers or the clinician can simply attach spacers made of 1-inch portions of sterile swabs or tongue depressors. The UVC energy should be delivered perpendicular to the wound bed to maximize delivery according to the cosine law.

Similar placement of the UVA and UVB lamp should be utilized to take advantage of the cosine law. However, treatment distances vary, with a general distance from UVA or UVB source to the skin surface being 30 inches.

Step-by-Step Guide to UVC Application

1. Cleanse face plate of UV lamp with antimicrobial agent per manufacturer's guidelines.
2. As client comfort permits, position client for maximal exposure of the wound.
3. Remove all dressings.
4. Cleanse wound with normal saline.
5. Remove excess wound fluid and loose particulate matter.
6. Drape periwound area or coat with nontoxic UV-blocking ointment (avoid getting it in the wound bed).
7. Protect clinician's and client's eyes from UV radiation with UV-protective goggles for the clinician and goggles or draping for the client.
8. Place UVC lamp source 1 inch or 2.5 cm from wound.
9. Irradiate wound according to UVC algorithm (see Figure 24-3).
10. Remove UV-blocking ointment and re-dress wound.

Step-by-Step Guide to UVA/UVB Application

1. Allow the UVA/UVB lamp adequate time to warm up according to manufacturers guidelines.
2. Determine MED or E_1 dose with erythrometer over a nonpigmented area such as the inner arm, starting with 30 seconds of exposure.
3. Follow steps 2–7 above.
4. Place UVA/UVB source 30 inches from wound bed.
5. Irradiate wound according to UVC algorithm (see Figure 24-3) using an E_1 dose initially to stimulate epithelialization and increase vascularity.
6. Remove UV-blocking ointment and re-dress wound.

Orient UV Lamp Parallel to Wound Bed

Observing cosine law, orient UV lamp parallel to wound bed with UV rays delivered perpendicular to the wound to maximize energy delivery.

Indications

As outlined in the preclinical and clinical studies sections, UV radiation appears to be indicated for the following:

1. Slow or nonhealing wounds
2. Necrotic wounds
3. Purulent or infected acute or chronic wounds

Contraindications

Commonly sited contraindications[22,24] to treatment include the following:

1. Diabetes
2. Pulmonary tuberculosis
3. Hyperthyroidism
4. Systemic lupus erythematous
5. Cardiac, renal, and hepatic disease
6. Acute eczema or psoriasis
7. Herpes simplex

Adverse Reactions

With any adverse reaction such as severe pain due to itching or burning, UV therapy should be discontinued. Hydrogel moist wound dressings or other products that have been shown to decrease the pain associated with radiation or burn wounds may increase client comfort and speed healing.

Self-Care and Teaching Guidelines

Administration of UV energy should be performed by a skilled individual licensed in the application of physical agent modalities. To prevent the occurrence of overexposure to the wound bed and inappropriate exposure to other skin areas, UVC treatment should not be administered by the individual receiving treatment or the responsible caregiver. Additionally, as with all physical agent modalities or procedures, the clinician should evaluate the necessity of using this modality on a frequent and regular basis to ensure optimum treatment outcomes.

CASE STUDY

Decontamination of a Wound Infected with MRSA Using UVC Radiation

Individual: M.G. **Age:** 79 **Start of Care Date:** 4/98

Medical History

M.G. was a 79-year-old nonambulatory female resident of a long-term care facility with a sacral wound. Her medical diagnoses included CHF with end-stage renal disease. She required mod-max assist of two therapists for all bed mobility. She had no prior history of pressure ulceration.

Reason for Referral

Client was referred to physical therapy due to impaired bed mobility and the presence of a nonhealing stage 3 sacral pressure ulcer.

FUNCTIONAL DIAGNOSIS AND TARGETED OUTCOMES

Wound Examination

The wound was a stage 3 pressure ulcer located over the sacrum. Wound margins were indurated and the periwound expressed moderate erythema. The periwound was also noted to be warmer than adjacent tissues. The wound bed was fully granulated and friable upon manual examination and a distinctive odor of ammonia was detected upon initial examination. Semiquantitative swab cultures of this wound indicated that it contained high numbers of methicillin-resistant *Staphylococcus aureus* (MRSA).

Functional Diagnosis

Impaired integumentary integrity secondary to full-thickness skin involvement and scar formation (from Guide to PT Practice, pattern 7D), chronic inflammation phase; *Targeted outcome*: Wound decontamination for progression through stages of wound healing and resolution of chronic inflammation.

Need for Skilled Services: The Therapy Problem

The client had a nonhealing stage 3 pressure ulcer and exhibited clinical signs of wound infection. Wound required decontamination and appropriate moist wound therapy to stimulate the healing process.

Treatment Plan and Outcome

A single application of UVC was applied to the wound bed to determine if one application of UVC for 30 seconds was effective in immediately reducing the bacterial load. The wound was initially cleansed with normal saline and then a semiquantitative swab culture was obtained using the 10-point culturing method. UVC was then applied to the wound bed with a V-254 halogen lamp with a calibrated output of 15 mW for 30 seconds. The periwound was completely covered with draping materials and the UVC lamp was placed parallel to the wound bed at a distance of 2.5 cm. Immediately after the UVC treatment, a second semiquantitative swab culture was performed. Both cultures were immediately sent for processing in the clinical laboratory. The laboratory report derived from the swab culture taken immediately prior to the UVC treatment showed high numbers of MRSA present. Results from the swab culture taken immediately post-treatment of the wound bed for 30 seconds with UVC demonstrated very low growth. This case study demonstrates the utility and immediacy of UVC in decontaminating the surface of the wound bed.

(Case study courtesy of Rhonda M. Jones, PT)

Documentation

Treatment times, duration, and angle of incidence should be documented along with the distance that the UV energy source is placed from the wound bed. Client position during treatment and specific lamp model and serial number should also be documented, as should treatment outcomes.

Lasers, LEDs, and SLDs

Biologic Effects of Lasers

The term photobiomodulation has been coined to describe the biologic/physiologic effects of low level or cold laser on living tissues.[3,61] Whether the target of the low-level laser is plant or animal, its effects are characterized as photobiomodulation since this modality has been shown to modulate biologic processes. Low-level laser may modulate biologic processes in either a stimulatory (photobiostimulation) or inhibitory (photobioinhibition) manner. The process by which this modulation occurs is via interaction of low-level laser light with naturally occurring chromophores (pigments located in plant and animal cells that absorb light). These chromophores are part of the powerhouses of the cell (mitochondria), and absorption of low-level laser light from the visible and infrared region of the EMS results in heightened cellular metabolism. Wavelengths of radiant energy between 600 and 1200 nm are capable of penetrating the dermis and interacting with chromophores in human tissues. Chromophores in cells that can absorb this low-level laser light include respiratory chain enzymes, melanin, hemoglobin, and myoglobin. Longer wavelengths of light (infrared) such as those produced by the gallium-arsenide (GaAs) laser can interact with a wide variety of cellular chromophores. In comparison, shorter wavelengths of light (visible and near infrared) such as those generated by the helium-neon (HeNe) laser interact with a limited number of chromophores (melanin, hemoglobin, and myoglobin).

The biologic effects of lasers, LEDs, and SLDs are numerous and varied.[30,31] Additionally, research indicates that compromised cells from damaged tissue are more responsive to these energies than their normal counterparts.[62] Tissues that are inflamed, edematous, and ischemic benefit from low-level laser energy. The cells in these tissues appear to have a lower threshold for excitation or energy transfer.

The effects of lasers, LEDs, and SLDs are seen primarily with photoenergy from the 600–900 nm range of the EMS.[3,30,31] Biologic effects produced by photoenergy in this wavelength range include increased cellular proliferation and differentiation, increased mitochondrial production of ATP, increased RNA synthesis, and increased release of chemotactic factors from mast cells. A number of other positive biologic effects of low-level laser have been identified that may enhance tissue healing. These effects include enhanced leukocyte infiltration, increased macrophage activity, increased fibroblast proliferation, increased growth fac-

tor release, enhanced epithelialization rates, and improved tissue tensile strength.[62,63,64]

Fibroplasia/Fibroblast Proliferation

A number of in vitro studies have demonstrated that low-level laser therapy facilitates the process of fibroplasia through stimulation of macrophages.[65,66] Three treatment wavelengths (660 nm, 820 nm, and 870 nm) were associated with enhanced synthesis and release of chemical mediators by macrophages that direct fibroblast proliferation. An additional study also demonstrated that fibroblast proliferation in cell culture was facilitated by treatment of co-cultured macrophage-like cells with laser using pulsing frequencies of 2.28, 18.24, and 292.30 Hz.[64,67]

Collagen Synthesis

Several in vitro studies have supported a role for low-level laser in stimulating collagen production.[66,67,68] In a study using human skin fibroblasts, irradiation with a HeNe laser produced increased collagen production up to four times that of controls when a treatment paradigm of four consecutive exposures at 24-hour intervals was utilized.[66] A second in vitro study involving human skin fibroblasts demonstrated that both the HeNe and GaAs lasers enhanced the proliferation of fibroblasts and the production of procollagen.[67] Findings from this study indicated that lower energy densities of the GaAs laser were required to augment fibroblast proliferation.

Muscle Cell Proliferation

The proliferative effects of low-level laser have also been demonstrated on muscle cells. Cell culture studies using muscle satellite/precursor cells and isolated muscle fibers in culture have shown an increased proliferative potential when exposed to low-level laser irradiation.[69] Low-level laser increased the number of satellite cells available for differentiation into muscle cells.

ATP Synthesis

Additional in vitro studies have also demonstrated a facilitatory effect of low-level lasers on adenosine triphosphate (ATP) production by mitochondria.[68,70] Cultured mitochondria from livers of Wistar rats were exposed to low-level laser irradiation by a HeNe laser. A 70% increase in ATP synthesis was found in mitochondria treated with 5 J/cm^2 compared with untreated controls. Upon further study, inhibition of the electron transport chain demonstrated that the augmentation of ATP synthesis by low-level laser treatment could be abolished. This finding led the authors of the study to conclude that the increased synthesis of ATP that was induced by low-level laser treatment may be the result of an increase in electron transfer in the inner membrane of mitochondria.

Immune System Stimulation

Another biologic effect of low-level lasers that has been documented in the research literature involves cells of the immune system. Low-level laser has been shown to increase the activity of T and B lymphocytes in vitro.[71] Researchers obtained blood samples from 50 individuals, with 20 normal donors and 30 donors suffering from breast cancer. Lymphocytes were separated from the blood samples and were irradiated in Petri dishes using either an argon laser at wavelengths of 488 or 514 nm or a HeNe laser at a wavelength of 633 nm. The energy density remained at 30 W/cm². The irradiation time was 3, 5, or 10 minutes, respectively. During each experiment, an increase in the number of active T cells was observed. With longer irradiation times, more active T cells could be identified. The maximum increase in percentage of T cells was identified at 10 minutes of irradiation time. Stimulation with the argon laser at 488 nm produced the largest increase in B cells when compared with controls. Data from this study indicate that both the argon and the HeNe lasers are effective in activating both T and B lymphocytes, which play a role in combating invading pathogens.[71]

Low-level laser irradiation has also been found to increase the ability of lymphocytes to bind pathogens.[72] Human peripheral blood lymphocytes irradiated with HeNe laser at an energy density of 5 J/cm² demonstrated an increased affinity for salmonella. Increased binding sites on lymphocytes for salmonella and an increased ability of lymphocytes to bind salmonella were observed.

Low-level laser irradiation has also been shown to inhibit growth of certain types of bacteria, including *E. Coli*,[73] indicating both a role for sensitizing the immune system to bacteria and fighting bacteria directly.

Biologic Effects of LEDs

Cells exposed to infrared LED lights have also been shown to grow 150% to 200% faster than untreated cells.[74] Infrared light produced by LEDs penetrates up to 23 cm and has been shown to stimulate a variety of cell types.[75] Human muscle cells treated with a infrared LED grew seven times faster than their untreated counterparts, compared with skin cells that grew five times faster.

Preclinical Studies

A number of studies have demonstrated a positive effect of low-level laser irradiation on the healing process in a variety of animal models.[3,63] Results from a recent meta-analysis indicate that research studies have demonstrated a greater positive effect of low-level laser treatment on healing in animal wounds compared with human wounds.[63] However, this larger positive effect observed with the animal studies may be simply due to the greater power associated with larger subject numbers.

Low-level laser therapy has been shown to enhance healing of experimentally induced wounds in cows, pigs, dogs, rabbits, rats, and mice. In a meta-analysis of these studies, the highest mean effect size was calculated for cows, followed by rats and then pigs.[63,76,77] Significant effects of low-level laser irradiation are more pronounced in loose-

skinned animals as compared with pigs, which have skin more similar to that of humans.

In animal wounds, low-level laser therapy has been shown to produce more rapid healing of wounds, faster rates of wound closure, enhanced formation of granulation tissue, improved alignment of collagen in tendons, increased tensile strength of tendons, and accelerated healing of fractures.[63] In these interventions, HeNe or GaAs laser treatments at 4 to 10 J/cm² produced positive effects.

The effects of low-level laser irradiation have also been studied in relation to prostaglandin production and mast cell activation and degranulation in animals.[63] Prostaglandins play an important role in the inflammatory process by increasing vascular permeability, and mast cells serve as a source of these chemical mediators. Mester et al in 1985 investigated the effects of HeNe laser at an energy density of 1 J/cm² on E- and F-type prostaglandins in dorsal rat wounds.[68] Four days post-injury, both types of prostaglandins significantly increased in laser treated wounds compared with controls. Induction of mast cell degranulation has also been demonstrated experimentally.[78] Irradiation of mast cells with a low-power laser using different pulsing frequencies demonstrated mast cell degranulation at 20 and 292 Hz.

LEDs have also been shown to enhance wound healing in animals. Whelan et al demonstrated an increase in wound healing in diabetic mice treated with infrared LEDS developed by NASA.[79]

Clinical Studies

Andre Mester was the first to demonstrate the effectiveness of lower power laser therapy in facilitating wound healing in chronic human ulcerations.[61,80] He purported to have achieved a 90% rate of healing in more than 1,000 patients using doses of 4 J/cm² or less. Positive effects of low-level laser therapy have been demonstrated on a number of wound types in humans. Low-level laser therapy has demonstrated increased rates of wound healing in surgical wounds, cutaneous fissures, and venous ulcerations, amongst others, by a variety of researchers.[63] A review of published studies by Belanger[61] found 14 studies of varying levels of evidence demonstrated a positive effect of low-level laser therapy on wound/ulcer healing. Of these studies, 12 of the 14 ranked at the highest levels of evidence (level I and II). In comparison, three studies with an evidence ranking of I or II found no benefit to low-level laser therapy in tissue healing.

Similar results were reported in a meta-analysis by Woodruff et al[63] in 2004. Aggregate analysis of the available data provided by both animal and clinical studies demonstrated a large overall positive effect of low-level laser on wound healing. The analysis also found that low-level laser therapy has a greater positive effect on healing in animal wounds (+1.97, mean effective size) than human wounds (+0.54, mean effective size). The greater average effect with animal studies may have been due to a number of reasons, including: (1) ease of controlling variables in the laboratory with genetically similar animals, (2) limited number of human studies available with computable effect sizes and whether the studies were representative of actual effects of laser on human wounds, and (3) the presence of a very large effect size with laser-treated bovine wounds. An additional consideration in interpreting the greater positive effect of low-level laser treatment on animal wounds is that the animal wounds examined in the research studies were acute in nature compared with the human wounds, which were all chronic. A direct comparison is difficult because of the appreciated intrinsic differences between acute and chronic wounds. Chronic wounds are known to differ from acute wounds biochemically.

In the meta-analysis by Woodruff,[63] the effect size for time to heal was also calculated. Nine studies met the inclusion criteria, with only one having a negative effect size. In this study, occluded wounds healed more quickly than control or laser-treated wounds. Wound management was not optimized in the laser-treated group. The other studies had positive effect sizes ranging from +0.06 to +9.10. Based on the calculated effect sizes, the researchers concluded that time to healing was the best representative measure of the effects of low-level laser therapy on wound healing. Additionally, results of the study also revealed that treatment of the wounds at or around day three resulted in the greatest acceleration of wound healing. This finding is congruent with other research findings that have demonstrated that low-level laser accelerates the inflammatory and proliferative phases of wound healing.

A question has remained as to the best type of low-level laser to use in treating wounds. In the meta-analysis by Woodruff et al,[63] data involving eight laser types were examined. All revealed a positive effect size, with the Krypton laser demonstrating the greatest effect on wound healing. However, the Krypton laser was represented in only one study. The argon, HeNe, and GaAs each produced high calculated effects of approximately the same size, +3.23, +3.05, and +3.02, respectively.

Clinical evidence to support the efficacy of LEDs in the treatment of human wounds is emerging. Whelan et al[81] has shown that infrared LEDs have the ability to rescue epithelial cells in children undergoing radiation and chemotherapy. The LEDs have prevented the development of oral mucositis and acute mouth ulcers in these children. Another LED technology that produces monochromatic infrared energy (MIRE) at 890 nm has also been shown to stimulate wound healing.[82,83] Horwitz et al[82] in 1999 treated individuals with chronic, nonhealing wounds that had failed traditional therapies with LEDs that delivered monochromatic infrared light at 890 nm. A significant enhancement in healing rates was reported in this case series. Treatment of individuals with this same light source has also been shown to increase sensation in individuals diagnosed with diabetic peripheral neuropathy and loss of protective sensation. Both uncontrolled and controlled clinical trials have reported similar results.[84-88]

The exact mechanism by which this technology augments wound healing in chronic wounds and facilitates the return of sensation in individuals with peripheral neuropathy is not well understood. However, it is thought that light energy stimulates the release of nitric oxide, a potent endogenous vasodilator, and thereby increases vasodilatation and enhances blood flow to treated tissues. One caution that the treating clinician must be aware of when using LEDs is the reported incidence of patient burns.[89] Caution is recommended along with on-going patient monitoring anytime a clinician works with a patient who has poor sensation.

Current Recommended Treatment Approaches for Laser

Procedure for Administration

One of the greatest limitations in interpreting current research and its relevance to clinical practice in the field of therapeutic lasers is the disparity in reporting of parameters in existing studies.[90,91] Future studies must accurately report laser parameters such as wavelength, pulsed vs. continuous, power density, exposure time, frequency, and total duration of the treatment so that these studies can be compared statistically.

Adding to the confusion, clinical cases and studies involving the use of SLDs routinely reference the findings of low-power laser studies. While these forms of photoenergy are similar to laser, they are not the same and therefore, should not be used interchangeably or compared while assuming they are equivalent. There are no published studies available comparing the effects of SLDs to laser. They both appear to have potential benefit for soft tissue healing; however, the therapeutic devices and research parameters should be clearly understood by the clinician using them and documented accordingly.

Equipment Selection. The primary characteristics that distinguish laser devices include a low-level power range of 10^{-3} to 10^{-1}W and a wavelength between 300 and 10,600 nanometers.[92] Several lasing mediums have been used to create lasers. These include gases such as helium and neon (632.8nm), ruby (694 nm), and argon (488nm). Newer laser technology employs semiconductor laser diodes, such as gallium arsenide (904nm) and gallium aluminum arsenide (830nm). Research has indicated that wavelength is the primary determinant of depth of penetration.[93] HeNe lasers have been shown to affect more superficial tissues, while gallium arsenide, which is longer in wavelength, appears to have effect up to 5 cm of depth (Exhibit 24-5). Whether a device is using continuous or pulsed mode also affects the average power output.

Several devices on the market now combine laser semiconductor diodes and superluminous diodes with claims that a more thorough treatment of both deep and superficial structures is provided. Every device should have a description of the types of light sources incorporated in the unit, wavelength, power output, pulse rate, intensity, and total irradiation time. Energy density is reported in joules per square centimeter.[3]

EXHIBIT 24-5

Laser Type	Helium Neon	Gallium Arsenide	Gallium Aluminum Arsenide
Lasing medium	Gas	Semiconductor	Semiconductor
Wavelength	632.8 nm	904 nm	830 nm
Electromagnetic spectrum	Red portion of visible light	Infrared	Infrared
Depth of absorption	2–5 mm	1–2 cm	3–5 cm

One key indication for using a low-level laser device versus another light therapy modality is the presence of an FDA warning label for class II or III devices.[93] If the device is truly a laser in its construction, it will carry a warning label.

Claims that a device produces temperature increases would also indicate that the device is not a low-power laser of the type that is currently approved for use by PTs in the rehabilitation setting. A low power laser, also known as a cold laser, does not produce a noticeable temperature increase in the tissue.

There are four classes of lasers based on power and their biologic effects. PTs and other wound care clinicians trained in physical agent theory and practice use class 3B lasers.[3,21] Laser classes include:

Class 1	< 0.5 mW	No hazards
Class 2	< 1 mW	Safe for momentary viewing
Class 3A	< 5 mW	
Class 3B	< 5 00mW	Photobiomodulation
		No photothermal effect
		No harm to skin or clothing
		Potential damage to the eyes
		Used by wound care clinicians/rehab
Class 4	> 500mW	Photothermal effects
		Harmful to skin, eyes, and clothing
		Use with extreme caution (medical use)

Preparation of Wound and Periwound. Prior to application of the laser, the wound and surrounding tissue should be cleansed thoroughly to remove loose slough and excess drainage. Presence of exudates diminishes laser penetration. A clear, transparent film should be placed over the wound to avoid contamination of the laser device.

CLINICAL WISDOM

A clear, transparent film should be placed over the wound to avoid contamination of the laser device.

Treatment Times. The more powerful the laser (intensity), the less time is needed to treat the area. For example, a 1-mW laser would take 1,000 seconds to deliver 1 joule of energy. A 10-mW laser would take 100 seconds to deliver the same energy. A 50-mW laser would take 20 seconds.[94] Most devices offer a preset time of exposure in seconds to create a programmed activation cycle. Overall dosage is based on the output of the laser in mW, the time of exposure in seconds, and the beam surface area of the laser in square centimeters. Depending on the device, some manufacturers recommend a rotation of the laser at several intervals to ensure thorough treatment of the target area. Studies have shown that larger doses or extended treatment times can be detrimental to healing.[93] Therefore, more is not necessarily better.

CLINICAL WISDOM

Studies have shown that larger doses or extended treatment times can be detrimental to healing.[93] Therefore, more is not necessarily better. Laser should be administered to the treatment area no more than once per day.

Treatment Distance. A common technique involves placing the head of the laser in direct contact with the transparent film covering the wound surface. The device is kept stationary for the prescribed treatment time. Sweeping motions are avoided to allow for maximal absorption of photons of light energy. Additionally, some clinicians advocate treatment with laser to the wound periphery.

Step-By-Step Application:

1. Cleanse the laser probe with 70% rubbing alcohol and a damp cloth or per manufacturer guidelines.
2. Position the client comfortably, while permitting adequate exposure of the wound.
3. Remove all dressings.
4. Cleanse the wound with normal saline.
5. Remove excess wound fluid and loose debris.
6. Cover the wound with a clear semipermeable film that extends at least 1/2 inch beyond the wound margins. If the wound has significant depth, press plastic wrap into the cavity to cover all open areas.
7. Protect the clinician's and client's eyes from laser radiation using laser protection goggles (Figure 24-6).
8. Place laser device in direct contact with the film over the wound bed. Maintain direct contact throughout the treatment (Figure 24-7).
9. Irradiate the area beneath the probe per manufacturer guidelines. If the wound is larger than the head of the device, move to the next untreated area and repeat the treatment until the entire wound surface is treated.
10. Remove the transparent film. Cleanse the wound with saline.
11. Redress with an appropriate wound dressing.
12. Cleanse the head of the laser with 70% rubbing alcohol and a damp cloth or per manufacturer guidelines.

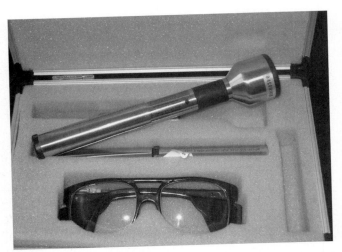

FIGURE 24-6. Protective eyewear.

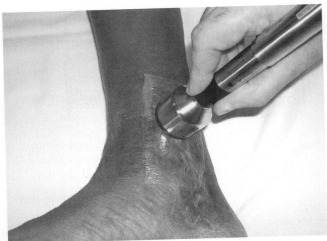

FIGURE 24-7. Low-level laser/cold laser system with protective eyewear

Indications[3]

Laser has not yet been FDA approved for use with wounds. Based on the available research related to wound healing, laser may be indicated for the following types of wounds:[92,94,95]

1. Acute or chronic wounds
2. Slow or nonhealing wounds
3. Infected or colonized wounds

Contraindications/Precautions[3]

1. Do not use over cancerous growths.
2. Avoid direct exposure to the eyes due to possible retinal burns. (Private treatment areas are recommended to avoid accidental eye exposure from reflected laser light.)
3. As a general precaution, do not use during the first trimester of pregnancy.
4. Do not treat over the thyroid gland.

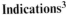

CLINICAL WISDOM

Avoid direct exposure to the eyes due to possible retinal burns.

Adverse Reactions

There have been no reported adverse reactions in the literature

Self Care

Administration of low-level laser therapy should be performed by a skilled individual licensed in the application of physical agent modalities. To prevent overexposure or inappropriate exposure to other areas, laser should not be administered by the individual receiving treatment or by the caregiver. The clinician should monitor the necessity of this intervention on a regular basis to ensure optimal outcomes.

Documentation

Location of the treatment, treatment parameters utilized, and response of the patient to the treatment should be documented. Wavelength, mode of treatment (pulsed vs. continuous), energy density or dose (power density × exposure time) should be documented, as well as frequency of application and total treatment sessions. Client position during treatment and wound preparation will be helpful for subsequent treating clinicians. Documentation of treatment outcomes may include but is not limited to changes in wound size, pain, and bioburden.

Conclusion

A high level of evidence supports the use of low-level therapeutic laser treatment for recalcitrant ulcers. Low-level laser treatment enhances the healing process through a plethora of mechanisms including facilitation of tissue synthesis by fibroblasts and other cells. Addition of this treatment modality to standard of care treatment approaches has been correlated with increased healing rates in both humans and animal wound models.

REVIEW QUESTIONS

1. What are the early cutaneous changes induced by ultraviolet radiation?
2. Describe the mechanism whereby UV radiation facilitates epithelialization.
3. What wavelength range has peak germicidal activity? In what band of UV radiation is this range found?
4. List two ways to protect the periwound from UV exposure.
5. Define the terms laser, LED, and SLD. How are they different?
6. What is the depth of penetration for lasers?
7. List and describe the biologic effects of lasers and LEDs.
8. Identify common indications and contraindications for laser application.

■ **CASE STUDY**

Promotion of Wound Closure with HeNe Laser Treatment

Individual: S.P. **Age:** 67 **Start of Care Date:** 12/05

Medical History

S.P. was a 67-year-old ambulatory male who lives with his wife on a small family farm. He has a diabetic, neuropathic wound (Wagner Grade 2) on the distal plantar surface of his left great toe. His medical diagnoses included diabetes, HTN, and mild CHF. He has a past history of diabetic neuropathic ulcers over the left first metatarsal head.

Reason for Referral

Client was referred to physical therapy due to impaired gait and balance with the presence of a nonhealing diabetic neuropathic ulcer.

FUNCTIONAL DIAGNOSIS AND TARGETED OUTCOMES

Wound Examination

The wound was covered with a thick callus except for a 1.0-cm opening that revealed a dry, pink granulation bed. No exposed bone or significant odor was detected. Upon saucerization of the callus, a dry pink granulation bed with minimal necrosis and exudate was revealed.

Functional Diagnosis

Impaired integumentary integrity secondary to full-thickness skin involvement and scar formation (from Guide to PT Practice, pattern 7D), Chronic inflammation phase; *Targeted outcome*: Wound stimulation for progression through stages of wound healing and resolution of chronic inflammation.

Need for Skilled Services: The Therapy Problem

The client had a Wagner stage 2 diabetic neuropathic ulcer that had failed to heal with traditional moist wound therapy and offloading. The wound required debridement, cleansing, appropriate moist wound therapy, and laser treatment to stimulate the healing process. Offloading continued with a diabetic walking boot.

Treatment Plan and Outcome

HeNe laser therapy was applied three times/week for 3 weeks until wound closure. Wound debridement was performed as needed along with wound cleansing prior to laser treatment. A transparent film dressing was placed over the wound and the wound was treated with the laser using a stroking method to produce a cross-hatch effect. A total treatment dose of 30 J/cm^2 was used at each treatment session. The wound closed with minimal scarring at the end of the third week.

REFERENCES

1. Licht, S. History of ultraviolet light therapy. In: Licht S ed. *Therapeutic Electricity and Ultraviolet Radiation*, 2nd ed. New Haven, CT: Elizabeth Licht; 1967: 191–212.

2. Licht S. History of ultraviolet therapy. In: Stillwell GK, ed. *Therapeutic Electricity and Ultraviolet Radiation,* 3rd ed. Baltimore: Williams & Wilkins; 1983:228–261.

3. Barham C D, Bounkeo J M, Brannon W M, Dawes K S Jr. and Woodruff L D. The efficacy of laser therapy in the treatment of wounds: A meta-analysis of the literature, Master's Thesis Graduate Program of Physical Therapy, North Georgia College and State University, Dahloneg, GA 30597 2003.

4. Hart D. Sterilization of the air in the operating room by special antibacterial radiant energy. *J Thorac Surg.* 1936;6:45.

5. Wu J, Barisoni D, Armato U. Prolongation of survival of alloskin grafts with no concurrent general suppression of the burned patient's immune system: A preliminary clinical investigation. *Burns.* 1996; 22(5):353–358.

6. Taylor GJ, Chandler L. Ultraviolet light in the orthopaedic operating theatre. *Br J Theatre Nurs.* 1997;6(10):10–14.

7. Moggio M, Goldner JL, McCollum DE, Beissinger SF. Wound infections in patients undergoing total hip arthroplasty. Ultraviolet light for the control of airborne bacteria. *Arch Surg.* 1979;114(7):815–823.

8. Berg M, Bergman BR, Hoborn J. Shortwave ultraviolet radiation in operating rooms. *J Bone Joint Surg* 1989;71(3):483–485.

9. Conner-Kerr TA, Sullivan PK, Gaillard J, Franklin ME, Jones RM. The effects of ultraviolet radiation on antibiotic-resistant bacteria in vitro. *Ostomy/Wound Management.* 1998;44(10):50–56.

10. Conner-Kerr TA, Sullivan PK, Keegan A, Reynolds W, Sagemuehl T, Webb A. UVC reduces antibiotic resistant bacterial numbers in living tissue. *Ostomy/Wound Management.* 1999;45(4):84.

11. Thai TP, Keast DH, Campbell KE, Woodbury MG, Houghton PE. Effect of ultraviolet light C on bacterial colonization in chronic wounds. *Ostomy/Wound Management.* 2005;51(10):32–45.

12. Sullivan PK, Conner-Kerr TA, Dixon S, Hamilton H, Webb A, Parrish E, Tefertiller C. The effect of UVC irradiation on wound closure. Presented at the 2000 Symposium on Advanced Wound Care & Medical Research Forum on Wound Repair, April 2000, Dallas, TX.

13. Enwemeka C, et al. The efficacy of low power lasers in tissue repair and pain control: a meta-analysis study. *Photomedicine and Laser Surgery.* 2004;22:323–329.

14. Http://einstein.stanford.edu/content/faqs/maser.html; February 2006.

15. Singer J.R. *Masers.* New York: John Whiley and Sons Inc.; 1959.

16. Http://inventors.about.com/gi/dynamic/offsite.htm?site=http://web.mit .edu/invent/iow/townes.html; February 2006.

17. Belanger AY. LASER. In: Belanger AY, ed. *Evidence-Based Guide to Therapeutic Physical Agents.* Philadelphia, PA: Lippincott Williams & Wilkins; 2003:191–221.

18. Mester E, et al. Effect of laser-rays on wound healing. *Am J Surg.* 1971;122(4):532–535.

19. Tunér J. 100 positive double-blind studies: enough or too little? *Proc SPIE.* 1999;4166:226–232.

20. Weisberg J. Electromagnetic spectrum. In: Hecox B, Mehreteab TA, Weisberg J, eds. *Physical Agents: A Comprehensive Text for Physical Therapists.* Norwalk, CT: Appleton & Lange; 1994:50.

21. Cameron M. Laser & Light. Seminar presentation. January 2005, Torrance, CA.

22. Weisberg J. Ultraviolet irradiation. In: Hecox B, Mehreteab TA, Weisberg J, eds. *Physical Agents: A Comprehensive Text for Physical Therapists.* Norwalk, CT: Appleton & Lange; 1994:377–378.

23. Moseley H. Sources of ultraviolet radiation. In: Moseley H, ed. *Non-Ionising Radiation: Microwaves, Ultraviolet and Laser Radiation.* Philadelphia, PA: IOP Publishing Ltd; 1988:110.

24. Hayes KW. Ultraviolet radiation. In: Hayes KW, ed. *Manual for Physical Agents,* 5th ed. Norwalk, CT: Appleton & Lange; 1999:

25. Schwarz T, Urbanski A, Luger TA. Ultraviolet light and epidermal cell-derived cytokines. In: Luger TA, Schwarz T. eds. *Epidermal Growth Factors and Cytokines.* New York: Marcel Dekker, Inc.; 1994:303.

26. Scott BO. Clinical uses of ultraviolet radiation. In: Stillwell GK, ed. *Therapeutic Electricity and Ultraviolet Radiation,* 3rd ed. Baltimore: Williams & Wilkins; 1983:228–261.

27. Stenback F. Health hazards from ultraviolet radiation. *Public Health Rev.* 1982;10:229.

28. Daniels F. Ultraviolet light and dermatology. In: Stillwell GK, ed. *Therapeutic Electricity and Ultraviolet Radiation,* 3rd ed. Baltimore: Williams & Wilkins; 1983:263–303.

29. van der Leun JC. On the action spectrum of ultraviolet erythema. *Res. Prog. Org. Biol. Med. Chem.* 1972;3:711–736.

30. Cameron MH. A shining light. *Adv Dir Rehabil.* April 2005;14(4):39–42.

31. Conner-Kerr T. Wound technology: The future is now. *ECPN.* October 2005;104:34–39.

32. Stein I, Shorey MM. Ultraviolet radiation in the treatment of indolent, soft-tissue ulcerations. *Physiother Rev.* 1945;25(6):272–274.

33. Willis EE, Anderson TW, Beattie BL, Acott A. A randomized placebo controlled trial of ultraviolet light in the treatment of superficial pressure sores. *J Am Geriatr Soc.* 1983;31:131.

34. Crous L, Malherbe C. Laser and ultraviolet light irradiation in the treatment of chronic ulcers. *Physiotherapy.* 1988;44:73.

35. Nussbaum EL, Biemann, Mustard B. Comparison of ultrasound/ultraviolet-C and laser for treatment of pressure ulcers in patients with spinal cord injury. *Phys. Ther.* 1994;74(9):812–825.

36. Taylor R. Clinical study of ultraviolet in various skin conditions. *Phys. Ther.* 1972; 52(3):279–282.

37. Harm W. UV carcinogenesis. In: Harm W, ed. *Biological Effects of Ultraviolet Radiation.* New York: Cambridge University Press; 1980:191.

38. Hensby CN, Plummer NA, Black AK, Fincham N, Greaves MW. Timecourse of arachidonic acid, prostaglandins E2 and F2 alpha production in human abdominal skin following irradiation with ultraviolet wavelengths (290–320 nm). *Adv. Prostaglandin Thromboxane Res.* 1980;7:857–860.

39. Brauchle M, Funk JO, Kind P, Werner S. Ultraviolet B and H_2O_2 are potent inducers of vascular endothelial growth factor expression in cultured keratinocytes. J. Biol. Chem. 1996; 271(36):21793-21797.

40. Holtz F. Pharmacology of ultraviolet radiation. *Br J Phys Med.* 1952; 5:201.

41. Kaiser MR, Davis SC, Mertz PM. The effect of ultraviolet irradiation-induced inflammation on epidermal wound healing. *Wound Repair Regen.* 1995;3:311–315.

42. Sauder DN, Kilian PL, McLane JA, Quick TW, Jakubovic H, Davis SC, Eaglstein WH, Mertz PM. Interleukin-1 enhances epidermal wound healing. *Lymphokine Re.* 1990;9(4):465–473.

43. Fan J, Schoenfeld RJ, Hunter RA. A study of the epidermal clear cells with special reference to their relationship to the cells of Langerhans. *J Invest Dermatol.* 1959;32:445–450.

44. Bergstresser PR, Toews GB, Streilein JW. Natural and perturbed distribution of Langerhans cells: responses to ultraviolet light, heterotopic skin grafting and dinitrofluorobenzene sensitization. *J Invest Derm.* 1980;75:73–77.

45. Wu J, Barisoni D, Armato U. Prolongation of survival of alloskin grafts with no concurrent general suppression of the burned patient's immune system: A preliminary clinical investigation. *Burns.* 1996;22(5):353–358.

46. Taylor GJS, Bannister GC, Leeming JP. Wound disinfection with ultraviolet radiation. *J Hospital Infection.* 1995;30:85–93.

47. High AS, High JP. Treatment of infected skin wounds using ultra-violet radiation: An in vitro study. *Physiotherapy.* 1983;69(10):359–360.

48. Norback I, Kulmala R, Jarvinen M. Effect of ultraviolet therapy on rat skin wound healing. *J Surg Res.* 1990;48:68–71.

49. Sullivan PK, Conner-Kerr T. A comparative study of the effects of UVC irradiation on select procaryotic and eucaryotic wound pathogens. *Ostomy/Wound Management.* 2000;46(10):44–50.

50. Sullivan PK, Conner-Kerr TA, Smith ST. The effects of UVC irradiation on Group A Streptococcus *in vitro.* *Ostomy/Wound Management.* 1999;45(10):50–58.

51. Taylor GJ, Leeming JP, Bannister GC. Effects of antiseptics, ultraviolet light and lavage on airborne bacteria in a model wound. *J Bone Joint Surg Br.* 1993;75(5):724–730.

52. El-Batouty MF, El-Gindy M, El-Shawaf I, Bassioni N, El-Ghaweet A, El-Emam A. Comparative evaluation of the effects of ultrasonic and ultraviolet irradiation on tissue regeneration. *Scand J Rheumatology.* 1986;15:381–386.

53. Das SK, Brantley SK, Davidson SF. Wound tensile strength in the hairless guinea pig following irradiation with pure ultraviolet-A light. *Br J Plast Surg.* 1991;44(7):509–513.

54. Davidson SF, Brantley SK, Das SK. The effects of ultraviolet radiation on wound healing. *Br J Plast Surg.* 1991;44(3):210–214.

55. Davidson SF, Brantley SK, Das SK. The reversibility of UV-altered wound tensile strength in the hairless guinea pig following a 90-day recovery period. *Br J Plast Surg.* 1992;45(2):109–112.

56. Basford JR, Hallman HO, Sheffield CG, Mackey GL. Comparison of cold-quartz ultraviolet, low-energy laser, and occlusion in wound healing in a swine model. *Arch Phys Med Rehabil.* 1986;67:151.

57. Morykwas MJ, Mark MW. Effects of ultraviolet light on fibroblast fibronectin production and lattice contraction. *Wounds.* 1998;10(4):111–117.

58. Mertz PM, Davis SC, Oliveira-Gandia M, Eaglstein WH. The wound environment: implications from research studies for healing and infection. *Wounds.* 1996;8(1):1–8.

59. Mertz PM. Interleukin-1 enhances epidermal wound healing. *Lymphokine Re.* 1990;9(4):465–473.

60. MacKinnon JL, Cleek PL. Therapeutic penetration of ultraviolet light through transparent dressing. *Phys. Ther.* 1984;64:204.

61. Belanger AY. LASER. In: Belanger AY, ed. *Evidence-Based Guide to Therapeutic Physical Agents.* Philadelphia, PA: Lippincott Williams & Wilkins; 2003:191–221.

62. Martin R. LASER-accelerated inflammation/pain reduction and healing. *Practical Pain Management.* Nov/Dec 2003:20–25.

63. Woodruff LD, Bounkeo JM, Brannon WM, et al. The efficacy of laser therapy in wound repair: a meta-analysis of the literature. *Photomed Laser Surg.* 2004;22(3):241–247.

64. Abergel RP, Lyons RF, Castel JC, et al. Biostimulation of wound healing by lasers: experimental approaches in animal models and in fibroblast cultures. *J Derm Surg Oncol.* 1987;13(2):127–133.

65. Young S, Bolton P, Dyson M, Harvey W, Diamantopoulos C. Macrophage responsiveness to light therapy. *Laser Surg Med.* 1989;9:497–505.

66. Rajaratnam S, Bolton P, Dyson M. Macrophage responsiveness to laser therapy with varying pulsing frequencies. *Laser Therapy.* 1994;6:107–11.

67. Abergel RP, Lam TS, Meeker CA, et al., Biostimulation of procollagen production by low energy lasers in human skin fibroblast cultures. *Clin Res.* 1984;32:567A.

68. Mester E, Mester AF, Mester A. The biomedical effects of laser application. *Laser Surg Med.* 1985;5:31–39.

69. Shefer G, Partridge TA, Heslop L, et al. Low energy laser irradiation promotes the survival and cell cycle entry of skeletal muscle satellite cells. *J Cell Sci.* April 1, 2002;115(Pt 7):1461–1469.

70. Passarella S, Casamassima E, Molinari S, et al. Increase of proton electrochemical and ATP synthesis in rat liver mitochondria irradiated *in vitro* by HeNe. *FEBS Lett.* 1984;175:95–99.

71. Kupin VI, Bykov VS, Ivanov AV, Larichev VY. Potentiating effects of laser radiation on some immunological traits. *Neoplasma.* 1982;29:403–406.

72. Passarella S, Casamassima E, Quagliariello E, et al. Quantitative analysis of lymphocyte-salmonella interaction and effect of lymphocyte irradiation by helium-neon laser. *Biochem Biophys Res Comm.* 1985;130(2):546–552.

73. Nussbaum EL, Lilge L, Mazzulli T. Effects of 630-, 660-, and 905-nm laser irradiation delivering radiant exposure of 1-50J/cm^2 on three species of bacteria in vivo. *J Clin Laser Med Surg.* December 2002;20(6):325–333.

74. Whelan HT, Smits RL, Buchman EV, et al. Effect of NASA light-emitting diode irradiation on wound healing. *J Clin Lasers Me Surg.* December 2001;19(6):305–314.

75. Marovino T. Cold LASERS in pain management. *Pract Pain Manage.* Sept/Oct 2004:1–5.

76. Lee P, Kim K, and Kim K. Effects of low incident energy levels of infrared laser irradiation on healing of infected open skin wounds in rats. *Laser Ther.* 1993;5:59–64.

77. Graham DJ, Alexander JJ. The effects of argon laser on bovine aortic endothelial and smooth muscle cell proliferation and collagen production. *Curr Surg.* 1990;47:27–30.

78. El Sayed SO, Dyson M. Comparison of the effect of multiwavelength light produced by a cluster of semiconductor diodes and of each individual diode on mast cell number and degranulation in intact and injured skin. *Laser Surg Med.* 1990;10:559–568.

79. Whelan HT, Buchmann EV, Dhokalia A, Kane MP, Whelan NT, Wong-Riley MT, Eells JT, Gould LJ, Hammamieh R, Das R, Jett M. Effect of NASA light-emitting diode irradiation on molecular changes for wound healing in diabetic mice. *J Clin Laser Med Surg.* 2003;21(2):67–74.

80. Mester E, Spiry T, Szende B, et al. Effect of laser rays on wound healing. *Am J Surg.* 1971;122:532–535.

81. Whelan HT, Connelly JF, Hodgson BD, Barbeau L, Post AC, Bullard G, Buchmann EV, Kane M, Whelan NT, Warwick A, Margolis D. NASA

light-emitting diodes for the prevention of oral mucositis in pediatric bone marrow transplant patients. *J Clin Laser Med Surg.* 2002;20(6):319–24.

82. Horwitz LR, Burke TJ, Carnegie D. Augmentation of wound healing using monochromatic infrared energy. Exploration of a new technology for wound management. *Adv Wound Care.* 1999 Jan-Feb;12(1):35–40.

83. Horwitz, LR, Burke TJ. Effect of monochromatic infrared energy on venous stasis ulcers. *Wound Care Institute Newsletter.* Jan/Feb 1999;4(1).

84. Kochman A. Restoration of sensation, improved balance and gait reduction in falls in elderly patients with use of monochromatic infrared photo energy and physical therapy. *J Geriatr Phys Ther.* 2004;27(1):16–19.

85. Kochman AB, Carnegie DH, Burke TJ. Symptomatic reversal of peripheral neuropathy in patients with diabetes. *J Am Podiatr Med Assoc.* 2002 Mar;92(3):125–130.

86. Leonard DR, Farooqi MH, Myers S. Restoration of sensation, reduced pain, and improved balance in subjects with diabetic peripheral neuropathy: a double-blind, randomized, placebo-controlled study with monochromatic near infrared treatment. *Diabetes Care.* 2004 Jan;27(1):168–172.

87. Powell MW, Carnegie DE, Burke TJ. Reversal of diabetic neuropathy and new wound incidence: the role of MIRE. *Adv Skin Wound Care.* 2004 Jul-Aug;17(6):295–300.

88. Prendergast JJ, Miranda G, Sanchez M. Improvement of sensory impairment in patients with peripheral neuropathy. *Endocrine Pract.* 2004 Jan-Feb;10(1):24–30.

89. Singleton E. FLA-0608 Warning Letter to Restorative Products, Inc. Department of Health and Human Services, Food and Drug Administration, December 2, 2005, www.fda.gov/foi/warning_letters/g5660d.pdf.

90. Reddy GK. Photobiological basis and clinical role of low-intensity lasers in biology and medicine. *J Clin Laser Med Surg.* 2004;22(2):141–150.

91. Calderhead RG. Watts a joule: On the importance of accurate and correct reporting of laser parameters in low-reactive-level laser therapy and photobioactivation research. Laser Therapy 1991;3(4):177-182.

92. Posten W, et al. Low-level laser therapy for wound healing: mechanism and efficacy. *Dermatol Surg.* 2005;31:334–340.

93. Mendez T, Pinheiro A, Pacheco M, Nascimento PM, Ramalho L. Dose and wavelength of laser light have influence on the repair of cutaneous wounds. *J Clin Laser Med Surg.* 2004;22(1):19–25.

94. Schindl M, Kerschan K, Schindl A, Schon H, Heinzl H, Schindl L. Induction of complete wound healing in recalcitrant ulcers by low-intensity laser irradiation depends on ulcer cause and size. *Photodermatol Photoimmunol Photomed.* 1999;15:18–21.

95. DeSimone NA, Christiansen C, Dore D. Bactericidal effect of 0.95-mW helium-neon and 5-mW indium-gallium-aluminum-phosphate laser irradiation at exposure times of 30, 60, and 120 seconds on photosensitized *Staphylococcus aureus* and *Pseudomonas aeruginosa* in vitro. *Phys Ther.* 1999;79:8039–8846.

Therapeutic and Diagnostic Ultrasound

Carrie Sussman and Mary Dyson

CHAPTER OBJECTIVES

At the completion of this chapter, the reader will be able to:

1. List the terminology used to describe the properties of therapeutic and diagnostic ultrasound, and explain the significance of each.
2. Analyze the current evidence of the physical and physiologic effects of therapeutic ultrasound as they relate to wound healing.
3. Evaluate whether ultrasound treatment is appropriate based on the patient, the wound, and the evidence.
4. Select the most appropriate therapeutic ultrasound device for the intended intervention and the most appropriate transmission medium to achieve the desired outcome.
5. Explain recent advances in the use of high-resolution ultrasound (HRUS) to monitor the extent of soft tissue injury and repair.
6. Apply ultrasound treatment interventions, if appropriately trained to do so.

The goal of this chapter is to present evidence of the physical and physiologic effects of ultrasound (US). High-frequency and low-frequency applications are presented. Clinical studies in which US has been used for the healing of animals and humans, as well as a metaanalysis report on the effect of US on chronic leg ulcers are included. For therapeutic US, the therapist is provided with sufficient information to select the most appropriate method of treatment for tissue repair in injuries of different etiologies and in different locations, as well as to clean and debride wounds using new US delivery systems. This chapter also describes recent advances in the use of high-resolution diagnostic US, to monitor the extent of soft tissue injury and its repair in a quantitative, objective manner.

Evaluating the Evidence

Ultrasound as a treatment for many disorders came into vogue about 1950. After an extensive review of the literature, Gam and Johannsen[1] identified over 300 published papers on US treatment appearing in the literature between 1949 and 1993, including clinical trials, experimental trials, and review articles. They identified two categories of treatment objectives that met the criteria for inclusion in a metaanalysis, namely the effect on pain associated with musculoskeletal disorders, and the effect on tissue repair in chronic leg ulcers. The authors subsequently performed and published a metaanalysis of the studies in each of these categories.[1,2] Their conclusion, based on the results of the pain metaanalysis, was that US used in the treatment of musculoskeletal disorders is based on empirical experience, but lacks firm evidence and well-controlled studies.[1]

One possible reason for the poor results shown in the metaanalysis for pain is the wide variety of musculoskeletal disorders evaluated in the studies, some of which were acute and others chronic. The metaanalysis included 22 trials in which 12 different musculoskeletal diseases were treated.[1] Similar findings were reported by Falconer, Hayes, and Chang[3] in a quantitative synthesis of the literature that addressed the effectiveness of US on pain in acute and chronic inflammatory conditions. Thirty-five studies were identified; of these, 28 (16 papers) were published before 1970, and five were published during the 1980s. All of the studies included human subjects with musculoskeletal disease. As with Gam and Johannsen's findings about pain, uncontrolled or unblinded studies more frequently reported positive outcomes.[1]

Johannsen and Gam's findings regarding the use of US for tissue repair in chronic leg ulcers were more positive, but still mixed.[2] Six studies met the criteria for this meta-analysis, which showed significant treatment effect versus placebo or other treatment after 4 and 8 weeks (16.9% mean difference after 4 weeks and 14.5% mean difference after 8 weeks). The investigators found that there was great variability in reporting and treatment methods in both the pain treatment and tissue repair categories. Most studies in both categories lacked proper descriptions of study dropouts, randomization methods, US apparatus used, mode of treatment delivery, description of sham apparatus, size of the treatment head, dosage, number of treatments, sonation time, methods of blinding, and so forth.[2]

Without well-designed controlled clinical trials, it is difficult to make definitive judgments about the efficacy of US. If a grade level can be assigned based on evidence of efficacy (following the Sackett scheme[4]), then a "B" would probably be appropriate for the use of US in the treatment of chronic leg ulcers, because efficacy has been demonstrated in several small randomized trials. The use of US in pressure ulcer treatment, on the other hand, shows mixed and limited supporting evidence. More about the evidence of these clinical trials is presented later in the chapter.

Both a 1993 review of the literature by the Agency for Health Care Research and Quality (formerly known as the Agency for Health Care Policy and Research) made in preparation for the 1994 publication of guidelines for treatment of pressure ulcers,[5] and Ovington's 1999 literature review and update of these guidelines,[6] considered US as an adjunctive therapy to accelerate or restart healing. The findings of both were that there was insufficient evidence to permit recommending the use of US for the treatment of pressure ulcers. Ultrasound was assigned a grade "C" recommendation in these studies.[5,6] A Cochrane review, performed in 2000, found that the evidence, although limited in scope, suggests US is beneficial in the healing of venous ulcers.[7] The literature about US therapeutic efficacy for human tissue repair is inconclusive. Further investigation with well-designed clinical trials is needed to resolve the questions. For now, the attention of the research community has shifted to the use of high-frequency MHz US for diagnostic purposes to determine the efficacy of wound-healing interventions and to diagnose the depth of tissue impairment, as well as the use of low-frequency kHz US for wound debridement and treatment. The new applications of kHz US show great promise and current information will be reviewed below.

Definitions And Terminology

Ultrasound

Ultrasound is a mechanical vibration transmitted at a frequency beyond the upper limit of human hearing (more than 20 kHz, where 1 Hertz = 1 cycle per second and 1 kHz = 1,000 cycles per second).[8] It causes the molecules of the media that can transmit it (e.g., biologic tissues) to oscillate or vibrate, and can be used therapeutically to accelerate wound healing, and diagnostically to assess the extent of soft tissue injuries and to monitor their repair in a quantitative manner.

Ultrasonic energy is produced when an ultrasonic electronic generator transforms AC line power to the US signal that drives a piezoelectric convertor/transducer. The electrical signal is then converted by the transducer to a mechanical vibration that is determined by the characteristics of the internal piezoelectric crystal. The mechanical vibration is then transmitted down to the piezoelectric crystal mounted in the applicator/handpiece which then expands and contracts. The amount of expansion and contraction is the amplitude and this is controlled by the amplitude knob of the device.[9]

Frequency

Many of the clinically relevant bioacoustic properties of US are related to its frequency (f). This is the number of times per second that a molecule displaced by the US completes a cycle of movement and returns to its original position. Frequencies are expressed in Hz, where 1 Hz = one cycle per second. The time taken to complete a cycle is termed a *period* (T).

High Frequency

Short-wave Megahertz US, typically between 0.5 and 3 MHz (i.e., between 0.5 and 3 million cycles per second), has been used for more than 40 years to stimulate healing, and for transdermal drug delivery. Thermal and nonthermal properties as well as cellular effects are related to this frequency. Depth of penetration is related to frequency as well. One MHz US penetrates tissues ≤5 cm , while 3 MHz penetrates tissue up to 1–2 cm.

Diagnostic US uses the range of 20–50 MHZ to image tissue. Current applications of Megahertz US to wound healing include imaging tissue so as to identify its structures and locate, diagnose, and monitor areas of tissue congestion and healing. The concepts of US scanning are detailed later in the chapter.

Low frequency

Kilohertz US, typically between 20 and 50 kHz, is also known as *long-wave US*. The therapeutic effects of kHz US have been identified over the last 20–30 years, and clinical technologies developed. Long-wave US has the ability to penetrate tissue much deeper than MHz US. Like MHz US, thermal or nonthermal effects as well as cellular effects occur depending on how it is applied. Applications of this new therapeutic frequency range are receiving a lot of interest for wound debridement, wound healing and for transdermal drug delivery.

Attenuation

Attenuation refers to the lessening of the force of a US wave as the sound energy is absorbed into, scattered, or reflected by the tissues. At higher frequencies, more of the energy is absorbed by superficial structures than penetrates into deeper structures. For example, US devices offering 3 MHz are now widely available and are used for wound healing when superficial tissues are to be treated. For decades, 1 MHz US has been useful for deep penetration into tissues. Kilohertz US, which has even less attenuation and therefore greater penetration of tissue, is now available for therapeutic purposes. These additional options provide opportunities to select devices with higher and lower frequencies for different treatment protocols and application to aide in tissue repair.

Half-Value Thickness

When US is transmitted through tissue, its intensity gradually decreases as a result of absorption, scattering, and reflection. The thickness of tissue necessary for the intensity to be reduced by one half is termed the *half-value thickness*. The intensity available at any depth within the tissue is inversely proportional to the depth of penetration (i.e., the greater the depth, the less will be the remaining available intensity). For example, if 1 W/cm^2 of 1 MHz US is applied to the skin at a depth of 5 cm, only 0.25 W/cm^2 would be available. Absorption, which is a major cause of attenuation (loss of intensity), is frequency-dependent. The greater the frequency, the shorter the wavelength, and the shorter the wavelength, the greater the absorption. The wavelength of a US beam at 3 MHz is shorter than at 1 MHz, and therefore absorption occurs more readily, reducing the half-value thickness by 3. In this example, the half-value thickness would be 5/3 = 1.7 cm. Three MHz is an efficient frequency to use to treat superficial regions, such as injured skin, but lower frequencies are indicated for deeper targets such as injured muscle or bone.

The amount of absorption varies with the composition of the tissues, as well as with the wavelength, which, as described above, is inversely related to frequency. Bone is more absorptive than highly proteinaceous tissues (e.g., dermis and muscle); protein is more absorptive than fat (e.g., adipose tissue); and fat is more absorptive than water-rich materials (e.g., plasma, edematous tissues). Because of this, the half-value thickness of bone is less than that of muscle, which is less than that of fat, which is less than that of edematous soft connective tissue. Ultrasound can, therefore, penetrate skin, fat, and edematous tissues to reach a deeply located injury in, for example, a joint capsule or a muscle. Low-frequency wavelengths are longer and consequently their depth of penetration is greater. With kHz US, even bone and metal can be penetrated, with sufficient energy remaining to have an effect on deeper injured tissues.

Wavelength

The *wavelength* (() is the shortest distance, measured parallel to the direction of wave propagation, between molecules that are at equivalent points of vibration in the repeated cycle of movement, which constitutes a wave. It is related to

the frequency and *velocity* (c) of the wave by the equation: (= c/f. The velocity of US in water, blood, interstitial fluid, and soft tissues is approximately 1,500 m/s. The higher the frequency, the shorter the wavelength. This is important diagnostically, because the shorter the wavelength, the greater the degree of resolution. A prototype soft tissue scanner developed at Guy's Hospital in London and tested at West Jersey and West Hudson Wound Healing Centers uses a frequency of 20 MHz, producing a wavelength that is sufficiently short to allow collagen fiber bundles and other components of intact and damaged soft connective tissues to be distinguished acoustically. This prototype provided the model for the Longport Digital Scanner, which is now being marketed in the United States.

In the realm of tissue treatment, high frequencies are more readily absorbed by tissues than are low frequencies and produce a greater thermal effect in the tissues. Lower frequencies produce cavitation and the microstreaming associated with it more readily than do higher frequencies; there is evidence that many of the biologic effects produced by therapeutic US are caused by cavitation and microstreaming.[1]

Equipment for Generating Ultrasound

The equipment used to produce therapeutic levels of both MHz and kHz US typically consists of a microcomputer-controlled high-frequency generator linked by a coaxial cable to an applicator (probe) or treatment head. The treatment head contains a disc of a piezoelectric material, such as lead zirconate titanate, which acts as a transducer to change one form of energy into another, in this case electrical energy into mechanical energy. When an alternating voltage is applied across such a disc, it expands and contracts at the same frequency as the oscillation, transducing the electrical energy into mechanical vibration, which determines the frequency of the US. The mechanical vibration produced is a function of the characteristics of the internal piezoelectric crystals. The vibration characteristics are amplified and transmitted to the applicator. The crystal within the amplifier contracts and expands creating a pressure wave referred to as acoustic streaming. The rapid vibration of the crystal causes cavitation, the formation and violent collapse of microscopic bubbles within a liquid. The acoustic streaming and cavitation properties of US are exploited for their bioacoustic effects, as explained below. Similar systems are used for MHz and kHz US, but the frequency of kHz vibration is much shorter and the wavelength therefore longer.

Kilohertz applications are currently being presented as new futuristic technologies for promoting wound healing and wound debridement. These new applications have been referred to as "breakthrough technology."[10] High-frequency MHz US is also being repackaged for diagnostic application. The novel delivery systems of these new technologies and their putative effects are presented throughout this chapter (Fig 25-1, 25-3 and Fig 25-6).

The Ultrasonic Field

The ultrasonic pressure field generated by the transducer depends on the size and shape of the transducer and on how it is mounted in the applicator. The pressure varies across the surface of the applicator, as well as with the distance from it. The pressure changes experienced by the tissues being treated, therefore, depend in part on their position relative to the applicator.

Ultrasound is emitted from a disc-shaped transducer as a beam, which is cylindric at its origin. This region is termed the *near field*, or *Fresnel zone* (generally within 10–30 cm of the sound head surface), and the energy distribution within it is extremely variable, meaning that the energy may

vary from little or no intensity to very high peak intensities. Beyond this, the beam starts to diverge and the energy distribution within it becomes more regular. This region is termed the *far field*, or *Fraunhofer zone*. The distance (d) from the transducer to the beginning of the far field is related to the radius (a) of the transducer and the wavelength (λ) of the US: $d = a^2/\lambda$. Transducers for kHz devices are very narrow but transducers used with MHz are of varying widths, and the following information needs to be interpreted with those differences in mind.

Unless the body part to be treated is immersed in a water bath in which the MHz transducer and target tissue can be separated by a distance sufficient for the target tissues to be in the far field, US therapy usually involves treatment of tissue in the nonuniform near field. The *beam nonuniformity ratio* (BNR) is a measure of this nonuniformity and is the ratio of the spatial peak intensity (I[SP]) to the spatial average intensity (I[SA]). These terms are defined below.

Applicators used to deliver MHz US have parameters affecting treatment results that are unique to each delivery system. Applicators with low BNRs have more homogeneous beam patterns that give more *predictable* results and are *safer* than those with higher BNRs, because the higher spatial peak intensities of the latter are potentially damaging.[11]

Equipment Selection

The selection of therapeutic MHz US equipment should be based on the following considerations:

1. Select a transducer with low BNR.
2. Select a transducer that is water immersible.
3. Select one transducer that is < 2 cm² and another 5 cm². Avoid large transducers with small effective radiating area (ERA).
4. Choose an ergonomically designed transducer that is comfortable to hold.
5. Select a unit with multiple frequencies for optimal treatment options, depending on desired depth of penetration.
6. Select a unit with a built-in feature that tests output performance every time the unit is powered up.
7. Recalibrate the unit at least twice a year. If there is significant drift, more frequent recalibration is required. If that does not take care of the problem, consider repair or replacement of the device.

Choice of kHz equipment is much more limited than MHz because it is new technology and as of this writing there are only a few products on the market that are approved by the FDA for medical use to treat wounds. Table 25-1 shows a comparison of three kHz products. More information about them is presented throughout the chapter, along with guidelines for their use.

Intensity

Intensity (I) is the amount of energy (in watts) per unit area per unit time. Applicators used for MHz transmission typi-

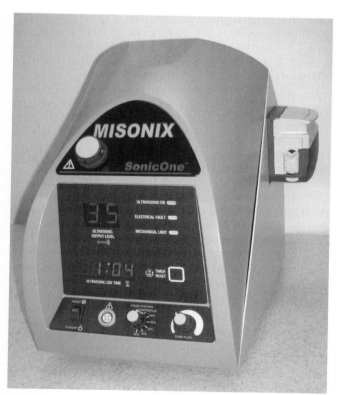

FIGURE 25-1 Misonix SonicOne Ultrasonic Wound Debridement System. (Misonex, Farmdale, NY.)

cally have an ERA of a few square centimeters. Kilohertz devices have a small effective radiating area (ERA). The ERA is always less than the size of the transducer surface, so the size of the transducer is not a true indicator of the actual radiating surface. Individual transducers should be scanned to ensure proper calibration of intensity in W/cm^2. The intensity can be averaged in space over the face of the applicator (termed *spatial average* [SA]) or in time (termed *temporal average*). When pulsed US is used, pulse average (PA) intensity (this is the TA during the period of the pulse) should be noted, as should the TA during the full pulse repetition cycle. The type of intensity should be specified as either I(SATA), if continuous, or both I(SATA) and I(SAPA), if pulsed. Information provided about the SATA is useful in comparing US dosages reported in studies. Exhibit 25-1 summarizes MHz US intensity terminology and gives examples.[12]

The movement of a device's piezoelectric crystal up and down is called its amplitude. The amplitude is controlled by the output control knob of the device. There is a direct relationship between amplitude and intensity, so that at low control settings there will be low amplitudes and low intensity sonication. To achieve the desired intensity for a particular therapeutic application, the output control setting is critical. Power has a variable relationship with amplitude and intensity. At a low control setting, the device will have a low wattage reading if it is sonicating water, but if it is sonicating viscose tissue then at the same setting there will be a higher wattage reading. The amplitude and intensity will be the same, but the power needed to drive the crystal to produce the same intensity and amplitude are greater. This is the concept of variable power.

Treatment application parameters are based on intensity reported in W/cm^2. Therapeutic applications generally operate in an intensity range from 0.1 to 2.0 W/cm^2, with the safe upper limit having been established by the World Health Organization (WHO) at 3.0 W/cm^2. Intensities over 3.0 W/cm^2 are used in surgical applications as ultrasonic scalpels and in tissue emulsification applications. Pulsing the US wave changes the average intensity and reduces the thermal effects because the acoustic energy is only applied for a portion of the treatment time per the formula shown in Exhibit 25-1.

Thermal and Nonthermal Effects

A medium intensity range of 1.0–2.0 W/cm^2 applied continuously for 5–10 minutes will elevate tissue temperatures to between 40 and 45°C.[11] This is acceptable only in adequately vascularized tissues. Temperatures above this cause thermal *necrosis* and must be avoided. Thermal effects occur with both 1 MHz and 3 MHz US when continuous wave US is applied, but at different tissue depths. In contrast, therapeutic kHz US can be used in continuous mode without physiologically significant heating. At a frequency of 3 MHz, energy absorption occurs mainly in superficial tissues (1–2 cm beneath the surface). At a frequency of 1 MHz, less energy is absorbed by the superficial tissues, provided that there is adequate output from the transducer. This frequency also penetrates into deeper tissues, with effective energy levels being available up to 5 cm below the surface. Nonthermal effects are reduced by pulsing the wave, because this reduces the average intensity over time. Whenever US is absorbed, heat is produced, but if the temperature increases less than 1° C, this is not considered to be physiologically relevant; in such circumstances, therapeutic effects are due primarily to nonthermal mechanisms. Kilohertz as well as MHz devices produce heat when used in the continuous mode. Fluid is used in conjunction with the kHz US delivery not only for conduction but also to dissipate the heat produced during the application. Pulsing the kHz wave reduces its heating effect.

Because many wounds occur in ischemic tissues, care must be used when applying thermal US in the presence of arterial occlusive disease. In these areas, there is reduced ability to dissipate heat, and burns can result. Ultrasound is contraindicated in the presence of arterial occlusion. Nonthermal application is safer over areas of impaired circulation.

Stable Cavitation and Microstreaming

The nonthermal effects of US occur at a low spatial average intensity. These effects can be achieved by pulsing at, for

---

EXHIBIT 25-1   Summary of Ultrasound Intensity Terminology

Intensity = total power output at a given setting of amplitude divided by the ERA in cm^2, measured in W/cm^2

Spatial average (SA) intensity: intensity averaged over the surface area of the transducer

Temporal average (TA) intensity: intensity average over the time of treatment

Pulse average (PA) intensity: temporal average during the period of the pulse

Spatial peak intensity (SP): peak intensity over the surface area of the transducer

Beam Nonuniformity Ratio (BNR): ratio of the spatial peak intensity to the spatial average intensity.

Most MHz units sold have BNR of 5:1 or 6:1 but may be as low as 2:1. Example: Transducer with BNR of 5:1 SA set at 1 W/cm^2 SP may be as high as 5 W/cm.^{2}

Spatial Average Temporal Peak Intensity (SATA): spatial average intensity of the US during the on time of the pulse. Clinical US units display the SATP intensity and the duty cycle.

Spatial Average Temporal Average Intensity (SATA): spatial average intensity averaged over the on and off time of the pulse (SATA = SATP _ duty cycle). Example: 1 W/cm^2 SATP at 20% duty cycle = 1 [[TIM]] 0.2 = 0.2 W/cm^2 SATA. SATA is amount of energy delivered to the tissues. For continuous US, the SATA is equal to the SATP.

Adapted with permission from Michelle Cameron, Ultrasound, *Physical Agents in Rehabilitation*, pp. 275–76, © 1999, W.B. Saunders Company.

TABLE 25-1   Kilohertz Ultrasound Device Comparison

Feature	Celleration MIST Therapy System 5.0	SÖRING/Sonoca 180	Misonix
Frequency	40 kHz	25 kHz	22.5 khz
FDA 510k Clearance Indications	K032378/K050129 Indications for use: The MIST Therapy System produces a low-energy ultrasound-generated mist used to promote wound healing through wound cleansing and maintenance debridement by the removal of yellow slough, fibrin, tissue exudates and bacteria. http://www.fda.gov/cdrh/pdf/k032378/K050129.pdf	K012753 Indications for use: selective ultrasonic dissection and fragmentation of tissue at the operation site during multi medical discipline surgery including: general surgery, neuro, thoracic, urology, and gastrointestinal modalities http://www.fda.gov/cdrh/pdf/k012753.pdf	K050776 Indications for use: Fragmentation and aspiration of both soft and hard tissue in the following surgical specialties: Neurosurgery, Thoracic surgery, Wound Care, Gastrointestinal surgery, Urological surgery, General surgery, Orthopedic surgery, Plastic and Reconstructive surgery, Gynecology http://www.fda.gov/cdrh/pdf5/k050776.pdf
Surgical Procedure	No Equivalent to stimulated autolytic debridement Selective	NO . Equivalent to advanced sharp debridement Tissue emulsification Soft tissue sparing selectively removes non viable / necrotic tissue types with minimal damage to or removal of healthy / viable tissue types. May be more effective and accurate than sharp debridement.	NO . Equivalent to advanced sharp debridement Tissue emulsification Soft tissue sparing: selectively removes non viable / necrotic tissue types with minimal damage to or removal of healthy/ viable tissue types. May be more effective and accurate than sharp debridement.
Clinician Qualification	Physician, podiatrist, physical therapist, advanced practice nurse Licensing requirements for sharp debridement equivalency Knowledge to appropriately use US	Physician, podiatrist, physical therapist, advanced practice nurse Licensing requirements for sharp debridement equivalency Training beyond needed for sharp debridement recommended Knowledge to appropriately use US	Physician, podiatrist, physical therapist, advanced practice nurse Licensing requirements for sharp debridement equivalency Training beyond needed for sharp debridement recommended Knowledge to appropriately use US
Intensity	Intensity (Therapeutic Range) 0.1 – 0.5 W/cm2 Intensity(Maximum) 1.25 W/cm2 The intensity is preset not variable. The dose is calculated by size of wound and the device selects the treatment time based on wound size. Intensities over 3.0 W/cm^2 are used in surgical applications as ultrasonic scalpels and in tissue emulsification applications	Adjustable treatment range: from 0.1 to 2.0 W/cm^2, Less than 3 W/cm^2 Amplitude adjustment from 20%–100%. Higher intensity may be needed for thicker tissues e.g. necrotic tissues. Intensities over 3.0 W/cm^2 are used in surgical applications as ultrasonic scalpels and in tissue emulsification applications	Adjustable Treatment range: from 0.1 to 2.0 W/cm^2 Less than 3 W/cm^2. Amplitude adjustment provided Higher intensity may be needed for thicker tissues e.g. necrotic tissues. Intensities over 3.0 W/cm^2 are used in surgical applications as ultrasonic scalpels and in tissue emulsification applications
Mode	Continuous	Continuous	Continuous and pulsed (50%–90% duty cycle choices)

(Continued)

TABLE 25-1 *(Continued)*

Feature	Celleration MIST Therapy System 5.0	SÖRING/Sonoca 180	Misonix
Fluid dispensing	Disposable single use product specific sterile saline bottle .	Fluid dispensing : Preset and variable by practitioner, Suction equipment can be attached to control fluid Fluid selection by physician order	Fluid dispensing: Increased amplitude allows the clinician to increase fluid output Suction equipment can be attached to control fluid Fluid selection by physician order
Fluid delivery mode	Mist,	Stream and Mist	Clinician can use exact amount of fluid from a fine spray to a steady stream
Control mechanisms	Control button on hand held applicator.	Foot control pedal	Foot control pedal
Duration of Treatment	3–5 minutes; wound size dependent.	Varies, usually 2–5 minutes patient tolerance, tissue quality, operator evaluation	Varies, patient tolerance, tissue quality, operator evaluation
Wound Bed Contact	No. Treatment distance 0.5–1.5 cm . Note: at greater distance more US energy will be attenuated.	Yes	Yes
Non-contact single Use Applicator	Yes	No	No
Selective Debridement	Yes , better for slough, softened necrotic tissue Use also for maintenance debridement	Yes, efficient	Yes efficient
Pain with treatment	No	Sometimes, Recommend use of lidocaine if needed	Sometimes. Sensitivity can be modulated with pulsed mode, recommend use of lidocaine if needed
Observation of Results	2–3 treatments slow effect	Immediate.	Immediate.
Potential for thermal tissue destruction with misuse	No thermal effects	Yes, through frictional heat. Heat dissipation with fluid	Yes, through frictional heat. Heat is dissipated in two ways: Use of a fluid and pulsed mode
Need to autoclave probe between patients	No, single use disposable applicator non contact	Yes, Probe life: not stated	Yes Probe life : approximately 300–400 uses
Aerosolization Potential	No	Yes	Yes
Infection control Requirements	No Aerosolization Disposable single use applicator Germicidal wipes provided for disinfecting the transducer handle, cable, generator, and cradle	Personal protection equipment recommended : masks, gloves, and gown being used Private Room, drapes, Wipe down of surfaces pre and post procedure of unit	Personal protection equipment required: masks, gloves, and gown being used Private Room, drapes, PPE, Wipe down horizontal surfaces
Products	Fig 25-3	Fig 25-6	Fig 25-1

Copyright C. Sussman, Sussman Physical Therapy, Inc.© Prepared from materials provided and evaluated by the companies listed.

example, a 20% duty cycle, and are attributed to two different mechanisms: *acoustic cavitation* and *acoustic streaming*. Acoustic Cavitation involves the production and vibration of micron-sized bubbles within the coupling medium and fluids within the tissues. The US beam affects small gaseous bubbles that move within the tissue fluids. As the bubbles collect and condense, they are compressed before moving on to the next area. The movement and compression of the bubbles can cause changes in the cellular activities of the tissues subjected to US. Stable cavitation occurs when the bubbles in the field do not change much in size. The effect of stable cavitation can result in diffusional changes along cell membranes, thereby altering cell function. Stable cavitation is potentially beneficial because of its ability to initiate cellular changes within the tissues. Unstable or transient cavitation refers to the collapse of the bubbles mentioned above. Transient bubbles implode, causing local mechanical damage and free radical formation. This is potentially very hazardous. It occurs at high intensities, particularly when the sound head is not moved during treatment and standing waves develop.

A second nonthermal effect of US is acoustic streaming. This is defined as the movement of fluids along the acoustic boundaries (e.g., bubbles or cell membranes) as a result of the mechanical pressure wave associated with the US beam.[11] Outcomes attributable to this effect include increased cell membrane and vascular wall permeability, and increased protein synthesis.

It has been suggested that stable cavitation and microstreaming are responsible for the stimulatory effects of low-intensity US, acting as a stimulus that reversibly modifies plasma membrane permeability, and thus modulates cellular activity. Transient cavitation and standing wave formation are potentially damaging, but are easily avoided by using low intensities and keeping the applicator moving during treatment.

High-Resolution Diagnostic Ultrasound

Ultrasound is widely used as both a diagnostic and a therapeutic modality. It has an excellent safety record and can be used with confidence to image sensitive structures such as a fetus, tumors, and granulation tissue. Originally developed to image macroscopic structures, high-resolution equipment that allows tissues to be viewed at the microscopic level is now available. This equipment uses higher frequencies of ultrasound than are available in lower resolution devices.

Imaging

Ultrasound imaging depends on the principle that different tissue components reflect and absorb US to varying degrees, depending on their acoustic properties, which, in turn, depend on their structure. For example, tissues rich in fat absorb less US than do tissues rich in protein. Reflection occurs at the interface between materials that differ in their acoustic properties, specifically in their acoustic impedance. Each reflection is termed an echo.

Piezoelectric materials not only transduce electrical signals into mechanical vibrations, but also transduce mechanical vibrations into electrical signals. In US imaging, the reflected US, i.e. each echo, is detected by the same transducer that produced it. The transducer listens for the echoes in the short intervals between the pulses of US emitted by the transducer. When a pulse of ultrasound travels through the tissues of the body it meets many targets (interfaces and scatterers) that generate echoes. The echoes return first from targets closest to the transducer, followed by echoes from targets further and further away from the transducer. The diagnostic US equipment determines the distance d of each target from the transducer by measuring the time t taken for the echo to return following the emission of the pulse (the go and return time), assuming a fixed value for the speed of sound c in human tissues (1540 ms^{-1}). The echo returns to the transducer after a total go and return time of $2d/c$. The distance or depth of each target is calculated as $d = ct/2$.

A two-dimensional *B-mode image*, *B-scan* or *brightness scan* typically consists of at least 100 adjacent pulse echo sequences (each termed a B-mode line) captured sequentially as the beam or pulse of ultrasound is moved across the tissues being scanned. A display spot on the viewing screen of the monitor moves from a point corresponding to the position of the transducer in a direction representing the path of the beam. Reflections, or echoes, increase the brightness of the spot. The stronger the reflection, the greater its amplitude and the brighter the spot.

The reflections or echoes received at each beam position are displayed as spots on the display screen of the scanner, the brightness of each spot being related to the echo amplitude as a grayscale display. The grayscale can be replaced by different colors to assist in visual interpretation of the image, the colors representing differing levels of echogenicity from different tissue components. The distance down the screen at which each echo is displayed indicates d, the depth of the target producing the echo.

The tissue components, and hence the pattern and brightness of the reflections from them, vary with tissue type and are modified by injury and during repair. When high-resolution diagnostic US is used, the resultant image, which superficially resembles a histologic section, can be thought of as a noninvasive biopsy produced in a nontraumatic, painless manner, with no damage to the tissues that interact with the high-frequency/low-intensity US.

Visual Details

The detail that can be visualized ultrasonically is dependent on the resolution of the imaging equipment used, and this depends mainly on the wavelength of the US, which is determined by the frequency; the higher the frequency, the shorter the wavelength and, therefore, the greater the resolution. There is an inverse relationship between frequency and depth of penetration, higher frequencies being less penetrative than lower frequencies. In one 1991 study, US at a frequency of 5 MHz (i.e., 5 million cycles of vibration per second) was described as providing "high resolution"[13] and was considered to be adequate to view, for example, the plantaris tendon, provided that this was at least 2 mm thick, when the aim was merely to demonstrate whether it was present and whether it was thick enough to be used as a graft.

More recently, improved instrumentation coupled with the use of higher frequencies and image analysis has resulted in the effective use of US to noninvasively visualize changes in tissue associated with the presence or development of injury and its repair. In 1993, O'Reilly and Massouh[14] published a pictorial essay in which they compared the ultrasonic appearance of normal and damaged Achilles tendons, using a real-time scanner equipped with a 7.5 MHz linear transducer and a 5 MHz sector transducer. They were able to detect and distinguish between tenosynovitis, acute and chronic tendinitis, peritendinitis, nodular tendinitis, and partial or complete tendon rupture on the basis of differences in echogenicity and measurements of tendon thickness, the changes detected ultrasonographically being confirmed invasively by fine-needle aspiration and histologic examination.

Higher frequencies, permitting greater resolution, can be used for more superficial structures, such as the components of skin, where less depth of penetration is required. In 1994, 20 MHz US was used by Karim et al[15] to image skin from various parts of the body, and it was demonstrated that mathematical algorithms could be used to characterize and classify the dermal monograms as to their site of origin. Two analytic techniques were investigated, fractal analysis and fast Fourier transform, the aim being to develop image analysis techniques sensitive enough to detect minute changes in the pattern of the ultrasonically produced images, and to avoid interobserver differences in interpretation of these images.

New High-Resolution Diagnostic Scanners

High-resolution diagnostic US (HRUS) equipment with increased sensitivity is now available commercially. This equipment has evolved from prototypes developed at the United Medical and Dental Schools of Guy's and St. Thomas's Hospitals in London. Marketed by Longport Inc. (Silchester, UK) as the Episcanner, it is currently in use in the United States, Europe, and Australia to monitor changes in soft connective tissues associated with damage and repair. A patent covering this equipment was applied for in 1995, the final version of the patent being provided by Dyson et al in 1996. The equipment is portable and is fitted with a polyvinylidene diflouride piezoelectric polymer transducer incorporated into a handset filled with distilled water. It emits a chain of single-cycle pulses at a frequency of between 10 and 50 MHz, although it is generally used at a center frequency of 20 MHz. This allows the production of images of the interfaces between acoustically different materials, with a resolution such that structures separated by approximately 65 μm (micrometers) in the direction of the US transmission can be distinguished. The transducer is moved within the probe by a stepper motor, producing pulses of US with a repetition frequency of 1 msec. The system has been designed to emit an ultrafast rise and fall time pulse of duration of less than 50 nsec. These sharp pulses allow excellent detection of reflected signals (echoes), which, after transduction, pass through a preamp unit in the probe before passing to the main unit. As with other US imaging devices, including those operating at lower frequencies, time-gain compensation is used to control for the attenuation that occurs as the US is reflected back to the transducer. Digitization of the reflected signals produces data that can be stored and used for statistical analysis.[16, 17] A digital scan converter stores information in the US scan format and displays it in the video format.

Practical Implications

High-resolution B-mode displays show the components of a slice of soft tissue, akin to a histological section, but without removal of these tissues for examination. The same region of the body can be scanned repeatedly, showing, for example, the speed of tissue healing.[18,19] Cross-sectional images of the skin produced by Longport's Episcanner have a very characteristic appearance. The hyperechogenic (highly reflective) keratinized layer of the epidermis can be distinguished from the less echogenic layers of living cells that collectively form the stratum malpighii. As shown with other high-resolution equipment, the interface between the epidermis and dermis can be identified as a hyperechogenic layer under the less echogenic layer.[20] The dermis shows variations in echogenicity; the pattern of echoes varying from a speckled appearance in the papillary zone of the dermis to a more linear appearance in its deeper reticular zone, where the collagen fiber bundles are thicker and more aligned. Hair follicles, blood vessels, tendon sheaths, tendons, ligaments, and adipose tissue can be identified, as can the interfaces between soft tissue and calcified tissue. Figure 25-2 shows images of dermal structures captured at 50 MHz. Fluid-containing spaces within the dermis are hypoechogenic, as is subcutaneous fat, although this produces some thin linear echoes that may represent strands of collagenous fibrous connective tissue that support the fat. The scanner allows changes in soft tissue associated with the repair of injuries to be monitored (*Color Plates 73* and *74*) and subjected to fractal analysis, as did earlier, less informative and versatile instrumentation.[21,22]

More recently, high-resolution B-mode US has been used to detect the dermal changes associated with exposure to pressure[23,24] and as a means of quantifying the irritant response.[25] Deeper soft tissue injuries, such as developing pressure ulcers, can also be detected at pressure points close to the bone before they become visible at the surface of the

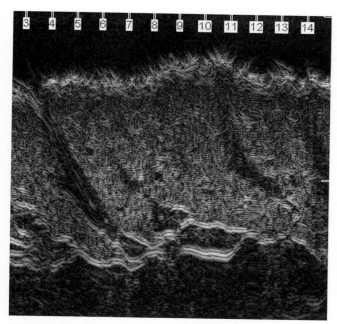

FIGURE 25-2 High-resolution ultrasound image of dermal structure captured at 50 MHz . (Courtesy of Paul Wilson, Longport, Inc.)

skin. High-resolution US (HRUS) is very sensitive in detecting fluid changes within tissues. It has been reported that HRUS can detect the edema associated with developing pressure ulcers 48 to 72 hours before there are clinical signs.[24] This edema is first recognisable in the subcutaneous tissue near the bone (*Color Plate 75A*). It then extends superficially, first into the reticular layer of the dermis (*Color Plate 75B*), and then into the papillary layer of the dermis (*Color Plate 75C*). Early detection of deep tissue injury allows pressure relief measures to be implemented before the ulcer breaks through the skin, with considerable reduction of suffering. A 3-year cost analysis of the use of high-frequency (high-resolution) diagnostic ultrasound technology's use in managing soft tissue injuries in a nursing home showed costs were reduced when HRUS was used as an addition to the current pressure ulcer risk assessment and management tool.[26] The ability of the highly sensitive Episcanner to detect and quantify muscle inflammation remains to be investigated. In 1990, Van Holsbeek and Introcaso[27] demonstrated echogenic differences between normal and inflamed muscle with less sensitive instrumentation.

Other uses of HRUS include monitoring changes in the thickness of the epidermis and underlying soft connective tissues, and in detecting lesions such as melanomas, potentially even those as small as 70 μm in thickness. As long ago as 1984, Shafir et al[28] indicated that what were then considered to be high-resolution US scanners could measure the thickness of melanomas. Accurate measurement of a melanoma's thickness can provide useful prognostic information, because this dimension is directly related to metastatic potential.[29] Also of importance is the potential of fractal

analysis of these high-quality images to provide quantitative data for comparison and assessment of the effectiveness of various therapies in the treatment of injured tissues. Fractal analysis may also be an aid to the diagnosis of a variety of skin pathologies, but this possibility remains to be examined critically.

One area of concern is the inability of clinicians to detect stage I pressure ulcers accurately in people with darkly pigmented skin[30-34]. This is due to the reliance for assessment on the parameter of color change, specifically redness (unblanchable erythema), for all patients, rather than considering the hues of blue-purple that may appear in people with darkly pigmented skin. Because the assessment of color is affected by the quantity and quality of the light source used, its value as the only indicator of stage I pressure ulcers in persons of color is questionable. Therefore, inclusion of other characteristics, such as skin temperature, stiffness, and sensation has been proposed,[33] together with the use of high-resolution US B-scans.[32,34]

Although the specific characteristics of early pressure-related injury are yet to be defined, awareness of the need to educate clinicians in culturally sensitive assessment techniques is growing.[17] Use of the HRUS as described above greatly increases both the sensitivity and specificity of correctly identifying stage I pressure ulcers, particularly in darkly pigmented skin. Furthermore, dependence on less accurate measures to identify stage I pressure ulcers, regardless of the skin's pigmentation, could be eradicated by the use of this equipment. The implementation of appropriate preventative measures and treatment, such as the use of the physical modalities described in this section, could significantly decrease the incidence of pressure ulcers in those at risk, leading to improvement in the quality of life and savings in the cost of health care. The effectiveness of these measures can now be assessed easily, objectively, and without damage or discomfort to the patient. [24,26,34]

High-resolution diagnostic ultrasound or ultrasound biomicroscopy is of considerable clinical importance that will grow as more uses are demonstrated for it. What is required now is more research of a high quality; this is currently being organized internationally.

CLINICAL WISDOM

The Longport Scanner is a portable device that can be used in many settings. The application of this technology and the resulting B scans, as seen in the color plates, take only a few seconds to produce, can be read immediately by a skilled clinician, transmitted for interpretation, or stored electronically, making them ideal for telemedicine applications.

Theory and Science of Ultrasound's Effect on Wound Healing

Cells close to stable bubbles are subject to bubble-associated microstreaming, which has been shown to increase their plasma membrane permeability to calcium ions, temporarily acting as a stimulus to cell activity (e.g., cell migration, proliferation, synthesis of intracellular and extracellular materials) and the synthesis and release of growth factors. All of these activities would be expected to accelerate wound healing. In cells treated in suspension, the suppression of cavitation also suppresses the stimulation of cellular activity. It should be noted that the ultrasonic stimulus is perceived by the cells and transduced by them; an amplified response then occurs of a type that varies according to the cell type involved.

Effect on the Phases of Healing

Wound recovery occurs as a series of overlapping biochemical responses to injury. Recovery normally concludes in approximately 21 days. Inflammation occurs in the first 72 hours. In these early hours, epithelial cells begin migration and reproduction to restore the skin integrity and to protect the body from infection or admission of foreign substances.

Inflammatory Phase

In normal wounding, the acute inflammatory state occurs following an initial clotting response that initiates a vascular response involving the arterial and venous systems. This, in turn, leads to vasodilatation and invasion of the area by a large number of white blood cells that release the growth factors necessary to initiate repair. (See Chapter 2 regarding the physiology of wound healing.) These white blood cells include macrophages, polymorphonuclear leukocytes, and mast cells. The mast cells degranulate, releasing histamine hyaluronic acid and other proteoglycans that bind with the watery wound fluid to create a gel. Coagulated wound gel will later be replaced by a dense, binding scar. The massive vascular incursion into the periwound tissues produces the symptoms associated with the inflammatory phase: calor, dolor, rubor, and turgor. This is a critical period of repair. Ultrasound delivered at this time stimulates the release of growth factors from platelets, mast cells, and macrophages, which, in turn, are chemotactic to the fibroblasts and endothelial cells that later form collagen-containing vascular granulation tissue. Early intervention with US accelerates the inflammatory phase, leading to more rapid entry into the proliferative phase of repair. It is not antiinflammatory, and therefore should begin as soon as possible, during the acute inflammatory phase.

Proliferative Phase

The proliferative phase follows the acute inflammatory phase, about 72 hours after injury, and overlaps the late inflammatory phase. The proliferative phase is divided into two stages, fibroplasia and contraction. New tissue has a pink granular appearance and is called *granulation tissue*. Granulation tissue builds on the collagen matrix laid down by the fibroblasts. Ultrasound stimulates fibroblast migration and proliferation. Dyson[36] reports that fibroblasts exposed to therapeutic levels of US in vivo were stimulated to synthesize more of the type of collagen that gives soft con-

nective tissue its tensile strength. Endothelial cells, responsible for vascularization of the granulation tissue, are also affected by US at this stage to produce more prolific growth. Under histologic examination, more angiogenesis is seen in granulation tissue that has been sonated at 0.75 MHz and 0.1 W/cm^2 than in untreated tissue.[36–38]

The late phase of proliferation is wound contraction. During this process, the wound is pulled together by the centripetal movement of the surrounding tissue. This results in less scar tissue formation. Fibroblasts transform into specialized contractile cells called *myofibroblasts* during this process. Myofibroblasts at this phase resemble smooth muscle cells. In some experiments, smooth muscle cells are reported to contract when treated with therapeutic levels of US. It has been postulated that myofibroblasts may be similarly affected. Ultrasound, applied during the inflammatory and early proliferative phases, may accelerate wound contraction both by causing those cells to develop earlier, and increasing their efficiency. At this time, however, the mechanisms by which this occurs are not fully understood. Dyson states that no reports have been found of excessive pathologic contraction (contracture) following treatment with therapeutic US.[36,38] Intervention with low-intensity, nonthermal US within 72 hours following injury can therefore be used to promote wound contraction, which results in a reduction in size of the resulting scar.[39]

Epithelialization Phase

Epithelialization begins concurrently with the inflammatory and proliferative phases. The epithelial cells begin moving and reproducing within a few hours of injury. These cells require an environment that is warm, moist, free of infection, and which provides a supply of nutrients and oxygen in order to move and to multiply.[40–42]

Ultrasound stimulates the release of growth factors necessary for the regeneration of epithelial cells. Ultrasound

Ultrasound and High-Voltage Pulsed Current for Dual Purpose

Ultrasound has been useful in the clinic to treat periwound tissue above undermined and tunneled areas because 1 MHz US can penetrate up to 5 cm. This treatment has been given in conjunction with high-voltage pulsed current (HVPC) to the wound bed. Response has been decreased depth and undermining measurements within 2 weeks of treatment's start. No adverse reactions occurred. This is a topic for further research. The protocol used involved 1 MHz, 0.5 W/cm^2 (SATP), 20% duty cycle, applied daily for 5 minutes to periwound area over a period of 2–3 weeks.[35] High-resolution diagnostic US can be used to visualize the extent of tunneling and its resolution.

has the capability of increasing the vascularity of the tissue, and may in this way improve nutrient and oxygen delivery. Ultrasound therefore appears to stimulate epithelialization and hasten it, by application to the periwound areas.

Remodeling/Maturation Phase

This phase is affected by low-intensity US *only if* treatment is commenced in the inflammatory phase. If so, the effects are more rapid entry into the remodeling phase, increased wound tensile strength, increased capacity to absorb energy without mechanical damage, increased elasticity, and deposition of collagen fibers in a pattern closer to that of intact tissue. Several researchers have reported that application of thermal US during the remodeling phase mechanically affects collagen extensibility and enzyme activity. Frieder et al[43] reported improved collagen organization, and Jackson et al[44] reported improved tensile strength in the tendon repairs of US-treated animals. Hart[39] demonstrated that treatment with low-intensity nonthermal US in the early inflammatory phase influenced the outcome of scar collagen density and organization. Later treatment is less effective.

Pain and Edema

Pain is a symptom associated with the inflammatory phase, and is due to the influx of blood, the release of chemicals such as histamine, prostaglandins, and bradykinin, and the associated pressure from posttraumatic edema on surrounding nerve endings. Reduction of pain is an essential part of wound healing, resulting in reduced muscle guarding and increased activity which, in turn, enhances circulation to the area of wounding. Pain also stimulates the sympathetic nervous system, producing a reactive hyperemia. The result is an increased area of inflammation. This enhances the metabolic requirements of the surrounding tissue for more nutrients and oxygen. Pain relief can reduce the area of involvement and decrease the bioburden.

It has been theorized that the pain threshold can be raised with thermal application of therapeutic US, decreased pain

being due to a rise in the nerve conduction velocity of C fibers.[45] However, after careful examination of the published reports, there is no conclusive theoretic explanation of how pain is relieved by US.[38] Pain is also a symptom of wound infection among most patients, including those with neuropathy.[46] The bactericidal effects of US, described later in this chapter, have been attributed to reduced pain after US treatment.

US for Skin Tears

Skin tears are a common problem for the elderly. They are often painful and surrounded with edema and ecchymosis. Application of nonthermal US with a conductive gel or lotion over a hydrogel transmission sheet or a transparent film dressing produces a reduction in pain and edema after one or two treatments, and dispersal of the ecchymosis within 6–10 sessions, depending on the size of the area involved. This method allows the dressing to remain in place between treatments, and will not disrupt the wound or cause skin damage. As healing progresses, expect the patient's mobility to increase. The protocol used involves 1 MHz, 0.5 W/cm^2 (SATP), 20% duty cycle, applied daily for 5 minutes to the periwound area. A setting of 3 MHz is preferable.[35]

Enhanced blood flow creates greater capillary pressure and fluid shift into the interstitial tissues, and this creates edema. Acoustic streaming may affect vascular permeability and help to control periwound edema. Edema-free and pain-free outcomes are highly desirable because they accelerate and decrease the duration of the inflammatory process.[7–11]

Circulation

Transcutaneous partial pressure of oxygen (tcPO$_2$) can be measured before and after treatment as a method of monitoring changes in blood flow (see Chapter 7). Byl and Hopf[47] found that, following pulsed low-intensity (0.5 W/cm^2) 1 MHz US, little increase in tissue temperature or oxygen transport occurred unless the individual was both well hydrated (three to four glasses of water), and receiving supplemental oxygen by nasal cannula. Well-hydrated subjects receiving supplemental oxygen had an increase in subcutaneous oxygen four times greater than that measured when breathing room air. Thermal application with high-dose (1.0 W/cm^2) low-frequency (1 MHz) US produced vasodilatation and raised tissue oxygen levels and temperature significantly. Care must be taken to avoid excessive thermal effects whereby circulation is diminished and heat cannot be dissipated rapidly.[47] Increased circulation brings nutrients and oxygen to the tissues and removes waste products that can impede healing. Because increased circulation and oxygen are such critical components of wound healing and are dose dependent, this needs to be considered in the use of protocols for healing.

Increasing Circulation with High-Dose US

Ischemic tissues surrounding a chronic wound which have not responded to other types of wound treatments may benefit from periwound US. If the wound bed is clean, expect increased serosanguineous exudate from the wound base to appear in 3–5 days. If the wound has necrotic tissue, expect to see lysis of the necrotic tissue, increased periwound erythema, and raised temperature due to the increased circulation associated with a change to the acute inflammatory phase. If this does not occur, repeat the single higher-intensity treatment and follow with lower-intensity treatments. Parameters of treatment are 1.0 to 1.4 W/cm^2 (SA, TP), 1 MHz or 3 MHz, and continuous 5- to 10-minute duration, depending on the size of the area. Reduce intensity to 0.5 W/cm^2 (SA, TP), pulsed 20%, applied 3–5 times per week after one treatment.[20]

Supplement Hydration and Oxygen

See that patients are well hydrated before US treatment. Add supplemental oxygen by nasal cannula at 5 L/min, which has been shown to prevent infection in surgical wounds[48] and to raise tissue oxygen levels when used in conjunction with US. Both will improve healing outcomes.

Thrombolysis and Fibrinolysis

Ultrasound has been described as increasing dispersal of the hemorrhagic material associated with bruising.[49] Acoustic cavitation appears be the mechanism that produces this fragmentation.[50] When US is passed through a liquid (e.g. blood or wound fluid) with alternating pressure, acoustic cavitation results in the formation of microbubbles. The microbubbles collapse rapidly. The mechanical forces resulting from the collapsing microbubbles appear to be sufficient to break the fibrin bonds in thrombi, inducing fragmentation—hence the use of the term fibrinolysis. At higher frequencies, more power is need to produce cavitation. The intensity of the collapsing force is diminished at >1 MHz, and not produced at >2.5 MHz.[51,50] There is a correlation of thrombus ablation with US and the elasticity of the arterial wall. A clot's low level of elasticity contributes to the fragmentation effect of the US, but the high elasticity of arterial walls resists damaging effects if high-power US is used. This is a key factor in the safety of US thrombolysis.[51] In the rabbit model, externally applied low-intensity US enhanced thrombolysis.[52] Investigations of the effect of combining US with pharmacologic thrombolytic agents (e.g. tissue-plasminogen activator [t-PA] or streptokinase) for enhanced thrombolysis report that there appears to be a synergistic effect on thrombus disruption that is not seen when US is used alone.[50,52, 53] Pulsed mid-kHz exposure is more effective for thrombolysis than continuous exposure. It minimizes the probability of heating, and improves absorption and the penetration of the sound wave into the tissues, all of which are beneficial in clinical applications.[10,53]

Bruising, Hematoma, and Deep Tissue Injury

In patients with wounds, often the initial insult is a deep tissue injury with extraversion of blood, followed by coagulation, hematoma and later by necrosis.[55] Initially this looks like a hematoma or bruise or purple pressure ulcer. With the extensive use of anticoagulation and antiplatelet therapy, incidence rates of hematoma related to pressure injury are likely to rise as time goes on (see Chapter 4). The onset of venous ulceration is often preceded by subcutaneous bleeding (*Color Plate 78*). Color plates 78–87 show two case examples, both before and after treatment, where pulsed US, 1 MHz, at low intensity was the only treatment used. Cases are presented at the end of this chapter. There was pronounced evidence of the absorption of hemorrhagic material following treatment of the peri-hemorrhagic area, and which was perhaps related to the thrombolytic effect of US. These were closed wounds, initially. By the time the skin sloughed off, the area of involvement was significantly reduced, and the open ulcers went on to heal in a timely sequence, which is not common.

Intervention with US appears to have been efficacious in resolution of a rectus sheath hematoma.[54] A patient receiving oral anticoagulant therapy developed a large hematoma of the rectus sheath, confirmed with sonography and CT scan. The hematoma was stabilized with pharmacological treatment. Since MHz US has the ability to increase blood flow (as described above), the physical therapy team believed that early intervention with US would pose a risk of new bleeding during the acute phase of the hematoma. Therefore, US application was delayed until the hematoma showed a predominantly hypoechoic image on sonogram, and coagulation parameters were within the correct range (INR=2–3.5). This status was achieved 9 days after onset. The use of pulsed 1 MHz US at 1.5–2 W/cm^2 around the hematoma was subsequently applied 5 days a week for 4 weeks (20 sessions). By the end of one week pain was negligible, and by the end of 2 weeks the hematoma was reduced 50% in size. By the end of 4 weeks it was barely palpable, and a follow up sonograph 2 weeks later showed that the hematoma had been resolved.

In all of these examples, the physical therapists used clinical reasoning based on their unique training and knowledge about the effect of US to safely and effectively treat the hematoma problems presented. The hypothesis that exogenous application of US to the adjacent skin can promote absorption and resolution of hematoma (deep tissue injury) or venous leakage needs further validation.

Bactericidal Effects

Bacterial infection is a common barrier to wound healing. Biophysical methods of bacterial control are useful in the treatment of resistant organisms and biofilms. The bactericidal effects of US appear to occur on several levels. On the tissue level, ultrasonic debridement has been shown to remove bacterial contamination.[56,57] Applying US for debridement of infected burn wounds was reported in 1980 by Schoenbach and Song.[58] In this animal study, rats were exposed to contact burns and a strain of *Pseudomonas aeruginosa*. The therapy group received daily tap-water bath with ultrasound while the controls received a daily tap-water bath without ultrasound. The treated group had a sharp reduction in colony counts while the controls all continued to have high colony counts. Cultures were also taken of the post treatment bath waters, which revealed high colony counts of *P. aeruginosa*. The rats in this study had no noted ill effects from the ultrasonic therapy. The researchers concluded that ultrasound was effective in reducing bacterial colony counts as well as allowing for initial healing to start.[58]

At the cellular level, ultrasound stimulates nitric oxide (NO) production and increases endothelial cell nitric oxide synthase activity.[59,60] Nitric oxide has been shown to kill pathogens when it reacts with peroxide oxygen ions, prevent replication of DNA viruses within cells, and serve as an immune regulator.[61] Chapters 2 and 3 have more information about the function of NO and nitric oxide synthase. Ultrasound has been shown to modify plasma membrane permeability and transport properties.[62] Marked disruption of bacterial cell membranes and reduced colony forming units (*Staphylococcus aureus*, *P. aeruginosa*, methicillin-resistant *S. aureus* [MRSA] and vancomycin-resistant Enterococcus [VRE]) was observed following application of US,[63] and was also effective in removing 99% of *P. aeruginosa*.[64] Bacterial death, measured by colony counts, was significant after application of the Sonoca 180(Söring Inc., Ft. Worth, TX) for a total of 120 seconds.[65] Niezgoda and Schulze presented information on cell death following treatment of cultured cells of *Escherichia coli*, *Streptococcus pyogenes*, *S. aureus*, and *P. aeruginosa* for 60 seconds with the Sonoca 180.[57,65] However, it is not clear whether these cellular studies were performed on planktonic or sessile bacteria in biofilms. Qian et al[66] found that there is a synergistic effect between US and 24 hour-old biofilms of *P. aeruginosa*. A significantly greater number of bacteria in a biofilm were killed by gentamicin when they were subjected to US at low frequency than when treated with either one alone.[66]

High- and low-frequency US have been used successfully for many decades for enhanced transdermal drug delivery.[67] The current term used for this application of US is sonophoresis, formerly phonophoresis. The mechanism of action is enhanced diffusion through the structural layers of the stratum corneum. Pretreatment or cotreatment of skin with US of various frequencies almost completely eliminates the lag time typically associated with transdermal drug delivery, and is sustained after the US is turned off. Pretreatment of a short application of US enables permeation of the skin prior to the drug delivery, and the skin remains in this state of high permeability for several hours, so that drugs delivered by this method have sustained release. Current applications include sonophoresis of lidocaine, insulin, and macromolecular drugs.[67] Information about use of US for transdermal application of antibiotics is available in Russian but not in English as of this writing. There are claims that the use of low-frequency US applications are bactericidal for biofilms, but that does not appear to be supported in the literature, unless delivered in conjunction with antibiotics. In a personal communication, Samir Mitragotri, an expert in sonophoresis, said that sonophoresis with antibiotics may be possible, but the issue may be that the sonophoresis may deliver too high a dosage.[68] More investigation about this concept could be useful.

Ultrasonic Wound Debridement

Early studies used a US device that delivered the sound waves in a water bath. Removal from wounds of necrotic debris, pus, and bacteria including biofilms is essential to prepare the wound bed for healing. Surgeons have used ultrasonic dissection to surgically débride tissue for many years. Now there are new ultrasonic tools available, that are just short of surgery, and are useful for bedside and clinical ultrasonic debridement of contaminated soft tissue. Ultrasound is reported to be less traumatic to tissue than abrasive scrubbing, high-pressure jet irrigation, or sharp/surgical debridement.[10,56,57,69] Ultrasound improves the outcome of bone debridement by maintaining the integrity of the directly involved bone trabecula, reducing contamination, preventing bacterial colonization, and decreasing possible infection.[56]

Technological advances have led to the development of tools like the MIST (Celleration, Eden Prairie, MN), Sonoca 180 (Söring Inc., Ft. Worth, TX), and Misonix SonicOne Ultrasonic Wound Debridement System (Misonex, Farmdale, NY). These devices deliver ultrasound coupled with a fluid system through a hand-held probe/applicator. These devices deliver 25–40 kHz low-frequency US. Intensity can be varied. They are approved for wound debridement and cleansing by the FDA. However, the delivery systems and their effects are not identical. MIST is a noncontact system. The Sonoca 180 and the Misonix Sonic One are used as contact instruments coupled with the wound fluid, or with the addition of saline, and have tips that push the fluid forward. The various tips provided offer a distinct advantage when necrotic tissue is located in hard to reach places, such as tunnels and undermined areas. These two devices offer a choice of fluid stream or mist applications (see table 25-1).

Clinically, the low-frequency US debriders have been used and tested in tertiary wound care centers for several years. Clinical case studies are just beginning to be presented and published.[10,57,65,70] The cases presented indicate favorable results of the treatment. Benefits reported include:

- selective removal of necrotic debris while there is preservation of granulation tissue
- bactericidal effects – reduced infection
- cleansing of deep tunneling and undermining is facilitated
- deep tissue penetration of ultrasonic vibration and energy

- excellent wound bed preparation for grafting or flap closure
- reduced use of narcotics to control pain
- minimal blood loss despite anticoagulation therapy
- rapid removal of fibrin

This advanced technology is not likely to become part of the wound care toolbox overnight, as it is very costly and requires high level of knowledge and skill to use correctly. It is not a benign intervention, even though negative effects are not well documented. In their multicenter study, Ennis et al[8] reported on 12 adverse events that were either possibly, probably, or definitely related to the use of the MIST device. These events included pain, erythema, blister, edema, ulcer enlargement and infection and additional ulcer development, and other unspecified. Policy and procedure guidelines for use of the Sonoca 180 in ultrasonic wound debridement was developed by Mary Verhege, who has extensive experience in the use of the Sonoca 180. Her policies and procedures are presented in the procedure section below. Clinical research is needed to determine the best treatment intervals, which wounds are candidates for treatment, and which will be most responsive to this treatment, and then compare the results with other debridement methods.[10,57]

Clinical Studies of Wound Healing

Animal Studies

Moderate-frequency 5 MHz US was selected to determine whether there was a beneficial effect from US when applied daily for short periods to postsurgical incisional wounds.[71] Subjects were Fischer F344 male rats. The US frequency was chosen because less than 20% of the power would penetrate deeper than 1 cm below the surface of the skin, so that most of the US energy would be absorbed in the vicinity of the wound. The chosen intensity for a 5-minute exposure was 0.05 or 0.075 W/cm^2. Several experiments were performed at different thermal intensities (ranging from 0.05 to 0.15 W/cm^2). Sonation was continuous. The extent of heat production by insonation and the effect on healing were the study variables. Measurements at all intensities following 5 minutes of continuous sonation showed an increase in subcutaneous tissue temperatures that were progressively larger with higher intensities of insonation.[71] At lower intensities (0.025 and 0.05 W/cm^2), 10 minutes of insonation produced only a small additional elevation in subcutaneous tissue temperature, indicating that a plateau in temperature had been approached by 5 minutes.[71]

Treatment of the surgically induced incisional wounds began on the fourth postoperative day, when clips could be removed. The clips would have interfered with the US beam, and, at that time, the wounds were entering the proliferative phase of healing. Expectation was that this was the optimal time to stimulate the fibroblasts to augment healing. Findings were that the breaking strength of the sonated wounds was equivalent but not greater than that of those treated by direct heating of the tissues. At the higher intensities (0.1 and 0.15 W/cm^2), healing was impaired, and dermal burns occurred.[71] In other studies, described below, treatment be-

---

▮ CASE STUDY

Debridement of Chronic Venous Ulcer

An ultrasonic device (Sonoca 180) was used over a 7 week period to treat a 45-year-old female patient with a chronic venous insufficiency ulcer of the left lower leg that she had suffered for approximately six months. For approximately 4 months prior to ultrasonic wound debridement, the patient had been treated with compression therapy, Unna Boots, and various other dressings as guided by the University of Virginia Chronic Wound Clinic, with little success. Initial wound assessment prior to ultrasonic therapy showed a large wound (7.8 cm × 6.6 cm = 51.48 cm^2) containing 80% well-adhered yellow slough, 15% pink moist tissue, and 5% dry black eschar in the center of the wound. The periwound skin was intact but was macerated at different points during therapy due to large amounts of exudate. When her skin appeared macerated, skin protectant was used. This was effective for maintaining periwound skin throughout therapy. As part of standard care, she wore an Unna Boot for compression, and had foam dressing over the wound to manage wound exudate between ultrasound sessions. Treatment goals were removal of necrotic debris and progression towards wound healing. Plan of care was to continue standard care and ultrasonic therapy once weekly for debridement. After two ultrasound treatments, the wound bed had improved, as indicated by reduction in yellow slough from 80% to about 20% without eschar, and was starting to granulate and contract. After seven treatments, the wound showed 90% granulation tissue, and wound contraction without slough or eschar. The wound size had decreased to 4.8cm × 5 cm = 24 cm^2. This was a 53% reduction in size in 8 weeks, demonstrating a positive healing trajectory. This patient required local application of lidocaine jelly for pain management during the first three or four treatments. By the end of the treatments, she no longer required pain medication.

The impression is that ultrasound debridement decreased the bioburden and restarted the healing process. Other patients treated at our clinic with the ultrasonic wound debridement therapy have not required any pain medications. The procedure used for this case study was supplied by Söring, Inc .

Acknowledgement: Thank you to Christine Newcomer, MSN, RN, WOCN, PhD Student University of Virginia, who supplied supporting information that is used in this section and kindly prepared the case study of her patient, who was treated with Sonoca 180 Wound debridement technology at University of Virginia. Thanks also to Catherine Ratliff PhD, APRM-BC, CWOCN , for arranging and mentoring this collaboration .

gan within 24 hours of surgery; signs of healing were reported by the fourth postoperative day.

In another study of burn-induced wounds in rats, two groups of animals were treated with pulsed (SATP 0.25 W/cm^2) and continuous (0.3 W/cm^2) US.[72] No stimulating effects were demonstrated in either US treatment group or against controls when evaluated by change in wound size and histologic examination. The investigators questioned the clinical benefit of treating burn wounds with US. There is no indication in the study report how soon after burn-induced wounding the US treatment commenced.

There is a lack of consensus on the dosimetry for treatment with US. To learn more about dosage and wound healing, Byl et al[73] made incisional wounds in miniature Yucatan pigs, and treatment was applied at different doses for different lengths of time. The tensile strength of wounds treated with different intensities, called *high-* and *low-dose US*, was tested. Two variables were evaluated, the breaking strength of the incision, and the deposition of hydroxyproline, which is a measure of collagen deposition. High-dose US was classified as 1.5 W/cm^2, continuous mode. Low-dose US was 0.5 W/cm^2, pulsed mode, 20% duty cycle. Both treatment groups received a frequency of 1 MHz for 5 minutes. The wounds were sonated for approximately 1.25 min/cm of incisional length, beginning 24 hours after surgery. The wounds were covered with a moisture- and vapor-permeable adhesive dressing (Tegaderm, 3M Medical-Surgical Division, St. Paul, MN) that was left in place for up to 1 week. The dressing was found to permit transmission of US energy and could be left in place, avoiding disruption of the wound between treatment sessions. Forty-eight wounds were made, and the wounds were divided into three groups: 12 for control and 18 each for high-dose US and low-dose US. The groups were subdivided into two groups of 12 that received low dose or high dose for 5 days and two groups of six that received high dose or low dose for 10 days.

The study found that the tensile strength for all treatment groups was significantly higher than that of the controls, but there was no difference in hydroxyproline deposition. A significant interaction was found between the number of days of treatment and the US dose. Hydroxyproline deposition was significantly higher and the breaking strength was higher for the low-dose group, compared with the high-dose group, after 10 days of treatment. The study findings suggest that during the first week, either low or high dose US will enhance wound breaking strength but, to facilitate collagen deposition and wound strength, low-dose US should be used if treatment is to continue for 2 weeks or more.[73]

A comparative study of the effect of US (0.1 W/cm^2 pulsed) and electrical stimulation (ES) (300 mA direct current, 30 minutes/day) on incisional wound healing in rats found that both modalities had positive effects on the proliferative phases of healing, but that ES was superior at the maturation phase.[74] Treatment was begun within 2 hours of the surgical procedure. Electrical stimulation treatment allowed wounds to move to the proliferative phase earlier than

in the US group, as indicated by the presence of more fibroblasts on the fourth day. Although the density and arrangement of collagen was greater in the US group on the seventh day, the collagen was more regular in the ES group on the same day. Breaking strength was higher in the US group than in the sham US group, but not as great as the ES group. Ultrasound affects the early phases of wound healing, but ES causes a beneficial effect on all phases. Ultrasound is more useful for the acute, uninfected, well-perfused wound, but ES is more useful for treatment of chronic or infected wounds, or wounds likely to be infected.[74]

Human Studies

Pressure Ulcers. In 1960, Paul et al[75] published a report of clinical observations of 23 patients with pressure ulcers which suggested that ultrasonic therapy is effective in reducing tissue congestion, cleansing necrotic tissue, and promoting healing and the return of skin function to a near normal state, and that a "scientifically controlled study would be richly rewarding."[75]

Twenty-five years later, based on the scientific evidence that nonthermal therapeutic US affects the biologic processes of repair through stable cavitation and/or acoustic streaming described above, a double blind randomized study was undertaken by McDiarmid et al[76] to determine whether these nonthermal therapeutic effects could be used to treat soft tissue wounds. Patients with partial-thickness skin loss caused by pressure ulcers, but not extending beyond the dermis, were selected. Forty patients were entered into the study and randomized into a US treatment and a sham US treatment group. Parameters for the US treatment were 3 MHz, 0.8 W/cm^2 (SATP), pulse duration 2 msec, duty cycle 20%, SATA intensity, 0.16 W/cm^2, effective radiating surface area 5.2 cm^2. Treatment duration was a minimum of 5 minutes for all pressure ulcers up to 3 cm^2. One additional minute was added for each 0.5 cm^2 area, for a maximum of 10 minutes. Frequency was three times per week. The insonated ulcers tended to heal more quickly, but the difference was not statistically significant. However, when comparing clean ulcers with infected ulcers, the mean healing time for the clean ulcers was 30 days versus 40 days for the infected ulcers. Although US had little effect on the healing of clean pressure ulcers, there appeared to be a statistically significant effect of US on the healing of infected pressure ulcers, implying that the major factor influencing healing is whether the ulcer is clean or infected. McDiarmid et al[76] speculated that, if the clean wound was already healing at an optimal biologic rate, the addition of a therapy such as US would not make a significant difference. On the other hand, slower-healing infected ulcers may benefit from the effect of US stimulation of the large number of macrophages—the pivotal cell of the inflammatory phase and repair—present in infected wounds, with a resulting release of "wound factors" from those cells and other repair cells.[76]

Nussbaum et al[77] conducted a comparison study of nursing care alone, nursing care with laser, and nursing care with an alternating protocol of US and ultraviolet C (UVC) on 20 spinal cord-injured patients with 22 pressure ulcers. Four of the initial subjects dropped out, leaving 16 subjects with 18 wounds to be considered for the analysis. Nursing care consisted of moist dressings and continuous pressure relief. The laser regimen was provided three times per week. The US/UVC regimen consisted of US treatment five times weekly, alternating the US and UVC daily, 5 days per week. If the ulcer had purulent drainage, the UVC was used three times per week; if not, US was used three times per week. Ultrasound protocol was frequency 3 MHz and intensity (SATA) of 0.2 W/cm^2 (1:4 pulse ratio) for 5 minutes per 5 cm^2 of wound area delivered to the periwound area. Results showed that the US/UVC treatment had a greater effect on wound healing than did the other treatment regimens.[77] The mean treatment time to wound closure was 4.1 weeks. The trend was for ulcers to heal faster in sites where wound contraction was the primary mode of closure (e.g., over the coccyx). The conclusion was that this regimen of US/UVC may decrease the healing time for spinal cord-injured patients with pressure ulcers.[77] This was a small study that combined two interventions, making it impossible to demonstrate the efficacy of either individually. Questions remain concerning whether the combination was essential, and what the effects of each treatment were.

Pressure ulcers were the subject of another study involving US by ter Riet et al.[78] Eighty-eight subjects were randomized into two groups, 45 for the treatment group and 43 for the control group. The trials lasted 12 weeks. Sixteen ulcers were stage IV, extending into muscle tissue, and 72 had less depth of tissue involvement. Treatment was given directly to the wound surface (although how this was accomplished for the stage IV ulcers is not described) and to an extended radius 0.75 cm beyond the wound edge. The treatment parameters were a frequency of 3.28 MHz, pulse duration of 2 msec, SATA 0.1 W/cm^2, and BNR less than 4. The minimum treatment duration was 3 minutes, 45 seconds. Wounds with treatment areas larger than 5 cm^2 were treated longer. A wound with an area of 10 cm^2 was treated for 7 1/2 minutes. Local wound care included once- or occasionally twice-daily cleansing or rinsing with sterile saline or chlorhexidine (0.1%) on gauze or in a syringe. Chlorhexidine is a cytoxic agent to cells of repair, and using it for wound cleansing may have affected treatment results. Four wound characteristics (color of surrounding skin, necrotic tissue, granulation tissue, and deepest tissue involved) were each marked on a scale, with grading from 1 = bad to 10 = excellent. Two outcome variables were end points: surface area reduction (in cm^2) and wound closure (yes or no). After 12 weeks, 40% of the ulcers (18/45) in the US group and 44% of the ulcers (19/43) in the sham US group were closed. The results showed a tendency for the US to be more effective in small wounds than in larger wounds, which could not be explained.[78] This multicenter clinical trial, published in 1996, did not support the hypothesis that US speeded up healing. However, examination of the methodology reveals that, although the US parameters were suitably controlled

and described, there was a large variation in ulcer size and depth, patient health, and wound cleansing methods. The surface area of the pressure ulcers varied at the outset from less than 1 cm^2 to more than 10 cm^2. Ulcer severity ranged from grade II to grade IV. The study sample had 16 patients with grade IV ulcers. Partial-thickness grade II ulcers heal faster than do full-thickness ulcers. To combine the two would bias the results. Furthermore, the patients were elderly (75–87 years); some were terminally ill and many incapacitated, those in the US-treated group being confined to bed from 14.4 to 24 hours per day, and those in the sham-irradiated control group from 14 to 20.5 hours per day. Therefore, it is perhaps unreasonable to expect a significant improvement in healing to occur following US therapy (or possibly any other type of physical therapy). Ideally, the variability of both treatment parameters and patient characteristics in such studies should be minimized, and the physical condition of the patients should be such that healing is likely to occur. Only then can the efficacy of procedures designed to speed up healing rather than initiate it be adequately assessed.

A pilot study of 5 subjects with 6 pressure ulcers was designed as a preliminary examination of the effects of MIST ultrasound on the size and appearance of pressure ulcers. The investigators found that after 4 weeks, ulcers receiving a 5–10 minute treatment 5–7 times weekly along with standard good wound care were 73% of their original size. Wound appearance based on the Photographic Wound Assessment Tool (PWAT) (see Chapter 5) improved significantly with healthy granulation tissue present.[79] These findings are promising, but a larger double-blinded multicenter study on pressure ulcers would be valuable.

Chronic Leg Ulcers. Ultrasound was used as a periwound treatment by Dyson et al[80] for a controlled trial among patients with chronic varicose ulcers. Two groups received either sonation or sham sonation three times per week for 4 weeks. Treatment parameters for the US treatment were 3 MHz, 1.0 W/cm^2 (SA, TP), pulse duration 2 msec, delivered to the tissues every 10 msec for up to 10 minutes. The treatment technique involved moving the head of the device over the skin immediately adjacent to the ulcer. At the end of 4 weeks, the experimental, sonated group had statistically significant reduction in wound size compared with the control group (experimental group 66.4% ± 8.8%; control group 91.6% ± 8.9%). No adverse effects of treatment were found.

Application of continuous 30 kHz US at an intensity (SATA) of 0.1 W/cm2 via a water bath for 10 minutes three times weekly showed significant healing of chronic venous leg ulcers when Peschen et al[81] treated 24 patients with chronic venous ulceration. All study and control patients were randomized and received either a conventional therapy of hydrocolloid dressings and compression or the conventional therapy plus US treatment. At the end of a 12-week period, the experimental group showed an average decrease in ulcer area of 55.4%, compared with only 16.5% in the control group—a highly significant decrease ($p = .007$). The water bath method of delivering therapeutic US has found acceptance in Europe, but not in the United States.[81]

Weichenthal et al [82] used an experimental device that consisted of a water bath and a transducer that produced 30 kHz US at intensity of 100mW/cm². Treatment was given for 10 minutes to the area of the ulcer in the water bath, which was heated to 32–34°C. Thirty-eight patients with chronic venous insufficiency who had leg ulcers were randomized into two groups. Both groups received standard wound care including compression bandaging, debridement, and antiseptics as needed. Results after 8 weeks of active and sham treatment were a decrease in ulcer area of 11% for the controls and 41% for the US group, a statistically significant result. Reported complications included minor transient pain during the treatment, mild to moderate but not pain-related erythema after treatment and persisting from 10 minutes to 2 hours. Wound debridement effects were not observed.

A metaanalysis of studies on the use of US therapy in the treatment of chronic leg ulcers was published in 1998.[22] Of the 14 studies found during a literature review, 6 were selected for inclusion. The metaanalysis demonstrated US therapy had a significant effect in decreasing ulcer surface area when compared with sham-irradiated controls. It was suggested, on the basis of the metaanalysis, that US had its best effect when delivered in "low doses" around the edge of the ulcer, but it was noted that further studies would be required to confirm this possible effect and to evaluate a possible dose–response relationship. The authors did not specify what they meant by a low dose. Of the six studies selected for inclusion, five used MHz US,[80,83–85] whereas the sixth used kHz US.[81] It should be noted that kHz US is more penetrative than MHz US, having the ability to pass through bone and metal, but it is less readily absorbed. The frequency of US used was not listed as a treatment variable in the metaanalysis. A statistically significant increase in the healing response, as demonstrated by a reduction in the surface area of the ulcers, was reported in four of the six studies. The authors of this chapter reviewed the two studies that found no significant effect with the following findings. The study of Lundeberg et al,[84] who used an unusual pulsing regimen (1:9), found no significant difference. The use of longer gaps between the pulses than were used in the other studies would reduce the temporal average intensity to 0.05 W/cm²; it is possible that such a low temporal intensity is below the level required to stimulate wound healing in chronic venous ulcers. Also, the study of Eriksson et al[19,86] failed to show statistically significant healing between controls and the US treatment group. Pulsed US was used, but pulsing ratio was not stated. The six studies are summarized in Table 25-2.

In a multicenter trial, Ennis et al[8] used the MIST therapy system to study the effects of US on wound healing . As stated earlier, MIST is a noncontact ultrasound device that has been approved by the Food and Drug Administration (FDA) for wound cleansing and debridement, and which has an expanded indication for "promoting wound healing."[8] (Figure 25-3) Like other US devices, electrical energy in the MIST system is transmitted to a piezoelectric transducer where it is changed into mechanical energy. The transducer operates at 40 kHz. The transducer horn vibrates longitudinally. The maximum transducer intensity delivered to the tissues through the applicator tip is 1.25 W/cm². The therapeutic intensity range is 0.1 to 0.5 W/cm². The sound waves are transferred to the tissue in a mist.

In Ennis' study, the duration of individual treatments was 4 minutes, delivered three times per week. Patients in the study all had diabetic foot ulcers. Patients who met the study's inclusion criteria were randomized into two matched groups, 27 in the treatment group, 28 in the control group. The total treatment period was up to 12 weeks or closure. Findings were that the MIST group had a 40.7% closure (epithelialization) rate compared to a 14.3% rate for the controls. Exudate diminished over time in the MIST group, but not among the controls. The use of US did not significantly decrease the number of sharp/surgical debridement events in the treatment group. Standard care was the same for both groups.

CLINICAL WISDOM

MIST and Pulsed Lavage with Suction

If a wound is grossly infected and the tissue is sloughy, definitely choose pulsed lavage with suction (PLWS) (see chapter 27). If the granulation tissue is poorly perfused, choose MIST because, although there appears to be an angiogenic effect with both, the MIST far exceeds the effect of the PLWS.

Teresa Conner-Kerr, personal communication, January 2006.

In an attempt to reproduce the results of the Pechen and Weichenthal studies, and to perform a clinical product evaluation, Johnson[87] treated 15 chronic venous ulcer patients with 30 kHz US, 100mW/cm², and reported the results of the uncontrolled clinical trial. Again a water bath heated to 32–34°C was used as the sound-conduction medium. Treatment was for 10 minutes, three times weekly over a 24 week period. All treated patients had reduction of wound size, exudate amount, and noticeable reduction in pain, with 50% achieving total healing. Clinical evaluation is an ideal way to apply and evaluate research results.

The body of evidence demonstrating the benefits of US for venous ulcer healing is slowly growing, but the trend is towards improved healing outcomes.[7] Clinical application to this patient population is warranted. Diabetic patients with foot ulcers appear to have potential benefit also, but the test group in the relevant study was so small that it is hard to generalize the results. What appears evident is that low-frequency US is a fresh approach with the potential to accelerate the healing process. At the time of this writing, the MIST device is the only low-frequency US device on the market in the United States with "promotes wound healing" as an indication.

TABLE 25-2 Protocols and Results of Studies Used in Metaanalysis[2xx2] of US Effects on Chronic Leg Ulcers[2]

Study Variable	Treatment	Roche and West[83]	Lundeberg et al[84]	Callam et al[85]	Dyson et al[80]	Ericksson et al[86]	Peschen et al[81]
Ulcer etiology		Venous	Venous	Venous predominately (94/108)	Venous	Venous	Venous
Method of randomization		Random allocate	Permuted blocks	Permuted blocks	Alternately	Alternately	Alternately
Number of subjects	Control	13	15	41 (15 dropouts)	12	13	12
	US	13	17	41 (11 dropouts)	13	12	12
Area treated		Periwound	Wound surface	Periwound	Periwound	Wound surface	Wound surface and periwound
Frequency of treatment		3 x/week	3 x/week	1 x/week	3 x/week	2 x/week	3 x/week
Frequency of device		3 MHz	1 MHz	1 MHz	3 MHz	1 MHz	30 kHz
Intensity		1.0 W/cm^2	0.5 W/cm^2	0.5 W/cm^2	1.0 W/cm^2	1.0 W/cm^2	100 mW/cm^2
Pulsed or continuous/duty cycle		1:4	1:9	Pulsed	1:5	Not stated	Continuous
Time		5–10 min	10 min	1 min/probe head area	5–10 min	Max 10 min	10 min
% Healing Results							
4 weeks	Control	↓ 28% SD 27.3	↓ 19 SD 9 1 healed	↓ 30% SD 61.6 5 healed	↓ 7.4% SD 8.9	↓ 27 SD 12 1 healed	↓ 8 SD 20
	US	↓ 35% SD 21.9	↓ 24 SD 12 2 healed	↓ 48 SD 49.8 6 healed	↓ 34% SD 8.8	↓ 35 SD 14 2 healed	↓ 27 SD 24
8 weeks	Control	↓ 7% SD 36.7	↓ 47 SD 10 3 healed	↓ 60 SD 41.9 6 healed	Not reported after 4 weeks	↓ 52 SD 13 4 healed	↓ 20 SD 24
	US	↓ 35.3 SD 30.1 # healed ulcers not reported	↓ 53 SD 8 5 healed	↓ 80 SD 24.6 14 healed	# healed ulcers not reported	↓ 68 SD 9 5 healed	↓ 40 SD 23 # healed ulcers not reported

Data from references listed in table.

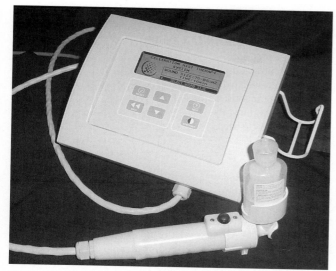

FIGURE 25-3 Noncontact Ultrasound MIST Therapy System. (Courtesy of Celleration, Eden Prairie, MN.)

RESEARCH WISDOM

Analysis of an air sample following use of the Non-contact Ultrasound MIST Therapy System showed no detectable production of aerosolized *P aeruginosa*. Protective clothing is therefore not required during treatment application. Penetration of the acoustic wave was at least 1 mm below the surface on agar plate. The surface temperature of agar-plated sample decreased by 1.9°C with 60 ml MIST.[64]

Scar. Ward et al[88] evaluated the therapeutic effects of US on scar contracture after burn injury, as well as the effect of standard burn physical therapy Consisting of stretching. Elongation of collagen tissue following a combination of stretching and heat has been reported to be greater than stretching alone. Therefore, the study investigators wanted to determine whether topical US would help patients with burns to progress to healed scar tissue. Joint range of motion and pain were the study variables chosen. The joints to be treated were randomized, and the patients and therapists were blinded to the treatment group. All treatments were performed every other day over a 2-week period with continuous US, 1 MHz, at 1 W/cm². Analysis of the data revealed no statistically significant differences in the two groups in either pain perception or joint range of motion. The lack of significance may be due to the fact that US has been demonstrated to be most effective during the inflammatory phase of healing, before scar formation is established, and to affect scar formation at that time by accelerating the healing response and the deposition and organization of the collagen. It is unlikely that US will be useful for healed scars.

TABLE 25-3 Intensity Levels for Therapeutic Ultrasound[1]

Intensity Levels	Range	Area
Low	< 0.3	W/cm²
Medium	0.3–1.2	W/cm²
High	> 1.2–3.0	W/cm²

Summary

The prior section of this chapter evaluates the efficacy of US. To summarize, the extant studies looked at seven important physiologic effects of US therapy that the healthcare professional should consider when selecting US intervention. Ultrasound has the following effects:

- It affects all phases of wound recovery at the cellular level if applied during the inflammatory phase.
- It accelerates the rate of progression through the phases of repair.
- It affects different tissue types differently, according to the tissues' ability to absorb energy. More tissue absorption requires lower-intensity application.
- It promotes absorption of hemorrhagic materials.
- It increases circulation and $tcPO_2$ if the patient is well hydrated and oxygenated.
* It is useful for the debridement of necrotic tissue and removal of biofilms.
- It enables noninvasive, nontraumatic treatment of either deep or superficial tissue, depending on frequency.

Following is a summary of three mechanisms of action by which US interacts with biologic tissue.[88] Absorption of sonic energy produces increased tissue temperature, followed by increase blood flow with high frequency US.

1. Mechanical vibration alters the tissue at the cellular or tissue levels.
2. The most important effect of US is cavitation, which has the ability to alter the cell membrane and noncellular structures.
3. Cavitation occurs most easily at lower frequencies.

Information about the effects of US on wound healing is less clear because of the limited number of clinical trials, the different parameters used for each study, the small sample sizes, and perhaps because the intervention was not appropriately applied. For example, it was applied to chronic wounds at intensities that would not restart the inflammatory phase of healing, leading to progression through the phases of repair. One study included two interventions, US and UVC, with good outcomes. Two studies included subjects who had pressure ulcers, whereas six studies included patients with chronic leg ulcers. The biologic effects described are independent of the wound etiology. The pressure ulcers ranged from partial-thickness to full-thickness, extending to tissue involvement at the level of muscle. The two types of wounds heal by way of different mechanisms, partial-thickness ulcers by reepithelialization, deep ulcers by contraction. The results for infected ulcers were better than those for clean ulcers. Infected ulcers are usually in an inflammatory phase of healing, which is when US is known to be most effective. Would a different protocol be better for a different phase of healing, and would that affect the outcome? More evaluation of the dosimetry parameters on the efficacy of US is still required. In the meantime, US may be the treatment of choice for some patients. Two examples are described in the case studies at the end of this chapter.

Choosing an Intervention: Clinical Reasoning

Candidacy for the Intervention

With any interactive treatment, the benefit to the patient must outweigh any possible risk. The physical therapist must, therefore, be able to assess both benefit and risk. The potential benefits have been described above. Knowledge of the mechanisms by which US interacts with tissue aids the PT in risk assessment. There is a long list of contraindications in the literature, and the excellent safety record of US owes much to the constraints on treatment that these have engendered (Exhibit 25-2). However, not all contraindications listed have been verified experimentally,[38] and it is possible that some patients who could have benefited from US treatment have been denied it. To ensure continued safe use, basic precautions must be considered (Exhibit 25-3).

Basic precautions start with the selection of the right candidate for treatment. A patient's medical history, the onset date, an injury's location and depth, and the size of the area to be treated will all guide the PT in deciding whether to use US. For example, one should review the medical history for information about the circulatory system. Information should be sought out concerning arteriosclerotic vessels, ischemia, and occlusion from reports

---

EXHIBIT 25-3   Precautions for Use of US[38]

> **EXERCISE CAUTION IN USE OF US**
> In acute infections
> Over subcutaneous bony prominences
> Over epiphyseal plates
> Over subcutaneous major nerves
> Over the cranium
> Over anesthetic areas

of vascular studies, or a noninvasive vascular examination planned. Ultrasound is not recommended over deep vein thrombosis or thrombophlebitis because of the risk of dislodging thrombi. Likewise, hemophiliacs should not be treated with US because of the risk of disturbing clot formation (thrombolysis). This should also be considered a precaution at the least, if not a contraindication, for patients on anticoagulant medications. Information about diabetes mellitus, type I or type II, should be sought out as well. Patients with type I diabetes are likely to have vascular and sensory impairments. Diabetes is an impairment to the repair process, and slower healing should be expected.

Ultrasound should be used in the pulsed mode over areas of poor circulation. A patient with loss of sensation due to a variety of pathologic causes (e.g., spinal cord injury or alcoholic neuropathy; see Chapter 18 for a more complete list) is not a candidate for thermal US. Treatment over anesthetic areas is a risk because malfunction of the equipment could lead to exposure to intensities that would normally induce pain and be indicative of tissue damage. The insensate patient will not be able to indicate pain during the treatment; therefore, pulsed low-dose US should be used for those cases.

If a patient has a history of spinal laminectomy, one should not treat with US over that area, because of the as-yet undetermined but potentially harmful effects on the spinal cord. A history of malignant or precancerous lesions or tumors in the area to be treated would be a contraindication, because therapeutic levels of US could stimulate cellular proliferation.[89] Injuries around the eye should *not* be treated with US because the sensitive retina may be affected.

Refrain from treating over the uterus during pregnancy to ensure that an embryo or fetus is not exposed to the intensities used in therapeutic US, which are higher than those used diagnostically. Do not treat over the gonads. Metal implants, including foreign objects, are often described in a medical history or directly by the patient, and only kHz US should be used over metal implants—although it is listed by kHz manufacturers as a contraindication. Clearly, more investigation is warranted so that the proper caveats are used when determining patient candidacy. In all cases, consider whether US therapy is indicated only after a thorough review. If in doubt, do not irradiate.

EXHIBIT 25-2   Contraindications for US[4,38]

> **DO NOT USE US**
> Over the uterus during pregnancy
> Over the gonads
> Over malignancies and precancerous lesions
> Over tissues previously treated with deep X-ray or irradiation
> On patients with vascular abnormalities
>   Deep vein thrombosis
>   Emboli
>   Severe atherosclerosis
> Over the cardiac area in advanced heart disease
> Over the eye
> Over the stellate ganglion
> For hemophiliacs not covered by factor replacement
> Over the spinal cord after laminectomy

Procedures

Protocol Considerations

High-Frequency (MHz) Treatment

Review the history for onset of the wound and prior treatment interventions. This will determine both the patient's candidacy and the appropriate treatment parameters. If the wound is acute, make use of the nonthermal effects of US. If chronic, consider a single upper-medium-intensity treatment and subsequent treatment at lower intensity. If the wound is located over a bony prominence, the PT must consider a method of sonation that will avoid increasing periosteal temperature. There are several ways to accomplish this objective: (1) select a high frequency (3 MHz), which is absorbed primarily in the more superficial tissues; (2) move the treatment head continuously to avoid standing waves; (3) treat through water for a more uniform far field; (4) for deeper wounds, select a lower frequency (1 MHz); (5) use pulsed mode. If the local circulation is poor, use pulsed US to avoid excessive heating because it will take longer for heat to be dissipated from the area. Assess the size of the area to be treated. Use this assessment to determine the duration of the treatment and the size of the applicator to select. Note that an applicator with a larger ERA will allow treatment of a large wound more rapidly than if an applicator with a smaller ERA is used. Small applicators, however, are very useful for being more selective in treating specific tissues. Select the coupling medium based on whether the skin is intact or broken (coupling media are described later). For acute conditions, the beam's intensity should be at the upper end of the low range; for chronic conditions, the middle range (see below). The anatomic location of the wound is a very important consideration when using US. For example, be aware of the location of major subcutaneous nerves, which absorb US energy very well and can become overheated. When treating young people, take into account epiphyseal plates, the growth of which may not be complete. This varies with the bone and sex, and there are racial differences as well.

To ensure the safe use of all frequencies of therapeutic US, the following basic precautions are recommended:

- Use US only if adequately trained to do so.
- Use US only to treat patients with conditions known to respond favorably to US therapy, unless it is being used experimentally with the understanding and approval of the patient, his or her medical advisors, and the local medical ethics committee or internal review board.
- Use the lowest intensity that produces the required effect, because higher intensities may be damaging. Burns, for example, occur when the intensity is too high or the frequency is low, and when the treatment head is not moved continuously or is moved too slowly.
- Move the applicator constantly throughout treatment to avoid the damaging effects of standing waves and, when treating in the nonuniform near field, of high intensity regions.
- Make sure that there is adequate coupling media and that it is free of air bubbles.
- Make sure that the equipment is calibrated regularly. A crystal may be broken, for instance, if the applicator head is dropped. Staff must report such incidents so that the applicator head can be tested before reuse. A faulty piece of equipment can result in inadequate treatment for the patient, or can produce shear waves and standing waves that can cause burns or other harmful effects.[38]

Expected Outcomes

Ultrasound is most effective when treating in the acute inflammatory phase of healing. During this phase, expect an acceleration of the inflammatory phase and early progression to the proliferative and epithelialization phases of healing (Exhibit 25-4). In chronic wounds, the first treatment outcome with MHz will be increased perfusion, observed as warmth, edema, and darkening of tissue color compared with adjacent skin color tones (Exhibit 25-5). In necrotic wounds, expect to see autolysis of the necrotic tissue; the outcome will be a clean wound bed. Wounds in two clinical trials progressed to closure in a mean time of 4–6 weeks.[76,77] Closure times could be longer for patients with intrinsic and extrinsic factors that limit healing. Published research is a valuable guide to the clinician in prediction of outcomes, but it must be supported by the experience of the program where the treatment is used.

Reassessment should confirm the predicted outcomes. If the wound does not change phase and/or reduce the size of surface area or overall size estimate within 2–4 weeks, the treatment regimen must change. There are several changes to US treatment to consider: enhance the inflammatory

---

EXHIBIT 25-4   Outcomes: Acute Wound

Wound healing phase diagnosis: acute inflammatory phase
Expected outcome:
    Skin color: change to that of surrounding skin
    Temperature: change to that of adjacent tissues or
      same area on corresponding opposite side of the body
    Edema free
    Necrosis free
    Wound progressed to proliferative phase

EXHIBIT 25-5   Outcomes: Chronic Wound

Wound healing phase diagnosis: chronic inflammatory phase
Expected outcome:
    Hyperemia: change in skin color to reddish blue or
      purplish, depending on color of surrounding skin
    Temperature: increased temperature of tissue, due to
      enhanced perfusion
    Edema: hardness, tightness, and shiny skin
    Wound progressed to proliferative phase

phase or restart it with the protocol for chronic wounds; change the frequency of the transducer; use a different size transducer for better ERA, or increase the treatment time; or recalculate the area if the wound has been debrided and become larger as a result.

Typical Protocol

Acute Wounds

Onset. Begin as soon as possible, ideally within a few hours of injury, but always during the inflammatory phase of healing. As mentioned previously, treatment with MHz US during this phase has been shown to result in the liberation of stimulatory growth factors from platelets, mast cells, and macrophages, with the result that the inflammatory phase is accelerated, the proliferative and remodeling phases occur earlier, and the scar tissue becomes stronger. (Exhibit 25-6) If treatment is delayed beyond the inflammatory phase, the strength of the scar tissue is not affected.[39]

Duration. Duration is usually based empirically on the surface area to be treated. The area is divided into zones, each 1.5 times the area of the ERA of the applicator, with 1–2 minutes being allowed for treating each zone. Some PTs recommend 1 min/cm². For the sake of the therapist, the maximum treatment time should be no longer than 15 minutes. If the wound is large, two sessions per day, one for each section of the wound, would be preferable. Three treatments per week have been found to be effective.

Intensity. In the interest of safety, the lowest possible intensity should be used. This is usually near the upper end of the low range (see Table 24-4). Note that, to obtain a significant increase in temperature, an I(SATA) of at least 0.5 W/cm² is required, but that primarily nonthermal effects can be achieved with lower SATA intensities, obtained by pulsing I(SATP) 0.5 W/cm² at, for example, 2 msec on, 8 msec off. Treatments should be pulsed if the local circulation is compromised and might be unable to dissipate heat efficiently.

Chronic Wounds

Onset. Begin as soon as possible.
Duration. Duration is the same as for acute wounds.
Intensity. Generally an I(SATA) at approximately the middle of the medium range is recommended (e.g., 0.5–1.0 W/cm² SA, TP). Pulsing should be used. Repair can be initiated by using *one* treatment at the upper end of the medium range (e.g., 1.2 W/cm²), after which lower intensities in the

medium range are used, as described above. It has been suggested that the higher intensity may produce local trauma, followed by acute inflammation, which is necessary to initiate healing in any postnatal wound. Note that this is a hypothesis that requires testing.

Frequency Selection

The PT should consider the following when selecting a frequency for treatment:

- If the lesion is superficial, a higher frequency is appropriate because high-frequency US is absorbed superficially.
- Although it is not readily available in many clinics, kHz US is another frequency in use in select wound care centers. The primary difference between kHz and MHz US is that kHz US is less attenuated, being less readily absorbed than MHz, and is readily transmitted through metal implants and bone; however, sufficient absorption occurs to produce a stimulatory effect.
- High frequencies (more than 1 MHz) are more appropriate than lower frequencies if thermal changes are required in the tissues.
- Lower frequencies (1 MHz or kHz) are more appropriate if primarily nonthermal effects, such as stable cavitation and/or microstreaming, are required. Equipment now on the market allows more flexibility to choose US frequencies and provides additional choices for the PT. The PT must know what each frequency is best suited to treat.

Coupling Media

Megahertz US requires a coupling medium that displaces air. This is essential because MHz US is reflected from air/water or air/tissue interfaces. The greater the difference in *acoustic impedance* (z) between the two materials forming the interface, the greater the amount of energy is reflected. The acoustic impedance of a medium is the product of its density (p) and the velocity of US through it (c). With MHz US, only a 0.2% reflection occurs at the interface between soft tissue and water, more than 50% between soft tissue and bone, and virtually complete reflection (99.9%) between soft tissue and air. Reflection reduces the amount of energy reaching the target tissues; if this falls below the stimulatory threshold (approximately 0.1 W/cm² I [SATA]), US will be ineffective. The ideal coupling medium would:

- have the same acoustic impedance as skin
- also act as a wound dressing
- be sterile, thixotropic, nonstaining, nonirritant, and chemically inert
- have slow absorption and evaporation rates
- be free from gas bubbles and other inclusions
- not break down when the US energy is transmitted through it
- be inexpensive

Hydrogel sheet and transparent film dressings are commonly used by PT clinicians for treatment of full- and par-

---

EXHIBIT 25-6 **Nonthermal US Protocol: Acute Inflammatory Phase**

Frequency	1 or 3 MHz
Pulsed duty cycle	20%–50%
Intensity	0.1–0.2 W/cm² (SATA)
Treatment frequency	3 times per week
Time	1 min/cm², max 15 min total

TABLE 25-4   Wound Dressing MHz US Transmission Rates

Dressing Product	US Transmission Rate
Hydrogels	
Nu-Gel	77.2% (±4.6%)
ClearSite	72% (±2.2%)
Aquasorb Border	45.3% (±2.1%)
CarraDress	42.8% (±5.9%)
Film Dressings	
CarraSmart Film	60.5% (±4.4%)
J & J Bioclusive	53.2% (±2.4%)
Tegaderm	47.1% (±2.3%)
Opsite Flexigrid	31.5% (±4%)

Reprinted with permission from Klucinec, B., et al., Effectiveness of Wound Care Products in the Transmission of Acoustic Energy, *Physical Therapy*, Vol. 80, No. 5, pp. 469–76, © 2000, with permission of the American Physical Therapy Association.

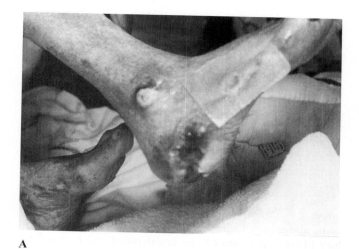

A

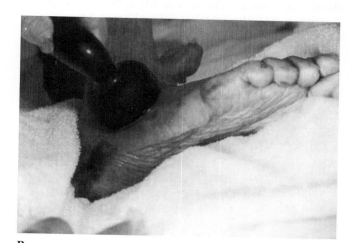

B

FIGURE 25-4 A and B. Application of MHz US through a Hydroscan.

tial-thickness wounds, and many US treatments are performed over these dressings. The ability of wound care dressings to transmit US affects the efficacy, efficiency, and cost of US treatment. A study of wound care products identified four sheet hydrogels and four transparent film dressings with different transmission rates.[90] Intensities from 0.2 to 2.0 W/cm^2 were tested at a frequency of 3.3 MHz. Ultrasound transmission gel was used on the skin and on top of the dressing to remove air. Plastic sheets that could have interfered with the sound energy transmission were removed from the tops and bottoms of the hydrogel sheets. Findings are listed in Table 25-4 and should help guide the clinician in selecting the dressing that will optimize treatment effects. For quick reference, sources for the dressing products are found in Appendix A at the end of this book.

Suitable coupling media that displace air and that can be used along the wound perimeter include commercially available US-transmitting gel, and over-the-wound, sterile, transparent, US-transmitting wound dressings with a high water content, e.g., Geliperm (Geistlich Sons Ltd., Newton Bank, UK) and Hydroscan (Echo Ultrasound, Reedsville, PA).Hydroscan (Figure 25-4A, B) is not labeled for use as a dressing, but is used for diagnostic US transmission and is an excellent transmitter of US energy, as long as there are no bubbles of air. (N. Byl, personal communication, 1994) Geliperm is available in Europe but not in the United States at this time.

Tegaderm, which was used in another study, was tested for transmission of US energy and found to transmit 40% of the acoustic energy.[73] Tests of the results of US stimulation on tcPO$_2$ measurements when energy was transmitted through Tegaderm showed no significant differences in the measurements, with or without the Tegaderm.[47] Tegaderm and similar transparent film dressings are useful for treating full-thickness wounds because the film will stretch down into the wound bed under the pressure of the US head. Make sure that the size of the film dressing is larger than the wound, so that the stress of the stretching doesn't pull the

adhesive away from the skin. Using US transmission gel on the surface of the film makes gliding of the head easier.

The method of using hydrogel sheets for transmission is as follows:

1. Place the dressing over the superficial-to-full thickness open area, ensuring that no air is trapped beneath the dressing.
2. Coat the surface of the dressing lightly with US transmission gel or lotion to ease the movement of the applicator head over the dressing surface.

Underwater application is a useful method for transmission of US. A metal whirlpool tank is a poor choice to hold the water because the metal reflects sound energy and increases the intensity in the body area near the metal. A plastic or rubber basin or tub would be acceptable. Air bubbles need to be eliminated by running the water and letting it stand for a few minutes before using it for US transmission. Underwater application is a good choice if the region to be treated is irregular and can be conveniently placed in the container. This includes the foot, ankle, hand, and elbow. Infection control requires proper disinfection of the water basin between uses. The applicator and the body part must be submerged throughout the treatment, and the applicator should not touch the skin. This would be advantageous if the area of treatment is painful. If possible, select a large container, such as a baby's plastic bathtub, where the target tissues can be placed a significant distance from the applicator. At that distance, the target tissues will be in the far field, where the spatial intensity is more uniform. It is recommended that the PT wear waterproof gloves that trap US reflecting air, so as to minimize exposure to the sound energy. In Europe, US at the kHz frequency is often delivered via a water bath so that the wound can be cleaned and debrided by it. Kilohertz US applied in a water bath stimulates the healing of chronic venous ulcers[81] and facilitates the debridement of bacteria- and particulate-contaminated wounds.[88,91]

Manipulation of the Applicator

Movement of the MHz applicator throughout treatment is essential to avoid exposing tissue to regions of high intensity. In the near field, where most treatments occur, the spatial peak intensity can be more than three times the SA. It is also essential to avoid excessive exposure to the peaks of pressure variation that occur in *standing wave fields* produced by the interaction of incident and reflected waves of US. Standing waves can damage tissue components, endothelial cells in particular, and exposure to them must, therefore, be avoided. The applicator should be moved either in short linear strokes a few centimeters long, ensuring that they overlap, so that the entire region is treated, or in small circular movements, also overlapping, so that the movement is essentially spiral.

Setup for Treatment

1. Explain the procedure to the patient and the caregiver.
2. Place the patient in a comfortable position that can be maintained for up to 15 minutes
3. Remove clothing from the area to be treated.
4. Warm US gel by placing it in a warmer or between folds of a hot pack—always test a drop for temperature before applying to the patient.
5. Remove the wound dressing, unless it is a film or hydrogel sheet that is to be left in place. Check for bubbles under the dressing and bleed them from the edges, if present.
6. Use either as a periwound treatment or direct application over a film or hydrogel sheet, as described above.
7. Treat deep wounds by a periwound application around the margins of the wound.
8. Keep the sound head perpendicular to the surface in complete contact with the surface area throughout the treatment.(See Figure 25-5.)

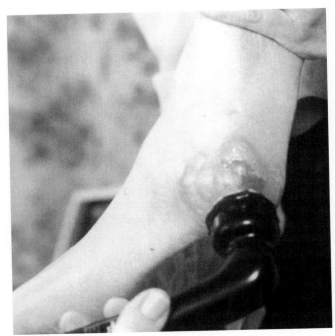

FIGURE 25-5 Periblister application of US gel.

CLINICAL WISDOM

Use US for Blisters

Treating blisters with US promotes absorption of the hemorrhagic material beneath the blister and healing of superficial and partial-thickness wounds. Absorption of hemorrhagic material may be due to enhanced macrophage activity via acoustic streaming and/or stable cavitation effecting thrombolysis. Use the protocol for acute inflammation and apply as a periwound application or in a water bath. Continue after the blister roof is removed as long as hemorrhagic material is absorbed. Hemorrhagic material should shrink in size daily; when it is no longer shrinking, it has probably necrosed and will need to be debrided. Color plates 79–82 and Case Study 2 illustrate a case in which US was the only treatment intervention, aside from a transparent film dressing, until it was determined that the focal area of necrosis needed debridement.

CLINICAL WISDOM

Sonation of Undermined/Tunneled Areas

One MHz US is a very useful means to treat undermined/tunneled areas surrounding wounds. These areas can be "mapped" on the skin surface with a marker pen (see Chapter 5 for more information about measuring undermining and tunneled areas) to guide the treatment. Imagine the wound with a grid over the area, or use a plastic screen with cm markings and divide the wound into quarters at the 12:00, 3:00, 6:00, and 9:00 positions. Depending on the size of the applicator, sonicate at the rate of 1 min/cm². For example, a 5 cm² applicator would be used to stimulate a 25 cm² wound area for 5 minutes. Undermined/tunneled regions can be visualized in high resolution US B-scans.

Aftercare

If the dressing is left intact, all that is required is to clean off excess US transmission gel/lotion. If a new dressing is to be applied, this should be done as soon as possible to avoid chilling of the wound tissues and slowing of epithelial migration and mitotic cell activity.

The US applicator must be handled carefully after use to avoid environmental contamination. After use, place the applicator in a rubber glove and transport it to a dirty sink area for cleansing with cold tap water and soap. Then place it in a cold disinfecting solution for the specified time, depending on the product used. This is usually from 5 to 20 minutes. It is useful to have two applicators, so that one can be used while the other is being disinfected, thus reducing down time.

Adjunctive Treatments

It is an essential part of clinical decision making to consider adjunctive treatments that may be given. Ultrasound may be the primary physical agent or it may be an adjunctive treatment, along with another biophysical agent. For example, for a deep wound, HVPC may be the treatment for the wound bed and US the treatment for the undermined peri-wound area. If this is the case, do the HVPC treatment first and leave the packing in the wound bed to keep it warm and clean while the US treatment is given.

Ultrasound may be given as an adjunctive treatment to whirlpool, when the whirlpool is used to soften necrotic tissue and the US is used to stimulate at the cellular level. Do the whirlpool first, then any debridement; flush out debris and any topical agents that could possibly be sonophoresed through the skin by the US. Ultrasound should follow the whirlpool because cells are stimulated by US to release chemotactic agents; those chemicals should not be washed out of the wound. As in the Nussbaum[77] study, US can be alternated with UVC (see Chapter 24).

Wound care products are part of the treatment regimen also, and should be considered in the treatment planning. Will the dressing be part of the US treatment, as described above, or will the dressing be removed and replaced when the US treatment is given? Will the dressing be changed every other day? Can it be changed in conjunction with the US treatment to minimize disruption of the wound healing environment? PTs need to check with nurses about the application of topical agents, such as petrolatum or petrolatum-based products, which will interfere with US transmission. This is another example of the importance of collaboration between nurses and PTs in order to avoid conflicting treatment approaches and to improve utilization management of services for the patient.

Other adjunctive US treatments include wound cleansing with the MIST device and debridement with the Sonoca. Information about use of MIST can be obtained from Celleration (www.celleration.com) A clinical policy and application procedures for Sonoca developed and used by Verhage is provided below and used here with her permission.

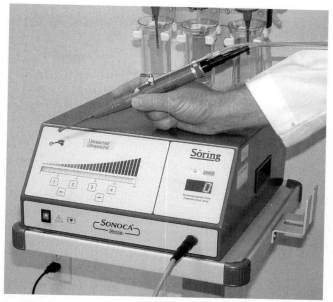

FIGURE 25-6 Söring Sonoca 180 ultrasonic wound debridement system. (Courtesy of Söring Inc., Ft. Worth, TX and Mary Verhage.)

Verhage Policy and Procedure for Use of the Sonoca 180 [92]

CLINICAL WISDOM

"The use of this modality for wound treatment is in its infancy and the 'pearls of wisdom' learned with repeated use are yet to be discovered."

Mary Verhage, personal communication, January 2006.

Purpose. To provide a method of wound debridement that produces optimal removal of nonviable tissue and enhances wound healing by stimulating the viable cell through the use of guided ultrasound. This policy will provide guidelines for ultrasonic assisted wound therapy and debridement with the Söring Sonoca 180. (Figure 25-6)

Policy.*

1. Ultrasonic-assisted wound therapy (UAW) is initiated by physician order including location to be treated and frequency of treatments (e.g. treatment of ulcer on right leg, PRN until necrotic tissue is removed).
2. Ultrasonic assisted wound therapy Söring Sonoca 180 treatment is only to be administered by trained, licensed providers; MD, PA, APNP, PT, and trained RN.
3. Wounds are considered contaminated, therefore UAW treatments are considered clean, not sterile. The only time UAW should be done using sterile technique is in the operating room when utilized prior to wound closure.

Policy and procedure are provided courtesy of Mary M. Verhage, RN, BSN, CWOCN. © Mary M. Verhage 2006.

4. The Söring Sonoca 180 user's manual is to be available for reference by the practitioner when the Sonoca is in use.

Equipment
- Söring Sonoca 180 and probe attachment (see Figure 25-6).
- Irrigation solution; 1000cc IV infusion bag of 0.9% NaCl, Ringer's lactate, or other premixed solution as ordered. Primary and secondary IV tubing with drip chamber.
- Personal Protective Equipment (PPE): gloves, fluid-resistant gown, face mask, eye protection, and shoe covers.
- Equipment protection: disposable plastic covers
- Disposable absorbent pads with impermeable layer
- Suction equipment
- Dressing change materials

Indications
- Locally infected wounds
- Wounds with impaired circulation
- Wounds with the need for debridement, irrigation, and topical treatment
- Pressure ulcers, diabetic foot ulcers, lower extremity diabetic ulcers, venous ulcers

Contraindications
- Untreated advancing cellulitis with signs of systemic response
- Wounds with metal components such as joint replacements, plates and screws, or implanted electronic devices within the treatment field
- Uncontrolled pain

Precautions
- The thermal effects of ultrasound are multiplied if the sound waves are allowed to reflect back up to the probe tip, creating a standing wave.
- Avoid putting the probe tip on intact skin without the fluid medium or it may create a burn
- The only irrigant that has been tested and approved for use with this device is 0.9% NaCL IV solution. Other potential choices such as antibiotics etc. have not been tested and could potentially induce harm.

Key Points/Information
- Physician to assess patient and wound status to determine wound treatment and write orders.
- Use the angled horseshoe-shaped probe for large flat surface areas or to wedge under the edge of thick necrotic tissue or eschar to lift and detach from viable tissue,
- Use double ball tip probe to treat tunnels, cavities, and undermining
- Use one standard irrigant, sterile 0.9% NaCl IV solution.
- Premedicate with systemic analgesic or local anesthetic e.g. lidocaine; use as directed prior to procedure, reassess pain frequently.
- Follow standard precautions include PPE for dripping, splashing, aerosolization of fluids.
- Follow infection control procedures if patient is in contact isolation for a resistant organism, follow precautions.

- Document predebridement wound condition; measure length, width, and depth; photograph.

Procedure
1. Obtain physician order as noted above.
2. Explain procedure to the patient.
3. Assess patient's comfort, current pain level, history of pain with debridement, and current analgesic regimen. Provide premedication for pain
4. Obtain appropriate Sonoca Sonotrode attachment from sterile processing.
5. Set up the Sonoca machine as illustrated in user's manual, hang irrigation solution, and prime IV tubing. Attach probe to ultrasound cable and tubing to probe.
6. Position patient, the wound, and the operator for comfort and accessibility.
7. Protect patient and clothing with absorbent pads (chux).
8. Provide adequate lighting.
9. Wash hands and apply PPE-gloves, mask, fluid resistant gown, eye protection, and shoe covers. Apply equipment-protective covering.
10. Prime ultrasound wand with irrigant, set drip rate and use to wet surface of the wound before the start of treatment. DO NOT OPERATE SONOCA WITHOUT IRRIGATION FLUID. In order for ultrasound waves to be transmitted, the probe tip must be in contact with fluid or moist wound. Fluid is also needed to dissipate heat.
11. Turn unit on and set intensity to begin treatment Activate ultrasound by depressing foot pedal.
    a. Start at low intensity and increase as patient tolerates. Power may be decreased to 20% or increased to 80% or 100% according to patient tolerance and tissue needs.
    b. Place probe in contact with wound bed/irrigant. Fluid placed on the wound bed will "bubble". This is not the same as boiling water. although heat will be produced. With probe in contact with fluid or wound bed, pass the probe tip with a slow continuous motion across the entire wound surface. DO NOT STOP IN ONE SPOT, sweep over and return for repeated treatment.
12. Continue the sweeping motion until treatment goals for the session are reached.
13. Treatment time: 20 seconds per cm^2 wound area
14. Limit the time of procedure to patient and clinician tolerance; discontinue if not tolerated due to pain, or when goals of treatment are achieved.
15. Turn off machine.
16. Gently wipe dry periwound tissue.
17. Assess patient condition and wound, measure and photograph as indicated.
18. Apply dressing or advanced therapy to wound as ordered.
19. Document procedure: location, treatment, dressing applied, intensity, duration, irrigation solution, patient tolerance, wound status after treatment. EXPECTED OUTCOME: Wound characteristics change with treatment

CLINICAL WISDOM

PRECAUTION: DO NOT TOUCH THE METAL TIP OF ANY OF THE LOW-FREQUENCY ULTRASONIC DEBRIDEMENT DEVICES MENTIONED HERE BECAUSE OF RISK OF BURNS.

Post-procedure

1. Remove equipment protection covering prior to moving it from area of use.
2. Wipe connector lines with facility-approved disinfectant.
3. Remove PPE and dispose of properly.
4. Have treatment room cleaned prior to next client use.
5. Remove Sonoca wand and probe tip.
6. Sterile process attachments per user's manual/facility recommendations

Color plates 76–77 show a venous ulcer before and after five minutes of debridement with Söring Sonoca 180.[70]

Self-Care Teaching Guidelines

Ultrasound should *not* be taught to a patient or a caregiver as a home treatment. Although it appears very innocuous, harm can be done by improperly trained and unsupervised individuals. To avoid harm, the many precautions listed earlier must be carefully considered. There are definite risks that are not readily apparent to the unskilled individual.

Documentation

The functional outcome report (FOR)[88] is an acceptable method to meet Medicare and other third-party payer guidelines for documentation of the need for physical therapy intervention for wound healing. The cases presented here are examples of how to use the FOR methodology. More information on the method is available in Chapter 1. Documentation of US treatment outcomes is extremely valuable. The cases documented below are examples of the value of recording on film those changes in wound healing that are produced by selected interventions. In both cases, US was the only intervention given. For example, it would be difficult to do a controlled, double-blind study of patients with new hematoma formation, as in Case Study 1. A single-subject design study would be one method of developing a body of knowledge about clinical outcomes. Case Study 2 was done as part of a student clinical affiliation project to determine how US affects hematoma formation under a blister. Photography was done every 2 days to track the change in the hematoma. There are many ways that the thoughtful clinician can present information about treatment interventions and advance clinical practice as part of the documentation process.

CASE STUDY 1

Venous Ulcer Treated with US

Patient: E.F.   Age: 82 years

FUNCTIONAL OUTCOME REPORT: INITIAL ASSESSMENT

Reason for Referral

The patient was referred to physical therapy for evaluation of ulceration of her left leg. The patient had a long history of Alzheimer's disease and was noncompliant with all attempts to keep the wound dressed. Nurses in the nursing home where she lived were concerned about infection and healing of the ulcer and wanted a physical therapist's opinion.

Medical History

The patient had a cardiac pacemaker and venous insufficiency. As a consequence of neurologic system changes associated with Alzheimer's disease, she was hyperactive and would not stay still for more than a couple of minutes at a time. Wound onset was 24 hours prior to referral.

Functional Diagnosis and Targeted Outcomes

Wound Examination   The wound is located above the left medial malleus. The surrounding skin is very friable, with extensive subcutaneous hemorrhaging and epidermal necrosis; petechiae surround the open area. There is mild edema, which is reactive to touching. The wound tissue is pink, with partial-thickness loss of the skin surface area

(see *Color Plate 76*).

Functional diagnosis   Impairment of the integumentary system; targeted outcome: wound closure; due date: 4 weeks.

Functional diagnosis   Impairment of the venous system (venous insufficiency); targeted outcome: absorption of hematoma; due date: 2 weeks.

Functional diagnosis   Acute inflammatory phase; targeted outcome: rapid wound contraction; due date: 4 weeks.

Psychosocial Examination   The patient removed dressings and would not tolerate any topical medications, compression stockings, or staying off her feet. She walked all day long and was very accomplished at removing passive restraints in a flash. She was totally noncompliant during the last episode of wounding.

Functional diagnosis   Impairment of mental functions. The functional loss causes undue susceptibility to venous ulceration of the legs and inability to heal without integumentary intervention. The patient has improvement potential and will heal after intervention, but she may continue to be at risk for venous ulceration.

Need for Skilled Services: The Therapy Problem

The patient has a history of recurrent ulceration above the left medial malleolus and impaired healing due to impairment

■ **CASE STUDY 1** *(Continued)*

of the venous system and impaired mental status. Ultrasound is indicated during the first 72 hours after injury during acute inflammation. Ultrasound would promote absorption of the hemorrhagic material and stimulate acceleration of the inflammatory phase, leading to rapid wound contraction.

TREATMENT PLAN

Periwound ultrasound will be applied at 1 MHz, at 0.5 W/cm^2 (SATP), 20% pulsed for 5 minutes five times per week for 4 weeks. The nurses will attempt to do a wound dressing with a transparent film as tolerated.

DISCHARGE OUTCOMES

Hemorrhagic material was significantly absorbed within 3 days. There was a change in wound shape and a reduction in size after 2 weeks. There was an 85% reduction in wound size at 4 weeks (see *Color Plates 67–69* for a pictorial review of the case).

DISCUSSION

Behavioral information as well as medical history were important considerations in choosing the intervention. From all perspectives, US was the most practical choice for this patient. However, because of her noncompliance with any other treatment, it was also an opportunity to evaluate the effects of the US. The absorption of the hemorrhagic material was unquestionable. The patient required constant engagement and diversionary activities by a physical therapy aide to tolerate the US by the physical therapist for even 5 minutes. By the end of 4 weeks she refused to comply further. Since the wound was closing, physical therapy was discontinued.

■ **CASE STUDY 2**

Blood Blister on the Heel Treated with US

Patient: M.M. Age: 83

FUNCTIONAL OUTCOME REPORT: INITIAL ASSESSMENT

Reason for Referral

The patient was referred to the physical therapist because the nursing staff had identified a blood blister on a heel.

Medical History

The patient had had a below-the-knee amputation on the other leg due to peripheral vascular disease. The limb was at risk for amputation, and early intervention was requested for limb salvage. Patient was alert/confused and nonambulatory. She could reposition but not consistently. She had had a prior episode of a cerebrovascular accident. The following medical problems are associated with this request for service.

Functional Diagnosis and Targeted Outcomes

Integumentary Examination   The surrounding skin was erythematous, edematous, and tender.

Functional diagnosis   Loss of function due to integumentary impairment; targeted outcome: accelerate the inflammatory response; due date: 2 weeks.

Wound Tissue Examination   The wound was covered with a bloody, fluid-filled blister. Bloody fluid suggests rupture of vessels beneath the blister.

Functional diagnosis   Wound in acute inflammatory phase; targeted outcome: debridement of blister, conservation of healthy tissue under the blister; due date: 2 weeks.

Associated impairment   Possibility of necrotic tissue beneath blister; targeted outcome: clean wound bed; due date: 4 weeks.

Functional diagnosis   Impairment of integument, depth to be determined; targeted outcome: exhibits granulation tissue; due date: 6 weeks.

Vascular Examination   Visual examination showed an inflammatory response to wounding. Palpation indicated weak but palpable pulses. Because of the prior vascular history, the presence of peripheral vascular disease was assumed.

Functional diagnosis   Vascular impairment; targeted outcome: enhanced perfusion; due date: 2 weeks.

Musculoskeletal Examination   The patient is nonambulatory, has limited mobility in bed, and needs verbal cues to reposition. Motor impairment from the stroke limits her mobility. Her Braden Risk Score is 15, indicating risk for pressure ulcers.

Functional diagnosis   Undue susceptibility to pressure ulceration; targeted outcome: pressure elimination; due date: immediately.

Evaluation

The patient's loss of function in these systems is responsible for the undue susceptibility to skin breakdown on the legs and inability to heal without integumentary intervention. The patient has improvement potential, and the wound will heal with intervention to bring perfusion to tissues and relieve pressure.

Need for Skilled Services

The patient has a prior history of failed wound healing leading to amputation. Intervention that will enhance wound tissue perfusion to conserve tissues underneath the blister and stimulate healing will be required. Wound dressings will not address these issues. The blister needs to be debrided to assess tissue damage. Absorption of hemorrhagic materials will conserve healthy tissues and result in a healed wound. Pulsed nonthermal US is the choice for tissue perfusion in the presence of peripheral vascular disease and for stimulation of macrophage activity to absorb clotted blood in the tissues.

TREATMENT PLAN

- Apply periwound nonthermal US to accelerate the inflammatory phase and promote absorption of hemorrhagic material (0.5 W/cm^2 [SATP] 1 MHz, 20% pulsed for 5 minutes).
- Sharply debride the blister roof.
- Continue US until the extent of the wound depth is determined.

OUTCOMES

Periwound US and debridement were begun on August 26. On August 31 the blister was debrided, and a large hemorrhagic/necrotic area was seen under the tissues; inflammation in the surrounding tissues was subsiding. On September 2, there was a 50% reduction in the size of the hemorrhagic area and resolution of the inflammation in the surrounding tissues. Minimal reduction in the area of the hematoma in next 2 weeks indicated that the tissues had necrosed and debridement had begun. On October 8 the wound was progressing to the proliferative phase; there was a small area of necrosis (see *Color Plates 79–82*). The US seemed to have had maximum benefit and treatment was changed to HVPC.

DISCUSSION

Removal of the blister roof identified an area of focal necrosis or hematoma. The only other treatment intervention was transparent film dressing. The size of the hematoma was reduced 50% with seven US treatments. Inflammation was accelerated, and the wound progressed to the proliferative phase. At this point treatment was changed to HVPC. Closure was achieved on November 2.

REVIEW QUESTIONS

1. Identify the physical properties of US with respect to frequency and intensity that affects its use for wound healing or diagnostic imaging.
2. Explain two physical effects of US that make it useful for wound healing.
3. What property of US makes it useful for thrombolysis?
4. Can US be used for bacteriacidal effects? How?
5. List 3 expected outcomes from an intervention with US.
6. What are the new uses for US technology?

REFERENCES

1. Gam AN, Johannsen F. Ultrasound therapy in musculoskeletal disorders: a meta-analysis. *Pain* 1995;63:85–91.
2. Johannsen F, Gam AN, Karsmark T. Ultrasound therapy in chronic leg ulceration: a meta-analysis. *Wound Repair Regen* 1998;6:121–126.
3. Falconer J, Hayes KW, Chang RW. Therapeutic ultrasound in the treatment of musculoskeletal conditions. *Arthritis Care Res* 1990;3(2):85–90.
4. Sackett D. Rules of evidence and clinical recommendations on the use of antithrombotic agents. *Chest* 1989;95(2):2s–4s.
5. Bergstrom N, Allman RM, Alvarez OM, et al. Clinical Practice Guideline: Treatment of Pressure Ulcers. U.S. Department of Health and Human Services (DHHS), Public Health Service (PHS) Agency for Health Care Research and Quality (AHRQ), formerly known as the Agency for Health Care Policy and Research (AHCPR). Rockville MD: AHRQ;. 1994.
6. Ovington LG. Dressings and adjunctive therapies: AHCPR guidelines revisited. *Ostomy Wound Manage* 1999;45(Suppl 1A):94s–106s.
7. Flemming K, Cullum N. Therapeutic ultrasound for venous leg ulcers (Review). *The Cochrane Database of Systematic Reviews.* 2000(4. Art.):No.: CD001180. DOI: 001110.001002/14651858.CD14001180.
8. Ennis WJ , Formann P, Mozen N, et al. Ultrasound therapy for recalcitrant diabetic foot ulcers: results of a randomized, double-blind, controlled, multicenter study. *Ostomy Wound Manage* 2005;51(8):24–39.
9. Misonex Inc. How Sonicators Work. Available at www.misonix.com. Last accessed January 6, 2006.
10. Stanisic MM, Provo BJ, Larson DL, Kloth LC. Wound debridement with 25 kHz ultrasound. *Adv Skin Wound Care* 2005;18(9):484–490.
11. Ziskin MC, Michlovitz SL. Therapeutic Ultrasound. In: Michlovitz SL, ed. Thermal Agents in Rehabilitation. Philadelphia: F.A. Davis, 1990.
12. Cameron MH. Ultrasound. In: Cameron MH, ed. Physical Agents in Rehabilitation. Philadelphia: WB Saunders, 1999.
13. Simpson SL, Hertzog MS, Barja RH. The plantaris tendon graft: an ultrasound study. *J Hand Surg* 1991;16:708–711.
14. O'Reilly MAR, Massouh H. Pictorial review: the sonographic diagnosis of pathology in the Achilles tendon. *Clin Radiol* 1993;48:202–206.
15. Karim A, Young SR, Lynch JA, Dyson M. A novel method of assessing skin ultrasound scans. *Wounds* 1994;6:9–15.
16. Gonzalez RC, Wintz P. Digital Image Processing. In: Gonzalez RC, Winter P, eds. Digital Image Fundamentals. Reading, MA: Addison-Wesley, 1987.
17. Bamber JC, Tristam M. The Physics of Medical Imaging. In: Webb S, ed. Diagnostic Ultrasound. Bristol, England: Adam Hilger, 1988.
18. Dyson M, Moodley S, Verjee L, et al. Wound healing assessment using 20 MHz ultrasound and photography. *Skin Res Technol* 2003;9:116–121.
19. Ebrecht M, Hextall J, Kirtley LG, et al. Perceived stress and cortisol levels predict speed of wound healing in healthy male adults. *Psychoneuroendocrinol* 2004;29:798–809.
20. Fornage BD, Deshayes JL. Ultrasound of normal skin. *J Clin Ultrasound* 1986;14:619.
21. Whiston RJ, Young SR, Lynch JA, et al. Application Of High Frequency Ultrasound To The Objective Assessment Of Healing Wounds. In: Proceedings of the Second Conference on Advances in Wound Management. London: Macmillan Press, 1992.
22. Young SR, Lynch JA, Leipins PJ, Dyson M. Ultrasound Imaging: A Non-Invasive Method Of Wound Assessment. In: Proceedings of the Second Conference on Advances in Wound Management. London: Macmillan Press, 1992.
23. Miller M, Dyson M. Principles of Wound Care. London: Macmillan Magazines Ltd., 1996.
24. Quintavalle PR. Getting a better view with high resolution ultrasound. *Podiatry Today.* 2002;15(10):30–36.
25. Liong JL. High Frequency Diagnostic Ultrasound as an Adjunct to Irritant Patch Assessment. Thesis. London: University of London UMDS, 1996.
26. Mertz P. Cost Analysis Of Utilizing High Frequency Ultrasound Technology To Manage Soft Tissue Injuries. Thesis. Kennedy-Western University, 2004.
27. Van Holsbeek M, Introcaso JH. Sonography of Muscle. In: Musculoskeletal Ultrasound. Chicago, IL: Mosby-Yearbook, 1990
28. Shafir R, Itzchak Y, Heyman Z, et al. Preoperative ultrasonic measurements of the thickness of cutaneous malignant melanoma. *J Ultrasound Med* 1984;3:205.
29. Breslow A. Thickness, cross-sectional areas and depth of invasion in the prognosis of cutaneous melanoma. *Ann Surg* 1970;172:902.
30. Graves D. Stage I pressure ulcer in ebony complexion. *Decubitus* 1990;3:4.

31. Bennett M. Report of the task force on the implications for darkly pigmented intact skin in the prediction and prevention of pressure ulcers. *Adv Wound Care* 1995;8:34–35.

32. Lyder C. Examining the inclusion of ethnic minorities in pressure ulcer prediction studies. *JWOCN* 1996;23:257–260.

33. Henderson C, Ayello C, Sussman C. Draft definition of stage I pressure ulcers: inclusion of person with darkly pigmented skin. *Adv Wound Care* 1997;10:34–35.

34. Dyson M, Lyder C. Wound Management With Physical Modalities. In: Morison M, ed. The Prevention and Treatment of Pressure Ulcers. Mosby 2001, Edinburgh.

35. Sussman C. Ultrasound for Wound Healing. Monograph. Houston: The Chattanooga Group. 1993.

36. Dyson M. Mechanisms involved in therapeutic ultrasound. *Physiother J Chartered Soc Physiother* 1987;73(3):8.

37. Dyson M, Young SR. Acceleration of tissue repair by low intensity ultrasound applied during the inflammatory phase. Presented at the meeting of American Physical Therapy Association and Canadian Physical Therapy Association; 1988. Toronto

38. Dyson M. Role Of Ultrasound In Wound Healing. In: McCulloch JM, Kloth LC, Feedar JA, eds. Wound Healing: Alternatives in Management. 2nd ed. Philadelphia: FA Davis, 1995.

39. Hart J. The Effect Of Therapeutic Ultrasound On Dermal Repair With Emphasis On Fibroblasts Activity. London: University of London, 1993.

40. Gillet JH, Mitchell JL. Acceleration of tissue repair of damaged skeletal muscle using ultrasound. *Orthop Prac* 1989;2(4):36.

41. Harding K. Wound Care: Putting Theory Into Clinical Practice. In: Krasner D, ed. Chronic Wound Care: A Clinical Source Book for Health Care Professionals. Wayne, PA: Health Management Publications, 1990.

42. Hardy MA. The biology of scar formation. *Phys Ther* 1989;69(12):1014–1023.

43. Frieder S, Weisberg J, Flemming B, Stanek A. The therapeutic effects of ultrasound following partial rupture of Achilles tendons in male rats. *J Orthop Sports Phys Ther* 1988;10:39–46.

44. Jackson BA, Schwane JA, Starcher BC. Effect of ultrasound therapy on the repair of Achilles tendon injuries in rats. *Med Sci Sports Exerc* 1991;23:171–176.

45. Consentino AB, Cross DL. Ultrasound effects on electroneuromyographic measures in sensory fibers of the median nerve. *Phys Ther* 1983;63:1788–1792.

46. Sibbald RG, Amstrong DG, Orstead HL. Pain in diabetic foot ulcers. *Ostomy Wound Manage* 2003;49(4A suppl):24–29.

47. Byl N, Hopf H. The Use Of Oxygen In Wound Healing. In: McCulloch J, Kloth L, Feedar JA, eds. Wound Healing: Alternatives in Management, 2nd ed. Philadelphia: FA Davis, 1996.

48. Knighton DR, Halliday B, Hunt TK, et al. Oxygen as an antibiotic: the effect of inspired oxygen on infection. *Arch Surg* 1984;119:199–204.

49. McDiarmid T, Burns P. Clinical applications of therapeutic ultrasound. *Physiother J Chartered Soc Physiother* 1987;73(4):14–21.

50. Luo H, Nishioka T, Fishbein MC, et al. Transcutaneous ultrasound augments lysis of arterial thrombi in vivo. *Circulation* 1996;94:775–778.

51. Hajri Z, Boukadoum M, Hamam H, Fontain R. An investigation of the physical forces leading to thrombosis disruption by cavitation. *Journal Thromb Thrombolysis* 2005;20(1):27–32.

52. Riggs PN, Francis CW, Bartos SR, Penney DP. Ultrasound enhancement of rabbit femoral artery thrombolysis. *Cardiovasc Surg* 1997;5(2):201–207.

53. Suchkova V, Carstensen EL, Francis CW. ultrasound enhancement of fibrinolysis at frequences of 27–100 kHz. *Ultrasound Med Biol* 2002;28(3):377–382.

54. Berna-Serna JD, Sanchez-Garre J, Madrigal M, et al. Ultrasound therapy in rectus sheath hematoma. *Phys Ther* 2005;85(4):352–357.

55. Parish CP. Decubitus ulcers: how to intervene effectively. *Drug Ther* 1983.

56. West BR, Nichter LS, Halpern DE, et al. Ultrasound debridement of trabeculated bone: effective and atraumatic. *Plast Reconstr Surg* 1994;93:561–566.

57. Breuing KH, Bayer L, Neuwalder J, Orgill DP. Early experience using low-frequency ultrtasound in chronic wounds. *Ann Plast Surg* 2005;55(2):183–187.

58. Schoenbach SF, Song IC. Ultrasonic debridement: a new approach in the treatment of burn wounds. *Plast Reconstr Surg* 1980;66:34.

59. Atland OD, Daleck D, Suchkova VN, Francis CW. Low-intensity ultrasound increases endothelial cell nitric oxide synthase activity and nitric oxide synthesis. *J Thromb Haemost* 2004;2:637–643.

60. Reher P, Harris M, Whitemea M, et al. Ultrasound stimulates nitric oxide and protaglandin E2 production by human osteoblasts. *Bone* 2002;31(1):236–241.

61. Witte M, Barbul A. General principles of wound healing. *Surg Clin North Am* 1997;77(3):509–528.

62. Dinno MA, Young SR, Mortimer AJ, et al. The significance of membrane changes in the safe and effective use of therapeutic and diagnostic ultrasound. *Phys Med Biol* 1989;34(11):1543–1552.

63. Kavros SJ, Wagner SA, Wennberg PW, Coclkerill FR. The effect of ultrasound mist therapy on common bacterial wound pathogens. Presented at the Symposium for Advance Wound Care, Baltimore, 2002.

64. Sullivan PK, Conner-Kerr T. Effectiveness of Non-Contact Mist Ultrasound Therapy (MUST) in Removal of *Pseudomonas aeruginosa* in vitro. Presented at the Symposium for Advanced Wound Care and Medical Research Forum on Wound Repair, Las Vegas 2001.

65. Niezgoda JA, Verhage MM, Walek D, Nelson KM. Clinical Experience Using Ultrasonic Assisted Wound Treatment. Presented at the Symposium for Advanced Wound Care, Las Vegas 2003.

66. Qian Z, Sagers RD, Pitt WG. The effect of ultrasonic frequency upon enhanced killing of P. aeruginosa biofilms. *Ann Biomed Eng* 1997;25:69–76.

67. Mitragotri S, Kost J. Low-frequency sonophoresis: a review. *Adv Drug Deliv Rev* 2004;56(5):589–601.

68. Mitragotri S, personal communication regarding sonophoresis of antibiotics, 2006.

69. Nicter LS, Williams J. Ultrasonic wound debridement. *J Hand Surg* 1988;13A(1):142–146.

70. Verhage MM, Niezgoda JA, Nelson KM, Walek D. Ultrasonic-Assisted Wound Tratment: A Novel Technique for Wound Debridement. Presented at the Symposium for Advanced Wound Care, Las Vegas, 2003.

71. Shamberger RC, Talbot TL., Tipton HW., et al. The effect of ultrasonic and thermal treatment on wounds. *Plast Reconstr Surg* 1981;68(6):860–869.

72. Cambier DC, Vanderstraeten GG. Failure of therapeutic ultrasound in healing burn injuries. *Burns* 1997;23(3):248–249.

73. Byl N, McKenze A, Wong T, et al. Incisional wound healing: a controlled study of low and high dose ultrasound. *Orthop Sports Phys Ther* 1993;18:619–628.

74. Taskan I, Ozyazgan I, Tercan M, et al. A comparative study of the effect of ultrasound and electrostimulation on wound healing in rats. *Plast Reconstr Surg* 1997;100(4):966–972.

75. Paul BJ, Lafrattta CW, Dawson RA, et al. Use of ultrasound in the treatment of pressure sores in patients with spinal cord injury. *Arch Phys Med Rehabil* 1960;41:438–440.

76. McDiarmid T, Burns P, Lewith GT, Machin D. Ultrasound and the treatment of pressure sores. *Physiotherapy* 1985;71(2):66–70.

77. Nussbaum EL, Biemann I, Mustard B. Comparison of ultrasound/ultraviolet C and laser for treatment of pressure ulcers in patients with spinal cord injury. *Phys Ther* 1994;74:812–825.

78. ter Riet G, Kessels AGH, Knipschild P. A randomized clinical trial of ultrasound in the treatment of pressure ulcers. *Phys Ther* 1996;76:1301–1312.

79. Thawer HA, Houghton PE, Keast DH, et al. A Pilot Study Examining the Effects of Ultrasound Mist Therapy (UMT) on the Size and Appearance of Chronic Pressure Ulcers. Presented at the Symposium for Advanced Wound Care, Baltimore, 2002.

80. Dyson M, Franks C, Suckling J. Stimulation of venous ulcers by ultrasound. *Ultrasonics* 1976;14:232–236.

81. Peschen M, Weichenthal M, Schopf E, Vanscheidt W. Low frequency ultrasound treatment of chronic venous leg ulcers in an outpatient therapy. *Acta Derm Venereol* 1997;77(4):311–314.

82. Weichenthal M, Mohr P, Stegman W, Breitbart EW. Low-frequency ultrasound treatment of chronic venous ulcers. *Wound Repair Regen* 1997;5:18–22.

83. Roche C, West J. A controlled trial investigating the effect of ultrasound on venous ulcers referred from general practitioners. *Physiotherapy* 1984;70(12):475–477.

84. Lundberg T, Nordstrom F, Brodda-Jansen G, Eriksson S, et al. Pulsed ultrasound does not improve healing of venous ulcers. *Scand J Rehabil Med* 1990;22(4):195–197.

85. Callam MJ, Harper DR, Dale JJ, et al. A controlled trial of weekly ultrasound therapy in chronic leg ulceration. *Lancet* 1987;2(8552):204–206.

86. Eriksson S, Lundberg T, Malm M. A placebo controlled trial of ultrasound therapy in chronic leg ulceration. *Scand J Rehabil Med* 1991;23(4):211–213.

87. Johnson S. Low-frequency ultrasound to manage chronic venous leg ulcers. *Br J Nursing* 2003;12(19 supp):s14–s24.
88. Ward RS, Hayes-Lundy C, Reddy R, et al. Evaluation of topical therapeutic ultrasound to improve response to physical therapy and lessen scar contracture after burn injury. *J Burn Care Rehabil* 1994;15(1):74–79.
89. Sicard-Rosenbaum L, Danoff JV, Guthrie JA, Eckhaus MA. Effects of energy-matched pulsed and continuous ultrasound on tumor growth in mice. *Phys Ther* 1998;78:271–277.
90. Klucinec B, Scheidler M, Denegar C, et al. Effectiveness of wound care products in the transmission of acoustic energy. *Phys Ther* 2000;80:469–476.
91. McDonald W, Nichter L. Debridement of bacterial and particulate contaminated wounds. *Ann Plast Surg* 1994;33(2):142–147.
92. Verhage, MM, Policy and Procedure for use of Sonica 180™, Personal Communication, Milwaukee WI January 2006

CHAPTER OBJECTIVES

At the completion of this chapter, the reader will be able to:
1. Grasp the physical principles and physiological effects of heating on body systems.
2. Present evidence of the putative effects of whirlpool for wound management.
3. Identify the candidacy of patients, the risks, benefits and disadvantages of whirlpool.
4. Apply best methods of using whirlpool that provide safe and effective wound treatment.

Hydrotherapy and use of warmth for wound healing is reported in the literature back to ancient times. In current physical medicine practice, whirlpool is often the hydrotherapy method selected. The rationale for selecting whirlpool to treat wounds includes its putative effects of:

1. Thermal effects
   - To increase local tissue perfusion to transport oxygen and nutrients to the tissues and remove waste products
   - To stimulate cellular activities for regeneration to facilitate neuronal mechanisms of analgesia for pain relief and increased mobility
2. Mechanical debridement
   - To reduce wound contamination, bioburden and infection by softening and removing debris and exudate

The physical principles of heat transfer, the putative effects and the efficacy of whirlpool for wound management and safe and effective methods of application of whirlpool are discussed in detail in this chapter.

Evaluating the Evidence

Whirlpool, a form of hydrotherapy, has been a standard treatment for chronic wounds and burns for many years. In 1994, the Agency for Health Care Policy and Research, now known as the Agency for Health Care Research and Quality (AHRQ), panel considered the evidence and, based on an absence of clinical trials, recommended a level "C" grade for this therapy (refer to the book *Introduction for the AHCPR Evidence Grading System* [1]). The AHCPR recommendation was "to consider whirlpool treatment for pres-

sure ulcers that contain thick exudate, slough, or necrotic tissue and to discontinue whirlpool when the ulcer is clean."[1] Feedar and Kloth recommended twice-daily (BID) hydrotherapy for most necrotic wounds and daily hydrotherapy if used in conjunction with other methods, such as wet-to-dry dressings, to facilitate debridement of wounds with slough.[2] The author has reviewed published research evidence about hydrotherapy treatment for healing that is presented later in this chapter under clinical studies.

Physical Principles and Physiological Effects of Whirlpool Therapy

In this section, the physical principles and physiological response to heat , which are the underlying bases for whirlpool therapy, necessary to achieve treatment objectives will be presented.

Physical Principles
Thermal Effects

Thermal effects of whirlpool that are involved in the safe and appropriate application of whirlpool therapy are: heat transfer, thermal regulation, circulatory effects, cellular effects, neuronal effects and the effects of different temperatures. Each of these topics are discussed here.

Heat Transfer

The body's ability to transfer heat is dependent on four factors: the area of body surface immersed, the temperature of the water, the duration of the application, and the ability to dissipate internal heat and maintain proper core temperature. Heat is transferred from the water to the body by conduction and convection. Conduction is the exchange of thermal energy between two surfaces. If there is a temperature gradient, the heat will be transferred from the warmer to the cooler surface, for example, from the water to the body.[3] Body fat will lessen and slow the conduction of heat to the body core. At the same time, high body fat content reduces the body's ability to dissipate heat and can cause body core temperature to rise to a dangerously high level. Obese persons may not be candidates for immersion of a large body area in the whirlpool because they are unable to dissipate heat well, so other methods of treatment should be considered.[3]

Submerged skin does not transfer heat from the surface; therefore, heat dissipation is shifted to the exposed body areas that can sweat and to the lungs. The greater the body surface area immersed, the less transpiration can take place on the skin surface. Respiration and heart rates increase as temperature of the water increases, most likely due to enhanced requirements for skin blood flow,[4] resulting in dehydration and increased cardiac output. Individuals with cardiopulmonary impairments or peripheral vascular disease are at risk in this situation.

Convection is a transfer of heat that occurs when there is circulation of a fluid, such as when water flows over the skin.[3] Heating occurs more rapidly by convection than by conduction. Surface body heat warms venous blood that is then carried toward the core, thus potentially raising core body temperature. As with conduction, this method of heat transfer stresses the cardiopulmonary system and peripheral vascular system. Again, caution should be used when considering immersion of persons with impairments of those systems. Together, conduction and convection bring the heat into and out from the body core to the surface. Radiation transfers the heat from the body surface to the atmosphere but cannot take place from immersed body areas, limiting heat dissipation and increasing the risk of hyperthermia.[3]

Physiological Responses

Thermal Regulation

The human body thermoregulatory system is centrally controlled by the hypothalamus to maintain a core temperature of about 37°C (98.6°F). Because of the effectiveness of the thermoregulatory defenses, body temperature rarely deviates more than a few tenths of a degree. The range of core temperature that does not trigger thermoregulatory responses is termed the *interthreshold range*.[5] Information from the skin surface, deep abdominals, thoracic tissue, spinal cord, and nonhypothalamic portions of the brain, as well as the temperature of the hypothalamus itself, each contribute roughly 20% of the information used by the hypothalamus for thermoregulatory control. The range of temperatures that does not trigger any thermoregulatory responses is only 0.2°C. Autonomic thermoregulatory defenses are not triggered unless the body temperature moves out of this interthreshold range.

Under normal conditions, the body maintains a temperature gradient between the core and periphery of 2 to 4°C.[6] Both systemic and local tissue temperatures are of considerable importance. If the hypothalamus receives a signal from the skin that there is a rise in temperature, the response is sweating. If the signal from the skin is cold, the response would be vasoconstriction and shivering. The object is a redistribution of body heat from the core to the periphery. All thermoregulatory responses are neuronally mediated. Nerve blocks prevent the normal activation of thermoregulatory defenses, such as sweating, vasoconstriction, and shivering. Peripheral inhibition of thermoregulatory defenses is a major cause of hypothermia during regional anesthesia.[6] Spinal cord-injured individuals and those with peripheral neuropathy also have peripheral inhibition of thermoregulatory defenses and are at risk for both mild hypothermia and thermal injury from immersion.

Nineteen percent of 104 control group postsurgical patients who experienced mild hypothermia during surgery developed postsurgical wound infection.[7] Mild hypothermia impairs the oxidative killing by neutrophils and decreases cutaneous blood flow, which reduces tissue oxygen and contributes to decreased wound strength by reducing the deposition of collagen. Heating core body temperature to 37°C, normothermia, during surgery in an experimental study group of 96 patients was found to reduce significantly the incidence of postsurgical wound infection and to increase significantly collagen deposition near the wound.[7]

Mild hypothermia also reduces platelet function and increases coagulation time.[8] These inhibitory effects were found to be completely reversible by rewarming the blood to 37°C.[9,10] There is a linear relation near 20% between mean skin temperature and core temperatures at the vasoconstriction and shivering thresholds; however, there is individual variability.[11] This function is accomplished by the shunting of blood from the arterioles to the venules and venous plexuses located in the hands, feet, and face.

CLINICAL WISDOM

Monitor Temperature

Use a thermometer to record tympanic membrane temperature during whirlpool treatment to monitor for changes in core body temperature.

Circulatory Effects

Heat is used to increase blood flow to the tissues.[12,13] Infection rates of tissues are inversely proportional to blood flow, and oxygenation of tissues is totally dependent on perfusion.[14,15] Application of heat for 20 minutes produces an immediate increase in blood flow, but the increase in blood flow is greater in the post-treatment period, with peak blood flow was reached an average of 46 minutes after terminating the application of heat. Longer exposure of up to two hours had no real effect on increasing the peak rise.[12] Local heating can increase local perfusion an average of threefold and is the simplest and most effective way of enhancing blood flow and increasing subcutaneous oxygen tension that is sustained, even after the heat source is removed.[14,16]

Tissues are totally dependent on blood flow to meet metabolic demands of inflammation. Increased oxygen tension makes tissue more resistant to infection.[16] Decreased tissue oxygen tension impairs the deposition of collagen and oxidative killing by the neutrophils.[15] Three different temperatures (38, 42, and 46°C) were tested in healthy adults to determine effects on local subcutaneous oxygen. Results of 100% increase in blood flow and 50% increase in subcutaneous oxygen were comparable for all three temperature,[17] thus showing how local warming can influence local blood flow.

Methods of applying heat include general body heating, local heating, and indirect heating. General body heating can be used to raise core body temperature if there is mild core hypothermia but can overtax the system if the patient is febrile. Mild core hypothermia can impair immune functions by vasoconstriction-induced hypoxia. Vasoconstriction-induced tissue hypoxia can decrease the strength of the healing wound because the process of collagen deposition and cross-linkages between strands of collagen is dependent on oxygen tension.[7] Full-body immersion in a whirlpool at normothermia could be used as an active way to raise core body temperature, induce peripheral vasodilation, increase blood flow and oxygen tension, and accelerate healing.[18] Exposure of a large body area to heat will also have systemic effects on the cardiovascular, respiratory and other organ systems. Initially, there will be a rise in blood pressure, followed by a decrease as peripheral vasodilation occurs. At 40°C, mean cardiac output and oxygen consumption increase, but not significantly, after a 20-minute session. Heart rate increases 1.3–1.5 times over the sitting or supine resting level, and mean blood pressure increases 1.1 times over the supine resting values. Such effects can have significant physiological consequences in compromised systems and require careful consideration before selection of whirlpool intervention. Risks are discussed below.

Direct heating has a direct relationship with increasing both superficial and deep tissue temperatures.[3] In many but not all situations, localized direct heating may have more advantages than generalized direct or indirect heating. For instance, direct heating of an ischemic extremity presents risk of thermal injury due to the rapid increase of tissue temperature and lack of adequate blood supply to dissipate and remove the heat. Indirect heating has been shown to increase blood flow and pulse rate at a distant area.[13] Application of heat to an extremity with impaired sensation likewise presents risk of burns because of lack of sympathetic nervous system input to mediate vasodilation needed to dissipate and remove the heat and/or lack of sensory input to warn of overheating[19] (Figure 26-1). Immersion of one upper extremity to produce indirect heating can be a useful way of applying heat and producing generalized vasodilatation. This will cause increased perfusion to the lower extremities with minimal fluid shift and is an alternative ap-

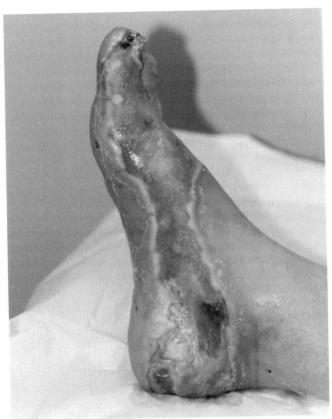

FIGURE 26-1 Burn resulting from putting neuropathic foot in hot water. (Copyright © Nancy Elftman)

proach that can be used to treat a wound in a patient with peripheral vascular disease or impaired lower extremity sensation. Since peripheral neuropath can also affect upper extremity euslante sensation before choosing this method. Indirect application of heat would also minimize exposure of an open wound to contamination and the risk of infection.

Indirect heating, also referred to as *reflex heating,* involves heating a distant body area. Local cutaneous thermoreceptors are stimulated by heat and carry impulses to the spinal cord and the thermoregulatory mechanisms of the hypothalamus. Core body temperature is also elevated when the lower body is warmed.[20] The warmed blood acts on constricted blood vessels of the skin, where a vasoactive mediator is released that stimulates vasodilatation. Vasodilation produces a mild inflammatory reaction through the release of histamine and prostaglandins. Bradykinin, a byproduct of an enzyme from sweat, is also released. Together, these chemical mediators enhance the permeability of the blood vessels. Increased blood flow following vasodilatation increases capillary hydrostatic pressure, producing fluid shift from the vessels into the interstitial spaces and resulting in mild edema and mild inflammation.[3] Mild inflammation can stimulate the biologic cascade of wound healing and restart healing.

Vasodilatation is a benefit for a patient with reduced perfusion, but it can be disastrous for a patient with venous insufficiency whose venous system has difficulty managing tissue fluids.[21] Fluid shifts also occur within the wound, with a loss of proteins, electrolytes, other nutrients, and growth factors found in wound fluid that pass out into the water. If the wound surface area is large, fluid shifts can lead to dehydration and depletion of nutrients needed for healing.[22] Use of saline instead of tap water will prevent loss of fluids. A saline whirlpool can be made by adding salt to the water. If fluid shift is of concern, perhaps another intervention would better meet the goals of treatment. Vasodilation is limited in the patient with calcified vessels and an ankle brachial index of >1.0 such as those with a history of diabetes mellitus. In this group the application of heat will at best have a muted response.

RESEARCH WISDOM

Whirlpool Implications for Venous Congestion

McCulloch and Boyd[21] reported that whirlpool treatment of a dependent leg resulted in increased hypotension and lower extremity vascular congestion, even in healthy individuals. The implications for the patient with a compromised venous system are very serious.

A further benefit of increased blood flow is improved delivery of oxygen, nutrients, antibodies, leukocytes, and systemic antibiotics to the tissues and removal of metabolites. In patients with comorbidities, such as diabetes, arterial occlusive disease, and limited mobility, there is a reduction of blood flow to the tissues. The impaired circulation compromises the effectiveness of antibiotics to control wound infection. Timing treatment to enhance perfusion and delivery of antibiotics to wound tissue is being tested with transcutaneous electrical stimulation.[23] Heat-induced perfusion in the whirlpool may be another way to enhance the delivery of antibiotic therapy. The physical therapists and nurses who administer the antibiotics should consider collaborating in scheduling whirlpool treatment time to coincide with optimal delivery of antibiotics circulating in the bloodstream to the tissues because it could enhance the benefits of both treatments. A clinical trial would test this hypothesis.

Cellular Effects

Studies on the effect of temperature on cells of tissue repair show contrasting results that may be cell specific. Warmth stimulates cell mitosis and enhances leukocytic activity. Research on pigs has shown experimentally that the speed of production of new epidermal cells is enhanced if the temperature is maintained at 37°C. Similar results have been reported following in vitro testing of human skin cultures. Leukocyte activity may fall to zero when wound temperature is cooled, such as during a dressing change. This will impair the phagocytic activity of the leukocytes.[24] It has been observed that it takes 40 minutes for a freshly cleaned wound to return to normal temperature and 3 hours for mitotic cell division to resume.[25,26]

Clotting factor activity is prolonged at temperatures below 35°C, resulting in decreased activation of the coagula-

tion cascade. More bleeding could be expected during debridement if a tepid whirlpool is used. Clotting function is restored with warming.[8] However, at 33°C, the proliferative capacity of endothelial cells was potentiated.[27] Fibroblasts treated with heat at 38°C have increased cell division and metabolic activity.[28] Chronic wound fluid is known to inhibit fibroblast activity. Heating of chronic wound fluid in a water bath showed that there was a temperature-dependent reduction in the inhibitory effect on fibroblasts. When the heated chronic wound fluid was added to fetal and adult fibroblasts, the fluid assisted in the growth of both fetal and adult fibroblasts.[29] Heating of wound fluid during whirlpool treatment may have a significant effect on restarting the growth of fibroblasts in chronic wounds.

Delayed phagocytosis and wound healing may be attributed to frequent changes in wound temperature. Therefore, the effect of temperature on cellular activity is an important consideration when choosing a treatment temperature for the whirlpool and in prompt aftercare. The effect of temperature changes on the cells of repair should also be considered an important factor when selecting the frequency of hydrotherapy treatment.

Neuronal Effects

Neural receptors for heat and cold are distributed all over the body. Signals from cold receptors travel along A-delta fibers and from warm receptors along C fibers. Neuronal mediation of thermoregulatory responses is the primary means of activation. Warm water has mild analgesic effects, reduces inflammation, is soothing, and relaxes muscle tension.[18,30,31] Patients experiencing severe pain or anxiety may find these effects soothing and analgesic. However, patients who are lethargic or semicomatose with already suppressed central nervous system function would be neurosuppressed to a point where they could become totally unresponsive. These patients should not be put in the whirlpool. Analgesia from the warm water is often reported, but some wound patients, especially those with ischemic limbs or burns, find that the agitation stimulates pain receptors. Treatment at a very gentle agitation level directed away from the wound tissue can be used to soothe, rather than stimulate, the nerves. Patient tolerance should be evaluated and treatment modified as required.

During whirlpool treatment, the patient should be encouraged to perform gentle exercise for muscle pump functions and strengthening. Both skin blood flow and sweating during exercise increase with a rise in water temperature and are notable at 35°C.[4] If exercise is to be performed during the wound treatment, consider the physiologic effects when choosing the water temperature and the extent of body area to be immersed. Joint range-of-motion extensibility is usually performed more easily and less painfully in warm water. The gentle stretching forces around the wound may stimulate tissue regeneration. Of course, stretching and exercise of a newly sutured wound should be avoided until the sutures are removed.

Physiologic Effects at Different Temperatures

The average skin temperature of the body is 34°C (93°F). The range of body indifference to temperature is 34–38°C (93–100.4°F). At 27–33.5°C (80–92°F), the temperature is tepid or nonthermal. At this temperature range, chilling with local vasoconstriction, decreased oxygen uptake, and tissue cooling that affects the cells of repair occurs.[12,28] Avoid mild core hypothermia at this thermal range by treating only a limited body area for a very short duration (e.g., 5 minutes) for cleansing or to soften dry tissue; keep the rest of the body and surrounding air temperature warm and slightly humid. Use a normothermic tap water rinse (35–37°C) immediately following the whirlpool to raise local wound temperatures.

Consider the tepid temperature choice for patients with venous disease in whom wound debridement and cleansing is the objective and where vasodilation would add blood volume and overload incompetent veins. The warm rinse would reduce shock to local cells of repair.

Neutral warmth is 33.5–35.5°C (92–96°F). Consider this temperature range for the patient with peripheral vascular disease, sensory impairment, or full-body immersion. Possibly the best choice of temperature to optimize cellular functions and enzymatic and biochemical reactions is at normal body temperature, or normothermia, defined as 98.6° F or 37° C ± 1° C.[32] The temperature range of 35.5 to 37°C is best when treating the patient with cardiovascular or pulmonary disease who would be stressed at a higher temperature.[3] At neutral warmth and normal body temperatures, tissues will be soaked, softened, and cleansed, and perfusion of the tissues will be increased.

Temperatures of 36.5–40°C (98–104°F) are acceptable for therapeutic heating.[3] Above 37°C or 98°F is classified as hot. Significant physiologic stress in the circulatory, nervous, and cardiopulmonary systems may occur under these conditions.[33] Water temperature choices are summarized as follows:[3]

- Nonthermal/tepid: 27–33.5°C or 80–92°F
- Neutral: 33.5–35.5°C or 92–96°F
- Normothermal: 37°C or 98.6°F
- Hot: 36.7–40°C or 98–104°F

Higher temperature levels are *not* recommended because of physiologic stress.

A tissue temperature rise of as much as 4°C at temperatures ranging from 37 to 42°C has been measured after immersion for 20 minutes in a whirlpool. As mentioned earlier, in a study of effects of the whirlpool on circulation, pulse rates increased 1.3–1.5 times over the sitting or supine resting level, and the mean blood pressure increased 1.1 times over the supine resting values.[3] Autonomic neuropathy and pulmonary dysfunction, which are common comorbidities with wounds, interfere with evaporative cooling. Limit the body surface area, lower the water temperature, and reduce the treatment time in the whirlpool for patients with cardiopulmonary and neuropathic diseases so that they are less physiologically challenged. If this is not practical, choose another treatment modality.

Temperature Precautions

As reviewed, water temperature modifies circulatory responses. Some treatment modification that the physical therapist (PT) should use to modify the heating effects of treatment follow:

- Water temperature should not exceed local skin temperature (usually 34°C) in the presence of peripheral vascular disease.
- Water temperature should not exceed 38°C in the presence of cardiovascular and pulmonary disease. The heat stimulates peripheral vasodilatation, with subsequent increased return of blood to the heart and increased cardiac output. The added load of blood volume can overtax a weak or decompensated heart muscle.[2]
- Water temperature of 32°C increases blood flow of 2.3 mL/dL of limb volume but will chill the wound and slow clotting and healing.[3,33]
- Extremes of temperature should be avoided in patients with sensory loss, such as those with alcoholic- or diabetic-related neuropathy or spinal cord injury, who cannot feel the temperature and respond to the heat. Loss of sensation can result in severe burns. Temperature sensation testing in a neuropathic patient is recommended before immersion in warm water. The procedure for testing is described in Chapter 4.

Evidence of the Effect of Whirpool on Wound healing

Many clinicians have moved away from use of the whirlpool since the release of the AHRQ *Pressure Ulcer Treatment Guidelines* because of a lack of evidence and cautions received from experts. The review of literature for other treatment interventions brought to light a number of studies in which whirlpool was used as either a co-treatment modality or the standard care treatment. Since the guidelines were published in 1994, one randomized controlled clinical trial of clean, surgically débrided pressure ulcers treated with whirlpool has been published.[34] Like most treatment intervention studies, the data from these studies often has gaps, such as treatment parameters used or the percentage of healing. The purpose of this review of the whirlpool reports is to look at which data have been reported and the evidence they provide for choosing an intervention with whirlpool hydrotherapy. Table 26-1 summarizes the data derived from the review and the following text outlines the studies more extensively.

Clinical Studies

A randomized clinical trial was performed to test the effect of whirlpool on surgically débrided, clean granulating, stage III and IV pressure ulcers.[34] Group A was treated with moist wound dressings and whirlpool hydrotherapy (N = 24) at 96–97°F and the control group B with moist wound dressings (N = 18). One 20-minute session was given daily. The whirlpool group showed a significantly faster rate of wound healing, mean rate 0.39 cm/week, in 58.33% of the whirlpool-treated ulcers, compared with a mean healing rate of 0.169 cm/week for 27.78% of the nonwhirlpool controls. Fewer wounds in the whirlpool group (9 versus 11) deteriorated during the course of treatment. However, the investigators were concerned that there were so many deteriorating wounds in both groups that could not be explained.

Whirlpool with povidone–iodine was chosen as the standard treatment for all patients in the two reports from Gogia. In a clinical report, two patients were treated with whirlpool and low-energy infrared cold laser (CL).[35] The patient in case study 1 had a 1.42 cm/week or 7.12% per week (99.7% healing) reduction in size after 14 weeks of therapy. The patient in case study 2 had weekly reduction in size of 1.5 cm/week or 5% per week (90% healing) in 18 weeks. Broad conclusions cannot be reached about use of these combined interventions. The second study was in a small controlled clinical trial (N = 12) of patients with pressure ulcers. The investigators followed a daily 20-minute whirlpool with povidone–iodine intervention with 20-minute electrical stimulation (ES) in half the patients, and the control half of the study received only a 20-minute treatment of whirlpool with povidone–iodine.[36] Both groups received aftercare with saline wet-to-dry dressings. The whirlpool control group in the ES study had a 5.23% per week reduction in wound area and 28.37% per week reduction in depth.

Gault and Gatens[37] found that a whirlpool control group had a 14.7% per week rate of healing. They designated one ulcer on each of six patients as a control and assigned that ulcer to a whirlpool control group. Results for those ulcers were a 14.7%/week healing rate.[37] However, the electrotherapy that was administered to the other ulcer may have had some systemic effect that influenced the rate of healing in the control ulcer.

Akers and Gabrielson[38] compared three treatment regimens: (1) whirlpool; (2) whirlpool with electrical high-voltage pulsed current (HVPC) stimulation; and (3) HVPC alone in the healing of pressure ulcers of 14 spinal cord-injured individuals. This controlled clinical trial reported that the whirlpool treatment was given once daily (QD), the

HVPC was given twice daily (BID), and the whirlpool given QD plus HVPC BID. The treatment parameters and the rate or percentage of healing were not reported. Results reported that there was no statistical significance between the three groups. The best outcomes were *achieved by the HVPC BID group, followed by the whirlpool QD group and the HVPC BID, and last, the whirlpool QD group. The study reported that numerous interval variations existed.*

Thurman and Christian[39] reported a case study of a patient with diabetes who was scheduled for surgical amputation of a foot with an infected abscess. The ulcerated foot was treated with a mixture of interventions including whirlpool and hexachlorophene for 10 minutes daily, followed by treatment with HVPC and other disinfecting agents and antimicrobials. Results were limb salvage, decreased infection, and exudate leading to wound closure in 4 months.

Carley and Wainapel's control group had a multitude of conventional dressing treatments, including mainly wet-to-dry dressings, gauze with Dakin's solution, or povidone–iodine.[40] Four were treated in the whirlpool. Results were not separated from the rest of the controls.

Wood et al[41] reported on results of a randomized controlled trial of 31 patients treated with whirlpool, saline wet-to-moist dressings, and compared the results with those of a group of 43 patients treated with low-intensity direct current. The whirlpool and dressing group had 3% healing or had increased wound size while the low-voltage microamperage direct current group had 58% healing. Perhaps some of the poor results in the whirlpool/saline wet-to-moist dressing group were due to the dressings drying out, resulting in repeated trauma during dressing changes.

In another study, whirlpool efficacy was compared with pulsed lavage by measuring the rate of formation of granulation tissue in a variety of chronic wounds.[42] Although the rate of granulation tissue formation was greater at 12.2% per week, for the pulsed lavage group, the whirlpool group had a granulation rate of 4.8% per week. Whirlpool and collagenase were both used throughout the course of treatment for ulcers of mixed etiologies, and 80% reached closure in a median time of 37 days (SD 27.5 days).[43]

Major abdominal surgery is often followed by pain because of increased tension on muscles and tissues. Results of these events have been attributed to causing anxiety, stress, and altered tissue regeneration. Findings of a controlled clinical trial of postoperative patients (N = 63) who had major abdominal surgery and who received an intervention with whirlpool after surgery showed reduced pain behavior, less signs of wound inflammation, and positive signs of healing over a 3-day period following surgery.[18]

Review of the results suggest that there were extrinsic factors that may have influenced the results of the treatment interventions, such as use of cytotoxic agents like povidone–iodine,[35,36,40] and hexachlophene and hydrogen peroxide.[39] Two studies[34,41] reported conscientiously avoiding chemical and mechanical trauma to the wounds treated with whirlpool, yet both reported significant deterioration of the whirlpool groups that was not explained.

TABLE 26-1 Clinical Studies Using Whirlpool

Investigators and Type of Study	Disease States Treated	Whirlpool	Electrical Stimulation	Other Treatments	Effects on Healing
Akers and Gabrielson[38] (N = 14) Controlled clinical trial-3 groups	Pressure ulcers (full or partial denervation of spinal cord)	1. Once daily	2. HVPC BID 3. WPL once and HVPC BID	Not reported	ES only best ES with whirlpool second best Whirlpool only least No statistical significance between 3 groups. Lots of internal variation.
Burke et al[34] (WPL N = 24 nonWPL N = 18) RCT	Pressure ulcers	Once daily, 20 min 96–98°F	N/A	Surgical debridement Saline wet-to-dry dressings	WPL group * 58.33% (14) mean 0.39 cm/week reduction in size 4.17% (1) no change 37.5% (9) deterioration NonWPL group* 27.78% (5) mean 0.169 cm/week reduction in size 11.11% (2) no change 61.11% (11) deterioration
Carley and Wainapel[70] (WPL N = 4 LIDC N = 30) RCT	indolent ulcers below knee or sacral	4–5 ×/week	LIDC Direct, 2 hrs BID, 5 x/week	Wet-to-dry dressings Dakin's or povidone-iodine, or hydrogel	WP group 45% healing (9%/week)* LIDC group 98.95% (19% week)* healing in 5 weeks
Gault and Gatens[37] (WPL N = 6 LIDC N = 6 subgroup) Controlled trial	Mixed	Once daily	LIDC Direct, 2 hrs BID or TID		LIDC 30%/week WP 14.7%/week, 2/6 increased in size
Gogia et al[36] (N = 6) Controlled trial	Mixed	Once daily 20 min with povidone-iodine, 100°F	HVPC 20 min Direct, 5 x/week	Saline wet-to-dry dressings	WPL 20 days 27.19% reduction in area (9.51%/week) 56.76% reduction in depth (19.86%/week) WPL and HVPC 20 days 34.73% reduction area (12.15%/week) 30.30% reduction in depth (10.6%/week)*
Gogia, Hurt, and Zim[35] (N = 2) Case Studies		Whirlpool with povidone-iodine	N/A	Infrared cold laser	Granulation, significant healing

(Continued)

TABLE 26-1 (Continued)

Investigators and Type of Study	Disease States Treated	Whirlpool	Electrical Stimulation	Other Treatments	Effects on Healing
Haynes et al[42] (WPL N = 15 PL N = 15) Controlled trial	Mixed	Whirlpool	N/A	Pulsed lavage Varied	PL 12.2% healing/week WP 4.8% healing/week
Juve[18] (N = 63) Controlled trial	Major abdominal surgery	Whirlpool daily 3 days postoperative	N/A	Probably dressings (type unstated)	Pain reduction Reduced wound inflammation Positive signs of wound healing
Thurman and Christian[39] (N = 1) Case study	Abscess, diabetes	Whirlpool with hexachlorophene detergent cleanser (pHisohex) 10 min	HVPC daily	Debridement Hydrogen peroxide soaks Antibiotic medication	Decreased infection, exudate, and wound size 6 months to closure
Vetra and Whittaker[43] Uncontrolled clinical trial (N = 140)	Mixed	Whirlpool 40°C daily		Collagenase daily	80% closure Mean time 37.0 days (SD 27.5 days) 7% good granulation and epithelialization 3% healthy granulation 10% reduction or cessation of drainage
Wood et al[41] (WPL N = 31 PLIDC N = 43) Randomized controlled trial	Pressure and venous ulcers	Whirlpool	PLIDC 3x/week	Cleansing Saline wet-to-dry dressings	Whirlpool and dressing group 3% healed or increased in size PLIDC 58% healed Data for whirlpool only, ulcers not reported

WPL = whirlpool, HVPC = high-voltage pulsed current, LIDC = low-intensity direct current, PLIDC = pulsed low-intensity direct current, BID = twice daily, TID = three times daily.

*Percentage healing per week calculated study data to transform data for comparison.

Data from references 30, 46, 47, 48, 49, 50, 51, 53, 54, 55, and 71.

Debridement, Cleansing, Wound Decontamination, and Infection

Debridement is the process for removal of devitalized tissue. It is now recognized as a key component for the management of chronic wounds and, as such, has become a standard of care to speed and achieve optimal wound healing. Debridement is differentiated from wound cleansing. The process of wound cleansing involves selecting a wound cleansing solution and a method of delivery that cleanses the wound with minimum chemical or mechanical trauma.[1] Whirlpool is a method of both mechanical debridement and wound cleansing. Other methods of debridement to manage necrotic tissue are discussed in Chapters 8 and 27.

Devitalized tissue in the wound prolongs the inflammatory process and delays the onset of the healing cascade and the healing process. When the body cannot rid itself of the bioburden of dead tissue and debris efficiently and effectively, as a result of compromised body systems or an excessive amount of debris, an intervention to speed the process must be considered. By performing a debridement procedure, the clinician minimizes the body's inflammatory response and removes a staging place for bacteria and fungi.

Use of mechanical force, such as turbulent water, to remove nonviable tissue is an invasive procedure that is nonselective and may cause damage to healthy as well as nonviable tissues. Trauma to granulation tissue and epithelial cells may occur if the wound is positioned too close to the high-pressure jets of the whirlpool.[2] Trauma from mechanical force prolongs inflammation and delays healing.[44] Therefore, care must be exercised during delivery of the whirlpool treatment to minimize trauma to healthy granulation tissue as well as to surrounding soft tissues, because even trauma distant from the wound site can influence the occurrence of local wound infection.[45] Trauma from shearing forces and turbulence can be avoided by adjusting the level of aeration from the jet to minimal or by turning off the aerator if tissues are very fragile, such as new skin grafts.[3]

The physical effects of immersion in water are soaking, saturating, loosening, and softening of loosely adherent necrotic tissue, which aids phagocytosis and deodorization. Whirlpool has little or no effect on densely adherent fibrous tissue, and other methods of debridement should be considered. Whirlpool as a debridement intervention is often followed by other debridement methods, for example, sharp, enzymatic, or autolytic.

Whirlpool-associated Risks

Risks to Cardiac, Vascular and Pulmonary Systems

In order for safe treatment to be given, medical history should be reviewed for medical problems. Cardiovascular problems to look for include the following: congestive heart failure so as to avoid cardiac overload, venous insufficiency to avoid local tissue congestion and for medications that alter cardiac function such as beta blockers that reduce blood pressure and heart rate because they will effect reaction to treatment. Even if such findings are not discovered in the medical history, if the patient is elderly it is important to be aware of changes in the cardiovascular system related to aging that affect cardiac and vascular performance including decreased vascular elasticity, decreased cardiac muscle compliance and performance and hypertension. Physiologic changes with ageing also involve the pulmonary system including diminished ventilation and gas exchange. There is risk of pneumonia especially in the elderly from airborne respirable water vapour droplets resulting from the agitation of the water in the whirlpool.[46] In all patients, vital signs including blood pressure, heart rate and respiration rates should be taken before, during and after treatment. In addition, all patients should be monitored closely during the treatment for: dizziness, feeling faint, or changes in mental status

CLINICAL WISDOM

Use of a face mask by the patient as well as personnel would reduce risk of inhalation of respirable droplets during the whirlpool treatment.

Risk of Tissue Damage

Surface environment of the skin is normally unfavorable to most microflora because its body surface pH is between 5 and 6.[47] Prolonged soaking supersaturates the wound tissue and surrounding skin, which may result in maceration, or the breaking down of the fibers of the skin and a change in the pH. During immersion, exudate is cleansed from the wound along with sweat and oils from the surrounding skin. Autonomic neuropathy impairs function of sweat and sebaceous glands, resulting in dry skin. Therefore, soaking of the neuropathic foot that has already impaired sweat and oil production and risk of maceration is not recommended.[4] Agitation is used to cleanse and débride the wound tissue by scrubbing it. The mechanical effects on circulation caused by agitation of the whirlpool are small.[5] It has been postulated that the mechanical stimulation of the cells stimulates granulation tissue formation.

Risk of Wound Infection

There is evidence that wounds treated with hydrotherapy are at risk for waterborne contamination and other complications. Reports in the literature demonstrate *Pseudomonas aeruginosa*-associated skin disease after immersion in whirlpool.[48–50] Factors that influence host susceptibility include the anatomic and physiologic defenses of the skin, the skin surface microecology wherein the skin humidity is altered, and intrinsic factors such as disease and age. The skin's relative dryness may be a defense mechanism to resist infection. The immersion in the whirlpool may negate the normal skin defenses. Chronic antibiotic therapy changes the normal flora of the skin and can lead to colonization and superinfection with organisms such as *P. aeruginosa*.[48]

A variety of intrinsic factors, such as diabetes, appear to increase host susceptibility to infection through the skin. Traumatic injuries such as burns and immunosuppressive therapies also increase host susceptibility to skin infection with *P. aeruginosa*.[48] Hydration of the skin and increased skin tissue temperature have been associated with *P. aeruginosa* infections as well, and most likely negates many of the skin's normal defenses. In experimental models, superhydration of the skin must be continued for several days before symptoms occur, and whirlpool usually offers considerably shorter exposure periods. Repeated immersion and exposure to the whirlpool water may lead to colonization of *P. aeruginosa* despite drying of the skin surface between sessions. There is potential for the bacteria to be harbored in the invaginations of the skin appendages, where they release proteolytic enzymes and exotoxins that result in an inflammatory reaction of the surrounding tissues.[5]

Wound decontamination and infection control are cited as reasons to use hydrotherapy, but evidence of their efficacy is mixed. Two studies compared the effects of whirlpool treatment and whirlpool treatment followed by vigorous rinsing. Neiderhuber et al[51] studied removal of bacterial load from the soles of the feet of 76 normal adults with intact skin. Factors considered in their investigation included water temperature, immersion time, agitation of the water versus soaking, spraying the part with clean water for 30 seconds, and agitation of the water during immersion, followed by spraying of the part with clean water for 30 seconds.[51] Findings showed that water temperature was not a significant factor in bacterial decontamination whereas duration of immersion was significant. There was a steady removal of bacterial load with longer duration treatment, 10–20 minutes being optimal. Agitation was best, compared with either soaking or spraying, in removal of skin surface bacteria, but the combination of immersion with agitation and spraying rinsed away 70% of the remaining contaminants, providing the best outcome.

Bohannon[52] studied a single subject with a venous ulcer and compared bacterial load following whirlpool with a low concentration of povidone–iodine without and with rinsing for 30–90 seconds at the maximum pressure tolerated by the subject. More than four times as many bacteria were removed with rinsing added than without. Both studies support the use of whirlpool with rinse to reduce bacterial colonies present on skin and wound surface. Considerable documentation in the literature shows that when the bacterial content of an ulcer exceeds 10^5 organisms per gram of tissue, healing is impaired.[1] However, neither the Neiderhuber nor the Bohannon study identifies the organisms isolated, nor do they use the threshold standard of an infected wound as 10^5 organisms per gram of tissue measured by wound biopsy or culture.[53] Only one patient with a wound was evaluated. Thus the strength of evidence based on these studies that whirlpool controls infection is poor.

Risk of infection for the patient with a burn or wound has been documented. Shankowsky et al[50] surveyed 202 burn units in the United States and Canada, with 158 (75.7%) responding, and found that these facilities regularly use hydrotherapy as part of burn care. Whirlpool was implicated as a cause of nosocomial infection leading to sepsis with *P. aeruginosa* (52.9%), *Staphylococcus aureus* (25.5%), and *Candida albicans* (5.2%).[50] Cardany et al[54] found that hydrotherapy did not reduce bacterial load on burned or normal skin, but the water contained heavy contamination with viable organisms that have the potential for contaminating clean wounds and for patient cross-contamination. A further documented complication is superhydration of the skin, which allows penetration of bacteria.[48,50] Water content of the skin may increase to 55–70% following a 20-minute immersion.[48] Intrinsic factors, such as immunosuppression, and diseases such as diabetes are known to increase susceptibility to infection. Hospitalized individuals, compared with healthy individuals, have a decreased resistance to infection and have the highest risk of secondary health effects.

Exposure to pathogens has been associated with many sources, including whirlpool tanks. Infectious organisms, particularly *P. aeruginosa*, have been identified in hydrotherapy equipment, despite rigorous efforts to disinfect properly and to monitor for cultures. For instance, Shankowsky et al[50] reported a lethal outbreak of aminoglycoside-resistant *P. aeruginosa* in a newly constructed burn center in which stringent methods of disinfection were used and despite routine bacterial surveillance. Control of the outbreak was achieved when the hydrotherapy tanks were used for closed wounds during rehabilitation.[50] The following reports show how different clinical settings interpreted and responded to data collected from studies of infectious organisms in hydrotherapy tanks.

Over a 4-week period, cultures were taken in the morning before treatment and at the end of the day from whirlpools in two institutions in a university medical center commonly used by diabetic dysvascular patients. Special attention was directed toward recovery of *S. aureus*, *P. aeruginosa*, and *Escherichia coli* organisms. Results of the testing were that only 11 of 96 cultures (11.5%) were positive for these prospective pathogens. The opinion of the study authors was that immersion in these whirlpool tanks was not likely to expose patients with open wounds to potential iatrogenic contamination.[55]

Seventeen whirlpool baths in sixteen nursing homes were examined for presence of *P. aeruginosa*. Large numbers of these organisms were found in water samples taken from whirlpool baths after agitation, but only 1 patient out of 253 residents was known to have a *P. aeruginosa* wound infection. Results of these findings led the Health Commission to advise the local survey team that, although the prevalence of known *P. aeruginosa* infection was low, the whirlpool baths should continue to be used only by continent residents with intact skin to avoid an infection hazard to the residents.[56]

Although the reports in the literature provide considerable evidence of risk of wound contamination, hydrotherapy is used in 94.8% of the surveyed institutions. Despite the reported high incidence of infection, hydrotherapy immersion continues to be used in 118 burn units. Only 27 respondents to the survey have discontinued immersion in favor of showers. Patients who are mechanically ventilated and/or invasively monitored are regularly immersed at 47.6% of the responding burn units.[50] Local treatment appears to reduce risk of lethal sepsis. Alternative measures of controlling wound infection with hydrotherapy using irrigation with sterile solution applied by a syringe or pulsatile lavage with suction are described in Chapters 8 and 27. Risk of infection due to immersion in hydrotherapy is becoming more widely recognized, but has not yet significantly changed clinical practice.

Summary

In the previous sections the physical principles and physiological effects and research evidence as well as risks of whirlpool intervention were reviewed. It was pointed out that it is critical for the PT to review the patient's medical history and do a systems review as guidelines for selection of an intervention with whirlpool.

Evaluation of study reports reviewed produced no evidence that whirlpool is harmful to granulation tissue. Good practice would be to take care that fragile granulation tissue or a new skin graft is protected from direct force of the whirlpool jet and that the force of the aeration is modified to avoid any problems. The same is true for patients on anticoagulant therapy who are at risk for deep tissue injury and hematoma.[57]

Whirlpool therapy will increase local blood flow for a sustained period of time after cessation of the treatment, increase subcutaneous oxygen, and stimulate the cells needed for healing. It is safe and effective to use, even after the wound is clean and free of exudate and necrotic debris.

Evidence of wound healing efficacy in treatment of patients with whirlpool is reported in two controlled clinical trials on pressure ulcers and surgical wounds,[18,34] as is evidence from studies in which it was the control treatment. Whirlpool may be the most efficient way to treat multiple or extensive wounds. It can be used to heat a large body area or a limited body area and raise core body temperature; it is useful to relax tissue tension and provide relief for painful wounds. Although the evidence is still limited, additional study would be helpful to identify the best frequency of treatment and temperature that best speed healing.

Choosing An Intervention: Clinical Reasoning

Candidacy

AHCPR *Pressure Ulcer Treatment Guidelines* state: "Heel ulcers with dry eschar need not be débrided if they do not have edema, erythema, fluctuance, or drainage. Assess these wounds daily for pressure ulcer complications."[1] It is the AHCPR panel's opinion that these findings indicate wound stability. The guidelines acknowledge that there is no research reported in the literature to support this recommendation. The recommendation does not take into consideration several issues. The expectation that eschar will be assessed daily is not realistic or practical in most care settings. The wound may appear stable, but the wound has an absence of inflammatory phase. Inflammatory phase may be suppressed for many reasons. Shouldn't the reason for suppressed inflammation be determined before deciding whether to debride the eschar?

Functional mobility is a key indicator of risk for pressure ulcers. Eschar on a heel limits the functional activity of the patient who is otherwise able, by limiting weight bearing on the eschar surface for transfers or ambulation. The patient with eschar on the heel cannot wear shoes and requires a special orthosis to remove pressure from the eschar. This precaution would be necessary until the wound heals. Leaving the eschar intact also means that the extent of the soft tissue injury cannot be determined. Wounds with eschar have the potential for healing or for deterioration. For example, documentation in the literature supports the potential for complete ulcer closure of heel wounds with eschar following debridement with hydrotherapy and collagenase.[43]

When should the eschar be left intact? When the patient has inadequate circulation or is in a state of health that will fail to support healing, eschar should not be soaked or débrided. For example, wounds and adjacent tissues that look like those in *Color Plate 52* should not be debrided of eschar. If there is no report of vascular studies in the medical record, the PT or nurse should consider performing noninvasive vascular testing or the patient should be referred to a vascular lab; then, candidacy for healing would be determined. For candidates, whirlpool is a quick and efficient way to soften eschar on the heels and enhance local tissue perfusion to facilitate debridement.

In the case study used to illustrate clinical decision making at the end of this chapter, circulatory status was evaluated in a patient with eschar on both heels and found to be adequate for healing. The patient was being positioned upright in a wheelchair, and significant pressure was being supported on the heels during transfer, creating risk of trauma to tissues already compromised. Whirlpool was used to soften and debride the eschar. As it turned out, the outer eschar concealed two smaller eschar areas, and these two needed to be softened and debrided, revealing deep tissue damage. Once that was accomplished, the wounds were treated by other means to closure. The patient's functional outcome after heels were healed was the ability to do a standing pivot transfer with one person to assist while weight bearing on both feet.

Patients with large amounts of necrotic tissue have a body system impairment of autolytic debridement and phagocytosis, and they need help from an intervention to hasten the process of removing the bioburden from the body. Whirlpool will hasten the softening of necrotic tissue and debridement. Wounds that contain debris, foreign bodies, and slough or that are highly exudative or malodorous and need intensive cleaning would benefit from whirlpool. Wounds of all tissue depths are treated in the whirlpool, but those that are deep, with undermining and tunneling, would be at greater risk for transmitting infection into the body. All wounds and surrounding skin should be vigorously rinsed with clean, warm tap water following removal from the whirlpool to remove deposits of debris and bacteria.

Patients with impaired vascular perfusion of the lower extremities have risk for impairment of healing and undue susceptibility to pressure ulceration. These individuals may be candidates for whirlpool intervention as a prevention strategy because of induced vasodilatation by direct and reflexive stimulation, as well as the enhanced perfusion by gravitational pull in the dependent position. A suggested method of preventive treatment strategy for individuals who have a high risk of pressure ulcers or those with intact stage I pressure ulcers includes daily whirlpool at 38–40°C to stimulate peripheral circulation. The improved circulation to the skin encourages skin growth and replacement, which makes the skin more elastic and less susceptible to shearing and pressure.[43,58] Patients with circulatory impairment who have wounds with extensive necrotic tissue to soften for debridement may benefit from this treatment. Vetra and Whittaker[43] found that patients with limited circulation and extensive necrotic tissue who most likely would have had to have limb amputation received benefit from the enhanced perfusion associated with heating in the whirlpool, combined with enzymatic debridement using collagenase.

In summary, the physical and mechanical effects of whirlpool are as follows:

Benefits

- Mechanical debridement:
  - Soaking and softening of eschar and other necrotic tissue
  - Scrubbing and loosening of necrotic tissue
  - Debriding by mechanical action of turbulence
  - Deodorizing the wound through cleansing
  - Soaking to remove dried dressings
- Removing excess antibacterial creams
- Increasing blood flow and tissue oxygen
- Increasing core body temperature
- Cellular effects:
  - Stimulating cell mitosis
  - Enhancing leukocytic activity
  - Speeding epidermal cell production
  - Bringing antibodies to wound area
- Fighting infection by improved oxygenation of tissue and removal of bacteria and debris
- Reducing pain through mild analgesia

Disadvantages

- Superhydrating and macerating skin
- Changing of skin pH changes skin surface environment
- Increasing risk of skin infection and wound infection

- Changing of mental status and possible dizziness
- Increasing heart and respiratory rates
- Increased cardiac output and possible inability to compensate
- Increasing edema in the dependent position
- Shifting fluids away from the body may lead to dehydration and nutrient depletion
- Traumatizing the wound or surrounding tissues by mechanical forces
- Traumatizing the tissues by overheating (burns) of insensate skin or ischemic tissue

Precautions

Historically, wounds of nearly every type are referred for hydrotherapy. Appropriate use versus overuse of whirlpools is an issue. There has been a definite pendulum swing from treating every wound in the whirlpool to avoiding whirlpool entirely or limiting use to only necrotic wounds. Whirlpool benefits for treating some specific wound-related problems (e.g., necrosis, thick exudate, circulation) have been described. The benefits and disadvantages must be carefully weighed. Whirlpool treatment can and should be modified to meet the intentions of the therapy.

Changing parameters are required if whirlpool is used. For example, if cleansing is the intention, tepid or neutral warmth (33.5–35.5°C or 92–96°F) will cleanse an ulcer in a patient with venous disease. Minimize the time in the dependent position (e.g., treat for 5 minutes, not 20 minutes). Follow with a warm water rinse, then apply compression therapy.[59] If the wounded limb is edematous or has friable skin around the wound and should not be immersed, perfusion can be enhanced by reflexive vasodilatation through immersion of the opposite lower extremity or an upper extremity.

Additional precautions should be considered to avoid potentially harmful effects when the following situations are present:

- Clean, granulating wounds: Clean, granulating wounds are easily traumatized by the force of mild agitation. Reduce aeration.
- Epithelializing wounds: Migrating epidermal cells may be damaged by even the least force. Shut off aeration.
- New skin grafts: Skin grafts will not tolerate high shearing forces and turbulence. Shut off aeration.
- New tissue flaps: New tissue flaps are very sensitive to shearing forces and vasoconstriction that can occur if the water or air temperature causes chilling. Shut off aeration, use normothermal temperature.
- Non-necrotic diabetic ulcers: Callus often surrounds diabetic ulcers and will be softened and macerated. Macerated tissue will not tolerate pressure, and the wound will be enlarged. Moisture retention under the callus may become a source of infection.
- Under certain circumstances, such as when a patient is on anticoagulation therapy or has hypertension, whirlpool should be used with caution. Consider not using the jet

because the force of the jet has the potential to traumatize the tissue and cause internal bleeding.[57]

Contraindications

Contraindications to use of whirlpool include the presence of any of the following:

- Moderate to severe extremity edema
- Lethargy
- Unresponsiveness
- Maceration
- Febrile conditions
- Compromised cardiovascular or pulmonary function
- Acute phlebitis
- Renal failure
- Dry gangrene (evaluate for ischemia)
- Incontinence of urine or feces (if whirlpool will be contaminated)

Patients who are not candidates for whirlpool therapy are those who are febrile, have cardiac or ventilatory pump failure or renal failure, are lethargic, or have venous system impairment. Even heating a single limb will raise core body temperature, which is already a problem with febrile patients. Local heating will increase cardiac output and respiration rate and can overload the cardiopulmonary system and renal system in those with impaired function.[3,22]

Patients with fetal posture contractures may not be able to be safely positioned in the whirlpool. Diabetics and spinal cord-injured individuals who have insensitivity of the feet may experience burns because of the inability to respond neurologically to thermal changes. Diabetics with callus formation on the plantar surfaces of the feet should *not* be treated in the whirlpool because the integumentary system is impaired, calluses will be softened, and subsequent exposure to pressure from standing on the foot will result in skin breakdown. The break in the skin will become a portal for infection.

Patients with dry gangrene should not have the tissues softened because the dry gangrene is nature's method of walling off the tissues and encapsulating the area. Softening of the tissue will reduce the barrier and allow infectious organisms to enter the body. Autoamputation of necrotic digits usually occurs anyway (see Chapter 8).

Personnel Safety

Standard precautions should always be followed by hydrotherapy personnel. The hydrotherapy personnel are exposed to airborne water vapor. Inhalation or contact dermatitis of water droplets containing bacteria and antiseptic or disinfection products presents health risks. Isolation of the patient with an open wound during treatment in the whirlpool may be beneficial because of aerosolization of infectious organisms and production of respirable droplets from the agitation of the water.[46,60] Staff should use protective gear. Policies and procedures should be developed for each health-care facility to minimize staff exposure.[46]

Masks, gowns, caps, and goggles are appropriate attire to use as barriers (see Chapter 28, Figure 28-2).

CLINICAL WISDOM

Whirlpool Bathing

One situation that needs clarification is the common referral of patients with wounds for whirlpool treatment and the expectation that this will serve as the patient's bath. The whirlpool is not a bathing pool or shampoo basin. The water in the tank is dirty with wound exudate and debris. Soap, shampoo, and disinfectants have ingredients that are harmful to wounds and may irritate delicate skin during soaking. For personal hygiene, a shower is preferable because all substances are flushed away from the wound and the skin. ∎

Delivery of Care

The survey of Thomson et al[61] found that in most burn units (100 units polled), nurses perform hydrotherapy procedures, although there is no consensus on who does it. Shankowsky et al[50] found that in most of the responding 118 burn units using immersion hydrotherapy, both debridement and rehabilitation/physical therapy treatments were included in a single hydrotherapy session (71.7%) and that hydrotherapy continued throughout the patient's length of stay. According to Medicare guidelines, whirlpool is considered a skilled physical therapy procedure when the patient's condition is complicated by disease processes, such as impaired circulation, areas of desensitization, open wounds (e.g., stage III and IV pressure ulcers), or other complications that require the skills, knowledge, and judgment of a PT. Diagnosis or prognosis is not the sole factor in deciding whether the service is skilled or not.[62]

Recently, some Medicare contractors have issued specific guidelines for physical therapy skilled services for wound care. The guidelines state that interventions that will increase function using treatment modalities specific to physical therapy require the skills of a PT (e.g., treatment of an open wound or burn over a joint while undergoing functional mobility training in the whirlpool). Wound care alone does not require the skills of a PT.[63] There is no consensus on who should deliver the hydrotherapy procedure. Whirlpool has long been considered a physical therapy procedure for patients with burns and wounds. Delivery of hydrotherapy services requires professional skills to select the appropriate candidate for and the best method of application of the therapy. As a health-care professional licensed in the use of physical agents, the PT would be expected to know the effects of hydrotherapy and thermal agents on the different body systems and the appropriate precautions to take.

Equipment

Whirlpool Tanks

Whirlpool tanks are used for immersion of either the full body or extremity and are sized accordingly. Large hydrotherapy tanks are called *Hubbard tanks* and may be used for aquatic exercise as well as for wound healing. They have either an attached turbine or a built-in turbine, or the turbine might be suspended from the side of a bathtub. The whirlpool is created by a mixture of water and air to create controlled turbulence. The more aeration, the greater will be the turbulence and pressure at the surface of the water.[3] The mixture is adjustable but varies from one piece of equipment to another. Force and directions of the agitation are usually adjustable. The tank may be made of stainless steel, Plexiglas, or tile (Figure 26-2).

Tank Selection

Select a whirlpool tank sized for the wound or body area to be treated. If a patient has multiple wounds, the water should cover those areas that need soaking, cleansing, or debriding. The full-body tank or tub will allow the patient to extend the legs fully and may be more comfortable. If the patient is contracted, select a tank in which the patient can be comfortably positioned. Hydraulic lift chairs and chaises or Hoyer lifts can be used to transfer a patient into the tank if the tank is too high or if the patient is nonambulatory. If the patient is seated on a chair for a leg whirlpool treatment, be sure there is no pressure under the thigh.

Procedure

Frequency and Duration

Frequency of hydrotherapy treatment has been traditionally tied to washing of burn wounds to remove topical creams

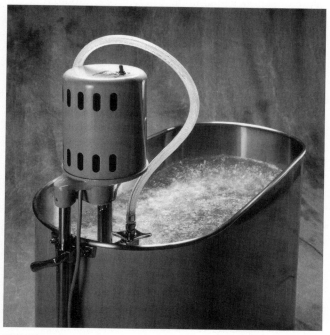

FIGURE 26-2 Whirlpool tank. (Courtesy of Whitehall Manufacturing/Acorn Engineering, City of Industry, California.)

used almost universally for patients in burn units. Protocols in burn facilities mandate washing the wound between each application of the topical agent. Soaking is also used to facilitate dressing changes. Topical agents commonly used to treat burns include silver sulfadiazine (Silvadene, Thermazene, SSD), Sulfamylon suspension, and silver nitrate used for bactericidal effects. Survey results of burn units show that hydrotherapy treatment is carried out at least daily (56.6%) and bi-daily (33.8%).[50] Although the same topical agents are used for other acute or chronic wounds, this is not universally the case. Therefore, the frequency of hydrotherapy treatment to cleanse the wound of topical agents should be modified to correspond to a different rationale of wound management. For instance, once daily 10- to 20-minute treatment for indicated wounds would be preferable in most cases to twice-daily 20-minute whirlpool treatments, which are still common. Once-daily or three-times-weekly whirlpool treatments minimize the frequency of dressing changes and exposure to infection, and maintain the wound temperature and the healing environment. Discontinue treatment when target outcomes are met, if the wound is not responding, or if other treatment options would better meet the needs of the wound and the patient.

Many whirlpool treatments are ordered twice daily. If wound cleansing and debridement are the reasons for selecting this intervention, once-daily treatment followed by application of moisture-retentive wound dressings or enzymes would be a good treatment protocol. Prompt wound dressing following the whirlpool/rinse treatment is needed. However, if enhancement of circulation and cellular effects are the reasons, a twice-daily treatment could be desirable. Intermittent heating at normothermia has been demonstrated to increase subcutaneous oxygen tension and presumably reduce infection.[16] Twice-daily treatments to the wound require twice-daily dressing changes and disrupt the wound environment twice. Dressings need to be selected that can safely and cost effectively be removed that frequently.

Wound dressing technology can now provide the healing wound with a scientifically controlled environment of temperature and wound fluid to promote healing. Infrequent dressing changes are now considered the method of choice to promote healing. Reimbursement should also be considered when selecting specialized dressings because they are expected to be left in place longer than gauze. Obviously, the PT, nurse, and physician must collaborate on making a dressing selection that will provide the best wound environment and that is appropriate for frequency of whirlpool.

Water Temperature

Select a water temperature based on the medical condition of the patient and the clinical objective of the treatment. All temperature ranges will soak, soften, and loosen necrotic tissue and cleanse the wound. Keep in mind that a temperature of 37°C is considered optimal for epithelial cell migration, mitotic cell division, and leukocytic activity.[48] Use the temperature closest to the optimal that will be consistent with the patient's medical status.

Monitoring Vital Signs

All patients not just those with a medical history of cardiopulmonary or cardiac disease, cerebrovascular accident, or hypertension should have their vital signs monitored before, during and after the whirlpool treatment. Record the patient's respiration and heart rate, and take blood pressure. Observe for change in mental status and any reports of lightheadedness. The latter is common with immersion of large body areas. The feeling of lightheadedness should go away after the patient sits for 5–10 minutes outside the hydrotherapy area. Also query the patient about the fifth vital sign, pain, before and after treatment. Many individuals find warm water soothing, and documentation of this vital sign should be noted.

Infection Control

A major concern about use of the whirlpool is infection. The following section presents pros and cons of using antiseptics in the whirlpool for treatment of infected wounds, comparison of clean tap water and saline on infection, and the value of vigorous rinsing after whirlpool treatment to control infection.

Use of Antiseptics

There is controversy about the use of antiseptic agents in the whirlpool. Most burn facilities use a disinfecting solution for hydrotherapy.[50,61] Bacterial resistance to antiseptics is documented. In addition, antiseptics have limited effectiveness in reducing bacteria when high bacterial counts are measured and are inactivated by organic matter, such as pus and wound exudate.[50,26] Research shows that the most commonly used antiseptic agents are harmful to the cells of tissue repair. AHCPR treatment guidelines for pressure ulcers state that antiseptic agents (e.g., povidone–iodine, iododophor, sodium hypochlorite solution [Dakin's solution], hydrogen peroxide, and acetic acid) should not be used to clean ulcers because of their cytotoxicity to fibroblasts.[1,63] No controlled studies document that repeated application of antiseptics to chronic wounds significantly reduces the level of bacteria in wound tissues.[1,64] All commonly used antiseptic agents that are used in the whirlpool have cytotoxicity, even at very low dilutions.[65]

Chemicals in antiseptics are absorbed through the wound tissue, and some patients develop toxicity or allergic responses to the chemical agents. As described above in the personnel safety section, water vapor is dispersed into the atmosphere during the agitation process. If the water in the whirlpool contains an antiseptic, the water vapour will also contain the antiseptic which will then potentially be inhaled by both patients and staff causing adverse respiratory effects.

Although using an antiseptic in the whirlpool is not generally encouraged, there are times when they should be used, such as for necrotic, heavily exudating wounds or when antibiotic-resistant organisms such as *P. aeruginosa* are found in a wound, and wound decontamination is required.

Rationale for using sodium hypochlorite solutions in whirlpool is to dissolve blood clots and that may be useful in solubilizing the clotted material that constitutes a considerable portion of necrotic tissue, but, as a consequence, delayed clotting may occur, and the wound exudate will become sanguineous.

A hydrotherapy burn unit tested different concentrations of chloramine-T (Chlorazene) to determine its effect on Gram-negative organisms.[66] Chloramine-T is an aqueous hypochlorite with a molecular structure that allows for slower release of free chlorine into the water, and this increases the bactericidal effects for a longer time.[67] Findings included negative cultures from patients and from the equipment after a 5-day treatment regimen using chloramine-T at a concentration of 200 parts per million (ppm). Patients' wounds, surrounding tissues, and staff reactions to the chloramine-T additive were carefully monitored, but no adverse side effects were found. Tank decontamination was achieved by running the turbine in the tank with the same solution after treatments. This reduced staff cleaning and disinfection time.

There has been heightened awareness of cytotoxicity to the cells of wound repair from antiseptics. Guinea pigs with an induced full-thickness wound were inoculated with *P. aeruginosa* to study the effects of chloramine-T on wound healing and wound decontamination.[68] One group of animals was immersed in tap water and the other set in water containing 300 ppm of chloramine-T solution at 36°C for 20 minutes. Results showed that, within 8–10 minutes of exposure to the chloramine-T solution, all microorganisms were killed. After immersion of the infected wounds in tap water on days 6–7 after wounding, there were a number of colony-forming units cultured from the water. There was no evidence of skin irritation in the chloramine-T group. Rates of wound healing of the full-thickness inoculated skin wounds were comparable in both the tap water and chloramine-T groups. After the 5 days, a wound culture, or clinical signs that show significant wound decontamination, the treatment should be changed to clear water, followed by vigorous rinse to rid the tissues of deposits of debris and bacteria. Longer use of the antiseptic agent may retard the healing process, due to the cytotoxic effects on the cells of repair.

Also consider other methods of wound decontamination, such as Photostimulation (described in Chapter 24) or electrical stimulation (described in Chapter 22). Chapter 11 includes additional information on the use of antiseptics, their actions, indications, precautions, directions for use, packaging, and effects on wound healing.

Be sure that the intention for using the antiseptic is clear, monitor carefully, and stop when the desired outcome is met (e.g., the wound is exudate free or necrosis free). Use at low concentrations. Some commonly used antiseptics in the whirlpool are as follows:

- Povidone–iodine
- Sodium hypochlorite
- Chlorhexidine gluconate (Hibiclens)
- Chloramine-T (Chlorazene)

Chloramine-T could be put into the water at the manufacturer-recommended dilutions and agitated for 10 minutes *following* removal of the wound to disinfect the tank. Then the tank can be emptied, scrubbed with a disinfectant, and refilled with fresh water.[3]

Use of Tap Water

Questions arise about the safety and efficacy of using plain tap water for wound cleansing and decontamination. A comparison study of 705 wounds looked at infection rates following wound cleansing with tap water and saline. It found that less infection occurred in wounds cleaned with tap water than with saline, and no bacteria were transferred to the wounds.[26] A comparison of normal saline and clean tap water wound irrigation used to remove bacteria from simple skin lacerations showed that both substances were comparable in reduction of bacterial counts.[69] Monitoring of local water supply for organisms has been useful in controlling nosocomial infection.[50]

Vigorous Rinsing

When a body or extremity is removed from the whirlpool, a layer of residue remains on the surfaces exposed to the water, just like the bathtub ring residue after a tub bath. This residue has many contaminants associated with it. A proven, safe method to reduce bacterial count is to follow whirlpool treatment with vigorous rinsing of the patient's skin and wound tissue with clean, warm water to remove the residue.[51,52] A shower may be the best method to cleanse a large body surface.

Aftercare

After the patient is removed from the whirlpool and rinsed with warm water, the wound should be debrided of any softened and loosened necrotic tissue, then rinsed again with warm tap water to remove loosened debris. After the final warm water rinse, the wound should be protected from cooling, contaminants, and desiccation. The best approach would be for the wound to be dressed immediately in the hydrotherapy area. If the setting does not allow for a complete dressing application while the patient is in hydrotherapy, a protective moist dressing, such as warm, saline-soaked gauze, should be placed in the wound and covered with a secondary dry dressing.

Infection Control for Whirlpool Equipment

The Centers for Disease Control and Prevention (CDC) and the American Physical Therapy Association (APTA) reviewed procedures for infection control in hydrotherapy and prepared a guide that is available through the APTA.[70] The procedures described here are adapted from the APTA guide. A copy of the guide would be valuable to all hydrotherapy departments.

Patients using whirlpools and other hydrotherapy tanks are often referred because of active infections. The infectious organisms and the organic debris are then deposited into the water. In warm water, steady temperature and agitation make it easy for bacterial pathogens to become harbored in the hydrotherapy equipment water pipes, drains, and other steel components associated with the device. These regions are difficult to clean and to disinfect or sterilize. In addition, the *Pseudomonas* bacteria has the ability to assume a sessile form, secreting a thick protective glycocalyx that colonizes the components described.[50] This increases the likelihood that highly contaminated water will contact the sites of open wounds, Foley catheters, and other percutaneous devices.

Besides the whirlpool tank and attached equipment, other equipment commonly used in the hydrotherapy department, such as Hoyer lifts, wheelchairs, and other transfer equipment, should be considered to be potential sources for colonization and transfer of infectious organisms.[70]

Procedure for Basic Cleaning of Hydrotherapy Equipment

Hydrotherapy equipment must be thoroughly cleansed to remove all foreign and organic materials from the object. Cleansing by vigorous manual scrubbing with detergents should precede disinfection procedures. The scrubbing should include the inside tank surfaces, the overflow pipes, the drains, the turbine shaft, and the thermometer shaft. The product chosen for cleaning should be an Environmental Protection Agency (EPA)-registered disinfectant.

- Because the cleaning procedures often involve actions that may cause splattering, the cleaner should wear gloves and goggles while cleaning. Follow precautions.
- Drain the hydrotherapy tank after each use.
- Rinse all inside tank surfaces with clean water.

Procedure for Disinfection of Hydrotherapy Equipment

An intermediate level of disinfection is recommended for all hydrotherapy equipment after treatment of patients with open wounds. Be sure that the exposure time to the disinfectant at label-recommended dilutions is equal to or not less than 10 minutes. Check with the housekeeping department for different choices of disinfection products that are in this category.

- Disinfection begins after the tank is cleaned and rinsed. Fill the tank with hot water, then add the disinfection product at the recommended dilutions. Expose all inside tank surfaces.
- The agitator needs to be disinfected also, which may be done separately by immersing it in a bucket with a solution of the disinfectant and running the agitator in the solution for 10 minutes.
- Following disinfection, drain and rinse the tank.
- Dry inside the tank with clean towels and keep the tank dry and covered until it is used again.
- Wipe all related hydrotherapy equipment surfaces with germicide after *each use.*[69]

Disinfection Products. A variety of disinfection products are on the market, and each formulation must be EPA-registered. These disinfectants are not interchangeable and should be reviewed for the varying performance characteristics of each.

Cleaning and Disinfection of Whirlpools with a Built-in Turbine Agitator. The procedure for cleaning and disinfecting whirlpools with built-in turbines/agitators differs slightly from the above listed procedures. The manufacturers of these whirlpools have specific instructions for spraying the internal turbine with a disinfecting solution. This disinfecting solution would need to remain in contact with the turbine for the time required, based on the product used. In all other respects, the cleaning procedure would be the same as that for other whirlpool tanks.

Culturing the Whirlpool and Related Equipment

Culturing is a controversial topic in the hydrotherapy area. One rationale for culturing is to prevent infection. To contribute to the prevention of infection, the results must be interpretable. The best definition of *interpretable* is that certain results lead to specific actions.[69] One school of thought is that if the best methods of disinfection are already accepted procedures, routine culturing of whirlpool and associated equipment is not going to cause a change in procedure and, therefore, is superfluous. Conversely, there are reports that careful monitoring of equipment and the water supply to identify potential sources of bacteria is useful in preventing outbreaks.[50]

Expected Outcomes

Prognosis for wounds treated by whirlpool is a change in tissue function in two to four weeks. Expect a wound treated for exudate and odor to be odor and exudate free in two weeks. Wounds that are treated for debridement should be necrosis free in two to four weeks, depending on volume of necrotic tissue present. Wounds that have a wound healing phase diagnosis of chronic inflammatory phase or absence of inflammatory phase should progress toward a wound healing phase of *acute inflammatory phase* in two weeks and to a wound acute proliferative healing phase in four to five weeks. The signs and symptoms of acute inflammation would include hyperemia, increased skin temperature, and mild edema, followed by a decrease in temperature by the end of the inflammatory phase and return to skin color to that of adjacent skin or comparable area on the opposite side of the body, progressing to a granulating, contracting wound in the proliferative phase, as seen in *Color Plates 1* and *2*.

The reported mean weekly healing rate from four studies in which whirlpool was used is 9.5% per week.[36,37,42,71] Burke et al[34] reported a 0.39 cm/week reduction in size but did not state the size of wounds; they also reported a 37.5% wound deterioration in the whirlpool group, with an overall outcome of healing for the treatment group and a 28% improvement and 61% deterioration in the nonwhirlpool group.[34] Payer's data from 1989 showed that wounds treated with whirlpool were usually treated for 3 months, with the presumed outcome a clean wound.[72] Wounds treated with other physical agents and advanced therapies have average lengths of treatment that range from 7.5 to 10.5 weeks, with closure as the reported outcome (see Chapters 22, 23, 24, 25). To be competitive, treatment with whirlpool must have comparable outcomes. If the wound is not progressing on the trajectory of healing, another intervention should be considered (see Table 26–1).

Self-Care Teaching Guidelines

After completing the diagnostic process, the PT may determine that hydrotherapy can be performed at home with a portable whirlpool unit attached to a bathtub. Grossly necrotic or purulent wounds are best not self treated until the necrosis and purulence are reduced to a level at which the patient and/or caregiver can manage them comfortably. Careful selection of the patient and caregiver must be made to have successful, safe and effective treatment results. The ability to understand and follow directions is critical. Bathtub cleansing and disinfection of the portable whirlpool is extremely important to avoid infection and sepsis. If in doubt about the ability to follow excellent disinfection procedures or if the patient is immune compromised (e.g. diabetic or on immune suppression drugs) do not recommend use of a portable whirlpool.

CLINICAL WISDOM

Instruct patients and caregivers to turn the home hot water heater down to 120°F and to always use a thermometer to test the water temperature before immersion to avoid burn injury.

- The patient and/or caregiver should be instructed in the correct water temperature, the duration of the immersion, how to rinse the wound after immersion, and the proper aftercare. A thermometer to take the water temperature should be used for safety to prevent burns. Some people believe that the water must be as hot as tolerable to be beneficial, and scald burns are common, especially in the elderly. Proper cleaning and disinfection procedures also must be taught for the tub and the portable agitator and thermometer.
- Patients with neuropathy should be instructed *never* to do home foot soaks or whirlpool because of the high risk of self-inflicted injury.
- Patients who are lethargic should have minimal soaking in tepid water, primarily for cleansing and softening of tissue, and this should be limited to single limb immersion
  - Instruct all patients and caregivers to monitor vital signs during the whirlpool treatment.
  - Teach the side effects of the treatment and how to respond to symptoms such as lightheadedness, dizziness, or lethargy.

- Explain the desired effects of the treatment and any symptoms that are undesirable. If the patient is being seen through a home care agency, a demonstration and return demonstration in the home, including repetition of instructions, is essential to ensure the correct care delivery. If this is not possible, perhaps a mock setup can be simulated in the hospital or clinic.
- Accountability is essential and encourages compliance. Set up a regular reporting schedule. A tracing of the wound by the therapist can be left with the patient, then laid over the wound for the patient or caregiver to compare changes in size and shape. It will also help to reinforce compliance with the treatment regimen. The changes can be reported to the PT by phone with periodic visits to monitor outcomes.

REVIEW QUESTIONS

1. What are five benefits of using whirlpool hydrotherapy?

2. How can temperature be used to modify therapeutic results?
3. How can risks of wound infection be mitigated?
4. What are 3 temperature precautions for using whirlpool hydrotherapy?
5. A diabetic patient has a neuropathic plantar ulcer over the 5th metatarsal head. Wound has callus of peri-wound tissue, granulation tissue in the wound bed with moist environment. There is no necrotic tissue or signs of re-epithelialization or infection. Ankle-brachial index is 1.2. Is this patient a candidate for whirlpool? Why?
6. A patient has chronic venous insufficiency with ulceration of the left tibia area proximal and superior to the medial malleolus. Wound originated following trauma. There is edema present and a grade II ulceration. There is minimal to no exudate, 100% granulation, no epithelialization, and no signs of infection. Ankle/brachial index is 1.0. Is this patient a candidate for whirlpool? Why?

■ CASE STUDY

Patient with Eschar on Both Heels

FUNCTIONAL OUTCOME REPORT

Patient Name: G.W.   Start of Care Date: 9/27

Medical History

84-yr-old, alert, confused black female. Nonambulatory resident of long-term care facility. Sits up in wheelchair and attends activity program. Medical diagnosis of Alzheimer disease, prior history of cerebrovascular accident (CVA). No prior history of pressure ulceration.

Reason for Referral

1. Dry, leathery eschar on both heels not responding to treatment with occlusive dressings. Indicates loss of healing capacity.
2. Need to determine severity of pressure ulcers on the heels.
3. Severely limited mobility and activity levels.

Systems Review and Exam

Circulatory System   Circulatory perfusion adequate for healing indicated by palpable pulses, warm feet, no significant leg edema, and ankle/brachial index (ABI) of 0.8, but produces inadequate response to wounding due to motor and joint impairment of lower extremities (loss of muscle pump function for circulation).

Musculoskeletal System   Musculoskeletal impairments of the lower extremities due to weakness, joint pain, and stiffness with contractures (10°) at the knees. Patient being positioned upright in wheelchair. Requires minimum assist to perform pivot transfer from bed to wheelchair. Weightbearing during transfer places stress on eschars. Unable to retain upright posture to ambulate and unable to reposition in wheelchair or bed for pressure relief.

Braden risk assessment scores each for activity and for mobility 2/4.

Neuromuscular System   Loss of volitional movements due to impaired neuromotor system. Loss of cognitive awareness of position. Loss of protective sensation to reposition (sensory impairment).

Cardiopulmonary System   No clinical signs of cardiopulmonary impairment. Probable diminished ventilation due to inactive mobility status and age.

Integumentary System   Adjacent and surrounding skin has normal skin color tones and turgor, compared with adjacent areas. No pain responses in wounded tissues.

Wound Healing Tissue Assessment   Bilateral heels crusted with hard dry eschar; impairment of integumentary integrity. No thermal changes at the margins of the eschars compared with adjacent tissues. No edema or erythema (color changes) signifies impairment of inflammation response. Unable to see the tissue status under the eschar; unable to determine extent/severity of tissue loss. Size: 25 cm² area of eschar on each heel.

Psychosocial   Patient unable to understand directions to reposition or exercise independently. Will follow guided movements. Needs caregiver intervention for repositioning, exercise, and transfers.

Functional Impairments and Functional Diagnosis   Loss of function in above systems causes the following:

1. Wound severity diagnosis: unable to stage impaired integumentary integrity associated with eschar on both heels. Removal of eschar needed to determine extent of wound depth.

(Continued)

■ **CASE STUDY** *(Continued)*

2. Wound healing phase diagnosis: absence of inflammatory phase and absence of proliferative phase. Needs restart of the inflammatory phase of healing after conversion to a clean wound that will progress through phases of healing.
3. Associated impairment of mobility and activity secondary to neuromuscular disability (Alzheimer disease and CVA).
4. Undue susceptibility to pressure ulceration on the feet due to motor and sensory impairment.
5. Low blood flow state but has adequate circulation to predict healing.

Short-Term Target Outcomes:		Due Date
Wounds:	Softening of eschar	3 days
	Debridement of eschar	7 days
	Shows evidence of inflammatory phase	14 days
	Shows evidence of proliferative phase	28 days
Mobility:	Nursing assistant will perform range-of-motion and guided exercise	3 days
	Therapeutic positioning in bed and wheelchair will be performed by nursing assistants all shifts	7 days
	Transfers with Multi-Podus-type splint	5 days

Prognosis: A clean stable wound with potential for closure in 28 days. Undue susceptibility to pressure ulcers on the feet due to impaired mobility and cognition will continue after wounds are healed. Wound closure in 90 days both heels.

Plan of Care with Rationale for Skilled Services

1. Multiple debridement methods required to hasten progression to clean wound bed

Procedures:
- Score eschar—to allow penetration of moisture
- Whirlpool to soak and soften tissue, enhance circulation daily
- Sharp debridement—incremental as tissue softens and loosens PRN
- Electrical stimulation—enhance microcirculation and stimulate cells leading to progression through phases of healing daily
- Enzymatic debridement daily—to hasten solubilization of necrotic tissues
- Autolysis with transparent film—to maintain moist wound environment to soften eschar
2. Therapeutic positioning to reduce risk of pressure and shearing to feet during transfers, in wheelchair, and in bed
3. Instruction of nurses' aides in range-of-motion and guided exercises to stimulate delivery of circulation to the tissues
4. Therapeutic exercise performed while in the whirlpool
5. Fitting of Multi-Podus-type splint

Target Outcomes Achieved at First Reassessment 10/1

Wound Status:
1. Eschar softened, partially debrided by day 4
2. Removal of outer eschar revealed two focal areas of necrosis covered by eschar
3. Wound has evidence of inflammatory phase: edema, increased warmth in surrounding tissues

Mobility:
1. Patient lying on pressure-relief support surface with pillows and Multi-Podus splint to relieve pressure
2. Patient sitting up in wheelchair with feet supported with Multi-Podus-type splint to relieve pressure during transfers
3. Range-of-motion and guided exercises by nurses' aide performed daily
4. Guided lower extremity exercise performed in the whirlpool

Reassessment 11/9

Wound Status:
1. Eschar free, yellow slough
2. Wound depth greater than 0.2 cm
3. Two interconnecting wounds (medial and lateral sides of heel with viable tissue connecting)
4. Wound healing phase progressed to proliferation phase—presence of contraction and granulation tissue

Mobility:
1. Patient is participating in daily exercise and range-of-motion regimen
2. Therapeutic positioning is in place for all shifts

Functional Impairments

1. Integumentary impairment secondary to full-thickness pressure ulcer on the heels
Target outcome: Clean proliferating and contracting wound—due date 21 days
2. Absence of epithelialization phase and sustained contraction
Target outcome: Progress to epithelialization phase and sustained contraction—due date 21 days

Revised Prognosis

Wound will heal to closure in 60 days.

Revised Treatment Plan and Target Outcomes

Need for Continuation of Skilled Services   Patient failed to respond to routine dressing and conservative management, is now responding to the treatment program. Treatment is done as a collaborative effort between the PT and nurse. Change in treatment interventions required due to change in wound status. Patient has demonstrated potential for healing following interventions but will continue to be at risk for pressure ulceration.

CASE STUDY _(Continued)_

Plan of Care (Intervention) with Rationale
- Discontinue whirlpool and sharp debridement tissue—neither needed to debride slough
- Continue electrical stimulation for microcirculation and stimulation of healing
- Discontinue enzymatic debridement—not needed to debride slough
- Change dressing to hydrogel and secondary dressing—to débride slough, for moist wound healing environment compatible with ES treatment regimen

Target Outcomes:

Clean wound bed	7 days
Proliferative phase: sustained contraction	14 days
Progress to epithelialization phase	21 days

Discharge Outcome
Wounds on both heels healed in 90 days from start of care.

Functional Outcome Reporting System methodology used with permission of Swanson and Co., Long Beach, CA.

REFERENCES

1. Bergstrom N, Bennett MA, Carlson C, et al. _Treatment of Pressure Ulcers._ Clinical Practice Guideline No. 15. Rockville, MD: Agency for Health Care Research and Quality (AHRQ), formerly known as the Agency for Health Care Policy and Research (AHCPR), U.S. Public Health Service (PHS), U.S. Department of Health and Human Services (DHHS); AHRQ Publication No. 95–0652. December 1994:45–65.
2. Feedar JA, Kloth LC. Conservative management of chronic wounds. In: Kloth LC, McCulloch JM, Feedar JA, eds. _Wound Healing: Alternatives in Management._ Philadelphia: FA Davis; 1990:135–172.
3. Walsh M. Hydrotherapy: the use of water as a therapeutic agent. In: Michlovitz S, ed. _Thermal Agents in Rehabilitation._ Philadelphia: FA Davis; third edition 1996:139–167
4. Shimizu T, Kosaka M, Fujishima K. Human thermoregulatory responses during prolonged walking in water at 25, 30 and 35 degrees C. _Eur J Appl Physiol Occup Physiol._ 1998;78(6):473–478.
5. Lopez M, et al. Rate and gender dependence of the sweating, vasoconstriction and shivering thresholds in humans. _Anesthesiol._ 1994;80(4):780–788.
6. Sessler DI. Mild perioperative hypothermia. _New Engl J Med._ 1997;336(24):1730–1736.
7. Kurz A, Sessler DI, Lenhart R. Perioperative normothermia to reduce the incidence of surgical-wound infection and shorten hospitalization. _New Engl J Med._ 1996;334(19):1209–1215.
8. Reed RL II, et al. Hypothermia and blood coagulation: dissociation between enzyme activity and clotting factor levels. _Circ Shock._ 1990;32(2):141–152.
9. Valeri CR, et al. Effect of skin temperature on platelet function in patients undergoing extracorporeal bypass. _J Thoracic Cardiovasc Surg._ 1992;104(1):108–116.
10. Michaelson AD, et al. Reversible inhibition of human platelet activation by hypothermia in vivo and in vitro. _Thromb Haemost._ 1994;71(5):633–640.
11. Lenhart R, et al. Relative contribution of skin and core temperatures to vasoconstriction and shivering thresholds during isoflurane anesthesia. _Anesthesiol._1999;91(2):422–429.
12. Abramson D, et al. Changes in blood flow, oxygen uptake and tissue temperatures produced by the topical application of wet heat. _Arch Phys Med Rehabil._ 1961;42:305–317.
13. Wessman HC, Kottke FJ. The effect of indirect heating on peripheral blood flow, pulse rate, blood pressure and temperature. _Arch Phys Med Rehabil._ 1967;48:567–576.
14. Rabkin JM, Hunt TK. Local heat increases blood flow and oxygen tension in wounds. _Arch Surg._ 1987;122:221–225.
15. Hopf H. _The Role of Warming and Oxygen Tension in Wounds._ Symposium on thermoregulation in wound care. Oxford, England: 1999.
16. Ikeda T, et al. Local radiant heating increase subcutaneous oxygen tension. _Am J Surg._ 1998;175:33–37.
17. Ikeda T, et al. The effect of three different local temperatures on subcutaneous oxygen tension. _Anesthesiol Analg._ 1997;84(2S).
18. Juve MB. Whirlpool therapy on postoperative pain and surgical wound healing: an exploration. _Patient Educ Couns._ 1998;33(1):39–48.
19. Hwang J, Himel H, Edlich R. Bilateral amputations following hydrotherapy tank burns in a paraplegic patient. _Burns._ 1995;21(1):70–71.
20. Kurz A, et al. Thermoregulatory response thresholds during spinal anesthesia. _Anesthesiol Analg._ 1993;77(4):721–726.
21. McCulloch JM, Boyd VB. The effects of whirlpool and the dependent position on lower extremity volume. _J Orthop Sports Phys Ther._ 1992;16:169.
22. Guyton AC, ed. _Textbook of Medical Physiology,_ 6th ed. Philadelphia: WB Saunders; 1981.
23. Alon G. _Antibiotics Enhancement by Transcutaneous Electrical Stimulation._ Presented at the Future Directions in Wound Healing Symposium; American Physical Therapy Association Scientific Meeting; June 1997.
24. Lock PM. The effect of temperature on mitosis at the edge of experimental wounds. In: Lundgren A, Soner AB, eds. _Symposia on Wound Healing: Plastic, Surgical and Dermatologic Aspects._ Sweden: Molndal; 1980:103–107.
25. Myers JA. Wound healing and the use of modern surgical dressing. _Pharm J._ 1982;229(6186):103–104.
26. Miller M, Dyson M. _Principles of Wound Care._ London: Macmillan Magazines Ltd; 1996:29–36.
27. Yang Q, Berghe D. Effect of temperature on in vitro proliferative activity of human umbilical vein endothelial cells. _Experientia._ 1995;51(2):126–132.
28. Xia Z, et al. Stimulation of fibroblast growth in vitro by intermittent radiant warming. _Wound Repair Regen._ 2000;8(2):138–144.
29. Park H-Y, Shon K, Phillips T. The effect of heat on inhibitory effects of chronic wound fluid on fibroblasts in vitro. _Wounds._ 1998;10(6):189–192.
30. Rush J, et al. The effects of whirlpool baths in labor: a randomized controlled trial. _Birth._ 1996;23(3):136–143.
31. Lenstrup C, et al. Warm tub bath during delivery. _Acta Obstet Gynecol Scand._ 1987;66(8):709–712.
32. Kloth LC, et al. Effects of normothermic dressing on pressure ulcer healing. _Adv Wound Care._ 2000;13(2):69–74.
33. Sussman C. The role of physical therapy in wound care. In: Krasner D, ed. _Chronic Wound Care: A Sourcebook for Health Care Professionals._ Wayne, PA: Health Management Publications; 1990:327–366.
34. Burke DT, et al. Effects of hydrotherapy on pressure ulcer healing. _Am J Phys Med Rehabil._ 1998;77(5):394–398.
35. Gogia PP, Hurt BS, Zirn TT. Wound management with whirlpool and infrared cold laser. _Phys Ther._ 1988;68(8):1239–1242.
36. Gogia P, Marquez R, Minerbo G. Effects of high voltage galvanic stimulation on wound healing. _Ostomy/Wound Manage._ 1992;38(1):29–35.
37. Gault W, Gatens PF. Use of low intensity direct current in management of ischemic skin ulcers. _Phys Ther._ 1976;56(3):141:145.
38. Akers T, Gabrielson A. The effect of high voltage galvanic stimulation on the rate of healing of decubitus ulcers. _Biomed Sci Instrum J._ 1984;20:99–100.
39. Thurman B, Christian E. Response of a serious circulatory lesion to electrical stimulation. _Phys Ther._ 1971;51(10):137–140.
40. Carley PJ, Wainapel S. Electrotherapy of acceleration of wound healing: low intensity direct current. _Arch Phys Med Rehabil._ 1985;66:443–446.
41. Wood JM, Evans PE III, Schallreuter KU, Jacobson WE, Sufit R. Newman J, et al. A multicenter study on the use of pulsed low intensity direct current for healing chronic Stage II and Stage III ulcers. _Arch Dermatol._ 1993;130(5):660–661.
42. Haynes L, et al. Comparison of Pulsavac and sterile whirlpool regarding the promotion of tissue granulation (abstract). _Phys Ther._ 1994;74(Suppl):S4.

43. Vetra H, Whittaker D. Hydrotherapy and topical collagenase for decubitus ulcers. *Geriatrics.* 1975;30:53–58.

44. Rodeheaver GT, Smith SL, Thacker JG, Edgerton MT, Edlich RF. Mechanical cleansing of contaminated wounds with a surfactant. *Am J Surg.* 1975;129(3):241–245.

45. Conolly WB, et al. Influence of distant trauma on local wound infection. *Surg Gynecol Obstet.* 1969;128(4):713–717..

46. Baron R, Willeke K. Respirable droplets from whirlpools: measurement of size, distribution and estimation of disease potential. *Environ Res.* 1986;39:8–18.

47. Highsmith AK, Kaylor BM, Calhoun MT. Microbiology of therapeutic water. *Clin Manage.* 1991;11(1):34–37.

48. Solomon SL. Host factors in whirlpool-associated *Pseudomonas aeruginosa* skin disease. *Infect Control.* 1985;6:402–406.

49. Jacobson JA. Pool-associated *Pseudomonas aeruginosa* dermatitis and other bathing-associated infections. *Infect Control.* 1985;6:398–401.

50. Shankowsky HA, Callioux LS, Tredget EE. North American survey of hydrotherapy in modern burn care. *J Burn Care Rehabil.* 1994;15:143–146.

51. Neiderhuber SS, Stribley RF, Koepke GH. Reduction of skin bacterial load with use of the therapeutic whirlpool. *Phys Ther.* 1975;5(5):482–486.

52. Bohannon R. Whirlpool versus whirlpool and rinse for removal of bacteria from a venous stasis ulcer. *Phys Ther.* 1982;62:304–308.

53. Swanson G. *Hydrotherapy Use in Standard Physical Therapist Practice Project.* Presented at class, University of Southern California, BKN 599. Los Angeles, CA; July 1997.

54. Cardany CR, Rodeheaver GT, Horowitz JH. Influence of hydrotherapy and antiseptic agents on burn wound bacterial contamination. *J Burn Care Rehabil.* 1985;6:230–232.

55. Stanwood W, Pinzur M. Risk of contamination of the wound in a hydrotherapeutic tank. *Foot Ankle Int.* 1998;19(3):173–176.

56. Hollyoak V, Boyd P, Freeman R. Whirlpool baths in nursing homes: use, maintenance and contamination with *Pseudomonas aeruginosa. Burn.* 1995;5(7):R102–R104.

57. Liefeldt L, Destanis P, Rupp K, Morgera S, Neumayer HH. The hazards of whirlpooling. *Lancet,* 2003:361(9356):534

58. Novotne J. Efficient bathing systems benefit patients and care givers. *DON.* July 1987:28–30.

59. McCulloch J. *Physical Modalities in Wound Management.* Preconference course. Presented at the Symposium on Advanced Wound Care; April 1995; San Diego, CA.

60. Loehne HB, et al. *Aerosolization of Microorganisms During Pulsatile Lavage with Suction.* In Combined Sections Meeting, American Physical Therapy Association; 2000; New Orleans, LA: APTA.

61. Thomson PD, Bowden ML, McDonald DK, Smith DJ Jr, Prasad JK. A survey of burn hydrotherapy in the United States. *J Burn Care Rehabil.* 1990;11(2):151–155.

62. Health Care Financing Administration. Coverage of Services, 3132.4. Woodlawn, MD: December 1987.

63. Blue Cross of North Carolina. Medicare Bulletin Number 98–9. December 1996, Part A Office, Durham, NC: 2–3.

64. Lineaweaver W, Howard R, Soucy D, et al. Topical antimicrobial toxicity. *Arch Surg.* 1985;120:267–270.

65. Kozol MD. Effects of sodium hypochlorite on cells of the wound module. *Arch Surg.* 1988;123:420–423.

66. Steve L, Goodhart P, Alexander J. Hydrotherapy burn treatment: Use of chloramine-T against resistant microorganisms. *Arch Phys Med Rehabil.* 1979;60:301–303.

67. Marquez RR. Wound debridement and hydrotherapy. In: Gogia P, ed. *Clinical Wound Management.* Thorofare, NJ: Slack; 1995:122–126.

68. Henderson JD, Leming JT, Melon-Niksa DB. Chloramine-T solutions: Effect on wound healing in guinea pigs. *Arch Phys Med Rehabil.* 1989;70(8):628–631.

69. Moscati R, et al. Comparison of normal saline with tap water for wound irrigation. *Am J Emerg Med.* 1998;16(4):379–381.

70. American Physical Therapy Association. *Hydrotherapy/Therapeutic Pool Infection Control Guidelines.* Alexandria, VA: American Physical Therapy Association; 1995:8–11.

71. Carley PJ, Wainapel S. Electrotherapy of acceleration of wound healing: Low intensity direct current. *Arch Phys Med Rehabil.* 1985;66:443–446.

72. Swanson G. Use of cost data, provider experience, and clinical guidelines in the transition to managed care. *J Insurance Med.* 1991;23(1):70–74.

Pulsatile Lavage with Suction

Harriett Baugh Loehne

CHAPTER OBJECTIVES

At the completion of this chapter, the reader will be able to:

1. List the indications and precautions of treatment with pulsatile lavage with suction.
2. Describe the benefits and outcomes of pulsatile lavage with suction.
3. Follow Occupational Safety and Health Administration, Centers for Disease Control and Prevention, and Federal Drug Administration guidelines for infection control.
4. Explain policies and procedures for treatment with pulsatile lavage with suction.
5. Describe the features of the products made by the three different manufacturers of pulsatile lavage with suction equipment.
6. Describe a device that provides jet lavage with and without suction.

Pulsatile lavage with suction (PLWS) is a method of wound care that provides cleansing and debridement with pulsed irrigation combined with suction. Battery-powered units are available, along with a selection of tips for cleansing and debridement of different wound configurations. The pulsed irrigant provides positive pressure, while suction provides negative pressure to remove the irrigant and debris to help reduce infection and to enhance granulation. This ultimately provides an improved foundation for wound healing.

Jet lavage via the Water Pik™ was first used by oral surgeons for soft tissue injuries in the Vietnam War.[1] Noting its efficacy, development of pulsed lavage with suction became a reality. Physicians have used these systems in the operating room since the early 1980s for irrigation in surgical procedures and to clean wounds of debris. Physical therapists (PTs) have used the systems since the late 1980s for irrigation and debridement to enhance healing of soft tissue wounds.

Theory and Science of the Therapy

Whirlpools traditionally have been the most common choice for hydrotherapy, with little demonstrable benefit.[2] Just as with whirlpool, there is limited research to support the use of PLWS for wound healing. There are numerous anecdotal reports and case studies of benefits, however.[3-5]

Haynes et al[6] reported that the rate of granulation tissue formation was 12.2% per week for wounds treated with PLWS and 4.8% per week for those treated with whirlpool. This study included six subjects as a control, using sterile whirlpool at one hospital, and seven subjects as an experimental group, using the Pulsavac (Zimmer Patient Care Division, Dover, Ohio) at another hospital. Photographs taken at initial evaluations and at discharge were entered into a computer for calculation of wound area and rate of wound closure. Data analysis used analysis of covariance. The increase in mean wound closure rate for all patients treated with whirlpool was 766.139 mm^2 per length of stay and for those treated with Pulsavac, it was 3373.690 mm^2. With the rate of wound closure significantly higher for those treated with Pulsavac versus sterile whirlpool, the authors state that PTs should consider that Pulsavac can decrease the healing time for a wound, as well as the hospitalization time required for the patient for wound treatment. The study concludes that, although there were many factors—both physiologically and environmentally—that could affect the rate of wound closure, the research suggested that treatment with PLWS promoted wound closure at a faster rate than did sterile whirlpool.

Other scientific and theoretic rationales for use of the therapy are as follows:

- It cleanses via gentle pulsatile lavage to stronger irrigation and debridement.
- It reduces bacteria and infection.

- It promotes granulation and epithelialization.
- Theory: The negative pressure of the suction stimulates granulation of clean wounds.

Management of Infection

Wound infection is a major concern in management of wounds. Dead and dying tissue, debris, clotted blood, and foreign bodies are predisposing conditions to wound infection. Rapid removal of these contaminants has been demonstrated to speed healing. Studies in the literature report that high-pressure pulsating irrigation in acute contaminated wounds decreases the presence of these contaminants and results in a lower incidence of wound infection.[7]

Debridement and irrigation are important methods for controlling infection in wounds. Different methods are described for irrigation of wounds, including bulb syringe, Water Pik, shower spray, spray bottles, and pulsatile irrigation/lavage. Irrigation pressures vary with use of these different devices. If the impact pressure is too low, below 4 pounds per square inch (psi), the lavage will not cleanse effectively. Safe, effective irrigation pressures range from 4 to 15 psi. Exhibit 27-1 includes the irrigation pressures obtained with these commonly used clinical devices.[8] A pressure of 8 psi has been found to be significantly effective in removing bacteria and infection.[9] Irrigation at 13 psi has been attributed to reduction of inflammation in traumatic wounds. Irrigation pressures exceeding 15 psi may traumatize tissue and drive bacteria into the wound tissues.[10,11] Stevenson et al[4] reportedly calculated and tested combinations of syringe and needle sizes to determine wound irrigating pressure. The pressure produced by a 35-mL syringe and a 19-gauge needle combination produced 8 psi. Irrigation pressure of a bulb syringe is 2 psi, which is not adequate to cleanse a wound.[8] The Water Pik ranges from 6 to more than 50 psi, which may cause trauma to a wound and drive bacteria into it.[10]

Comparison studies among gravity flow irrigation, bulb syringe, and jet lavage on removal of bacteria and foreign bodies in wounds showed that the number of bacteria in the jet lavage group was comparable with the 10^5 levels attributed to the body's ability to manage infection.[12] The pulsatile lavage systems, described later in this chapter, allow the psi to be adjusted. The psi treatment setting chosen will depend on the amount of necrotic tissue/exudate, the location of the wound, and the patient's comfort. Pulse rate, as well as psi, has been demonstrated clinically to effect granulation formation and epithelialization of clean wounds.[3]

The medical community has been concerned that high-pressure irrigation may drive bacteria and contaminants into a wound and adjacent tissues. Bierbaum[12] reviewed several studies that looked at this problem. A high pressure of 70 psi delivered 3 cm from the surface in moderately contaminated wounds was found to spread the fluid laterally, rather than beneath the wound surface; however, it also impaired tissue defenses. In heavily contaminated wounds, there was a 100-fold reduction in bacterial count after high-pressure irrigation.

Part of clinical decision making involves weighing the risk/benefit ratio. Sometimes multiple risks have to be considered when selecting a treatment intervention. For example, will the benefit of high-pressure cleansing of a highly contaminated wound outweigh the known risk of tissue trauma and have a better outcome than an inadequate response? PTs would not use high-pressure irrigation unless under the direct supervision of a physician. If the assessment indicates that high-pressure irrigation needs to be considered, it is a criterion for referral to the physician.

Pulsed jet lavage has been used for treatment of traumatic wounds in operating rooms and in the military for decades.[13] Delivery of vancomycin-, streptomycin-, and tetracycline-water solutions with pulsating jet lavage eliminated or reduced bacteria as early as the second day, with earlier healing, less tissue loss, and reduced scarring. Infected diabetic foot lesions treated with pulsatile lavage and topical antibiotics had infection controlled, and the wounds were able to be closed surgically with grafts or flaps. Reduced inflammation has been reported following pulsed lavage treatment and was correlated to the extent of foreign material remaining in the tissues. Early cleansing with this therapy accelerated wound healing.[12]

Wound cleansing with battery-powered, disposable pulsatile irrigation devices modeled after operating and emergency room equipment received favorable mention as an alternative to whirlpool therapy to minimize cross-contamination, decrease treatment time, speed healing, and shorten length of hospital stays. Additionally, these devices were recommended for their versatility and the ability to personalize treatment to provide a best outcome for the patient and the wound.[14] However, in a review of evidence,

EXHIBIT 27-1 Irrigation Pressures Delivered by Various Devices

Device	Irrigation Impact Pressure (PSI)
Spray bottle—Ultra Klenz	1.2
Bulb syringe	2.0
Piston irrigation syringe (60 mL) with catheter tip	4.2
Saline squeeze bottle (250 mL) with irrigation cap	4.5
Water Pik at lowest setting (1)	6.0
Irrijet DS syringe with tip	7.6
35-mL syringe with 19-gauge needle or angiocatheter	8.0
Water Pik at middle setting (3)	42
Water Pik at highest setting (5)	> 50
Pressurized Cannister-Dey-Wash	> 50

Reprinted from Bergstrom N, Bennett MA, Carlson CE, et al. *Treatment of Pressure Ulcers*, Clinical Practice Guideline No. 15, December, 1994, U.S. Department of Health and Human Services, Public Health Service, Agency for Health Care Policy and Research, AHCPR Publication No. 95-0652.

there were no controlled clinical trials to support efficacy for wound healing.[14]

Luedtke-Hoffmann and Schafer[15] reviewed the literature for effects of PLWS on wound cleansing and attempted to compare it with more traditional methods. Research comparing the effectiveness was scant. Pulsed lavage following whirlpool was more effective at removing bacterial contamination than was pulsed lavage alone.[16,17] They concluded that PLWS is a safe method of cleansing. Research shows no evidence of bacteremia after lavage applications, regardless of pressure, but until more research is done, impact psi should remain between 4 and 15 psi.[15]

Mechanical Debridement

Irrigation is an effective mechanical debridement method to loosen and flush out debris and bacteria from contaminated wounds. Fluid dynamics play an important role in expelling the loosened debris with the high-flowing irrigation stream. The incidence of wound infection is decreased as the amount of irrigation fluid increases.[12]

Pulsed stimulation of the tissue is also thought to affect wound debridement. The pulse phase rapidly compresses the tissue; then, during the interpulse phase, the tissue decompresses. This may be a mechanism for mechanically loosening debris. There is increased ease of sharp debridement after the treatment, due to the loosened and softened necrotic tissue.

PLWS is considered a strategy of debridement. There are no licensing boards in the United States that prohibit PTs from performing debridement (except for surgical debridement, which is outside the scope of practice of all PTs). Physical therapist assistants (PTAs) should get a ruling from their state boards as to the legality of their using PLWS.

Treatments with PLWS are coded with the rehab codes 97597 and 97598, the codes for sharp/selective debridement, which include PLWS. The codes are assigned according to the total size of the wound(s) treated. Total treatment areas of less than 20 sq cm are coded 97597; areas of more than 20 sq cm are coded 97598. Each code can be used only once per treatment session, regardless of the number of different types of selective debridement utilized. Whirlpool is not included in these codes and cannot be charged if utilized for "debridement."

CLINICAL WISDOM

CPT Codes

New CPT codes 97597 and 97598 for selective debridement, which include PLWS, were effective in January 2005.

Negative Pressure

Concurrent suction with pulsatile lavage appears to stimulate production of granulation tissue in "clean" wounds as a result of the negative pressure.[18] Negative pressure applies noncompressive mechanical forces to the tissues and dilates arterioles. Dilatation allows increased blood flow and tran-

scutaneous oxygen delivery to the tissues.[19] Suction also removes debris, bacteria, and irrigant. This theory of negative pressure by the author is based on the work of Argenta and Morykwas in the development of the V.A.C.™

Indications for Therapy

The author's clinical experience includes use of PLWS for both clean and infected wounds of many etiologies. Wounds that have benefited from this therapy are included in the list shown in Exhibit 27-2.

Patient Benefits

Patients derive many benefits from treatment by PLWS. Frequently, the patient can be treated by the PT instead of the physician in the operating room, with significant cost savings. Treatment has contributed to the salvage of limbs.[3] Periwound maceration is avoided with site-specific treatment. There is improved safety with no transfers into/out of the whirlpool, as well as improved comfort with no change in temperature and the ability to control the pressure of the fluid on the wound.

A retrospective study by Ho et al in 2004 examined charts of patients treated with PLWS from January 2001 to April 2003. Charts of 27 patients with pressure ulcers treated with PLWS were reviewed to determine the safety profile of this treatment. The results indicated a favourable safety profile, with no documented complaint of pain, moderate or severe bleeding, significant wound infection, or autonomic dysreflexia due to treatment.[20]

Patient benefits are summarized as follows:

- PLWS offers cost savings if operating room is not needed.
- It has contributed to salvage of limbs.
- It has improved safety.
- It offers improved comfort.
- Periwound maceration is avoided.
- It can be used for treatment of tracts, tunnels, and undermining (Figure 27-1).
- Treatment is possible if whirlpool treatment is contraindicated.
- Treatment is possible if whirlpool treatment is inaccessible.

CLINICAL WISDOM

Irrigation and Debridement of Tracts and Tunnels

Pulsatile irrigation is an excellent choice for irrigation and debridement of tracts, tunnels, and/or undermining.

Patients who would benefit from hydrotherapy but are contraindicated for whirlpool should be considered for pulsatile lavage, such as those who are unresponsive, have cardiopulmonary compromise or venous insufficiency, a diagnosis of diabetes/neuropathy, and/or those who are febrile or incontinent. Pulsatile lavage also can be offered to patients who cannot be placed in the whirlpool because of contrac-

EXHIBIT 27-2 **Examples of Indications for Pulsed Lavage**

Type or Wound/Patient History	Rationale
Venous insufficiency ulcer A patient with a history of chronic leg wounds hit the pretibial area of his right lower extremity on a table leg 6 months ago. He has had open wounds on the lower extremity since then. The lower extremity is also edematous and there is periwound maceration. The patient is using a compression stocking.	If pulsed lavage with suction is used, the wounds can be treated with the lower extremity elevated to avoid increased edema. Treatment is site-specific, so periwound maceration is not increased. Granulation and epithelialization can be stimulated, possibly by negative pressure of the suction.
Neuropathic ulcer A patient with diabetes and loss of protective sensation in both feet has an ulcer on the plantar surface of his left heel. He has a callus with a fragile area in the center at the head of the 5th metatarsal.	Instead of soaking the foot in a whirlpool, pulsed lavage with suction will offer site-specific treatment that will not compromise the callus and fragile area. In addition, the patient's lower extremity will not be in a dependent position, thereby avoiding edema, and the patient's skin will not be burned due to loss of sensation (a risk with whirlpool).
Pressure ulcer A paraplegic patient with bowel and bladder incontinence has a large sacral pressure ulcer.	An incontinent patient cannot be immersed in a whirlpool, but incontinence is not a contraindication to pulsed lavage with suction. Even if the patient were not incontinent, his wound would be difficult to treat in a whirlpool because he would have to lie on his sacrum, putting pressure on the wound site. In addition, he would have to be transported to physical therapy on a hard stretcher. This is not necessary with pulsed lavage because it is a bedside procedure.
Sternal wound Following coronary artery bypass graft surgery, a patient develops a wound infection and dehiscence. She is on a cardiac monitor and ventilator in the intensive care unit.	This patient's wound can be irrigated and debrided at the bedside using pulsed lavage with suction. Whirlpool immersion is not an option because of her medical equipment—cardiac electrodes cannot be placed in water.
Perineal wound A patient has Fournier's gangrene with multiple deep, narrow tunnels; there is purulent drainage with a foul odor. The patient is septic with a temperature of 105°F.	Whirlpool is contraindicated for a febrile patient. Pulsed lavage with suction is the alternative, using a product with a flexible tip to allow irrigation and debridement of the tunnels and to decrease the bacterial count.
Partial-take split-thickness skin graft A patient with pyoderma gangrenosum has had a split-thickness skin graft on the right lower extremity. There has been only partial take, with eschar and necrotic slough at the failed site.	Because pulsed lavage with suction is site-specific, it can be used to treat only the failed portion of the graft without compromising the remainder of the graft. Eschar will be hydrated enough to allow sharp debridement (escharotomy) following pulsed lavage.
Fasciotomies A patient with multiple fractures to his left lower extremity secondary to a motor vehicle accident is in skeletal traction. Medial and lateral fasciotomies have been performed, due to edema, and now there is periwound erythema and purulent drainage from tunnels and undermining.	Traction can be maintained and the wounds can be treated without disturbing the hardware if pulsed lavage with suction is used. The tracts can be irrigated using a device with a long, flexible tip.

Used with permission from *Advances in Skin and Wound Care* 2000 May/June 13 (3): 133–134, © Springhouse Corporation/ www.springnet.com.

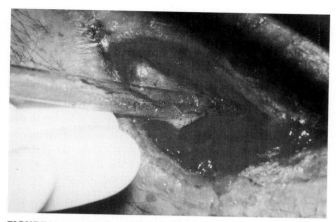

FIGURE 27-1 Gunshot wound with tunnel.

tures; ostomies; incisions with intact sutures; IV placement; skeletal traction; casted extremities; obesity; confinement to the intensive care unit (ICU), intermediate care unit (IMCU), burn unit, or isolation (negative pressure room); or combativeness/restraints.

Treatment is possible for the following conditions if whirlpool treatment is contraindicated:

• Unresponsiveness
• Cardiopulmonary compromise
• Venous insufficiency
• Neuropathy/diabetes
• Fever
• Incontinence if body whirlpool is required

Treatment is possible in the following circumstances if whirlpool treatment is inaccessible:

• Contractures—difficult body placement
• Ostomies
• Closed incisions with sutures intact
• IV placement
• Skeletal traction
• Casted extremities
• Obesity exceeding weight limit for stretcher/whirlpool
• Patient combative/restrained
• Patient in ICU, IMCU, burn unit, or isolation (negative pressure room)

PT Benefits

The PT is able to use time more efficiently and effectively when performing PLWS as compared with whirlpool. A pulsatile lavage treatment can take 15 to 30 minutes, compared with 45 to 60 minutes of the therapist's time for a whirlpool treatment. It is convenient because there is no need to fill, drain, and clean a whirlpool. Clean up is minimized because all supplies are disposable. This makes it possible for the PT to schedule more treatment visits. The design of the devices used for PLWS provides the PT with the ability to control the intensity of the treatment, in pounds per square inch, and to select the correct tip for specific ef-

fects, leading to optimal results while safeguarding tissue. Some units allow greater control than others. Therefore, it is important that the PT be aware of parameters and the limitations of the available equipment.

Sharp debridement is significantly easier after PLWS treatment because of the presence of loosened, softened debris and necrotic tissue. PT benefits are summarized as follows:

• There is no destruction of granulation tissue if 4–15 psi impact pressure is used.
• There is increased efficiency with increased productivity.
• The PT has the ability to control psi.
• Ease of sharp debridement is increased after treatment.
• Treatment is convenient.
• Clean up is minimized.

Facility Benefits

In an acute care facility, PLWS contributes to a decreased length of stay because of the rapid rate of granulation and epithelialization. Patients can be discharged home with dressing changes sooner than if not treated with PLWS. Wounds treated with PLWS are ready for grafting/flap surgery more quickly. Physician and staff time is saved if the patient is treated with PLWS by the PT and does not have to be taken to the operating room for irrigation and debridement by the surgeon. Cross-contamination is virtually eliminated because all supplies are disposable. This is especially important with infection control issues for blood-borne pathogens (BBP) and the spread of methicillin-resistant *Staphylococcus aureus* (MRSA) and vancomycin-resistant enterococci (VRE). There are potential cost savings by using pulsed lavage with suction compared to whirlpool that include: no need to buy whirlpools, the disinfectant to clean them, the water and the power to heat the water, and the staff to maintain them. Facility benefits are summarized as follows:

• The length of stay is decreased because of the rapid rate of granulation and epithelialization.
• Physician and operating room staff time is saved.
• Cross-contamination is eliminated.
• Cost savings are gained with elimination of whirlpools.

Precautions

The most important three words to remember when treating a patient with PLWS are: ***know your anatomy!*** As with any method of debridement, it is imperative to have a strong anatomy background, enhanced by cadaver dissection, and to have an illustrated textbook in close proximity. Just as important is awareness of the possibility of anomalies. When unsure of specific anatomy, it is recommended that the patient's surgeon be contacted for edification regarding exposed and nearby structures. This is especially true when irrigating tracts and undermining.

There are no known absolute contraindications to treatment with PLWS. As with any wound care treatment, however, certain precautions should be observed. These precautions apply to treatment of the following:

- Insensate patients
- Those taking anticoagulant medication
- Those with wounds with tracts, tunnels, and/or undermining

Experienced therapists will treat wounds that require extra attention to the entire procedure (see *Color Plate 83*). These include the following:

- Wounds near major vessels (e.g., in the groin or axilla)
- Wounds near a cavity lining (e.g., pericardium or peritoneum)
- Bypass graft sites, anastomoses
- Exposed vessel, nerve, tendon, bone
- Grafts, flaps
- Facial wounds

Certain wounds should be assessed carefully before being treated in a facility or home where a physician and emergency medical aid are not immediately available. Careful decision making is needed before treating wounds near major vessels, cavity linings, and bypass graft sites outside of an acute care hospital or hospital outpatient setting.

Outcome Measures

Clinical decision making involves evaluation of intervention choices to achieve a desired outcome. PLWS is a very versatile treatment choice. As discussed earlier, it can be used for all wounds in which the expected functional outcome is infection free, necrosis free, inflammation free, exudate free wound base filled with good granulation, in preparation for closure by secondary intention or surgery.

Wound closure by secondary intention or preparation for surgical closure and limb salvage with an intention of PLWS are reported in case studies.[3,12] Surrounding skin is protected from maceration. Because there are no controlled clinical trials of this therapy to compare, they cannot be used as a guide to length of time to achieve an expected outcome. Clinical judgment of the author suggests that the clinician should expect a decrease in necrotic tissue in 1 week and an increase in granulation/epithelialization in 1 week (see *Color Plates 82* and *83*). Following are some additional expected clinical outcomes:

- Odor and exudate free: 3–7 days
- Necrosis free: 2 weeks
- Progression from chronic inflammatory phase to acute inflammatory phase: 1 week
- Progression from acute inflammatory phase to proliferation phase: 2 weeks

A clinical outcome is one type of expected outcome. Another type of outcome to be considered is cost. The cost of an outcome includes many factors, such as labor, supplies, and length of stay. For example, the average treatment time with pulsatile irrigation is 15–30 minutes, compared with 45–60 minutes for a whirlpool treatment. Infection control costs are minimal because of single-use, disposable components. Cross-contamination is virtually eliminated. These are very important cost-management factors in facilities that must work continuously to control contamination with BBP, MRSA, and VRE. Debridement with pulsatile irrigation with suction can be performed as a physical therapy procedure, rather than as a surgical procedure. This reduces surgeon and operating room costs.

Patient and caregiver satisfaction surveys monitor perceptions of how patients feel about the treatment they received and how it has affected function. Patients want to feel safe, secure, and comfortable during the treatment procedure. They may be scared about the consequences of failure to heal. Some are unable to attend a therapy session in the PT department. Treatment with pulsatile lavage can be given at the bedside with no need for lifts and transfers. Because of its portability and disposable components, it is an ideal modality for home treatment.

Frequency and Duration

Patients are usually treated once a day. If the wound has more than 50% necrotic/nonviable tissue with purulent drainage/foul odor, and especially if sepsis is present, treatment twice a day is reasonable. Treatment two or three times a week is recommended if there is a full granulation base, no odor, and no purulent drainage. If the wound is being treated with negative pressure wound therapy (NPWT), such as the vacuum-assisted closure (VAC, Kinetic Concepts, San Antonio, TX [described further later in the text] device), PLWS is used with each VAC change, usually two or three times a week. PLWS should be discontinued when the wound is closed, there is no increase in granulation/epithelialization in 1 week, or there is no decrease in necrotic tissue in 1 week (Exhibit 27-3).

Cautions

Treatment should be stopped if the patient complains of increased pain or is unable to tolerate treatment because of pain. A premedication order may be needed from the patient's physician. With an arterial bleeder, treatment must be stopped immediately and the physician called immediately. Any other bleeding not stopped with pressure within 10 minutes requires a physician consultation. If an abscess other than the one being treated is opened or a bone/joint disarticulation occurs, the physician also should be notified. Cautions are summarized as follows:

- Stop treatment when the following occurs:
  1. Patient complains of increased pain.
  2. Patient is unable to tolerate treatment because of pain.
- Stop and call physician in any of the following circumstances:
  1. Patient has an arterial bleeder; notify physician immediately.

EXHIBIT 27-3   Frequency and Duration of Treatment

Frequency	Daily	Twice Daily	Three Times/Week	Discontinue
Most wounds	X			
> 50% necrotic		X		
Purulent drainage		X		
Sepsis		X		
Full granulation base			X	
VAC being used			X	
Duration				
No increased granulation for 1 week				X
No decreased necrotic tissue for 1 week				X
Wound closed				X

2. Bleeding has not stopped after 10 minutes of pressure.
3. Abscess is opened.
4. Joint is disarticulated.

CLINICAL WISDOM

Prevent Disruption of Clot Following Pressure to Stop Bleeding

After applying pressure over gauze packing to stop bleeding and bleeding has stopped, leave the bottom layer of gauze in place to avoid disruption of the clot and restarting of the bleeding. Cover with the prescribed dressing.

Vacuum-assisted Closure

KCI's VAC is a device that uses a pump, attached by tubing to a foam dressing placed in the wound, to create a vacuum to remove fluid. The negative pressure on the wound helps to reduce edema, increase blood supply, and decrease bacterial colonization. The procedure increases tension among the surrounding cells, which encourages cell growth and division, drawing the edges of the wound to the center and assisting wound closure. It provides a moist wound environment to promote more effective cellular activity; it also helps to prevent contamination of the wound site from outside bacteria. Other NPWT devices are being manufactured.

Details and use of the VAC are described in Chapter 12. There is frequently confusion among patients and clinical personnel due to the similarity in the names *VAC* (originally called *Decubivac* and *Dvac*) and *Pulsavac*. These are two entirely different interventions for wound management, though, indeed, they complement each other. The combination of the VAC and pulsed lavage has healed wounds four times faster than nontreated wounds, producing extraordinary cost savings.

CLINICAL WISDOM

NPWT and PLWS

NPWT and PLWS used in conjunction with each other provide an optimal intervention for management.

Performance of PLWS

Procedures for PLWS

Procedure Setup

Most patients ideally are treated on a high-low stretcher, bed, or treatment table adjusted to a height that ensures the therapist's proper body mechanics. Treatment may be delivered in a private treatment room in the physical therapy department or elsewhere, or at bedside in the patient's private room. A fluid-proof or fluid-resistant pad is placed under the body part with the wound, and clean towels are strategically placed around the wound and covering adjacent body parts, IV sites, and other portals of entry. An aseptic field is set up, with treatment and dressing supplies in easy reach. A strong light source is important during pulsatile lavage and debridement.

Outpatients with lower extremity wounds can be treated while seated in a wheelchair with an elevating footrest, with towels padding the footrest. The therapist sits on a low footstool in front of the patient and in easy reach of the aseptic field setup of treatment and dressing supplies. A basin can be placed under the foot to catch any overflow of irrigant.

An aide is invaluable for efficiency and assistance with difficult body placement in treatment of some wounds. Duties vary, depending on the system used. Connecting the tubing to the suction source, warming and spiking the bags of fluid, and emptying and replacing the filled suction canisters and new fluid bags are common procedures that can be done by the aide, saving the therapist time and from having to change gloves during treatment. After the treatment is completed, the aide also can dispose of the personal protective equipment, old dressings, and disposables while the therapist completes the documentation.

Infection Control

Standard Precautions. Protocols should adhere to each facility's policy, which can be more, but not less, stringent than Occupational Safety and Health Administration (OSHA) guidelines.[21] The importance of hand hygiene, including hand washing at the sink or use of an alcohol-based hand sanitizer, before and after the use of gloves cannot be overemphasized.[22]

In 2003 there was an outbreak of a multidrug-resistant bacteria in a hospital in the United States that was traced to patients being treated with PLWS. Some of the patients died. The spread of the bacteria was apparently due to environmental contamination attributed to PLWS being utilized without proper personal protective equipment (PPE) and other infection control techniques. As a result the CDC and FDA investigated and made recommendations for infection control guidelines for treatment with PLWS, based on the following information, which has been included in this chapter since the first edition. Additional recommendations were made and are discussed below.[23,24]

Due to aerosolization of microorganisms during treatment, as evidenced in a study by Loehne et al,[25] the patient should be treated in a private room with walls and doors that shut, not privacy curtains or open areas. On admission to the facility, if wound management with PLWS is anticipated and PTs provide the treatment at bedside, the patient should be assigned a private room as a medical necessity. This should be included in the facility's policies and procedures. (Exhibit 27-4.)

If the patient is treated at the bedside, all visitors should leave the room during treatment. If treated at home, family members/visitors should leave the room during treatment. All IV sites and other portals of entry on the patient, as well as wounds not being treated, should be covered with a clean towel.

All exposed linen used to control splash should be placed in a clear plastic biohazard bag after treatment for transport to the laundry. Disinfect the stretcher/wheelchair after each treatment if it is used to transport and treat the patient. Do not use a mattress or cushion with tears in the protective covering. Use basins to contain the irrigant overflow with treatment of extremity wounds. Disinfect the basin after each use. Clean the dressing cart with an approved disin-fectant solution after each use. Reusable face shields should be cleaned with a disinfectant that has been approved as effective against HIV, hepatitis B, and tuberculosis. Dispose of all disposables in the appropriate waste stream per OSHA guidelines.

Additional guidelines include considering use of a surgical mask for the patient during treatment. Thoroughly clean and disinfect all horizontal surfaces that can be touched by hand (e.g., bed rails, pumps) after treatment. There should be no supplies in open shelves or cabinets; do not open drawers during treatment. Cover any exposed supplies or personal articles with a clean towel. Do not reuse single use only items.

Personal Protective Equipment. Secondary to aerosolization and splashing, all staff present during treatment must wear personal protective equipment, consisting of the following:[26] (Figure 27-2):

- Surgical masks
- Hair covers (with ears covered)
- Face shields
- Fluid-proof (not fluid-resistant) gowns
- Fluid-resistant shoe covers (at the therapist's discretion for the aide)
- Nonsterile/sterile gloves with extra long cuffs to cover cuffs of gown

---

CLINICAL WISDOM

Follow Infection Control Guidelines for Treatment with PLWS

To avoid spreading bacteria with resultant morbidity and mortality, follow the suggested guidelines for infection control procedures while treating patients with PLWS.

Single Use Only. All disposables except two discussed below are marked for single use only. The FDA and OSHA mandate compliance. In fact, if used more than one time, Medicare and other payers consider the occurrence investigational and not reimbursable. Legal liability is possible if disposables are reused.

Davol (Figure 27-3) and Stryker each have suction diverter tips that allows the same handpiece to be used multiple times with the *same* patient, with a new tip being utilized at different treatment times. This is due to the fact that the suction mechanism is diverted from the interior mechanism of the product. Otherwise, units cannot be cleaned without damaging the product or being assured that all contaminants and/or disinfection material is removed.

The handpieces used with suction diverter tips must be properly stored between treatments on the same patient. The irrigation port must be plugged, the IV tubing spike capped, and all placed in a storage bag and labeled with the patient's name, medical record number, and date. The facility sets the maximum time to be used before disposal of the handpiece, usually one week or five treatments. Remember that with

---

EXHIBIT 27-4   Summary of Infection Control Guidelines for Treatment with PLWS

1. Treat patient in private room, appropriately ventilated, with walls and doors that close
2. Cover any exposed supplies or patient's personal items
3. Cover any exposed tubes, ports, etc., and any wounds not being treated
4. Consider masking the patient
5. No family or visitors in room during treatment
6. Observe standard precautions, including hand hygiene
7. Staff must wear appropriate PPE
8. Dispose of disposables in appropriate waste stream
9. Discard suction canister or liner as appropriate, after each treatment
10. Do not reuse single use only items
11. After treatment, thoroughly disinfect all environmental surfaces touched

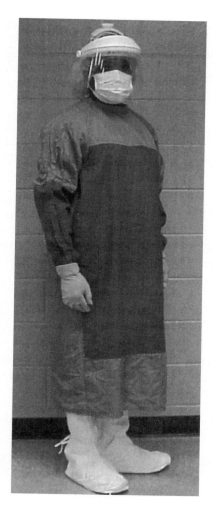

A

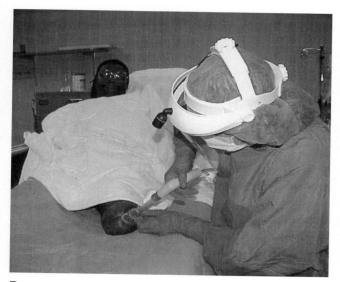

B

FIGURE 27-2 Personal protective equipment for hydrotherapy treatment.

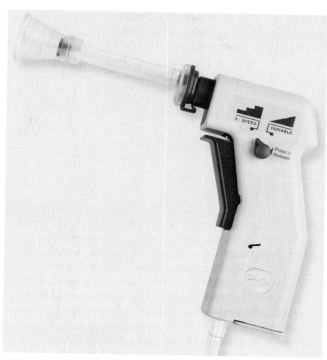

FIGURE 27-3 Simpulse® VariCare® System. (Courtesy of Davol, Inc., Cranston, Rhode Island.)

continued usage, the battery strength will be diminished, and therefore so will the PSI.

Even with FDA approval, this author has reservations about the ability to disinfect the external components of the product, such that the device can be stored and reused without concern for contamination. It also requires time, products, and space to disinfect and store. It precludes sterile procedure except for the first usage. The Davol VariCare now has a protective sleeve to cover the handpiece during treatment, which increases protection from contamination. The sleeve and a storage bag are provided with each tip package.

> ### CLINICAL WISDOM
> #### Single Use Only
> Use of PLWS products only one time with disposal after use ensures no cross-contamination between patient treatments.

Latex Content

All battery products used (Exhibit 27-5) are latex-free. Therefore, latex-sensitive and latex-allergic patients, especially those with myelodysplasia, may be treated with PLWS.[27] The latex-allergic therapist is not at risk even if latex were a part of the product, as gloves are worn during treatment.

Equipment Needed

Power Unit. All products are powered by batteries, and the products are completely disposable. (Exhibit 27-6). The

EXHIBIT 27-5 Latex Content of Products

Latex	Davol	Stryker	Zimmer
Not present	VariCare	SurgiLav InterPulse	Pulsavac Plus LP

EXHIBIT 27-6 Products Available and Power Source

Power Source	Davol	Stryker	Zimmer
Batteries—unit disposable	VariCare	SurgiLav Plus InterPulse	Pulsavac Plus LP

batteries in the Davol product can be removed easily without contamination and can be recycled. The batteries in the Stryker and Zimmer products cannot be easily removed from the battery case and should be discarded. Stryker offers also a rechargeable battery option. A rechargeable power pack, charger station, and rechargeable handpieces are available.

Tips. Sterile debridement tips include a small splash shield for soft tissue debridement and general irrigation, and long, flexible tips for undermining, tracts, and tunnels (Exhibit 27-7). Multiple other tips are available, depending on the manufacturer; however, most of these are utilized by physicians in the operating room. The PT needs only the small splash shield and the long, narrow, flexible tips, although new tips are in product development.

If using the Zimmer Pulsavac Plus LP small splash shield, the hard shield covering the soft shield should be retracted and not used during treatment. The small, pliable splash shield on all products placed in total contact with the tissue is recommended to obtain adequate suction for negative pressure, unless in undermining or tunnels. The flexible tips have measurement markings in centimeters to allow for safe and accurate measurement of extensive undermining, tracts, and tunnels. The flexible tips should be inserted and retracted continuously during treatment to irrigate and débride the entire area of the wound. The same tip can be used for treating multiple wounds on the same patient in the same treatment session, if the least necrotic wounds are treated first. Figure 27-4 shows a wound view with an irrigation tip.

All products have hand controls and tubing for spiking the saline bag (Figure 27-5).

Irrigation Fluid. Normal saline (0.9% sodium chloride) is preferred. Antibiotics can be added with a physician's order.

Water is not recommended because it is not physiologic. Antiseptic agents or skin cleansers (povidone-iodine, iodophor, sodium hypochlorite, hydrogen peroxide, and acetic acid) should not be used due to cytotoxicity to normal and/or wound tissue.[10]

Saline bags should be warmed to 39–41°C with a fluid warmer or in hot tap water. The number of bags used depends on the number and size of the wounds, the amount of necrotic tissue and exudate, and the patient's tolerance of the procedure.

Suction. Either a wall suction or portable pump is necessary for this modality. Equipment includes canisters, a regulator, and connecting tubing, which is required if the suction source is too far away from the wound with the tubing provided.

The suction removes debris, bacteria, and the irrigant, and provides negative pressure to increase the rate of granulation tissue.[8] Parameters are usually 60–100 mm Hg of continuous suction. It should be decreased if there is bleeding, if the wound is near a vessel or cavity, or if the patient complains of pain.

CLINICAL WISDOM

Importance of Impact Pressure

It is very important for the therapist to control and to know the *impact* pressure at all times during the treatment. ∎

Pressure

Pressure is measured in psi. If the pressure is too high, bacteria and foreign matter can be forced into viable tissue, and granulation and epithelial tissues can be damaged. The Agency for Health Care Research and Quality (formerly

EXHIBIT 27-7 Most Often Used Tips for Soft Tissue Wound Care

Tip	Davol	Stryker SurgiLav	Stryker Interpulse	Zimmer
Fan spray with splash shield	Yes	Yes	Yes	Yes
Retractable splash shield	Yes	No	No	No
Fan spray without splash shield	No	No	No	Yes
Shower with splash shield	No	Yes	No	Yes
Shower without splash shield	No	No	No	Yes
Open tract	Yes	No	No	No
Narrow open tract	Yes	No	No	No
Flexible, narrow open tract with suction	Yes	No	Yes	Yes
Flexible, narrow open tract without suction	No	No	Yes	No
Suction diverter tips	Yes	Yes		No

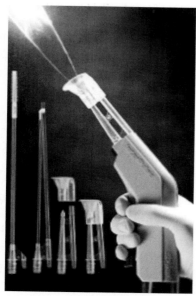

FIGURE 27-4 SurgiLav with a tip. (Courtesy of Stryker Instruments Kalamazoo, MI.)

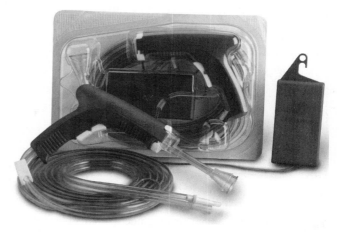

FIGURE 27-5 Pulsavac Plus LP, hand controls, and tubing pack. (Courtesy of Zimmer, Inc.)

known as the Agency for Health Care Policy and Research) guidelines recommend a treatment range of 4 to 15 psi.[8]

Initiation of treatment is usually 4 to 6 psi, with a typical range of 8 to 12 psi. A setting of 4 to 6 psi is advised for tracts, tunnels, and undermining, due to inability to visualize the wound base and nearby structures. Treatment with greater than 15 psi should be undertaken only if the physician is present and with a specific written order (Exhibit 27-8).

During treatment, psi should be increased in the presence of tough eschar and excessive necrotic tissue. It should be decreased if the patient complains of pain, if bleeding occurs, or if the tip is near a major or exposed vessel, nerve, tendon, or cavity lining. Exhibit 27-9 provides the pressure range and control available on various pressure products.

Jet Lavage

Although not providing pulsed lavage, it is worth noting that recent products on the market—Jetox™-ND without suction and Jetox™-HDC with suction (DeRoyal)—provide through jet lavage a relatively painless wound cleansing and debridement without a power source. The device was developed in Israel in the 1990s and patented in the United States in 2001. It uses compressed oxygen with a small amount of saline (1.5 ml /min) solution to administer a gentle jet stream. Saline recommended is 0.9% sodium chloride. The microdrops are between 5–100 microns and are accelerated up to 200 meters per second. A desensitizing effect is created due to the air generated through the oxygen source, making it beneficial for those patients whose wounds are hypersensitive.

Easily portable, this latex-free device can be used in the clinic, at bedside, or in the home, requiring only an oxygen source. Proper personal protective equipment is required for treatment with jet lavage, as with all lavage therapies. The shield should be placed against the treatment area to maintain optimum treatment distance. PSI is listed in Exhibit 27-10. Treatment with Jetox-ND is utilized until loose debris and exudate are sufficiently removed. It is single use only and completely disposable. There are at present no published studies addressing the efficacy of Jetox-ND treatment.

EXHIBIT 27-8 Pressure Used

Pulsatile Lavage with Suction					
PSI	**4–6 psi**	**4 psi**	**8–12 psi**	**15 psi**	**16+ psi**
Initiation	X				
Tracts/undermining	X				
Minimum effective		X			
Typical range			X		
Maximum—PT				X	
With physician present					X

EXHIBIT 27-9　Pressure Range and Control Available (On/Off Control on All Handpieces)

Product	PSI Range	Adjust at Source	Vary at Hand Control
Davol VariCare	Small splash shield: o Low: 3.8 o Medium: 9.6 o High: 11.2 o Variable: 0–11.3 Flexible: 2–6	No	Dial controls—Variable and three settings: low, medium, high
Stryker SurgiLav Plus	Shower: 8–14 Fan: 2–4 Concentrated spray: 4–6	No	Switch with two settings
Interpulse	Fan: 4–6 Coaxial fan: 4–8 Soft tissue: 10–12 Flexible with suction: 6–9 Flexible no suction: 12–14	No	Trigger with variable control
Zimmer Pulsavac Plus LP	Fan: 6.3–12.6 Shower: 3.2–5.8 Flexible: 8.6–12.2	No	Trigger control

EXHIBIT 27-10　PSI with Jetox-ND, Determined by Oxygen Setting

L/MIN	PSI
9 L/min	4
11 L/min	6
13 L/min	9
15 L/min	12

Conclusion

PLWS is an optimal strategy for debridement and irrigation for all wounds. With control of impact psi; site-specific treatment; the ability to treat tunnels, tracts, and undermining; enhancement of sharp debridement; avoidance of cross contamination; and an increased rate of granulation and epithelialization, PLWS offers the PT a valuable intervention for wound management. Treatment with PLWS, resulting in decreased length of stay and avoidance of facility-acquired infections with increased rate of wound closure, contributes to cost-effective treatment.[6]

How to Use Different Equipment Models

Davol Simpulse VariCare Procedure

Begin Treatment

1. Attach the suction canister to the regulator on the suction source.
2. Adjust suction to the appropriate mm Hg continuous.
3. Hang the saline bag(s) on an IV pole.
4. Remove the handpiece, tubing, dual spike adapter and the tip from the package; place on aseptic field.
5. Connect the dual spike adapter to the pump spike, if desired.
6. Attach the tip to the handpiece.
7. Spike the irrigation bag.
8. Connect the tubing to the suction connection on the handpiece and to the suction source.
9. Remove the lock pin on the handpiece to release the trigger, and the blue retaining ring, if the tip with the large splash shield is used; discard pin and ring.
10. Squeeze the trigger with the mode selection switch set to continuous variable mode to fill the tubing with solution. The bag may be squeezed to facilitate priming.
11. Place the tip in/on the wound and pull the trigger. The delivered pressure varies with the amount of pressure on the trigger.
12. Two modes of use are available: continuous variable control or three-step variable control for low, medium, or high psi.

When Treatment is Completed

1. Turn off suction and remove the tubing from the suction source.
2. Release the latch on the bottom of the handpiece, pull out the battery compartment, and remove the batteries. Batteries can be recycled if not contaminated.
3. Follow manufacturer's directions for disinfecting and storage of reusable equipment if suction diverter tip is used.
4. Dispose of all other equipment in a white biohazard bag.
5. Empty the suction canister into a hopper or commode if that is facility policy.

6. If disposable, place the empty canister in an appropriate biohazard bag. If glass, place in a clear biohazard bag to be sent for resterilization.

Stryker SurgiLav Plus and InterPulse Procedure
Begin Treatment

1. Attach the suction canister to the regulator on the suction source.
2. Adjust suction to the appropriate mm Hg continuous.
3. Hang the bag of saline on an IV pole.
4. Remove the handpiece, tubing, and the tip from the package; place on aseptic field.
5. Insert the tip into the handpiece by depressing the tip locking mechanism.
6. Spike the bag of saline with the battery pack.
7. Connect the suction tubing to the suction canister.
8. Squeeze the trigger to fill the tip with solution.
9. Place the tip in/on the wound and pull the trigger.
10. Adjust speed for desired psi—varies with the tip; only two pressures are available with each tip for the SurgiLav.

When Treatment is Completed

1. Turn off suction and remove the tubing from the suction source.
2. Recharge batteries if using rechargeable handpiece and batteries.
3. Follow manufacturer's directions for disinfecting and storage of reusable equipment if suction diverter tip is used.
4. Dispose of all other equipment in a white biohazard bag.
5. Empty the suction canister into a hopper or commode if that is facility policy.
6. If disposable, place the empty canister in an appropriate biohazard bag. If glass, place in a clear biohazard bag to be sent for reprocessing.

Zimmer Pulsavac Plus LP Procedure
Begin Treatment

1. Attach the suction canister to the regulator on the suction source.
2. Adjust the suction to the appropriate mm Hg continuous.
3. Hang the saline bag(s) on an IV pole.
4. Remove the handpiece, tubing, battery pack, and tip from the package; place on aseptic field.
5. Retract the locking ring by pressing up.
6. Attach the tip to the handpiece.
7. Lock the debridement tip in place by depressing locking ring.
8. Attach the battery pack to the IV pole.
9. Spike the irrigation bag with the irrigation tubing; a dual spike adapter is available.
10. Connect the suction tubing to the suction source.
11. Depress the top of the toggle trigger to prime the system.

12. Place the tip in/on the wound and turn the handpiece on.
13. Depress the top of the toggle trigger for high-speed fluid delivery. Depress the bottom of the toggle trigger for low-speed fluid delivery. Center the toggle trigger for no fluid delivery.
14. To change tips during treatment, retract the locking ring for tip removal.
15. To limit suction at the handpiece, activate the clamp at the base of the handpiece on the suction line.

When Treatment is Completed

1. Turn off suction and remove the tubing from the suction source.
2. Dispose of batteries per facility policy.
3. Dispose of the entire unit in a white biohazard bag. It may not be reused.
4. Empty the suction canister into a hopper or commode if that is facility policy.
5. If disposable, place the canister in an appropriate biohazard bag. If glass, place in a clear biohazard bag to be sent for reprocessing.

DeRoyal Jetox-ND Procedure
Begin Treatment

1. Connect the oxygen tube to the oxygen source.
2. Assure that the Jetox-ND valve is in the closed position.
3. Open the Jetox-ND package.
4. Screw the other end of oxygen tube to the Jetox's luer connection.
5. Insert the spike into the solution bag. The bag may be placed near the treated area.
6. Affix the shield sleeve onto the Jetox-ND nozzle up to the grooves, to maintain the optimum treatment distance.
7. Open the valve.
8. Hold the wand with nozzle end away from the clinician and patient.
9. Open the oxygen source to appropriate setting for desired PSI.
10. The shield should be in contact with the wound area to begin treatment.

When Treatment is Completed

1. Close the Jetox-ND valve.
2. Close the oxygen source.
3. Dispose of the product per facility policy.

DeRoyal Jetox-HDC Procedure
Begin Treatment

1. Connect the oxygen tube to the oxygen source.
2. Assure that the Jetox-HDC valve is in the closed position.
3. Attach the other end of oxygen tube to the Jetox-HDC's luer connection.

4. Affix the suction tubing to the connector on the Jetox-HDC.
5. Insert the spike into the solution bag. The bag may be placed near the treated area.
6. Open the valve.
7. Hold the wand with tip end away from the clinician and patient.
8. Open the oxygen source to desired flow setting for appropriate PSI.
9. Turn on the suction source. Adjust per patient tolerance and amount of wound debris.
10. The tip of the wand should be in contact with the wound area to begin treatment.

When Treatment is Completed

1. Close the Jetox-HDC valve.
2. Close the oxygen source.
3. Turn off the suction.
4. Dispose of the wand and tubing per facility policy.

Documentation

The following case study uses the diagnostic process described in Chapter 1 to document the need for skilled PT intervention using PLWS. The methodology of the functional outcome report is provided.

■ **CASE STUDY**

Gunshot Wound Treated with Pulsatile Lavage with Suction

Patient ID: W.S. **Age:** 29 **Onset:** January 2

INITIAL ASSESSMENT

Reason for Referral

The patient was referred for a blasted shoulder wound with buckshot, necrotic tissue, tunnels, and undermining in the wound.

Medical History and Systems Review

The patient, previously fully functionally independent with no prior medical history, suffered a self-inflicted gunshot wound to the left shoulder. On the day of the injury and admission to the hospital, January 2, 1995, he had surgical exploration of the blasted shoulder wound. The humeral head was resected; fragments were resected from the laterally pulverized clavicle. There was no injury to the brachial plexus or axillary vasculature. The left upper extremity was placed in traction with pins. He had subsequent surgical incisions and drainage of the wound in the operating room on January 3, 4, 5, and 6, with closure of the shoulder capsule on January 6 (see Figure 27-4).

Evaluation

The patient was admitted to the burn unit after the initial surgery because of the severity of the wounds and the complicated dressing changes required. The presence of necrotic tissue, purulent exudate, buckshot, and numerous tunnels and undermining were indications for treatment with pulsatile lavage with concurrent suction.

EXAMINATION—JANUARY 13

Joint Integrity

The left humeral head has been resected. The left upper extremity is in skeletal traction with pins, with shoulder abducted to 90°. The lateral clavicle is pulverized.

Circulation

There is no injury to the axillary vasculature; there is edema in the left upper extremity.

Sensation

There is no injury to the brachial plexus.

Mobility

The patient is restricted to the supine position.

Integumentary

The left shoulder has a through-and-through wound, with the shotgun entrance wound on the anterior and the exit wound on the posterior.

Size

- Anterior border—118.75-cm surface open area
- Posterior border—50.0-cm surface open area
- Medial depth—2.0 cm
- Lateral depth—1.75 cm
- Tunneling and undermining cannot be measured because of proximity of vessels

Tissue Assessment The wound has red granulation with scattered areas of yellow and brown necrotic tissue; there is buckshot present. The periwound tissue is erythematous and edematous.

Wound Healing Phase The wound is in acute inflammatory phase.

FUNCTIONAL DIAGNOSIS

- Soft tissue injury
  1. Absence of proliferative phase
  2. Absence of epithelialization phase
  3. Undue susceptibility to infection caused by debris in wound
- Functional loss of mobility associated with shoulder injury leading to inability to perform self care and undue susceptibility to pressure ulcers

Need for Skilled Services

Pulsatile lavage with suction by PT is indicated in an attempt to avoid another surgical incision and drainage and

CASE STUDY *(Continued)*

to prepare the wound for a subsequent skin graft. Increased mobility will be allowed with an accelerated healing process. Therapeutic positioning is necessary to avoid pressure ulcers.

Targeted Outcomes

- The wound bed will be clean, including tunnels and undermining.
- The wound will progress through the phases of healing from inflammatory to epithelialization.
- The patient will be properly positioned to remove pressure.

Treatment Plan

- Irrigate and mechanically débride the wound with the Pulsavac System, including tunnels and undermining. Remove the buckshot. Treat with 1 L of normal saline, 4 to 12 psi, 80 mm Hg suction.
- Perform sharp debridement of necrotic tissue with forceps and scissors.
- Maintain moist wound bed and obliterate dead space with dressing changes of wet to damp Dakin's solution–soaked gauze; cover with a 5 9-inch gauze pad and secure with dry gauze and paper tape. Tunnels and undermining will be loosely packed.
- Perform therapeutic positioning.

Prognosis

There will be no necrotic tissue and no debris. The wound will have a red granulation base and be ready for skin grafting by the physician.

Target Date   Two weeks.

Frequency   Once a day, 6 days per week.

REEXAMINATION BY PHYSICAL THERAPY ON JANUARY 20

Size

- Anterior wound—68.25-cm surface open area
- Posterior wound—28.75-cm surface open area
- Medial depth—1.5 cm
- Lateral depth—1.0 cm

Tissue Assessment   The wound has no necrotic tissue. There is a full red granulation base and increased epithelialization. There is no periwound erythema. Tunneling and undermining are present only in the proximal portion of the anterior wound.

Wound Healing Phase   Proliferative phase.

Intervention

Physical Therapy   Six treatments of pulsatile lavage with suction, followed by sharp debridement as needed.

Physical Therapy and Nursing   Dressing changes.

Physicians   On January 19 the pins are removed and traction is discontinued. The patient is transferred from the burn unit to a regular room.

Revised Prognosis

Closure of the wound by secondary intention.

DISCHARGE OUTCOME

The patient's wounds not only required no further surgical incisions and drainage, but also had a significant increase in granulation and epithelialization with no necrotic tissue present. Anterior and posterior wounds had a decreased surface open area of 42%. Medial depth decreased 25% and lateral depth decreased 43% within 7 days. The physicians decided to allow the wound to close by secondary intention rather than a skin graft. The patient was discharged home January 21, to continue dressing changes by his mother. Future surgical procedures were anticipated to replace the shoulder joint. He was lost to follow-up.

CASE STUDY

Complex Pressure Ulcers Treated with Pulsatile Lavage with Suction

Patient: female   **Age:** 53 y/o   **Onset:** 04/17/01.

INITIAL ASSESSMENT

Reason for Referral

The patient was referred for management of complex pressure ulcers.

Medical History and Systems Review

The patient was transferred to our facility June 7, 2001, following gastric bypass surgery April 17, 2001, at an outside hospital, with resultant severe pressure ulcers from time in surgery.

Several days post-op she developed tachycardia, fever, and low blood pressure. A pulmonary embolus was ruled out,

but and upper GI series indicated a contained leak at the proximal anastomoses. She underwent an urgent re-exploration with repair. She subsequently developed florid sepsis, was hemodynamically unstable, and developed acute renal insufficiency with acute tubular necrosis, which lead to acute renal failure.

Two large wounds developed: a stage III-IV pressure ulcer on the sacrum and lower back, and dehiscence of the abdominal wound. Her wound management consisted of pulsatile lavage with suction, wet-to-dry dressings, and Silvadene.

She had multiple courses of antibiotics, including Primaxin, Diflucan, Methixene, Ancef, and vancomycin. There was slow advancement of diet with the last noted prealbumin 4.9 on 5/24/01. Increased protein was provided by Promod, Arginaid, and a pureed diet.

(Continued)

■ **CASE STUDY** *(Continued)*

Her past medical history included morbid obesity, hypoventilation syndrome (Pickwickian syndrome), obstructive sleep apnea, gastroesophageal reflux disease, asthma, diverticulosis, hyperthyroidism, DJD, bladder incontinence, fibromyalgia, depression, chronic migraine headaches, CHF, IBS, and a large ventral hernia.

Her past surgical history included gastric bypass with Roux-en Y, urgent re-exploration for anastomotic leak, debridement of pressure ulcers, cholecystectomy, multiple bilateral knee surgeries, esophageal dilatation, TAH-BSO, and blood transfusions.

Medications included Lasix, Synthroid, Zestril, and Zaroxolyn. Allergies included penicillin, sulfa drugs, and NSAIDs.

The patient was a medically retired secretary, single, and lived with one of her children and her family. She did not use tobacco or alcohol. She denied use of controlled substances, THC, alternative, or herbal medications.

The admitting plan per the physician was:

- Wound care consult for advanced wound care
- Serial prealbumin twice weekly
- Dietary consult
- Low air loss bariatric bed
- PLWS
- NPWT
- Possible future skin grafts

Wound Care Evaluation

The patient was morbidly obese, had massive pressure ulcers posteriorly, and an abdominal wound dehiscence. All resulted from a complicated post-op bariatric surgery course.

EXAMINATION, JUNE 8, 2001
Joint Integrity

There is limitation of motion of both knees following multiple surgeries.

Circulation

The patient has venous insufficiency, HTN, and CHF.

Sensation

Sensation is WNL.

Mobility

The patient is reluctant to participate with PT. She is ambulatory in her room.

Integumentary

Left buttock/low back wound, stage IV
- 36 × 23 × 8 cm deep
- 1 cm side area extends 4 cm length
- undermining proximally ~ 7 cm

Satellite lesion distal to above
- 5.5 × 1 cm

Tissue assessment

The posterior wounds are ~ 90% granulation, with convolutions and finger-like projections of hypergranulation. There is ~10% slough.

Drainage

The drainage is moderate, both serous and purulent, and has a mild, distinct odor.

Right buttock
- several large areas reddened/blistered tissue
- ? Stage II pressure ulcers vs. tape burns

Abdominal - surgical dehisced wound
- 23 × 11 × ~5 cm deep
- undermining: 7–5 o'clock, 1–4 cm
- tract: 6 o'clock, 12+ cm
- tract: lower third wound, 5.5 cm distally

Tissue assessment

The abdominal wound is ~85% red granulation, ~15% yellow slough, and has exposed sutures.

Drainage
The drainage is moderate, serous, and has no odor.

Wound Healing Phase

- Chronic inflammatory

Functional Diagnosis

- Impaired integumentary integrity
- Muscle weakness

Need for Skilled Services

PLWS by the PT is indicated to irrigate and débride the wounds, and to reduce the bacterial burden. NPWT is indicated to increase granulation and decrease the need for large skin grafting/flap. Therapeutic positioning is of paramount importance to prevent further deterioration of present pressure ulcers, and to prevent other pressure ulcers. Mobility will be increased with accelerated healing of wounds and will contribute to wound healing. Strengthening is important for mobilization and self care. Nutrition intervention is mandatory for optimal healing of wounds and to follow gastric bypass precautions.

Targeted Outcomes

- Clean wounds
- Progress from chronic inflammatory to proliferative phase
- Increase granulation and contraction to prep for grafts
- Pressure relief
- Increase mobility and strength for functional ADL
- Optimize nutrition

Treatment Plan

- Irrigate and debride, promote granulation and epithelialization with PLWS
- Sharp debridement with forceps and scissors prn

■ **CASE STUDY** *(Continued)*

- Right buttock wounds: dressing with foam and transparent film
- NPWT to control exudate, enhance contraction, promote granulation
  - Back wounds: black foam, 125 mm Hg suction, continuous
  - Abdominal wound: white foam (change to black foam with increased granulation), 75 mm Hg suction, continuous
- Bariatric low air loss mattress, frequent therapeutic positioning
- Physical therapy for mobilization and strengthening, begun 06/11/01
- Nutrition intervention to optimize intake to meet protein calorie needs within post-gastroplasty restrictions

Prognosis

There will be no necrotic tissue, no purulent drainage, increased granulation tissue, no undermining/tunnels, and increased contraction. The wounds will be prepared for STSG per MD. She will develop no new pressure wounds. Her ambulation and strength will be increased. Nutrition will be optimal for wound healing.

Target date:

8 weeks

Frequency

- Wound treatment: every other day per physical therapy wound specialist
- Mobilization and strengthening: every day per physical therapy
- Positioning: every two hours per nursing staff
- Nutrition: per dietitian

RE-EXAMINATION, 07/08/01

Size

Left buttock/low back

- ~26.4 × 17 × 6.2 cm deep
- extended area re-epithelialized
- undermining proximally 4.2 cm
- undermining distally to right buttock 6.6 cm

Satellite lesion distally

- 3.8 × 0.8 cm

Tissue Assessment

The wound is ~98% granulation with minimal areas of convolutions and hypergranulation, and ~2% slough.

Drainage

Drainage is moderate and serous.

Right buttock
- Reddened/blistered areas improved
- New undermining of large wound in this area

Size

Abdominal wound
- 18.8 × 5.6 × ~3 cm deep
- Undermining 9–1 o'clock, 0.3–3.8 cm
- Tract at 6 o'clock closed
- Tract lower third wound distally: 2 cm
- VAC dressing changed to black foam 07/02/01

Tissue Assessment

The abdominal wound is ~95 % red granulation and ~5 % yellow slough with exposed sutures.

Drainage

Drainage is moderate, serous, with no odor.

Wound Healing Phase

Proliferative

Interventions

- 07/10/01, excisional debridement of wounds
- 07/19/01, TPN infusions begun—88 days, through 10/16/01
  - prealbumin 06/07/01: 6.6; 10/04/01: 17.6mg/dl [N:20-40]
- Multiple unsuccessful trials at enteral feeds
- Multiple central and PICC lines
- 07/31.01, transfusion of packed cells
- 08/04/01, transfer to ICU
- 08/04/01, thoracostomy tube right , pneumothorax
- 08/04/01, endotracheal tube intubated
- 08/10/01, tracheostomy
- mechanical ventilation continued throughout admission
- 09/05/01, patient made DNR
- 09/06/01, 10-4-01, femoral vas cath
- 09/06/01, hemodialysis begun
- 10/01/01, nursing began abdominal wound dressing changes
  - calcium alginate, foam , transparent film prn
  10/08/01, PT began PLWS, NPWT dressing changes posterior wounds twice a week
  10/16/01, care withdrawn per patient and family wishes
  10/16/01, patient expired
  Even though the patient did not survive her multiple morbid conditions, the wounds themselves improved, in spite of the multiple co-morbidities. PLWS was an important contributing factor to that improvement.

REVIEW QUESTIONS

1. A patient three weeks status post coronary artery bypass graft (CABG) has a dehisced, infected sternal wound and has undergone a sternectomy. The pericardium is exposed and there is undermining at the margins. What is the treatment strategy of choice for PT wound management?

2. A patient is readmitted from an extended care facility, 4 weeks status post right total hip replacement. The dehisced wound has purulent drainage with a foul odor, from a narrow tunnel that probes to the joint. How this is wound best treated by physical therapy?

3. A patient with paraplegia is admitted with a stage III–IV? sacral pressure ulcer. What is the treatment of choice for wound management?

4. An outpatient who is a heavy smoker is referred to physical therapy for treatment of venous insufficiency ulcers on both lower extremities. He cannot tolerate sharp debridement of the necrotic tissue in the wounds. What is the ideal treatment plan?

REFERENCES

1. Keblish DJ, DeMaio M. Early pulsatile lavage for the decontamination of combat wounds: historical review and point proposal. *Mil Med.* 1998;163:844–846.
2. Hess CL, Howard MA, Attinger CE. A review of mechanical adjuncts in wound healing: hydrotherapy, ultrasound, negative pressure therapy, hyperbaric oxygen, and electrostimulation. *Ann Plast Surg.* 2003:51:210–218.
3. Loehne HB. Enhanced wound care using Pulsavac System: Case studies. *Acute Care Perspect.* 1995;9:13–15.
4. Morgan D, Hoelscher J. Pulsed lavage: promoting comfort and healing in home care. *Ostomy Wound Manage* 2000;46:44–49.
5. Mustoe T. Understanding chronic wounds: a unifying hypothesis on their pathogenesis and implications for therapy. *Am J Surg.* 2004;187:65S–70S.
6. Haynes LJ, Handley C, Brown MH, Ho L, Merrifield HH, Griswold JA. *Comparison of Pulsavac and Sterile Whirlpool Regarding the Promotion of Tissue Granulation.* Lubbock, TX: University Medical Center and Methodist Hospital; 1994.
7. Saxe A, Goldstein E, Dixon S, et al. Pulsatile lavage in the management of postoperative wound infections. *Am Surg.* 1980;46:391–397.
8. U.S. Department of Health and Human Services. Treatment of pressure ulcers. *AHCPR Clin Pract Guideline.* 1994;15:50–53.
9. Stevenson TR, Thacker JG, Rodeheaver GT, Bacchetta C, Edgerton MT, Edlich RF. Cleansing the traumatic wound by high pressure syringe irrigation. *JACEP.* 1976;5(1):17–21.
10. Bhaskar SN, Cutright DT, Gross A. Effect of water lavage on infected wounds in the rat. *J Periodont.* 1969;40:671.
11. Wheeler CB, Rodeheaver GT, Thacker JG, Edgerton MT, Edlich RF. Side effects of high pressure irrigation. *Surg Gynecol Obstet.* 1976;143:775–778.
12. Bierbaum B. *High Pressure, Pulsatile Lavage in Wound Management: A Literature Review.* Cranston, RI: Davol, Inc.; 1986.
13. Bhaskar SN, Cutright DE, Hunsuck EE, Gross A. Pulsating water jet devices in debridement of combat wounds. *Mil Med.* 1971;136:274–276.
14. Rodeheaver GT. Pressure ulcer debridement and cleansing: a review of current literature. *OstomyWound Manage.* 1999;45(Suppl):80S–85S.
15. Luedtke-Hoffmann KA, Schafer DS. Pulsed lavage in wound cleansing. *Phys Ther.* 2000;80:292–300.
16. Niederhuber SS, Stribley RF, Koepke GH. Reduction of skin bacterial load with use of the therapeutic whirlpool. *Phys Ther.* 1975;55:482–486.
17. Bohannon R. Whirlpool versus whirlpool and rinse for removal of bacteria from a venous stasis ulcer. *Phys Ther.* 1982;62:304–308.
18. Morykwas MJ, Argenta LC. Use of negative pressure to increase the rate of granulation tissue formation in chronic open wounds. Presented at the annual meeting of the Federation of American Societies of Experimental Biology; March 28–April 1, 1993; New Orleans, LA.
19. Argenta LC, Morykwas M, Rouchard R. The use of negative pressure to promote healing of pressure ulcers and chronic wounds. Presented at the joint meeting of the Wound Healing Society and the European Tissue Repair Society; August 22–25, 1993; Amsterdam, Netherlands.
20. Ho CH, Bogie KM, Banks PG, et al. Pulsatile lavage for pressure ulcer management: safety profile. Poster presentation at SAWC. April 2005.
21. Occupational Safety and Health Administration. Bloodborne pathogen standard. *Federal Register.* 1991;56(235):64175–64182.
22. Maragakis L. Multidrug-Resistant (MDR) Acinetobacter. Johns Hopkins websitehttp://hopkins-heic.org/infectious_diseases/acinetobacter.html 07/03/2005
23. Maragakis LL, Cosgrove SE, Song X, et al. An outbreak of multidrug-resistant *Acinetobacter baumannii* associated with pulsatile lavage wound treatment. *JAMA.* 2004;292:3006–3011.
24. Fuller J. Cover up and clean up to prevent deadly infections. *Nursing 2005.* 2005;35:31.
25. Loehne HB, Streed SA, Gaither B, Sherertz RJ. Aerosolization of microorganisms during pulsatile lavage with suction. *OstomyWound Manage.* Abstract. 2002;48:75.
26. Goodman CC, Boissonnault WG. *Pathology: Implications for the Physical Therapist,* 2nd ed. WB Saunders; 2003;Philadelphia, Pennsylvania
27. U.S. Food and Drug Administration. Allergic reactions to latex-containing medical devices. *FDA Med Bull.* 1991;July 2–3.

Management of the Wound Environment with Negative Pressure Wound Therapy

Allen Gabriel, Elizabeth Hiltabidel, Adela Valenzuela, and Subhas Gupta

---

CHAPTER OBJECTIVES

At the completion of this chapter, the reader will be able to:
1. Describe the science behind negative pressure wound therapy (NPWT).
2. Describe applications of V.A.C.® Therapy based on peer-reviewed literature.
3. Explain indications for the use of V.A.C.® Instill therapy.

With advances in medical technology, patient life expectancy has increased in the past 20 years. Management of acute and chronic wounds, which can develop in the setting of many diseases, is a major challenge to society because of its magnitude, complexity, and cost. Every day newer adjuvant wound products are introduced in an effort to further stimulate and enhance wound healing. Many benefits of these products are anecdotal, with minimal scientific evidence.

More than 2.8 million patients in the United States with chronic wounds are treated at a cost of billions of dollars per year.[1] Chronic, open, nonhealing wounds pose a continual challenge in medicine because the treatment is variable and there are no documented consistent responses.[2] Clinically, chronic wounds may be associated with pressure, trauma, venous insufficiency, diabetes, vascular disease, or prolonged immobilization. The treatment is variable and costly, demanding lengthy hospital stays or specialized home care requiring skilled nursing and costly supplies. Rapid healing of chronic wounds could result in decreased hospitalization and earlier return of function. Many different types of conventional and traditional treatments have been recommended to enhance wound healing. During the past decade, especially, technological advances have contributed in the explosion of products used in management of acute and chronic wounds.

Negative Pressure Wound Therapy

One adjunctive therapy is negative pressure wound therapy (NPWT), also known as Vacuum-assisted closure (V.A.C.®). In 1995, the Federal Drug Administration (FDA) approved and introduced the V.A.C.® Therapy System, (KCI®, San Antonio, Texas) which has become a widely utilized therapy among multiple surgical and non-surgical specialties. Indications for NPWT were expanded in 2000 to include a variety of wound types (Table 28-1). V.A.C.® therapy received FDA clearance in 2002 for use in partial-thickness burn wounds. The most recent development in NPWT is the V.A.C.® Instill, an innovative combination of negative pressure and the intermittent instillation of various solutions or suspensions into the wound bed.

Many specialties utilizing NPWT have adopted this new system and have successfully treated a wide variety of wounds, including complex injuries that cannot be closed primarily, soft tissue avulsions, crush injuries, degloving injuries, and infected/contaminated wounds, as well as preplanned surgical incisions.

V.A.C.® is a NPWT product manufactured by Kinetic Concepts Incorporated (KCI ®) for the management of acute and chronic wounds. The therapy involves placing an open-cell foam dressing into the wound cavity and applying controlled negative pressure, typically 125 mm Hg below ambient pressure.

NPWT provides a negative pressure that is distributed over the wound surface by an airtight thin-film secondary dressing (drape). The VaCuum sealing facilitates the drainage of excessive fluid and debris, which has been shown to lead to a decline in bacterial counts, decreased interstitial edema, and increased capillary blood flow. The technique provides both adequate wound drainage and a humid environment necessary for wound healing, and thus combines the benefits of both open and closed (moist) wound healing.

TABLE 28-1 General Indications for V.A.C.® Therapy

Grafts
Flaps
Pressure ulcers
Diabetic ulcers
Dehisced surgical wounds
Chronic wounds
Acute wounds
Traumatic wounds
Partial-thickness burns

History of NPWT

The use of negative pressure has been used for thousands of years in China as an adjunct to acupuncture techniques.[3] A technique called cupping, wherein a heated glass sphere is applied to the skin, is a method of applying pressure to a specific acupuncture site. It was in the 17th century that the first report of the presence of V.A.C.uum was made by Galileo's Italian assistant, Evangelista Torricelli.[3] This discovery was followed by the creation of the syringe by the Frenchman Blaise Pascal and the V.A.C.uum pump by Dutchman Christian Huygens.[4]

The application of negative pressure to an open wound was first described by several Russian studies starting in the 1970s[5] and 1980s.[6-13] The understanding of their literature was limited due to the paucity of English abstracts, and thus it was difficult for English-speaking clinicians to evaluate these studies critically.

At the same time, Fleishman et al were the first German group to report on V.A.C.uum sealing, which is similar to what is known as NPWT in the United States.[14] Subsequent studies continued to describe the success of V.A.C.uum sealing in treatment of open wounds.[15-18] Fleishman et al was also the first group to describe a new dimension of V.A.C.uum sealing, which included instillation of antiseptics and antibiotics to infected wounds.[19, 20] These papers described the successful treatment of infected wounds with up to 14 months of follow up. This technology is known as V.A.C. Instill in the United States.

All of the non-U.S. studies were performed using wall suction devices or surgical V.A.C.uum bottles. Those devices can cause problems with appropriate delivery, control, and maintenance of negative pressure.[21]

It was in 1993 when Louis Argenta and Michael Morykwas presented the first animal studies involving use of negative pressure therapy.[22] Following these investigations, Morykwas and colleagues postulated that multiple mechanisms might be responsible for these observed effects.[23, 24] Since then, this technology has received FDA approval for its use in the treatment of wounds, and it has been licensed to and made commercially available from KCI.

The Wound Environment

Wound healing is a complex and dynamic process that includes an immediate sequence of cell migration leading to repair and closure. Repair and closure begins with removal of debris, control of infection, clearance of inflammation, angiogenesis, deposition of granulation tissue, contraction, remodeling of the connective tissue matrix, and maturation.[21,25] As growth factors, cytokines, proteases, and cellular and extracellular elements all play important roles in different stages of the healing process, as alterations in one or more of these components could account for the impaired healing observed in chronic or compromised wounds. Levels of various matrix metalloproteinases (MMPs), including (MMP-1 (collagenase), MMP-2 (gelatinase A), and MMP-9 (gelatinase B), and serine proteases are markedly increased in fluids from chronic wounds,[26] whereas they are decreased in wounds undergoing deposition of granulation tissue.[27] Other proteases, such as neutrophil elastase, have also been observed to be significantly higher in chronic wounds.[28] Elevated levels of serine proteases degrade fibronectin, an essential protein involved in the remodeling of the extra cellular matrix (ECM).[26, 29]

In compromised wounds, because of underlying pathogenic abnormalities and the altered biochemical and cellular environment, necrotic tissue and slough tends to accumulate continually.[30] The main pathophysiology of necrotic tissue formation is the result of inadequate local blood supply. The necrotic tissue contains dead cells and debris that are a consequence of the fragmentation of dying cells. Conversely, some wounds contain a yellow fibrinous tissue that mostly consists of fibrin and pertinacious material. This is frequently referred to as slough. The accumulation of necrotic tissue or slough in a wound promotes bacterial colonization and prevents complete repair of the wound. This halts wound progress to the next stage, and the wound remains in the inflammatory stage indefinitely because the continued presence of bacteria in a wound leads to production of pro-inflammatory mediators such as IL-1, TNF-_, prostaglandin E2, and thromboxane.[31] Although inflammation is part of normal wound healing, healing may be prolonged if inflammation is excessive.[32]

Not all bacteria in a wound have deleterious effects, and therefore they can be divided into three distinct categories: contamination, colonization, and infection. Both contamination (presence of nonreplicating organisms) and colonization (replicating organisms without tissue necrosis) do not produce a host response, whereas a severe infection produces a host response that has deleterious effects to wound healing. It is also important to be cognizant of age as a factor in wound healing, since the biochemical and cytokine milieu that is present as age increases is similarly present in chronic wounds. In animal models, a delayed inflammatory response has been observed after acute wounding in middle-aged and aged as compared with young mice.[33, 34]

Additionally, cellular and molecular characteristics of aged skin can impede the healing process. There is up-regulation of MMP-2 in normal aged skin, and MMP-2 and MMP-9 in acute wounds in aged skin in comparison with young adults.[33,34] This alteration in the cytokine profile is similar to that seen in chronic wounds in younger patients.

These factors may combine to predispose the remodeled wound to recurrent breakdown.

Theory and Science of NPWT Therapy

The physiologic and molecular biologic mechanisms by which NPWT accelerates wound healing are to a large extent unknown. Three factors responsible for accelerated wound healing with this therapy have been postulated and studied scientifically in animal studies.[35]

Wound healing involves a complex series of events that begins at the moment of injury and continues for months to years. After wounding, edema and interstitial fluid create an oxygen-poor environment due to the collapse of microcirculation. The thin-walled capillaries collapse because of an increase in intersitial fluid and pressure exerted on the vessels. This leads to the collapse and back up of the microcirculation, leading to localized thrombosis and a poor wound healing environment.

With the advent of NPWT, improved healing has been shown both in animal studies and clinically.[35-37] The proposed mechanism involves reduction in localized edema, increased blood flow, decreasing bacterial colonization, removing inhibitory agents, promoting granulation tissue formation, promoting a moist wound healing environment, enhancing epithelial migration, and promoting wound contraction.[38] To understand the benefits completely, a thorough review of the scientific basis of NPWT is warranted. The seminal scientific evidence can be divided into five areas: blood flow, granulation tissue formation, bacterial clearance, flap survival, and cytokine milieu.

Blood Flow

All tissues need oxygen and nutrients for metabolism and cell turnover. Any impediment to the localized blood flow has deleterious effects to wound healing. To understand the mechanisms involved in improving blood flow, a brief review of physiology is needed.

The movement of fluid and accompanying solutes between compartments (mostly water, electrolytes, and smaller molecular weight solutes) is governed by physical factors such as hydrostatic and oncotic forces. These forces are normally balanced in such a manner that the fluid volume remains relatively constant between the compartments. When the fluid volume within the interstitial compartment increases, this compartment will increase in size, leading to tissue swelling (i.e., edema). In most capillary systems of the body, there is a net filtration of fluid from the intravascular to the extravascular compartment. In other words, capillary fluid filtration exceeds reabsorption. This would cause fluid to accumulate within the interstitium if it were not for the lymphatic system, which removes excess fluid from the interstitium and returns it back to the intravascular compartment. Circumstances, however, can arise in which net capillary filtration exceeds the capacity of the lymphatics to carry away the fluid (i.e., net filtration > lymph flow). When this occurs, the interstitium will swell with fluid, thereby becoming edematous. Some of the precipitating factors of edema that can be related to wound healing include decreased plasma oncotic pressure (as occurs with hypoproteinemia), increased capillary permeability caused by proinflammatory mediators (e.g., histamine, bradykinin) or by damage to the structural integrity of capillaries so that they become more "leaky" (as occurs in tissue trauma, burns, and severe inflammation);,and lymphatic obstruction.

In the first series of experiments, the role of NPWT on blood flow was evaluated in the back wounds of anesthetized swines.[35] Deep circular defects, 2.5 cm in diameter, were dressed with open-cell polyurethane-ether foam with a pore size ranging from 400 to 600 um connected to a subatmospheric pressure device. Laser Doppler technique was employed to measure blood flow in the subcutaneous tissue and the muscle surrounding the wounds, as these structures were exposed to increasing levels of negative pressure, applied continuously at 25-mm Hg steps. The results indicated that flow increased with increasing levels of negative pressure, peaking at 125 mm Hg. While an increase in blood flow equivalent to four times the baseline value occurred with negative pressure values of 125 mm Hg, blood flow was decreased with higher levels and completely inhibited by negative pressures of 400 mm Hg and above.[35] A negative pressure value of 125 mm Hg was therefore selected for use in subsequent studies.

The same study also evaluated the effect of an intermittent negative pressure mode with 5 minutes on and 2 minutes off on the local blood flow. Results showed that this intermittent mode maintained local blood flow at four times the baseline blood flow after 2 minutes in the off mode. Thus, the intermittent mode is considered to be the optimal mode for certain wound characteristics. Table 28-2 presents guidelines for intermittent versus continuous NPWT. The proposed mechanism for improved blood flow entails removing the intersitial fluid from the tissues immediately surrounding the wound and decompressing the microcirculation and restoring blood flow.

One recent study re-evaluated the role of NPWT on blood flow in a different animal model involving skin wounds on white rabbits.[39] Investigators found that NPWT promoted a significant increase in capillary blood flow velocity and capillary blood volume.[39] It was also shown that NPWT stimulated endothelial proliferation and angiogenesis, narrowed endothelial spaces, and restored the integrity of the capillary basement membrane.[39] This study confirms the hypothesis of edema reduction with use of NPWT, as seen with restoration with the basement membranes leading to less leaky capillaries. This is also directly related to the change in the cytokine milieu that we see with use of NPWT, which will be discussed in detail later in this chapter.

Granulation Tissue Formation

Granulation tissue is a mix of small vessels and connective tissue in the wound base. The base forms a nutrient-rich matrix that can support the migration of epidermal cells across the wound bed. A well-granulated wound provides an opti-

TABLE 28-2 **Guidelines for V.A.C.® Therapy Intermittent Versus Continuous Mode**

Continuous Mode	Intermittent Mode
Flaps	Minimally exudating
Difficult dressing application	Large wound
Highly exudating	Small wound
Meshed grafts	Stalled progress
Painful wounds	
Tunnels or undermining	
Unstable structures	

mal bed for epidermal migration and for skin graft, as the newly formed capillaries support the inhibition or diffusion of exudates through the host bed that provide nutrients and dispose of waist products.

The rate of granulation tissue production under negative pressure was determined using the original swine model by measuring the reduction in wound volume over time.[35] Full-thickness wounds were created on the dorsum of anesthetized swine. One wound was treated with wet-to-moist saline dressings, one with continuous V.A.C.uum, and the third with intermittent V.A.C.uum (5 minutes on and 2 minutes off). The animals were anesthetized daily and wound volume was determined by measuring volume displacement of casts of each wound made with dental impression material. Compared with control wounds dressed with saline-soaked gauze, significantly increased rates of granulation tissue formation occurred with both continuous (mean 63.3%, +/- standard deviation [SD] 26.1%) and intermittent (mean 103%, SD 35.3%) application of negative pressure.[35]

The observation that intermittent or cycled treatment appears more effective than continuous therapy is interesting, although the reasons for this are not fully understood. Philbeck et al had two possible explanations.[40] They suggested that intermittent cycling results in rhythmic perfusion of the tissue, which is maintained because the process of capillary auto-regulation is not activated. They also suggested that because cells that are undergoing mitosis must go through a cycle of rest, cellular component production, and division, constant stimulation may cause the cells to "ignore" the stimulus and thus become ineffective. Intermittent stimulation allows the cells time to rest and prepare for the next cycle. For this reason it is suggested that cyclical negative pressure should be used clinically, although some authors[41] suggest that this may follow a 48-hour period of continuous V.A.C.uum, which can be applied to exert a rapid initial cleansing effect. Not every wound should be treated in the intermittent mode, but wounds needing granulation tissue should be treated in this setting (Table 28-3).

Moykwas et al evaluated the granulation tissue rate formation between different negative pressure settings, ranging from 25 mm Hg to 500 mm Hg.[42] The original hypothesis was confirmed with this study, in that wounds treated with a 125-mm Hg V.A.C.uum exhibited a significant increase in the rate of granulation tissue formation as compared with treatment at 25 mm Hg or 500 mm Hg. In addition, recently Saxena et al confirmed the original belief that tissues subjected to mechanical forces result in a higher amount of tissue growth.[43] The application of micromechanical forces may be a useful method with which to stimulate wound healing through promotion of cell division, angiogenesis, and local elaboration of growth factors.

The effect of the mechanical suction force of the V.A.C.uum device on wound healing is not surprising. This fundamental role of mechanical force in regulating tissue growth, repair, and remodeling was recognized by Julius Wolff more than a century ago and in 1911, the use of mechanical forces on wounds was thought to result in angiogenesis and tissue growth.[44] Tissue adaptation to changing physical stresses is a basic requirement for growth and survival of living systems. The extensive use of tissue expanders and the Ilizarov bone distraction technique in the past 20 years demonstrate how tissue moves and grows in response to the application of mechanical force, with viscoelastic flow, increased mitotic rate, and angiogenesis.[45-46] Recently, Saxena et al studied this theory through a computer model (finite element) of a wound and simulated V.A.C.® application.[47] The finite element model showed that most elements stretched by V.A.C.® application experienced deformations of 5 to 20 percent strain, which are similar to in vitro strain levels shown to promote cellular proliferation. Importantly, the deformation predicted by the model also was similar in morphology to the surface undulations observed in histologic cross-sections of the wounds. Therefore the application of forces stimulate wound healing through promotion of cell division, angiogenesis, and local elaboration of growth factors.[47] NPWT moves distensible soft tissue by an effect similar to tissue expansion. At the same time, it stimulates more rapid wound healing with increased rates of granulation tissue formation.

Bacterial Clearance

The definition of clinical infection is equivalent to greater than 10^5 organisms per gram of tissue. It has been postulated that the microorganisms consume the nutrients and oxygen that would otherwise be directed toward tissue repair. In addition, they release enzymes that break down protein, which is a crucial part of wound regeneration. Recently, Schmidtchen et al showed that elastase-producing bacterial isolates were shown to significantly degrade plasma proteins and extracellular products of human skin and fibroblasts, and inhibit fibroblast growth.[48] These effects, in conjunction with the finding that proteinase production was detected in wound fluid ex vivo, suggest that bacterial proteinases play a pathogenic role in chronic wounds. Reducing the bacterial load of a wound improves its healing capacity because the body can then concentrate on healing rather than on fighting invasion of microorganisms.

A swine study was conducted deliberately infecting wounds (*Staphylococcus aureus* and *Staphylococcus epi-*

TABLE 28-3   Recommended Guidelines for Treating Wound Types

Wound Type	Cycle	Subsequent Cycle	Target Pressure (Black Foam)	Target Pressure (Versa Foam)	Dressing Change Interval
Acute–traumatic	Continuous first 48 hrs	Intermittent (5 min ON/2 min OFF) for rest of therapy	125 mm Hg	125–175 mm Hg; titrate up for more drainage	Every 48 hrs (every 12 hrs with infection)
Pressure ulcers	Continuous first 48 hrs	Intermittent (5 min ON/2 min OFF) for rest of therapy	125 mm Hg	125–175 mm Hg; titrate up for more drainage	Every 48 hrs (every 12 hrs with infection)
Surgical wound dehiscence	Continuous first 48 hrs	Intermittent (5 min ON/2 min OFF) for rest of therapy	125 mm Hg	125–175 mm Hg; titrate up for more drainage	Every 48 hrs (every 12 hrs with infection)
Meshed grafts & bio-engineered tissues	Continuous for duration of therapy		75–125 mm Hg	125 mm Hg; titrate up for more drainage	Remove dressing after 3–5 days (drainage should taper prior to removal)
Chronic ulcers	Continuous first 48 hrs	Intermittent (5 min ON/2 min OFF) for rest of therapy	50–125 mm Hg	125–175 mm Hg; titrate up for more drainage	Every 48 hrs (every 12 hrs with infection)
Flaps	Continuous for duration of therapy		125–150 mm Hg	125–175 mm Hg; titrate up for more drainage	Fresh = every 72 hrs Complicated = every 48 hrs (every 12 hrs with infection)

The V.A.C.®– V.A.C.®Therapy Clinical Guidelines, January 2003, KCI USA, Inc.

dermidis) and measuring the number of colony-forming units per gram of tissue over time from both wet-to-moist treated wounds and V.A.C.uum-treated wounds. No antibiotics were used to treat the infection. NPWT-treated wounds showed a significant decrease in the number of bacterial colony-forming units from 10^7 organisms per gram of tissue to 10^4 by the 5th day of treatment.[35]

The proposed mechanism for this reaction is twofold. First, NPWT reduces the amount of stagnant infected fluid in the wound, such as slough, which may be harboring bacteria as previously discussed. Second, there is improved local blood flow, which can supply the necessary immunomodulators to eradicate clinical infection.

Flap Survival

Clinical observation shows that jeopardized flaps with poor venous outflow have been rescued with the use of NPWT if they were applied within 6 hours of clinical deterioration.[49, 50] The posterior compartment of rabbit hind limbs was crushed for 4 hours with 15-kg weights. Following removal, fasciotomies were made and NPWT was applied to the wounds of four rabbits. Serum samples for myoglobin in control animals showed a rapidly rising level versus the treated group, which remained at baseline.[51]

Moykwas et al also examined flap survival in their original swine study. The best results were seen with wounds that were pretreated and post-treated with NPWT, resulting in 72.2% flap survival rate. This was a significant increase of 21% survival rate with NPWT treatment compared with controls in random pattern flaps. The proposed mechanism is once again the increased blood flow locally that is observed in these flaps.

Cytokine Milieu

Treatment of wounds continues to be a challenge in the health-care community. Research is now focusing on the biochemical components of chronic wounds. There is growing support for the concept that a chronic wound is "stuck" in the inflammatory phase of healing.[52, 53] There is evidence that mitogenic cellular activity decreases in chronic wound fluid, whereas acute wound fluid promotes DNA synthesis.[54, 55] Research also has been directed in evaluating the cytokines found in wound fluid. Harris et al showed that higher levels of cytokines were found in nonhealing ulcers, and, interestingly, cytokine levels decreased when a chronic wound began to heal.[54] However, it is important to differentiate the different cytokines in the different wound healing stages.

Wound healing proceeds through three basic phases (inflammatory, epithelization, and proliferative) with different cytokines predominating in each phase. Cytokines mediate cellular function by binding cell membrane receptors. Recently, a study evaluated the change in concentration of cytokines during NPWT of traumatic wounds of the lower extremity.[56] There was a significant decrease in inflammatory cytokines tumor necrosis factor-alpha (TNF-_), platelet-derived growth factor (PDGF), and transforming growth factor-beta (TGF-_); and a significant increase in epithelization cytokines: endothelial growth factor (VEGF), IGF, PD-ECGF, and in proliferative cytokines: transforming growth factor-alpha (TGF-_), basic fibroblast growth factor (bFGF), and EGF compared with baseline.[56] These results indicate a decreasing concentration of inflammatory cytokines and an increasing concentration of proliferative and maturational cytokines with the use of NPWT. This correlated with the clinical appearance of wound healing.[56]

Chronic wounds have also shown higher levels of matrix metalloproteinase (MMP) than do acute wounds.[28, 57-63] This response is supported by recent studies showing that higher levels of MMP degrade proteins and the exogenous growth factors needed for wound healing.[62, 63] Shi et al evaluated the changes of MMP 1, 2, and 13 in granulating wounds after the treatment of NPWT in humans. Their results showed that NPWT promotes healing of chronic wounds through depressing the expressions of MMP-1, 2, 13 mRNA and protein synthesis, depressing the degradations of collagen and gelatin.[64] Tang et al explored the influence of NPWT on expression of Bcl-2 and NGF during wound healing in Sprague-Dawley rats. They concluded that the application of NPWT during wound healing increases the expression of the apoptotic modulation-related protein Bcl-2 and affects the expression of NGF/NGF mRNA, which promote the wound healing process.[65]

The ability of locally applied topical negative pressure in improving wound healing is continuously being evaluated, with more basic science research supporting its benefits.

Indications for Therapy

NPWT therapy enhances healing and promotes closure in a variety of open wounds. Chronic full-thickness wounds, such as pressure ulcers, along with venous, arterial, and neuropathic ulcers have all been proven appropriate for NPWT. Acute wounds, including burns, dehisced incisions, split-thickness meshed skin grafts, and muscle flaps, have also been shown to benefit from NPWT therapy.[66, 67]

The authors have successfully used V.A.C.® conservatively on select wounds complicated by fistulae, as an off-label application, and wounds with exposed mucosa, bone, tendon, and/or orthopedic hardware (Table 28-4).

V.A.C.® Instill therapy is an innovative combination of negative pressure and the intermittent instillation of various solutions or suspensions into the wound bed. It is indicated for patients who would benefit from NPWT, drainage, and controlled delivery of topical wound treatment solutions over the wound bed. In addition to the common types of wounds listed above, instillation therapy may also be beneficial in decreasing wound pain and/or decreasing the bacterial burden of infected wounds.

Contraindications for Therapy

Contraindications for treatment with NPWT include necrotic tissue, untreated osteomyelitis, malignancy in the wound, and high output fistulae to organs or body cavities. Precautions to consider include active bleeding, anticoagulant use, and difficult wound hemostasis.[68] When vital organs are exposed, precautions such as the placement of absorbable Vicryl mesh or its equivalent should be considered.[66]

NPWT enhances the body's natural capability to heal by accelerating the formation of granulation tissue, improving perfusion through removal of excess interstitial fluid (edema), and reducing bacterial colonization. A multifactorial approach in evaluating the candidacy of a patient must take place.

Expected Outcomes

The first use of NPWT in humans was reported by Argenta et al in 1997.[36] They included 300 wounds: 175 chronic

TABLE 28-4 Recommended Guidelines for Foam Use

Indications	V.A.C.® Polyurethane (Black Foam)	V.A.C.® VersaFoam® (White Foam)	Either
Deep, acute wounds with moderate granulation tissue present	X		
Deep pressure ulcers	X		
Flaps	X		
Exquisitely painful wounds		X	
Superficial wounds		X	
Tunneling/sinus tracks/undermining		X	
Deep trauma wounds			
Wounds that require controlled growth of granulation tissue			X
Diabetic ulcers			X
Dry wounds			X
Postgraft placement (including bioengineered tissues)			X
Shallow chronic ulcers			X

The V.A.C.®–V.A.C.® Therapy Clinical Guidelines, January 2003, KCI USA, Inc.

wounds, 94 subacute wounds, and 31 acute wounds. These were treated until completely closed or could be covered with a split-thickness skin graft, or were suitable for surgical reconstruction by rotating a flap onto the healthy granulating wound bed. Overall, 296 wounds responded favorably to treatment, and the authors concluded that V.A.C.® is an extremely efficacious modality for treating chronic and difficult-to-heal wounds.[36]

Since this sentinel clinical study, numerous other papers have described the effective use of V.A.C.® in the treatment of a variety of wound types, including extensive degloving injuries,[69, 70] infected sternotomy wounds,[41, 71-75] infected complex deep spinal wounds with exposed instrumentation,[76, 77] complicated diabetic foot and lower extremity wounds,[17, 78-87] and various soft tissue injuries or defects prior to surgical closure, grafting, or reconstructive surgery.[88, 89] NPWT has also revolutionized the way open abdominal wounds are treated. In a retrospective review, Smith and colleagues described the successful use of NPWT over a four-year period in 93 patients who required open abdomen management for a variety of conditions.[90,91] Several recent studies have described the use of NPWT as an important adjunct to managing open abdominal wounds.[92-94]

V.A.C.® has also been used in conjunction with split-thickness skin grafts in the treatment of burns and degloving injuries[69, 70, 95-97] and is claimed to be particularly useful for body sites with irregular or deep contours such as the perineum, hand, or axilla.[67, 98] In all these situations the V.A.C.uum helps to hold the graft securely on the wound bed, thus preventing pooling of tissue fluid, which would otherwise make the graft unstable. Contoured wounds needing closure with skin grafts are often located in complex anatomic regions or are in unusual positions, which make conventional skin graft stabilization techniques cumbersome and ineffective.

In 1998, Blackburn et al described the use of NPWT as a bolster for split-thickness skin grafts.[99] They concluded that its use was efficacious, with increased graft take due to total immobilization of the graft, thereby limiting shear forces, elimination of fluid collections, bridging of the graft, and decreased bacterial contamination.[99] Molnar et al[100] described how they used V.A.C.® in conjunction with skin grafts to treat four patients with full-thickness loss of the scalp following a burn injury or excision of an extensive carcinoma. Recently, the effective use of NPWT as a bolster to split-thickness skin grafts was reinforced in vulvo-vaginal and lower extremity reconstructions.[101, 102]

In addition to improving skin graft take, Molnar et al showed that NPWT improved the take rate and time to vascularization of Integra (Ethicon, Inc., Somerville, N.J.), compared with previous published results, even with complicated wounds.[103] In a manner similar to that of composite or full-thickness skin grafts, a critical factor in the success of this product is that the collagen/glycosaminoglycan matrix becomes vascularized and metabolically incorporated into the body.

NPWT was used for eight patients (age range 2 to 60 years) with complex wounds. Bone was exposed in 62.5% of cases, joint in 50%, tendon in 37.5%, and bowel in 25%. The estimated Integra take rate was 96%. No adverse side effects were observed with this technique. It was concluded that this technique may be a practical alternative to flap closure.[103] Similarly, the use of NPWT in conjunction with SIS (small intestinal submucosa) (Cook Surgical, Bloomington, Ind.) to facilitate incorporation has also been documented successfully in neonates.[104] This, however, was not the first report of NPWT in the pediatric population. In 2000, Mooney et al reported the efficacy of V.A.C. therapy in the pediatric population leading to decreased complex microvascular surgeries.[105] Recently a large series reported successful management of various tissue defects by V.A.C. therapy in children.[106] In addition, Arca et al showed that NPWT was also safe in premature neonates weighing less than 1500 g.[107]

Numerous case histories describing the successful use of V.A.C.® in a variety of nonhealing or chronic wounds have been published.[66, 83, 108-111] There is also growing evidence for the benefits of NPWT in pressure ulcer treatment.[1,4,21,112-115] Gupta et al described the first literature-supported guidelines for managing pressure ulcers with NPWT.[1]

As described, the V.A.C.® device can be applied over any type of tissue or material, including dermis, fat, fascia, muscle, tendon, blood vessels, bone, Gortext graft, synthetic mesh, hardware, and synthetic skin substitutes.[87] This makes almost any wound a candidate for V.A.C.® therapy; however, there are three prerequisites. All wounds must be devoid of necrotic tissue, devoid of fibrotic tissue, and have localized blood supply to the wound bed, prior to application of NPWT. With the increasing number of geriatric and polymorbid patients, NPWT has become an alternative treatment modality to more complex reconstructive operations. As some patients are not candidates to undergo prolonged anesthesia, NPWT has become a temporizing tool in complicated wounds to bridge between debridement and final closure.

Cost of Therapy

In a study by Philbeck et al,[40] records for 1,032 Medicare home-care patients with 1,170 wounds that failed to respond to previous interventions—and subsequently treated with the V.A.C.®—were reviewed. Reductions in wound area were compared with rates reported by Ferrell et al[116] in 1993, and costs were analyzed. Ferrell reported trochanteric and trunk pressure ulcers averaging 4.3 cm², treated with a low-air-loss (LAL) surface and saline-soaked gauze closed at an average of 0.090 cm² per day. For comparison with Ferrell's outcomes, Philbeck et al analyzed stage III and IV trochanteric and trunk wounds treated with LAL and the NPWT. The V.A.C.® treated group averaged 22.2 cm² decrease in the area and closed at an average 0.23 cm² per day. The average 22.2 cm² wound in the Philbeck study, treated as described by Ferrell, would have taken 247 days to heal, with a treatment cost of $23,465. Using V.A.C.®, the wound would have healed in 97 days with a treatment cost of $14,546. The cost comparison took into account the costs of materials—including equipment rental—and home-care nursing visits. Philbeck concluded that V.A.C.® therapy is an efficacious and economic treatment modality for a variety of chronic wounds.[40]

In an independent analysis of the same patient data used in Philbeck's study, the Weinberg group[117] considered only wounds that were more than 30 days old and had failed previous interventions (n = 979). Once treated with V.A.C.® therapy, 77% of those wounds closed or were progressing toward closure after 60 days. Weinberg concluded that, on average, V.A.C.® therapy would successfully heal more chronic wounds than would standard therapies and that V.A.C.® treatment would cost $1,925 less per patient.[117]

Research and case studies have demonstrated that the use of V.A.C.® therapy can decrease hospital stays, office visits, and/or home visits. Costs for V.A.C.® equipment rental and dressing supplies will vary among institutions and geographic locations. Caregivers need to stay abreast of Medicare, state aid, and managed care contracts regarding the reimbursement of V.A.C.® therapy because these contracts are continuously being reviewed and revised.

Application of Therapy

Several V.A.C.® systems are available for NPWT(Figure 28-1). The type of unit used is dependent on the amount of exudate and on patient mobility. The application of the system is a simple technique, with equipment that is user friendly.(Table 28-5) The digital readout on the pump guides the user through different options, such as pressure settings and problem solving. Equipment that is unfamiliar to healthcare providers can be intimidating; therefore, the authors recommend that institutions develop a technique for the use of the V.A.C.® system,[35, 36] such as the one outlined in Table 28-6. Complete application of therapy is described in detail in Table 28-5. Users should be educated on the equipment,

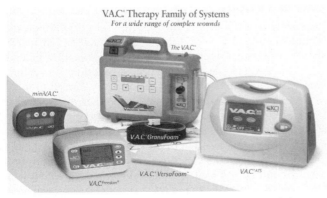

FIGURE 28-1 Examples of negative pressure wound therapy devices with KCI V.A.C.®

application, removal, and monitoring of the therapy to achieve positive patient outcomes. Once health-care professionals are comfortable with the therapy, the cost benefits, including time savings and improved patient outcomes, will be realized.

To function optimally, the transparent adhesive drape must cover the foam dressing as well as an additional 3–5 cm border of intact periwound skin and form an airtight seal. Obtaining such a seal can be particularly difficult near the anus or vagina or where the surrounding skin is moist. These problems can sometimes be overcome by the use of a hydrocolloid dressing, which is first applied around the wound and used as a base for the adhesive membrane.[36] Some of the practical problems associated with the application of the V.A.C.® system have been discussed previously by Greer et al,[83] who developed techniques to allow it to be used successfully on sacral pressure ulcers close to the anus and on multiple large ulcers on the lower extremities.

V.A.C.® Instill™

NPWT instillation has been recently introduced to the acute care market as an evolutionary addition to standard NPWT. It combines the mechanisms of action of standard NPWT with timed, intermittent delivery of an instilled topical solution. NPWT instillation is indicated for patients who would benefit from vacuum-assisted drainage and controlled delivery of topical wound treatment solutions and suspensions over the wound bed. It is also intended for use with aqueous solutions in a physiologic pH range defined as 6.0–7.4. Alcohol-based solutions and solutions that contain alcohol are contraindicated because of their potential negative effect on the foam dressing. Hydrogen peroxide solutions are also contraindicated for instillation.

NPWT instillation set-up differs from the standard NPWT devices in that it has an additional set of ingress tubing that allows gravity feed of solutions into the dressing. An intravenous pole that accommodates standard intravenous fluid bags is attached to the device. A mechanical clamp opens and closes the intravenous tubing. Instillation time can be set from 1 second to 2 minutes, and the hold time, or period of time the fluid sits in the wound, can also be programmed (1 second to 1 hour). The programmed negative pressure resumes at the end of the hold time to remove the remaining instilled topical solution and wound exudate, as well as collapse the foam. Because the solution is gravity fed, the intravenous bag must be at or slightly above the level of the wound.

In his published case series exploring the use of NPWT instillation using V.A.C.®, Wolvos concludes that culture-directed antibiotic wound irrigation appears to effectively decrease the bacterial burden of infected wounds, change the apearance of some wounds from infected to clean, and convert wound culture data from positive cultures to no growth or normal flora.[118, 119]

An initial paper describing the combined effects of NPWT and instillation of antiseptics or antibiotics was pub-

TABLE 28-5   Procedure for V.A.C.® ATS Application

Method	Key Points
Preparing patient:	
a. Explain procedure to patient	
b. Assist patient into correct position	Position will depend on location of wound
Don gloves	Follow standard precautions
Remove old dressings and dispose of dirty dressings and gloves	
Don gloves	
Clean wound and remove gloves	Use wound cleanser or normal saline
Dry and prepare periwound	Shave hair on border around wound, if applicable
Open dressing assembly package	
Place the V.A.C.® unit on a level surface or hang on the footboard, turn machine on, and set appropriate settings	Use the green button located above the electrical cord on the left side of the unit to turn machine on; settings must be ordered by an MD
Insert the canister into the V.A.C.® unit	
Cut foam to fit within the wound	Make sure the pattern cut is slightly smaller than the wound, fitting the size and shape of the wound, including tunnels and undermining areas
Don gloves	
Place the foam to fit into the wound cavity	Foam dressing should not extend onto intact periwound skin
a. Size and cut drape to cover the foam dressing	The drape should be cut larger than the wound with an additional 3–5 cm extending beyond the foam covering intact skin
Remove drape backing exposing the adherent side	Layer indicated with a # 1
Place the transparent drape over the foam	For fragile periwound skin, use skin prep before drape application or frame the wound with a hydrocolloid
Remove the top layer of the drape	Indicated with a # 2
Cut a 2-cm hole into the drape over the central area of the foam dressing	Fluid will pass through the opening
Remove backing on T.R.A.C. pad to expose adhesive backing and apply over cut hole	
Apply gentle pressure around the T.R.A.C. pad to ensure complete adhesion	
Connect the T.R.A.C. tubing end to the canister tubing end and release clamps (2)	Clamps are to be used when disconnecting patients from suction
Turn therapy on	Therapy on/off button is located on the face of the machine
Check for air leaks	Apply a second piece of transparent film dressing; the foam should appear like a raisin if suction has been established

DOCUMENTATION

1. Date, time, procedure
2. Assessment of the wound
3. Patient tolerance of procedure
4. Settings of the KCI V.A.C.® system
Nurse's signature and initials

lished by Fleischmann et al[19] in 1998. Fleischmann is generally credited for pioneering the NPWT instillation technique in orthopedic medicine. Among the 27 patients with acute infections of bone and soft tissues, chronic osteomyelitis, or chronic wounds treated with NPWT instillation, the authors found only one instance of recurrence of infection in a patient with chronic osteomyelitis in 3 to 14 months of follow up.[19]

In a recent series, NPWT instillation demonstrated a significant reduction in the mean time to infection clearance, wound closure, and hospital discharge compared with traditional advanced wound care methods.[120] Patient tolerance and compliance with the therapy is enhanced with the decreased time to closure and quicker hospital discharge occurs as well. The improved outcomes also affect indirect costs such as loss of work days, recovery time, and mortality. Additional studies with larger patient samples are needed to further substantiate the results of this novel wound treatment therapy.

TABLE 28-6 Sample V.A.C.® ATS Technique

Personnel Who Typically Perform Technique:

MD, RN, PA, NP, PT

Equipment Needed

Gloves	V.A.C.®ATS therapy unit
Scissors	V.A.C.® ATS canister kit; includes canister and tubing
Wound cleanser	V.A.C.® ATS dressing assembly; foam dressing, film drape, and T.R.A.C. pad with tubing

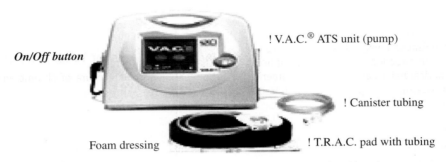

On/Off button

! V.A.C.® ATS unit (pump)

! Canister tubing

Foam dressing
! T.R.A.C. pad with tubing

< Film dressing (drape)

NOTE:

1. The KCI V.A.C.® therapy unit (pump) must be rented, and disposables purchased from KCI®.

2. The following are wound contraindications for use of the V.A.C.® Therapy: malignancy in the wound, necrotic tissue with eschar present, untreated osteomyelitis, non-enteric and unexplored fistula, exposed blood vessels or organs.

3. Closely monitor patients on anticoagulants.

4. The pressure setting (mm Hg) and interval of dressing changes must be ordered by the physician. Protocols for dressing changes as described by KCI® should be followed.

V.A.C.® GranuFoam™ Silver™

Ionic silver has long been recognized as an effective antimicrobial against a broad spectrum of pathogens and is considered to be biocompatible with mammalian tissue.[121-126] The resurgence of interest in silver products for wound care stems from the increase in the level of bacterial resistance to traditional antibiotics. For example, rates of methicillin-resistant *Staphylococcus aureus* (MRSA) increased steadily over the past decade from about 30% in 1989 to approximately 40% in 1997 among ICU patients.[127] Unlike traditional antibiotics, ionic silver has multiple mechanisms of action, such as inhibiting cellular respiration, denaturing nucleic acids, and altering cellular membrane permeability.[128,129] Appropriately high concentrations of silver coupled with the various mechanisms of action make it difficult for microorganisms to develop resistance to silver because they would have to undergo several mutations to develop defense mechanisms against the multipronged attack of silver. Silver also has low mammalian cell toxicity and is now known to have potent anti-inflammatory properties when delivered at the appropriate concentrations.[130]

The new silver dressing is an FDA-cleared, open-celled, reticulated polyurethane foam that has been microbonded with metallic silver via a proprietary metallization process. This dressing is specifically designed to be utilized with the V.A.C.® therapy device to combine antimicrobial activity with the existing mechanisms of action of NPWT. The silver is microbonded to the dressing in such a way that it retains the same porosity and structure of traditional V.A.C.® GranuFoam® dressings to simulate the same micromechanical effects. The porous nature of the foam in a negative pressure environment also allows for compression and conformability to the entire wound surface. Research indicates that the ability of a silver-containing dressing to conform to the contours of a wound is important to reduce areas of noncontact where bacteria may proliferate.[131]

In a recent series, the NPWT–silver dressing combination significantly reduced time needed to clear infection, time to patient discharge, and time to wound closure when compared with current standards of advanced wound care. The combination of NPWT with the antimicrobial action of ionic silver makes the GranuFoam Silver dressing a useful addition to the armamentarium of wound therapies.

■ CASE STUDY

This is a 71-year-old male admitted to the hospital for left hip chronic wound with drainage. He was post-op, open reduction internal fixation (ORIF) for left hip fracture 1 month prior to admission. He had no known allergies and was on several routine medications. He was admitted for incision and drainage (I&D) of the hip wound. The surgery showed a large hematoma, with infection down to the hardware. Infection was cleaned up, and part of the fascia lata was débrided because of the infection. Eight days later, he developed another infection and was taken to the operating room again for a subsequent I&D. Previous wound care treatments had been wet-to-moist normal saline packing two to three times a day and pulsatile lavage. His medical history was significant for insulin-dependent diabetes, peripheral vascular disease, and pericardial calcification. His surgeries in the past included pericardial calcium resection, left below-the-knee amputation, and back surgery.

Wound Assessment

V.A.C.® therapy was initiated 4 days after surgery. The wound was anatomically vertical along the left lateral thigh. The wound bed was 80% beefy red granulation tissue, with 20% exposed tendon and hardware (Table 28–7). Drainage was clear serous fluid with no odor noted. Periwound was nonerythematic with wound edges attached. Measurements were 25 cm × 7 cm × 3 cm, with a 5-cm depth at the 2:00–5:00 position. Client had been on a course of vancomycin hydrochloride (Vancocin) IV piggyback and was on rifampin (Rifadin) orally. Client complained of excruciating pain on palpation of wound and was medicated with hydromorphone hydrochloride (Dilaudid) IV during dressing changes. There were no special support surfaces on the patient. Physical therapy (for strengthening) and nutritional services were following the patient at this time.

Indications/Goals for V.A.C.® Therapy

Nonhealing wound. Closure of chronic wound and/or preparation for flap/skin graft.

Review of Clinical Course with V.A.C.® Therapy:

After 3 weeks of therapy, there was significant progress in wound filling and contraction (Figures 28-2A and B). The patient was discharged home on V.A.C.® therapy, with the expectation of complete wound closure.

TABLE 28-7 Case Study Review of Left Hip Wound Clinical Course with V.A.C.® Therapy

Date	Length	Width	Surface Area	Depth	Undermining	Color	Hardware Exposed	Odor
7/24/00	25 cm	7 cm	175 cm²	3 cm	5 cm between the 2:00 and 5:00 position	80% beefy red	20% hardware and tendon exposed	none
7/26/00	25 cm	5 cm	125 cm²	3 cm	6 cm @ the 4:00 position	95% beefy red, 5% yellow	minimal hardware exposed	none
7/28/00	24 cm	5.5 cm	132 cm²	1 cm	2 cm @ the 4:00 position	90% beefy red	10% exposed hardware	none
8/9/00	24 cm	4 cm	96 cm²	0	2 cm @ the 3:00 position	95% beefy red	5% exposed hardware	none
8/16/00	24 cm	3 cm	72 cm²	0	1 cm @ the 3:00 position	97% beefy red	3% exposed hardware	none
8/19/00	Discharged to home on the V.A.C.® therapy.							

After 3 weeks of therapy, there was significant progress in wound filling and contraction. The patient was discharged home on V.A.C.® therapy, with the expectation of complete wound closure.

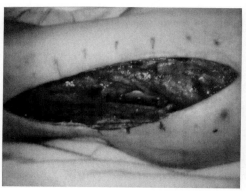

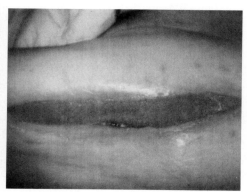

FIGURE 28-2 Progress in wound filling and contraction with V.A.C.® therapy. **A.** 7/24/00 left hip wound with exposed hardware. **B.** Clean, healthy granulation tissue after treatment with V.A.C.® therapy.

A

B

Conclusion

Closure of any wound is evaluated with a reconstructive mindset that includes the following goals: close wound, prevent infection, provide stable and robust coverage, minimize donor defect, and maximize function. Taking those factors into account, plastic surgeons use what is called the *reconstructive ladder*, shown in Figure 28-3, which proceeds through the various levels of intervention used to close wounds.[132, 133] The ladder consists of basic principles of wound closure along with more complex closures such as using local, distant, and free flaps. As such, the reconstructive ladder is similar to an elevator, as presented in the literature.[132,133] At some point along that elevator, clinicians must be able to make "stops" to introduce the high-tech tools and devices now available, for example, NPWT, which can be used at any level of the reconstructive elevator whether treatment is moving up or down levels of intervention.[132,133]

Deciding which tools to use and how to adapt navigation of the elevator to each patient is far more important to understand. The patient's overall condition, in terms of critical care issues, malnutrition, and immunosuppression, is key, as is determining what class of wound needs treatment. The main goal in wound reconstruction is to replace like with like. Therefore, NPWT has revolutionized wound care and serves both as a temporizing therapy to bridge to the final step as other factors are maximized (e.g., nutrition) and as a final therapeutic technology.

REVIEW QUESTIONS

1. 19-year-old female presents with a 5 × 4 cm forearm wound. The wound has a good base of granulation tissue and is progressing well. Granulation tissue mainly consists of:
   a. fibrinous tissue
   b. mix of small vessels and connective tissue
   c. MMPs
   d. collagenase
2. The original scientific studies involving negative pressure wound therapy by using the V.A.C.® were in:
   a. adult patient population
   b. pediatric patient population
   c. swine
   d. rabbits
3. The effect of the mechanical suction force of the vacuum device on wound healing was first noted in:
   a. 1995
   b. 1911
   c. 1993
   d. 1984
4. Ilizarov bone distraction technique demonstrates:
   a. how tissue moves and grows in response to the application of mechanical force
   b. an increase in angiogenesis
   c. an increase in mitotic figures
   d. all of the above
   e. none of the above

REFERENCES

1. Gupta S, Baharestani M, Baranoski S, et al. Guidelines for managing pressure ulcers with negative pressure wound therapy. *Adv Skin Wound Care*. 2004;17(Suppl 2):1.
2. Brown KM. Harper FV, Aston WJ, et al. vacuum-assisted closure in the treatment of a 9-year-old child with severe and multiple dog bite injuries of the thorax. *Ann Thorac Surg.* 2001;72:1409.
3. Banwell PE, Teot L. *Topical Negative Pressure (TNP) Therapy*. Focus Group Meeting. London, UK, 2003.

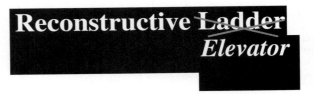

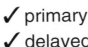

FIGURE 28-3 Reconstructive ladder.

4. Banwell PE, Teot L. Topical negative pressure (TNP): the evolution of a novel wound therapy. *J Wound Care*. 2003;12:22.

5. Zhivotaev VM. Vacuum therapy of postoperative infected wounds of the urinary bladder. *Klin Khir*. 1970;5:36.

6. Davydov Iu A, Larichev AB, Men'kov KG. Bacteriologic and cytologic evaluation of Vacuum therapy of suppurative wounds. *Vestn Khir Im I Grek*. 1988;141:48.

7. Davydov Iu A, Larichev AB, Smirnov AP, et al. Vacuum therapy of acute suppurative diseases of soft tissues and suppurative wounds. *Vestn Khir Im I I Grek*. 1988;141:43.

8. Davydov Iu A, Larichev AB, Kozlov AG. Pathogenetic mechanisms of the effect of vacuum therapy on the course of the wound process. *Khirurgiia (Mosk)*. 1990;42.

9. Davydov Iu A, Larichev AB, Abramov A. Substantiation of using forced early secondary suture in the treatment of suppurative wounds by the method of vacuum therapy. *Vestn Khir Im I I Grek*. 1990;144:126.

10. Davydov Iu A, Larichev AB. Plastic surgery of the choledochus using full autologous vein transplant. *Khirurgiia (Mosk)*. 1991;125.

11. Davydov Iu A, Abramov A, Larichev AB. Vacuum therapy in the prevention of postoperative wound infection. *Vestn Khir Im I I Grek*. 1991;147:91.

12. Davydov Iu A, Larichev AB, Abramov A, et al. Concept of clinico-biological control of the wound process in the treatment of suppurative wounds using vacuum therapy. *Vestn Khir Im I I Grek*. 1991;146:132.

13. Davydov Iu A, Larichev AB, Abramov A. Wound healing after vacuum drainage. *Khirurgiia (Mosk)*. 1992:21.

14. Fleischmann W, Strecker W, Bombelli M, et al. Vacuum sealing as treatment of soft tissue damage in open fractures. *Unfallchirurg*. 19983;96:488.

15. Fleischmann W, Becker U, Bischoff M, et al. Vacuum sealing: indication, technique and results. *Eur Orthop Surg & Trauma*. `1995:37.

16. Fleischmann W, Russ M, Marquardt C. Closure of defect wounds by combined Vacuum sealing with instrumental skin expansion. *Unfallchirurg*. 1996;99:970.

17. Fleischmann W, Lang E, Kinzl L. Vacuum assisted wound closure after dermatofasciotomy of the lower extremity. *Unfallchirurg*. 1996;99:283.

18. Fleischmann W, Lang E, Russ M. Treatment of infection by vacuum sealing. *Unfallchirurg*. 1997;100:301.

19. Fleischmann W, Russ M, Westhauser A, et al. Vacuum sealing as carrier system for controlled local drug administration in wound infection. *Unfallchirurg*. 1998;101:649.

20. Moch D, Fleischmann W, Westhauser A. Instillation vacuum sealing—report of initial experiences. *Langenbecks Arch Chir Suppl Kongressbd*. 1998;115:1197.

21. Banwell P, Withey S, Holten I. The use of negative pressure to promote healing. *Br J Plast Surg*. 1998;51:79.

22. Whitworth I. *History and Development of Negative Pressure Therapy*. Topical Negative Pressure Proceedings. London UK, 2003;1:22.

23. Morykwas M J, Argenta LC. Nonsurgical modalities to enhance healing and care of soft tissue wounds. *J South Orthop Assoc*. 1997;6:279.

24. Fabian TS, Kaufman HJ, Lett ED, et al. The evaluation of subatmospheric pressure and hyperbaric oxygen in ischemic full-thickness wound healing. *Am Surg*. 2000;66:1136.

25. Banwell P. Topical pressure therapy in wound care. *Journal of Wound Care*. 1999;8:79.

26. Yager DR, Zhang LY, Liang HX, et al. Wound fluids from human pressure ulcers contain elevated matrix metalloproteinase levels and activity compared to surgical wound fluids. *J Invest Dermatol*. 1996;107:743.

27. Cook H, Davies KJ, Harding KG, et al. Defective extracellular matrix reorganization by chronic wound fibroblasts is associated with alterations in TIMP-1, TIMP-2, and MMP-2 activity. *J Invest Dermatol*. 2000;115:225.

28. Grinnell F, Zhu M, Parks WC. Collagenase-1 complexes with alpha2-macroglobulin in the acute and chronic wound environments. *J Invest Dermatol*. 1998;110:771.

29. Wlaschek M, Peus D, Achterberg V, et al. Protease inhibitors protect growth factor activity in chronic wounds. *Br J Dermatol*. 1997;137:646.

30. Falabella AF, Carson P, Eaglstein WH, et al. The safety and efficacy of a proteolytic ointment in the treatment of chronic ulcers of the lower extremity. *J Am Acad Dermatol*. 1998;39:737.

31. Ladwig GP, Robson MC, Liu R, et al. Ratios of activated matrix metalloproteinase-9 to tissue inhibitor of matrix metalloproteinase-1 in wound fluids are inversely correlated with healing of pressure ulcers. *Wound Repair Regen*. 2002;10:26.

32. Davey ME, O'Toole GA. Microbial biofilms: from ecology to molecular genetics. *Microbiol Mol Biol Rev*. 2000;64:847.

33. Ashcroft GS, Horan MA, Herrick SE, et al. Age-related differences in the temporal and spatial regulation of matrix metalloproteinases (MMPs) in normal skin and acute cutaneous wounds of healthy humans. *Cell Tissue Res*. 1997;290:581.

34. Ashcroft GS, Herrick SE, Tarnuzzer RW, et al. Human ageing impairs injury-induced in vivo expression of tissue inhibitor of matrix metalloproteinases (TIMP)-1 and -2 proteins and mRNA. *J Pathol*. 1997;183:169.

35. Morykwas MJ, Argenta LC, Shelton-Brown EI, et al. Vacuum-assisted closure: a new method for wound control and treatment: animal studies and basic foundation. *Ann Plast Surg*. 1997;38:553.

36. Argenta LC, Morykwas MJ. Vacuum-assisted closure: a new method for wound control and treatment: clinical experience. *Ann Plast Surg*. 1997;38:563.

37. Argenta PA, Rahaman J, Gretz HF III, et al. Vacuum-assisted closure in the treatment of complex gynecologic wound failures. *Obstet Gynecol*. 2002;99:497.

38. Lambert KV, Hayes P, McCarthy M. Vacuum assisted closure: a review of development and current applications. *Eur J Vasc Endovasc Surg*. 2005;29:219.

39. Chen SZ, Li J, Li XY, et al. Effects of vacuum-assisted closure on wound microcirculation: an experimental study. *Asian J Surg*. 2005;28:211.

40. Philbeck TE, Jr, Whittington KT, Millsap MH, et al. The clinical and cost effectiveness of externally applied negative pressure wound therapy in the treatment of wounds in home healthcare Medicare patients. *Ostomy Wound Manage*. 1999;45:41.

41. Tang AT, Okri SK, Haw MP. Vacuum-assisted closure to treat deep sternal wound infection following cardiac surgery. *J Wound Care*. 2000;9:229.

42. Morykwas MJ, Faler BJ, Pearce DJ, et al. Effects of varying levels of subatmospheric pressure on the rate of granulation tissue formation in experimental wounds in swine. *Ann Plast Surg*. 2001;47:547.

43. Saxena V, Hwang CW, Huang S, et al. Vacuum-assisted closure: microdeformations of wounds and cell proliferation. *Plast Reconstr Surg*. 2004;114:1086.

44. Thoma R. Ueber die Histomechanik des Gefasssystems und die Pathogenese der Angioskleroose. *Virchows Arch F Pathol Anat*. 1991:204.

45. Olenius M, Dalsgaard CJ, Wickman M. Mitotic activity in expanded human skin. *Plast Reconstr Surg*. 1993;91:213.

46. Urschel JD, Scott PG, Williams HT. The effect of mechanical stress on soft and hard tissue repair; a review. *Br J Plast Surg*. 1988;41:182.

47. Saxena V, Hwang CW, Huang S, et al. Vacuum-assisted closure: microdeformations of wounds and cell proliferation. *Plast Reconstr Surg*. 2004;114:1086.

48. Schmidtchen A, Holst E, Tapper H, et al. Elastase-producing *Pseudomonas aeruginosa* degrade plasma proteins and extracellular products of human skin and fibroblasts, and inhibit fibroblast growth. *Microb Pathog*. 2003;34:47.

49. Marks MW, Schneider AM, Capizzi M, et al. *Muscle Flap Survival After Complete Venous Occlusion by Application of a Negative Pressure Device*. 66th Annual Meeting of the American Society of Plastic and Reconstructive Surgeons. San Francisco, CA, 1997.

50. Morykwas MJ, Schneider AM, Templeton TW, et al. *Isolated Muscle Flap Survival with Complete Venous Occlusion: Varying Delay in External Application of Sub-atmospheric Pressure*. 67th Annual Meeting of the American Society of Plastic and Reconstructive Surgeons. Boston, MA, 1998.

51. Morykwas MJ, Howell H, Bleyer AJ, et al. The effect of externally applied sub-atmospheric pressure on serum myoglobin levels following a prolonged crush/ischemia injury. *Trauma*. 2002;53:537.

52. Ayello EA, Cuddigan JE. Conquer chronic wounds with wound bed preparation. *Nurse Pract*. 2004;29:8.

53. Ayello EA, Cuddigan JE. Debridement: controlling the necrotic/cellular burden. *Adv Skin Wound Care*. 2004;17:66.

54. Harris IR, Yee KC, Walters CE, et al. Cytokine and protease levels in healing and non-healing chronic venous leg ulcers. *Exp Dermatol*. 1995;4:342.

55. Katz MH, Alvarez AF, Kirsner RS, et al. Human wound fluid from acute wounds stimulates fibroblast and endothelial cell growth. *J Am Acad Dermatol*. 1991;25:1054.

56. Bennett D, Gabriel A, Komorowska-Timek E, et al. Characterizing the changing gene statement of chronic wounds. *PSRC*. 2002:45A.

57. Bullen EC, Longaker MT, Updike DL, et al. Tissue inhibitor of metalloproteinases-1 is decreased and activated gelatinases are increased in chronic wounds. *J Invest Dermatol*. 1995;104:236.

58. Wysocki AB, Staiano-Coico L, Grinnell F. Wound fluid from chronic leg ulcers contains elevated levels of metalloproteinases MMP-2 and MMP-9. *J Invest Dermatol*. 1993;101:64.

59. Wysocki AB. Wound fluids and the pathogenesis of chronic wounds. *J Wound Ostomy Continence Nurs.* 1996;23:283.

60. Shinoda C, Takaku S. Interleukin-1 beta, interleukin-6, and tissue inhibitor of metalloproteinase-1 in the synovial fluid of the temporomandibular joint with respect to cartilage destruction. *Oral Dis.* 2000;6:383.

61. Mulder GD, Vande Berg JS. Cellular senescence and matrix metalloproteinase activity in chronic wounds. Relevance to debridement and new technologies. *J Am Podiatr Med Assoc.* 2002;92:34.

62. Watelet JB, Demetter P, Claeys C, et al. Neutrophil-derived metalloproteinase-9 predicts healing quality after sinus surgery. *Laryngoscope.* 2005;115:56.

63. Watelet JB, Claeys C, Van Cauwenberge P, et al. Predictive and monitoring value of matrix metalloproteinase-9 for healing quality after sinus surgery. *Wound Repair Regen.* 2004;12:412.

64. Shi B, Chen SZ, Zhang P, et al. Effects of vacuum-assisted closure (V.A.C.) on the expressions of MMP-1, 2, 13 in human granulation wound. *Zhonghua Zheng Xing Wai Ke Za Zhi.* 2003;19:279.

65. Tang SY, Chen SZ, Hu ZH, et al. Influence of vacuum-assisted closure technique on expression of Bcl-2 and NGF/NGFmRNA during wound healing. *Zhonghua Zheng Xing Wai Ke Za Zhi.* 2004;20:139.

66. Mendez-Eastman, S. Negative pressure wound therapy. *Plast Surg Nurs.* 1998;18:27.

67. Genecov DG, Schneider AM, Morykwas MJ, et al. A controlled subatmospheric pressure dressing increases the rate of skin graft donor site reepithelialization. *Ann Plast Surg.* 1998;40:219.

68. Kinetic-Concepts-Incorporated. V.A.C.® recommended guidelines for use, wound closure. *Physician & Caregiver Reference Manual,* San Antonio, TX: Kinetic Concepts, 1999.

69. Meara JG, Guo L, Smith JD, et al. Vacuum-assisted closure in the treatment of degloving injuries. *Ann Plast Surg.* 1999;42:589.

70. DeFranzo, AJ, Marks MW, Argenta LC, et al. Vacuum-assisted closure for the treatment of degloving injuries. *Plast Reconstr Surg.* 1999;104:2145, 1999.

71. Clubley L, Harper L. Using negative pressure therapy for healing of a sternal wound. *Nurs Times.* 2005;101:44.

72. Song DH, Wu LC, Lohman RF, et al. Vacuum assisted closure for the treatment of sternal wounds: the bridge between debridement and definitive closure. *Plast Reconstr Surg.* 2003;111:92.

73. Tang AT, Ohri SK, Haw MP. Novel application of vacuum assisted closure technique to the treatment of sternotomy wound infection. *Eur J Cardiothorac Surg.* 2000;17:482.

74. Obdeijn MC, de Lange MY, Lichtendahl DH, et al. Vacuum-assisted closure in the treatment of poststernotomy mediastinitis. *Ann Thorac Surg.* 1999;68:2358.

75. Fleck TM, Fleck M, Moidl R, et al. The vacuum-assisted closure system for the treatment of deep sternal wound infections after cardiac surgery. *Ann Thorac Surg.* 2002;74:1596.

76. Mehbod AA, Ogilvie JW, Pinto MR, et al. Postoperative deep wound infections in adults after spinal fusion: management with vacuum-assisted wound closure. *J Spinal Disord Tech.* 2005;18:14.

77. Antony S, Terrazas S. A retrospective study: clinical experience using vacuum-assisted closure in the treatment of wounds. *J Natl Med Assoc.* 2004;96:1073.

78. Ballard K, McGregor F. Use of vacuum-assisted closure therapy following foot amputation. *Br J Nurs.* 2001;10:S6.

79. Clare MP, Fitzgibbons TC, McMullen ST, et al. Experience with the vacuum assisted closure negative pressure technique in the treatment of non-healing diabetic and dysvascular wounds. *Foot Ankle Int.* 2002;23:896.

80. Eginton MT, Brown KR, Seabrook GR, et al. A prospective randomized evaluation of negative-pressure wound dressings for diabetic foot wounds. *Ann Vasc Surg.* 2003;17:645.

81. Eldad A, Tzur T. Vacuum—a novel method for treating chronic wounds. *Harefuah.* 2003;142:834.

82. Espensen EH, Nixon BP, Lavery LA, et al. Use of subatmospheric (V.A.C.®) therapy to improve bioengineered tissue grafting in diabetic foot wounds. *J Am Podiatr Med Assoc.* 2002;92:395.

83. Greer SE, Duthie E, Cartolano B, et al. Techniques for applying subatmospheric pressure dressing to wounds in difficult regions of anatomy. *J Wound Ostomy Continence Nurs.* 1999;26:250.

84. Moch D, Fleischmann W, Russ M. The BMW (biosurgical mechanical wound treatment) in diabetic foot. *Zentralbl Chir.* 1999;124(Suppl 1):69.

85. Petrie N, Potter M, Banwell P. The management of lower extremity wounds using topical negative pressure. *Int J Low Extrem Wounds.* 2003;2:198.

86. Armstrong DG, Boulton AJ, Banwell P. Negative pressure wound therapy in treatment of diabetic foot wounds: a marriage of modalities. *Ostomy Wound Manage.* 2004;50:9.

87. Venturi ML, Attinger CE, Mesbahi AN, et al. Mechanisms and clinical applications of the vacuum-assisted closure (V.A.C.®) device: a review. *Am J Clin Dermatol.* 2005;6:185.

88. Avery C, Pereira J, Moody A, et al. Negative pressure wound dressing of the radial forearm donor site. *Int J Oral Maxillofac Surg.* 2000;29:198.

89. Greer SE, Longaker MT, Margiotta M, et al. The use of subatmospheric pressure dressing for the coverage of radial forearm free flap donor-site exposed tendon complications. *Ann Plast Surg.* 1999;43:551.

90. Barker DE, Kaufman HJ, Smith LA, et al. Vacuum pack technique of temporary abdominal closure: a 7-year experience with 112 patients. *J Trauma.* 2000;48:201.

91. Smith LA, Barker DE, Chase CW, et al. Vacuum pack technique of temporary abdominal closure: a four-year experience. *Am Surg.* 1997;63:1102.

92. Scott BG, Feanny MA, Hirshberg A. Early definitive closure of the open abdomen: a quiet revolution. *Scand J Surg.* 2005;94:9.

93. Kaplan M. Managing the open abdomen. *Ostomy Wound Manage.* 2004;50:C2.

94. Miller PR, Thompson JT, Faler BJ, et al. Late fascial closure in lieu of ventral hernia: the next step in open abdomen management. *J Trauma.* 2002;53:843.

95. Josty IC, Ramaswamy R, Laing JH. Vacuum assisted closure: an alternative strategy in the management of degloving injuries of the foot. *Br J Plast Surg.* 2001;54:363.

96. Morykwas MJ, David LR, Schneider AM, et al. Use of subatmospheric pressure to prevent progression of partial-thickness burns in a swine model. *J Burn Care Rehabil.* 1999;20:15.

97. Banwell PE. Topical negative pressure wound therapy: advances in burn wound management. *Ostomy Wound Manage.* 2004;50:9S.

98. Schneider AM, Morykwas MJ, Argenta LC. A new and reliable method of securing skin grafts to the difficult recipient bed. *Plast Reconstr Surg.* 1998;102:1195.

99. Blackburn JH II, Boemi L, Hall WW, et al. Negative-pressure dressings as a bolster for skin grafts. *Ann Plast Surg.* 1998;40:453.

100. Molnar JA, DeFranzo AJ, Marks MW. Single-stage approach to skin grafting the exposed skull. *Plast Reconstr Surg.* 2000;105:174.

101. Carson SN, Overall K, Lee-Jahshan S, et al. V.A.C.uum-assisted closure used for healing chronic wounds and skin grafts in the lower extremities. *Ostomy Wound Manage.* 2004;50:52.

102. Dainty LA, Bosco JJ, McBroom JW, et al. Novel techniques to improve split-thickness skin graft viability during vulvo-vaginal reconstruction. *Gynecol Oncol.* 2005;97:949.

103. Molnar JA, DeFranzo AJ, Hadaegh A, et al. Acceleration of Integra incorporation in complex tissue defects with subatmospheric pressure. *Plast Reconstr Surg.* 2004;113:1339.

104. Gabriel A, Moores D, Gupta S, et al. Management of complicated abdominal wall defects with small intestinal submucosa (SIS) and vacuum assisted closure (V.A.C.®). *J Pediatr Surg. in press,* 2006.

105. Mooney JF III, Argenta LC, Marks MW, et al. Treatment of soft tissue defects in pediatric patients using the V.A.C.® system. *Clin Orthop Relat Res.* 2000;26.

106. Caniano DA, Ruth B, Teich S. Wound management with vacuum-assisted closure: experience in 51 pediatric patients. *J Pediatr Surg.* 2005;40:128.

107. Arca MJ, Somers KK, Derks TE, et al. Use of vacuum-assisted closure system in the management of complex wounds in the neonate. *Pediatr Surg Int,* 2005;21:532.

108. Deva AK, Buckland GH, Fisher E, et al. Topical negative pressure in wound management. *Med J Aust.* 2000;173:128.

109. Deva AK, Siu C, Nettle WJ. Vacuum-assisted closure of a sacral pressure sore. *J Wound Care.* 1997;6:311.

110. Baynham SA, Kohlman P, Katner HP. Treating stage IV pressure ulcers with negative pressure therapy: a case report. *Ostomy Wound Manage.* 1999;45:28.

111. Hartnett JM. Use of vacuum-assisted wound closure in three chronic wounds. *J Wound Ostomy Continence Nurs.* 1998;25:281.

112. Banwell PE. Topical negative pressure therapy in wound care. *J Wound Care.* 1999;8:79.

113. Smith N. The benefits of V.A.C.® therapy in the management of pressure ulcers. *Br J Nurs.* 2004;13:1359.

114. Jones SM, Banwell PE, Shakespeare PG. Advances in wound healing: topical negative pressure therapy. *Postgrad Med J.* 2005;81:353.

115. Ford CN, Reinhard ER, Yeh D, et al. Interim analysis of a prospective, randomized trial of vacuum-assisted closure versus the healthpoint system in the management of pressure ulcers. *Ann Plast Surg.* 2002;49:55.

116. Ferrell BA, Osterweil D, Christenson P. A randomized trial of low-air-loss beds for treatment of pressure ulcers. *Jama.* 1993;269:494.

117. Weinberg-Group. *Technology Assessment of the V.A.C.® for In-home Treatment of Chronic Wounds.* Washington, DC: The Weinberg Group; 1999.

118. Wolvos T. Wound instillation with negative pressure wound therapy. *Ostomy Wound Manage.* 2005;51:21.

119. Wolvos T. Wound instillation—the next step in negative pressure wound therapy. Lessons learned from initial experiences. *Ostomy Wound Manage.* 2004;50:56.

120. Gabriel A, Heinrich C, Shores JT, et al. Negative Pressure Wound Therapy with Instillation: Case Series Describing a New Method for Treating Infected Wounds. *Ann Plast Surg.* submitted, 2006.

121. Vanscheidt W, Lazareth I, Routkovsky-Norval C. Safety evaluation of a new ionic silver dressing in the management of chronic ulcers. *Wounds.* 2003;15:371.

122. O'Meara SM, Cullum NA, Majid M, Sheldon TA. Systematic review of antimicrobial agents used for chronic wounds. *Br J Surg.* 2001;88:4.

123. White RJ. An historical overview of the use of silver in wound management. *Br J Nurs.* 2001;10:S3.

124. Demling RH, DiSanti L. The role of silver technology in wound healing: Effects of silver on wound management. *Wounds.2001;*13:15.

125. Burrell RE, Heggers JP, Davis GJ, Wright JB. Efficacy of silver-coated dressings as bacterial barriers in rodent burn sepsis model. *Wounds.1999;*11:64.

126. Tredget EE, Shankowsky HA, Groeneveld A, Burrell R. A matched-pair, randomized study evaluating the efficacy and safety of Acticoat silver-coated dressing for the treatment of burn wounds. *J Burn Care Rehabil.* 1998;19:531.

127. Fridkin SK, Gaynes RP. Antimicrobial resistance in intensive care units. *Clin. Chest Med.* 1999;20:303.

128. Ovington LG. The truth about silver. *Ostomy Wound Managemen.* 2004;50:1S.

129. Driver VR. Silver dressings in clinical practice. *Ostomy Wound Management.* 2004;50:11S.

130. Wright JB, Hansen DL, Burrell RE. The comparative efficacy of two antimicrobial barrier dressings: in vitro examination of two controlled release of silver dressings. *Wounds.* 1998;10:179.

131. Jones S, Bowler PG, Walker M. Antimicrobial activity of silver-containing dressings is influenced by dressing conformability with a wound surface. *Wounds.* 2005;17:263.

132. Bennett N, Choudhary S. Why climb a ladder when you can take the elevator? *Plast Reconstr Surg.* 2000;105:2266.

133. Dunn R, Watson S. Why climb a ladder when you can take the elevator? *Plast Reconstr Surg.* 2001;107:283.

INDEX